Stone's Plastic Surgery Facts

A Revision Guide
Fourth Edition

D1355020

Stone's Plastic Surgery Facts

A Revision Guide
Fourth Edition

Tor Wo Chiu

Director of Burn Service, Head of Plastic Reconstructive
and Aesthetic Surgery, Department of Surgery, Prince of Wales Hospital,
Shatin, Hong Kong

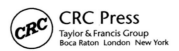
CRC Press
Taylor & Francis Group
Boca Raton London New York

CRC Press is an imprint of the
Taylor & Francis Group, an **informa** business

CRC Press
Taylor & Francis Group
6000 Broken Sound Parkway NW, Suite 300
Boca Raton, FL 33487-2742

© 2019 by Taylor & Francis Group, LLC
CRC Press is an imprint of Taylor & Francis Group, an Informa business

No claim to original U.S. Government works

Printed on acid-free paper

International Standard Book Number-13: 978-1-138-03170-8 (Paperback)
International Standard Book Number-13: 978-1-138-59673-3 (Hardback)

Visit the Taylor & Francis Web site at
http://www.taylorandfrancis.com

and the CRC Press Web site at
http://www.crcpress.com

To my family

Contents

Preface to the fourth edition

I remember buying the first edition of *Plastic Surgery: Facts* by Christopher Stone. I was not alone in appreciating the easy-to-read format, and the fact that it was born out of the author's revision notes made it all the more useful for those of us studying for our own exit examinations in plastic surgery.

I had the privilege of taking over the project for the previous (third) edition. The production of each new edition has added a large amount of new information. I focused on arranging the material for clarity and readability, and also to follow the syllabus of the Intercollegiate Surgical Curriculum Programme as closely as possible – the chapter layout is based on the Key Topics. There is also the excellent e-LPRAS resource that I have had the privilege of being able to contribute to.

Obviously, discussion of everything on the plastic surgery syllabus is not possible in a book of this size, nor is this intended to be the scope of this book. Each revision takes a great deal of time and effort; however, I was greatly encouraged to continue updating this book by the feedback from plastic surgery trainees. I was gratified to hear their comments and their appreciation of the philosophy of the book – it is very dense with information and deep insights. It is most useful after some prior reading of the subject.

The book has been thoroughly updated to include new materials including the surgical management of lymphoedema, the eighth edition of the 2018 Staging for Melanoma, updates in melanoma management such as PD1 protein inhibitors and inclusion of newer flaps such as the SCIP and MSAP. I have expanded the scope of the book somewhat to cover materials relevant to the US board exam. The article summaries have been a favourite feature of the book and have been retained and updated. Every reference has been rechecked and reviewed. I hope that new readers find this book useful.

Foreword

Taking the board exams marks the finale of a long training journey. During the preparation, it will probably be the last time you dive in deep to the whole broad spectrum of plastic surgery. It is during this time your general concept and understanding of plastic surgery is organised and stored as part of your knowledge. After this period of in-depth studying, you will be most likely to focus on a single or a couple of subspecialties in plastic surgery. At this time, your knowledge of that subspecialty field will continuously grow and expand, whilst the rest of the general knowledge stays dormant. My current work focuses on reconstruction of trunk and lower extremity, and the experience accumulated from this work allows me to evolve and provide new ideas and approaches. However, when a patient walks through the door, it is your job to notice the clues other than the subspecialties you focus on. This is when your fundamental knowledge of plastic surgery kicks in to observe the patient as a whole and not to miss obvious or hidden clues. That is why this opportunity to build your fundamentals and organise your thoughts and knowledge on plastic surgery is important as this will be the foundation of your future practice.

Dr Tor Chiu practices a wide spectrum of plastic surgery in one of the most prestigious training facilities in Hong Kong. His experience from the United Kingdom and Hong Kong allows him to have a wide exposure to plastic surgery, and lets him adapt to the new trends in this field. By training residents, he understands what is more essential in today's practice and how the fundamentals of plastic surgery evolve. He has added these new trends in this book, which gives you the opportunity to study and organise new topics as well as current knowledge in plastic surgery.

This book will help you develop and organise your knowledge in plastic surgery. It will guide you in your board exams; most of all, it will help you build your fundamentals in plastic surgery, which you can take along with you in your journey as a clinician.

Joon Pio Hong, MD, PhD, MBA
Professor
Department of Plastic Surgery
Asan Medical Center, University of Ulsan
Seoul, South Korea

Wound care

A. WOUNDS AND WOUND HEALING

I. WOUND HEALING AND TISSUE TRANSPLANTATION

WOUND HEALING

Wound repair proceeds through several stages that overlap somewhat:

- Inflammation (haemostasis, then increased vascular permeability and cell infiltration)
- Proliferation (re-epithelialization, fibroplasia)
- Remodelling (maturation)

INFLAMMATORY PHASE (DAYS 0–6)

Haemostasis – this phase is immediate, short-lived (lasting minutes) and characterised by **vasoconstriction** and **coagulation**. Haemostatic cascades lead to the formation of a thrombin–platelet plug (clot) that is adherent to type II collagen exposed by endothelial disruption. This clot has several functions:

- The **fibrin** acts as a scaffold for incoming cells and concentrates cytokines and growth factors such as platelet-derived growth factor (PDGF), transforming growth factors (TGF), α and β at the site.
  - It traps more platelets to perpetuate the cycle.
  - Fibrin is an essential component of wound healing.
- It releases chemotactic factors such as interleukin 2 (IL-2), tumour necrosis factor (TNF)-α, TGF-β.

Inflammation – this phase (lasting 3–5 days) is defined by the **vasodilation** (due to inflammatory mediators such as **histamine,** kinins, complement), **increased vascular permeability** and **cell infiltration. Cells** clear debris and initiate the proliferative phase; close regulation is needed to avoid overactivity (SIRS) or underactivity (chronic wounds – wounds that do not heal in an orderly set of stages in a timely manner, usually within 3 months; these are characterised by persistently elevated levels of matrix metalloproteinases, MMPs).

- **Neutrophils**
  - Within 12 hours of wounding, cells appear in the wound, attracted by chemotaxins including fibrin degradation products (FDPs), complement proteins, IL-1s, TGF-β, TNF-α, platelet factor 4 (PF4) and PDGF. Translocation of marginating neutrophils (at 24–48 hours) through capillary endothelium and basement membrane is facilitated by collagenase.
  - Neutrophils produce inflammatory mediators and cytokines, and remove debris; the response and population decline after a few days, whereupon the function of debris removal is taken over by macrophages. Neutrophils are not essential for wound healing.
- **Macrophage**s arrive after 48–96 hours and begin to phagocytose debris and release cytokines and growth factors, thus coordinating and promoting healing. They are **vital to wound healing**.
- **Fibroblasts** become the dominant cell type 1 week after injury, with a key role in the production of collagen. TGF-β promotes migration and proliferation of dermal fibroblasts.
- **T-lymphocytes** migrate into wounds after the macrophages (at 5–7 days) and persist for up to 1 week – a reduced response may lead to inferior wound healing. Their primary role seems to be to mediate in fibroblast recruitment and activation.
- **Keratinocytes** – differentiated cells are converted to immature cells that migrate over the wound surface.

PROLIFERATIVE PHASE (4 DAYS TO 3 WEEKS)

Re-epithelialisation begins within hours of wounding with migration of marginal keratinocytes over the matrix due to **loss of contact inhibition**, staying beneath the eschar. There is a phenotypic conversion of differentiated keratinocytes into non-polarised cells expressing basal cytokeratins similar to cultured cells; increased mobility comes from dissolution of anchoring junctions and reorganisation of the cortical actin cytoskeleton to form lamellipodia. Cells stop migrating when they form a contiguous layer (contact inhibition). As the basement membrane is reconstituted, the cells are induced to adopt their previous morphology and form anchoring junctions with fibronectin. A **moist environment** increases the rate of (re)-epithelialisation.

- **Epidermal growth factor** (EGF) – mRNA levels increase rapidly after wounding to promote re-epithelialisation. Abnormalities of EGF expression are thought to impair wound healing; glucocorticoids suppress EGF expression in cutaneous wounds but have less effect on EGF receptor levels.
- **Growth-related oncogene α** (GRO α), originally called 'melanocyte growth-stimulating activity' due to its mitogenic activity on melanocytes, is also a chemoattractant for neutrophils that is more potent than IL-8. Both GRO α and IL-8 stimulate keratinocyte proliferation in vitro; both are maximally expressed on day 1 after injury and subside after wound closure.
- **Insulin-like growth factor-1 (IGF-1)** and IGF-binding protein-1 have been demonstrated to act synergistically to accelerate the healing of adult skin wounds; exogenous IGF-1 increases myofibroblast expression in rat wound models (Achar RA, *Acta Cir Bras*, 2014). IGF-1 levels seem to be predictive of the response of diabetic foot ulcers in patients treated with HBO (Aydin F, *J Diabetes Res*, 2013).

Fibroplasia – there is an influx of fibroblasts over the fibronectin scaffold; they are activated by PDGF and TGF-β. These cells synthesise type **III collagen**, which with ongoing neovascularisation forms **granulation tissue**. Wound tensile strength increases during the fibroblastic phase.

- **Activin** is strongly expressed in wound skin. Overexpression in transgenic mice improves wound healing and enhances scar formation; activin A has been implicated in stimulating formation of granulation tissue whilst activin B mRNA has been localised to hyperproliferative epithelium at the wound edge.
- Secretion of glycosaminoglycans (GAGs) such as hyaluronic acid (HA), chondroitin sulphate and dermatan sulphate, which become hydrated to form an amorphous ground substance within which fibrillar collagen is deposited.
- Zinc, vitamins A (retinoids) and C are also required for normal collagen synthesis.

Angiogenesis – low oxygen tension in the wound leads to secretion of vascular endothelial growth factor (VEGF); MMPs degrade the extracellular matrix (ECM) to facilitate the passage of newly formed vessels.

REMODELLING PHASE (3 WEEKS TO 18 MONTHS)

The ECM appears to modulate fibroblast activity through changes in composition during healing. When fibronectin initially predominates, fibroblasts actively synthesise HA and collagen, but in a maturing wound, when collagen becomes abundant, fibroblast proliferation and collagen production then cease – irrespective of any stimulation by TGF-β. At this point, the wound becomes a relatively acellular scar. This phase ends with the formation of the final scar.

- **Collagen remodelling.** Residual fibroblasts mature into myofibroblasts and form cell–matrix and cell–cell contacts that contract the wound (scar contracture). Type III collagen is gradually replaced by type I collagen by the activity of MMPs released by macrophages, keratinocytes and fibroblasts, slowly returning to the normal type I/III ratio of 3:1.
  - Collagen is initially disorganised but then becomes lamellar (and aligned along lines of stress).
- **Peak wound tensile strength** is achieved at ~60 days and is a maximum of ~80% of unwounded skin strength.
- **Vascular maturation.** The abundant capillaries regress.

CYTOKINES AND GROWTH FACTORS

Cytokines

Cyto, from Greek *kyttaro*, which means 'cell', and kines, from Greek *kinisi*, which means 'movement'.

Cytokines are small molecules (peptide, protein or glycopeptide) that are secreted predominantly by immune cells (mostly lymphocytes and macrophages) and affect the behaviour of other cells. They are important in cell-to-cell signalling and mediate in protective and reparative processes and also regulate cell growth and maturation. Interferon α (IFN-α) was the first cytokine to be discovered in 1957.

Cytokines tend to be pleiotropic (affects many different cells) and redundant (many do the same thing); they can be synergistic or antagonistic. One can try to classify them broadly according to their function:

- Non-specific (innate) immunity and inflammation – mostly made by macrophages, mast cells and endothelium.
  - Chemokines (chemotaxis)
  - TNF and IL-1
  - IFN-γ and Il-12 (chronic inflammation)
- Specific (acquired/adaptive) immunity – most are made by T-helper (TH) cells.
  - IFN- γ and IL-5 (cell activation)
  - IL-2 and IL-4 (lymphocyte proliferation)
- Haematopoiesis – made by endothelium, macrophages, etc.
  - Colony stimulating factors causing haematopoietic cell proliferation

Tumour necrosis factor-α

TNF-α is released by macrophages/monocytes when stimulated by pathogens, tumour cells and toxins. It appears at wound sites 12 hours after wounding and peaks at 72 hours.

- Mediates in chemotaxis of inflammatory cells.
- Up-regulation of cellular adhesion molecules on endothelium.
- Other effects on collagen synthesis; may impair wound healing if it persists at high levels beyond natural peak, and excess TNF-α is associated with multisystem organ failure.

Interleukin-1

Interleukins (ILs) are cytokines, classically made by leucocytes **that act on other leucocytes**. Interleukin-1 (IL-1) is produced by macrophages/monocytes as well as keratinocytes at wound sites. It is detectable at wound sites after 24 hours, peaking around day 2 with levels rapidly declining thereafter.

- Neutrophil activation and chemotaxis
- Increased collagen synthesis and keratinocyte maturation
- Similar action to TNF-α; also activates T helper cells
- High levels in chronic non-healing wounds; also called endogenous pyrogen and causes fever

Interleukin-2

Interleukin-2 is produced by T lymphocytes.

- Sustains the post-injury inflammatory response via T-cell activation
- Promotes fibroblast infiltration at wound sites

Interleukin-6

Interleukin-6 is released by macrophages/monocytes, polymorphs and fibroblasts.

- Promotes stem cell growth and B- and T-cell activation, and mediates in hepatic acute phase protein synthesis
- Stimulates fibroblast proliferation
  - High IL-6 increases scarring and high systemic levels have been described as a marker of **wound severity in major burns** and a poor prognostic indicator (Modi S, *Indian J Med Microbiol*, 2014).
  - Low IL-6 in elderly patients with impaired wound healing and at scar-less foetal wound sites.

Interleukin-8

Interleukin-8 is released by macrophages and fibroblasts at wound sites.

- Neutrophil chemotaxis, adhesion and activation
- Promotes keratinocyte maturation and migration
- High levels in patients with psoriasis and low levels at foetal wound sites

Interferon γ

Interferons **interfere** with viral replication. Interferons α and β are type 1 and interferon γ is type 2. Interferon γ is produced by T-helper cells primarily, but also by Tc and macrophages. It has many functions in both specific and non-specific immunity.

- Macrophage and polymorph activation
- Mediates in wound remodelling; reduces wound contraction
- Possible role for decreasing scar hypertrophy but may decrease wound strength

Interleukin-4

Interleukin-4 is produced by T-cells, mast cells and B-lymphocytes.

- Promotes B-cell proliferation and IgE-mediated immunity and inhibits the release of pro-inflammatory cytokines by macrophages.
- Promotes fibroblast proliferation and collagen synthesis at wound sites.
- High levels are found in patients with scleroderma.

Interleukin-10

Interleukin-10 is produced by activated macrophages and T-cells; it has mostly **inhibitory** actions.

- Inhibits production of pro-inflammatory cytokines at acute wound sites
- Persistently high levels at chronic wound sites, e.g. venous ulcers; contributes to impaired wound healing

Growth factors

Growth factors are polypeptides whose primary role is in regulation of cell growth and maturation.

Platelet-derived growth factor

PDGF is released from platelet α granules and by macrophages.

- Recruitment and activation of immune cells and fibroblasts in the early post-injury phase.
- Later stimulates the production of collagen and GAGs; reduced levels are found in non-healing wounds.
- Three isomers of PDGF (2 polypeptide chains 'A' and 'B'):
  - AA – elevated at acute wound sites
  - BB – most useful clinically, used for chronic and diabetic ulcers (**Regranex®**, see below)
  - AB

Transforming growth factor β

TGF-β is released by macrophages, platelets and fibroblasts; it has mostly **inhibitory** actions.

- Blocks macrophage activation; inhibits the action of other cytokines on neutrophils and endothelium.

- Fibroblast maturation, collagen and proteoglycan synthesis.
- Inhibition of proteases.
- There are three isomers – TGF-β1, TGF-β2 and TGF-β3.
  - TGF-β1 and TGF-β2 are associated with hypertrophic and keloid scarring, and neutralising antibodies decrease scarring at rat wound sites (Shah M, *J Cell Sci*, 1994).
  - Low TGF-β levels at foetal wound sites.
  - TGF-β3 shown to decrease scarring.
  - Ratio of TGF-β1 and β2 – TGF-β3 determines nature of scar.

Fibroblast growth factor

Fibroblast growth factor (FGF) is released from fibroblasts and endothelial cells.

- Regulates angiogenesis and keratinocyte migration at wound sites.
- Two main forms – acidic FGF (or FGF-1) and basic FGF (or FGF-2) that binds to the same receptors as aFGF but is 10 times more potent.
- Application of exogenous bFGF to wound sites accelerates re-epithelialisation.
- Eight other isoforms – FGF-7 is keratinocyte growth factor (KGF) 1, which is low in diabetics and steroid immunosuppression. Recombinant KGF has been shown to improve wound re-epithelialisation.

Epidermal growth factor

EGF is released from keratinocytes.

- EGF promotes epithelialisation.
- Promotes collagenase release from fibroblasts (for remodelling).
- Inhibits wound contraction at foetal wound sites.

Vascular endothelial growth factor

VEGF is mainly released from keratinocytes; there is a minor contribution from macrophages and fibroblasts.

- Promotes angiogenesis at wound sites.
- Mediates in the formation of granulation tissue.

Insulin-like growth factor

At wound sites, IGF is released by macrophages, neutrophils and fibroblasts; levels rise to a peak within 24 hours of wounding and persist for several weeks.

- Promotes fibroblast and keratinocyte proliferation, with possible role in angiogenesis.
- Two isoforms – IGF-1 and IGF-2.
- Low IGF levels are observed in diabetic and steroid-suppressed wounds.

COLLAGEN

Collagen forms about one-third of the total protein in the human body. It is a triple helix formed from three α-helical chains; 25 different α-chains have been identified, each encoded by a separate gene. There are at least 16 different types of collagen. Their structural differences determine the ability of their helical and non-helical regions to associate, form fibrils and sheets or cross-link different collagen types; 90% of body collagen is type I. In normal skin, the ratio of types I/III = 3:1. See Table 1.1.

- Type I – most common and predominates in bone, tendon and skin
- Type II – hyaline cartilage, cornea
- Type III – immature scar, blood vessels, bowel, uterus
- Type IV – basement membrane
- Type V – foetal and placental tissue

The initial product is the pro-α-chain. Post-translational hydroxylation of proline and lysine residues (requires vitamin C and iron) is important for structural strength and stability by cross-linking the triple helix, as well as being necessary for its export from the cell.

- Procollagen – three polypeptide chains in a triple helix form tropocollagen. All types contain a repeating Gly-Pro-X sequence that allows folding.
- Tropocollagen units form collagen filaments.
- Filaments form fibrils, which form fibres with enormous tensile strength. The typical 'fibrous' collagens are I, II, III and V.

Early collagen is thin and randomly orientated parallel to the skin surface; collagen that is laid down during the later stages of wound healing is thicker and lies along stress lines, thus increasing wound strength.

- Initially, type III collagen production is high and then type I replaces type III until a ratio of 3–4:1 is achieved.

Table 1.1 Common types of collagen

Number	Distribution	Disorders
I	Bone, skin, tendon, ligaments, cornea	Deficient in osteogenesis imperfecta
II	Cartilage, vitreous humour of eye	Deficient in chondrodysplasia
III	Skin, blood vessels, intestines, uterus	Excessive: early wound, early Dupuytren's contracture, hypertrophic scar Deficient: Ehlers–Danlos syndrome
IV	Basal laminae, lens	Deficient in vascular Ehlers-Danlos syndrome (EDS type IV - 13 types described in 2017)
V	Associated with type I	Found in active stage Dupuytren's contracture

- Myofibroblasts cause wound contraction that reduces the wound size (not the same as a contracture that is excessive scar contraction across a mobile surface). There is gradual decrease in vascularity.

See 'Syndromes associated with altered healing'.

FACTORS AFFECTING WOUND HEALING

Discussions generally divide factors into patient factors and wound factors.

Wound factors

- **Hydration** increases the rate of epithelialisation, hence the rationale for occlusive dressings (see 'Moist wound healing'). The mechanisms proposed for this improved healing include thermal insulation, altering wound oxygen/carbon dioxide/pH, maintaining growth factors as well as acting as a physical barrier.
- **Infection** – the presence of $>10^5$ organisms (or lower concentrations of β-haemolytic streptococcus) **prolongs the inflammatory phase.** Endotoxins reduce tissue oxygenation and stimulate phagocytosis and the release of collagenases and radicals that may damage normal tissue. **Taking swabs of open wounds is generally pointless;** colonisation does not equate to infection and would not normally inhibit wound healing.
- **Foreign bodies** (or necrotic tissue) prolong the inflammatory phase, are obstacles to healing and are nidi for bacteria.
- **Ischaemia** – energy in the form of glucose and oxygen is required for proliferation (cell replication and protein synthesis) as well as fibroblast and neutrophil activity. Reduced oxygen tension causes inefficient keratinocyte migration. Fibroblasts, in particular, are oxygen-sensitive and an oxygen tension of >40 mmHg augments fibroblastic activity and is required for the hydroxylation of proline and lysine in the collagen α-chain. Oxygen also facilitates cell-mediated killing of pathogens in the wound. **Ischaemia and reduction of local oxygen tension may be a component of other processes**:
  - Oedema – reduces tissue perfusion and leads to capillary closure.
  - Protein extravasation forms a diffusion barrier.
  - Radiation – direct DNA damage, impaired inflammatory response, endarteritis obliterans.
  - Diabetes mellitus (DM).
  - Smoking.
- **Tissue expansion** – increased rate and strength of healing.
- **Low serum protein** – prolonged inflammatory phase and impaired fibroplasia.
- **Increased ambient temperature (30°C)** – accelerates wound healing.

Patient factors

- **Age** – there is a reduction in the cellular multiplication rate with age. Tensile strength and wound closure rates also decrease with age – the various stages of wound healing are all protracted.
- **Nutrition** (see 'Nutrition') – malnutrition is associated with impairment of fibroblast function and reduced wound tensile strength.
  - Protein malnutrition especially deficiencies of arginine and methionine compromises wound healing.
  - Vitamin C – essential for hydroxylation of collagen.
  - Vitamin E – antioxidant actions neutralise lipid peroxidation (and thus cell damage) caused by ionising radiation, for example.
  - Minerals – many are cofactors in collagen production, e.g. zinc influences re-epithelialisation and collagen deposition.
- **Systemic illness** – such as anaemia or pulmonary disease may impair oxygen delivery and collagen synthesis.
- **Smoking** (multifactorial) – the nicotine in one single cigarette causes vasoconstriction that lasts 90 minutes, cyanide impairs oxidative enzymes whilst carbon monoxide (CO) impairs the oxygen-carrying capacity of haemoglobin. Stopping smoking will ameliorate the effects of
  - CO after >12 hours.
  - Free radicals (1 week).
  - Nicotine effects (10 days).
  - CDC recommends quitting 4 weeks before surgery, but there is no consensus. The highest risk is in surgeries where tissues may have reduced vascularity, e.g. composite grafts/replants, extensive tissue undermining, e.g. facelifts.
  - There is no evidence that nicotine replacement therapy affects wound healing, but it is probably prudent to avoid in high-risk surgery.
- **Diabetes mellitus** (see 'Diabetic ulcers') – multiple factors are at work in addition to the microvascular disease that reduces oxygenation. These patients are prone to infections that should be treated aggressively. However, with adequate glycaemic control, most surgical wounds should heal satisfactorily.
  - Glycosylation of proteins may alter functions, e.g. glycosylated haemoglobin has a higher affinity for oxygen, which impairs oxygen delivery to the tissues.
  - Increased blood glucose impairs cellular function.
    - Sorbitol by-products are toxic.
  - Sensory neuropathy decreases protective reflexes and increases vulnerability to ischaemia.
  - Autonomic neuropathy leads to anhydrosis (dry skin) and arteriovenous shunting.
  - Reduced fibroblast numbers and immune dysfunction.
  - Vascular disease and ischaemia.
- **Drugs.**

- **Steroids** – anti-inflammatory actions affect wound healing in many ways including **impaired macrophage and fibroblast** function, reduced angiogenesis and contracture. Vitamin A is usually said to reverse steroid effects and increases collagen synthesis.
- **Non-steroidal anti-inflammatory drugs (NSAIDs)** – almost halve collagen synthesis in some studies, which is related to the reduction in prostaglandin production.
- **Chemotherapy** – e.g. cyclophosphamide is anti-inflammatory whilst methotrexate potentiates infections.
- **Syndromes associated with altered healing**
  - **Ehlers–Danlos** – a group of patients with defects in collagen metabolism (e.g. lysyl oxidase) commonly affecting **type III collagen**, though some have deficiencies of types I and V. The skin is really stretchable and recoils without wrinkles. Patients exhibit joint hyper-extensibility with tissue fragility and **poor healing** with post-operative bleeding, wound infections (defective immune response) and wider atrophic scars. Non-essential surgery is not recommended.
  - **Cutis laxa** – variable modes of inheritance. There is an elastin defect causing the skin to be thin and stretchable (but does not recoil due to the lack of elastin), with easy bruising; joints are normal. **Essential surgery can be** performed, though there is an association with cardiorespiratory disease.
  - **Homocystinuria** – autosomal recessive (AR) inherited deficiency of cystathionine synthase that is needed to metabolise methionine. Accumulated homocysteine initiates the clotting cascade, and causes arterial sclerosis, thrombosis, poor perfusion and platelet malfunction. There is a high risk of developing cardiovascular disease.
  - **Osteogenesis imperfecta** – patients have a **defective collagen I gene**, and wounds typically heal with wide scars.
- **Dystrophic epidermolysis bullosa** is a hereditary disease of skin and mucosa that causes blistering after trivial trauma and heals by scarring. It is associated with mutations of **collagen VII**, which form anchoring fibril-specific proteins. Typically, there is cocooning of the digits in an atrophic scar – pseudosyndactyly and flexion contracture; the digits are generally quite mobile despite the deformity, but surgical release is generally not rewarding as recurrence is almost inevitable. Exsanguination during any surgery should be performed by elevation and not bandaging; tourniquets need extra padding. Grafts can be taken with hand knives; both donor and recipients heal fairly well, but haemolytic streptococcal colonisation is not uncommon. Patients generally die young (third decade) from squamous cell carcinoma (SCC).

ADJUNCTS TO HEALING

There are a plethora of modalities and products put forward for enhancement of wound healing. The strength of evidence is variable but overall is fairly low.

- **Hyperbaric oxygen** therapy (HBOT) increase oxygen delivery to wounds but its use in wound healing in general is controversial. It may be useful in selected wounds, e.g. ischaemic (acute arterial insufficiency, crush injuries), radionecrosis, necrotising fasciitis (NF)/gas gangrene and diabetic ulcers. Medicare covers its use if there are 'no measurable signs of healing for at least 30 days of standard wound therapy'.
- **Negative pressure** – the exact mechanism is unclear but reportedly removes interstitial fluid and oedema to improve oxygenation, removes deleterious inflammatory mediators, reduces bacterial counts and speeds up formation of granulation tissue (see 'Negative pressure wound therapy').
- **Growth factors** – some are commercially available and used in some localities, e.g. PDGF, GM-CSF and KGF2. However, the evidence is generally not that convincing, and their use is regarded as mostly experimental. Recombinant PDGF B-chain (becaplermin) is marketed as Regranex®, the only agent shown to be efficacious in double-blind studies. It has FDA approval; however, there is a warning that there is an increased cancer mortality in patients who use three or more tubes. Recombinant human EGF is used in South Korea for wound healing; one product has been used to reduce radiation dermatitis (Kang HC, *Radiat Oncol*, 2014).
  - Apligraf® is a bioengineered product, initially marketed as a skin substitute. Although some wounds did heal, it became evident that the material was not actually incorporated – it acted as a wound stimulator – in chronic wounds, there would be outgrowth of previously dormant keratinocytes at the wound edges (see below). Activskin® is a similar product made in China (CRMI).
- **Electrostimulation (ES)** therapy – the premise is that there is an endogenous electric field in wounds and that cells are sensitive to and respond to an applied field. Multiple animal studies seem to have demonstrated some efficacy, but good clinical evidence is lacking; some attribute this to a paucity of uniform protocols/products (e.g. DC or pulsed current at low frequency or high voltage, pulsed EM field, etc.). There were weak recommendations from the pressure sore advisory panels (NPUAP, EPUAP and PPPIA) in 2014.
  - NICE 2015 does not recommend ES as an adjunctive treatment for diabetic foot problems unless as part of a clinical trial.
  - Cochrane reviews (Aziz Z, *Cochrane Database Syst Rev*, 2010, updated in 2015) demonstrated a lack of level 1 evidence.

- **Lasers** – low-level laser therapy (LLLT), aka 'biostimulation', is said to increase cellular activity especially of fibroblasts and keratinocytes. Light is administered at wavelengths of 680–890 nm, over several applications; it does not generate heat and is thus often referred to as 'cold' laser.
  - LLLT was introduced in the 1960s by Mester E. Devices have FDA approval (1994) for relief of minor muscle and joint pain and improvement of superficial circulation. The consensus seems to be that it is not more effective for temporary pain relief than heat therapy; most insurance companies do not cover its use.
  - There seems to be some evidence for a role in reducing post-irradiation oral mucositis (Kumar SP, *Indian J Palliat Care*, 2013).
- **Ultrasound** (low frequency, i.e. ~20 kHz, traditionally used to relieve muscular spasms). Cavitation (gas bubbles) and streaming (unidirectional steady mechanical force) seem to alter the characteristics of cell membranes.
  - Use in venous ulcers and pressure sores yields inconsistent results.
    - Systematic reviews in *BMJ Clinical Evidence* (2007) deem it to be of 'unknown effectiveness'.
    - NICE 2011 stated that there was promise but the low level evidence, and lack of comparisons, meant that its use in the NHS was not supported.
  - Most insurance companies will not cover its use.

See other chapters for healing of bone, tendon and nerves.

WOUND MANAGEMENT

Management of wounds involves a comprehensive assessment of the patient as a whole, as well as the wound itself. This includes looking for conditions/factors that can affect healing, and also the nutritional status.

NUTRITION

Whilst there has been much research on the subject, as yet, there is no simple, single reliable method of assessing nutritional status. Criteria that have been used for this include the following:

- **Clinical**, e.g. recent weight loss, signs of loss such as muscle wasting/loss of fat, oedema. Unplanned weight loss of more than 10% over 6 months is associated with a poor response to injury.
  - BMI < 18.5 implies nutritional impairment whilst BMI < 15 is associated with significant mortality.
  - Skin fold thickness of triceps, mid-arm circumference.
- **Biochemical markers** – transferrin, retinol binding protein but most commonly prealbumin. **Prealbumin**

has a half-life of 2–3 days and is thus a better measure of protein nutrition than albumin (half-life 20 days, and may be reduced by sepsis/inflammation as well as malnutrition). Closure of surgical wounds is more successful if the albumin is >30).
- Nutrition Risk Index = (1.519 × albumin g/L) + 0.417 × (present weight/usual weight × 100). A score below 100 indicates malnutrition.
- Lymphocyte function and body nitrogen are primarily research tools.

NICE recommends nutritional support for patients who have 5 days or more of reduced intake, or those with poor absorption, high losses or increased requirements. Nutrition can be supported by various means:

- Oral supplements – over and above a normal hospital diet, is simple and relatively effective.
- Enteral feeding for those with inadequate oral intake, is cheaper and safer than parenteral feeding and numerous studies have shown benefit.
- Parenteral feeding (peripheral or central) is reserved for those with non-functioning gut, e.g. short bowel, high output fistula. Some trials show that preoperative TPN reduces complications but not mortality in malnourished patients; there is less support for the use of post-operative TPN and it may actually be harmful.

Whilst many **micronutrients** are important in healing, replacement is only indicated in deficiency states.

- **Vitamin A** is one of the exceptions to this rule. Administration reverses most of the steroids' effects on inflammation, except for infections and wound contraction. It may be considered in those on chronic steroid therapy.
- Vitamin E supplements do not have any beneficial effects on wound healing, and large doses may actually inhibit healing (decreased tensile strength).
- Taking large doses of vitamin C does not improve healing.
- The benefit of glutamine is most well studied particularly in burns; arginine seems to have mixed effects.

SPECIFIC WOUND MANAGEMENT

The fundamentals of wound management are usually summarised with the acronym TIME (or DIME).

- Tissue management (or Debridement)
- Infection control
- Moisture balance
- Edge advancement

Debridement

Debridement of necrotic, non-viable tissue, which also reduces bacterial load, bioburden (**and biofilm**) is an important part of wound management. The word comes from the French *debridement* (old French *desbrider*), meaning to take away the bridle, and the procedure is usually attributed to Napoleonic war surgeons (Desault). The aim is to convert a chronic wound into an acute wound.

- Non-selective
  - **Mechanical**, which includes
    - Wet-to-dry dressings – characteristically painful
    - Scrubbing
    - Hydrotherapy
  - **Hydrogen peroxide** (usually 3%) – this is a source of reactive oxygen species that when applied to tissues bubbles due to the reaction with tissue catalase releasing water and oxygen. Staphylococci tend to be catalase-positive whilst Streptococci do not have catalase and are thus said to be more susceptible to peroxide. It is commonly used as a wound antiseptic, and whilst it shows broad in vitro activity, the few clinical studies generally show that it is relatively ineffective in reducing bacterial load, though it does appear not to delay wound healing. The AMA (Roderheaver GT, *Chronic Wound Care: A Clinical Source Book for Healthcare Professionals*, 2nd Edn, 1997) suggested that the effervescence may have some mechanical benefit in loosening debris and necrotic tissue.
  - **Antiseptics** such as chlorhexidine (works within 20 seconds but lasts only 6 hours), povidone iodine 10% (equivalent to 1% availability, needs 1 minute to work), alcohol, etc. have a wide spectrum of activity and low risk of resistance, but may damage healthy cells.
  - **Topical antimicrobials** include the usual antibiotics mupirocin, fucidic acid and neomycin, but some include silver, honey and cadexomer iodine (Iodosorb, Smith and Nephew). They do not harm healthy tissue, but antibiotics should only be used for 1–2 weeks due to concerns over sensitisation and resistance.
- Selective debridement
  - **Surgical** (some would put this in the non-selective category). This is the most common method and involves blades/curettes, etc.; some use more complicated systems such as the Versajet®.
  - **Enzymatic** – selectively digest dead tissue/slough. Iruxol Mono® is a collagenase, clostridiopeptidase A, but takes several days to work. Others such as Nexobrid® (bromelain, derived from pineapple stems) may work quicker (Rosenberg L, *Burns*, 2004) but is not widely available.
    - **Autolytic** – the combination of moist dressings, e.g. hydrocolloids and endogenous proteolytic enzymes, can lead to the liquefaction of necrotic tissue that then separates. It can be enhanced with hydrocolloids/hydrogels/occlusive films and products such as medical honey.

- **Biological** – **maggots** of certain species, e.g. *Lucilia sericata*, can cause benign myiasis, i.e. the larvae only digest dead tissue, extracorporeally through chymotrypsin-like enzymes (note that some species cause malignant myiasis, damaging healthy tissue). There are reports of an antimicrobial action and promotion of healing. There may be pain after 2–3 days, supposedly due to alkaline secretions, whilst other secretions may cause irritation/excoriation of normal skin
    - Maggots have been used in military wounds for a long time. Crile demonstrated that soldiers with maggot-infested wounds actually did better. Following the increasing use of antibiotics, maggot therapy declined, but it has had a resurgence since the 1980s. In the United Kingdom, they can be prescribed and used in the community. They are useful in infected necrotic wounds including diabetic ulcers and pressure sores, particularly those unfit for surgery. One study showed healing of 90% of MRSA-infected wounds after one to two maggot applications over 4–6 days.
    - Maggots take 10–14 days to pupate, requiring a dry place; thus, it is important to keep them in the wound and to dispose of them quickly.

Infection control

- **Contamination** – there are low numbers of non-replicating bacteria.
- **Colonisation** – bacteria are replicating but are not provoking an inflammatory response. It does not normally inhibit normal wound healing.
- **Infection** – there are a large number of bacteria that are invading wound tissue and are provoking an inflammatory reaction.

Taking wound swabs for bacterial culture is a very common practice but not that useful; swabbing open wounds is particularly pointless. Quantitative analysis of tissue biopsy is the gold standard; $>10^5$ is regarded as significant.

- **Biofilms** are polymeric glue-like structures with collections of bacteria within them. Their significance is that the bacteria are relatively protected from the immune system as well as simple wound care. They often require physical removal, e.g. debridement, as well as topical antiseptics/antimicrobials or systemic antibiotics; Prontosan® (betaine-polyhexanide) uses electrostatic disruption/surfactant action to disrupt a biofilm.

Moisture balance

There are many wound dressings available; but in simple terms,

- If the wound is dry, add moisture with hydrogels, hydrocolloids or films.
- If the wound is too wet, remove moisture with foams or alginates.

MOIST WOUND HEALING (WINTER G, *NATURE*, 1962)

This concept is a mainstay of modern wound healing and is promoted by occlusive dressings such as hydrocolloids, hydrogels and films.

- Maintains hydration and temperature
- Prevents scab/eschar formation
- Promotes epithelialisation
- Autolysis
- Slightly acidotic environment
- Growth factors more active

EDGE ADVANCEMENT

The wound edge may be undermined or rolled due to excessive proliferation. Failure of wound edge migration may be due to persistent/inadequately debrided slough, prolonged wound inflammation or senescent cells.

ULCERS

An ulcer is a breach in the epithelium and there are multiple causes. The ulcer characteristics, particularly the edge and base, provide important information. The surrounding tissues specifically skin condition, circulation and sensation (e.g. glove and stocking neuropathy) also provide clues. Long-standing ulcers should be biopsied to exclude malignancy (**Marjolin's ulcer**); other problems to consider include vasculitis/autoimmune disease, sickle cell, infection or

- **Hydroxyurea** (an antineoplastic agent used to treat haematological malignancies) can cause painful leg ulcers (usually after prolonged use) that are refractory to local care until the drug is discontinued.
- **Pyoderma gangrenosum** is a necrotising cutaneous vasculitis that may be associated with inflammatory bowel disease or rheumatoid arthritis. Histological findings are non-specific and the diagnosis is clinical. Ulcers in IBD patients may improve when the bowel disease improves. Surgery is contraindicated.

VENOUS ULCERS

This is the commonest cause of leg ulcers in developed countries (70%–90%), affecting 1.7% of the elderly in the United Kingdom and costing 600 million GBP a year in health costs. A minority will also have an arterial component.

- Typically a painless (unless infected) ulcer over medial malleolus (**gaiter area** – a gaiter being a protective item that covers the ankle to the instep area. They also cover the lower trouser, differentiating them from spats). Aching and swelling at the end of the day are improved by elevation.
- The typical skin changes are lipodermatosclerosis (scarring) and pigmentation due to haemosiderin deposition.

- Valvular dysfunction leads to **venous hypertension;** a history of DVT was found only in 28% (Moffat CJ, *QJM*, 2004). This leads to protein extravasation and formation of a perivascular fibrin cuff. Duplex ultrasound studies have shown that superficial venous incompetence is found in most patients with venous ulceration (Magnusson MB, *Eur J Vasc Endovasc Surg*, 2001), sometimes with deep venous reflux, but isolated reflux in deep or perforating veins is uncommon.
- There are many dressings to choose from, and there is little evidence that any one product demonstrates superiority to the others, though hydrocolloids/foams may help reduce pain.
  - **Pentoxifylline** (Trental®), normally used for intermittent claudication through increases in microcirculatory blood flow, may be more effective than placebo, with or without compression (Jull AB, *Cochrane Database Syst Rev*, 2012). Most of the side effects were gastrointestinal. SIGN (2010) suggests that it may be used; however, it is an unlicensed indication.
- **Compression therapy** (to counteract venous hypertension) by trained nurses is a key treatment. There are some regional preferences but results are similar.
  - Four-layer bandaging (4LB) is popular in the United Kingdom; full healing is achieved in 8 weeks.
  - Short stretch bandaging is preferred in Europe.
  - Unna boots made from zinc oxide and calamine-impregnated bandages, changed once every 1–2 weeks, are common in the United States. They facilitate ambulation.
- **Superficial vein surgery** (various forms of venoablation including high ligation and GSV stripping, sclerotherapy and RFA or endovenous laser) is much more beneficial for ulcer healing/recurrence than deep vein surgery, which has significant complications. The evidence for subfascial perforator ligation in ulcer healing remains unconvincing. Venous surgery/referral to a vascular surgeon does not need to be delayed in patients with healthy granulating ulcers with no evidence of infection. The **ESCHAR trial** (2004) found no difference between compression alone (89% at 3 years) vs. compression with surgery for superficial reflux (93%), but the latter group has a reduced recurrence rate and more 'ulcer-free time'.
- **Surgery to the ulcer** can be considered if conservative treatment fails. Skin grafts work reasonably well, but recurrence is almost inevitable without dealing with the venous insufficiency; flaps are a major undertaking but import vascularity.

DIABETIC ULCERS

Approximately 15% of diabetic patients suffer from ulcers. The aetiology is often mixed: one-third are purely neuropathic, one-third are neuropathic and ischaemic whilst one-fourth is purely ischaemic. **Neuropathy** is important and has anatomic, ischaemic and metabolic contributing factors:

- Elevated blood sugar levels reduce sodium pump activity and increase intracellular sorbitol, leading to nerve swelling and intraneural compression.
- Alterations in microcirculation lead to focal nerve loss.
- May have 'double crush' phenomenon, e.g. concomitant carpal tunnel, cubital tunnel syndrome.
- Sensory neuropathy leads to loss of protective sense.
- Autonomic neuropathy – anhidrosis, dry cracked skin from AV shunting.

Wound care in diabetics is a particular challenge.

- **Off-loading** is very important.
- **Increased infection risk** (usually Staphylococci or Streptococci) due to impaired lymphocyte function and impaired phagocytosis. Antibiotics should be used judiciously; some countries have banned the use of topical antibiotics in diabetic wounds due to resistance problems.
- **HBOT** reduces amputation rates and is covered by Medicare if ulceration has been unresponsive to 30 days of standard treatment.
- **Apligraf** (see later) use is covered in non-responsive diabetic and venous ulcers, though insurers have recently cut back on the reimbursement per treatment.

Microangiopathy does not contribute significantly to the development of ulcers in diabetics; thus, vascular reconstruction can be beneficial. It may be more useful for foot ulcers compared to calf ulcers. Diabetic patients have atherosclerosis similar to non-diabetics but often with different distributions – they tend to have tibioperoneal disease with long segment occlusion and calcification, whilst any femoral disease tends to be diffuse. The peak flow improvement occurs 1 week after a bypass but takes up to 1 month after an endovascular intervention; the latter also has a higher rate of short-term failure.

- **Amputation** – toe fillet, plantar VY, ray/transmetatarsal amputation are choices for gangrenous toes; >½ of all amputations performed are secondary to diabetic disease.
- **Reconstructions** may be 'simplified' with the use of negative pressure wound therapy (NPWT) to reduce bacterial counts, improve the formation of granulation tissue especially over non-favourable wounds with exposed tendons, bones and joints and improve the take of skin grafts.
- The current consensus is to aggressively postpone the need for amputation:
  - 1/3 need a more proximal amputation due to poor healing.
  - 1/2 have a contralateral limb amputation within 5 years.
  - The 5-year survival after amputation is 40%.

Diabetic foot reconstruction using free flaps increases 5-year survival rate. (Oh TS, *J Plast Reconstr Aesthet Surg*, 2013)
A retrospective review of 121 reconstructive procedures in diabetic foot wounds. A variety of free perforator flaps (ALT, SCIP, anterior or upper medial thigh flaps) were used with 91.7% success, with overall limb salvage rate at 5 years being 86.6%. Statistical analysis shows improved 5-year survival in patients who had foot reconstruction compared to those who had an above ankle amputation (86.8% vs. 41.4%).

TISSUE TRANSPLANTATION

- **Immunology**
- **Skin grafts**
- **Bone grafts**
- **Tendon healing and tendon grafts**
- **Tissue allografts, xenografts and alloplasts**

IMMUNOLOGY

Major histocompatibility antigens (MHC, also called human leucocyte antigens – HLA, in humans) are found on the surface of cells.

- Type 1 – all nucleated cells and platelets
- Type 2 – antigen-presenting cells (APCs): Langerhans cells, macrophages and lymphocytes

RESPONSE TO MHC-ALLOANTIGENS

- APCs present alloantigen to T-cells and express IL-1.
- IL-1 causes T-helper (CD4+) to produce IL-2.
- IL-2 causes clonal expansion of T-helper cells and B-lymphocytes.
- IL-2 also activates Tc-cells and NK cells (cellular immunity).
- B lymphocytes mediate antibody-mediated cell lysis (humoral immunity).

ALLOGRAFT REJECTION

Unmatched tissue grafts from another patient, i.e. allografts, will be rejected; skin is the most allogenic tissue – rejection in hand/face transplants is first manifested as a blotchy rash.

- **Acute rejection** occurs after 7–10 days due to T-cell infiltration (cellular immunity). It may be delayed in immunocompromised patients until the immunodeficient state has passed, e.g. recovery from a severe burn or stopping immunosuppressant drugs.
- **Late rejection** is due to antibody-mediated cell lysis (humoral immunity).
- **Hyperacute rejection** is due to preformed antibodies and the rejection response begins immediately.

- **Graft versus host reaction** occurs when allograft containing lymphoid tissue reacts against an immunocompromised host, and is a particular risk in bone marrow transplant.

Immunosuppressant drugs are needed to block rejection in allotransplantation:

- Cyclosporin blocks IL-2, which blocks clonal expansion of Tc-cells.
- Azathioprine inhibits T-cell-mediated rejection by preventing cell division.
- Prednisolone blocks the generation and release of T-cells.

BIOMATERIALS

These are biological materials used to replace or augment tissues in the human body and can be classified as

- Autograft – living tissue from host
- Isograft – from a genetically identical twin
- Allograft – tissue from same species
- Xenograft – tissue from different species
- Alloplast – derived from synthetic material.

The biological reactions to a foreign body include

- Immediate inflammation with early rejection
- Delayed rejection
- Fibrous encapsulation
- Incomplete encapsulation with continuing cellular reaction
- Slow resorption
- Incorporation

TISSUE ALLOGRAFTS, XENOGRAFTS AND ALLOPLASTS

Tissue allografts

These generally do not contain living cells due to processing to reduce antigenicity, though bone allograft may have osteoconductive and osteoinductive properties. They are usually incorporated into host tissues providing a structural framework for the ingrowth of host tissues.

- Their advantages include a plentiful supply; a donor site is not required and operation time is usually reduced.
- Disadvantages include a potential for infection/disease transmission, and they demonstrate a variable amount of resorption.

Examples include

- Lyophilised fascia (dura mater, fascia lata) – risk of Creutzfeldt–Jakob disease (CJD) transmission in the former. Typically there is a 10% resorption rate.
- Homologous cartilage – greater tendency for resorption, replacement with fibrous tissue, ossification and more infection compared with autologous tissue. A tissue

is said to be homologous if it performs the same basic function in the recipient as the donor.
- Homologous bone – acts generally as scaffold for formation of new bone; slower to become incorporated and revascularised.
- AlloDerm® (Lifecell Corp) – cadaveric dermis that has been processed to remove cellular elements, allowing incorporation into the host.
- Glyaderm® (Euro Skin bank) is a glycerolised acellular human dermis, which can be used as a dermal substitute, which is then covered by a thin autograft.

SKIN 'ALLOGRAFTS'

Cadaveric skin was first used as temporary cover in burns by Brown in 1953. It has not been satisfactorily used as a skin transplant (i.e. a true allograft) in major burns (Mahdavi-Mazdeh M, *Int J Organ Transplant Med*, 2013).

- The skin must be retrieved within 24 hours of death from a refrigerated cadaver under aseptic conditions (screening serology for hepatitis B and C viruses, human immunodeficiency virus and skin samples for culture of bacteria, yeast and fungi). It is stored in nutrient media at 4°C for up to 1 week ('fresh') or sterilised (e.g. irradiation) and cryopreserved (controlled freezing at 0.5–5°C/min to –196°C with liquid nitrogen and a cryoprotectant solution). When needed, it is rapidly rewarmed to 10–37°C (~3–4 min). Alternatively it can be processed with 85% glycerol (Euro Skin), which is a slow-acting but effective bactericide.
- Donor exclusion criteria – high-risk categories for HIV, i.e. male homosexuals, drug abusers, those with tattoos, prostitutes and haemophiliacs, those with infection/sepsis, neoplasia and autoimmune disease. Only two cases of viral transmission in 3 million tissue transplants (including skin) have been described.

Cadaveric skin is the best **biological dressing** for areas of full thickness skin loss; however, it is temporary due to rejection through HLA-DR and Langerhans cells; thus, they are strictly not allografts. Burns patients are immunosuppressed so rejection may be delayed – some cases demonstrate up to 85% viability at 1 year (see 'Burns').

- Coverage of areas of full thickness skin loss, e.g. after burn debridement, in the face of inadequate donor skin. The cadaveric dermis will adhere tightly to the (fibrin of the) wound bed and keep it clean and reduce losses, whilst the donor sites heal and become available for a second harvest.
- It can also be laid over widely meshed autograft to reduce wound desiccation (Alexander/sandwich technique).
- Some use cadaveric skin or porcine skin as 'test grafts' to see if a wound bed is ready to support autografts, e.g. in debrided chemical burns.

CULTURED EPITHELIAL AUTOGRAFT

Epithelial culture (Rheinwald JG, *Cell*, 1975) begins with a full thickness skin biopsy of several square centimetres taken from the patient. After culturing for 2–3 weeks, there will be enough cells to cover a 1.8 m² sheet five cells thick. The cells take by adhesion more than revascularisation; overall take is 80% under favourable conditions, though late loss can occur.

- Cultured epidermal cells express fewer MHCII/HLA-DR antigens and thus *allogenic keratinocytes* could potentially be used. Animal studies have shown temporary take contributing to wound closure, but the cells do not persist for more than a week – they may accelerate wound healing by interaction with host cells, and through cytokines and growth factors. The results so far have been too costly and time-consuming to be clinically useful.

TISSUE XENOGRAFTS

Animal-derived wound dressings have been used as early as 1500 BC. The dressing dries and falls off as the burn heals; they are 'ejected' rather than rejected, and thus the term 'xenograft' should be avoided for these materials. Similarly, whilst other animal-derived products are used for permanent incorporation, they are acellular after significant processing, and probably do not qualify as true xenografts.

- **Surgisis®** (Cook) – derived from pig small intestine submucosa (SIS); an updated product Biodesign was released in 2008. It is often used for fascia replacement; the acellullar matrix allows tissue ingrowth; it received FDA clearance in 1988 as a hernia repair material.
- Similar products include – Cellis®, Strattice® (Lifecell) and Permacol® (Covidien). There are no good clinical data for its effectiveness over other biological meshes or standard mesh. Some of these are being promoted for use in (covering) breast implants; however, it is much less elastic than human ADMs and is associated with higher seroma rates.

TISSUE ALLOPLASTS

Alloplasts have abundant supply without donor site morbidity, but tend to be expensive and elicit a host reaction of some sort as they are foreign materials. Silicone and Medpor® are the commonest types of implant materials used in the face.

- **Silicone** is a silicon polymer and its physical state depends on the amount of cross-linking. It is generally inert, which means it tends to be encapsulated rather than incorporated.
- **Medpor®** (high-density porous polyethylene) – allows vascular ingrowth and reduced tissue reaction, but it is expensive and can be difficult to remove.

- **Hydroxyapatite** – a calcium phosphate salt available in dense (high-pressure compaction) or porous hydroxyapatite. A natural source of hydroxyapatite comes from coral. It allows a degree of vascular ingrowth but is brittle and can be difficult to shape. It is also available for use as a tissue filler (Radiesse®).
  - Nanocrystalline hydroxyapatite (NanoBone®) – new bone formation is seen after 5 weeks. There is a size limit; clinical studies suggest that (cranial) defects larger than 4–5 cm will be incompletely ossified. Such materials are unable to tolerate load bearing. Note that autologous bone is prone to resorption in the absence of load bearing, and thus would offer a few advantages over biomaterials under these circumstances.
  - Calcium carbonate also derived from coral (but without additional conversion to phosphate) is resorbed and totally replaced. However, it is not very strong.
- **Gore-Tex®** – expanded polytetrafluoroethylene (ePTFE) – is available in many different forms. It provokes a weaker foreign body reaction and reduced ingrowth in comparison to polypropylene mesh, and thus is said to have weaker interface with tissues (almost no capsule formation) with potentially more herniation but fewer adhesions and fistulae. However, major differences are not evident in studies.
- **Metals**, e.g. stainless steel, vitallium alloy, titanium alloys (10 times stronger than bone and well tolerated but has low fatigue tolerance).
- **Polylactide compounds**, e.g. Lactosorb® plating system used in craniofacial surgery, poly-L-lactic acid (PLLA) tissue fillers (Sculptra®). These are completely resorbed and thus have fewer long-term risks.
- **Polyglactin** – is available as a suture (Vicryl), film or mesh.

BONE AND BONE HEALING

Bone is composed of 35% organic material (mostly type I collagen), 60% mineral (mainly hydroxyapatite) and 5% trace elements.

TYPES OF BONE

Developmental classification

- Endochondral bone – laid down as cartilage first, usually at an epiphysis, followed by ossification. This occurs in long bones.
- Membranous bone (skull, facial, clavicle) – osteoid is laid down directly by osteoblasts without a cartilaginous stage. Also occurs in primary bone healing.
  - Membranous bones are said to undergo less absorption than endochondral when used as onlay grafts on facial bones (Zins JE, *Plast Reconstr Surg*, 1983).

Structural classification

- Cortical – concentric lamellae around a Haversian canal.
- Cancellous – made up of lamellar bone but in loosely woven spicules/trabeculae. It is not the same as immature/woven bone.

Fracture healing

Normal bony union/healing occurs at 4–8 weeks in adults. A good **blood supply and stability** of the bony ends is essential for healing. The blood supply to bone comes from:

- Nutrient artery, which enters the medulla and usually supplies the inner two-thirds of the cortex
- Periosteal artery, which supplies the outer third of the cortex
- Metaphyseal, apophyseal (at tendon/ligament attachments) and epiphyseal supplies.

Bony union

- **Primary union** – healing without an intermediate cartilage phase. The bone forms directly at the opposed Haversian canals at the fracture surfaces by osteoclastic action and osteocyte osteoid formation with little or no external callus reaction. This type of healing requires tight apposition and compression of bone ends, e.g. if a fracture is anatomically reduced and immobilised by rigid compressive fixation, e.g. AO system of facial fracture fixation.
  - It takes about 6 weeks, i.e. typically longer than secondary bone healing; also known as membranous union and is less common.
- **Secondary union** has an endochondral phase with hyaline cartilage deposition. This type of healing occurs in fractures that are not rigidly fixed or have a small gap. There are four phases similar to wound (skin) healing described above:
  - **Haemorrhage, inflammation and proliferation** (1–7 days) – activation of clotting cascade to form a fibrin coagulum (fracture haematoma) between the bone ends, which is invaded by neutrophils, then by macrophages and fibroblasts to form granulation tissue/collagen, whilst osteoclasts resorb necrotic bone.
    - Acid tide
    - Alkaline tide ~day 10 with increased alkaline phosphatase coinciding with the production of woven bone
  - **Soft callus stage** (3–4 days) – capillaries from the periosteum invade the fibrin clot. Periosteal activity peaks at 24–36 hours; undifferentiated periosteal mesenchymal cells differentiate to become chondrocytes that form a **cartilaginous** external or bridging callus, with further differentiation of chondrocytes into osteoblasts with endochondral ossification of the callus to form woven bone. The hard callus stage occurs about 3 weeks after injury.
  - **Remodelling** (years) of woven bone to mature lamellar bone, orientated along lines of stress.

Abnormal union

- Non-union – permanent absence of histological osteogenic material between fracture ends
  - Fibrous/fibrocartilage
  - Pseudoarthrosis with fibrocartilage cap
  - Persistence of fracture ends with no cartilage (which implies excessive mobility)
- Delayed union – slow but will eventually heal to acceptable union. It differs from non-union by the potential for consolidation after proper immobilisation and reduction.
- Malunion – non-anatomic union exists, which can either be normal or fibrous.

CAUSES OF POOR UNION:

- Local
  - **Inadequate fixation**/immobilisation is the most common cause of poor bony union. There is 'eburnation' (rounded osseous ends) and medullary blood vessels fail to bridge the gap leading to an avascular zone and potentially osteogenic material turns into a fibrous scar.
  - Inadequate blood supply, which also predisposes to infection.
  - Infection – **non-union may be the only sign of infection**.
  - Recurrent trauma.
- Systemic
  - Age (children can heal in 3 weeks or less, but the elderly may take 8 weeks or more).
  - Medication, e.g. steroids.
  - There is mixed evidence that NSAIDs have adverse effects on fracture healing.
  - Malnutrition and general metabolic disorders (renal failure, deficiency of vitamins ACD).
  - Bone disease (Paget's, osteogenesis imperfecta).

HEALING OF BONE GRAFTS

Bone that is transferred without its blood supply from one region to another will 'heal' in various ways. The relative contributions of osteoconduction, osteoinduction and osteogenesis depends on the composition of bone.

- **Osteoinduction** – pluripotential cells in the recipient site (pericytes) are **'induced' to become bone cells**; this is controlled by growth factors called bone morphogenic proteins (BMPs). Some products include recombinant human BMPs for 'highly osteoinductive bone grafts'.
- **Osteoconduction** – bone graft acts as a scaffold for the ingrowth of cells and capillaries. Old bone is

reabsorbed and new bone deposited, i.e. **'creeping substitution'**. Most bone fillers fall into this category, e.g. cancellous auto/allografts, demineralised bone matrix, hydroxyapatite, etc.

- **Osteogenesis** – new bone is produced by cells that survive within well-vascularised parts of the bone graft. Cancellous autograft (and bone marrow) will have enough osteoprogenitor cells to be considered osteogenic.
- **Osteointegration** is often mentioned in this discussion. It is the capacity of bone to **bind directly** to the surface of an implant (usually titanium alloy) without a fibrous layer, making it very rigid.
  - Titanium is useful being very strong yet bendable, and well tolerated; however, as there is no bone growth, extrusion is always a risk.

The most basic requirement for a bone graft to work is for it to be **osteoconductive**, whilst osteoinduction and osteogenesis will theoretically promote faster integration of the graft. All bone grafts undergo some degree of absorption; it is dependent on the **microarchitecture** (more than embryological origin). Stability is another major determinant. See Table 1.2.

- **Cortical bone** tends to form a non-viable scaffold matrix. The osteocytes within lacunae die leaving an intact Haversian canal system and graft take occurs by **osteoconduction**, i.e. the bone graft is a surface to 'conduct' cells at the recipient bone ends, which migrate into it, proliferate and carry out their functions. Osteoclastic resorption and osteoblastic deposition lead to eventual replacement of the graft. Characteristically, there is initially high strength that decreases with bone resorption and is regained after remodelling is complete.
- **Cancellous bone** graft generally consists of morcellised pieces of bone that are readily vascularised by surrounding tissues, whilst the presence of viable osteoblasts in the graft allows **osteogenesis** and contributes to new bone growth. **Osteoinduction** can occur by factors such as BMPs that cause undifferentiated mesenchymal cells to differentiate along osteoblastic pathways. Cancellous bone offers **more reliable take** due to the larger surface area of contact and can be used to stimulate healing, provide bulk or bridge small gaps, but offers little structural support initially; but this increases as more bone is incorporated.

Vascularised bone grafts (VBGs), i.e. bone flaps, are superior to bone grafts in terms of incorporation time, mechanical strength and retention of mass, and thus are recommended for defects larger than 5–6 cm. Most cells in the lacunae are actually non-viable, dying before neovascularisation. VBGs are more resistant to irradiation and infection. In contrast to simple fractures, they can still take over a year for stable union.

- Distraction osteogenesis can be used for selective bony defects.

Bone graft materials are generally classified as autograft, allograft, alloplast and xenograft. They can be fresh (with greater risk of disease transmission), fresh frozen or freeze-dried. **Autografts are the gold standard**.

- Blood (soaked sponge) is the best wrapping for a bone graft, wrapped again in a saline gauze. Antibiotic solutions are harmful; even crystalloid solutions have harmful effects after long exposures. High temperatures and exposure to air kill osteocytes.

Allografts function as a scaffold and are generally slower to incorporate/vascularise than equivalent autograft; they are widely available in a number of forms.

- Exogenous BMPs can lead to new bone growth through conversion of osteoprogenitors into osteoblasts.
- Rh-BMP2 and rh-BMP7 are FDA-approved for spine surgery, fractures and alveolar clefts.
- BMP9 is most potent.

FACTORS AFFECTING HEALING OF BONE GRAFTS

In general, take can be improved by **ensuring good contact**, rigid fixation, increasing the cancellous/cortical ratio and retaining periosteum.

- Patient factors, e.g. age, nutrition, immunosuppression, diabetes, obesity, drugs, etc. (see 'Wound healing')
- Bone graft factors
  - Intrinsic properties – there is usually less resorption if the periosteum is intact and possibly in membranous bone. Processing of allografts such as freeze-drying reduces immunogenicity and the risk of disease transfer, compared to fresh bone.
- Recipient site – irradiation, infected or scarred.
- Fixation – rigidity of, (see 'Bone and bone healing')
- Mechanical stress – physiological loading speeds up union and creeping substitution.

Table 1.2 Characteristics of types of bone grafts related to their healing and strength over time

	Vascularised bone	Cortical graft	Cancellous bone
Osteoinduction	+/–	+/–	++
Osteoconduction	+	+	++++
Osteoprogenitor cells	++	–	+++
Immediate strength	+++	+++	–
6-month strength	+++	+++	++
12-month strength	+++	+++	+++

BONE GRAFTS VS. CARTILAGE GRAFTS

- **Bone autografts**
  - Can be incorporated without host reaction and is relatively resistant to infection.
  - Donor site morbidity is a problem, as is the variable resorption rate in the graft – cortical grafts maintain their volume better than cancellous (see above).
- **Cartilage autografts**
  - Relatively easy harvest and less donor site morbidity; infection and resorption are rare but grafts may calcify.
  - Have a **tendency to warp** and memory is very difficult to overcome.
  - Quantities are quite limited (septum, rib, conchal).

TENDON HEALING IN THE HAND

Tendons consist of a dense network of spiral collagen fibres that are predominantly type I; there is some type III collagen, some ground substance and a small amount of elastin.

- Ground substance (~60% water) provides support and spacing to the collagen.
- Elastin facilitates recoil and recovery.
- Smooth gliding is facilitated by lubricin (proteoglycan 4).
- They are relatively acellular – mostly (~95%) specific tendon cells (tenoblasts and tenocytes); the remainder include fibroblasts and synoviocytes. The low metabolic/anaerobic activity of mature cells is suited for the tensional stresses, but makes repair slow. Tendon stem/progenitor cells (TSPC) were found (Bi Y, *Nat Med*, 2007), but their role is uncertain.

The **endotenon** envelops tendon fascicles and binds them together. It also supports the sparse vessels and nerves; it is continuous with perimysium and periosteum. The **epitenon** is a vascular, cellular outer layer of a tendon, which runs through a synovial sheath (zones 1 and 2 in the hand), whilst in zones 3 and beyond, where there is no tendon sheath, the outer vascular layer is called **'paratenon'**.

BLOOD SUPPLY AND HEALING

The blood supply in zones 1 and 2 of the hand comes via mesenteries ('mesotenons') called the **vinculae** – long and short, that enter the dorsal surface of the tendons from the transverse digital arteries at the level of the cruciate pulleys. Synovial fluid also contributes to nutrition via imbibition and is an important source in the hand; in the forearm, tendon nutrition is mainly derived from vessels in the paratenon.

Tendon healing occurs by processes analogous (to skin healing) of inflammation (with cellular response), proliferation (fibroplasia) and remodelling. The early vascular response in particular seems to be important and ensures the survival of the new fibrous material.

- **Extrinsic healing** by cells recruited from synovial sheaths and surrounding tissues forming adhesions.
- **Intrinsic healing** by cells within the tendon itself.
- The two occur together and in cooperation.
  - Early collagen production is predominantly type III and 'random'.
  - Remodelling begins 6–8 weeks after injury (consolidation phase) and lasts up to 2 years (maturation phase).
  - In most, the tendon does not regain full 'strength' – it usually thickens and stiffens to partly compensate.
- Studies have demonstrated that the strength and rate of healing are maximal in a tendon that is moving and stressed. A repaired tendon is weakest during the period of collagen lysis at about days 10–14.
- Strategies to improve tendon healing include
  - Growth factors – animal experiments seem to indicate a role for VEGF, TFGβ, PDGF and bFGF.
  - **Platelet-rich plasma** (PRP) as a source of autologous growth factors was popular for awhile. Systematic reviews did not show any improvement in the healing of tendinopathy (de Vos RF, *JAMA*, 2010).
  - Mesenchymal stem cells (MSCs) including marrow and adipose derived (ADSCs).
- **Biomaterials** to avoid autologous tendon transfer/graft.
  - Xenografts, e.g. Permacol™, and allografts, e.g. GraftJacket™, have been used in rotator cuff and Achilles tendon repairs (Lee DK, *J Foot Ankle Surg*, 2008).
  - Collagen gels, often with bone marrow MSCs, have been used in animal studies only.
  - Scaffolds composed of cell-loaded collagen I nanofibres/composites (Kishore V, *Biomaterials*, 2012); these have been used in animal studies but have been difficult to scale up to humans.

Autologous platelets have no effect on the healing of human Achilles tendon ruptures: A randomized single-blind study. (Schepull T et al., *Am J Sports Med*, **2011)**
Despite the vogue for PRP, this RCT provides level 2 evidence that PRP is not useful for the treatment of Achilles tendon ruptures.

The risk of fluoroquinolone-induced tendinopathy and tendon rupture. (Del Rosso JQ, *J Clin Aesthet Dermatol*, **2010)**
Levofloxacin, ciproxin and ofloxacin are antibiotics of the fluoroquinolone (FQ) class. After the first report of Achilles tendinopathy in 1983, many other cases followed. In 2008, the FDA mandated a black box warning of increased adverse events including tendon rupture – based on epidemiological studies, there is a 3.8× risk compared to other antibiotics. FQs have a high affinity for connective tissue and inhibit tenocyte metabolism including proliferation and collagen synthesis. Age >60 and concurrent steroids

seem to increase the risk; half of cases occur within 1 week of administration.

The Achilles tendon is affected in 95% of FQ-related cases in a literature review (Lewis T, *J Athl Train*, 2014); rupture of finger and thumb tendons, shoulder, hip and knee tendons have been reported less frequently.

II. NECROTISING FASCIITIS

NF was first described by Wilson in 1952. It is a potentially life-threatening infection (up to 53% mortality) that progresses along fascial planes and subcutaneous tissues.

CLASSIFICATION

- **Type I. Mixed/polymicrobial** (80%) – anaerobes (*Escherichia coli, bacteroides*) and aerobes (*Staphylococcus aureus, Streptococcus pyogenes, Enterococcus faecalis*). In most cases, *streptococci* and/or *staphylococci* are the initiating agents; anaerobic bacteria proliferate in areas of local hypoxia such as traumatic/surgical wounds or medical compromise. Type I NF is more common in the elderly or those with illness such as diabetes, alcoholism and malignancy.
  - *Vibrio vulnificus* (Latin *vulnus,* a wound and *facere,* to make) is often seen in those with chronic liver disease and may follow raw seafood ingestion as well as injuries in fishmarkets. This type of disease sometimes called **saltwater NF** classically demonstrates subcutaneous bleeding.
- **Type II. Monomicrobial.** Although more recently methicillin-resistant *Staphylococcus aureus* (MRSA) has been implicated, the causative agent is usually group A β-haemolytic *streptococci* (e.g. *Streptococcus pyogenes*) carried in the nose/throat of 15% of the population. This is the classic 'flesh-eating bacteria'; it can also contribute to type I infections. Type II NF can affect all age groups and the healthy (up to a half); there is an association with varicella zoster and NSAIDs. The (lower) extremity is affected most often. There are a number of **virulence factors**:
  - Exotoxin, e.g. streptococcal pyrogenic exotoxin A (SpeA); this **superantigen** (antigens that cause non-specific activation of T-cells resulting in polyclonal T-cell activation and massive cytokine release) causes systemic upset.
  - Streptokinase that activates plasminogen and fibrinolysis.
  - Hyaluronidase.
  - Haemolysins.
  - M proteins that inhibit opsonisation by an alternative complement pathway.
- **Type III. Clostridial** 'gas gangrene' with myonecrosis, is due to *Clostridium perfringens* (Gram-positive rods) in 80%, although it can be caused by other species, e.g. novyi and septicum. It often follows trauma/surgery; local tissue hypoxia leads to activation of spores with

α (exo)toxin, i.e. lecithinase production that breaks down cell membranes.
  - Classically there is characteristic surgical emphysema (crepitus, also found in some forms of non-clostridial gangrene) and 'dishwater' exudate. Myonecrosis may give rise to deeper pain.
  - Cases with bloody blisters contain *Clostridium welchii* if aspirated.
  - High mortality – aggressive surgical approach needed with some evidence to support role of HBOT.

Meleney's synergistic gangrene is rare but rapidly progressive due to synergism between aerobic haemolytic *staphylococci* (*aureus*) and microaerophilic non-haemolytic *streptococci*. It was described in 1924 by Frank L. Meleney, a US surgeon working mostly at Columbia University in New York, but saw the cases in China; he was also one of the first to use bacitracin.

Jean-Alfred **Fournier** described five cases of perineal gangrene of (then) unknown cause in 1883; Baurienne had described idiopathic gangrene of the male genitalia over 100 years earlier. It has since been recognised as a polymicrobial NF, i.e. type I, originating possibly from local abscesses or urogenital tract infections. Diabetes and other causes of immune impairment are risk factors. Infection spreads along the potential spaces bounded by the fascial layers; thrombosis of the **external pudendal arteries** compromises the circulation of the scrotum. There is early skin necrosis due to thin subcutaneous tissue; the corporoa, testes and cord structures are usually spared.

RISK FACTORS

- Surgery and even intravenous infusions or intramuscular injections have been associated with NF.
- Insulin-dependent DM (IDDM).
- Cirrhotic liver disease (Hung TH, *Singapore Med J,* 2014).
- NSAIDs, e.g. ibuprofen.
- Varicella zoster virus infections.

CLINICAL FEATURES

A high index of suspicion is required to act quickly on the early signs (disproportionate sepsis and pain).

- Local swelling and redness, **intense pain out of proportion** to the appearance. There is very rapid spread **subcutaneously**; the dissemination of infection through tissue planes causes thrombosis of blood vessels and violaceous skin changes with dusky/grey hues and haemorrhagic bullae, with **crepitus** (in less than 10%) and anaesthetic zones due to nerve necrosis. The underlying fascial necrosis is more extensive than overlying skin changes, which are **secondary**.
- **Systemic toxicity** – apathy, confusion and septic shock, that is classically **out of proportion** to the skin disease. The elderly may be unable to mount a pyrexial response.

MANAGEMENT

The early stages of the condition may be difficult to recognise, but diligence is required as it can develop rapidly; early treatment is vital – those who present in shock have the worst prognosis. NF remains a largely clinical diagnosis; imaging may help in delineating the extent or excluding other processes. Early debridement is the key and should not be delayed for radiology or other studies.

- **Tissue biopsy** – rapid Gram stain of deeper tissue – surface biopsies may detect other bacteria that do not actually contribute to the disease.
  - There are rapid streptococcal diagnostic tests and PCR for Spe.
  - The so-called **'finger test'** via a 2 cm incision is said to demonstrate the loosened tissue planes, cloudy or 'dishwater' exudate and lack of bleeding but is very much dependent on the experience of the physician.
  - Hans Christian Gram (1853–1938) was a Danish bacteriologist who developed the staining technique.
- **Radiology** – subcutaneous gas may be seen on plain X-rays but is usually of little value.
  - The use of Doppler ultrasound has also been described. Sharif (*Am J Roentgenol*, 1990) found CT and MRI to be more useful than ultrasound or plain X-rays.
  - Computed tomography (CT) with contrast may help (see below) but can be normal in early stages.
  - **Magnetic resonance imaging** (MRI) can demonstrate fascial necrosis by T2 hyperintensity in the deep fascia, and a variable pattern of gadolinium enhancement on T1 – in general, the sensitivity of MRI exceeds its specificity. Studies have not demonstrated significant superiority over contrast CT – the latter is a much more efficient way to screen cases, but (contrast) CT may be contraindicated due to acute renal failure.
  - Imaging should be used cautiously; non-diagnostic tests may hinder/delay diagnosis and treatment.

TREATMENT

- Resuscitation including ICU supportive therapy – ventilation/oxygenation, inotropic support and dialysis where necessary.
- **Intravenous antibiotics**, e.g. **clindamycin** (stops the production of toxins and M proteins), gentamicin (covers Gram negatives), third-generation cephalosporins (covers Gram negatives) and imipenem. Immunoglobulins may be given to those with *streptococcal* toxic shock syndrome.
  - Many propose **gentamicin with clindamycin** as standard coverage, adding ampicillin if Gram stain shows enterococci.
  - Anaerobes suggested by 'foul-smelling' lesions are covered by clindamycin or metronidazole.

- Radical surgical debridement to healthy tissues, with a 'second look' at 24 hours. Several debridements are often needed. McHenry (1995) found that survivors had surgery after a mean of 25 hours after admission, whilst in non-survivors, this interval was 90 hours.
- HBOT has been proposed for clostridial NF.

Necrotizing fasciitis and its mimics: What radiologists need to know. (Chaudhry AA, *Am J Roentgenol*, 2015)
The finding of gas tracking along fascial planes in an ill patient is almost pathognomonic, but imaging is often not needed and can delay treatment. The diagnosis is still primarily clinical.

- **CT** may show dermal thickening, soft tissue attenuation and inflammatory fat stranding, but the hallmark is soft tissue air with deep fascial fluid collections.
- **MRI** will show dermal and soft tissue thickening with increased signal on fluid-sensitive sequences. Late stages will demonstrate gas collections in the fascial layers seen as hypointense foci. IV gadolinium increases sensitivity but is not essential. MRI is the modality of choice for soft tissue infection, but acquisition is time-consuming and its availability is often more limited than CT.

III. CLOTTING AND HAEMOSTASIS

There are four components to clotting and haemostasis.

- **Vasoconstriction** – contraction of vascular smooth muscle both as a local reflex and in response to thromboxane release from platelets.
- **Activation of platelets** – with disruption of the endothelium, platelets adhere to the underlying tissue and the intrinsic pathway is activated. Aggregated platelets promote local thrombin and fibrin generation.
- **Coagulation** – intrinsic (involves normal blood components) and extrinsic (requires tissue thromboplastin from damaged cells) pathways both activate factor X. Most coagulation factors are made in the liver except for VIII and thromboplastin.
- **Fibrinolysis** – i.e. fibrin removal, which is the result of the action of plasmin (plasminogen activators from endothelial cells promote conversion of plasminogen to plasmin).

DISORDERS OF COAGULATION

- **Congenital**
  - Haemophilia A – factor VIII deficiency that is X-linked.
  - von Willebrand's disease – autosomal dominant (AD) deficiency of von Willebrand factor (vWF) that will also reduce factor VIII somewhat (as it normally protects VIII from breakdown).

It is the commonest inherited abnormality of coagulation and is actually a collection of conditions with vWF deficiency rather than a single disease entity.

- **Acquired**
  - Vitamin K deficiency inhibits the synthesis of II, VII, IX and X; warfarin also inhibits the production of these (as well as protein C and S).
  - Liver disease – reduced synthesis of clotting factors and reduced/abnormal fibrinogen.
  - Disseminated intravascular coagulation (DIC) – simultaneous coagulation and fibrinolysis, causes reduction of platelets and fibrinogen, but increase in FDPs.

DISORDERS OF HAEMOSTASIS

- Thrombocytopaenia – due to reduced production, increased destruction or abnormal function of platelets, e.g. aspirin (blocks platelet cyclo-oxygenase) and clopidogrel (reduces platelet aggregation by inhibiting adenosine diphosphate [ADP] binding).
- Blood vessel abnormalities, e.g. due to Cushing's syndrome/steroids, Henoch–Schönlein purpura (HSP).

HYPERCOAGULABILITY STATES

Between 5% and 15% of venous thromboses are caused by inherited deficiencies. Some causes include

- Activated protein C resistance (APC) (factor V Leiden mutation) – APC normally inactivates factors V and VIII. This is one of the most common inherited causes.
- Antiphospholipid antibody.
- Homocysteinaemia.
- Elevated factors VIII and XI.

HAEMOSTASIS IN PLASTIC SURGERY

See also 'Burns'.

ADRENALINE

Adrenaline causes vasoconstriction by binding to post-synaptic α-2 adrenoreceptors on vascular smooth muscle. It is often used to reduce bleeding in plastic surgery (see also 'Liposuction') and thus improves surgical visibility. It also prolongs the effect of lidocaine.

- Many textbooks state that adrenaline is contra-indicated for local infiltration/nerve blocks of the extremities due to the 'end' arteries. A literature review (Denkler, *Plast Reconstr Surg*, 2001) found 48 cases of necrosis after digital blocks reported in 1880–2000; most cases occurred prior to the 1950s and none involved lidocaine. They were probably related to the use of acidic procaine–epinephrine.

- Similarly, there have been no reports of finger necrosis in accidents with EpiPens® – there may be some minor local necrosis, but the main side effect has been 'reperfusion' pain. Adrenaline has a plasma half-life of 2–3 minutes (compare that to the warm ischaemia time for a digit), though the end effects on vascular smooth muscle will last for longer. There are no evidence-based remedies, but the use of phentolamine seems logical; some report that it reduces the incidence of pain afterwards.

There have been several literature reviews supporting the safety of adrenaline use in the digits, including a Cochrane review in 2015, and a big case series (Lalonde D, *J Hand Surg Am*, 2005) with 3110 consecutive cases of surgery on the digits using lidocaine with adrenaline.

The general advice is to use the lowest possible effective concentration of adrenaline – whilst adrenaline will still have a vasoconstrictive effect at dilutions up to 1 in 1,000,000, it will take longer to work. It is important to wait 4–5 minutes before making the incision; there can be increased blood flow in the first minute or so presumably due to the vasodilatory effects of lidocaine. Maximal vasoconstriction occurs after ~20–25 minutes.

- Use of 1 in 100,000–200,000 adrenaline seems to be safe for digital blocks.
- Other recommendations include the following:
  - Do not inject >20 mL of 1 in 200,000 solutions within 10 minutes.
  - Caution in patients with severe hypertension, phaeochromocytoma, etc.

Adrenaline with lidocaine for digital nerve blocks. (Prabhakar H, *Cochrane Database of Syst Rev*, 2015)
They found four eligible studies on ring blocks for digits. There were no reports of adverse events such as ischaemia, but also no cost analysis or benefits – one study had weak evidence to suggest that adrenaline prolonged the duration of anaesthesia. Two studies suggested a reduced incidence of bleeding with the use of adrenaline. The authors concluded that there was limited evidence to recommend use or avoidance of adrenaline in nerve blocks.

HAEMOSTATIC AGENTS

There is a range of tools to stop/reduce intra-operative bleeding, such as radiofrequency, argon beam coagulators, lasers, harmonic scalpels as well as the usual cautery, clips and sutures. Other products can be classified as follows:

Passive agents – these rely on clotting factors of the patient. They need blood/bleeding in order to work – they absorb blood, activate platelets and induce coagulation. There are a variety of products:

- Cellulose (oxidised), e.g. Surgicel®. Note that it has a rim-enhancing appearance on CT that may mimic an abscess.

- Gelatin sponge, e.g. Gelfoam®, made from purified pork skin gelatin – the mechanism of action is not fully understood.
- Collagen (microfibrillar), e.g. Avitene®.
- Chitosan (shrimp shells), e.g. Celox rapid® – also causes vasospasm, attracts platelets, sticks to wound.
- Zeolite (from lava) Quikclot® – non-biodegradable, and thus has potential for foreign body reaction.
- Kaolin (a clay mineral) – 'Combat gauze', promotes clot formation.

ACTIVE AGENTS

- **Thrombin products.** Human thrombin–gelatin sponge mix, e.g. Floseal®, a combination of active and passive haemostatics. Initial products used bovine material and led to coagulopathy due to the formation of inhibiting factor V antibodies. There is a theoretical risk of disease transmission including JCD, which is minimised in recombinant products.
- **Fibrin sealants** – these produce fibrin independent of the patient's coagulation – e.g. Tisseel® (Baxter) that consists of human pooled fibrinogen and thrombin, as well as synthetic aprotinin (antifibrinolytic). They are better **sealants** than haemostatics; they adhere to collagen on damaged tissues and can deal with minor diffuse bleeding. They are reabsorbed after a week or two. Fibrin sealants can be used to aid the placement on skin grafts on wounds particularly in burn patients.
  - There are some theoretical concerns over disease transmission; Crosseal® is made entirely of non-animal components.
  - An alternative is to use the patient's own blood – Vivostat® machine is used to prepare autologous fibrin sealant from 120 mL of whole blood.
  - TachoSil® is an absorbable fibrin sealant patch.

B. PRESSURE SORES

I. AETIOLOGY AND RISK ASSESSMENT

'Pure' pressure sores begin with tissue necrosis near a bony prominence leading to a cone-shaped area of tissue breakdown with its apex at the skin surface. Affecting this is the additional impact on the soft tissue from moisture, infection and shear forces, etc. (see below). Acute sores are often 'iatrogenic' in the sense that there is an episode of prolonged unrelieved pressure, whilst chronic sores tend to be seen in those with spinal cord injury or chronic debilitation. The latter tend to have multiple recurrences; thus, flaps should be planned in a way to allow re-elevation or not to interfere with other flaps.

- ~10% of patients in acute care facilities develop pressure sores (mainly sacral); up to 24% in chronic hospitalised patients.

- 66% of elderly patients with neck of the femur (NOF) fractures and 60% of quadriplegic patients develop pressure sores.
- Supine patients develop sacral, heel and occipital sores (~40–60 mmHg of pressure); whilst the wheelchair/chair bound develop ischial sores (~100 mmHg when sitting).
- Lying on one side causes trochanteric sores.

RISK ASSESSMENT

Many different systems that stratify the risk of developing a pressure sore have been described. In the end, whilst it is the standard of care that will have the greatest contribution, it is not fair to blame all pressure sores on 'poor' care, as not all can be prevented in the susceptible.

- Norton Scale for elderly patients.
- Waterlow score – pressure sore risk assessment chart (at risk/high risk/very high risk depending on scores) – the higher the score, the higher the risk.
  - Body mass index (BMI)
  - Continence
  - Mobility
  - Nutrition
  - Skin changes/type
  - Sex/age
  - Adverse wound healing factors/tissue malnutrition
  - Neurological deficit
  - Major surgical intervention(s)/trauma
  - Drugs (steroids, cytotoxics, anti-inflammatory)
- **Braden Scale.** This is one of the most commonly used scoring systems, and like all systems should be used together with clinical judgement. The scale stratifies the risk according to six parameters: sensory perception, skin moisture, activity, mobility, friction, shear and nutritional status. The lower the score, the higher the risk. Starting from a maximum value of 23 (no risk), the risk of developing a sore comes at a threshold value of 18 (originally 16), whilst those with a minimum score of 6 have the highest risk. Inter-rater reliability is fairly high at 0.83–0.99. **Identification of risk should lead to action.**

NECESSARY ACTIONS (THE 3 R'S)

- Redistribute surfaces (pressure relieving surfaces)
- Remobilise
- Reposition
  - Avoid higher pressure positions such as lying on the side, semi-recumbent; instead choose 30° lateral or elevating the head of the bed (up to 30°, as a compromise between sacral pressure and respiratory function/protection)
  - Change up to Q2H, supplementing with small shifts

PATHOGENESIS

In simple terms, prolonged unrelieved pressure will lead to ischaemic necrosis if the tissue pressure is greater than perfusion pressure; the damage is proportional to the pressure and its duration. Many believe that lower pressure for longer periods does more damage than high pressure for shorter periods.

- **Muscle is more susceptible** than skin to pressure necrosis. Animal studies (pigs) demonstrated that 500 mmHg for 2 hours or 100 mmHg for 10 hours caused muscle necrosis, but it took 11 hours of 600 mmHg to cause skin ulceration.
- Kosiak found that continuous pressures of 70 mmHg (in dogs) produces irreversible necrosis after 2 hours, but this could be prevented by relieving the pressure every 5 minutes.

In reality, there are many other factors that contribute to the pathogenesis:

- Altered sensory perception, as well as
  - **Incontinence** and exposure to moisture (skin maceration and breakdown).
  - **Friction and shear force** – traction on perforator vessels to the skin causing vessel angulation may occlude flow, subcutaneous degloving.
  - **Infection** – apart from causing tissue damage by itself, infection increases susceptibility to pressure, whilst pressure also increases susceptibility to infection.
- Intrinsic factors may also contribute to
  - Ischaemia, sepsis and peripheral vascular disease (PVD), DM, smokers, etc. reducing perfusion
  - Loss of protective sensation
  - Malnutrition and reduced wound healing

GRADING OF PRESSURE SORES

Grading was originally described by Shea in 1975 and has been modified/updated into various sets of guidelines. There were separate European and American systems, the European Pressure Ulcer Advisory Panel (EPUAP) grading system and the National Pressure Ulcer Advisory Panel (NPUAP) system, respectively. The many similarities led eventually to a combined International NPUAP/EPUAP classification system (2009, then 2014).

- **Stage I** – Intact skin with **non-blanchable redness** of a localised area, usually over a bony prominence. Darkly pigmented skin may not have visible blanching; its colour may differ from the surrounding area.
  - The area may be painful, firm, soft, warmer or cooler as compared with the adjacent tissue.
  - Generally, this would be expected after about an hour of sustained pressure.
- **Stage II – Partial thickness loss** of dermis presenting as a shallow open ulcer with a red-pink wound bed, without slough. It may also present as an intact or ruptured serum-filled blister.
  - This stage should not be used to describe skin tears, tape burns, perineal dermatitis, maceration or excoriation.

- **Bruising** indicates suspected deep tissue injury.
- **Stage III – Full thickness tissue loss.** Subcutaneous fat may be visible, but bone, tendon or muscle are not exposed. Slough may be present but does not obscure the depth of tissue loss. There may be undermining and tunnelling.
  - The depth of a stage III ulcer varies by anatomical location. The occiput and malleolus do not have much subcutaneous tissue, and stage III ulcers can be shallow. In contrast, areas of significant adiposity can develop extremely deep stage III pressure sores.
  - Generally follows >6 hours of pressure.
- **Stage IV** – Full thickness tissue loss with **exposed bone, tendon or muscle.** Slough or eschar may be present on some parts of the wound bed; there is often some undermining and tunnelling.
  - They can extend into muscle and/or supporting structures (e.g. fascia, tendon or joint capsule) making **osteomyelitis** possible. Exposed bone/tendon is visible or directly palpable.

However, it is important to appreciate that the surface appearance does not reliably reflect the underlying extent of the sore.

- **Suspected deep tissue injury (depth unknown)** – purple/maroon localised areas of discoloured intact skin or blood-filled blister due to damage of underlying soft tissue from pressure/and or shear. This may be preceded by stage I type changes.
  - Deep tissue injury may be difficult to detect in individuals with dark skin tones. Evolution may include a thin blister over a dark wound bed, or this may further evolve and become covered by thin eschar.
  - **Evolution may be rapid** exposing additional layers of tissue even with optimal treatment.
- **Unstageable (depth unknown) –** Full thickness tissue loss in which the base of the ulcer is obscured by slough and/or eschar.
  - Until the obscuring layer has been removed (at least partly) to expose the base, the true depth, and therefore stage, cannot be determined.
  - Stable eschar (dry, adherent, intact without erythema or fluctuance) on the **heels** serves as 'the body's natural (biological) cover' and should not be removed.

Unavoidable pressure injury: State of the science and consensus outcomes. (Edsberg LE, *J Wound Ostomy Continence Nurs*, 2014)
The formation of a pressure ulcer is a multifactorial process that at times cannot be prevented even with excellent prevention and management. A consensus conference in 2014 came to the conclusion that main risk factors were impaired cardiopulmonary status/tissue oxygenation, hypovolaemia and sepsis, oedema and PVD. Manoeuvres such as elevation of the head of the bed >30° significantly increase risks.

II. MANAGEMENT

PRESSURE ULCER MANAGEMENT

National Clinical Guideline Centre. *Clinical guideline* 179 April 2014

- **Pressure relief** – Use high-specification foam mattresses, or consider a dynamic support surface.
- **Ulcer measurement** – Record and document wound dimensions including undermining using validated measurement techniques where possible.
  - **Wound measurement** is notoriously difficult and 'standard' methods such as using tape measures or grids are prone to error. Photography needs to be standardised in terms of lighting and angle; the latter can cause apparent increases or decreases in size.
- **Debridement** – promote autolysis by dressing choice, unless it would take too long – in which case, choose sharp debridement (or larval therapy).
- **Nutrition** – supplements should not be routinely offered for patients without identified deficiencies.
- **Dressings** – many choices of dressings that promote warm moist healing in stage II–IV sores.
- **Antimicrobials** – not indicated without clinical signs of infection.

TREATMENT

A multidisciplinary team environment is desirable and should include nursing staff, physiotherapists, occupational therapists, dieticians and community nurses.

GENERAL

- Assess and **optimise nutrition** including correction of anaemia, optimise blood glucose; patients should stop smoking. Patients are often chronically malnourished, though the direct association has not been demonstrated. Whilst nutritional support of those with adequate intake has **not** been shown to prevent the development of sores (NICE 2014), there is low-quality evidence that **protein-rich** nutritional support may improve healing.
  - In the absence of a deficiency, there is limited evidence for additional supplementation of micronutrients. The role of zinc supplementation is unproven, whilst vitamin C has no effect beyond 10–20 mg/day according to RCTs, i.e. no role for 1 g dosage.
- **Treatment of infection** (commonly *Staphylococcus aureus*, *Proteus*, *Pseudomonas*, *Bacteroides*) with oral antibiotics.
  - Colonisation is common (swabs represent surface contamination only; do not treat positive wound cultures alone) – proof of actual tissue infection requires a deep biopsy. A pressure sore may cause sepsis, but it is **most commonly due to a UTI**.
- According to NICE, systemic antibiotics are not indicated unless there is clinical evidence of sepsis, spreading cellulitis or underlying osteomyelitis. There is also no evidence for the routine use of topical antimicrobials/antiseptics.
- Osteomyelitis must be actively sought for (see below); bone biopsy is most sensitive.
- Adjuncts to healing.
  - The role of HBOT is largely unproven, whilst LLLT or ultrasound has been shown to be not useful.
  - Direct contact capacitative electrical stimulation (**strength A-3** EPUAP NPUAP. Treatment of pressure ulcer: Quick reference guide 2009). NICE does not recommend electrotherapy, but some suggest that it can be considered for recalcitrant stage III–IV sores.
  - The role of growth factors has not been fully elucidated, though some studies have shown improved healing with bFGF and PDGF.
- Catheterise if incontinent.
- Relieve spasm (common in spinal cord injury); otherwise, sores will inevitably recur – baclofen, diazepam or dantrolene may be useful but some may require botulinum toxin, surgical release, amputation or neurosurgery, e.g. cordotomy/rhizotomy.

RELIEVE PRESSURE

The effect of relieving pressure by regular turning and using a suitable bed has been confirmed by three RCTs; it is also important to take care during transfer and pad pressure points prophylactically.

- Effective pressure relief for 5 minutes every 2 hours (seated patients should lift themselves every 10 minutes). Reducing head elevation, i.e. 30° or less, will reduce sacral shear forces/pressure.
- Repositioning every 4 hours on an appropriate support surface is as good as every 2 hours (**strength A-1** EPUAP-NPUAP 2009).

NICE 2014 recommends high-specification foam mattresses as a cost-effective treatment in patients with pressure sores as well as in prevention, and if inadequate, an electronic mattress should be considered.

- Electronic mattresses
  - Pegasus – **alternating pressure system** for periodic offloading.
  - Nimbus – dynamic flotation system. Seems to be more comfortable for patients.
  - Cochrane Review (McInnes, *Cochrane Database Syst Rev*, 2015); the relative merits of constant low pressure vs. alternating pressure are unclear. Medical-grade sheepskins reduce the risk of ulcer development.

- Beds
  - **Clinitron** – ceramic beads fluidised by warm air, i.e. air fluidised bed – aims for pressures <20 mmHg. The forced warm air reduces skin moisture, but this, in turn, may cause excessive fluid and electrolyte losses from those with large wounds. These beds lose their effectiveness if the patient sits up 45° or more. In addition, they are rather bulky; turning of patients may be difficult and pulmonary toilet may be impaired in those with breathing problems.
  - **Mediscus** low air loss beds, made of groups of cells that inflate and deflate independently; unlike the Clinitron, there is little/no drying effect, but there is a tilting mechanism to allow the patient position to be altered. The contact surface area is maximised; it aims to exert <25 mmHg at any one point.
- Those in wheelchairs are suggested to have 8 cm thick cushions and to relieve the pressure for 10 seconds after every 10 minutes.

DRESSINGS

Many dressings for pressure sores have been described; generally there are few substantial differences as long as they promote moist wound healing. Negative pressure (NPWT) dressings can be used in larger defects, particularly those with excessive exudate, or after debridement until the patient is ready for definitive surgery – the wound can be improved or reduced in size, but only a minority of cases will avoid surgery in this way. Patient acceptance of a dressing regime is affected by

- Leakage and odours that affect social interaction
- Length of time between changes for convenience
- Pain especially during dressing changes

INVESTIGATIONS

- Blood – albumin, FBC, ESR, LFT, RFT, glucose.
- Wound swabs (see above), tissue biopsy.
- **Osteomyelitis** is associated with a higher risk of wound breakdown and the development of sinuses and deep abscesses. It needs to be actively excluded using a combination of investigations including ESR, white cell count and X-rays (to identify sequestra); bone scans and CT are not particularly sensitive. **Bone biopsy** is the single most useful test with a specificity of 96% but a low sensitivity of 73%. MRI may be better than CT (97% sensitive, 89% specific, Huang AB, *J Comput Assist Tomogr*, 1998) but not quite as good as bone biopsy; PET is prone to false positives.
  - Some suggest a two-stage plan to wait for the results of bone biopsies taken at debridement before embarking on formal reconstruction, whilst others, in general, aim empirically for 'healthy' bleeding bone with further therapy dependent on results.

III. SURGERY

PRINCIPLES

Surgery is best suited to the well-motivated patient (able to adhere to post-operative measures) with a stable condition (or liable to improve). Proper patient selection is particularly important – the wound must have the capacity to heal. Heel sores are generally best healed by secondary intention. Faecal diversion may be helpful in selected patients.

- 'Oncological' debridement of the sore, i.e. **'pseudotumour technique'** – some use methylene blue or a betadine pack inserted into the cavity to guide the completeness of excision. All devitalised tissue should be removed, along with osteomyelitis and the pseudobursa.
- Excision of bony prominences (caution with ischial tuberosities).
- The choice of flap/closure depends on the site of the sore (see below) and may be modified by the patient's ambulatory status.
  - A range of local flaps have been described; it is important to maintain future flap options as the pressure sore is likely to recur. Flaps should be designed to be as large as possible. Muscle flaps are good for filling in **dead space**, but muscle is vulnerable to ischaemia and tends to atrophy; furthermore, sacrifice may affect ambulation; fasciocutaneous (FC) flaps are durable but generally offer less tissue bulk.
  - **Wounds should be closed at maximum stretch**; tension should be judged in various positions; closures that depend on positional changes are doomed to failure.
  - Free flaps, e.g. latissimus dorsi to the superior gluteal artery, are usually a last resort for large defects or where local options have been exhausted.
  - Avoid having suture lines in the areas of pressure. Sutures should be left for 3 weeks.

POST-OPERATIVE CARE

There is a high rate of recurrence (40%–60%) that may be reduced to 25% by optimising post-operative rehabilitation, which is a long process.

- Skin care optimised (start pre-operatively with general management measures mentioned above).
- Take care with transfers as surgery is often performed with the patient prone, and patients need to be flipped over for extubation and transfer. **Avoid pressure on the reconstructed area for at least 2 weeks** post-operatively with the patient position prone/decubitus for weeks with low-pressure mattress/bed, followed by limited sitting protocols, e.g. three 4-hour periods of sitting per day with pressure-relieving manoeuvres every 15 minutes.

- **Use of drains** and antibiotics (quantitative cultures recommended by some). Timing of drain removal is variable; some wait until there is only scant drainage, whilst others wait at least 2 weeks.
- Patient education. Patients should be discharged only after home assessment and necessary facilities, e.g. low-pressure mattress, are in place.
- Outpatient support – to maintain patient motivation, to reinforce need to modify risk factors (both clinical and social), to maintain wound closure.

Common complications include haematoma, infection, dehiscence and recurrence. The published literature shows a wide range of success rates. Overall short-term surgical results are good, but sores may recur (**scarred tissue has only about half of the original strength**) especially in young paraplegics and the compromised elderly (70%–80%), compared to single figures in the non-paraplegics. In the largest published series, the best results are 20% recurrence after 4 years. There was no association found with the number of previous surgeries; second sores were found in other sites in >½ of cases. Studies have shown that patients with pressure sores are more likely to die, but this seems to be related to the generalised state rather than the ulcer itself, i.e. it is an indirect marker for malnutrition, coexisting illness, etc.

SPECIFIC PRESSURE SORES

Ischial pressure sores (28%)

These are the commonest sores in **paraplegics** who sit in wheelchairs. They are usually quite large, and thus are the most difficult type of sore to treat. Ischial sores have a slightly **higher recurrence rate** than sacral sores – using flaps that can advance again is advantageous. Some surgeons prefer to use the flaps from the leg rather than the gluteal region, and vice versa (Kua EH, *J Plast Reconstr Aesthet Surg*, 2011). Patients are not allowed to sit for 3–6 weeks after surgery; thereafter, sitting is allowed for short periods with a wound check each time for dehiscence or erythema (should not last for more than 30 minutes).

- **Muscle (hamstring) VY flaps** have decent bulk. Whilst a single muscle flap (e.g. long head of biceps) may be sufficient in the ambulatory, a larger posterior thigh flap (VY hamstring, Hurteau JE, *Plast Reconstr Surg*, 1981) with biceps, semimembranous and semitendinous can be used in paraplegics. The muscles, supplied by branches of the profunda femoris, have their origins and insertions divided. These flaps can be readvanced if the sore recurs; these flaps do not seem to heal as well as gluteal flaps.
- **Posterior thigh FC flaps** (medially or laterally based) can be used as rotational or transposition flaps with SSG to the donor site. This is similar to the **(inferior) gluteal thigh flap** described by Hurwitz (*Plast Reconstr Surg*, 1981) based on the

inferior gluteal artery (IGA) branch that runs close to the posterior femoral cutaneous nerve and thus could be sensate. The thigh flap should be broadly based; although it is usually an axial pattern flap, the occasional absence of the artery means that it may be largely random.

- **Tensor fascia lata** (TFL) is a type 1 flap based on the ascending or transverse branch of the lateral circumflex femoral artery (LCFA). The muscle arises from the anterior superior iliac spine (ASIS) and greater trochanter of the femur and inserts as fascia lata/iliotibial tract to the lateral tibial condyle, and thus helps to maintain lateral knee stability.
  - The axis is from ASIS to lateral patella with the pedicle entering about 6–10 cm from the ASIS. A myocutaneous flap can be harvested with a skin paddle reaching up to 8 cm above the lateral femoral condyle. However, the **distal (and the important) part is unreliable** and may not reliably cover ischial defects. Some have suggested delaying the distal end (Zufferey J, *Eur J Plast Surg*, 1988) 3 weeks before. The flap can be made sensate by including the lateral femoral cutaneous nerve. It is also a suitable option for reconstruction of perineal and lower abdominal/groin defects; dividing the proximal attachments can increase the arc of rotation. The inferior part of the donor site often needs to be grafted.
- **Gracilis** – a relatively flimsy flap that may be used in smaller defects, with relatively little donor morbidity.
- **Gluteal** FC/musculocutaneous (MC) flap especially based on the IGA (see below), as large rotation/transposition flaps (see below).
  - A more elegant option, particularly for small defects, is to use local propeller flaps based on nearby perforators ('freestyle'). Some describe the existence of enlarged perforators by the edge of a chronic wound (Wound Edge Based Perforator Flaps, WEBP flaps) (Kelahmetoglu O, *Plast Reconstr Surg*, 2015).
- **Anterolateral thigh** (ALT) is a versatile flap with a long pedicle and significant mass particularly when a portion of the vastus lateralis is included. It is a bit of a reach to the ischial region; the flap can travel medially (Yu P, *Plast Reconstr Surg*, 2002) or laterally (Kua EH, *J Plast Reconstr Aesthet Surg*, 2011), usually subcutaneously, though a route through the muscles has been described (Lee JT, *J Plast Reconstr Aesthet Surg*, 2007).

Ischial pressure sores: A rationale for flap selection. (Foster RD, *Br J Plast Surg*, 1997)
The inferior gluteus maximus (GM) island flap was the most commonly used flap for reconstruction in this series, with the highest success rate, which was attributed to less tension with hip flexion. The use of this flap was first reported in 1979 (Mathes SJ, *Clinical Atlas of Muscle and*

Musculocutaneous Flaps) and modified subsequently by Scheflan (*Plast Reconstr Surg*, 1981) and Stevenson (*Plast Reconstr Surg*, 1987).

Mean time to healing was 38 days with complications in 37% including wound infection, edge dehiscence and partial flap necrosis. Necrosis was most common in TFL flaps (nearly half) and least in V–Y hamstring flaps.

- Predictors of poor outcome included large sore size, previous surgery and adverse wound healing factors.

Trochanteric sores (19%)

Patients with trochanteric sores often have hip/leg contractures – making closure more difficult and less reliable. There may be significant undermining due to the tissue mobility over bone.

- **TFL – probably the most commonly used**. The flap is usually moved as a transposition flap but can be VY, hatchet, bipedicled, etc. The flap can be potentially sensate in those with intact L3.
- **Vastus lateralis** (type 1) based on descending branch of the LCFA (10 cm from ASIS) can cover greater trochanter, pubis and lower abdomen.
- **Lateral thigh fasciocutaneous flap** (first lateral perforator of the profunda femoris artery) can be posteriorly or anteriorly based.
- **Rectus femoris flap.**

Sacral sores (17%)

Sacral sores tend to be quite painful. If the sore is small and due to a reversible short illness, direct closure/grafting/conservative management can be considered – particularly in those who will be ambulatory and are sensate. These methods may have a recurrence rate up to 70%.

- **Gluteal rotation flap**(s) (FC or MC) are most commonly used. They are straightforward and reliable to use; they can be raised again and advanced further if the sore recurs. Bilateral flaps can be used. The trend is to use perforator-based flaps, reserving myocutaneous flaps for larger cavities, particularly with osteomyelitis.
  - **V–Y GM** myocutaneous flaps 'burn bridges' as they cannot be (easily) elevated again.
- **Lumbar perforator flaps** can be based on any of the four perforators, but the second is largest (Kato), whilst others suggest using two perforators.
- Smaller defects can be filled with 'freestyle' islanded perforator flaps/WEBP flaps.

GLUTEAL FLAPS

The GM muscle is parallelogram-shaped and can provide a 24 × 24 cm, type II muscle flap that is supplied largely by the superior and gluteal arteries (SGA and IGA), with extensive anastomosis with the lumbar perforators. The gluteal region can be used in many ways, e.g. MC, muscle or FC flaps

(see below). The muscle can be quite atrophic in quadriplegic patients.

GLUTEAL MUSCLE/MYOCUTANEOUS FLAP

The GM MC flap has high shear resistance and can cover a large area. The muscle origin is divided off the gluteal surface of the ilium and the edge of the sacrum to allow rotation into the defect; the arc of rotation may be limited by the superior gluteal vessels, but these can be divided and the flap will survive on the inferior gluteal vessels alone. The muscle insertion on the femur can be detached to allow the muscle to be reflected as a turn-over flap into the sacral defect (and can also close lower lumbar defects). Harvesting the entire muscle may lead to some loss of hip stabilisation; the muscle can be split and the upper part can usually be used in ambulatory patients with relatively few problems.

GLUTEAL FASCIOCUTANEOUS/PERFORATOR FLAPS

The skin of gluteal flaps is supplied by 20–25 perforators (1–2 mm in diameter) from the gluteal arteries, but will survive on one or two decent-sized perforators; 50% of perforators are superior to the piriformis, 30% inferior and the remainder in the middle. SGA perforator (SGAP) flaps are type C (Mathes and Nahai) FC flaps; Koshima (1993) described their use in sacral sores. Morbidity is reduced as muscle is not sacrificed; hip stability is maintained and thus can be used in ambulatory patients.

- The surface marking of the SGA is a point 5 cm inferior to PSIS and 5 cm lateral to midline (or at the junction of proximal and middle one-thirds of a line from PSIS and the apex of greater trochanter), with the IGA 3 cm below that. During surgery, the buttocks are strapped apart and the exit point of SGA on skin is marked and a handheld Doppler used to find the main perforators, which are usually inferolateral to this point and above piriformis.
  - **Piriformis** is the key muscle that runs between the gluteal arteries and lies along the middle third of a line that runs from the middle of a line joining the posterior superior iliac spine to the coccyx, to the greater trochanter.
- Harvest a flap that is as large as possible even for apparently small defects. The first incision is made along the superior border to the subfascial level to search for a suitable perforator from medial to lateral; if a substantial vessel is not found, then it can be converted into a random rotation flap. Laterally placed flaps tend to have a longer intramuscular course that needs to be dissected out, but the extra pedicle length will allow greater flap movement. Flaps should be rotated less than 180°; torsion is the main cause of problems, i.e. venous congestion. Using a single large perforator is preferable to several smaller ones.

Long-term outcome of pressure sores treated with flap coverage. (Yamamoto Y, *Plast Reconstr Surg*, 1997)
The generally accepted view is that ischial sores typically have large dead spaces and are more likely to need muscle flaps, whilst sacral sores have smaller dead spaces and can be closed with FC flaps. However, in this series, sores reconstructed with FC flaps seem to exhibit less recurrence than with MC/muscle flaps:

- Muscle flaps provide good early cover, but the muscle becomes atrophic.
- Muscle is more susceptible to ischaemia (all pressure points in the body are naturally covered by skin fascia, not muscle).

Their conclusion was that muscle flaps are actually inadequate for the surgical management of sores **in the long term**.

Management of pressure sores by constant tension approximation. (Schessel ES, *Br J Plast Surg*, 2001)
The authors describe their management of chronic pressure sores:

- By wound excision with partial suturing and continued dressings to residual wounds.
- The remainder of the wound is closed by using a constant low-grade tension with a Proxiderm® device that acts on subcutaneous tissues, based on the principle of 'internal tissue expansion'.

Time to healing in a mixture of wounds was 5–42 days with a success rate of about 70%–80%. The advantages put forward include the avoidance of major surgery in debilitated patients. Contraindications include an inflamed wound, wounds with excessive discharge or contamination (faeces) or a deep cavity.
A refinement is to use NPWT in combination with the tension devices/sutures. Some call this arrangement vacuum-assisted dermal recruitment (VADER, van der Velde, *Ann Plast Surg*, 2005). There seems to be some synergy – the negative pressure reduces oedema, removes inflammatory exudate and relieves some of the localised tension forces that can develop around tension sutures/devices.

Perforator-sparing buttock rotation flap for coverage of pressure sores. (Wong CH, *Plast Reconstr Surg*, 2007)
The authors describe their experience with buttock FC rotation flaps based on visualisation and preservation of the perforators from superior or inferior gluteal arteries. The flaps were used for sacral, ischial and trochanteric sores.

- Other papers have suggested similar approaches to pressure sore coverage, perforator based or at least perforator-aware flaps may represent a shift in the way pressure sores are managed.

- **Seyhan T**, *Ann Plast Surg*, **2008.** This team from Ankara describes their experience with gluteal perforator flaps, though they used them as islanded perforator flaps (like Kim YS, *J Plast Reconstr Aesthet Surg*, 2009 and Jakubietz RG, *Microsurgery*, 2009 who modified it further by taking a plug of muscle [where needed] along with the distal perforator, which they thought would hopefully be supplied in a retrograde fashion).
- **Lin PY**, *Microsurgery*, **2012.** They describe the use of superiorly based gluteal FC rotation flaps for ischial sores – the main pedicles are perforators from the SGA, but other perforators from the IGA are preserved, with intramuscular dissection to facilitate flap movement. Conversely, an inferiorly based rotation flap in a similar manner is used to cover sacral sores. These flaps were successfully elevated again when sores recurred. They offered a simple algorithm for flap choice:
  - Sacral – large gluteal rotation flap; they stress the need for a large flap even for small defects.
  - Trochanteric – TFL.
  - Ischial – posterior thigh flap or gluteal rotation flap without muscle.

IV. NEGATIVE PRESSURE WOUND THERAPY

NPWT is used on a variety of wounds particularly pressure sores (stages III and IV). The principle is that **negative pressure** (strictly it is a pressure lower than atmospheric rather than actually being 'negative') can improve the state of a wound, converting it into one that may be healed by a lesser surgical procedure.
Suggested mechanisms of action include the following:

- **Wound fluid** that inhibits fibroblast and keratinocyte activity and contains MMP responsible for collagen breakdown is removed. **Reduction of oedematous fluid** in the tissues also facilitates oxygen delivery.
- Encourages wound contraction – analogous to tissue expansion relying upon creep; exerts **mechanical deformational forces** upon the ECM and upon cells, which promotes growth factors, modifies apoptosis and stimulates mitosis.
  - Some call this microstrain, distinguishing it from macrostrain, which is the contracting foam causing the wound edges to come closer together.
- Encourages formation of granulation tissue.
- Increases **local blood flow**.
- **Decreases bacterial colonisation**. In one study, it reduced bacterial count to below 10^5 quicker (5 days instead of 11) than with dressings alone, but others have shown little effect. One study showed that whilst Gram negative bacilli counts decreased, *Staphylococcus aureus* increased; sepsis and TSS have been reported with NPWT probably due to inadequate debridement. Overall, the effects on wound microbiology per se are probably minor.

- Some research done recently suggests that the polyurethane (PU) foam itself increases angiogenesis possibly related to a foreign body effect, inducing a better quality granulation tissue and reducing the bacterial count.
- NPWT is not a substitute for debridement.

The basic setup consists of

- Evacuation tube placed within PU foam dressing that has been tailored to fit the wound that is relatively clean
- Airtight seal created by covering the wound and sponge with an occlusive dressing
- Vacuum pump connected via a canister/trap for collection of wound 'effluent'
  - 75–125 mmHg subatmospheric pressure is commonly used (more 'negative' pressures supposedly cause collapse of vessels and decreased blood flow). Intermittent therapy (5 minutes on/ 2 minutes off) is supposedly more effective at promoting granulation tissue, but tends to cause more discomfort.
    - Some systems use a cyclical mode (Curavac®), which is meant to incorporate the advantages whilst reducing the pain involved with intermittent vacuum.
  - Dressings are changed every 48–72 hours depending on the clinical situation. This, in addition to the enclosed nature of the dressing, offers major advantages over conventional dressing in complex wounds. NPWT can be used in the community with portable/home machines.

The list of indications for the use of NPWT is increasing and includes the following:

- **Secure skin** grafts particularly in awkward areas, e.g. perineal or in complex wounds; lower pressures are used, i.e. continuous 50–75 mmHg for 4–5 days.
  - NPWT can also be used to secure dermal scaffolds such as Nevelia® and Integra®.
- **Sternotomy wounds** – NPWT has been a useful option in treating this difficult problem. Apart from improving the wound condition, they also stabilise the chest, improving the mechanics of ventilation (Harlan JW, *Plast Reconstr Surg*, 2002).
- **'Burst abdomen'** from acute loss of abdominal wall tissue or wound dehiscence, swollen viscera – the dressing should not be placed directly on abdominal viscera: an intervening layer should be used; there are dedicated dressings, e.g. Vivano® abdominal kit (Hartmann), whilst a cheap alternative is a split IV fluid bag (Bogota bag).
- **Wounds with *small* areas of bare bone** (DeFranzo AJ, *Plast Reconstr Surg*, 2001)/tendon/cartilage, or exposed orthopaedic metalwork, mesh (de Vooght A, *Plast Reconstr Surg*, 2003) or other prosthetics; NPWT allows granulation tissue to cover the defects whilst keeping the wound clean and moist.

- **Venous ulcers** generally need lower pressures ~50 mmHg in continuous mode with or without adjuvant therapy such as cultured keratinocytes or SSG.
- **Vulnerable suture lines** – may be supported/ protected with lower-pressure NPWT, e.g. Prevena®, Pico®, with reduced surgical site events compared to conventional dressings. Sometimes called incisional or preventive NPWT (Pellino G, *Int J Surg*, 2014).
- **Sponges**
  - Black PU sponge (400–600 μm) supposedly encourages formation of granulation tissue.
  - White polyvinyl sponge denser with smaller pores, said to be gentler and can be used over fragile structures.
  - Silver impregnation.
  - It is important to remember that NPWT sponges are not designed to have an intervening layer of tulle/non-adherent dressing, which alters the mechanics of the setup, the exceptions being use with skin grafts or overexposed bowel.

The first commercial system was the VAC® (vacuum-assisted closure) from KCI (Kinetic Concepts, Inc.). The patents, based on the work of Dr Argenta and Mr Morykwas at Wake Forest University who published two papers in the same issue of *Annals of Plastic Surgery* in 1997, have been fiercely protected. Other manufacturers eventually produced alternative systems citing earlier examples of the use of subatmospheric pressure in wounds, particularly from Russia. There were many rounds of litigation particularly from 2005 onwards. Presently, KCI has ended its litigation with both Smith and Nephew as well as Wake Forest University – having stopped paying royalties in 2011 after an unfavourable judgement in the United States.

In 2009, the Agency for Healthcare and Research Quality reviewed the literature concerning devices from 11 manufacturers with no evidence of significant differences. Some systems include modifications, such as using cyclical pressure modes, e.g. Curavac®, or silver impregnated sponges or an instillation system (VAC Veraflo®) that allows for wound irrigation with saline, Prontosan or 0.5% silver nitrate or antibiotic/antiseptic solutions.

PRECAUTIONS

NPWT is not an alternative to adequate debridement; nonviable material should be debrided away **before** NPWT. Where NPWT is used before closing a larger complex cavity, e.g. sternal/abdominal dehiscence, the **CRP count** can be used to monitor progress and suitability for definitive surgical closure. CRP levels rise and peak at 72 hours, presumably due to surgical trauma, and fall again afterwards. A persistently high or increasing CRP level suggests wound infection.

- **Residual tumour** in the wound is the main contraindication to therapy as increased blood flow may cause accelerated growth.

- **Exposed vessels** – patients have died after NPWT was used on groin wounds after femoral endarterectomy. Caution is required with the bleeding risk in patients on anticoagulation, particularly after dressing change/ removal. Overgranulation is a risk associated with leaving dressings in situ for too long.
- **Fistulae** used to be a contraindication, but studies have shown that NPWT can be used in selected cases to treat explored fistulae with a piece of foam fitted to the fistula opening; a lower pressure, e.g. 75 mmHg, is usually used. Remember to take a note of the number of sponge pieces inserted.

COMPLICATIONS

FDA issued a preliminary public health notification in 2009 regarding serious complications with NPWT – there were six deaths reported in 2 years (associated with bleeding) and 77 injuries including infection and dressing retention. It was updated in 2011 with six further deaths. Less serious complications include

- Pressure necrosis of adjacent skin if the patient lies on the tubes.
- Maceration of surrounding intact skin if the sponge inadvertently overlaps it.
- Pain (mainly in venous ulcers).
- Overgranulation with ingrowth into sponge – this leads to traumatic dressing changes with bleeding. This can be related to leaving dressings in situ for too long; some suggest using a non-adherent layer such as paraffin gauze or silicone dressings, e.g. Mepitel®, but generally the systems are not designed for use with an additional layer.
- Large volumes of exudate may be lost from larger acute wounds – monitor fluids and electrolyte balance as necessary.
- Air leaks encourage wound dehydration and may cause the wound condition to deteriorate. If a leak cannot be sealed with Tegaderm, etc., either do it again from scratch or change to conventional dressings; a leaking system should not be allowed to remain in situ.

Despite the common usage of NPWT, well-designed trials are lacking. Cochrane reviews have **failed** to find strong supporting evidence for

- Healing of **chronic wounds** compared to hydrocolloids, hydrogels and alginates (2001 and 2008).
- Healing of selected acute surgical wounds such as sternal wounds or incisions on obese patients; there were reports of 'blistering'. Rates of graft loss were lower, but 'homemade' systems performed similarly (2014).
- Partial thickness burns (2014).
- Pressure sores, when compared to 'moist wound healing' (2015).

- Leg ulcers (2015), except perhaps in combination with a skin graft.

There is some preliminary evidence that suggests NPWT used in diabetic wounds (Dumville JC, *Cochrane Database Syst Rev*, 2013) may show improved healing compared to other treatments.

Negative-pressure wound therapy with instillation: International consensus guidelines. (Kim PJ, *Plast Reconstr Surg*, 2013)
NPWT with instillation (NPWTi) is the introduction of solutions such as Prontosan®, Lavasept® in a volume sufficient to saturate the sponge and held for 10–20 minutes before resuming NPWT, i.e. **not irrigation**. The consensus committee reviewed available evidence and suggested that it can be used in infected/contaminated wounds, including those with exposed bone/osteomyelitis or exposed prosthesis, and diabetic and pressure ulcers. However, it cannot replace debridement.

Kim (*Plast Reconstr Surg*, 2015) suggested that normal saline is as effective as antiseptics in NPWTi.

Meta-analysis of negative-pressure wound therapy for closed surgical wounds. (Hyldig N, *Brit J Surg*, 2016)
The authors reviewed 10 studies and concluded that there was a significant reduction in wound infection (relative risk 0.54) compared with standard care. There was no significant reduction in wound dehiscence.

C. SCAR MANAGEMENT

I. SCAR FORMATION

REGENERATION VS. REPAIR

Cells can be classified according to their proliferative potential:

- **Labile cells** divide and proliferate throughout life (M to G1 of the cell cycle), e.g. epithelia, bone marrow haematopoietic cells.
- **Stable cells** are normally quiescent but can be stimulated to replicate (G0 to G1), e.g. hepatocytes, endothelium, mesenchymal cells, e.g. osteoblasts.
- **Permanent cells** have left the cell cycle and cannot undergo mitosis (postnatally) and thus are never regained after loss, e.g. neurones, cardiac muscle.

Repair can be regarded as equivalent to healing. **Regeneration** is the formation of lost tissue without scarring. In tissues with labile or stable cells, true regeneration requires an intact supporting network. Thus, adult tissues tend to heal with some degree of scarring (healing by fibrous tissue, or gliosis in brain), except perhaps following parenchymal cell death in the liver (e.g. after exposure to hepatotoxic chemicals) or very superficial skin/mucosal wounds (above the basement membrane).

Fetal wound healing. (Rowlatt U, *Virchows Archiv*, 1979)
This was the first report of scar-free healing in humans.

The term 'foetal wound healing' is used to describe the regenerative process that occurs with minimal or no scar formation; it only occurs in the skin and bone of the foetus, but not nerve or muscle, i.e. it is organ specific. There is a wound size limit for scarless healing, which decreases with gestational age.

The ability to repair is also age-dependent. In humans, scarring of cutaneous wounds will begin from about 24 weeks gestation, depending in part on the size of the wound. The exact reasons for this are unclear, though some have postulated on the significance of various findings including the following:

- **Environment** – sterile intrauterine environment, amniotic fluid rich in HA and growth factors. However, early studies have shown that the intrauterine environment is neither necessary nor sufficient for scarless repair, i.e. it is a property intrinsic to foetal skin.
  - Lorenz (*Development*, 1992) showed that foetal skin transplanted into adult athymic mice healed scarlessly.
- Wounds are conspicuous by an **absence of inflammation** and angiogenesis; healing is largely controlled by **fibroblasts** rather than macrophages. **It is not true regeneration per se, but it is well-organised healing.**
  - Rapid increase in HA and receptors on fibroblasts.
  - Type III collagen deposition is more organised.
  - Reduced levels of TGF-β, PDGF, bFGF.
  - More fibromodulin (inhibits TGF-β), less decorin.
  - More adhesion proteins, e.g. fibronectin and tenascin (modulator of cell growth and migration in foetal wounds).

NORMAL SCAR FORMATION

Dermal injury triggers a cascade that results in the deposition of a vascular collagen matrix that, as it accumulates, becomes a red, raised scar – fibrous connective tissue formed when healing by repair. As the matrix matures and remodels, the scar will become flatter, less vascular and paler after ~9 months (takes longer in children and in those with more darkly pigmented skin).

CLASSIFICATION OF SCARS (MUSTOE TA, *PLAST RECONSTR SURG*, 2002)

- **Immature** – red and lumpy, itchy or painful, eventually matures to become paler and flatter (occasionally hyper- or hypopigmented).
- **Linear hypertrophic** – arises within weeks of surgery and grows over 3–6 months to a rope-like appearance with maturation within 2 years. They are possibly due to excessive tension or delayed wound healing; external taping is proposed by some surgeons as a preventative measure, but the efficacy is unknown/doubtful.
- **Widespread hypertrophic** – widespread raised, red itchy scar; typically a **burns scar** that remains within the borders of the injury.

- **Minor keloid** – focally raised, red, itchy scar that extends beyond the borders of the original injury. It may take up to a year to develop and fails to resolve; excision is typically complicated by recurrence. There may be genetic and anatomical influences.
- **Major keloid** – as for minor keloid but may continue to extend over years. These typically occur over the anterior chest wall.

FACTORS PROMOTING A FINE SCAR

Surgical Factors

- Atraumatic technique. This may sound obvious, but it is important to respect the tissues and blood supply.
- Eversion of wound edges. Wound inversion leads to a difficult to correct scar deformity.
- Placement of the scar – adjacent to or within contour lines (e.g. nasolabial fold), within or adjacent to hair-bearing areas (e.g. facelift, Gillies lift) and parallel to **relaxed skin tension lines** (RSTL, Borges 1962 'facial wrinkles' that were made obvious by squeezing the skin), that usually lie perpendicular to the axis of the underlying muscles.
  - **Langers (cleavability) lines**. Karl Langer (1861). Dots of ink pushed into the skin surface with a 2 mm awl were seen to form lines (spaltbarkeit) – does not always correspond to generally accepted best lines particularly in scalp, forehead, periorbital areas, etc.
  - **Kraissl's 'wrinkle lines'** – similar to Borges but described for the whole body.
- Shape of the scar – 'U'-shaped scars tend to become pincushioned/trapdoor, e.g. bilobed flap. Trapdoor scars can be difficult to correct; W-plasty/multiple Z-plasty is usually recommended. Flap thinning rarely helps.
- Ellipse (strictly fusiform) length should ideally be 4× its width to avoid dog-ears.

CHOICE OF SUTURE

- Cutting versus non-cutting needle.
- Monofilament vs. braided. Skin sutures are usually monofilaments; braided sutures are more 'traumatic' and may increase infection risk. There are antibiotic-coated sutures on the market, e.g. Vicryl plus® with Triclosan.
- Absorbable vs. non-absorbable: absorption by proteolytic enzymes; non-absorbable sutures tend to cause less tissue inflammation.
  - Vicryl is polyglactic acid – tensile strength gone by 30 days, absorbed by 90 days. It is braided.
    - Vicryl rapide® (irradiated) is absorbed more rapidly (7–10 days of support) and is useful for skin closure in children.
    - Catgut (actually sheep intestine) is a good temporary suture but is not available in all localities due in part to BSE concerns (Japan, Europe). The sutures were withdrawn in the United Kingdom and Hong Kong.

- PDS is a polydioxanone monofilament – loses tensile strength at 60 days, absorbed by 180 days, i.e. both double that for vicryl.
- Staples are often used for speed, particularly on the scalp or for securing skin grafts. Animal studies have shown mechanical equivalence with sutures (Roth JH, *Can J Surg*, 1988). Cochrane review (Anderson ER, *Cochrane Database Syst Rev*, 2004) and a meta-analysis (Clay FS, *Am J Obstet Gynecol*, 2011) showed no demonstrable difference between staples and sutures for closure of caesarean section wounds.

PATIENT FACTORS

- Age – infants (1–3 months) and the elderly tend to have good scars, whilst children are prone to have hypertrophic scars (HTS).
- Region of the body. The presternal and deltoid regions seem prone to develop problem scarring.
- Skin type – glabrous skin seems to be more prone to scar hypertrophy.
- Individual's scar-forming properties – some patients seem to be more prone to form hypertrophic/keloid scars; 'keloid families' have been described.

FACTORS THAT CONTRIBUTE TO SUTURE MARKS

It is important to note that the suture itself is not the most important variable. Suture marks are partly due to epithelialisation of the suture track; in some cases, it may be related to local pressure necrosis or infection including 'stitch abscesses'.

- **Length of time** the suture is left in place – sutures removed within 5–7 days usually do not leave stitch marks whilst sutures removed at 14 days will.
- **Tension** on the wound edges/skin sutures tied too tightly. Skin wound tension can be relieved by placing deeper stitches to bring the skin edges together in apposition, obviating the need for tight skin sutures.
- **Region of the body** – the hands are rarely affected by stitch marks, whilst trunk, upper extremities more likely to be affected.
- **Infection** – braided sutures are more likely to harbour bacteria (*Staphylococcus*); some have antimicrobial activity. In general, minimise the number and weight of sutures used to close a wound.
  - Degradation by proteolysis (e.g. catgut) is likely to cause more tissue reaction than degradation by hydrolysis (e.g. Vicryl®).

II. HYPERTROPHIC AND KELOID SCARS

The history is an important key to differentiating between HTS and keloids. Both types of scarring can coexist within one scar, e.g. a largely hypertrophic midline laparotomy scar may have some keloidal parts.

HYPERTROPHIC SCARS

See also 'Burn scars', Chapter 2, **Section D.I.**

- HTS are raised scars **limited** to the initial boundary of the injury, including burns.
  - More contractile component – there are myofibroblasts, with actin expression.
- They may be related to wound factors such as tension and delayed wound healing.
  - Meyer (*Br J Plast Surg*, 1991) demonstrated areas of high tension in the presternal area.
    - Pull in one direction causes a stretched scar.
    - Pull in multiple directions causes a hypertrophic scar.
- They tend to **occur soon after injury** and show **spontaneous regression** over months/years.

KELOID SCARS

Alibert (1817) coined the term *cheloides* from the Greek word for crab claws.

- These **extend beyond** the boundary of the original injury. Histologically, there are large collagen bundles with less cross-linking and more disorganisation than HTS.
- They tend to appear after a longer time interval following the injury (months/years).
  - These first two criteria are the most useful clinically.
- They do not show any significant regression without treatment.
- They seem to be more closely correlated with dark skin colour (15× more common in dark-skinned people).
- Patients with keloid scars tend to be of a younger age, and there are instances of a familial tendency.
  - A survey of 32 patients with ear keloids after piercing demonstrated that the risk of developing a keloid was higher (80%) if they were pierced at or after the age of 11, compared to 23.5% if they were pierced before that age (Lane JE, *Pediatrics*, 2005). Some speculate that this may be related to hormonal factors; there may be accelerated growth of keloids during pregnancy, and some may resolve after menopause.
  - There seem to be sites of predilection including anterior chest, shoulders and deltoid. Some suggest that this is related to skin stretching tension, which is greatest at the outer edges (Akaishi S, *Ann Plast Surg*, 2008), but keloids can also develop in places that do not seem to be under tension – e.g. earlobes. It is apparent that not all keloids behave in the same way; for example, ear keloids are more amenable to surgery than sternal keloids, further complicating any discussion that lumps all scars altogether.

- Some believe ear keloids to be caused by an immune response to sebum and thus may be secondary to damage of pilosebaceous structures. High piercings are more likely to get infected, and also develop keloids.

On macroscopic examination, both keloids and HTS are raised erythematous scars, characterised by an excessive disordered accumulation of collagen, particularly type III. Some describe heavily hyalinised collagen nodules called 'keloidal collagen' and less blood vessel density in keloids. However, even histological examination may be inconclusive. It was once thought that **α-smooth muscle actin (SMA)** expression was found in HTS but not keloids (Ehrlich HP, *Am J Pathol*, 1994), but this has been disputed – keloid myofibroblasts do express α-SMA but less often than HTS (Lee JY, *Am J Dermatopathol*, 2004;26:379).

When interpreting the literature, it is important to note their shortcomings: many studies do not properly distinguish between HTS and keloids, do not distinguish between excision and debulking/intralesional surgery or have follow-up times that are too short to study recurrence rates in keloids (see imiquimod studies). Finally, there is a failure to refer to original articles – many articles are fond of stating that the recurrence rate after surgery alone for keloids is **45%–100%** whilst listing the following references:

- Mathangi Ramakrishnan K. Study of 1000 patients with keloids in South India. *Plast Reconstr Surg* 1974;53:276–280.
  - This Indian study included 108 cases treated with surgery with 80% recurrence, with no mention of adjunctive treatments, histological evidence or follow-up period.
- Cosman B. Correlation of keloid recurrence with completeness of local excision. *Plast Reconstr Surg* 1972;50:163–166.
  - This study of 18 keloid surgeries only had 4 that did not also have post-operative radiotherapy, with one recurrence in the average follow-up period of 1 3/4 years, i.e. 25%.
- Cosman B. The surgical treatment of keloids. *Plast Reconstr Surg* 1961;27:225.
  - This retrospective review had 340 cases of keloid over 1932–1958 with an overall recurrence rate of 38.5%, whilst the 25 cases that were excised with no post-operative radiation had a 54% recurrence rate.
- Conway H. Differential diagnosis of keloids and hypertrophic scars by tissue culture technique with notes on therapy of keloids by surgical excision and decadron. *Plast Reconstr Surg* 1960;25:117–132.
  - This study investigated the adjunctive effect of dexamethasone. The recurrence rate with surgery alone was 45%.

Thus, articles quoting a recurrence rate with **surgery alone** with these references must be referring to a study of Indian patients in 1974 ($n = 58$, 80%) or American patients in 1972 ($n = 4$, 25%), in 1961 ($n = 25$, 54%) and in 1960 (45%). Several other commonly quoted papers do not actually include patients treated with surgery alone (Darzi MA, *Br J Plast Surg*, 1992; Lawrence WT, *Ann Plast Surg*, 1991).

The link between hypertension and pathological scarring. (Huang C, *Wound Repair Regen*, 2014)
The authors discuss the potential association between hypertension and the development of pathological scarring. Previous articles by the senior author have shown that Japanese patients with multiple or large keloids were more likely to have hypertension than those with small keloids, and that hypertensive patients were more prone to bad scars after surgery. There are some speculative ways keloids could be connected with hypertension including fibroblast function and ECM remodelling. The connection may explain why ACE inhibitors (Ardekani GS, *Plast Reconstr Surg*, 2009) and calcium channel blockers (D'Andrea F, *Dermatol*, 2002) have been reported to be useful in keloid treatment.

Update on scar management: Guidelines for treating Asian patients. (Kim S, *Plast Reconstr Surg*, 2013)
Asians have three times risk for hypertrophic scarring compared to Caucasians; even 'normal' scars tend to have prolonged erythema and pigmentation. Asian skin is thicker, particularly the dermal layer, which has greater collagen density, and a more vigorous fibroblastic response. Asian skin also has increased melanin content and sebaceous gland numbers.

According to this and other literature reviews, the following therapies could be considered for (routine) therapy. Again, it is stressed that properly controlled studies are lacking.

HYPERTROPHIC SCARS

These scars have a tendency to regress with time.

Silicone therapy – Silicone gel with or without pressure therapy is often the first-line treatment for HTS. If used for close to 24 hours a day for 3 months (an arbitrary 'course'), the response rate is approximately 65%–88%. There is little evidence for its use in the **prevention** of problem scarring.

- There are various formulations of silicone gel. Clear gel sheeting (Cica Care®) may be more effective than liquid gel (Dermatix Ultra®) for reducing scar height, itch and erythema; however, compliance is much improved when using the latter, making the overall effect similar.
- The mechanism of action is uncertain. One theory is that in a scar even with a grossly intact epidermis, the barrier to water loss is disrupted and this increases **transepidermal water loss (TEWL)**, resulting in keratinocyte dehydration that alters their behaviour with upregulation of pro-fibrotic cytokines fibroblasts, e.g. IL-1β and down-regulation

of anti-fibrotic (TNF-α), that leads to increased TFG-β and fibroblastic activity (Mustoe T, *Aesthet Plast Surg*, 2008). Cytokines may act via the IL-8 effect on MMP-9 (Xu W, *J Invest Dermatol*, 2014). The theory is that silicone would work by reducing TEWL by occlusion and improving hydration, rather than by any effect intrinsic of silicone.

- Other forms of occlusion, e.g. polyurethane films, also work.
- Some patients will report 'allergy' to silicone. True allergic is extremely rare; what is more likely is an intolerance to the occlusion.

Pressure therapy – pressure garments can be fitted as soon as the wounds have healed and should be used continuously, i.e. >23 hours/day, until wound maturation, i.e. 6–12 months. Obviously compliance may be an issue (~41%).

- Pressure may work through local tissue hypoxia/ischaemia causing decreased collagen synthesis and increased collagenase activity. Optimal pressures have not been scientifically established, though it is commonly believed that compression pressure should be higher than capillary pressure (25 mmHg); but the literature can be contradictory. Some suggest 15–24 mmHg can still be effective, whilst higher pressures are faster-acting; but others say that high pressures are harmful and uncomfortable (particularly if 30–40 mmHg).
- The fit should be reassessed regularly (oedema settles and children grow) and garments replaced as necessary. Pockets can be made to accommodate additional padding, but it can still be difficult to apply pressure to concave and flexor areas.
- Some suggest they should be used prophylactically in wounds that take more than 2 weeks to heal, but prospective data suggest that the use of pressure garments has no effect on the speed of maturation of burn scars (Chang P, *J Burn Care Rehabil*, 1995).
  - It is much less effective in older scars.

   Laser – there seems to be a role for laser therapy, but it is not well defined.

- Alster (*Plast Reconstr Surg*, 1998) demonstrated that 585 nm pulsed dye lasers (PDL) may improve scar pliability, erythema and texture (though not everyone has had similar results); multiple treatments with lower fluences may reduce dyspigmentation, particularly in patients with Asian skin. It is more useful for early scars (Dierickx C, *Plast Reconstr Surg*, 1995).
- Intense pulsed light (IPL) with a 590 nm filter can also be used to treat vascular/immature scars, with improved mVSS (Sarkar A, *Indian J Plast Surg*, 2014). It has deeper penetration and is more painful than PDL. There is less purpura.
- Fractional ablative lasers, i.e. carbon dioxide, e.g. Ultrapulse DeepFx/SCAAR Fx®, can be used for **mature burn scars** (Shumaker PR, *Trauma Acute Care Surg*, 2012). The thin pillars of ablation heal quickly with collagen remodelling in the surrounding zone.

This can be combined with topical medications, e.g. triamcinolone or 5-FU, to increase bioavailability, i.e. laser-assisted drug delivery (LAD).
- Nd:YAG may be helpful in acne scarring.

Onion extract (*Allium cepa*) – a randomised trial did not find any improvement compared to standard therapy (Chung VQ, *Dermatol Surg*, 2006) for surgical wounds, although it seemed to help in reducing scars in darker skinned patients undergoing laser tattoo removal (Ho WS, *Dermatol Surg*, 2006).

- Quercetin is a derivative of *A. cepa* and has antihistamine effects.

KELOID SCARS

Steroid injection, e.g. triamcinolone, is first-line treatment for keloids (Al-Attar A, *Plast Reconstr Surg*, 2006). The exact mechanism of action is unclear, but it may act to decrease collagen synthesis, stimulate collagenase production and reduce inflammation. Triamcinolone has been shown to reduce levels of α-1 antitrypsin and α-2 macroglobulin that are high in keloids. Side effects include dermal atrophy, telangiectasia and depigmentation; systemic side effects are rare. The current use of intralesional steroid (concentration, dosages and timing) is mostly based on the empirical findings of Ketchum (1974). There are very little data to support variations in practice such as

- 10 mg/mL vs. 40 mg/mL
- Mixing with lignocaine to reduce pain

   Cryotherapy – scar cryotherapy was first proposed by Shepherd in 1982 with delivery by spray or surface contact. The proposed mechanism was vascular damage (thrombosis) whilst leaving the collagen matrix intact, supposedly reducing scarring. The area around the contact point consists of the **lethal zone** (temp < –22°C) with cryonecrosis and the **recovery zone** (–22°C to 0°C) with cells that tend to survive. With surface cryotherapy, the dermis lies in the recovery zone (thus perhaps less efficacious), whilst with intralesional therapy, the epidermis (with its melanocytes) is in the recovery zone and explaining the supposed reduced rate of hypopigmentation.

- Early reports suggested an average 51.4% scar volume reduction after one session with reduction of symptoms (Har-Shai Y, *Plast Reconstr Surg*, 2003). Early equipment consisted of lumbar puncture needles connected to a liquid nitrogen canister (Gupta S, *Int J Dermatol*, 2001), but has evolved to more sophisticated systems such as dedicated machines (Intralyze®) that offer quicker and more precise freezing.

Surgery. Surgery alone may be contemplated for localised lesions in certain locations, e.g. ear keloids that tend to respond better; however, in most cases, recurrence risk should be reduced by combining surgery with other treatments such as post-operative radiotherapy (25% recurrence surgery plus radiotherapy, surgery alone >50% recurrence), steroids or 5-FU.

- **Fillet flap** (Kim DY, *Plast Reconstr Surg,* 2004) – this skin-preserving debulking concept has been described to reduce recurrence rates for ear keloids with '5 As and 1B': asepsis, atraumatic, absent raw surface, avoid tension, accurate approximation and bloodless surgery, i.e. 'good surgical technique'.
  - There are proponents for either total excision vs. intralesional excision/debulking. Supporters of the former suggest that it is easier to prevent than treat keloids.
- Scar revision can be contemplated in HTS with a definite history of problems with wound healing or in scars that have crossed skin tension lines.

  Radiotherapy – the exact mechanism is unclear, but it seems to be related to damage of keloid fibroblasts; in vitro studies showed an increase in apoptosis (Ogawa R, *Ann Plast Surg,* 2007). In 2015, the Royal College of Radiologists said that although there is no robust type 1 evidence, it seemed that administering RT after keloid excision is associated with a reasonably low recurrence rate (grade C) and should be used within 24–72 hours after excision (grade D). It can be considered in situations with high risk of recurrence, e.g. in Asians, in areas such as the sternum. Radiotherapy alone (i.e. without surgery) is not recommended. The use of post-operative radiotherapy is much higher in Japan than the United Kingdom.
- Different RT regimes exist depending on local practices. It seems that the higher the dose, the greater the risk of problems such as dyspigmentation and malignant disease. The risk of carcinogenesis is low when surrounding tissues, e.g. thyroid and breasts, are adequately protected (Ogawa R, *Plast Reconstr Surg,* 2009)
  - Kovalic (*Int J Radiat Oncol Biol Phys,* 1989) gave 12G in three fractions over 3 days, which halved the recurrence rate in 113 keloids compared to surgery alone (73% control rate). There was a greater risk of recurrence if the keloid was >2 cm, had previous treatment or occurred in men. The authors said that delivery within 24 hours made no difference.
  - Van Leeuwen (*Plast Reconstr Surg Glob Open,* 2015) conducted a systematic review with 33 studies, with the 6 best graded level II evidence.
    - High-dose-rate brachytherapy is better than low-dose-rate brachytherapy or external irradiation. Single dose regimes are effective.
    - Short time interval (<24 hours) more effective.
    - Recurrences occurred at a mean of 15 months.

Postoperative electron-beam irradiation therapy for keloids and hypertrophic scars. (Ogawa R, *Plast Reconstr Surg,* 2003)

A total of 147 keloids were excised followed by 15 Gy electron beam post-operatively. The overall recurrence rate at 24 months was 32.7%, being higher in 'high stretch tension' areas such as chest wall, scapula and suprapubic regions compared to neck, earlobes and lower limbs. Side effects included hyperpigmentation (45.6%) and hypopigmentation (2%), and were mostly mild and temporary.

OTHER TREATMENTS

More recently, there has been a plethora of intralesional treatments suggested for keloids (and HTS) that are largely case reports/small case series, i.e. low evidence level. Some have combined fractional ablative CO_2 laser with topical steroids, 5-FU, etc. (Laser-Assisted Delivery LAD).

- **5-fluorouracil (5-FU)** – this is an antimetabolite (pyrimidine analogue) that is antiproliferative with widespread actions on cell growth. It is cytotoxic, but the doses used in keloids (intralesional injection of up to 50 mg of 50 mg/mL per session) are supposedly subtoxic; some propose a lower dose regime (<10 mg/mL) particularly in combination therapy, e.g. with steroids. Overall, the evidence is equivocal, but there may be a role in lesions refractory to steroid injections.
  - Uppal (*Plast Reconstr Surg,* 2001) – 11 Afro-Caribbean patients had 5-FU applied after lesions were removed; control scars (patients were self-controls) were soaked with saline. Biopsies showed reduced markers (ki-67, vascular cell adhesion molecule VCAM1, TGFβ-1,) but not CD68; fibroblasts in 3/5 treated patients had reduced contractile capacity.
  - A literature review in 2016 by Shah VV suggested that 5-FU monotherapy achieves good scar improvement in 45%–78% of patients, whilst **combination with triamcinolone** (average 1–4 mg steroid vs. 45 mg 5-FU) increases the response rate to 96% of patients. Systemic side effects were not seen; some studies reported local erythema, ulceration and dyspigmentation.
- **Imiquimod** 5% cream has been used to prevent recurrence after surgery (see below). It is an immune response–modifying agent; chemically, it is an imidazoquinolone compound that stimulates the production of interferon α, TNF and IL-2 by binding to surface receptors (e.g. Toll 7) on macrophages and other inflammatory cells including T-cells.
  - When applied once daily for 8 weeks following excision of keloid scars in 12 patients, no recurrence was observed at 24 weeks (Berman B, *J Am Acad Dermatol,* 2002). The study was supported by an educational grant from 3M Pharmaceuticals, manufacturers of Aldara®.
  - Side effects included pain, irritation and mild hyperpigmentation. Others found that keloids recurred after the cream was stopped (Malhotra AK, *Dermatology,* 2007), usually by the 12th week after surgery (Cacao FM, *Dermatol Surg,* 2009).

- **Antimetabolites/cytotoxics:**
  - **Interferons, 5-FU, Bleomycin, mitomycin, retinoic acid.** Wang (*Ann Plast Surg*, 2009) and Shridarani (*Ann Plast Surg*, 2010) found substances of 'promise/potential'. However, the studies, in general, suffer from problems with methodology (small numbers, short follow-up) with most patients having had other therapies in addition to the one of interest.
- **Others** include doxorubicin, verapamil, tacrolimus, tamoxifen, TGF-β, interleukins and vitamin E. Topical vitamin E is popular, but without supporting evidence; it can cause allergic dermatitis.
- **Botulinum toxin (BTX)** – The theory is that tension vectors acting on the edge of wounds affect the synthesis of immature collagen fibres and lead to widened/abnormal scars. BTX would reduce scar formation by reducing wound tension.
- One of the first reports used BTX A in eyelid surgery (Choi JC, *Ophthal Plast Reconstr Surg*, 1997) to reduce wound complications such as dehiscence. Some papers suggested an improvement in scarring.
- Ziade (*J Plast Reconstr Surg*, 2013) – a prospective trial where facial wounds were randomised to BTX A (mean 20U) or no injection within 72 hours. Although assessment of photographs after 1 year suggested an improvement in the scar, there were no differences in PSAS, OSAS and VSS.
- A meta-analysis of nine RCTs by Zhang (*PLoS One*, 2016) showed differences in scar width, patient satisfaction and VAS.

2
Burns

A. ACUTE BURNS

I. RELEVANT ANATOMY

- Skin surface area ~0.2–0.3 m² in the newborn and 1.5–2.0 m² in the adult.
- Thickness of epidermis from 0.05 mm (eyelids) to 1 mm (sole of the foot).
- Dermis is approximately 10× thicker than epidermis, site for site.

The skin has many different functions:

- Mechanical barrier to bacterial invasion
- Control of fluid loss
- Thermoregulation
- Immunology and metabolism, e.g. vitamin D
- Neurosensory and social interaction

EPIDEMIOLOGY

- 0.5%–1% of the UK population sustains burns each year. Approximately 10% of these will require hospital admission, and of these, 10% are life threatening.
- 45% of admissions in the United States are scalds in children <5 years of age.
- Burns sustained during road traffic accidents have a high incidence of concomitant injury.
- The **burn LD50** is strongly influenced by the age of the patient: Bull (*Ann Surg*, 1954) found the LD50 to be 46% and 49% in the 0–14 and 15–44 groups, respectively, compared to 27% in the 45–64 group and 10% in the group 65 years and above. The LD50 has increased with multiple improvements in burn care. Data from 2007 showed 98%, 78%, 70% and 35% in these four groups, respectively.

- **Baux score** (1961) **Age + TBSA – the 'futility score'**, where predicted mortality is 100%, has changed with improvements in care.

  - Revised Baux (Osler T, *J Trauma*, 2010) – inhalational injury adds 17 to the score.
  - American Burn Association National Burn Registry 2012 Baux score with 50% fatality was 108 overall; men seemed to have a survival advantage.
  - Roberts (*J Trauma Acute Care Surg*, 2012) **futility score should be reset to 160**, LD50 to 110.

Pathophysiologic response to burns in the elderly. (Jeschke MG, *EBioMedicine*, 2015)
Burn mortality has been in the elderly group and has changed little over the last few decades (1995–2015). The overall mortality rate was 29%; the authors report increased incidence of sepsis, inflammation, infections, hypercatabolism and organ failure. BSA was a major influence – for burns over 20% TBSA, mortality in the elderly was >70% compared to <15% in adults.

OUTCOME

- There are many different formulae that calculate the risk of mortality following burns. Most of these are based on statistical analysis of an institution's retrospective data – thus will be most applicable to that institution's demographic and local practice. Outcome predictors are not as useful as they sound; they should be applied with caution to clinical care of patients; clinical decision-making particularly the withdrawal of treatment should be based on the clinical response to treatment rather than calculated figures.
- The most consistent risk factors are **burn size** (it could be argued that burn volume would be more accurate), **age** and **inhalational injury**. Other factors include premorbid disease, co-existent trauma and pneumonia.

The improvements in the mortality rate have been due to multiple factors including

- Early and effective resuscitation through improved protocols
- Control of sepsis, antibiotics/antimicrobials
- Improved management of inhalation injury
- Early wound excision and grafting
- Development of alternative wound closure materials

BLISTERS

Damage around the dermo-epidermal junction will lead to the leakage of plasma from heat-damaged vessels causing the epidermis to separate from the dermis, i.e. form a blister. Osmotically active particles within the blister fluid contribute to its progressive enlargement with time.

Some choose to leave intact blisters alone (Herndon), whilst others, myself included, tend to prefer to have blisters de-roofed – after all the overlying skin has lost the normal functions of skin, it obscures the view of the burn itself and tense blisters can be painful. There seems to be no convincing evidence either way regarding the effect of blister fluid on wound healing. It may contain growth factors (Ono I, *Burns*, 1995), but potentially harmful inflammatory mediators have also been found.

- Increased adenosine concentrations, which have potent anti-inflammatory action (Shaked G, *Burns*, 2007). Yuryeva (*Biochem Moscow*, 2014) found that stimulation of adenosine receptors on myeloid cells enhances leukocyte migration at the site of burn injury.
- Burn blister fluid decreases keratinocyte replication and differentiation (Garner WL, *J Burn Care Rehab*, 1993), whilst others have found EGF and IL-8 that stimulate re-epithelisation and FGF2 as well as angiogenin that encourages neovascularisation (Pan SC, *J Burn Care Rehab*, 2015).

ESCHAR

Again, an eschar-covered wound can be regarded as an open wound because it retains none of the normal functions of skin. In addition

- It is a medium for bacterial growth.
- It is a hindrance to wound healing.
- It is a source of inflammatory mediators and toxins, which may compromise distant organ function and exacerbate immunosuppression.
- It consumes clotting factors, fibrinogen and platelets.

A circumferential limb eschar may impede distal circulation, whilst truncal eschar may compromise ventilation; decompression may be necessary.

- **Pseudoeschar** may form in deeper burns after the use of topical antimicrobials, which react with the wound exudate; this includes silver sulphadazine (SSD; some suggest that it is due to the polypropylene glycol carrier)

and flammacerium (SSD plus cerium nitrate, a more leathery dry pseudoeschar). It can lead to confusion over the depth of the burns in inexperienced hands.

II. ASSESSMENT, RESUSCITATION AND INITIAL MANAGEMENT OF BURNS

First aid at the scene:

- **Stop the injury**, which depends on the type of injury, i.e. extinguish any flames ('stop, drop and roll'), switch off/interrupt electrical power source, dilute acids and alkali by irrigation (rather than neutralisation), remove affected clothing, etc.
- **Cool the burn wound** (but keep the patient warm) to reduce the tissue damage. Timely cooling reduces direct thermal trauma and stabilises mast cells, reducing the production of lactic acid and the release of histamine and other inflammatory mediators such as thromboxane. The **EMSB** (emergency management of severe burns) course suggests using running cold tap water **for 20 minutes** ~15°C (avoid ice or iced water, which will cause vasospasm and further compromise of tissue perfusion) (Sawada Y, *Burns*, 1997). Though this is most useful in the first half hour, it is still worth considering even **up to 3 hours** post-burn and will also reduce pain. Hydrogel dressings are not as useful (for cooling) but can be used when running water is not available.

PRIMARY SURVEY

In the emergency department (ED), the approach is basically the same in principle as for any trauma patient, i.e. **ABC**. It is important to remember that seriously burnt patients may suffer additional injuries aside from the burns due to the original incident such as an explosion/car crash or events afterwards such as jumping out of windows to escape from a house fire. The following sequence applies to a 'major' burn:

Airway with C-spine control. A simple check for airway patency is to talk to the patient (and get a response).

- Open airway with chin lift/jaw thrust manoeuvre. Use a Yankhauer sucker to remove debris from the mouth and secure the airway with
  - Guedel airway (size approximately with nose to angle of mandible distance)
  - Nasopharyngeal airway (exclude cribriform plate or base of skull fracture)
  - **Endotracheal tube** – adults size 7 (female) or 8 (male) on average; children – a formula may be used: (age/4) + 4 uncuffed (3 cuffed) or size of nostril/little finger nail.

Breathing (look, feel, listen) – provide 100% oxygen through a non-rebreathing mask.

- Exclude life-threatening chest injuries such as tension pneumothorax.
- Emergency chest decompression (escharotomy) if circumferential full thickness burns are limiting

respiratory movements (elevated ventilation pressures will drop rapidly with appropriate decompression). This is rarely required during the primary survey.

Circulation with haemorrhage control.

- Apply pressure to actively bleeding wounds.
- Insert and secure two large-bore cannulae preferably through unburned skin – consider intraosseous infusions in children <2 years of age. Commence crystalloid infusion according to fluid deficit as gauged by clinical condition (peripheral and central pulses and BP), e.g. full rate Hartmanns, and adjust to resuscitation formula after the primary survey.
- Take blood for FBC, LRFT, glucose, group and save/cross-match, ABG and carboxyhaemoglobin.

Disability: AVPU is a simple method of assessing the approximate level of response:

- Alert
- Responding to voice
- Responding to pain
- Unresponsive

Exposure with environmental control

- A **full inspection** – remove all clothing but keep the patient warm; perform a log roll to check the back. Hair may need to be trimmed to aid assessment as well as to make dressings easier; this is particularly important in chemical burns. Remove all jewellery particularly those that may potentially cause constriction.
- 'Estimate' the size of the burn **(% TBSA)** according to
  - **Wallace rule of nines** – described by Pulaski and Tennison in the late 1940s; it was passed around largely by word of mouth and not published until Wallace referred to it in 1951.
    - Alex Burns Wallace was a Scottish physician.
    - Serial halving can be used in EDs.
  - **'Patient's palm'** (the palmar surface of both the anatomical palm and the closed fingers) is taken as 1% of the total body surface area, and although this is only an approximation, it is a good method for patchy burns. Recent studies with 3D scanners have calculated that the palm is 0.89% (men 0.92% and women 0.87%); this figure varies with stature.
  - **Lund and Browder chart** (1944). Burns charts are more accurate, but more time consuming; they are often used for 'definitive' assessment. They allow documentation of the distribution, as well as whether a burn is full or partial thickness; they offer a useful pictorial record.
    - However, they do still represent a best fit model based on average patients with average builds; 'anomalies' such as amputees, pregnant patients, etc. do not fit well. As such, some are utilising **3D cameras** and software to provide individualised and accurate TBSAs.

- Remember not to include **erythema**; this is a sign of an epidermal injury, e.g. sunburn. It is red, is very painful and blanches/refills quickly but without blisters or other change in the skin surface. It is a reversible hyperaemia that will fade over several hours and has little/no pathophysiological consequences in terms of a significant inflammatory response.

Estimate depth by clinical characteristics (see below).

At this stage, the EMSB course describes 'FATT' for

- Fluid – give resuscitation fluid according to the Parklands formula (see below)
- Analgesia – 0.05–0.1 mg/kg iv morphine, titrating to response
- Tests – blood tests as above, imaging such as cervical spine X-rays, etc.
- Tubes – (re)assess need for urinary catheter, IV, endotracheal tube, etc.

Secondary survey

- AMPLE history (allergies, medications, past medical history, last meal and events and environment of injury)
- Head-to-toe examination for non-life-threatening injuries; assess need for decompression (see below)

Burn depth assessment

The depth of a burn is related to the contact time and the temperature – according to Moritz (*Am J Pathol*, 1947) who performed series of experiments on pigs and humans, it would take 6 hours for irreversible damage to occur at 44°C, but only 1 second for *transepidermal necrosis* at 70°C. The important distinction to make is whether the injury is full thickness or not.

- Superficial partial thickness
  - Painful with blisters.
  - Skin is red, blanches and refills.
  - Hair follicles are still intact.
- Deep partial thickness
  - May be less painful/sensitive.
  - Small or no blisters.
  - Fixed staining in tissues.
- Full thickness
  - Waxy white or charred eschar.
  - Insensate, less pain (there is some pain due to reaction around full thickness burns).
  - No blisters.

Clinical assessment is only accurate in 64%–76% of cases even for experienced surgeons (Heimbach D, *J Trauma Acute Care Trauma*, 1984). Tissue biopsies, looking at denatured collagen and vessel patency on H&E or immunohistochemical identification of vimentin are often regarded as a gold standard, but are expensive and leave scars, and thus impractical for use in clinical practice. **Laser Doppler imaging** (LDI) is the closest to a practical standard for burn depth assessment with high positive (95%–97%) and negative predictive values when used to identify burns that will heal within 3 weeks (Pape SA, *Burns*, 2001). It is useful in reducing unnecessary surgery/costs and provides an objective measurement that is vital for research. Newer technologies such as laser speckle imaging seem promising. The following are mostly of research interest only:

- **Dyes**
  - Early work with radioisotopes (32P) was encouraging in animals (Bennett JE, *Plast Reconstr Surg*, 1957) but proved to be poorly reproducible and too cumbersome.
  - Goulian used non-fluorescent dyes, e.g. Evans blue (1961) and bromophenol blue (1968), to assess the areas of viability with intact circulation, but they are fairly indiscriminate when it came to determining burn depth and thus were of low clinical utility.
    - Some paint methylene blue on preoperatively and excise the stained portions – the theory being that live tissues will metabolise the dye (Manjulabai M, *Indian J Appl Res*, 2015)
  - Fluorescent dyes proved to be of limited use due to a lack of quantification and a large degree of variability.
    - **Indocyanine green** is the most recently studied, and the strength of the signal is proportional to blood flow (Sheridan R, *J Burn Care Rehab*, 1995) but is hindered by dye leak at a time when the capillaries are very permeable. Recent improvements in technology may allow it to be revisited.
- **Thermography**. Deeper burns would appear cooler (>2°C is the usual threshold) due to a decreased perfusion. However, this could be confounded by evaporative cooling (partly counteracted with clingfilm). Newer technologies provide cheaper and more sensitive detectors; dynamic thermography as well as infrared thermography may improve the predictive value.
- **Ultrasound** – high-frequency ultrasound (20–200 MHz) with a contact probe allows assessment of dermal features such as hair follicles and sweat ducts; non-contact methods with pulse wave Doppler ultrasound have been used in human studies and found 96% correlation with prediction of healing within 3 weeks (Iraniha S, *J Burn Care Rehab*, 2000).
  - Photo-acoustic imaging to demonstrate zone of stasis.
- **Microscopy**
  - In vivo videomicroscopy to visualise dermal capillary integrity (Mihara K, *Burns*, 2012)
  - In vivo confocal microscopy (Altintas MA, *Burns*, 2009)
  - Optical measurement, e.g. optical coherence tomography that measures the reduction of collagen birefringence
- **Others**
  - **NIRS** (near-infrared spectroscopy) to look at tissue oxygen saturation (Seki T, *Int J Burn Trauma*, 2014)
    - Hyperspectral imaging (Chin MS, *Plast Reconstr Surg Glob Open*, 2015) is an alternative way to look at tissue perfusion.

- Terahertz imaging – similar technology used in body scanners

Initial management of the burn wound, i.e. in the ED.

- Toilet the wound with saline (antiseptics such as chlorhexidine are not necessary except in grossly contaminated wounds).
- The wound can be dressed with clingfilm or saline-soaked gauzes prior to transfer to the definitive unit. Specific burns dressings should only be used after consultation with the receiving unit – **silver sulphadiazine** (SSD) can compromise accurate wound assessment; it should only be considered if the burn wound is contaminated or a significant delay in transfer is anticipated.
  - SSD is contraindicated in pregnant or nursing mothers and children <2 months due to the risk of kernicterus from the sulphonamide moiety. Although its role in reducing burns infection is undoubted, there is evidence that it actually impedes re-epithelialisation (i.e. decreased speed of healing by an adverse effect on keratinocyte DNA) and may increase scarring due to pro-inflammatory effects.
- Tetanus prophylaxis should be considered as per protocols, but antibiotics are not usually required.
- Criteria for transfer to a burns unit (local criteria may vary):
  - Burns >10% in children or 15% in adults
  - Burns at extremes of age unless minor
  - Full thickness (FT) or deep partial thickness (PT)
  - Inhalation injury
  - Burns of special areas – face, perineum and hands/feet
  - Electrical or chemical burns
  - Burns requiring decompression

III. RESUSCITATION REGIMENS

RESUSCITATION

Intravenous resuscitation is given for burns >15% BSA in adults (10% in children) – remember that the threshold is somewhat arbitrary, but has been clinically validated. They correspond roughly to the size of burns expected to produce a significant systemic response. The volume given is calculated according to formulae such as the **Parkland** formula:

- **2–4 mL/kg body weight/% TBSA**
  - Give half (Hartmann's/Ringer's lactate) in the first 8 hours, calculating **from the time of the injury** (replacing deficits as quickly as practical, usually taken to be 2 hours) and the remaining half over the next 16 hours.
  - It is common to give more fluid (50% more) if there is an inhalational injury or with electrical injuries. More fluid may also be needed in those with pre-existing dehydration, e.g. due to a substantial delay in transfer or concomitant injury causing loss of circulating volume. Beware

of **fluid creep** (see below), which is a significant risk if >0.25 L/kg has been infused.

- Give some colloid in the second 24 hours usually in the form of 5% albumin, 0.5 mL/kg in addition to maintenance crystalloid.
- Children will need **maintenance fluid** in addition to the resuscitation volume in the first 24 hours; dextrose saline is usually used, but hypoglycaemia (due to low hepatic glycogen stores) and hyponatraemia may occur. Use half normal saline if transfer is delayed.
  - 100 mL/kg up to 10 kg
  - 50 mL/kg up to 20 kg
  - 20 mL/kg up to 30 kg
- The formula is named after **Parkland Memorial Hospital in Dallas**. It is (unfortunately) associated with the assassination of JF Kennedy in 1963 – the president died there, and his assassin Lee Harvey Oswald died there after being shot by Jack Ruby who in turned died there in 1967 due to a pulmonary embolism.
- The formula was described by **Dr Charles Baxter** (1929–2005) based on canine studies showing that it could restore extracellular volume to within 10% of control, followed by use in burn patients. He was the director of the Emergency Room at Parkland Hospital when JFK was shot.

Remember that, in the end, whatever fluid formulae you use, these are only guides and provide a starting point for fluid administration – it is important to monitor the effectiveness of resuscitation constantly and to respond accordingly and speedily. The trend is to begin at the lower end, e.g. 2 mL/kg/% TBSA, to reduce the risk of **fluid creep** (clinicians are much better at increasing fluids for low urine output than reducing them for high urine output) with 'colloid rescue' typically 12–24 hours after the burn.

MONITORING IN MAJOR BURNS

- Pulse, BP, respiratory rate and core temperature.
- Pulse oximeter (beware CO poisoning).
- ECG if necessary.
- **Urine output** is the single most sensitive non-invasive parameter; insert urinary catheter for hourly monitoring in major burns. **Urine output is not a reliable indicator of the volaemic state in the second 24 hours (see below)**.
  - 0.5–1.0 mL/kg/hour in adults.
  - 1.0–2.0 mL/kg/hour in children; weighing nappies is an alternative to catheterisation in infants.
  - If output falls, then consider administering a fluid challenge of 5–10 mL/kg and to increase the rate of fluids in the next hour by 150%; avoid overhydration.
  - Manage haemoglobinuria by encouraging a high urine output, e.g. forced alkaline diuresis:
    - 12.5 g/L mannitol
    - 25 mmol/L NaHCO$_3$

- Goal-directed resuscitation using parameters such as lactase base deficit has not been shown to improve outcomes in burns and may be associated with more fluid creep.

The phenomenon of 'fluid creep' in acute burn resuscitation. (Saffle J, *J Burn Care Res*, 2007)
Fluid creep is a significant problem in modern burns care. It occurs when burns patients receive more resuscitation than predicted by the Parkland's formula, and more than is actually required. The increased fluid has been related to progressive oedema (including lungs and brain) and serious complications such as **abdominal compartment syndrome**.

The reasons put forward for fluid creep include the following:

- Parkland formula is not that accurate in large burns.
- Clinicians are slow/reluctant to reduce fluid infusions when urine output is high.
- Delayed presentation increases fluid requirements; regionalisation of burn facilities may contribute to this.
- Opioid creep – opiates have significant cardiovascular effects including partial antagonisation of the adrenergic stress response.
- Influence of goal-directed resuscitation – it is not needed in all patients but tends to lead to overresuscitation.

Overall, the aim is to give **the least amount** of fluid required to maintain tissue perfusion and prevent burns shock, to minimise the dangers and complications of overresuscitation. Greater vigilance is required, as well as further studies into

- Better endpoints of resuscitation, e.g. invasive monitoring of cardiac output and/or tissue perfusion
- Pharmacological manipulation, e.g. block/reduce oedema formation at capillary level, high-dose vitamin C (positive results in Japan have not been reproducible) or plasma exchange/plasmapheresis (to reduce cytokine levels)

CHOICE OF RESUSCITATION FLUIDS

Although the Parkland formula calls for crystalloid, there are many other formulae in use that seem to work equally well.

- **Crystalloid**, e.g. Hartmann's solution in Parkland formula, is recommended by the BBA and is the most commonly used resuscitation fluid.
  - Hartmann's – Na$^+$ 130 mmol, K$^+$ 4, Ca^{2+} 1.5, Cl$^-$ 109, lactate 28. The original solution was described by Sydney Ringer (British physician and physiologist, 1836–1910), and lactate was added as a buffer, i.e. lactated Ringer's or Ringer's lactate; currently there is slight variability in the composition between different manufacturers.
  - Normal saline – 154 sodium and 154 chloride.
  - 5% dextrose – 50 g glucose in 1 L of water.

- **Colloid**, e.g. Muir and Barclay formula:
  - % TBSA × weight kg/2 = one ration.
  - Give one ration 4 hourly in the first 12 hours; then give one ration 6 hourly in the next 12 hours and give the final ration over 12 hours.
  - There are concerns that the protein may leak out of the circulation and potentiate third space losses (although non-burned tissues re-establish normal permeability quickly after injury).
- **Others**
  - **Hypertonic saline** regimes have been described (Monafo WW, *J Trauma*, 1970) with the aim of reducing the volume of fluid required and thus may be of value in **patients with large burns (over 40%) and inhalational injury (Warden GD, World J Surg, 1992)**. However, it will cause a shift of intracellular water to the extracellular space, and intracellular dehydration. The clinical significance of this is uncertain, but less hypertonic solutions are probably safer; complications include excessive Na^+ retention and hypernatraemia, and Huang (*Ann Surg*, 1995) found an increased incidence of renal failure and death. Central pontine myelinosis is extremely rare and is usually associated with hypertonic saline being used to correct profound hyponatraemia (too quickly). Close monitoring including daily serum sodium levels is required. Although clinical studies have been equivocal, there may be a role for hypertonic saline, but its use should probably be reserved to experienced practitioners.
  - **Dextran** is a high-molecular-weight polysaccharide (polymerised glucose) available in different sizes, e.g. 40, 70 and 150 kDa molecules; 40% is excreted in the urine whilst the remainder is slowly metabolised. It is not commonly used in burns resuscitation, and there are problems associated with its use.
    - Dextran 40 improves flow by reducing red cell sludging (and is thus sometimes used in microsurgery), whilst dextran 70 causes more allergic reactions and compromises blood grouping.
  - **Fresh frozen plasma** can be used in children (hypoproteinaemia develops rapidly in paediatric patients), being particularly useful in treating **toxic shock**. It delivers passive immunity, though there is a risk of viral transmission.
  - **Enteral feeding** can be used to provide fluid maintenance in selected cases with 10%–15% burns (e.g. cooperative patient without nausea and vomiting) with the advice that the potassium requirement be doubled and that free access to plain water should be discouraged. Fluid resuscitation regimens should also replace sufficient salt (lost into burn tissue from the extracellular fluid), though this is usually a secondary issue in practice. Enteral protocols are

of greatest value in the Third World and after major disasters.
  - Proctoclysis ('Murphy's drip' 1913) is rarely used in developed countries.

ALBUMIN DEBATE

There is a frequently quoted report in the *British Medical Journal* (July 1998) from the Cochrane Injuries Group reporting on a meta-analysis of 30 studies comparing albumin with crystalloid resuscitation fluid in the three groups of hypovolaemia, burns and hypoproteinaemia. They found that the risk of death was higher in albumin-treated groups – for every 17 patients treated with albumin, there is 1 additional death (6 for every 100).

- Relative risk for hypovolaemia was 1.46.
- Relative risk for burns was 2.40.

This has often been used as justification for regarding colloids as being dangerous in burns resuscitation. However, there are several important criticisms of the report:

- The studies used in the meta-analysis were very dissimilar, and the indications and regimens for giving albumin in these studies were not standard policy in UK burns units.
- Only three burns studies were included (1979, 1983, 1995) with less than 150 patients included in total.
- There has been a generally good experience with the use of albumin in the United States, where reports demonstrate that 80% of paediatric burns >95% TBSA given albumin survive.
- Vincent (*Crit Care Med*, 2004) performed a meta-analysis looking at 71 trials and found that albumin resuscitation in patients critically ill from a variety of causes resulted in decreased morbidity and mortality.
- Another Cochrane review (Perel P, *Cochrane Database Syst Rev*, 2013;2:CD000567) found no difference in survival in critically ill/injured patients but stated that the cost of albumin made its use over crystalloid difficult to justify.

FLUID REPLACEMENT AFTER 24 HOURS

By this point, the peak increase in capillary permeability/tissue oedema has passed, and there is a need to restore serum albumin. If crystalloid was given (in large volumes) in the first 24 hours, then protein **(0.5 mL/kg/% TBSA of 5% albumin)** may be given. Some suggest changing Hartmanns to D5W; maintenance fluid can often be given via enteral feeding (double K+ requirements to 120 mmol/24 hours).

- The urine output during this period is a **less reliable guide** to volaemic status due to the problems listed below. It may be better to monitor hydration by plasma sodium and urea levels.
  - Glucose intolerance (due to anti-insulin stress hormones) causes hyperglycaemia, then glycosuria leading to osmotic diuresis.

- Disturbances of ADH secretion (inappropriate ADH, diabetes insipidus).
- High respiratory water loss.

BURN WOUND DRESSINGS AND TOPICAL AGENTS

The ideal burn wound dressing does not yet exist. Desirable properties of a burn dressing would include

- Protection against trauma and infection
- Reduction of evaporative heat and water loss
- Absorption of wound exudate
- Pain relief

The most basic dressings aim to absorb exudate and keep the wound dry, e.g. paraffin gauze or tulle gras (named after Tulle, France, a region famous for making nets), which may be impregnated with various antiseptics/antibiotics:

- Jelonet (plain paraffin gauze) vs. Mepitel® (non-adherent silicone net dressing)
- Bactigras® (0.5% chlorhexidine)
- Xeroform® (3% bismuth tribromophenate)
- Sofratulle® (framycetin)

To reduce colonisation/infection, the burn wound eschar should be cleansed with diluted aqueous chlorhexidine at each dressing change. Common organisms affecting burn wounds include *Staphylococcus aureus*, Gram-negative bacteria including *Proteus* and *Klebsiella* and mixed anaerobes including *Escherichia coli*. Common burns dressings include the following:

- **Non-silver**, e.g. fusidic acid, neomycin and bacitracin.
  - **Bactroban®** (mupirocin 2%) is a topical antibiotic that has wide activity against skin infections; increasing resistance has led some territories to return it to prescription only. It needs to be applied several times a day; polyethylene glycol absorption may be an issue in large wounds and thus should be used cautiously in those with renal impairment.
  - **Sulfamylon®** (mafenide acetate) has relatively poor activity against Gram-negative bacteria and has limited activity against *Staphylococci* including methicillin-resistant *S. aureus* (MRSA) – it is mainly bacteriostatic. It can be **painful** (twice daily application), which is attributed to the high osmolarity of the 10% cream; a 5% solution is said to be less painful and can be used as wet gauze soaks every 6–8 hours; 5% of patients suffer from a rash. It may cause **metabolic acidosis** due to inhibition of carbonic anhydrase.
- **Silver**
  - Silver ions bind to and disrupt bacterial walls; the anions also bind to and inhibit bacterial enzymes. The multifaceted mechanisms of action are said to reduce the risk of resistance, but it has been described in some *Pseudomonas* species.

However, the nonspecific effect also means that it can harm healthy tissues.
  - **Agyria** – silver is absorbed (at a greater rate in open or more vascular wounds such as a partial thickness burn) and excreted in the urine (Rosemary Jacobs was a patient who famously became grey after taking colloidal silver); it is certainly much less common with modern silver products and, if present, is usually transient.
- **0.5% silver nitrate** is active against *Staphylococcus*, *Pseudomonas* and other Gram-negative bacteria; concentrations >0.5% are more toxic to normal cells. It usually comes as a solution used to wet gauze dressings; there is a risk of toxicity by systemic absorption, but this is limited by its insolubility. It is an effective burn wound dressing. However,
  - Leaching of electrolytes, especially sodium, may occur from the burn wound, and supplements may be needed especially in children to avoid hyponatraemia.
  - It may rarely cause methaemoglobinaemia.
  - It stains fabric brown/black.
- **Silver sulphadiazine** (SSD) has a broader spectrum of antimicrobial activity compared with silver nitrate; sporadic resistance to *Pseudomonas aeruginosa* has been reported. The cream is applied daily and leads to the formation of a **pseudoeschar** resembling a deeper burn, which may complicate wound depth assessment. It should therefore only be used once a decision has been made regarding burn depth and the need for surgery. It penetrates burn eschar poorly and, like silver nitrate, it is used mainly for prophylaxis – it is **not suitable for treating** invasive infection. Side effects include the following:
  - Transient neutropenia (5%–15%) may occur after 2–3 days; the neutrophil count recovers even if SSD is continued and increased infection rates have not been reported. White cell counts should be monitored.
  - Maculopapular rash (5%).
  - Haemolytic anaemia in patients with G-6-PD deficiency.
  - It can cause kernicterus (due to the sulphonamide moiety) in children <2 months old and should also be avoided in pregnant and breastfeeding women.
  - **Methaemoglobinuria** is a rare side effect, where the Fe^{2+} (ferrous) form of haemoglobin is oxidised to Fe^{3+} (ferric), which is inactive. Normally, 3% of all haemoglobin is composed of methaemoglobin and is converted back by methaemoglobin reductase (an inherited deficiency of this enzyme has been described). It can be treated with 1 mL/kg 1% methylene blue.

- It may inactivate enzyme-debriding agents if used concurrently.
- Wasiak (2013, *Cochrane Review, Dressings for superficial and partial thickness burns*) found that in burns less than 15%, SSD actually delayed healing and increased pain compared to other dressings such as biosynthetic silicone-coated and silver dressings; hydrogels were associated with better outcomes.
- Currently, due to the pro-inflammatory effects and the potential for greater scarring, it is not used on the face and is no longer first line in modern burn units, but can be useful for burns of the perineum.

- **Flammacerium** is SSD with cerium nitrate. Cerium is a 'rare earth' metal, which is not that rare; it displaces calcium ions, but how this relates to its activity is unclear. It is **bacteriostatic** – it leads to metabolic inhibition after it is taken up by micro-organisms. There is supposed 'synergy' with SSD, but most clinical studies show little in the way of additional antibacterial action. Its most obvious effect is on the physical characteristics of the burn wound, which hardens to a green-yellow eschar with leathery consistency that is adherent to the underlying wound (as opposed to SSD, which tends to macerate the wound). This is said to reduce bacterial colonisation and to sequester burn toxins preventing them from entering the circulation, and has been shown in some studies to reduce mortality in severe burns. More recent randomised studies have clarified early contradictory results with demonstrable improvement in epithelialisation times and reduced length of hospital stay.
  - Severe side effects are rare, but there is a risk of methaemoglobinaemia, haemolytic anaemia, and kernicterus as for SSD. Some experience a stinging sensation.
- **Silver dressings.** There are a large number of dressings that have silver in them; they are generally reserved for burn wounds that are infected or at high risk of infection.
  - **Acticoat®** is a nanocrystalline (greater surface area) silver-impregnated dressing that aims to deliver silver ions continuously to the wound. The dressing needs to be kept moist by sterile water rather than saline, which would inactivate the silver ions.
  - **Aquacel silver®** – rather than release silver into the wound, this hydrofibre dressing is said to absorb exudate and bacteria into it, supposedly reducing side effects.
  - **Cochrane reviews**.
    - Storm-Versloot (*Cochrane Database Syst Rev,* 2010) found that studies were generally of low quality, and that there was insufficient evidence to suggest that silver dressings can promote healing or prevent wound infection.
    - Vermeulen (*Cochrane Database Syst Rev,* 2007). Only three trials of sufficient quality could be identified; one study (Jorgensen B, *Int Wound J,* 2005) showed that ulcers healed at a quicker rate when dressed with a silver foam, but the final time to healing was not significantly different.

Biological dressings (see 'Recent advances') such as porcine skin and amniotic membrane (AM) have significant advantages in non-infected partial thickness burns by virtue of their adherence to the wound till it has healed. This greatly simplifies wound care and reduces the pain of dressing changes.

BURNS INFECTION

The pathophysiology of the burn wound increases the risk of infection:

- Disruption of barrier
- Necrotic tissue in eschar
- Use of invasive devices

Burns are also associated with a decrease in both cellular and humoral immunity; serum from burn patients is immunosuppressive in vitro and prolonged survival of allografts is seen in vivo. There is

- Decreased numbers of lymphocytes.
- Reduction of immunoglobulin levels.
- Increased macrophage activity – these are major producers of inflammatory cytokines after a burn and also responsible for its cytotoxic and cytostatic effects including lymphocyte suppression (Schwacha MG, *Burns*, 2003).

Generally, the presence of bacteria at a level $>10^5$ reduces the success of graft take, although lower levels of β-haemolytic Streptococcus, e.g. *S. pyogenes,* are also a contraindication for skin grafting (Wilson GR, *Ann Roy Coll Surg Engl,* 1988) due to fibrinolysis. However, it can be effectively managed with antibiotics. The presence of *P. aeruginosa* also doubles the risk of graft loss, and antibiotics tend to be less effective (Hogsberg T, *PLoS One,* 2011). The presence of a **biofilm** as well as finding bacteria penetrating deeper into the wound (Fazli M, *J Clin Microbiol,* 2009) limits the efficacy of many treatments.

- **Prophylactic systemic antibiotics** are usually not warranted; antibiotics do not penetrate eschar and indiscriminate use promotes resistance. Antibiotics should be guided by clinical assessment and microbiological results.
- **Sepsis should be suspected** if there is a change in temperature, blood glucose or the acute onset of heart failure, pulmonary oedema, acute respiratory distress syndrome (ARDS) or ileus.
- **Toxic shock syndrome** (TSS) due to *S. aureus* TSS toxin is a rare but severe complication in children.

BIOFILM

The phenomenon was found on rocks in a Canadian stream that had a slippery slime with a bacterial population that grossly outnumbered the bacteria in the water. The term 'biofilm' is used to describe these aggregations of bacteria embedded in a self-produced extracellular polymeric substance (EPS) that adhere to surfaces (living or dead), particularly those in contact with water. They are not removed by gentle rinsing, and the bacteria within are relatively protected from antimicrobial agents.

Management includes

- **Debridement** – curettage/'scrub' to physically remove the biofilm, with or without chemical rinses, e.g. betaine in Prontosan®, Lavasept®, etc.). The biofilm will grow back quickly unless other steps are taken.
- **Topical antimicrobials/antiseptics**, e.g. silver, iodine, polyhexamethylene biguanide (PHMB). Most topical agents by themselves have limited action on biofilm; some advocate the use of detergent-type products such as xylitol and EDTA, but convincing clinical evidence is lacking.

Prophylactic antibiotics for burns patients: Systematic review and meta-analysis. (Avni T, *Br Med J*, 2010)
This literature review included 17 trials and demonstrated that prophylactic systemic antibiotics reduced overall mortality. There was a decrease in pneumonia and wound infections. However, the reviewers commented that the overall methodological quality of the included trials was poor, and they do not recommend antibiotic prophylaxis in severe burns except perioperatively.

IV. MECHANISMS OF BURN INJURY

BURN WOUND

Jackson's burn wound model (Jackson D, *Br J Surg*, 1953) has been used to describe the different zones (or volumes) of injury occurring in a burn wound.

- **Zone of coagulation** – the central part closest to the point of contact, has the severest damage and is characterised by coagulative necrosis, which is irreversible.
- **Zone of stasis** – the surrounding area is characterised by decreased tissue perfusion.
  - It is potentially salvageable and the aim of effective resuscitation is to allow this zone to recover by restoring capillary microcirculation and thus re-establish tissue perfusion, limiting the production of free radicals.
- **Zone of hyperaemia** – burns that are >25% BSA will involve the **whole of the body** in the zone of hyperaemia due to large amounts of circulating inflammatory mediators.

SYSTEMIC EFFECTS OF A MAJOR BURN

A major burn (>20%–30%) will affect the whole body (hence 'systemic') and can have many serious effects including the following:

- **Reduced cardiac output** due to
  - Decreased myocardial contractility – a myocardial depressant factor has been proposed, but its nature/ existence is controversial. This reduced function can persist despite adequate resuscitation.
  - Decreased venous return and inadequate preload.
  - Increased afterload – increased systemic vascular resistance.
- **Increased systemic vascular resistance**
  - Catecholamines and sympathetic activity.
  - ADH and angiotensin II, neuropeptide Y.
- **Pulmonary oedema**
  - Increased pulmonary vascular resistance.
  - Increased capillary pressure and capillary permeability.
  - Left heart failure.
  - Hypoproteinaemia.
  - Direct vascular injury following inhalational injury.
- **Downregulation of cell-mediated and hormonal immune responses**
- **Renal** – decreased renal perfusion, increased antidiuretic hormone (ADH) and aldosterone and increased sodium and water retention
- **Metabolism** – catabolic response
- **Liver/pancreas**
  - Glucose intolerance.
  - Increased metabolic rate.
  - Protein catabolism especially muscle.
  - Growth inhibition.
- **Gastrointestinal** (see below)
  - Stress ulceration – Curling's.
  - Gut stasis, ischaemic enterocolitis (rare) and bacterial translocation (treat/prevent with selective gut decontamination).
  - Gall bladder and acalculous cholecystitis.

BURNS OEDEMA

Normal Starling's forces demonstrate a slight net filtration pressure, with this being matched by lymphatic drainage back to the venous system. In an acute burn, this near-balance is disturbed and soft-tissue oedema develops due to

- **Increased capillary hydrostatic pressure** (due to vasodilation and venoconstriction)
- **Increased capillary permeability** (due to inflammatory mediators, peaking at 3–6 hours), leading to
- **Decreased plasma oncotic pressure** (due to loss of albumin from the circulation into the tissues)
- **Increased tissue oncotic pressure** (albumin accumulates into the tissues and then the large proteins break up into more osmotically active units)

- **Decreased tissue hydrostatic pressure** (unfolding of damaged macromolecules causes a loosening effect)
- **Generalised impairment in cell membrane function** leading to increased swelling of cells

The nature of the oedema also depends on the depth of the burn:

- In partial thickness burns, 90% of oedema (mostly in dermis) is present at 4 hours, peaking at around 12 hours.
- In full thickness burns, the oedema (mostly in subcutaneous fat) peaks at about 18 hours and 25% is still present at 1 week, i.e. persists for longer, supposedly due to poor lymphatics and perfusion.
- With larger burns, severe and sustained oedema also develops in non-burned tissues (see above). Oedema contributes to **tissue hypoxia.**

Inflammatory mediators underlie the development of oedema. There can be local (e.g. histamine and prostaglandins, kinins) and systemic factors (e.g. catecholamines, angiotensin). Whilst treatments such as vitamin C, heparin and inhibitors of kinin and prostaglandin production have been suggested, their clinical benefit is still unproven.

HISTAMINE

Histamine is released from mast cells in heat-injured skin and is responsible for the following:

- Early phase of increased capillary permeability (first hour of oedema).
- Arteriolar dilatation and venular constriction.
- Pain (and itch).
- Histamine and its derivatives stimulate xanthine oxidase pathways in the endothelial cell membrane (hypoxanthine to xanthine) and generation of oxygen free radicals with reperfusion (see below).

PROSTAGLANDINS, LEUKOTRIENES AND THROMBOXANES

These are products of the arachidonic acid pathway and act primarily at a local level. Prostaglandins and leukotrienes are released from neutrophils and macrophages. Neutrophil-blocking antibodies given post-burn have been shown to reduce oedema in animal studies (Hansbrough JF, *Crit Care Med*, 1996).

- **PGE2 is the most important prostaglandin in** the pathogenesis of burn wound oedema and increases vascular permeability.
- PGI2 is a vasodilator and also increases capillary permeability.
- TXA2 is produced locally by platelets; it is less important in oedema formation, but through vasoconstriction, it may extend the zone of coagulative necrosis. Increased serum TXA2/PGI2 ratios have been found in burn patients. Systemic ibuprofen in sheep reduces post-burn tissue ischaemia by blocking TXA2 production but has little effect on burn wound oedema.

FREE RADICALS

Oxygen radicals are moieties with unpaired electrons and consequently are strong oxidising agents. These include the superoxide anion ($O_2\cdot$), H_2O_2 and hydroxyl ion ($OH\cdot$).

- Hydroxyl ion is the most damaging ($Fe^{2+} + H_2O_2 \rightarrow Fe^{3+} + 2OH\cdot$).
- Catalase neutralises H_2O_2 whilst superoxide dismutase neutralises $O_2\cdot$, and iron chelators (desferrioxamine) may be protective against $OH\cdot$ formation.

Reperfusion injury results as flow is re-established to a zone of stasis, providing oxygen to drive renewed free radical production through a variety of mechanisms:

- Phospholipase A2 acts on free phospholipids (from cell injury), converting them along arachidonic acid pathways to products that are chemotactic to neutrophils. These cells are a source of oxygen free radicals that further injure membrane lipids and stimulate further phospholipase A2, etc.
- Xanthine oxidase catalyses the conversion of hypoxanthine to xanthine in endothelial cells with free radicals released as by-products. Histamine stimulates xanthine oxidase, and hence cromoglycate, H2 receptor antagonists and allopurinol (inhibits xanthine oxidase) may be beneficial.

ANGIOTENSIN II AND VASOPRESSIN

- A fall in renal perfusion pressure stimulates the release of renin from juxta-glomerular cells (afferent arteriolar cells) that monitor renal perfusion. Renin converts a circulating α-globulin, angiotensinogen, to angiotensin I, which is in turn converted in the circulation (mainly by pulmonary endothelial cells) by angiotensin-converting enzyme to **angiotensin II** (AII).
  - AII acts upon the hypothalamus to release ADH (which is also released from the hypothalamus due to stimulation of osmoreceptors monitoring plasma osmolality), which promotes water re-absorption from the collecting ducts.
  - AII acts at the adrenal cortex (zona glomerulosa) to release aldosterone (also released due to sympathetic efferent discharge), which then increases sodium (and water) retention at the distal convoluted tubule.
  - AII causes vasoconstriction including the efferent renal arterioles.
  - AII induces thirst.

NITRIC OXIDE

Nitric oxide (NO) is produced by many types of cells including vascular endothelium through the oxidation of L-arginine by NO synthetase. It has been demonstrated to be an important regulator of vasomotor tone as well as

- Increasing capillary permeability
- Inhibiting platelet aggregation
- Systemic effects as a neurotransmitter

NO reacts with superoxide free radicals to produce the highly reactive **peroxynitrite** molecule. It is required for leukocyte-mediated killing and may contribute to resistance to infection and wound healing at later stages of inflammation (Rawlingson A, *Burns*, 2003). It has been implicated in both the local burn wound inflammation and the systemic inflammatory response to a major burn including pulmonary and cardiovascular dysfunction; dysregulation of NO production is associated with multiple organ failure.

OTHERS

- Bradykinins increase capillary permeability.
- Serotonin causes vasoconstriction and increases permeability.
- Catecholamines are part of the stress response (along with glucagon, ACTH and cortisol). The resultant systemic vasoconstriction affects vessels in non-burned skin, muscle and viscera. The use of inotropes, e.g. in ICU, can adversely affect burn healing.

V. CAUSES OF BURN INJURY

The commonest cause of a burn is heat. Other causes include

- Electrical
- Cold injury
- Chemical and extravasation

ELECTRICAL BURNS

Approximately 1000 deaths occur per year due to electrical injury in the United States, including 80 due to lightning.

- **The Joule effect** (or Joule's first law) is the conversion of electrical energy into heat: $J = I^2RT$, where J is the heat produced, I is the current, R is the resistance and T is the duration of current.

  Hence, more heat occurs when electrical energy passes along tissues of high resistance, e.g. bone (nerve and blood vessels have least resistance).

  A limb will tend to 'cook' from inside out; **FDP and FPL** are affected the earliest as they are closest to the bone of the forearm. Other important parameters include the frequency of the current and the pathway taken through the body. Wet skin or jewellery such as rings also affects current flow (which is more important than the voltage per se).

- **Cardiovascular effects** – cardiac dysrhythmias (RBBB, SVTs and ectopics) are diagnosed in up to 30% of high-voltage injuries. If cardiorespiratory arrest occurs, prolonged resuscitation may be worthwhile. Data extrapolated mostly from animal testing suggest that as little as 17 mA AC travelling across the chest could induce fibrillation in humans. In industry, 30 V is generally regarded as a conservative threshold for dangerous voltage.
- **Neurological effects** – repeated or severe injuries that are not fatal often cause neuropathic sequelae. With

current travelling through the head, there is a rapid loss of consciousness (electrical stunning), a fact that is made use of in slaughterhouses (250 V or above).

Classification of electrical burns

Low voltage (<1000 V)

This tends to cause local tissue necrosis similar to thermal injury. Due to its alternating nature, injury with an AC power supply can cause cardiac arrest/VF at a much lower current than a DC. AC of about 10 mA through a 68 kg person can produce continuous muscle contractions ('let go threshold') that may lead to deeper injury, as the victim cannot let go (stronger flexors overpower the extensors to sustain the grip).

High voltage (>1000 V)

This often causes deep muscle injury and **compartment syndrome**, leading to haemochromogenuria. There are usually **entry and exit wounds** (areas of full thickness necrosis) on the skin surface.

- Cardiorespiratory arrest
- Fractures/dislocations
- Bowel perforation or paralytic ileus
- Physiological spinal cord transection in up to 25%

Lightning injury (very high voltage, very high current, short duration)

Victims of a strike may have fractures/dislocations and corneal injury and tympanic perforation.

- **Direct strike** (from the highest point to the ground).
- **Ground splash** (lightning hits a relatively poor conductor first, e.g. a tree or the ground, and then the discharge jumps to make secondary contact with the victim).
- **Stride potential** (when lightning strikes the ground and spreads laterally, it induces a potential difference between the legs of a victim on the standing on the ground, and causes current to briefly flow).
- **Lichtenberg figures** ('lightning flowers') are fern-like patterns on the skin and are pathognomonic of a lightning strike.

  Thermal injuries in electrical burns can occur

- **At entry and exit points** (contact and grounding point; this is actually a misnomer of sorts because in AC, the flow is back and forth – with very high voltages, there may be multiple exit sites)
- **Due to arcing** (up to 80% of injuries related to electricity are due to the arc flash)
- **Due to thermal burns** following ignition of clothing

General Management

- **ABC**
  - ECG. Continuous cardiac monitoring for 24 hours is usually suggested for those with high-voltage injuries particularly where current has passed

through the chest/heart, e.g. hand-to-hand current flow has greater risk than hand-to-foot. Transcardiac current may have sustained effects on the conducting system of the heart, predisposing to late/delayed arrhythmias.

- Monitor for haemochromogenuria (haem in urine that is either due to haemoglobin or myoglobin) and compartment syndrome. Muscle necrosis and its sequelae can be life-threatening.
- Debridement and definitive wound closure after 24–72 hours.
  - Salvage of devitalised tissues with emergency free flaps that bring in additional blood supply. Consider vein grafts to ensure that anastomoses are performed outside the zone of injury.
  - CURA (comprehensive urgent reconstruction alternative) (Zhu ZX, *Burns*, 2003):
    - Early (70% within 1 hour of admission) conservative wound debridement, preserving vital structures (nerves, tendons, bone) even where viability is in doubt
    - Flap cover (including vascularised nerves, etc.) within 48 hours with continuous irrigation of the wound bed beneath the flap with lidocaine and chloromycetin in saline for up to 72 hours.
  - Amputation where necessary.

Cardiac monitoring always required after electrical injuries? (Kramer C, *Med Klin Intensivmed Notfmed*, 2016)

This is a single centre retrospective study with 169 patients over 15 years. In the high voltage group, one died due to open intracranial injury and cardiac arrest; of the remaining six, five had normal ECGs and one had sinus tachycardia. They concluded that asymptomatic stable patients with a normal admission ECG do **not** need inpatient cardiac monitoring.

Most literature supports this view, i.e. asymptomatic patients with a normal initial ECG do not require cardiac monitoring if there has been no loss of consciousness and if the voltage was less than 1000 V, even if transthoracic (Bailey B, *Emerg Med J*, 2007). However, the evidence for high-voltage injury is unclear.

Delayed complications

- Cardiac dysrhythmias.
- Neurological problems.
  - Central (from 6 months) – epilepsy and encephalopathy
  - Brainstem dysfunction
  - Cord problems including progressive muscular atrophy, amyotrophic lateral sclerosis and transverse myelitis
  - Peripheral (from months to up to 3 years) – progressive neural demyelination
- Cataracts (from 6 months) occur in up to 30% of patients with high-voltage electrical burns involving the head and neck.

COLD INJURY

Cold injury can either be local (frostbite) or systemic (hypothermia, body core temperature of <35°C). The latter is usually due to exposure of the body to cold temperature with lowering of the core temperature, whilst the former is usually due to focal exposure of body parts to cold (slow cooling) or agents such as dry ice or liquefied gases (fast cooling), e.g. liquid nitrogen.

Predisposing factors for hypothermia

- Extremes of age
- Alcohol (causes peripheral vascular dilatation)
- Mental instability
- Low ambient temperature with strong air currents (wind chill).

Predisposing factors for frostbite (by slow cooling)

- Temperature, wind chill factor and duration of contact
- Pre-existing hypoperfusion (atherosclerosis, etc.) and smoking (vascular spasm)
- Moisture content versus oil content of the skin

Four phases of cold injury

- **Prefreeze** (3–10°C). Before ice crystals have formed; there is increased vascular permeability.
- **Freeze–thaw** (–6 to –15°C). Extra- and intra-cellular ice crystals form at –4°C, i.e. when the skin is supercooled, which is necessary owing to the generation of background metabolic heat. At –20°C, 90% of all available water is frozen.
- **Vascular stasis** with dilatation and coagulation, thus shunting blood flow away from the affected part.
- **Late ischaemic phase** with cell death and gangrene.

The mechanisms of tissue damage include a combination of the following:

- Mechanical injury from oedema and distension.
- Direct damage – ice crystal damage causes apoptosis and altered gene regulation from non-random DNA cleavage. It has been demonstrated in vitro, but the in vivo significance is unclear.
- Vascular injury and reperfusion injury with free radical lipid peroxidation.

Effects of thawing

- Initial reversible vasoconstriction then hyperaemia with restoration of the dermal circulation.
- Endothelial cell damage and formation of microemboli leading to distal occlusion and thrombosis (no reflow) and oedema.
  - With larger vessels, the internal pressure keeps them open whilst healing occurs, but in the long term, there is narrowing from subsequent intimal hyperplasia and smooth muscle proliferation. Smaller vessels tend to collapse and remain closed due to lack of opening pressure.

- Liberation of inflammatory mediators and oxygen free radicals, which contributes further to the frostbite injury causing oedema and formation of blisters and, later, an eschar.

Common acute symptoms of cold injury are coldness and **numbness with pain on rewarming;** part of the damage comes after the temperature drop. Specific symptoms may have predictive value and favourable features include

- Intact pinprick sensation
- Indentable skin (indicating elasticity)
- Normal colour
- Larger blisters with clear fluid

Management

The depth of a cold injury is usually more difficult to judge than thermal burns; thus, initial treatment tends to be conservative. Avoid rewarming if there is a risk of refreezing as the eventual damage will be much worse (supposedly multiplicative, not additive). There is a period of vascular instability/spasm for several days after.

- **Avoiding rubbing** frozen parts. Necrosis is reduced by rapid rewarming through immersion in circulating water at 40–42°C for ~30 minutes with **analgesia** (NSAIDs).
- **Afterdrop phenomenon** – peripheral vasodilation on rewarming allows the cold blood from the extremities to return to the centre, causing hypothermia.
- Leave blisters alone; elevate and splint extremities.
- There are no specific medications or dressings that have been proven to alter the course of a cold injury.
    - Intravascular heparin/tPA may reduce vasospasm and microvascular thrombosis; some studies suggest reduced amputation rates, but this is controversial.
    - Heparin, warfarin, steroids, vitamin C and HBOT have doubtful efficacy.
- Tetanus and antibiotic prophylaxis is advisable.
- Surgery is usually delayed once the depth of injury has become obvious. Investigations such as NMR, radionuclide scans, laser Doppler, etc. have been found to be not useful.
    - Amputation is often delayed as demarcation may take weeks.

There is usually good long-term recovery, but possible sequelae include

- Residual burning sensations for weeks, usually precipitated by warming
- Cold intolerance/Raynaud's phenomenon
- Localised areas of bone resorption, and joint pain and stiffness
- Nerve injury
    - Permanent sensory loss.
    - Hyperhidrosis as a manifestation of altered sympathetic activity.

- **Skin refrigerants** such as ethyl oxide make use of this cooling effect to produce topical anaesthesia, e.g. for vaccinations in children, due to the fact that cooling decreases nerve conduction in C and A delta fibres. Studies show them to be as effective as EMLA for minor surgery, providing temporary numbness for up to 1 minute. May temporarily relieve muscle spasm pain.
- Nerve injuries are usually temporary in the 0–5°C range, whilst colder temperatures (–15 to –20°C) will cause long-term functional loss. Some return is likely if the nerve sheaths are intact.

Cryotherapy

This was first used for tissue ablation in the 1960s with probes for internal tumours and cardiac conducting system; it has been used mainly in dermatological practice. The severity of the injury depends on factors such as

- Temperature
    - Short exposure (0°C to –10°C) causes minimal necrosis, with little/no ice crystal formation.
    - At cooler temperatures (less than –15°C)/longer exposure, crystals form, first extracellularly then intracellularly.
    - At –40°C to –50°C, destruction is practically certain.
- Rate of cooling
    - Slow cooling causes more extracellular ice formation along with cellular dehydration.
    - Faster cooling causes more intracellular damage.

There is an inverse 'U' curve of viability, with low viability at very high and very low rates of cooling. Even at very low temperatures, a small proportion of cells particularly at the periphery will survive, which underlies the rationale for **cycles** of freeze–thawing and/or using adjuncts, e.g. chemotherapy.

Studies demonstrate that whilst cells and glands/hair follicles may die from freezing injury, the fibrocollagenous matrix and fibroblasts are more resistant and thus preserved, potentially allowing more favourable healing. Damaged collagen tends to be resorbed and replaced, and wound contraction is rare.

CHEMICAL BURNS

Chemical injuries constitute approximately 3% of burn admissions with most being work-related (depending on the local population), affecting men and the upper extremities more frequently.

- Civilian chemical burns – mainly acids and alkalis
- Military chemical injuries – mainly white phosphorus
- Industrial
    - Acid burns are common in plating or fertilising industries.
        - Nitric acid (engravers acid, also used in electroplating) burns have a characteristic **yellow staining**.

- Hydrofluoric (HF) burns – glass etching, petroleum refinement and wheel cleaners/rust removers.
- Alkali burns.
  - Sodium and potassium hydroxide in oven, drain cleaners, soap manufacture.
  - Hypochlorite – bleach.
- Phenol – dye, fertiliser, plastic and explosives manufacture.

Tissue damage

A feature of chemical burns is that there is usually continued tissue damage long after the initial exposure. The severity of the injury is related to

- Concentration and strength of the agent (these are not equivalent).
- Duration of exposure. Some chemical remains in the tissue, even after repeated irrigation.
- Type of chemical.
- Site affected.
  - Industrial exposures in particular may have an inhalational component.
  - Eye injuries can be devastating.
- Systemic effects.

Emergency management

- Removal of contaminated clothing and copious lavage with **running water** (care with 'run-off' injuries) whilst avoiding hypothermia. In the industrial setting, 'decontamination' procedures are usually of a high standard; thus, injuries often tend to be less severe than household injuries where the problem may be 'ignored' (due to lack of awareness and lack of protective measures) until it is too late.
  - **Dilution** rather than neutralisation (which causes an exothermic reaction and requires positive identification of the agent) is the aim; 5% acetic acid neutralisation of sodium hydroxide burns has been used to reduce damage in animal models without detectable increases in temperature. Surface pH (tested with strips) is often used, but its usefulness has not been properly assessed.
    - Some contraindications to water (see below)
    - Diphoterine® – polyvalent ring molecule that can bind/sequester a number of different moieties without generating heat
  - Trim fingernails/remove jewellery.
- If necessary
  - Urgent eye consultation for any ocular involvement.
  - Check blood pH/gases for acid base balance.
  - Encourage diuresis with mannitol to prevent renal complications, with agents that have systemic absorption/effects.
  - Conventional treatment dictates that the wounds are allowed to demarcate – the theory being that

debriding and grafting too early may lead to graft loss due to the presence of residual chemical.
- Waiting longer obviously risks deeper damage; thus, emergency debridement aiming to reduce the chemical load and the final damage is emerging as an alternative in selected injuries. Wounds can be covered with biological dressings as a 'test graft' of sorts before using autograft.
- A more active protocol is particularly relevant in extravasation injuries, (cyto)toxics and HF.

There are certain situations in which **water should be avoided**:

- Alkali metals (sodium, potassium and lithium) undergo exothermic reactions with water. The material should be covered with oil before gently wiping it away.
- The penetration of phenol increases with dilution (see below).
- White phosphorous (also known as yellow phosphorous because it is yellow – it also smells like garlic) is a military agent but is also found in fertilisers. It self-ignites in air and can cause cutaneous burns. It oxidises to phosphorous pentoxide, which combines with water to produce **phosphoric acid**; 1% copper sulphate solution turns the phosphorous black (a film of cupric oxide), increasing its visibility for removal.
  - Cochrane review (Barqouni L, *Cochrane Database Syst Rev*, 2014) suggested that there was no evidence that use of copper sulphate improves outcomes, and there is some evidence that its systemic absorption may be harmful. The US military recommends bicarbonate neutralisation as first aid, with identification by either smoking on air exposure or fluorescence in the dark.
  - ECG monitoring is advised in cases with electrolyte imbalance.
  - Red phosphorous is non-toxic.

Alkalis, e.g. NaOH, KOH, lime

Alkalis are more common at home (drain cleaner, oven cleaner or bleach); they tend to cause less immediate damage but more eventual damage.

Mechanism of Injury

- Saponification of fat – **liquefactive necrosis**, which means that alkalis are capable of deep penetration.
- Protein denaturation – corrosive action produces a soft eschar with or without shallow ulceration, e.g. hypochlorite (bleach) or phenol.

Cement, i.e. calcium oxide

There is an exothermic reaction with water, e.g. sweat to form CaOH, which is an alkali (pH 12–13); it is capable of full thickness burns after 2 hours. The typical injury involves cement getting inside the victim's boots, and because the early symptoms usually consist of mild irritation, it is often ignored leading to prolonged contact with significant desiccation injury.

Drain cleaners

The common drain cleaners found in supermarkets are usually composed of alkalis (sodium or potassium hydroxide, with or without bleach); some are enzyme-based (usually marketed as eco-friendly). Acid drain cleaners are also available but primarily intended for use by plumbers due to the violent reaction with water; they are amongst the most hazardous household chemicals available to the public. Unfortunately, they also seem to be the agent of choice in chemical assaults.

Sulphur mustard

This is an amber oily agent that penetrates skin easily. It binds to DNA and causes cell death; vesicle formation is a common feature. Rapid decontamination is desirable, e.g. passive means with Fuller's earth ('clean dirt' also used to clean the Taj Mahal). Injuries tend to be painful but usually do not require surgery, as they tend to heal within a week or two.

ACIDS

Mechanism of Injury
Tissue damage occurs mainly by **coagulative necrosis.**

- Desiccation – dehydration of tissues. The reaction is often exothermic, e.g. sulphuric and concentrated hydrochloric acid (HCl).
- Reduction – binding free electrons in tissues. Often exothermic also.
- 'Protoplasmic poisons' – block cell viability/function through, e.g. binding vital ions, such as calcium in the case of HF.

Sulphuric acid

This is found in **lead acid batteries** and is also used in industry. It is a desiccant and its reaction with water is highly exothermic; it can cause full thickness burns after 1 minute. The eschar is typically leathery bronze, covering a deep ulcer.

Formic (methanoic) acid

This pungent chemical is found in industrial descalers and is used in dye and textile industries. The wound typically has a greenish colour with blistering and oedema. Systemic absorption may lead to metabolic acidosis, haemolysis and haemochromogenuria; serious sequelae such as blindness (due to optic nerve damage from systemic absorption), ARDS and necrotising pancreatitis may result.

Hydrofluoric acid

This chemical is used in the glass industry for dissolving silica. It is capable of causing severe injury.

- F^- binds to Na^+/K^+ ATPase resulting in K^+ efflux from cells and hyperkalaemia.
- F^- complexes with cations including Ca^{2+} and Mg^{2+}; binding intracellular Ca^{2+} leads to **cell death**.

- There is desiccation, corrosion, protein denaturation, **liquefactive necrosis** and bone decalcification; unrecognised injuries inevitably progress to extensive tissue destruction. Systemic hypocalcaemia leads to cardiac dysrhythmia; refractory (fatal) VF may be induced by the action of F^- on the myocardium. Even 2% TBSA involvement may be fatal.

MANAGEMENT

Emergency management of HF burns

The risk of systemic toxicity increases with the size of the burn (>5% BSA, any concentration) and the concentration (>1% BSA if >50% concentration); toxicity may develop rapidly and should be treated urgently **without waiting** for biochemical results, if necessary.

- **Dilution by copious irrigation.**
- **Chelation** of F^- with calcium preparations, with pain as a guide.
  - **Topical** calcium gluconate gel – a 'home-made' remedy can be made by mixing lubricating jelly 4:1 with 10% calcium gluconate solution. Repeat every 30 minutes until the pain has gone.
  - **Injection** of the burn with 5% calcium gluconate, $0.5 \, mL/cm^2$ with a 27-gauge needle, from the periphery inwards, repeated as necessary. Note that calcium solutions themselves can cause 'extravasation'-type injuries (the risk is lower with gluconate compared to chloride), and excessive volumes may cause a pressure effect.
  - **Infusing** intra-arterial 10% calcium gluconate diluted 1:5 with 5% dextrose at a rate of 15 mL/hour every 4 hours. This is reserved for severe hand burns. The use of intravenous infusion with Bier's type block has also been described. Fasciotomy may be required.
  - **Inhalation/ingestion** is rare but can be treated by nebulised and oral calcium, respectively.
- **Elimination of fluoride** may be improved by
  - **Sodium bicarbonate** – alkalinises urine to promote excretion.
  - **Haemodialysis**.
  - **Urgent wound debridement**/excision.
- **Correct systemic hypocalcaemia and hypomagnesaemia**; ECG/cardiac monitoring is needed – beware of prolonged QT interval.
  - **Intravenous fluids** may be needed as calcium administration causes polyuria.

Hydrocarbons

The skin injuries are usually superficial, but systemic absorption of the compounds can lead to respiratory depression. Petrol exposure has three potential mechanisms of injury:

- Lipid solvent action causing endothelial cell membrane injury with erythema and blistering.
- Lead absorption (binds CNS lipids).
- Ignited petrol causes thermal injury.

Phenol

Otherwise known as carbolic acid, phenol is used commonly as a disinfectant (Lister 1865) but is a component of deep facial peels as well as tar.

- Contact can cause dermatitis and depigmentation, whilst prolonged exposure may lead to (coagulative) necrosis.
- It tends to be **relatively painless** due to nerve demyelination and destruction of nerve endings.
- It is highly lipid soluble (aromatic hydrocarbon) and is easily absorbed. It can cause haemolysis, cerebral oedema and **dysrhythmias**. It binds irreversibly to albumin and ingestion of 1 g may prove fatal.
- Whilst stronger solutions lead to the formation of an eschar (barrier), **dilution in water facilitates dermal penetration**. Therefore, treat with caution – irrigation with water requires copious volumes, preferably followed by wiping with polyethylene glycol, glycerol or even vegetable oil.

Hot bitumen burns

Bitumen is a mixture of petroleum-derived hydrocarbons, mineral tars and asphalt. It is primarily used in road construction and waterproofing. It needs to be heated to 100–200°C before use; thus, it can cause thermal and chemical injury.

- Cool the burn wound at the scene; the bitumen becomes hard as it cools quickly. There is some debate regarding whether adherent bitumen should be removed **urgently** as this may cause additional trauma; however, in most cases, (gentle) removal is advised as it does allow early evaluation of the injury.
- There are numerous methods described such as liquid paraffin, which slowly dissolves the bitumen.
  - Sunflower oil (Turegun M, *Burns*, 1997).
  - Baby oil (Juma A, *Burns*, 1994).
  - Butter (Tiernan E, *Burns*, 1993).
  - Neomycin with Tween 80 (polyoxyethylene sorbitan; Demling RH, *J Trauma*, 1980).
  - Mineral Oil Fleet Enema (Carta T, *Burns*, 2015).
  - De-solv-it® (Iuchi M, *Burns*, 2009) was better than petrolatum, olive oil, salad oil, butter, Neosporin ointment in terms of dissolution in vitro.

DIFFERENCE BETWEEN BITUMEN AND TAR

Tar looks like bitumen but is derived from coal, thus the term 'coal tar'. It is cheaper but more temperature-sensitive, and is more hazardous to health compared to bitumen (>5% crude coal tar is a Group 1 carcinogen). It is not used as often in modern construction.

Articles often refer to 'tar' when they actually mean bitumen.

EXTRAVASATION INJURY

The escape of fluid/drugs from the veins into subcutaneous tissues is a well-known adverse event associated with intravenous therapy. The extent of the resultant damage depends on the concentration, volume and chemical composition of the infusate; in particular, radiological contrast media, hypertonic solutions and cytotoxic drugs especially doxorubicin may cause extensive soft tissue necrosis. Loth (*J Hand Surg Am*, 1986) described the 'necrosis interval' (NI) from exposure to necrosis; patients seen after this should be treated conservatively.

- Osmotic/hypertonic (NI 6 hours), e.g. calcium, 10% dextrose, contrast, total parental nutrition (TPN)
- Vasoconstrictors (4–6 hours)
- Cytotoxicity (up to 72 hours), e.g. doxorubicin
- Infusion under pressure

CLASSIFICATION

- Painful (Grade 1)
- Moderate oedema (Grade 2)
- Skin cool and blanched (Grade 3)
- Skin necrosis, absent distal pulses and capillary refill >4 seconds (Grade 4)

Patients at the extremes of age are at most risk. The dorsum of the hand and the foot are most frequently affected, as they are more likely to be dislodged with movement. Older studies suggest that up to 11% of children and 22% of adult patients receiving IV fluids experience some form of extravasation injury; significant injuries occur in approximately 0.1%–6% of patients receiving intravenous chemotherapy. Cancer patients are inherently at high risk due to the following:

- Systemically unwell including malnutrition.
- Veins are thin and fragile.
- Often require multiple venepuncture sites, and optimal sites may be unavailable due to previous chemotherapy, or changes secondary to radiotherapy, surgery or lymphoedema.
- **Cytotoxic agents** generally cause two types of local cutaneous reactions:
  - Irritants – cause a short self-limited phlebitis with a tender, warm, erythematous reaction at the site.
  - Vesicants – e.g. doxorubicin and mitomycin. The reaction is often called chemical cellulitis: initially it resembles irritation but may worsen, depending on the amount of extravasation, and necrosis may follow. The wound usually heals poorly and surgery may be necessary in some cases.

MANAGEMENT

Neonatal units (and oncology units) should have a local protocol in place.

- Stop the infusion promptly.
- Attempt aspiration of residual drug through the cannula before removing it. Avoid applying pressure.
- Mark the affected area and elevate the limb.
- Substance-specific measures:

- Local cooling may help in preventing ulceration with cisplatin, doxorubicin or paclitaxel. On the other hand, warm compresses are recommended for the vinca alkaloids, calcium/potassium/sodium.
- 'Antidotes' are controversial as some may themselves be harmful, and any benefit may be related to dilution – e.g. injection of saline has some success.
  - Hyaluronidase for vinca alkaloids
  - Thiosulphate for mechlorethamine cisplatin
  - Phentolamine for vasopressors
- Others:
  - Local injection of steroid – variable success (which may be expected as reactions with antineoplastics are not usually associated with significant inflammation).
  - Local injection of GM-CSF has been used for mitomycin injury (Shamseddine AI, *Eur J Gynaecol Oncol*, 1998).
  - Topical DMSO (free radical scavenger; Bertelli G, *J Clin Oncol*, 1995).
  - Early local excision may be favoured with more harmful chemicals.

Not all extravasations lead to necrosis; the vast majority heal without serious sequela – deep damage is rare. Conservative treatment is often suitable for most extravasation injuries (particularly grades 1 and 2); it can be difficult to predict how they will heal. Evidence for the usefulness of irrigation and liposuction is limited to case reports/series but can be considered in selected cases.

Extravasation injuries. (Gault DT, *Br J Plast Surg*, 1993)
The paper describes two techniques, liposuction and saline flush-out – skin incisions around the area are made with a no. 11 blade: 1500U hyaluronidase in 10 mL normal saline is infiltrated followed by irrigation of a further 500 mL saline via a cannula. Analysis of the flush-out confirmed the presence of the agent, i.e. being removed from the injury site. In this way, 86% healed without soft tissue loss.

RCT animal studies suggest that using hyaluronidase only works if used within 12 hours (ideally 1 hour); saline irrigation is effective only before obvious necrosis develops.

Liposuction and extravasation injuries in ICU. (Steinmann G, *Br J Anaesth*, 2005)
The article presents two cases of extravasation injury (thiopentone and contrast media) treated with liposuction within 6 and 2 hours of the injury, respectively. Both healed uneventfully.

STEVEN JOHNSON SYNDROME/TOXIC EPIDERMAL NECROSIS (SJS/TEN)

There is widespread necrosis of the superficial epidermis, with separation at the dermal–epidermal junction and bullae formation. The **Nikolski sign** is separation of the epidermis with slight lateral pressure.

- There may be a non-pruritic macular rash that develops into blisters/necrosis; an erythematous patch often develops a purple or necrotic centre.
- The skin lesions appear about 1 week after the first dose of antibiotics (anticonvulsant-related disease may be delayed for 1–2 months).
- These patches represent partial thickness defects that heal quickly within 1–2 weeks unless superinfected.
- Further lesions can appear; areas may become confluent to form large wounds.
- Mucosal involvement, e.g. eyes, oropharyngeal, urogenital, etc.

Although some use SJS and TEN interchangeably, strictly patients with SJS have <10% BSA involvement whilst in TEN it is >30%, with intermediate level **involvement termed SJS/TEN overlap**. Differential diagnoses include pemphigus/pemphigoid and acute GVHD. It was previously believed to be related to erythema multiforme as different points on the same spectrum, but now most regard them as distinct diseases. Some caution is needed in interpreting older literature that did not make this distinction.

- Stevens and Johnson were paediatricians who described the condition in children following drug treatment.
- In 90%, it is associated with drugs especially sulphonamides (co-trimoxazole), allopurinol, NSAIDs and phenytoin, but almost any drug can be the cause – it is idiosyncratic/unpredictable. On average, it occurs a week after antibiotics but up to 2 months after phenytoin.
  - A definitive cause is not found in ~20%.
- The underlying pathology seems to be related to an immune complex disorder with type IV delayed hypersensitivity. In some cases, symptoms may be delayed for up to 8 weeks. There may be HLA associations: HLA-B 5801 with allopurinol-related disease (Dean L, *Genotype*, 2013) and HLA-B 1502 with carbamazepine (screening is recommended in Han Chinese, Thai and Malaysians, but not Japanese). In the latter, when the drug is bound to the HLA molecule on the APC, the complex is able to activate the TCR on cytotoxic T cells.
  - A 'Swiss cheese' risk model has been used to explain the association of the structure of the drug (after metabolism) and the HLA alleles.
  - There is a significant cytokine response: TNFα, IFNγ, etc.
- A minority of cases are associated with an infection, commonly viral, e.g. coxsackie, herpes simplex, but a connection with group A β-haemolytic *Streptococcus* infection has also been described. These cases tend to be associated with immunosuppression, and the overall course is less severe.
- Overall mortality is 3%–15%, but is higher in TEN (up to 40%).

TREATMENT

Treatment is largely supportive. Sepsis is the main concern and significantly affects the prognosis.

- Wounds can be treated simply – biological dressings such as porcine skin or biobrane may be useful. SSD has a sulphonamide moiety and thus theoretically could exacerbate the problem, but there has been no convincing evidence to support this view. Prophylatic systemic antibiotics are not indicated.
- Subcutaneous oedema and metabolic derangements typical of a burn are not seen; thus, the acute fluid requirements are titrated to clinical parameters. Burns type resuscitation is not needed.
- Early feeding, taking care with mucosal involvement.

Active Treatment

- **Steroids** – although early administration (within 48 hours) may be beneficial, there are significant risk of side effects, e.g. infections, inhibition of wound healing, and it may mask signs of sepsis. There are no RCTs, but it is often used in Germany.
- **Immunoglobulin** (IVIG) – results have been inconsistent. IVIG is said to block the CD95/Fas receptor; there is Fas overexpression in TENS, and binding to the receptor leads to keratinocyte apoptosis. It is rather expensive and side effects may be severe, e.g. renal failure, anaphylaxis or aseptic meningitis.
- **Less commonly used**:
  - Plasmapheresis
  - Thalidomide to reduce TNF-α overexpression
  - Cyclophosphamide, cyclosporin A

VI. PAEDIATRIC BURNS

There are many differences to consider. Scalds are much more common, and children will have fewer but very different premorbid conditions, e.g. more asthma, no IHD. A child with an uncomplicated 95% burn has ~50% chance of survival. There should be a high index of suspicion for non-accidental injuries (NAI).

- The skin is thinner and hence burns for a given energy insult will be deeper.
  - At 55°C and above, children will burn four times quicker than adults (Feldman KW, *Pediatrics*, 1983).
  - Moritz (*Am J Pathol*, 1947) says that water at 70°C and 60°C causes **transepidermal** necrosis in 1 and 5 seconds, respectively. Some quote this as full thickness injury, which is not strictly true.
  - In many countries, water heaters are limited to a maximum of 50°C (the concern that Legionnaire's disease may increase has not been borne out).
- The surface area will need to be considered differently due to the altered body proportions (larger head and smaller lower limbs), using either a modified Rule of nines, patients palm method or a Lund and Browder chart.

- Modified rule of nines – for a 1 year old (see below), then for each year over, take 1% from head and neck and add half to each lower limb.
  - Head and neck 18%
  - Lower limb 14%
  - Upper limb 9%
  - Anterior trunk 18%
  - Posterior trunk 18%

AIRWAY

The airway in children is narrower – the tongue is larger and the pharynx is narrower relative to the size of the oral cavity. There may also be partial occlusion by enlarged tonsils and adenoids, and the trachea is less rigid and narrower - thus, the paediatric airway develops more resistance for a given degree/thickness of swelling compared with adults. Children have a shorter, larger floppy epiglottis; they are more prone to laryngomalacia and bronchial irritability and thus spasm.

BREATHING

Children rely more upon diaphragmatic respiration, and hence thoracoabdominal burns, even if not circumferential, may still require decompression.

CIRCULATION

The relative paediatric circulating volume is larger at ~80 mL/kg compared with the adult, 60 mL/kg.

- The heart rate is less reliable as an indicator of volaemic status. Children normally have a lower resting BP than adults (~100 mmHg systolic), which is well maintained until late when, e.g. up to 25% of circulating volume has been lost. Delayed refill, pallor, sweating and obtunded consciousness are ominous late signs.
- Difficult intravenous access – an intraosseous infusion may allow delivery of up to 100 mL/hour of fluid; the low marrow fat content means that fat embolus is rare.
- Hypoglycaemia is more common due to less stored glycogen.
- Hyponatraemia is more common due to lack of renal medullary concentrating capacity, which may cause cerebral oedema. Hypokalaemia and hypophosphataemia may also result from the diuresis.

Resuscitation should start at 4 mL/kg/% TBSA along with maintenance fluid – 5% dextrose or **half dextrose/half saline** (0.45% saline and 4% glucose – 77 mmol sodium, 77 mmol chloride and 50 g glucose).

- First 10 kg – 100 mL/kg
- Second 10 kg – 50 mL/kg
- Thereafter – 20 mL/kg

Some use formulae based on the body surface area, e.g. Galveston Shriner's, where the total volume (24 hours) = 5000 mL/m²/BSA burn + 2000 mL/m²/total BSA. BSA is calculated from formula or nomograms based on height and weight. It is important to avoid volume overload, which may easily precipitate right heart failure or pulmonary oedema. The kidneys are immature with less concentrating ability, and **urine output continues despite hypovolaemia**. A urine output of 1–2 mL/kg/hour is the lowest acceptable figure in children.

DEFICIT AND EXPOSURE

The larger surface-area-to-volume ratio means that children lose heat more quickly. They have less of a thermoregulation response (no shivering reflex in neonates), less insulating fat, poorly developed piloerection, etc. Thus, it is important to perform dressing changes quickly and efficiently to reduce exposure times, whilst maintaining an ambient temperature of ~30°C. The tendency towards hypothermia (note that burn patients 'normally' have a temperature ~38°C) may lead to

- Ventricular arrhythmias, CNS and respiratory depression
- Oxyhaemoglobin dissociation curve shifted to the left

ANALGESIA

Adequate analgesia is important but sadly is often underused in paediatric burns. (Singer A, *J Burn Care Rehab*, 2002)

- Paracetamol 10–15 mg/kg four times daily, maximum 5 doses a day.
- Ibuprofen 5–10 mg/kg three times a day, maximum 40 mg/kg/day.
- IV morphine is useful but underutilised:
  - 0.1 mg/kg IV – 10 minutes before dressing, titrating with boluses
  - 0.2 mg/kg IM – if only a single dose anticipated
- Morphine 0.2–0.5 mg/kg orally – 60 minutes before (dressing). However, it is difficult to titrate, bioavailability is less predictable and there is usually prolonged sedation afterwards – making it less suited for outpatient dressings.
- Entonox® (50% nitrous oxide, 50% oxygen) has been used in many units for dressing changes for many years (Baskett PJF, *Postgrad Med J*, 1972). There is some anxiolysis but probably limited analgesia – patients usually need to have other forms of analgesia on board. Common side effects include dry mouth, dizziness and nausea.

OTHER SEQUELAE

Longer-term considerations in children include the following:

- Inhibition of growth for several years post-burn without compensatory catch-up. After inhalation injury, the respiratory reserve is reduced for up to 2.5 years post-burn.

- Breast development may be unimpaired, even with burns involving the nipple–areolar complex. Do not overdebride burns over the breast area; release contractures early.
- Joint contractures appear to be more of a problem in children than adults, supposedly more so where excision has been to fascia rather than fat.
- Psychosocial problems.

NON-ACCIDENTAL INJURIES

Non-accidental (or intentional) burns mostly occur in children as a form of child abuse but may also occur in the elderly, including those in institutional care. There may be clues pointing to a NAI, but there is no single feature that can be relied upon. Injuries may be due to 'neglect' rather than 'abuse' per se. Some distinguishing features include the following:

- Intentional scalds are often due to forced immersion affecting extremities or the buttocks/perineum.
  - Immersion injuries have clear upper margins instead of splashes (Maguire S, *Burns*, 2008). **'Sparing'** has been described as the pattern of injury, e.g. child making a fist when their hand is being forced into hot water. Similarly, when a child is being forced buttock down into hot water, there will be sparing of abdominal creases due to flexing up, a 'doughnut pattern' on the buttock due to close contact with the bathtub and sparing of the soles of the feet.
- Contact burns will mirror the object being used for 'branding'; accidental injuries tend to be less complete, less well circumscribed, randomly placed and more superficial.
- There may be associated or old injuries such as fractures or other unrelated injuries.

Other clues include the following:

- Explanation offered is not compatible with the injury sustained, often blaming a sibling.
- Unexplained delay in presentation.
- Apparent lack of parental concern.
- Apparent lack of parent–child bonding.
- Passive, introverted child.

PSYCHIATRIC CONSIDERATIONS

Established psychiatric disturbances may have led to the initial burn injury, e.g. suicide attempt, or altered perception due to substance abuse or withdrawal may have contributed to the injury. In addition, delirium may be a psychological reaction to injury or a manifestation of metabolic derangement, e.g. hypoglycaemia, hypoxia, sepsis or pain. The following problems have been described:

- Psychosis, delusions, hallucinations or paranoia (rare in children)
- Post-traumatic stress syndrome

- Poor sleep, hypervigilance, flashbacks, nightmares
- Depression, panic attacks, guilt (e.g. sole survivor)
- Longer-term problems
  - Self-consciousness and poor self-esteem
  - Phobias and anxiety

Children and adolescents appear to become well adjusted eventually.

Is there still a place for comfort care in severe burns? (Platt AJ, *Burns*, 1998)

With the improvements with burn care, even those with massive burns may survive. This was a questionnaire-based survey of 'comfort care' policy in the United Kingdom and found that priorities for determining suitability for resuscitation were

- Age and % TBSA
- % TBSA full thickness burn (including special areas)
- Smoke inhalation
- Preburn morbidity

Suicidal intent was not an important factor in decision-making. Although patients' wishes were taken into account, often treatment had already been initiated including sedation and intubation. The choice for 'comfort care' was usually a joint decision between the consultant and the relatives.

The authors specifically state that it is important to emphasise that 'comfort care' does not equate to 'no care'. In most 'borderline' cases, a trial of full resuscitation to assess the patient response allows time for the family to become involved in a decision 'in the light of day'.

B. SURGICAL MANAGEMENT OF BURNS

I. BURN SURGERY

In simple terms, the aim is to remove non-viable tissues, which are a source of inflammatory mediators and a nidus for bacteria, and to close the wounds with autograft in a timely manner. The concept of a 'burn toxin' (Rosental SR, *Burns*, 1959) formed by the application of heat to skin was popular up to the early 1990s.

There are many variables to consider in burn surgery.

TIMING OF BURN SURGERY

- Immediate – escharotomy/decompression, tracheostomy if required as an emergency.
- Early – burn excision and grafting – the definition of early is rather arbitrary but most would agree on **no more than 5 days** if possible.
  - Excision before 48 hours reduces wound colonisation and infection.
- Late, e.g. release contractures, late burn scar reconstruction

DECOMPRESSION VS. ESCHAROTOMY

It is often said that an escharotomy is needed to manage external restriction on ventilation or perfusion to the extremities. However, using the concept of 'decompression' is more useful in many ways – the aim of the intervention is made clear, and not just limited to a specific procedure, i.e. incising the burn eschar that in itself may be inadequate to relieve/abort impending compartment syndrome due to muscle oedema. In the latter scenario, a 'fasciotomy' would be needed.

It is also often said that an escharotomy can be done by the bedside with a scalpel as it is painless and bloodless. Except in dire emergencies, it is preferable to perform the procedure in a controlled environment with diathermy and pain control (i.e. under GA, in an operating theatre).

The forearm is usually decompressed with two incisions along the preaxial and postaxial borders, taking care to avoid damaging the ulnar nerve at the elbow. The alternative single volar S incision may be inadequate in ~50% of cases, and an additional longitudinal dorsal incision may be needed. It is important to evaluate the adequacy of the decompression afterwards.

EARLY BURN EXCISION

The trend has been to favour early excision, and this is associated with

- Improved survival rate.
  - Herndon (*Ann Surg*, 1989) – in patients aged 17–55 with TBSA >30%, there was a 9% mortality with early surgery vs. 45% with conservative management (grafting after eschar separation).
  - Tompkins RG at Boston Shriners (*Ann Surg*, 1986) practically eliminated mortality in children with burns under 70% BSA (Tompkins RG, *Ann Surg*, 1988).
- Reduced blood loss. Blood loss is least when burns are excised within 24 hours (0.4 mL/cm^2) vs. 0.75 mL/cm^2 between 2 and 16 days post-burn, with wound colonisation and the so-called **inflammatory phase** (Desai MH, *Ann Surg*, 1990).
  - Higher blood loss with surgery between days 2 and 7 (Barret JP, *Burns*, 1999) or between days 3 and 15 days (Hart DW, *Surgery*, 2001).
- Fewer metabolic complications.
- Decreased hospital stay and expenditure.

This, in combination with other improvements in critical care, antibiotics, nutrition, etc. have improved burns survival – the LD50 was 30% TBSA in the 1930s (Rose JK, *Burns*, 1997) and 70% in 2010 (Taylor S, *J Burn Care Res*, 2014).

SCALDS

Hot water scalds in children are an exception of sorts to the rule of early excision; the depth of the burn is often mixed and indeterminate in the early stage. Thus, to reduce the excision of viable tissue, the decision for surgery can often be delayed for a week or so. At this stage, it will be easier to determine which areas are truly non-viable, and by allowing some healing to occur, a smaller area needs to be grafted. This will reduce blood loss by avoiding the inflammatory phase, but will increase the risk of forming hypertrophic scars.

LEVEL OF EXCISION

Tangential excision was first described by Zora Janzekovic from Slovenia (1918–2015) in the 1960s, though her work was initially met with disbelief. The surgery basically involves shaving off layers of eschar until viable/bleeding tissue is reached. It offered better results over full thickness, but the major drawback is excessive bleeding, and graft take over fat can be subpar. Bleeding can be reduced through the following:

- Cautery and adrenaline-soaked gauzes (1 in 10,000 to 1,000,000) – regular changing is needed; otherwise, they tend to 'stick'.
- Adrenaline can be injected subcutaneously (with or without hyalase) before excision of eschar (or graft harvest), or limbs can be shaved under tourniquet control. These measures may hinder judgement of the adequacy of excision.
- Pressure/bandaging and elevation after debridement may help in the limbs.
- **Fascial excision** is indicated where the burns are deep, i.e. at least full thickness and the fat layer is deeply involved. There is less bleeding with this technique and graft take is good. However, the cosmetic appearance is poor and lymphoedema can be a long-term problem.
- Skin grafts are somewhat haemostatic, but will not stop brisk bleeding.
- Avoiding the 'inflammatory phase' (see above).
- Staging was recommended in the past, and whilst the concept is still valid, the criteria have been modified by all round improvements. Proposed limits included
  - 20% BSA burn each time (Herndon D.).
  - 2 hours OT time (i.e. avoid areas that need intra-operative turning).
  - 10 units transfusion.
  - Hypothermia below 35°C.
  - Whilst the hands are a priority, in a large surface area burn, the priority is to close up large surfaces quickly, e.g. lower limbs; the face is often left until later except for the eyelids.

Alternatives to surgical excision include the following:

- Versajet® 'hydrosurgery' (Smith and Nephew) uses a 'cutting' hand piece that consists of a pressurised jet of saline passing across a gap that 'cuts' and sucks in debris by the Venturi effect. Unlike pulsed lavage systems, there is much less 'spray' involved, and the small size of the probe makes it useful for debriding burns of the eyelids, hands and perineum that would be difficult with conventional knives. It does not work well with thicker burns or flamazine eschars. The consumables are rather costly.
- Chemical debridement (see 'Burns dressings').

GENERAL INTRA-OPERATIVE PATIENT CARE

- Monitor core temperature – keep ambient temperature high, which can make it somewhat hot and uncomfortable for the surgeons.
- Avoid hypo- or hypervolaemia – monitor urine output; consider CVP monitoring and arterial lines.
- Blood loss should be reduced as much as possible with meticulous haemostasis (see above). Loss should be accurately assessed.
  - Some propose a policy of **restrictive transfusion,** with a threshold of 7 g/dL instead of 10 g/dL (Kwan P, *J Burn Care Res*, 2006); the old '10/30' rule was to transfuse below 10 g/dL or haematocrit below 30. RCTs show non-inferiority with some showing reduced mortality. Contraindications include patients with pre-existing cardiovascular disease.
- Donor sites are traditionally dressed with Kaltostat (calcium alginate – there is exchange for tissue sodium and the released calcium activates haemostasis). As alginates dry out and become difficult/painful to remove, some suggest that they should be exchanged for a less adhesive dressing once haemostasis has been achieved.

Evidence base for restrictive transfusion triggers in high risk patients. (Spahn DR, *Transfus Med Hemother*, 2015) Blood transfusions are not trivial; known sequelae include increased mortality, organ dysfunction, longer hospital stay as well as transfusion reactions and the risk of infection. Seven RCTs compared restrictive (7–8 g/dL) vs. liberal transfusions (9–10 g/dL). There was a reduction in the use of red cells that was safe as well as saving money. Two of the studies demonstrated reduced mortality. A trigger of 7 g/dL is suggested; 8 g/dL for those with ACS.

WOUND CLOSURE

Closure of the burn wound has the following benefits:

- Reducing water, electrolyte and protein losses
- Reducing pain and wound infection

AUTOGRAFTS

Burn wounds are generally closed with autografts. Full thickness skin grafts (FTSGs) are superior to partial thickness or split skin grafts (SSGs) but are limited by the donor site. Thus, in most scenarios, SSG is used as a reasonable compromise – however, wounds of the face (especially the eyelids) and/or the fingers are probably better covered with FTSG or, at least, thick SSGs; donor sites can then be covered with SSGs or ADM with thin SSGs. It is common to harvest SSGs from the lateral thighs; the scalp is a very good donor site for smaller burns, particularly in children, and for the face.

To maximise the donor graft, a number of strategies can be used:

- **Mesh** – a machine makes multiple linear cuts in the graft to allow it to be stretched out in one direction; this increases the area that can be 'covered' and improves conformity and drainage. Note that the wound bed that is not directly covered by the graft will heal from the edges (of the graft); with wider meshing (more than three times), the interstices are prone to desiccation and rarely provide aesthetically acceptable cover. The performance of widely meshed skin can be improved by being covered with cadaveric skin (sandwich technique) with or without cultured keratinocytes.
  - Kamolz (*Ann Burns Fire Disasters*, 2013) found that skin meshers do not achieve their stated ratios – 1:1.5 was 1:1.27 (85%) and 1:3 was 1.59 (53%). Meek micrografting was much more consistent with claimed ratios.
- **Reharvesting** – SSG can be harvested from the same donor sites after they have healed (2–3 weeks). However, as the dermis does not regenerate, there is a limit to the number of times skin can be harvested from one site, with donor morbidity increasing with each time.

Meshing and reharvesting this cannot adequately deal with wounds more than 50%–60% BSA (Mcheik JN, *Plast Reconstr Surg Glob Open*, 2014). A number of strategies can be used for such wounds, but the results are relatively poor/inconsistent.

- **Meek skin grafting.** This was originally described by American surgeon Meek CP in 1958 and offered large expansion ratios by cutting the graft into spaced out small (3 × 3 mm) squares. However, it was rather technically demanding, and meshing became more popular (Tanner JC, *Plast Reconstr Surg*, 1964). Modified Meek techniques were easier to use and led to a resurgence (Kreis RW, *Burns*, 1993); 1:9 Meek expansion performs as well if not better than 1:6 mesh. Peeters (*Burns*, 1988) found that expansion was about twice as efficient as meshing, achieving 99.8% and 93.8% in 1:3 and 1:9 expansion, respectively.
- **Micrografting.** Historically, Reverdin JL described 'epidermic grafting' in 1869 where small pieces of skin were lifted up with a needle, cut off with a scalpel and then placed on the wound bed; 'pinch grafting' described by Davis was similar but included some of the dermis. These were largely forgotten until some surgeons reported success with cutting up thin skin grafts into small pieces (under 1 mm) with scissors, food processors, double meshing at right angles or dedicated machines etc. – achieving expansion ratios of 10:1 or more. Although it is popular in certain centres in China and India, it has seen limited uptake elsewhere for various reasons including reports of increased scar contracture.
  - Intermingling micrografting – autograft is mixed with cadaveric or porcine skin.

- **Cultured epithelial autografts** (CEAs) – the patient's keratinocytes can be cultured over 3–4 weeks from a 2 × 2 cm skin biopsy to form sheets 5 cells thick (type I/epidermal skin substitute) large enough to cover the whole body. The efficiency of culture is reduced in older patients. The in vitro process was first described by Rheinwald and Green in 1975 with its first clinical application in burn patients in 1981 by O'Connor.
  - **Epicel® (Genzyme)** and Holoderm® (Tego Science, Seoul Korea) are commercial preparations: a skin biopsy is sent to the manufacturer for culture and 1.8 m² is delivered in sheets after ~4 weeks. They are expensive but may offer better consistency than most in-hospital facilities.
  - Take comes from adhesion and not revascularisation as in normal skin grafts and varies from 15% to 95%. Results are better (60%–70%) in fresh wounds particularly those with some residual dermis or when allograft has been used to cover the excised wound bed first (increase capillary density and reduce infection).
  - **Sensitivity to infection** – CEA is very vulnerable to bacterial proteases and cytotoxins. These can cause complete loss of CEA at levels harmless to SSGs; thus, it should be avoided in infected wounds. Wounds should be prepared properly with meticulous debridement and haemostasis, or covered with cadaveric skin whilst waiting for the culture.
  - **Healed CEA skin is more fragile** than SSG, and large bullae/blisters on shearing can occur for up to 6/12; these bullae contain high levels of thromboxane A2 (TXA2) and prostaglandin E2 (PGE2) suggesting on-going inflammation (Desai MH, *J Burn Care Rehab*, 1991). Electron microscopy has demonstrated a lack of anchoring fibrils for dermal attachment; it can take up to 5 years before it resembles normal skin. This may hamper/delay rehabilitation with pressure garments, increasing the risks of long-term problem scarring.
  - Using CEA is very labour-intensive and requires significant resources. The long preparation time is one of several significant limitations of the technique. Efficient logistics are important – surgery and coverage should be staged to manageable sizes.
  - Even with these limitations, CEA is still regarded as potentially life-saving by offering wound closure in situations where conventional treatment would fail or have very poor results, e.g. 65%–70% FT burns, with the caveat that it is not suitable for **long-term coverage**. A 30%–50% burn is often regarded as threshold to consider using CEA, whilst some suggest a lower threshold for children, e.g. 20%.
  - The current trend is to use CEA in different ways:
    - **Combination** with a dermal component, e.g. a two-stage technique with either Integra or dermal substitute.

- - **Preconfluent cells** – there is a trend not to use sheets of cells but to use preconfluent cultured cells in suspension that are easier and quicker (14–16 days) to produce than sheets.
- A variant (mixed cell 'culture' – ReCell®) is said to reduce dyspigmentation in partial thickness injuries as they heal. They have been used for resurfacing flaps after dermabrasion to improve colour match (Hivelin M, *J Plast Reconstr Aesthet Surg*, 2012). ReCell may speed up healing of donor sites (Hu Z, *Br J Surg*, 2017;104:836) but claims that it is an alternative to skin grafting are based on weak evidence.
- Cultured epidermal cells express fewer MHCII/HLA-DR antigens and thus **allogenic keratinocytes** could potentially be used (see above 'Skin allografts').

II. RECENT ADVANCES

It is important to define terms to avoid confusion:

- **Wound cover** – this means primarily to restore barrier function and its temporary nature is implied. In practice, these would be used for clean superficial partial thickness burns or split skin donor sites, e.g. (biological) dressings.
- **Wound closure** – permanent closure of wound involves adhesion, ingrowth of host tissues and/or integration of materials. The Holy Grail is a product that can reconstruct both dermis and epidermis in one procedure, instead of using autograft.

These terms along with 'skin substitute' have been used interchangeably and inconsistently, leading to some confusion. Generally, 'skin substitutes' should be taken to refer to substitutes for *autograft*, i.e. wound closure, that may be used where the patient's own skin is in short supply. Thus, it aims to replace or substitute skin *permanently*, and it can be considered as epidermal, dermal or composite (types I, II and III, respectively).

WOUND COVER

There are many commercial products available and their efficacy is probably very similar – studies often use no treatment as control. The choice of products used by a particular unit depends on many factors:

- Wound factors
  - Size and depth of the wound
  - Level of contamination
  - Vascularity of the wound bed
- Unit factors
  - Experience of the unit
  - Resources available

CADAVERIC SKIN

Cadaveric skin is regarded as the best biological dressing but has limited availability due to a paucity of donations, whilst religious and cultural considerations can further complicate its use. Girdner used fresh cadaveric skin in 1881 to cover shoulder wounds on a young boy struck by lightning, but after a period of apparent healing, it was eventually rejected. Fresh cadaveric skin will be rejected through HLA-DR and Langerhans cells, by a combination of cytotoxic antibiotics and sensitised lymphocytes and will become necrotic by 2 weeks, with a heavy cell infiltration and some damage to the graft bed by cell-mediated immunity. Longer 'survival' in severe burn patients is possible due to the state of relative immunosuppression.

- **Human allograft** is a term widely used in the literature but should be restricted to situations where the skin is being used as a definitive transplant, but not when it is used as a temporary dressing where the term 'cadaveric skin' is more appropriate. There have only been a few reports of use of allografts with immunosuppression as a skin transplant (Achauer BM, *Lancet*, 1986); it has not been used satisfactorily in major burns.
- **Adhesion** to the wound bed is one of the most important factors for a successful skin substitute and is usually due to the interaction of fibrin in the wound to the elastin in the dermis of the cadaveric skin. **Tight adhesion reduces the loss of fluid, electrolytes and protein, and the cover reduces inflammation, energy loss, pain and wound infection**. Wound healing is accelerated. The epidermis may slough off whilst the dermis remains adherent, still maintaining its function. Small portions of biological dressings may be incorporated into the wound but will remodel rapidly; these are best seen as 'collagen dressings'.
  - **Rejection** then occurs by progressive desiccation and slow separation from the host bed; with non-viable cadaveric skin, there is a foreign body reaction rather than an immune response.
- Fresh cadaveric skin performs the 'best', but its supply is limited by the short storage life and it tends to be more antigenic due to its cellularity along with a greater risk of disease transmission such as hepatitis B and C and HIV. Preservation (e.g. cryopreservation and glycerolisation) improves availability and reduces immunogenicity by removing cell components.
- The main clinical use of cadaveric skin is to temporarily cover debrided (burns) wounds when there is insufficient donor site to allow time for healing and reharvesting. Another relatively common use is to overlay widely meshed autograft, i.e. a sandwich graft (Alexander technique).

PORCINE SKIN

Animal-derived wound dressings have been used as early as 1500 BC; Canaday described the experimental use of lizard skin in 1682, whilst in the nineteenth century,

Reverdin and Lee used bovine skin (1869) and porcine skin (1880), respectively. Frogskin and bovine skin (Kollagen®) are currently used in Brazil and India, respectively, but porcine skin has been the most widely used biological dressing for decades.

- The term 'xenografts' is to be avoided for these biological dressings for reasons discussed above.
- Potato peel and banana leaves are organic materials sometimes used in developing countries; however, these behave very differently. They need to be changed regularly and technically should not be classed as skin substitutes.

Porcine skin is often said to be the closest in structure to human skin, and as a dressing seems to act in a qualitatively similar fashion as cadaveric skin through adhesion to the wound bed, though it seems to be **quantitatively less effective**. Porcine skin dressings usually consist of the dermal layer only and are most commonly used on partial thickness burns. They do not demonstrate the immunological rejection seen with fresh cadaveric skin; the dressing dries and falls off as the burn heals; they are **'ejected'**. The prevailing view has been that 'take' or vascularisation does not occur in porcine skin used in this way; the porcine dermis is not invaded by human capillaries, though there may be a neutrophilic infiltration after a week.

AMNIOTIC MEMBRANE

The AM is the thin semi-transparent innermost layer of the foetal membrane. It had been used as a wound dressing since 1910, until it was largely replaced by porcine skin. There has been a recent resurgence in the use of this resource that is usually discarded, e.g. commercial products such as Amniofix® (Mimedx).

There is a risk of contamination and disease transmission with the use of fresh amnion, and thus it is harvested in a controlled manner similar to transplants from carefully screened donors and then processed, preserved (e.g. with cryopreservation, glycerol or γ-irradiation) and batch-tested for sterility. AM has some immune privilege; thus, it demonstrates limited immunogenicity and has some anti-inflammatory effects. AM has a good barrier function, whilst the transparency allows easy wound surveillance. It is also very conforming, and thus very useful for superficial PT burns of the face and other difficult to dress areas, as well as donor sites.

SYNTHETIC

Biobrane®

Biobrane® (Smith and Nephew) is a synthetic bilaminar material: one layer consists of a fine nylon mesh coated with type I **porcine** collagen, and the second layer is silicone. As the nylon scaffold is not biodegradable, the aim is not to allow tissue ingrowth, which would require surgical removal; rather it is used as a temporary wound cover, i.e. a **dressing**. Biobrane is a reasonable substitute for units without access to porcine skin or AM.

It has been used since 1979, with a large body of experience that demonstrates a reduction in pain and faster healing times in partial thickness burns (though mostly compared to SSD). It is used in many UK Trusts, and Christian, Islamic, Jewish and Hindu leaders have accepted the use of the product after discussions. There have been some studies demonstrating problems such as a significant infection rate, but are probably related to improper application, e.g. using it on deeper burns, on contaminated or inadequately debrided wounds.

Transcyte®

This product consists of a nylon polymer mesh coated with neonatal human fibroblasts, and bonded to a silicone membrane. As the fibroblasts proliferate, they produce components of ECM such as collagen, matrix proteins and growth factors. After freeze–thawing, the cellular component becomes inactive, and as such, it may be viewed as being similar to Biobrane, but with growth factors. It was usually promoted as an alternative to cadaveric skin, but like Biobrane, it is meant to function as temporary wound cover and definitive wound closure is still required. Results have been similar to Biobrane with one study showing a slight reduction in the healing time and need for autografting compared to Biobrane and Silvazine. However, it is much more expensive and thus has found a limited market; it is currently owned by Organogenesis.

WOUND CLOSURE

Two-Staged Closure

For reasons discussed previously, it has been imperative to develop ways of closing large full thickness burn wounds satisfactorily. The strategy most commonly used is to cover the wound immediately with a dermal scaffold; the scaffold is initially avascular but becomes vascularised over a period of weeks, and can then support an epidermal layer usually in the form of a thin SSG. This provides a bilayer reconstruction similar to full thickness skin but with much reduced donor site morbidity. A wide range of materials have been used **as dermal scaffolds**, and in most cases, even when the material has a structure similar/identical to dermis, this scaffold is ultimately remodelled by the patient's own fibroblasts. Early wound closure with dermal scaffolds has beneficial effects such as reducing nutritional requirements in the severely burnt child (King P, *Burns*, 2000).

- **Allogenic dermis** is a commonly used dermal scaffold in the United States and Europe; the combination of cryopreserved allodermis with pre-confluent CEA results in 45% engraftment. **Alloderm®** (LifeCell) is a commercially available acellular dermal allograft, which is mainly marketed for use in abdominal wall reconstruction or as an acellular dermal matrix (ADM) used with breast implants. There have been a few reports of its use in deep burns as a dermal substitute with SSG applied at a second stage (Yim H, *Burns*, 2010).

- **Integra®** (Integra LifeSciences) is the most widely used synthetic skin (dermal) substitute for burn wound closure. It was developed in 1981, gaining FDA approval in 1996. It is a synthetic bilaminar composed of a layer of **bovine** matrix collagen with (shark) chondroitin-6-sulphate, covered by a silicone film. The matrix allows the ingress of fibroblasts and capillaries, producing a vascularised dermal equivalent after ~3 weeks, that can then support an **ultrathin skin graft** (as long as basal cells are included). There is no evidence of survival benefit in acute burns; it can be used for moderately large areas of full thickness burns, but it is probably most useful in non-acute situations such as burn scar reconstruction. The low nutritional needs allowing for slow revascularisation means that Integra can be used to cover/bridge small portions of avascular structures such as bone, cartilage and irradiated structures, where autografts may be otherwise contraindicated.
  - There is a significant learning curve, but the main disadvantages are its cost and its susceptibility to infection, which should be managed aggressively. RCTs show that in major burns, the average Integra take is 80% compared to 95% for SSG but with better pliability, less mesh patterning and less hypertrophic scarring. Using negative pressure wound therapy (NPWT) may improve outcomes; some case studies/series have described a one-stage approach with a thin dermal scaffold, thin skin graft and NPWT, but the results have been inconsistent.
- **Nevelia®** (Symatese) received CE marking in 2013; it has a bovine collagen I layer on a porous matrix covered by a silicone layer that is polyester mesh-reinforced making the silicone layer less prone to tearing on suturing/stapling compared to Integra and can better withstand meshing. Furthermore, it does not include GAGs (found in Integra) which may have inhibitory actions on fibroblasts, keratinocytes and on angiogenesis (De Angelis B, *Int Wound J*, 2018) though the clinical significance of this is unclear.
- **Matriderm®** (Skin and Health Care AG) is a matrix of bovine type I collagen with elastin that is similar to the matrix layer of Integra; there is no silicone layer. Studies in rat models demonstrated similar patterns of vascularisation and graft take.

Single-stage closure

Two-staged procedures are the current standard of care due to their reliability; some have tried to condense this combination into a single stage, but this generally requires a much thinner ADM layer (<1 mm) to be reliable. Vascularisation is the limiting factor.

The Holy Grail in skin replacement is to have a bilayer tissue assembly that can be transferred in a single stage; however, thus far, there has been a lack of consistent results beyond animal studies or case studies.

- Studies describing the pre-construction of a bilayer have often used cultured cells to seed scaffolds and are examples of a '**top-down**' approach. The dermal equivalent/scaffold such as collagen-glycosaminoglycans can be produced beforehand, preferably with functional autologous fibroblasts. Autologous keratinocytes are preferred for the top layer, but the time required for expansion and maturation is a problem, and such methods are difficult to 'scale up' for industrial production. Revascularisation of the top layer is the major hurdle; scaffolds >1 mm revascularise poorly.
- '**Bottom-up**' approach – cells are used to produce constructs without use of a discrete scaffold, usually using a bio-ink with a cell suspension, bio-paper for temporary support and a bio-printer. One can theoretically prefabricate the vasculature and deposit multiple cell types.

There seemed to be many promising potential products at the turn of the last century but were not successful. Currently, there are no commercial products that can permanently replace both dermis and epidermis in a single stage.

- **Apligraf®** (Organogenesis) is a bilayer of bovine type I collagen gel and **living neonatal fibroblasts** covered with a cornified epidermal layer from neonatal **keratinocytes** (MHC type II antigens are lost after 7 days of culture). Sometimes referred to as a type III/composite skin substitute, this product comes ready to use but has a short shelf life of 5 days (due to the cells) and thus needs to be ordered (from the United States) when needed. It was intended to be a skin equivalent, but subsequent clinical experience found that although wounds would heal, the donor cells themselves were not viable beyond 4–8 weeks. It is now regarded as a source of growth factors and extracellular matrix to the wound bed ('wound modulator'), and its primary indication with FDA approval, is for chronic wounds that do not respond to a month of standard therapy. Cost benefit analyses have shown advantages including decreased costs and more time in the healed state when compared to conventional treatments in both venous ulcers and diabetic ulcers. However, recently, insurers have cut back significantly on the amount refunded.
- **Dermagraft®** (Organogenesis) consists of living allogenic dermal fibroblasts that are cultivated on a degradable scaffold to generate a neodermis. It was initially intended as a dermal substitute, but it was found that the fibroblasts die a few weeks later; thus, like Apligraf it probably acts primarily to deliver growth factors. It is more expensive, and whilst the product is cryopreserved and has a longer shelf life, this means local cryostorage facilities are needed. It has been difficult to market.

- **Cultured skin substitute (CSS),** developed by Boyce at the University of Cincinnati, is a combination of autologous cultured epithelium with a collagen fibroblast implant that aimed to produce a skin substitute with both epidermal and dermal components that could be applied in a single stage (Harriger MD, *Transplantation*, 1995). Early results were encouraging and led to grants from the military and attempts at commercialisation (as Permaderm®). However, trial irregularities resulted in an FDA clinical hold in 2007. Despite this, and legal action between various stakeholders, the FDA granted Orphan Drug designation in 2012. Amarantus acquired the product in 2015 (now ESS), and its status was changed to a corporate-sponsored investigational new drug (IND) effectively wiping away old study results; a new phase 2a clinical study (NCT01655407) into its use in deep partial or full thickness burns >50% vs. meshed autograft was initiated. New sets of results are awaited.

Thus, tissue-engineered bilayers have not shown clinical success. The fate of these products demonstrates that despite receiving clinical approval or undergoing clinical trials, tissue-engineered skin equivalents have not lived up to the (over)expectations that led to a glut of commercialisation. It was also found in many cases that what seemed to work in the laboratory did not translate simply to a successful product; scaling up products of research was costly, particularly as the production processes had usually not been optimised. In the end, many products underperformed or did not behave as intended when used clinically. Even with viable products, gaining worldwide approval proved to be torturous and time consuming. In the end, many tissue-engineered products did not sell in sufficient volume in approved applications to generate enough return for the investment.

HAND BURNS

The hands are crucial for function (prehension and expressing emotions) and cosmesis (being very visible). **Prolonged immobilisation is detrimental** to long-term hand function. To preserve as much function as possible, hand burns require 'aggressive' therapy – which includes both surgery and physiotherapy (splintage, elevation and movement). Ideally, therapists should assess the hands at every dressing change, so changes can be made if necessary. Rehabilitation is as important as the actual surgery, if not more so, in determining the final outcome for the patient.

- Burn injuries commonly involve the dorsum, where oedema can be much more pronounced due to the looser subcutaneous tissues, and can limit metacarpophalangeal joint (MCPJ) flexion and thumb adduction leading to the **'position of comfort'**.
  - The palms are usually protected by reflex closure and the thicker skin rarely needs grafting.
- During healing, it is vital to splint the hand in the **position of function** with MCPJ 70° flexed, interphalangeal joints (IPJs) extended, thumb abducted and wrist extended 20°.

- Physiotherapy – active and passive movements, whilst avoiding precipitation of heterotopic bone formation by over-aggressive mobilisation, particularly of shoulder and elbow. Regional anaesthesia (brachial plexus block) to encourage movement may be needed.

SURGERY

- For **partial thickness** hand burns, pay attention to positioning and exercises during healing. Those that heal within 2 weeks usually do well.
- **Intermediate depth** burns represent a more complex management problem. Different approaches include the following:
  - **Aggressive** – excise and graft early, with less hypertrophic scarring and **more predictable results** in most cases, but at the expense of 'over-treating' a proportion of patients.
    - Mobilise before surgery.
    - Wider sheet grafts (reducing the number of seams) are preferred, avoiding seams across joints. Splint in the position of function whilst waiting for graft take. The hands should be re-examined on the fourth post-operative day in theatre, with thorough cleaning and touch-up surgery, if needed.
    - Early mobilisation.
  - **Conservative** – dressings for 2 weeks and graft residual areas. Vigorous physiotherapy is continued throughout. Functional results are similar to above.
  - **In between** – reassess injuries on the fifth post-injury day. Continue with conservative treatment if there is healing, or proceed to surgery if still indeterminate.
- **Deeper burns** often feel cool, tense and swollen with clawing. Decompression may be necessary: the digits should be released along the line joining the flexion crease tips that lies dorsal to the neurovascular bundles and volar to the extensor mechanism. The dorsum of the hand is also decompressed along two of the intermetacarpal spaces. Full thickness burns will need early excision and skin grafting.
  - Small areas of exposed tendon, bone or joint (most commonly PIPJ) may be allowed to granulate and then grafted later, and although in the long term this may leave thin and unstable skin, it can always be replaced electively. Larger areas should be covered with flaps or placed into abdominal/groin pockets.

BURN STIFFNESS

Stiffness of burnt hands is not uncommon and is usually joint-related.

- **Early phase stiffness** (before 6 weeks) may be treated non-surgically with aggressive mobilisation.
- **Late stiffness** is more problematic. Stiffness that remains **after** a vigorous regime of joint mobilisation

will probably need joint treatment, e.g. MCPJ capsulectomy, as long as the intrinsic muscles are working. Tendons are released as needed with joints fixed in the position of function with K-wires. Thin flaps can be considered when there is a reasonable expectation of improved function; there are many choices, but flaps with a fascial base, e.g. lateral arm or temporoparietal flaps, may allow better tendon gliding, at least in theory.

- The joint condition can be assessed by 'passive motion testing' (expect **at least 30°** of PIPJ flexion and not the painful minor degrees of movement seen in severe fibrous/bony ankylosis).
- Tendon integrity (assessed with active motion testing) will make the patient a better candidate for joint surgery.
- Skin replacement and tenolysis are pointless if the joint is already fixed.

BURNS IN SPECIFIC AREAS

- Ear – chondritis should be treated aggressively, i.e. debridement to avoid late deformation. Mafenide is traditionally regarded as a good antimicrobial for ear burns due to its ability to penetrate cartilage; the general advice is to avoid bulky dressings and soft pillows to reduce compression.
- Eyelids – skin grafts either FTSG or thicker SSG – it is important to warn the patient that further surgery should be expected, but the final results are usually acceptable.
- Face – a decision should be made by the end of the first week, and burns that are not expected to heal within 2–3 weeks should be debrided and grafted. Scalp grafts offer a reasonable colour match and an inconspicuous donor site.
- Perineal burns – usually managed conservatively.
- Lower limb – remember to elevate. Foot burns are treated aggressively due to the risk of infection.

C. COMPLICATIONS OF BURNS

I. PATHOPHYSIOLOGY OF SMOKE INHALATION AND EFFECT ON RESPIRATION

INHALATIONAL INJURY

Eighty percent of fire-related deaths are due to inhalation injury (IH).

- Maximum upper airway oedema and narrowing occur ~24 hours post-injury.
- IH in an adult increases mortality rate by 40%; mortality increases further if the patient also develops pneumonia.
- IH is also an independent predictor of mortality in burn patients; adds 17% to Revised Baux score (see above).

Injured lungs may become secondarily infected; the common sequence is for acute insufficiency (0–48 hours), pulmonary oedema (48–72 hours) and bronchopneumonia (3–4 weeks). Burn injury lungs are often less compliant due to the overlying burn eschar as well as the loss of surfactant; thus, positive end pressure ventilation (PEEP) is often needed and is more vulnerable to colonisation with subsequent infection, particularly if intubated. Survivors commonly have long-term sequelae with reduced pulmonary capacity, increased airway reactivity, bronchiolitis obliterans or bronchiectasis.

CLASSIFICATION

These three categories correspond roughly to thermal, chemical and metabolic mechanisms of lung injury, respectively.

- **Supraglottic** – primarily thermal injury to the upper airways above the larynx.
- **Subglottic** – primarily chemical injury to alveoli due to dissolved acidic products of combustion. Due to the large expansion of the cross-sectional area, damaging heat rarely gets beyond the larger airways, except for superheated steam.
- **Systemic** – primarily toxic effects of inhaled poisons especially CO and cyanide.

DIAGNOSIS

A high degree of suspicion is required based on the history (fire in an enclosed space), signs and symptoms.

Symptoms

- Shortness of breath/dyspnoea
- Brassy cough and wheezing
- Hoarseness/change in voice

Signs

- Circumoral soot and burns
- Increased respiratory rate and effort of ventilation
- Stridor
- Altered consciousness

Pathophysiology

Injury leads to release of inflammatory mediators causing

- Increased pulmonary artery blood flow
- Bronchoconstriction (TXA2) and increased airway resistance

  In turn, this leads to

- V–Q mismatch.
- Decreased pulmonary compliance (increases risk of barotrauma if ventilated).
- Interstitial oedema, fibrin casts within the airways act as a culture medium promoting infection and cause distal atelectasis.

Later on

- Formation of a pseudomembrane during the healing phase ~18 days post-injury
- Permanent airway stenosis/fibrosis

CARBON MONOXIDE TOXICITY

Carbon monoxide (CO) is a colourless, odourless, poisonous gas produced by the incomplete combustion of hydrocarbons. It has a 200–250× greater affinity for haemoglobin (Hb) than oxygen and shifts the Hb–O_2 dissociation curve to the left.

- The half-life of COHb is ~250 minutes in a patient breathing room air but is reduced to 45 minutes with the administration of 100% oxygen; HBOT further accelerates the breakdown of COHb (20–30 minutes at 3 ATM) and facilitates clearance from cytochromes.
  - HBOT may reduce neurological sequelae, though the evidence is not strong; wider use is limited by logistical factors.
- COHb levels >5% (>10% in smokers) are indicative of IH but do not provide an accurate measure of the severity. The time elapsed since exposure is important; nomograms can be used to extrapolate exposure levels. Toxic symptoms generally appear at levels >20% (headache) with progressive deterioration until death at levels >60%.
- CO also directly binds cytochrome c oxidase, i.e. sick cell syndrome (reduced Na^+/K^+ pump function). Cytochrome-bound CO is washed out after ~24 hours causing a secondary rise in serum COHb and possibly post-intoxication encephalopathy.
- Late myocardial and neurological deterioration has been described.

HYDROGEN CYANIDE TOXICITY

Cyanide compounds are released when certain plastic materials burn. They bind to and inhibit cytochrome oxidase, thus uncoupling oxidative phosphorylation. It is rapidly fatal at inspired concentrations >20 ppm and serum levels >1 mg/L (smokers have background levels of ~0.1 mg/L). Cyanide level measurements are not widely available/tested; there should be a high degree of suspicion, particularly in patients with concomitant CO poisoning who fail to improve with oxygenation.

- ST elevation on ECG.
- Increased ventilation via stimulation of peripheral chemoreceptors makes toxicity worse.

TREATMENT

- 100% O_2.
- The safest option is probably hydroxycobalamin 5 g infused over 15 minutes (Cyanokit®), which acts as a chelating agent that complexes free cyanide to aid its renal excretion.

- Sodium thiosulphate and sodium nitrite are no longer commonly used for CO poisoning; the latter carries a risk of hypotension and methaemoglobinaemia.

Other toxic gases include
- HCl – alveolar injury and pulmonary oedema
- NO – pulmonary oedema, cardiovascular depression
- Aldehydes – irritant leading to mucosal sloughing and systemic inflammatory response

However, it seems that gases in IH primarily act through simple **asphyxiation** by displacing oxygen at the alveolar level, rather than through toxicity per se.

INVESTIGATIONS IN SUSPECTED INHALATIONAL INJURY

- **Arterial blood gases** with COHb.
  - PaO_2/F_IO_2 ratios.
  - Mean alveolar–arterial oxygen gradients.
- **Fibre-optic bronchoscopy (FOB)** – closest to a 'standard' investigation for IH. Check for soot deposition, swollen mucosa or frankly burnt tissues; FOB cannot access the distal/smaller airways.
  - There have been some attempts to grade/quantify findings.
- **Chest X-ray** – there are typically few early signs. CT chest may complement FOB, allowing the assessment of parenchymal radiological changes, such as the thickness and calibre of bronchioles.

GENERAL MANAGEMENT OF INHALATIONAL INJURY

Treatment of IH is largely supportive. IH increases the fluid resuscitation requirement for concomitant cutaneous burns.

- Humidified O_2 followed by chest physiotherapy, sputum culture and bronchoalveolar toilet.
  - There should be a **low threshold for intubation** – prophylactic intubation decreases pulmonary-related mortality (Venus B, *Crit Care Med*, 1981).
- Mechanical ventilatory support may be needed, but is challenging in the context of thermal lung injury and aggressive fluid resuscitation. It is important to try to avoid barotrauma even if it means that the $PaCO_2$ is slightly high. Avoid tracheomalacia and long-term tracheal stenosis by ensuring cuff pressures of <20 cm H_2O and conversion from ET to tracheostomy if the period of supported ventilation is prolonged.
- A variety of treatments have been described:
  - Aerosolised or systemic bronchodilators (β2-adrenergic agonists), muscarinic antagonists or epinephrine.
  - Aerosolised acetyl cysteine is a powerful mucolytic and may mop up reactive oxygen species (ROS), but its exact role is not defined.
  - Anticoagulants, e.g. nebulised heparin, fibrinolytics to ameliorate fibrin casts.

- **ECMO** (extracorporeal membrane oxygenation) can be considered in those with severe but potentially reversible cardiorespiratory failure, not responding to maximal conventional therapy (>7 days of high-pressure ventilation according to O'Toole (*Burns*, 1998).
- Treat only recognised infective complications rather than prophylactically.
  - The commonest source of infection is either from ET tube or opportunistically from the patient's GI and skin commensals. Over-use of antibiotics will predispose to over-population with opportunistic organisms.
  - Stress ulcer prophylaxis with either sucralfate or H2 receptor antagonists does not affect pneumonia rates (Cioffi W, *J Trauma*, 1994).

Extracorporeal membrane oxygenation in burn and smoke inhalation. (Asmussen S, *Burns*, 2013)
This was a systematic review of articles on ECMO and IH pre-2012. There were only a few studies, but the available data suggest that use of ECMO in IH confers no survival benefit. Patients with scalds tended to do better than flame burns, whilst shorter ECMO times (arbitrary threshold 200 hours) were correlated with survival. The authors conclude with the statement that with the improvements in ECMO technology and expertise, further research is worthwhile.

II. DIETETICS AS RELATING TO BURN-INJURY METABOLISM

PHASES

- **Ebb/Shock phase** – there is attenuated metabolism and decreased tissue perfusion in the first 24 hours; this responds to the period of fluid resuscitation.
- **Flow/recovery phase** – gradual increases in cardiac output, heart rate, oxygen consumption and supranormal temperature (about 2°C above normal). This hypermetabolic and hyperdynamic phase peaks 14 days after injury, slowly returning to normal as wounds heal.
  - Metabolic perturbations such as elevated basal metabolic rate (BMR) and negative nitrogen balance may persist for up to 2 years after a severe burn. There may be growth delay in children.

CATABOLISM

Driven by inflammatory mediators, catecholamines and counter regulatory hormones, burn patients will continue to catabolise protein during the first week post-burn **despite** aggressive feeding.

- Loss of 10% total body mass leads to immune dysfunction.
- Loss of 20% – decreased wound healing.
- Loss of 30% – severe infections.
- Loss of 40% – death.

Thus, it is important to try to reduce this hypercatabolic response. Strategies include (Herndon DN, Tompkins RG, *Lancet*, 2004) the following:

- **Prevent infection**
- **Early wound closure**, preferably autograft but also includes biosynthetic skin substitutes (staged closure) and cadaveric allograft (temporary closure)
- **Raising the ambient temperature** to 33°C for example, so heat for evaporation derives from the environment and less is used by the patient in trying to maintain an elevated body temperature

NUTRITIONAL SUPPORT OF THE CATABOLIC RESPONSE

Objectives

- Initiate (enteral) feeding within 24 hours – preferably 8 hours – of injury (with caution in the critically ill).
- Maintain weight within 5%–10% of baseline (see above).
- Avoid micronutrient deficiency.
- Minimise hyperglycaemia and hypertriglyceridaemia.

The BMR increases dramatically during the acute injury phase, 50% in a 25% burn and 100% or more for burn injuries >40% TBSA. Oxygen consumption and CO_2 production steadily increase over the first 5 days post-injury:

- Associated increase in protein, fat and glycogen catabolism.
- Post-receptor insulin resistance.
- Enhanced glucose delivery to cells including fibroblasts, inflammatory cells and endothelial cells at the burn wound. Carbohydrate metabolism is greatly altered with increased glucose uptake and gluconeogenesis.

Route

Continuous **enteral feeding** is preferred; parenteral feeding is considered when there is a prolonged ileus or intolerance of enteral feeding. Early feeding will minimise net protein loss and protect the gut from bacterial translocation, reduce gastric ileus and avoid Gram-negative septicaemia.

- **Enteral nutrition** preserves mucosal integrity, protects against bacterial translocation in the gut and is associated with improved regulation of the inflammatory cytokine response (Andel H, *Burns*, 2003).
  - Some are opposed to the use of TPN in burn patients. TPN is associated with up-regulated expression of TNF-α, which adversely affects survival.
  - However, TPN is tolerated in the severely ill and, when utilised properly, is useful and safe in those undergoing frequent surgery. Some centres use it in combination with enteral nutrition (Sheridan RL, *J Burn Care Res*, 2000).

- **Gastric feeding.** Mortality is reduced in patients who can be fed successfully via the enteral route; a delay of >18 hours reduces the chances of successful enteral feeding. Metoclopramide and cisapride can be used to assist gastric emptying. There are some concerns with aspiration, and generally the feed needs to be discontinued for surgery. Postburn ileus tends to affect the stomach and colon the most.

  - With established gastric ileus, tubes may be sited post-pylorically. Some surgeons advocate routine **duodenal feeding** over gastric feeding; as there is less feed regurgitation, it may reduce aspiration pneumonia and can be continued during surgery. However, it is technically more demanding and approximately 30% develop diarrhoea. Furthermore, hormonal stimulation of the liver and pancreas is greatly reduced when the feed is not placed in the stomach (Raff T, *Burns*, 1997), and the efficacy of ulcer prophylaxis is reduced.

- Caution is still needed with either method of enteral feeding:

  - **Overfeeding** with high calorie enteral nutrition should be avoided – it may lead to impairment of splanchnic oxygen balance in septic burn patients and hyperglycaemia. Overfed patients are more difficult to wean off ventilators.
  - **Feeding induced bowel necrosis** has been reported in the critically ill (Marvin R, *Am J Surg*, 2000), particularly in those with sepsis, and those requiring significant amounts of vasopressors. It is sensible to begin feeding at low infusion rates (check absorption by aspirating).

FORMULAE TO CALCULATE DAILY CALORIE REQUIREMENTS

A dedicated and experienced burns nutritionist is essential. Most advocate a moderately **high carbohydrate regimen** – 52% carbohydrate, 28% fat, 20% protein – which stimulates protein synthesis and improves lean body mass. Inadequate protein intake compromises wound healing, muscle function and the immune system; greatest nitrogen losses occur between days 5 and 10. Children have less body fat and a smaller muscle mass, and hence need proportionately more carbohydrates. Many different formulae have been proposed:

- **Curreri formula for adults** – 25 kal/kg (usual body weight) + 40 kcal/% BSA per day (Curreri PW, *J Trauma*, 1971). This can be applied to burn patients with BSA up to 50%; although it is commonly used, some feel that it tends to overestimate (more than most). Some have also modified this into a 'Curreri Junior' formula for children.
- **Hildreth formula for children** – 1800 kcal/m^2 body surface area + 1300 kcal/m^2 burn area (surface area can be extrapolated using nomograms) per day (Hildreth

MA, *J Burns Care Rehabil*, 1990). This is applicable for children up to 12 years old. Older formula from the author were slightly different.

- **Sutherland formulae** (Sutherland AB, *Burns*, 1976):
  - Adults – 20 kcal/kg + 70 kcal/% TBSA
  - Children – 60 kcal/kg + 35 kcal/% TBSA
- **Harris–Benedict formula** – the BMR is calculated with formulae derived from measurements in healthy volunteers, and an injury factor of 2.1 is recommended for burns. More recent studies have shown that resting energy expenditure (REE) rarely exceeds the Harris–Benedict predicted BMR by more than 50% in burns of >45% BSA when treated with modern techniques.
- Some more modern formula are finding favour:
  - Toronto formula – based on multiple regression analysis of many calorimetric studies
  - Schofield formula (might underestimate, thus usually rounded up)

TYPES OF FEED/SUPPLEMENTS

- It is common (as well as cheap and convenient) to use standard enteral feeds. Speciality formulae may be of benefit; it is common to give supplements of micronutrients, e.g. vitamins, trace elements, zinc, copper and selenium, but the evidence for benefit is not that strong.
  - High carbohydrate and low fat diets supposedly reduce proteolysis and shorten hospitalisation compared to high fat diets. However, there is the significant risk of hyperglycaemia that is potentially deleterious in the critically ill.
  - **Glutamine** is the preferred fuel for dividing cells; it is usually abundant but becomes a conditionally essential amino acid after severe trauma when demand exceeds supply. Glutamine supplementation is relatively well studied; it is safe with moderate benefits seen. Optimal regimes/dosages are uncertain.
    - Arginine requires further study – one concern is that the effect on NO production may be detrimental.
  - Cochrane review (Wasiak J, *Cochrane Database Syst Rev*, 2006) found that early nutrition may ameliorate the hypermetabolic response in adults with a burn injury, but there was no evidence to suggest that it was any different with late (after 24 hours) enteral nutrition.

PHARMACOLOGICAL MEASURES

- Hormonal administration (Herndon DN, *Lancet*, 2004). The hormonal response can be modulated by provision of anabolic hormones such as growth hormone (GH).
  - rhGH (0.2 mg/kg/day) reduces wound healing time.

- rhGH (0.05 mg/kg/day) in children improves growth for up to 3 years post-burn.
  - Side effects include hyperglycaemia with one-third requiring insulin (Singh KP, *Burns*, 1998) though not in children.
  - A multicentre European study of critically ill (mainly post-operative cardiac surgery) patients demonstrated a doubling of mortality with hGH.
- Other potentially useful hormones:
  - **Oxandrolone** (weak testosterone analogue with anabolic effects) restores lost lean mass and improves wound healing (Demling RH, *J Burns Wounds*, 2005). It may cause a variable level of liver dysfunction – usually a transient elevation in aminotransferases.
  - Insulin, IGF-1.
  - β-Blockade with propranolol (to block the raised catecholamine response) lowers heart rate and thus the oxygen requirement.
  - rhGH costs US\$490 per day (in 2002) vs. US\$21 for oxandrolone (and ~US\$3 for insulin and propranolol).

Non-pharmacological measures include physical exercise, which as part of post-burn rehabilitation has also shown to improve muscle mass.

MONITORING NUTRITION

The normal tools are of limited use in a critically ill burn patient, and no single test is fully reliable. Trends in a series of measures are more useful:

- Weight – confounded in the acute phase by fluid changes.
- Acute phase proteins, e.g. pre-albumin, CRP can be measured twice weekly. Peak drop in pre-albumin occurs at about 1 week; persistently low levels are associated with reduced survival.
  - Prealbumin $t_{1/2}$ 3 days vs. albumin 20 days.
  - Albumin is a poor marker in the acute phase but is useful in the rehabilitative phase.
- Urinary urea nitrogen.
- Indirect calorimetry provides the most accurate measure of energy expenditure but is costly and not widely available. It measures the respiratory quotient (RQ), which is the ratio of CO_2 production to O_2 consumption, and the normal fasting ratio is 0.70–0.85. The recommendation is for measurements to be made one to two times per week to assess nutrition started at 120–130% of measured REE. Whilst it is difficult to link indirect calorimetry with improved outcomes, it does reduce the risk of **overfeeding** (which is inherent in most formula) with its complications of fatty liver, hyperglycaemia, fluid overload and accumulation of fat vs. muscle.
- Increased RQ results from an increased CO_2 production, i.e. increased carbohydrate metabolism, which may complicate respiratory function.
- Decreased RQ usually indicates an inadequate calorie intake.

ESPEN endorsed recommendations: Nutritional therapy in major burns. (Rousseau AF, *Clin Nutr*, 2013)

A group of Burn specialists evaluated trials between 1979 and 2011 and came up with the following:

Strong recommendations

- Early enteral feeding, using the gastric route first
  - Provision of elevated protein requirements – adults 1.5–2 g/kg in adults, 3 g/kg in children
  - Limit glucose delivery to a maximum of 55% energy and 5 mg/kg/hour
- Early provision of trace element and vitamin supplementation
- Attenuate hypermetabolism by pharmacologic (propanolol, oxandrolone) and physical means (early surgery and thermoneutral rooms)

Suggestions

- Use indirect calorimetry; otherwise, use the Toronto formula (Schofield in children) to reduce overfeeding.
- Maintain fat administration equal or less than 30% of total energy delivery.

III. BURNS SHOCK AND SEPSIS

BURNS SHOCK AND OEDEMA

See 'Burns oedema'.

BURNS SEPSIS

Infection accounts for over 50% of the deaths in major burns (Edwards-Jones V, *Burns*, 2003). It may be difficult to distinguish infective complications from the hypermetabolic response to the burn injury.

- **Risk of infection increases with burn surface area.** There is significant immunosuppression (both cellular and humoral) especially with burns >30% TBSA, which when coupled with a warm moist environment leads to increased infection risk in the open wounds.

To counteract this, most burns units advocate early wound excision and grafting for deep burns, and wound dressings with antimicrobial agents.

- *S. aureus* accounts for up to 75% of infections.
  - Damage from collagenases and proteinases, enterotoxins A, B and C and exotoxin, e.g. toxin shock syndrome toxin-1 (TSST-1)
- MRSA – increasing resistance to vancomycin being seen.
- *P. aeruginosa* is found in up to 25% of burn wounds. It produces a toxin pigment pyocyanin as well as exotoxin A.
- Other pathogens
  - *Streptococcus pyogenes*
  - Coliform bacilli
  - Fungi including *Candida* and *Aspergillus*

TOXIC SHOCK SYNDROME

TSS was originally described in 1978; some patients may have a genetic predisposition. The condition is related to the production of TSST-1 toxin that causes an overstimulation of the immune system. The toxin is produced by many strains of *S. aureus* including MRSA. Most people develop the antitoxin by age 30 due to exposure throughout life. Symptoms of TSS include

- Pyrexia and rash
- Diarrhoea and vomiting
- Hypotension

It is not related to size of burns and has been reported in small burns (<10%) in children. Mortality rates of up to 50% have been reported; thus, treatment has to be rapid and focused:

- Early targeted antibiotic therapy.
- Anti-TSST-1 immunoglobulin/pooled γ-globulin/FFP contains the antibodies against the toxin. Patients treated rapidly will improve quickly.

METHICILLIN-RESISTANT *S. AUREUS*

MRSA was first identified in 1961 and currently accounts for up to 50% of all nosocomial infections in the United States (Cook N, *Burns*, 1998) and about 25% of *S. aureus* in burns patients (Lesseva MI, *Burns*, 1996). Strain typing can be useful to monitor spread of infection and response to treatment. MRSA carries a **mec-A gene** encoding bacterial cell wall penicillin-binding proteins with reduced affinity for β-lactams. Different strains have different mec genes (I-VI).

MRSA is a common cause of nosocomial infection in burns patients, probably due in part to a combination of the open wounds and relative immunosuppression, and also indiscriminant use of quinolone antibiotics and ciprofloxacin. There is a high incidence of environmental contamination in burns units; close proximity to infected patients and inadequate hand washing by healthcare personnel are other risk factors for spread. The prevalence of MRSA in different burns units varies significantly, but the exact reasons for this are not clear.

Burn wound infection may lead to graft loss or systemic sepsis; some strains produce an enterotoxin leading to TSS. Infected burn patients should be screened and barrier-nursed.

- Hand washing and alcohol hand rubs (act by protein denaturation and are rapidly bactericidal in vivo with slow regrowth).
- Environmental decontamination (disinfection).
- Isolation of infected patients and decolonisation with 5 day course of nasal bactroban, chlorhexidine throat gargle, bactroban wound ointment and triclosan skin cleanser daily.
- Prevalence refers to the proportion of the overall population that has the condition at a certain time

vs. **incidence** that looks at a disease rate within a time period, i.e. prevalence looks at all disease, whilst incidence looks at new disease.

TREATMENT

It is important to eradicate *S. aureus* infection regardless of methicillin sensitivity or resistance.

- Early wound closure – the presence of MRSA *per se* is not a contraindication to wound closure by SSG or other means.
- Topical **mupirocin** is a standard for decolonisation of nasal MRSA, but there is increasing incidence of resistance associated with its use, and also a significant relapse rate. There is no convincing evidence that it reduces the risk of surgical infection (NICE 2008).
  - Topical **SSD** performs well in vitro but is less effective than mupirocin, clearing less than 50% of wounds.
- Systemic **vancomycin** alone or in combination with fucidin/rifampicin. Vancomycin has been the antibiotic of choice for MRSA for decades, but increased use of the antibiotic and a high spontaneous mutation rate have led to development of resistance.
  - Ciproxin and other FQs, and macrolides are not optimal because resistance is common.
    - Clindamycin – risk of *Clostridium difficile* overgrowth/infection.
    - Tetracyclines.
    - Linezolid – may cause myelosuppresion, neuropathy and lactic acidosis.
    - Rifampicin may be used in combination with other agents but never alone due to resistance; drug interactions are common.

IV. OTHER COMPLICATIONS

ACALCULOUS CHOLECYSTITIS

This is a very rare complication (<0.5% of burned patients with an average burn size ~50%) with a high mortality and presents typically as fever, right upper quadrant pain and tenderness, and a raised white cell count 2–4 weeks post-burn. The diagnosis can be made by ultrasound and is treated by cholecystectomy.

CURLING'S ULCER

This condition occurs more frequently in the presence of sepsis.

- Only one-third report pain and patients usually present with haematemesis; 12% perforate. Gastric ulcers tend to be multiple whilst duodenal ulcers are solitary.
- The risk can be reduced from 86% to 2% with effective fluid resuscitation, enteral feeding and prophylaxis with antacid therapy/mucosal protectants, e.g. sucralfate.

ISCHAEMIC ENTEROCOLITIS

This condition is characterised by mucosal ischaemia and bacterial translocation, and is associated with a high mortality rate. Some suggest selective digestive tract decontamination (SDD), e.g. with cefotaxime, tobramycin, polymixin or amphotericin B, but this may increase colonisation by Gram positives including MRSA.

SUPPURATIVE THROMBOPHLEBITIS

This occurs mainly at peripheral cannulation sites and is related to duration of placement. It is usually occult and only one-third show clinical signs presenting as sepsis/positive cultures with 'unknown' source. Commonly involves

- Non-burns patients – *Staphylococcus*, *Klebsiella*, *Candida*
- Burns patients – same as those cultured from the burn wound

Heterotopic ossification after severe burns. (Richards AM, *Burns*, 1997)

By definition, heterotopic ossification (HO) is the formation of lamellar bone in soft tissues where it does not normally form. Myositis ossificans (MO) is HO in muscles and other soft tissues, and strictly it is a misnomer and should be termed fibrodysplasia ossificans progressiva (FOP). It can occur with or without previous injury. FOP is a rare AD disease that begins at age 5 on average. Non-hereditary MO is uncommon in children and occurs from direct muscle trauma with ossification confined to the muscle. Ectopic calcification is mineralisation but histologically is not bone.

The overall incidence of HO in burns is approximately 1%–3% and the exact aetiology is unclear, though it is more common in patients with >20% TBSA. It occurs most commonly close to the olecranon. It seems to be related to movement, and joints underlying areas of FT burn may be at increased risk; it may be associated with aggressive–passive mobilisation of shoulder and elbow.

- The typical time of onset is between 3 weeks and 3 months.
- Serum calcium and phosphate are usually unchanged; alkaline phosphatase may rise but is an unreliable indicator.
- The calcification increases as long as wounds remain open. Early radiographic signs may be reversed by effective burn wound closure.

Once matured (decreased activity on bone scan, usually >12 months), excision typically does not lead to recurrence and is the treatment of choice (Chen HC, *Burns*, 2009).

- NSAIDs such as indomethacin, COX2 inhibitors, may help – possibly by preventing osteoblastic differentiation of mesenchymal cells, and may be indicated in high-risk cases.
- Bisphosphonates bind calcium and phosphates to prevent hydroxyapatite crystallisation, and thus bone matrix is not mineralised; however, it does become mineralised after treatment is stopped. It is controversial, there are significant side effects and routine use is probably not indicated.
- Radiation therapy – exact therapy unknown.

MARJOLIN'S ULCER

See Chapter 8 **Section** C. III 'Squamous cell carcinoma'.

HYPOPIGMENTATION

Management of hypopigmentation following burn injury. (Grover R, *Burns*, 1996)

Hypopigmentation after a burn is usually permanent; supposedly the post-burn scar is a barrier to melanocyte migration and melanosome transport from melanocyte to keratinocyte. Treatment options include

- Dermabrasion with wound bed covered by
  - Ultrathin SSG
  - Particulate grafting – morcelised skin graft (Harashina technique 1985)
  - Melanocyte transplantation – melanocytes (and keratinocytes) cultured from a trypsinised skin biopsy
- Tattooing/camouflage make-up/natural dyes, e.g. henna, especially for Asian skin

D. BURNS RECONSTRUCTION AND REHABILITATION

I. BURN SCAR MANAGEMENT

See also 'Hypertrophic scars', Chapter 1, **Section** C.II.

A scar will result whenever a wound heals by the process of repair, but scars can be normal or abnormal. Over a period of months, normal scars go through a sequence where the scar may appear red, raised and firm as the vascular matrix accumulates before a plateau period that is followed by remodelling/maturation to become softer, flatter and paler.

PRINCIPLES OF BURN SCAR MANAGEMENT

There is a distinction between scar minimisation and scar treatment.

SCAR MINIMISATION

- Optimise timely healing – appropriate dressings or early burn excision and wound closure
- Maintain a full passive range of movement and optimise active joint mobilisation
  - Even in the critically ill, passive ranging should be possible particularly at dressing changes; remember to give adequate analgesia.
- Splint in position of function throughout treatment and rehabilitation

SCAR TREATMENT

- Early ambulation and exercise, to maintain joint movement, muscle mass and bone density
- Massage and pressure garments
- Topical treatments such as steroid injections, silicone and laser
- Avoid permanent joint changes by early scar release

HYPERTROPHIC SCARS

The hypertrophic scar is a common consequence of burn injury; it follows a qualitatively similar process as the normal scar, although both the accumulation of the matrix and the duration of abnormality are much greater. These scars have an abundance of disorganised type 1 collagen and a high TGF-β3/TGF-β1 and TGF-β 2 ratio. Post-burn hypertrophic scarring generally becomes apparent 6–8 weeks after grafting. They tend to develop at sites of delayed wound healing, e.g. deeper burns, infected wounds or those allowed to heal by secondary intention. For management, see Chapter 1 Section C. II 'Hypertrophic and keloid scars'.

Pulsed dye laser in burn scars. (Parrett BM, *Burns*, 2010)
This is a review of the use of the PDL (either 585 or 595 nm) for hypertrophic scars. The erythema associated with these scars may be due to dilated microvessels occluded by endothelial cells; vascular proliferation plays a key role. PDL causes photothermolysis; laser energy absorbed by haemoglobin causes coagulation, and the tissue hypoxia leads to collagen realignment and remodelling. Clinical studies have demonstrated that PDL flattens/decreases scar volume, increases pliability, reduces erythema and improves texture, usually after two to three treatments, and recurrence is usually not seen. The most common side effect is purpura for a week, whilst pigmentation problems may occur in darker-skinned patients. Both acute and established hypertrophic scars are suitable for treatment, but PDL is less effective in thick scars, though it can be combined with other modalities. The authors suggest that PDL should be considered before surgical excision.

II. BURN RECONSTRUCTION

Rehabilitation is the process by which a person attains his or her maximal potential following injury; it involves both surgical and non-surgical treatments (see above). Priorities include

- Prevention of deformity
- Restoration of active function
- Restoration of cosmesis

TIMING OF RECONSTRUCTION

- **Emergency**. Urgent surgery is needed, i.e. before discharge, when vital structures are exposed, e.g. the cornea.

- **Essential**. Problems that are not urgent but will significantly improve the patient's final function or appearance if performed early, e.g. contractures that prevent the activities of daily living, limiting range of movement and not responding to non-surgical measures. Similarly, scarring in children adversely affecting growth should be treated early. Microstomia or other perioral scarring that limits dietary intake is another example.
- **Elective**. Most cases of burn scarring will fall into this category; many will be focused primarily on aesthetics, and surgery will generally occur after scar maturation.

Reconstructive surgery in burn patients is characterised by an often severe lack of donor sites, and having to operate on scarred tissues with altered vascularity that would affect options such as tissue expansion, local flaps or skin grafts.

Reconstructive surgery using an artificial dermis (Integra): results with 39 grafts. (Dantzer E, *Br J Plastic Surg*, 2001)
This is a review of patients who underwent Integra grafting for functional reconstruction of a scarred area. The authors state that treated areas were supple, were not adherent to underlying structures and had uniform skin colour and texture, with little or no hypertrophic scarring.

The authors suggest that for best results, a well-vascularised wound bed with good haemostasis is needed. Meshing was avoided and fenestration by hand was preferred when drainage was needed. The Integra was secured with stitches or staples with a tie-over dressing for mobile sites. Ultra-thin SSGs replaced the silicone layer after a mean of 22 days. The most common complication was infection (5/31); however, the transparent silicone allows easy identification of infected areas, which are excised and antibiotics started.

RECONSTRUCTION OF SPECIAL AREAS

Head and neck

Facial burns are generally treated conservatively at least initially due in part to their superior healing potential.

- Reconstruction should follow aesthetic units either with FTSG where required or thick unperforated sheet SSG, e.g. from the scalp. Quilting and exposed grafting are useful techniques – inspect grafts twice daily and aspirate haematomas as required. Pressure therapy should be started early.
- Useful FTSG donor sites are pre-/postauricular area, supraclavicular fossa, upper eyelid and nasolabial folds. The preference is for skin from above the clavicle ('blush zone'); other sites tend to produce colour/texture mismatch.
- Commissural burns/contracture are a very difficult problem – start splinting early and continue for 6 months; however, many still need (repeated) surgery.

BURN CONTRACTURES

Contraction versus contracture

Contraction is a physiological process that is part of wound repair related to **myofibroblast** activity (these normally undergo apoptosis in normal maturing scars). Contracture is a pathological process occurring in a scar that has already re-epithelialised and 'healed', which causes shortening, deformity and limitation of movement. Their incidence is somewhat inversely proportional to the quality of acute burn care available. They can affect concavities such as the neck, axilla, web spaces and flexor surfaces of joints.

- **Myofibroblasts** are the source of contraction in wounds; they are found dispersed throughout granulating wounds and appear on the 3rd day, peaking on the 10th day. They are specialised fibroblasts with contractile myofilaments and cellular adhesion structures, and their action leads to contraction of the entire wound bed.

Intrinsic vs. extrinsic contracture

The best example is ectropion that may be due to scarring of the eyelid (intrinsic) or a relatively normal eyelid being pulled down by a cheek/chin/neck scar (extrinsic). With intrinsic contracture, all lamellae/layers need to be addressed.

Neck contractures

Neck contractures are one of the most common burn contractures. They lead to obliteration of the chin neck angle (CNA), and eventually the anterior neck space as the chin is brought down to the manubrium. The soft tissues of the lower face are deformed downwards. There are various ways of grading the contracture according to the functional disability, e.g. having to tilt the body back or persistent upward gaze to make eye contact, whilst the contracture may be classified according to its position.

- Intubation can be difficult.
- The defect after scar release can be very substantial.

Correction of neck contractures

- **Grafts**
  - Thicker SSGs or FTSGs from the abdomen. FTSG donor sites can be pre-expanded depending on the amount of tissue needed, or grafted with SSG or Integra®/Nevelia® (dermal matrices, DM).
  - DM to resurface the neck wound defect.
  - Post-operative splinting is important to slow down recontracture.
- **Pedicled flaps**
- Previously, burnt skin can still be used despite altered blood flow/microcirculation. An excessively increased rate of complications and necrosis has not been borne out in studies/clinical experience.

- **Random neck flaps** including Z-plasties may be used for narrow web/bands.
- **Supraclavicular artery flap** (Lamberty BG, *Br J Plast Surg*, 1979) is based on branches of the transverse cervical artery (TCA) that originates in the triangle between the posterior edge of sternomastoid, external jugular vein and clavicle. The vessel can be marked out preoperatively with handheld Doppler. The flap territory runs from its origin to the shoulder tip and is usually sufficient to reach the chin. Tissue expansion can be used to aid donor site closure.
- **Trapezius flap** – Early descriptions in the literature often had conflicting vascular anatomy. The muscle is supplied superiorly by the descending branch of the TCA and inferiorly by the dorsal scapular which may be a (deep) branch from the TCA (25%) or directly from the subclavian (75%); studies have demonstrated functional anastomoses between the two systems. The vessel is marked out with handheld Doppler preoperatively, and the flap is harvested with the patient positioned laterally/prone.
  - **The muscle bulk at the base of the flap** can be disfiguring but should not be reduced until at least 6 weeks later. Leaving the superior portion of the muscle intact tends to reduce functional deficits, i.e. shoulder weakness, but also reduces the arc of rotation of the flap. By contrast, the function of the inferior part (below C7 prominens and tip of scapula laterally) can be taken over by other muscles including serratus, and thus harvesting it is said to have few functional consequences.
  - **Extra long trapezius flap** can be raised with typical markings up to iliac crest (about 40 cm in length and 8–10 cm in width). Under the trapezius, a small muscle cuff can be kept when the flap pedicled is back.
- **Free flaps** especially thin perforator flaps, e.g. ALT flap, which can be thinned intra-operatively or post-operatively; blunting of the CNA usually requires secondary revision.

Axillary contractures

It is difficult to maintain the arms in abduction in an acute burn; thus, axillary contractures are not uncommon. The adduction deformity can be quite debilitating particularly in conjunction with reduced elbow motility.

- IA   Anterior axillary fold
- IB   Posterior axillary fold
- II   Both anterior and posterior axillary folds
- III   Both folds and the dome of the axilla

Incisional release and grafting are options particularly for types I and II contractures. Type III contractures benefit from tissue replacement often in the form of local flaps, e.g. parascapular/bilobed flaps, LD/TDAP or free flaps.

Total face reconstruction with one free flap. (Angrigiani C, *Plast Reconstr Surg*, 1997)

The authors present their experience with this technique in five patients with severe facial burns. Bilateral extended scapular–parascapular free flaps were used to reconstruct five full thickness full-face burns (nose required separate technique). Bilateral microvascular anastomoses of superficial circumflex scapular arteries to facial vessels were performed. The donor area on the back required grafting.

Pre-expanded ultra-thin supraclavicular flaps for (full) face reconstruction with reduced donor-site morbidity and without the need for microsurgery. (Pallua N, *Plast Reconstr Surg*, 2005)

The authors present their experience of facial reconstruction in 12 patients. Large tissue expanders were placed under the area of the flaps, from the TCA to the shoulder. They were able to harvest thin flaps up to 30 × 14 cm.

SCALP ALOPECIA

Burns to the scalp often lead to areas of hair loss. Serial excision can deal with alopecia up to 15% of total scalp. For larger areas of loss, tissue expansion is a useful technique; the scalp can be expanded to twice its area before noticeable reduction of hair density occurs.

MCCAULEY CLASSIFICATION

- Type I – single alopecia segment
  - a – <25% – single expander
  - b – 25%–50% – single expander with over-inflation
  - c – 50%–75% – multiple expanders
  - d – >75% – multiple expanders
- Type II – multiple areas of alopecia amenable to tissue expansion correction
- Type III – multiple areas of alopecia not amenable to tissue expansion
- Type IV – total alopecia

TRUNK AND GENITALIA

Burns to the nipple–areolar complex in adolescence may disturb breast growth; however, the breast bud lies quite deep and so is often preserved. Nevertheless, scar contractures may impair development, and typically, the burned breast tends to be flatter and lacks natural ptosis necessitating scar releases and possibly mastopexy of the uninjured side.

- Implants, if required, should be placed subpectorally.
- Nipple reconstruction can be considered with local flaps such as skate flap, though the risk of necrosis is increased due to scarring.
- Tissue expansion for trunk reconstruction works better than for extremities burns (~30% complication rate).

Reconstruction of the burned breast with Integra. (Palao R, *Br J Plastic Surg*, 2003)

Childhood-burn breast scars were reconstructed using Integra®. The authors recommend careful preservation of the inframammary fold, and overlapping of Integra® to avoid scar hypertrophy. Standard antibiotic prophylaxis was given. Unmeshed autografts were used for the second stage on ~day 28 on average. The authors reported 100% take with no infections with this technique and concluded that it provided good aesthetic reconstruction and improved scar quality.

Adnexal structures do not regenerate, so some patients complain of dryness but it can be managed by moisturising creams. Integra that has 'taken' can be expanded like normal skin, though the mechanism for this is unclear (Tsoutos D, *J Burn Care Res*, 2007).

UPPER LIMB

Joint flexion contractures, in general, should be released early before secondary contractures of the joint(s), tendons, etc. occur. X-rays to rule out HO are useful. Common options are

- Skin grafts in conjunction with scar release or excision. The defect is often unexpectedly large.
- Dermal substitutes and thin skin grafts.
- Flaps.

HANDS

Although coverage of the hands is a high priority compared with other body sites, with a life-threatening major burn, the priority is to close as wide an area as possible, i.e. trunk and lower limbs. Delayed healing of hand burns may lead to dorsal skin contracture and syndactyly. Sometimes the thick scarring makes assessment of joints/tendons difficult; often the final assessment is made during surgery.

- **Stiffness** is common (see 'Hand burns').
- **Dorsal scar contracture** can be treated by full scar excision, extensor tenolysis and soft tissue coverage with thin flaps such as lateral arm or radial forearm free flap.
  - Vigorous post-operative physiotherapy and appropriate splinting, avoiding wrist hyperextension (and compression neuropathies) is important.
- **Burn syndactyly** most commonly affects the first web. In the fingers, there is usually web reversal with the dorsal web being more distal, and there may be limitation of abduction. Unlike congenital syndactyly, skin grafts are almost always needed due to a lack of tissue laxity. Treatment options include Z-plasty type flaps: jumping man flap, VM-plasty or 4-flap-plasty, etc. Recurrence is not uncommon despite splintage.

III. BURNS ITCH

Pruritis is a common complaint that can be used as a rough surrogate of scar maturation. It tends to begin around the time of healing, peaking at ~2–6 months, but can persist for a long time – in one study, 29% had persistent itch at 4 years and 5% at 12 years. It seems to be more common in burns of the lower limbs and burns that take >3 weeks to heal. It is poorly understood and can be difficult to treat.

Itch is transmitted by C-fibres, though it may involve a separate subset distinct from pain fibres; some say that itch is conveyed by epidermal fibres, whilst pain goes by the dermal fibres. There are many substances that are said to be involved including histamine, as well as serotonin, proteases, kinins and neuropeptides including substance P. Overall, the evidence base is rather scanty. Clinical psychologists may have a role, teaching better coping strategies to patients.

STRATEGIES

- **First line** – **antihistamines** (chlorpheniramine, diphenhydramine, cyproheptadine – using non-sedatives during day, piriton at night) in combination with
  - Emollients, e.g. simple moisturisers and aloe vera
- Pressure garments (may decrease histamine release)
- Opioids and sedatives as needed
- **Second line** – it is perhaps sensible to choose simple methods with a few side effects even if they may not work that well, e.g. massage, silicone (may take 3 months or more), TENS, hypnosis, capsaicin cream (Axsain, inhibits substance P), topical silver, etc.
- Some have reported good results with PDL.
- **Third line** – use possibly more efficacious treatments but with side effects that may persist, e.g.
  - Antihistamines
    - Topical, e.g. Anthisan, a cream for bites.
    - H1 and H2 antagonists – some studies suggest synergy.
  - Topical steroids (inhibition of collagen production causes skin thinning).
  - TCA creams.
    - Doxepin – effect probably partly due to the affinity of doxepin for H1 and H2 receptors and action on muscarinic receptors. It may cause a slight burning sensation.
    - Dothiepin.
  - Gabapentin works in some but may cause behavioural problems in children.
  - Tacrolimus.

3

Head and neck

A. PRINCIPLES OF DIAGNOSIS AND MANAGEMENT OF MAXILLOFACIAL TRAUMA

I. GENERAL

The most common aetiological factors in head and neck trauma are assault (nasal > mandible > zygoma) and road traffic accidents (RTAs), though the introduction of seatbelts has reduced facial injuries from 21% to 6%. Important points in the history to take note of include

- Degree and direction of force
- Loss of consciousness, if any
- Previous maxillofacial injuries, eyesight and occlusion

GENERAL EVALUATION

The ABC (primary survey) system is used to detect life-threatening injuries, in particular **airway obstruction**:

- Segmental mandibular symphyseal fractures may fall backwards into the oropharynx along with the tongue due to the unopposed action of geniohyoid and digastric muscles.
- Haemorrhage from fractures (especially Le Fort) involving pterygoid plexus of veins, maxillary or ethmoidal arteries, or rarely from the internal carotid artery into the tonsillar fossa.
  - Rarely life threatening (see below).
  - Most cases can be managed with nasal packing; sometimes, immediate fracture reduction, angiography and selective embolisation or ligation may be needed.
- Oedema.
- Altered consciousness.

Definitive airways are more likely to be needed if there is significant head injury, particularly with complex fractures (difficult to stabilise, large amounts of swelling and bleeding).

- Endotracheal intubation should be undertaken by experienced staff, with a surgical airway (cricothyroidotomies/tracheostomies) as a backup should it fail.

Breathing – there may be coexistent severe chest injuries such as tension pneumothorax, haemothorax or flail chest.

Circulation – profuse bleeding from fractures sufficient to cause haemodynamic compromise is unusual; associated injuries may contribute to blood loss (internal or external).

Specific assessment of the fracture(s) is part of the **secondary survey**:

- Look, feel and move – examine in sequence, either up-down or down-up.
  - Fractures cause bruising, swelling and tenderness ± loss of function. Remember to check intra-orally – inspect and palpate maxillary buttresses.
  - Look for asymmetry.
  - Feel for step deformities and crepitus.
  - Move mandible (and eyes).

Upper face

- Forehead/forehead sensation
- Crepitus indicating frontal sinus fracture
- CSF rhinorrhoea (anterior cranial fossa fracture)

Mid-face

- Orbits
  - Ocular dystopia, restricted eye movement
  - Exorbitism or enophthalmos
  - Pupil size and reactivity

- Diplopia/field defects
- Raccoon eyes (anterior cranial fossa fracture)
- Zygoma
  - Malar flattening, best viewed from above; palpable step along inferior orbital rim
  - Trismus
- Nasal bones
  - Palpable deformity, check specifically for septal deviation/haematoma
- Maxilla
  - Infraorbital nerve numbness.
  - Malocclusion.
  - Increased mobility (grasp anterior maxilla whilst fixing the face at the nose); however, impacted fractures may not move.
    - Maxillary alveolus moves but nasofrontal area does not – Le Fort I.
    - Maxillary alveolus and nasofrontal area move – Le Fort II.
    - Entire mid-face moves – Le Fort III.

Lower face

- Mandible
  - Sublingual bruising suggests a fracture.
  - Malocclusion, abnormal bite and trismus.
  - Lower lip numbness due to inferior alveolar nerve (IAN) injury.

Others

- Laryngotracheal injuries – cricoid/thyroid cartilage fracture.
- Ears.
  - Haemotympanum and signs of middle cranial fossa fracture, i.e. CSF otorrhoea, Battle's sign (postauricular bruising = base of skull fracture until proven otherwise)
  - Conductive or sensorineural hearing deficit
- Loose teeth may be reinserted (and stabilised with wires to adjacent teeth) but success depends on the timing (poor if >30 minutes) and the condition of the roots. Teeth should be gently cleaned without damaging root surface and transported in milk, balanced saline or buccal vestibule.
- Soft tissue injuries.
  - Examine for facial nerve injury.
  - Parotid duct division.
  - Tear duct division.

ASSOCIATED INJURIES

Many trauma patients with obvious facial injuries will be assigned to the plastic surgeons without adequate multisystem evaluation (a finding borne out by studies – significant additional **undetected** injuries were found in up to 12%–25%). It is vital that the plastic surgeon receiving the patient performs a full assessment as a matter of routine.

- 25% of orbital fractures have globe injuries.
- 15%–20% of facial fractures have cervical injuries.
- X-rays including CXR in patients with damaged or missing teeth.
- Neurological injuries.
  - Primary – due to initial injury.
  - Secondary – due to response to injury, e.g. hypotension, hypoxia.
  - Skull base fracture may be indicated by CSF rhinorrhoea or epistaxis.

INVESTIGATIONS

Computed tomography (CT) scan is the investigation of choice for all maxillofacial trauma except perhaps for isolated mandibular injuries.

- Orthopantomogram (OPG)
- AP mandible open and closed
- Reversed Towne's view for the condyles
- OM views for mid-facial injury

PRINCIPLES OF SURGICAL MANAGEMENT

- Early one-stage repair with access to all fracture fragments
- Rigid fixation with immediate bone graft if needed
- Definitive soft tissue cover

II. FRONTAL SINUS FRACTURES

The frontal sinus drains via the nasofrontal duct to the middle meatus. It is absent unilaterally in 10%, bilaterally in 4%. The anterior table is thick and **severe force is needed** for the frontal region to be fractured. There is a CSF leak in up to 20%. There may be a palpable deformity and paraesthesia of the forehead. X-ray may demonstrate a fluid level, but CT (axial and coronal) is usually needed to delineate the fracture clearly. Late complications include sinusitis, mucocoeles and meningitis; thus prophylactic antibiotics are often given.

- Anterior wall (thicker)
  - **Non-depressed fractures** do not usually need specific treatment, unless associated with NOE fracture or supraorbital rim fracture (risk of extension to duct). If the fracture is above the level of the sinus floor, the duct is probably spared.
  - Depressed, but not comminuted – elevate via subbrow/butterfly incision and fix with low profile plate/wire; some have used cyanoacrylate glue.
  - Depressed and comminuted – may need (cranial) bone graft. If there is extensive disruption of mucosa, it may be better to obliterate the sinus (parietal bone, abdominal fat or temporalis fascia). Some suggest that filling with non-vascularised material is no better than leaving it unfilled (Rohrich RJ, *Plast Reconstr Surg*, 1995).

- **Posterior wall fracture.** CSF rhinorrhoea (β2-transferrin test or bedside ring test) and pneumocephalus may follow; urgent neurosurgical consultation is needed.
- The duct lies medial and posterior and is thus more likely to be involved with posterior wall fractures. If the mucosa and duct (test drainage with **methylene blue**) are undamaged, then surgery may not be needed.
  - Serial X-rays to check aeration of the sinuses.
  - Complications may not manifest for several years. Patients should be educated about symptoms.
- When the nasofrontal ducts are injured, it may be necessary to remove the mucosa, block off the duct (fat, bone or pericranial flap) and cranialise the sinus; if only one nasofrontal duct is injured, removing the midline septum may help.

III. ORBITAL FRACTURES

The orbit is composed of seven bones, with the thinnest part being the lamina papyracea of the ethmoid bone that forms the lower part of the medial wall. There is up to 20% risk of an associated ocular injury, and though most ocular injuries are minor, careful screening is needed.

GENERAL SYMPTOMS AND SIGNS

- **Ocular dystopia** refers to the position of the **globe** and in trauma results more commonly from a change in the orbital volume of the orbit.
  - **Enophthalmos** is due to a discrepancy between ocular tissue and orbital volume causing the globe to sink in, e.g. blow-out fracture increasing the orbital volume.
    - 1 mm of bony displacement results in 1 mL of volume change; up to 2–3 mm is acceptable and non-deforming.
  - Compare this to **exophthalmos** which is usually the result of increased ocular tissue but normal orbital volume, e.g. classically, Graves/hypothyroidism, less commonly tumours or malformations.
  - **Exorbitism** (proptosis) is the result of normal ocular tissue but decreased orbital volume – which may be associated with craniosynostosis or not (non-syndromic).
  - Shifts in the AP position of the globe may be detectable by an increased distance between corneal surface and the lateral orbital rim and objectively measured with a Hertel exophthalmometer (normal is 16–18 mm and discrepancy <3 mm), but this will not be useful if the lateral orbit (reference point) has been fractured/displaced.
- **Orbital dystopia** – the bony orbits either do not lie on the same horizontal plane (vertical dystopia) or too close/far (hypotelorism/hypertelorism), and this is usually the result of craniofacial developmental anomalies.

- **Hypertelorism** may be due to encephaloceles, craniosynostosis, facial clefts or bone disorders. Globe repositioning is usually delayed until 4–6 years of age (after consolidation of bones to reduce comminution) unless there are visual problems.
- **Hypotelorism** (like that infamous statue of Cristiano Ronaldo) does not usually affect vision, and because there are few psychosocial issues, treatment is not usually required.
- **Telecanthus** – inner canthi are widely separated (>35 mm, normal 30–32 mm though obviously this depends in part on the size of the patient), which may or may not be associated with hypertelorism.
  - Check the medial canthal tendon (MCT).
- Bruising, oedema, subconjunctival haemorrhage (may be due to bleeding from fracture site if the posterior extent cannot be seen).
- Diplopia and ophthalmoplegia, e.g. inferior rectus tethering.
- The **afferent pupillary defect** is an important clinical finding – if the optic nerve is damaged, then its consensual response (which remains intact) will overcome its direct response and will cause paradoxical dilatation when light is shined in the affected eye (and not in the normal eye which causes a consensual dilatation). Also known as Marcus Gunn pupil.
- Rupture, vitreous and anterior chamber haemorrhage and lens dislocation; these require urgent assessment by an ophthalmologist.

INCISIONS

The major concern is to avoid causing lower eyelid retraction, ectropion or entropion.

- **Subciliary** (just below lashes) gives better exposure medially, but also has the highest risk of retraction.
  - Stepped skin flap (Converse JM, *Plast Reconstr Surg*, 1981) with incision 2–3 mm below the lash line. The skin is raised off the muscle which is incised 2–3 mm below the level of the skin incision, i.e. just below tarsal plate. The dissection is followed down to the orbital rim. The periosteum is incised anteriorly on the orbital rim to avoid vertical lid shortening. Stair stepping is said to reduce scar inversion, but there is still ~10% risk of transient ectropion and 30% of permanent scleral show.
  - Skin only flap – the muscle is divided at the level of the orbital rim. There is a higher incidence of skin necrosis, bruising and ectropion.
  - Skin-muscle flap – the muscle is incised at the same level as the skin i.e. non-stepped.
- **Transconjunctival approach** – internal incision just below the level of the tarsal plate (may need lateral extension) has cosmetic advantages; 3% risk of permanent scleral show vs. ~28% in subciliary incision.

- **Subtarsal** incisions cause less ectropion/scleral show at the expense of a more obvious scar with oedema. It can be a good option in older patients with prominent lower lid wrinkles.

LOCATION OF ORBITAL FRACTURES

- **Medial wall fractures** often result from assault/RTAs, and commonly involve the medial wall alone (type I) or with the adjoining orbital floor (type II), and sometimes with wider injury to the zygoma or frontoethmoidal complex (types III and IV, respectively). CT is important for diagnosis, though visual symptoms/enophthalmos may provide clues. Type I fractures can be treated conservatively or, if necessary, repaired with mesh through a frontoethmoid approach, whilst type II requires subciliary/transconjunctival incisions.
- **Lateral wall** fractures – usually associated with a zygoma fracture.
- **Orbital roof** fractures are rare and almost never occur in isolation in adults, usually occurring in the context of multiple fractures particularly with frontal sinus fractures. Urgent CT scan and neurosurgery consultation are needed; large displaced fractures will need to be reduced. In children, isolated fractures may occur as the frontal sinus is not well developed and cannot disperse the forces as effectively.
- Orbital floor fractures.
  - Surgery may be required to correct increased orbital volume/**enophthalmos**, **muscle entrapment** or ocular dystopia. There may be suspensory ligament and inferior rectus injury.
  - Access to the orbital floor is gained via lower lid, subciliary or transconjunctival incisions (with lateral canthotomy). The herniated tissue is carefully reduced and the orbital floor is reconstructed with **alloplastics** (Medpor, titanium mesh, silastic, Supramid) or bone. They have the same risk of early infection but alloplasts also have a 2% long-term risk of infection and late extrusion.

BLOW-OUT FRACTURE

This is a particular fracture pattern, with wall displacement away from the globe that increases orbital volume and thus causes enophthalmos (although in the acute phase, superimposed haemorrhage and oedema may cause exophthalmos).

- Indirect conduction of force along the bone vs. direct transmission by intraorbital contents (hydraulic mechanism). Bone recoils quicker than the soft tissue and thus may trap it.
- Blow-in fractures are rare and when wall displacement decreases orbital volume, exorbitism may result. There may be impingement on the recti, which can be tested for with the forced duction test.

Indications for surgery include

- **Floor defects** >2 cm² especially posterior to the globe equator.
- Low vertical position of globe (dystopia/ptosis).
- **Enophthalmos** may result from as little as 5 mm displacement of the orbital rim; good imaging is vital (Grant MP, *Clin Plast Surg*, 1997). Surgery requires good access with several incisions; reposition the rim before the internal walls and pay attention to soft tissue repair/re-attachment.
- **Muscle entrapment** is an absolute indication – early release (1 week, see below) aims to avoid ischaemia. However, the diagnosis is not always clear cut – **forced duction testing** (FDT) has a significant false-positive rate, and it is less reliable within the first week.
  - FDT – grab insertion of the inferior rectus after topical LA.
  - Diplopia does not equate to entrapment as it may be partly caused by oedema, muscle contusion or prolapse. Thus, it may be worthwhile waiting, particularly if FDT is negative.
    - Diplopia may also be due to prolapse (>5 mm downward displacement).
  - As some cases of entrapment may resolve spontaneously, surgery is **not** necessarily urgent.
    - Diplopia that lasts for >2 weeks is more likely to be due to entrapment.
    - Delaying treatment for >2 weeks is less likely to be successful. One-third of cases of diplopia will be permanent if untreated.
- The need to treat other fractures especially zygomatic.

IMAGING OF ORBITAL FRACTURES

CT is the mainstay investigation, particularly fine cut coronal views (which can be reconstructed from axial data in modern machines). They are particularly useful in visualising the orbital floor and can be used to estimate orbital volumes. Commonly used X-rays include OM, Waters' and Caldwell views (Figures 3.1 and 3.2), but these are rarely used in isolation.

- Medial orbital wall fractures are virtually undetectable on plain X-ray.
- Anterior orbital floor fractures may have a teardrop sign, but many of these can be treated conservatively – only the posterior floor fractures mandate treatment (for enophthalmos).
- Endoscopic evaluation – uncommon.

LINES OF DOLAN

- Line 1 (orbital line, from lateral to medial) – fractures of the lateral orbit or diastasis of the frontozygomatic suture, fracture of the orbital floor.
- Line 2 (zygomatic line) – fractures of the lateral orbit and zygomatic arch.
- Line 3 (maxillary line) – fractures of the lateral wall of maxillary sinus and zygomatic arch.

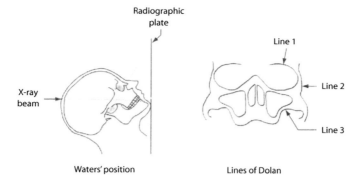

Radiographic plate

Line 1

Line 2

Line 3

X-ray beam

Waters' position

Lines of Dolan

Figure 3.1 Waters' view. The arrow shows the direction of the X-ray beam. Inclination brings the petrous bones below the floor of the maxillary sinus. This provides the single most comprehensive projection with good views of the maxilla, maxillary sinuses, zygoma (and arches), orbital rims and nasal bones. Lines of Dolan (see main text). Charles Alexander Waters (1888–1961), American radiologist.

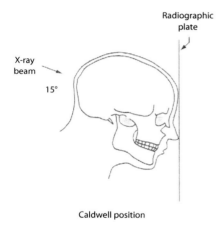

Radiographic plate

X-ray beam

15°

Caldwell position

Figure 3.2 Caldwell position. The arrow shows the direction of the beam. The inclination removes the petrous ridges from a view of the orbital structures and is thus useful for imaging fractures of the orbital margins, frontal bone and zygomaticofrontal sutures.

POST-OPERATIVE COMPLICATIONS

- **Persistent diplopia** – 10% have diplopia at presentation and up to half will become persistent (usually affecting upward gaze only). It may be due to entrapment of the inferior rectus muscle, but may be due to nerve/muscle injury or **scarring (i.e. unknown).** Persistent diplopia should be followed closely and a CT may be required.
- **Blindness** (0.3%) is thankfully rare. It may be due to bone fragments, haematoma or oedema impinging on the optic nerve or retinal detachment. Orbital exploration in the presence of globe rupture or hyphaema can exacerbate injury. Traumatic optic neuropathy is rare (1%–2%) and often goes undetected, as the mildest form may cause only slight colour blindness; steroids are often used (see below).
- **Ectropion** – typically due to scarring especially with subciliary incisions even though the (cutaneous) scar itself tends to heal well. Initial management includes

prevention with Frost sutures, eyecare, lid massage and taping; most cases resolve. A transconjunctival scar release or a skin graft may be necessary.
- **Enophthalmos is rare** (3%), but can be severe, particularly if it involves the posterior part of orbital cavity. Although it is often due to increased orbital volume, it can occur even after the fracture has been anatomically reduced, when it may be due to scarring, loss of ligament support, etc.
  - Anterior volume changes have little effect, whilst middle volume changes usually cause superior–inferior displacement.
  - Treat by osteotomy or augmentation of volume along with release of periorbital tissues; 1.5 mL of augmentation advances the globe 1 mm. Overcorrection is needed to compensate for the effects of perioperative swelling.

EYE INJURIES

Superior orbital fissure syndrome

- Structures passing through this fissure are cranial nerves III (also has some parasympathetics), IV and VI to extraocular muscles, V1 and ophthalmic veins. Fracture, oedema or haemorrhage causes pressure within the muscular cone formed by the recti.
- Symptoms include exorbitism, ophthalmoplegia, dilated pupil (due to loss of III parasympathetic constrictor tone leading to unopposed sympathetic dilator activity), ptosis (due to loss of sympathetic supply to Müller's muscle that travels with lacrimal branch) and anaesthesia in V1 territory.
- Fracture reduction may be needed with gradual recovery in weeks to months.

Orbital apex syndrome

Fractures through the optic canal with division of the optic nerve at the apex of the orbit may cause neuritis, papilloedema or blindness. Early steroid therapy may be indicated;

surgical decompression is increasingly popular in the context of fractures.

Traumatic optic neuropathy

This is the loss of vision without external or internal ophthalmoscopic evidence of eye injury – the optic atrophy appears weeks later and is usually said to be secondary to a direct globe injury, followed by retinal vascular occlusion, orbital compartment syndrome and injury to proximal neural structures. Treatment is usually conservative; the 1999 International Optic Nerve trauma study (Levin LA, *Ophthalmology*, 1999) demonstrated no clear benefit of high-dose steroids or optic canal decompression – there was an increase in acuity in 32%, 52% and 57% of surgery, steroid and observation groups, respectively, but it was non-randomised.

Sympathetic ophthalmia

The problem (an inflammatory response) affects both eyes and may cause complete blindness. The aetiology is unknown but may occur secondary to a penetrating eye injury or after intraocular surgery. Some speculate on a cell-mediated response (to melanin-containing structures from the retina) and prevention by enucleation of severely injured and sightless eyes within 2 weeks is suggested; evisceration is cosmetically more pleasing but may be less effective.

Traumatic carotid cavernous sinus fistula

A fracture may cause tears in vessels and formation of a fistula, which leads to proptosis, injection and chemosis. There may be an ocular bruit and a dilated ophthalmic vein on CT angiography. There may be embolic or ischaemic events (due to steal phenomenon). Some fistulae may close spontaneously, but others may need either carotid ligation or coil placement to obliterate the fistula.

IV. MAXILLARY FRACTURES

ANATOMY

The body of the maxilla contains the maxillary sinus that is fully formed by 15 years of age. The bone has four main processes: alveolar, frontal, zygomatic and palatine.

There are **four vertical pillars** of the face that transmit forces from the maxilla to the skull base and are the best areas for bony fixation:

- Nasomaxillary (canine) buttress – alveolar process of maxilla (opposite to the canine) to the frontal process of the maxilla and nasal bones, i.e. medial to the orbit
- Zygomatic buttress – alveolar process of the maxilla (opposite first molar tooth) to the zygomatic process of the frontal bone, i.e. lateral to the orbit
- Pterygomaxillary buttress – posterior body of the maxilla to the skull base via the sphenoid (including the pterygoid plates)
- Mandibular buttress – ascending ramus to the skull base via the temporo-mandibular joint (TMJ)

And **five horizontal buttresses**:

- Supra-orbital bar
- Infraorbital rim
- Zygomatic arch
- Palate
- Body of the mandible

LE FORT FRACTURE CLASSIFICATION

The existence of thick buttresses that are interspaced with thinner areas means that distinct patterns of fractures are seen.

Le Fort II is most common > I > III; Le Fort fractures rarely occur in isolation (Figure 3.3).

- **Le Fort I** – a horizontal fracture that separates the alveolar and palatine processes from the body of the maxilla. Note that the pterygoid plates are usually affected in Le Fort I fractures but are left intact in Le Fort I osteotomies (pterygomaxillary disjunction). There may be **anterior open bite** from posteroinferior displacement of the maxilla, which may or may not be clinically mobile.
- **Le Fort II** – a pyramidal fracture similar to I, but the fracture line passes through the zygomaticomaxillary suture/maxillary antrum, the orbital floor, medial orbital wall and across the nasofrontal area. It incorporates the nasal skeleton (nasal bones and septum) and the infraorbital foramen (nerve may be injured).

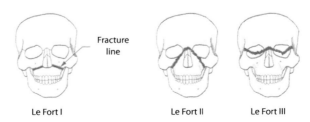

Le Fort I   Fracture line   Le Fort II   Le Fort III

Figure 3.3 Types of Le Fort fractures.

- Disruption of the medial canthal ligament, attached to the frontal process of the maxilla, may lead to telecanthus.
- There may be mobility at the nose, when manipulating the maxilla.
- **Le Fort III** – a transverse fracture that passes through the frontomaxillary junction, orbit and zygomaticofrontal (ZF) junction to separate the whole of the maxilla and mid-face from the skull base (craniofacial disjunction) with a 'free-floating' maxilla with mobility at the ZF suture and nasofrontal region.
  - There is an anterior open bite as for II and anaesthesia of maxillary teeth, which usually resolves.

CLINICAL PRESENTATION

Maxillary fractures usually present with **malocclusion**, malar flattening and loss of height. Mid-face fractures are often comminuted; some may be dentoalveolar only, involving a row of teeth with their supporting bone only. Particular examination points include

- **Bite/malocclusion.** This underlies the decision to operation.
  - Look for palatal fractures. Palatal fractures can be plated submucosally or top of the mucosa and removed 12 weeks later. Other options include intermolar wiring.
  - **Cracked tea-cup sign** – percussion of an upper tooth with an instrument may produce a distinctive note (compared with a solid metallic resonance) if a tooth is broken or if the maxilla is fractured. This should be used with caution as it may cause more damage.
- With one hand on the maxilla and nasal root, a floating palate **without nasal** movement is usually due to a Le Fort I fracture.
  - Cheek anaesthesia – usually Le Fort II.
- About one-third of Le Fort II/III fractures are complicated by CSF rhinorrhoea due to fractures of the naso-ethmoid area (**cribriform plate**, meaning like a sieve – Latin cribrum, not cribiform); 95% resolve within 3 weeks, but antibiotic prophylaxis of meningitis is advisable. Persistent leaks may need repair of the dural tear via craniofacial approach.

SURGICAL TREATMENT

Nasotracheal intubation will allow access to the lower mid-face and teeth, and facilitate the possible need for IMF; otherwise, a tracheostomy may be needed. The first step is to re-establish bite; if the mandible is also fractured, it is usually fixed first to provide a stable base. A superior gingival sulcus incision is used to expose the fracture line in a Le Fort I fracture – taking care to identify and preserve the infraorbital nerve; an additional subciliary incision exposes the infraorbital rim in Le Fort II fractures. In Le Fort III fractures, a bicoronal incision may be needed as an alternative to a combination of lateral brow, subciliary and/or nasofrontal incisions to fix the ZF and nasofrontal regions.

- Reduction
  - Rowe or Tessier disimpaction forceps are used to move the maxillary fragment, being watchful for haemorrhage from descending palatine arteries.
  - IMF may be needed to reduce fractures and restore/maintain occlusion.
- Fracture fixation
  - Intra-osseous wires or miniplates (1.5–2.0 mm) – aiming for four points of fixation (bilateral medial and lateral buttresses). Bone grafts may be needed to fill defects and restore height.
  - External fixation may be required in those requiring anterior traction, or cases with severe comminution, with concomitant fracture or dislocation of both condyles.

Complications include malocclusion, mal-/non-union or maxillary sinusitis. Le Fort III fractures may also be complicated by eye problems – blindness, epiphora, hypertelorism or CSF leak.

V. ZYGOMATIC FRACTURES

The zygoma contributes to the lateral orbital rim at its articulations with the sphenoid and frontal bones, and also contributes to the orbital floor where it articulates with the maxilla. Zygomatic fractures are tetraploid rather than 'tripod':

- Infraorbital rim, to the floor, often through the infraorbital foramen
- Lateral orbital wall – zygomaticofrontal suture
- Zygomaticomaxillary (ZM) buttress
- Zygomatic arch – usually at the thin part posterior to the zygomaticotemporal (ZT) suture

The articulations of the zygomatic bone with its neighbouring bones need to be assessed; high-energy injuries may cause comminution. The ZF suture is the strongest and is generally the last of the articulations to fracture completely – thus, as a simple rule, if it is disrupted, then ORIF is indicated. Undisplaced fractures may be treated conservatively (with regular re-evaluation); however, the fracture is usually unstable due to the pull of the masseter and the vast majority need fixation to avoid **late deformity** (malar flattening and face widening).

CLASSIFICATION – KNIGHT AND NORTH

This is one of the most commonly used systems.

- Undisplaced
- Arch fracture
- Depressed body fracture
- Depressed body fracture with medial rotation
- Depressed body fracture with lateral rotation
- Comminuted fracture

EXAMINATION

- Look.
  - Swelling, bruising and lateral conjunctival haemorrhage.
  - **Malar flattening** when viewed from above – the zygoma tends to be displaced inferiorly (and medially and posteriorly), which may lead to descent of the lateral canthus (and Whitnall's tubercle) and a **downsloping palpebral** fissure.
    - Facial widening
  - Dystopia.
  - There may be **enophthalmos** with an associated blow-out fracture.
- Feel – tenderness, fracture mobility and step-off. Infraorbital nerve **paraesthesia**. A significant amount of swelling often makes examination difficult.
- Move – trismus may be present.

IMAGING

- **Facial CT** – the basis of most operative decisions.
- X-rays
  - Submentovertex (SMV, for zygomatic arches).
  - Occipitomental (OM) views.
  - Reverse Waters is a 30° below horizontal AP with more bone magnification.

Zygomatic fractures should generally be fixed to optimise appearance as the bone is central to facial projection. Fixation would reduce facial widening and late displacement and late enophthalmos (3%); the masseter is a strong deforming force. Two-point fixation may create an axis, about which the zygoma can rotate under powerful contractions of masseter.

ACCESS TO THE ZYGOMA FOR ORIF

Closed reduction of displaced fractures (e.g. via a Gillies lift) may be suitable for a very selective set of patients, but is usually an uncommon option. However, there may be a resurgence with the greater availability of intraoperative CT (Rabie A, *J Craniofac Surg*, 2011), though without fixation stability can be uncertain. It is important to **avoid chewing** and thus masseter contraction in the early post-operative period. Incisions and dissection may cause numbness in the distribution of ZT and ZF nerves.

Severe high-energy injuries may need a coronal incision for greater exposure.

- **Lateral brow/upper lid incision** – access to the temporal process and supraorbital rim, i.e. ZF suture. It is the most important landmark to ensure accurate reduction.
- **Subciliary incision** – access to the sphenoid process (infraorbital rim) and arch. The skin incision is made 2 mm below the ciliary (lash) line.
  - Lid incisions offer easy access, but are usually avoided because of the obvious scar and the risk (albeit low) of lower lid oedema and retraction.
  - Transconjunctival incision.
- **Buccal sulcus incision** – access to the maxillary process to visualise the ZM buttress. The need/indications for fixation are somewhat controversial; bone grafting may be needed in complex and comminuted fractures.

ORIF COMPLICATIONS

- Early
  - Diplopia (usually resolves within 24 hours).
    - Note that monocular diplopia indicates an ocular problem and requires urgent attention.
  - Bleeding including retro-orbital haematoma.
  - Nerve injury.

- Late
  - The most common cause of post-reduction enophthalmos is inadequate fracture reduction.
  - Scars and cicatricial ectropion. Tissue descent and bony migration are more common with comminuted fractures; they may be reduced by periosteal suspension and fixation, respectively.
  - Plate infection, extrusion, migration, failure.
  - Bone healing problems – delayed, malunion, non-union.
  - Sinus problems.

GILLIES LIFT

This is the standard approach to **zygomatic arch fractures,** which cause mainly aesthetic problems with visible/palpable contour deformities (typically 'W'-shaped), with or without trismus.

- A 3 cm incision is made in the hairy temple; 4 cm superior to the zygomatic arch and 2–3 cm posterior to the temporal hairline (alternatively, 1 inch forward and 1–2 inches up from the top of tragus). The incision is angled so that it is perpendicular to the line of your instruments.
- The superficial temporal fascia (temporoparietal fascia) is continuous inferiorly with the SMAS and superiorly with the galea. The deep temporal fascia splits to encircle the zygoma; thus, access needs to be gained to the plane under this fascial layer. The muscle fibres should be visible through the incision.
- A Rowe's elevator is inserted and tunnelled deep to the zygomatic arch and a lifting action used to reduce fracture whilst the head is stabilised.
- It allows reduction only; fixation is usually unnecessary. A transoral approach has also been described (Keen approach; alternatively, a Carole Girard screw is useful for manipulating bone fragments).

- The same approach can be used to disimpact the zygoma in a zygomatic complex fracture, placing the elevator behind the anterior attachment of the arch behind the body of zygoma.

VI. MANDIBULAR FRACTURES

The mandible is fractured in more than half of all facial fractures (only nasal bone fractures are more common); mandibular fractures are three times more common than zygomatic fractures. Most fractures are open (into the mouth); fractures near the root of a tooth are also considered open. Antibiotics active against *Staphylococcus aureus* and anaerobes as well as antiseptic mouthwashes are recommended.

CLASSIFICATION ACCORDING TO ANATOMICAL LOCATION

Where the mandible tends to break depends in part on the nature/cause of the trauma, e.g. RTA, sport or assault – the relative frequencies of these often vary between different populations (see below). The most common sites of fracture are partly explained by **pre-existing areas of weakness** of the mandible.

- **Condyle** (30%–40%) – the condylar neck is thin; accounts for ~2/3 of fractures in those <10 years of age.
- Angle (20%) – the root of the wisdom tooth leads to a weak area. These injuries are often due to interpersonal violence.
- Parasymphysis (10%–15%) – often where the long canine root is lined up with the mental foramen (MF).
- The body fractures more often in the elderly as it thins due to resorption.
- Ramus and coronoid process fractures are rare – 3% and 2%, respectively.
- The mandible is in effect a 'ring bone', and whether it fractures in one place or two depends on how flexible or stiff the system is, respectively. As it is, the TMJs imbue some flexibility and thus there is an average of 1.5–1.8 fractures per mandible fracture. The 'second' fracture should be actively sought for/excluded.

- **Guardsman's fracture** – one of the commonest multiple fractures, is caused by a fall or blow to the middle of the chin resulting in bilateral condylar fractures and a para/symphyseal fracture. It is seen in the elderly, epileptics and occasionally in soldiers who faint on parade. The mandible may be retracted with an anterior open bite. Generally the symphysis is fixed along with only one condylar fracture after IMF is used to regain proper occlusion. IMF is left in place for 2 weeks to treat the other condylar fracture.

FRACTURE CLASS

- I – Teeth on both fragments
- II – Teeth on one fragment
- III – Edentulous

Class I fractures may be stable and treated with closed reduction/fixation, e.g. IMF, whilst class II (if displaced) and III fractures usually require open treatment due to less stability and support from the dentition.

Other classifications include open vs. closed, displaced vs. non-displaced, favourable vs. unfavourable and single vs. multiple.

MUSCLE ACTION ON THE MANDIBLE

Depending on the configuration of the fracture, muscle forces may act to distract or compress a fracture site.

Parasymphyseal fragment is

- Pulled down by geniohyoids
- Pulled down and laterally by the digastrics
- Pulled backwards by genioglossus

Body of the mandible is

- Pulled up by masseter
- Pulled up and backwards by temporalis
- Pulled backwards by the pterygoids

Unfavourable fractures (Figure 3.4) are those that are likely to become displaced due to muscle action on the fracture fragments. The angle, in particular, is a 'lever' area

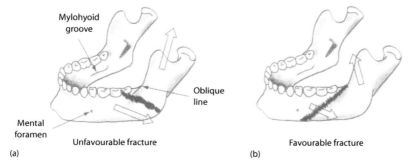

Figure 3.4 Mandibular fracture. (a) Unfavourable fracture. Displacement is likely. Upward arrow represents pull of the temporalis, masseter and medial pterygoid muscles, whilst the downward arrow represents the digastric and mylohyoid muscles. (b) Favourable fracture. Displacement is unlikely as muscle forces tend to compress fragments together.

biomechanically; this leads to **the highest complication rate**. The dynamic forces have important implications for the biomechanics:

- Compression forces along the inferior border
- Tensile forces (tending to pull apart) along the superior border
- Torsional forces between canines

EXAMINATION

Look for

- Pain, swelling, **intra-oral haematoma** – the mental nerve exits the MF below the first and second premolars, about halfway down in the dentulous mandible. The nerve may course a few millimetres below the MF before exiting; damage may cause paraesthesia to the teeth anterior to the forarmen as well as the skin of the lower lip and chin.
  - Mandibular fractures may often be 'open' into the oral cavity but rarely compound to the skin. Mouthwash and antibiotics are suggested.
- Assess excursion and occlusion
  - **Trismus** (normal 3.5–5 cm – first 2 cm is rotatory; the next 2 cm is a combination of rotation and translation and the final 2 cm is translation).
  - **Malocclusion**, open bite (inability to close the gap between jaws completely), missing/loose teeth.
- **Chin deviation** in those with a fractured condyle.

PALPATE

- Bimanual examination of mandible stability/mobility and focal tenderness, step deformities.
- The condyles can sometimes be palpated between fingers in the preauricular region and external auditory meatus (EAM).

X-RAYS

- **OPG** (Panorex) provides the most useful information in a single X-ray.
  - OPG requires a cooperative patient to sit up.
  - OPG only has an 86% sensitivity, i.e. it **may miss** fractures especially in the symphyseal region due to overlap with C-spine, and the condylar/subcondyle/ramus regions are not as well visualised. OPGs provide good alveolar ridge/dental detail.
- Mandibular series
  - PA (Caldwell) shows symphysis and angle.
  - Reversed Towne's offers good views of condyles.
  - Oblique view shows ramus to condyles.
- CT provides useful information on the mandible and teeth including those in the line of the fracture and easy visualisation of fracture displacement. It is useful for planning surgery.
  - 3D reconstruction

TREATMENT

- Patients should be nursed head up to reduce swelling.
- Antiseptic mouthwash.
- Oral antibiotics are recommended if the fracture is open, though the actual benefit is debatable; prompt surgical management is more important in the prevention of infection.
  - Role of perioperative antibiotics has proven benefit (Zallen RD, *J Oral Surg*, 1975).
  - Role of post-operative antibiotics unproven (Abubaker AO, *J Oral Maxillofac Surg*, 2001; Miles B, *J Oral Maxillofac Surg*, 2004).
  - 1 shot/day prophylaxis similar/better than 7 days (Andraesen JO, *J Oral Maxillofac Surg*, 2006).

The choice of treatment depends in part on several factors including patient age, site of fracture and the state of the dentition. Patients with maxillofacial injuries sustained after high-velocity trauma will often have other major injuries including neurosurgical damage causing coma. There has been a tendency to delay treatment of facial fractures in these multiply injured patients, but it seems that the perceived advantages of delay have been inappropriately emphasised. Early definitive surgical management poses no additional risks yet results in better function and aesthetics. It is difficult to be accurate with the (neurological/neurosurgical) prognosis early on, but for patients with coma of duration >1 week, ¼ die, ¼ are disabled and the remainder return to useful work. In particular, flaccidity and persistently raised ICP are poor prognostic factors.

Most fractures require some form of reduction and immobilisation, but some can be treated **conservatively** (soft diet, etc.) – checking for displacement with repeat imaging 2 weeks later (when healing will not be evident):

- Undisplaced fractures including the condyle
- Greenstick fractures
- Normal occlusion with minimal trismus

The choice of surgery

- **Closed treatment** with IMF is suitable for most condyle, coronoid and ramus fractures.
- **ORIF** is recommended for displaced, unstable fractures (particularly those of the **angle to symphyseal area**).

Airway or bleeding issues aside, most cases of mandibular fracture are **not urgent.** Whilst it was often thought that fractures should be fixed somewhat urgently, e.g. within 12 hours (Champy) or at least within a few days, a literature review by Ellis (*Oral Maxillofac Clin North Am*, 2009) found no evidence to suggest that delay increases complications. Operating early (<48 hours) may reduce the infection rate, but otherwise there is little difference when delayed for 1–2 weeks, though fractures in the young heal quicker.

Sometimes delay is due to practical concerns – it is often not possible to arrange the necessary investigations and the operating time before the swelling becomes significant; consequently, surgery may need to be delayed until the swelling settles.

CLOSED TREATMENT

Intermaxillary fixation (IMF) is regarded as non-rigid fixation. It is usually not used by itself except for condylar fractures (see below); it can be used to stabilise dentoalveolar fractures. However, it is a significant undertaking for the patient: it requires meticulous oral hygiene and a liquid diet for the duration. Some technical tips are as follows:

- Prestretch wires.
- Stop turning when a secondary twist develops or it will break.
- Molar to molar is sufficient.

    Complications include

- Damage to gums and teeth, which may lead to loosening; avoid using incisors over a long period. In children, piriform rim and circummandibular wiring are alternatives to arch bars and IMF screws. In edentulous patients, gunning splints can be used, held in place with wires passed around the mandible and through the maxillary sinus.
    - Fracture deviation – there is a tendency to twist fragments towards the tongue.
    - Occlusion should be checked once or twice a week, changing to elastics as necessary.
- Airway problems are unusual, but wire cutters should be kept by the patient, particularly just after surgery.
- Healing will take about 4–6 weeks, but this needs to be balanced against the negative effects on TMJ function; there is a trend to use IMF for shorter periods.

OPEN TREATMENT

ORIF allows direct visualisation, for precise fracture reduction and the best restoration of occlusion. Most importantly, it allows early mobilisation that reduces TMJ stiffness.

   IMF may be applied first to aid restoration of occlusion and definitive fixation (see below). At the end of the procedure, the occlusion is reassessed, and depending on the result, the IMF can be removed or kept. Gear (*J Oral Maxillofac Surg*, 2005) actually found that experienced surgeons are more likely to dispense with IMF before ORIF.

   There are two main systems for definitive fixation in use:

- **Rigid fixation** (as espoused by the Association for Osteosynthesis/Association for the Study of Internal Fixation [AO/ASIF] school, i.e. AO technique, which is popular in the United States) to produce **primary bone healing** under absolute stability can be achieved by
    - **Interfragmentary compression plates** (with slight inclines built into the screw holes) – a small tension band plate with monocortical screws on the alveolar border neutralises tensile forces, whilst the larger (2.4 or thicker) inferior border stabilisation plate with bicortical screws neutralises compression and torsion stresses. They should be overcontoured slightly to avoid distraction on other surface with dynamic compression plates, which may be a bit

tricky. Complications of infection and malocclusion are more common than miniplates, and there is more stress shielding.
    - **Reconstruction plates** – locking screws to the plate rather than compressing bone to the plate. This is a load bearing (as opposed to load sharing) fixation system; it is desirable in situations such as comminuted fractures, bilateral fractures or fractures with loss of continuity.
    - **Lag screws** (two) can be used for oblique fractures of the para/symphyseal region, but the fracture needs to be precisely reduced first. It is very effective with the minimal amount of implant material; however, it is an exacting technique and not for the occasional operator.
- **Adaptive systems/monocortical miniplates (Michelet FX, *J Oral Maxillofac Surg*, 1967; Champy M, *Zahn Mund Kieferheilkd Zentralbl*, 1975).** The underlying concept is that only tensile stress (stress leading to expansion) is harmful to fracture healing; excessive mobility will lead to bone resorption and ingrowth of fibrous tissue. It is technically less demanding, quicker and cheaper. Monocortical fixation reduces the risk of root damage, particularly in children. They are classed as **semi-rigid** – rigid fixation is generally not needed in facial fractures; functional fixation/stability is sufficient. It is popular in Europe and Australasia.
    - **Concept of ideal lines of osteosynthesis (~internal fixation):**
        - Two plates anterior to the MF to stabilise against complex muscle pull – larger inferior and smaller superior plates, 4–5 mm apart.
        - One plate at the angle that must be on the upper border (oblique line) since this is the tension side of the fracture that tends to pull open. Many actually use a dual miniplate technique (superior and inferior) at the angle but still call it 'Champy'.
    - More experienced surgeons (performing >10 a year) tend to move away from AO/ASIF to Champy (Gear AJ, *J Oral Maxillofac Surg*, 2005).
    - The major complication rate with miniplates is lower than rigid fixation, whilst minor complications such as screw/plate failure may be higher. It is important to avoid excessive periosteal stripping, but bony stability is always the priority; careful cooling during drilling is advised to reduce bone necrosis and screw loosening.
- **In practice, successful fixation is probably more related to operator technique and bone quality than the plating system per se.** Proper stable fixation is important to allow healing; excessive mobility leads to resorption and fibrosis, and in the presence of metalwork, more resorption and infection.

   Resorbable plates (poly-L-glactic acid, PLLA) are available but have a limited shelf-life, cost more and have a higher profile than titanium plates, with an increased risk of erosion (newer plates are slimmer). They may be considered for use in children and for mid-face fractures in particular. A Cochrane review of their use in orthognathic surgery showed no statistically significant difference in post-operative discomfort, level of patient satisfaction, plate exposure or infection for fixation using either titanium or resorbable materials. How this translates to their use in fractures is unclear. In particular, there is concern regarding their sturdiness for use in mandibular fractures, though there is an increasing body of literature supporting their use (Ongodia D, *J Maxillofac Oral Surg*, 2014; Lim HY, *J Korean Assoc Oral Maxillofac Surg*, 2014). Potential complications included infection (~9%), inflammatory reactions and partial resorption.

COMPLICATIONS

The mandible is the **only articulating** skull bone, and this means that complications are more like to arise in mandibular fractures compared to other facial fractures. In particular, >¼ of the complications occur with angle fractures.

- Infection (6%) is the most common complication and may lead to non-union, delayed union (3%) and pseudoarthrosis. Good fixation is the best protection against infection.
- Nerve injury (2%–8%), especially the IAN.
- Ankylosis due to excessive immobilisation; arthroplasty or joint replacement may be needed.
- Plate removal (5%–10%); the most common indication is infection followed by exposure and 'discomfort', i.e. partly subjective, and in one study, one-third of plates were removed for this reason.

CONDYLAR FRACTURE

Condylar fractures are relatively common; restoring occlusion and maintaining TMJ function are the main aims of treatment.

Selected fractures can be adequately treated by conservative means; a simple protocol may be as follows, if there is:

- **No malocclusion** – soft diet and analgesia (25%) observe for developing malocclusion, which then requires IMF (with elastics, see below).
- **Malocclusion** – closed reduction (IMF, ~50%) except for lateral **anterior open bite**, which probably requires ORIF, especially if **displaced**, if bilateral or if there are panfacial fractures (see below).

Those who have ORIF will usually have a brief period of IMF followed by early mobilisation (7–10 days). In general, open treatment results in good alignment, but surgery is often regarded as being difficult – the limited access, the risk of facial nerve injury and the small fracture fragments make surgery challenging. **Joint stiffness is actually more common with ORIF**.

A comparison of open vs. closed treatment in 2002 found no overall functional difference, though patients who had open treatment tended to have more severe injury and more surgical complications. Closed treatment results in good movement but poor alignment; in particular, there may be shortened height with jaw deviation on mouth opening. Although maximal mouth opening tends to be similar in the medium to long term, those who had closed treatment had more problems with **late malocclusion** (anterior open bite). Consequently, there has been a recent trend to move away from conservative treatment.

The main issues/complications with condylar fractures are

- Malocclusion (usually contralateral posterior open bite, whilst bilateral fractures may cause anterior open bite)
- Deviation of chin with mouth opening
- TMJ ankyloses, trismus

CLOSED TREATMENT

IMF for 2 weeks or so is the current trend (definitely no more than 2 weeks in children). Controlled mobilisation at 2 weeks can be considered if the fracture geometry is favourable:

- 2 weeks of elastics to pull the mandible up and forward, with jaw of range of motion training and night-time elastics. A shorter wait is suggested for children ~7–10 days; the condyle is vascular and prone to burst-type injuries rather than fracture, with ankylosis and growth disturbances because of the growth centre in condyle as potential consequences.
- Complications include ankylosis (that often follows intra-articular fractures with haemorrhage leading to fibrosis), shortening and malocclusion that may need subsequent surgery.

OPEN REDUCTION

Muscle relaxation may facilitate surgery. Routes of access include the following:

- **Preauricular/transparotid** – allows direct visualisation of condyle but there is limited access for fixation. Rarely used alone – high fractures of the condyle/ramus are usually approached via a Risdon incision combined with a preauricular incision.
- **Submandibular/Risdon** – good for low subcondylar fractures, but poor access to medially displaced fractures.
- **Retromandibular** – good access to inferior condyle/ramus.
- **Endoscopic**.

The absolute indications for ORIF were described by Zide (1983 and modified in 1989).

- **Inability to maintain occlusion** with 2 weeks of IMF
- Dislocation into middle cranial fossa or EAM
- Lateral extracapsular displacement
- Open joint with foreign body or gross contamination

In practice, the relative indications for surgery depend on the preference of the individual surgeons, and additional indications often quoted include

- Where IMF is contraindicated, e.g. head-injured patients/mental retardation and unable to tolerate/cooperate with IMF, or where IMF is not possible:
  - Bilateral fractures, particularly in those with no dentition for IMF
  - Bilateral fractures with comminuted mid-facial fractures
  - Bilateral fractures with associated orthognathic problems
- Severe shortening, angulation or lateral displacement of >30° with severe malocclusion.
- Patient has panfacial fractures that require open fixation to re-establish vertical height.
- Low fractures are candidates for surgery because of reasonable access.
- It is often said that if the fragment is large enough to fit two screws, then operate. Placing only one screw leads to hinge motion.

POST FRACTURE REHABILITATION IS IMPORTANT

In all cases – conservative treatment, IMF or ORIF, early active ROM exercises are needed to rehabilitate the TMJ. Physiotherapy is important in recovering joint function; the patient is asked to practice in front of a mirror – stretching exercises include active opening and lateral excursions, progressing to active and digitally assisted jaw levering. Stacking wooden tongue depressors can be useful to increase the range of mouth opening; alternatives include the Therabite® device.

- Openly fixed fractures – move as comfort allows
- Closed unilateral – single class II elastic band, i.e. upper canine back downwards to first molar/second premolar
- Closed bilateral – heavy elastic bands for 2 weeks

TEETH IN FACIAL FRACTURES

Nomenclature

Position:

- 'Mesial' describes the position towards the central incisors, i.e. towards the midline.
- 'Distal' describes the position away from the midline.

Surfaces of a tooth:

- Buccal vs. lingual
- Occlusal vs. apical

Dental involvement

The management of teeth that have been exposed/involved in fractures has long been debated. Reasons for removal of a tooth during ORIF include

- Grossly mobile/complete displacement from socket
- Root fracture or exposed at apices, lack of support (bone and gum) in socket
- Pre-existing issues, e.g. periodontal disease, evidence of periapical lucency
- Functionless tooth, i.e. absence opposing tooth

Generally, it has become less of a concern and a tooth can usually be retained if it is otherwise healthy; **the repair fixation is stable and prophylactic antibiotics given**, as long as one accepts the increased risk of complications, e.g. plate removal.

EDENTULOUS FRACTURES

The most common site for fractures in edentulous patients lies in the body near the angle – there is a pivot at the angle with no teeth to buffer the impact. The management of (mandibular) fractures in this group has its own set of challenges.

- Definition
  - The risk of complications increases with the degree of atrophy especially if <**10 mm** tall; there is little cancellous bone and minimal potential for healing.
- The lack of teeth compromises the accuracy of reduction.

TREATMENT

- Stable fractures can be treated conservatively (soft diet), whilst those with minimal displacement can be managed with closed reduction with splints and dentures.
- For open treatment, circumferential/circummandibular wiring is usually the technique of choice.
  - Bone grafts may be needed (primary or secondary).
  - Reconstruction plates may be needed in more complex fractures, e.g. those with multiple segments.

FRACTURES IN CHILDREN

Paediatric facial fractures are fairly uncommon. They are more likely to be greenstick whilst condylar fractures are often treated conservatively with analgesia and soft diet. Fractures that require reduction should be operated on quickly as they can become fixed within a week.

CAUTIONS IN CHILDREN

- IMF is often not stable enough (mixed dentition with missing teeth, small teeth).
- Mini/micro-plates need to be used cautiously – screws may disrupt permanent tooth buds.
- Absorbable plates may be considered (see above). Minor degrees of imperfect restoration of occlusion tends to self-correct over ~2 years.

VII. NASAL AND NASO-ETHMOID FRACTURES

NASAL FRACTURES

These are the commonest facial fractures; the nose is a prominent feature and a frequent recipient of trauma due to either interpersonal violence or personal injuries such as falls, sports or RTA. The nasal bones usually fracture in their lower half where the bone is thinner. Experiments by Clark in 1970 showed that the nasal bones are more likely to break (i.e. less force required) from a lateral blow than a frontal blow. Numbness at the tip of the nose indicates anterior ethmoidal nerve injury. Diagnosis may be difficult if the patient presents whilst tissues are oedematous. It is important to rule out a nasoorbitoethmoid (NOE) fracture.

> **Stranc and Robertson classification** of lateral injuries (relating to increasing forces) (Stranc MF, Robertson GA, *Ann Plast Surg*, 1979):

- Plane I – **only the ipsilateral bone**, with a depression usually at the junction of the upper two-thirds and lower one-third (fracture site in 80%).
- Plane II – **ipsilateral depression with contralateral nasal outfractured** and/or impacted into the frontal process of maxilla.
- Plane III – forces sufficient to fracture the frontal process of maxilla and lacrimal bone with possible lacrimal duct injury. There may be multiple fragments.

Manipulation under anaesthetic (MUA) should be performed within 2 weeks:

- Asch forceps for correction of septal deviation.
- Walsham forceps for in-/out-fracture of nasal bones, release/disimpact.
  Post-operatively:
  - Nasal packs may be used to splint fracture fragments and septum.
  - Nasal POP/splint used to maintain position after reduction of fracture.
  - Late correction will need formal rhinoplasty; secondary reconstruction should be delayed for at least 6 months.

NOE FRACTURES

These fractures involve the area between the medial canthi (Figure 3.5).

- **Telecanthus** occurs as the MCTs are displaced laterally/rupture – **elicit with bowstring test.** It may not be evident in acute phase.
  - Normal intercanthal distances:
    - Male 28 ± 4 mm
    - Female 25 ± 3 mm
- Loss of dorsal nasal projection (saddle nose), with periorbital oedema and ecchymosis.

- **Lower orbital rim step-off** – the medial segment is lower due to the fragments sinking under gravity (compare this with zygomatic fractures where lateral segment is pulled down by the masseter).
- Enophthalmos, +/– diplopia.
- Subconjunctival haemorrhage.

Markowitz classification based on central fragment bearing MCT:

- Type I – single central fragment without MCT disruption
- Type II – comminuted central fragment without MCT disruption
- Type III – severely comminuted with disruption of MCT

MANAGEMENT

It is a difficult fracture to repair and you only really get one good chance; it is difficult to revise subsequently. It is important to reconstruct the intercanthal relationship as well as the nasal dorsal projection and internal orbital structures.

- Access via laceration, coronal flap (best) or medial orbital (Lynch) incision. Upper buccal incision and subciliary/transconjunctival incisions may also be needed.
- Fracture stabilisation with miniplates if possible.
  - MCT reconstruction with **transnasal wiring** (transnasal canthopexy). Type III fractures often need bone grafts.
  - **Calvarial cantilever bone graft** for nasal dorsum.
- Redrape soft tissues paying particular attention to the nasoorbital valley.
- The nasolacrimal system should be inspected for damage and managed appropriately.

IX. SOFT TISSUE FACIAL INJURIES

SIMPLE LACERATIONS INVOLVING SKIN ONLY

Direct pressure is the preferred method of controlling bleeding in the ED; 'blind' clamping is discouraged, as it may damage important structures.

- Irrigation of the wound with copious amounts of saline is a vital step and should be performed as soon as possible; its importance is often underestimated and omitted by emergency staff.
- High-pressure irrigation has been shown to be more effective in reducing bacterial numbers than low-pressure irrigation, but it may increase tissue damage; using a 20–50 mL syringe with a 16–19 G cannula is sufficient in most cases. Antiseptics such as chlorhexidine are not necessary except perhaps in grossly contaminated wounds and may actually damage viable tissues.
- It is preferable to close wounds within 6 hours, but the good vascularity of facial soft tissue means that a slight delay is still acceptable (up to 24 hours), as long as they

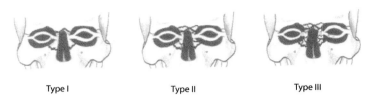

Figure 3.5 Types of naso-ethmoid fractures.

have been cleaned (see above). Most 'civilian' wounds can be closed after debridement with the exception of delayed presentation, bites, crush/avulsions and those with impaired wound healing.

WOUND CLOSURE

Debride skin sparingly; even 'questionable'-looking tissue may still heal in the face and hands due to the good blood supply, but trim grossly irregular or 'shelved' edges. Conservative debridement is particularly important around the lip, commissures, eyelid and distal nose where defects may be difficult to reconstruct.

- Abrasions are superficial wounds and will heal quickly, but need to be scrubbed thoroughly to avoid permanent **traumatic tattooing** that would be difficult to treat subsequently.
- Meticulous closure of lacerations in layers – deeper absorbable sutures should allow skin closure with precise apposition without tension – use anatomic landmarks to aid proper alignment.
  - Regional blockade is preferred to direct/local infiltration of LA to reduce distortion.
- With tissue loss, complex flaps are not indicated at the initial stage due to unreliable survival of flaps and wound edges especially in crush/avulsion injuries.
  - Suture displaced tissues into their normal positions (Gillies and Millard principle) whilst avoiding distortion; undermining tends to be less useful than you think, as tissue mobility depends mostly on the tissue redundancy.
  - Areas that cannot be closed primarily are most appropriately treated with skin grafts or dressings; areas with residual dermis may be given a chance to heal.
- Avulsion-type injuries are more problematic with damage to the microvasculature that may not be immediately evident and if sutured back into place may lead to necrosis. In the face and hands, larger areas should be revascularised (microsurgery) if at all possible; in other areas, harvesting the skin from the flap to be used as skin grafts may be considered before the tissue dies.

The wound is waterproof after 48 hours. Clean the wound several times a day rather than allow clots/crusts to form; the value of antimicrobial ointments in clean incised wounds is not proven but is a common practice.

- Antibiotics are not needed unless the wound is contaminated or grossly infected; a lower threshold is sensible in those with immunosuppression, e.g. those taking steroids or in diabetics. Prophylaxis has been shown to be effective (Cochrane review) at reducing infections in dog, cat and human bites with Augmentin being adequate in most cases.
- Sutures should be removed early (after 5 days for the face, after 3–4 days for the eyelids).

Alternatives to sutures include the following:

- **Tissue adhesives** (cyanoacrylates such as Histoacryl® or Dermabond®) are useful, particularly in children, but it is important not to get the glue into the wound, which is less about its minimal cytotoxicity and more about potential tattooing of the blue indicator dye. Histoacryl® is N-2-butylcyanoacrylate and sets after 30 seconds. Several studies have demonstrated efficacy, e.g. a controlled study with paediatric facial lacerations with low tension (Quinn JV, *Ann Emerg Med*, 1993).
  - Some say that Histoacryl is stronger than Dermabond (octylcyanoacrylate), though this is disputed. A Cochrane review (Farion KJ, *Cochrane Database Syst Rev*, 2002) found no differences between the two in clinical use; with regards to dehiscence, glues have a **number needed to harm** (NNH) of 40, i.e. 1 out of 40 wounds closed with glue will dehisce, a 2.4% additional risk compared to standard closure.
- **Steristrips.** Avoid traction when applying the strips (applies to adhesive dressings in general); otherwise, erythema (may be mistaken for 'allergy') or blistering may occur, particularly in the elderly.
  - Some emphasise that strips should be touching/ slightly overlapping so that even distribution of force occurs across the incision as fibroblast activity is sensitive to direction of stresses (Eastwood M, *Proc Inst Mech Eng H J Eng Med*, 1998).
  - Others suggest that strips should be placed along, rather than perpendicular to, the incision. This reduces the number of strips needed, and also reduces the risk of pulling the wound apart when removing them.

- Steristrips are not as strong as sutures or glue, and come off easily when wet and are thus not suited for lacerations around the mouth.
- Maximal wound strength (80%) is reached at 8 weeks, but at the time of suture removal, it is only 5%–10% of normal skin strength. Some recommend steristrip support after suture removal, but the actual efficacy is unknown.

DEEPER LACERATIONS

Knowledge of the underlying anatomy is invaluable for the plastic surgeon dealing with trauma:

- Cut muscle bellies can be apposed with a modified Kessler or similar stitch without excessive tension that would otherwise strangulate the tissues or 'cut through'. Muscle healing with subnormal but useful function has been demonstrated in animal models: segments that are denervated undergo variable atrophy and fibrosis, with 50% tension and 80% shortening at 12 weeks after total transection, but this is much better than no repair.
- The parotid duct lies along the middle third of a line joining the tragus to the midpoint of the philtrum; it travels with the buccal branch of the facial nerve (which is often damaged as well) and the transverse facial artery. It pierces the buccinator at the upper third molar and enters the oral cavity at upper second. In cases of suspected duct trauma, the duct can be cannulated for injection of air or methylene blue (may stain tissues); alternatively, use a thick prolene suture. The duct should be repaired with fine sutures (8'0 or 9'0) over a stent that is either looped out of the mouth, taped to the face or cut short and secured intra-orally (which is as difficult as it sounds). The stent is left in place for 5–7 days. If the duct cannot be repaired
  - Stump ligation is recommended for proximal injuries. This will lead to temporary painful swelling with a small risk of infection; the gland atrophies after a couple of weeks. In general, the use of vein grafts to reconstruct the duct has been unsuccessful.
  - In distal transection, the duct stump can be diverted to another part of the oral cavity, but it is a difficult and often unrewarding procedure.
- Isolated parenchymal lacerations can be repaired; pressure dressings and glycopyrrolate can be used if needed. Some say that parenchymal lacerations do not need to be sutured – salivary fistulae are rare and tend to close conservatively within a few days/weeks.

B. HEAD AND NECK MALIGNANCY

The AJCC divides head and neck cancers into the following categories:

- Lip and oral cavity
- Pharynx
- Larynx
- Paranasal sinus
- Salivary gland
- Thyroid
- Oesophagus

Head and neck cancers form 7% of all cancers; one-third of these patients will die from their tumours whilst one-fifth will have synchronous tumours. It occurs in males more frequently; smoking and alcohol increase the risk of squamous cell carcinomas (SCCs) by up to 15 times.

I. PREMALIGNANT CONDITIONS

These are skin/mucosal lesions that are not malignant but may become malignant.

LEUKOPLAKIA

Schwimmer first used this term in 1877, though Paget was the first to recognise the malignant potential of the lesion. Oral lesions are strongly associated with smoking and betel nut chewing, less so with intra-oral sepsis (caries), drinking spirits and chronic irritation (which is less important now and the classic chronic cheek bite lesion does not transform). In other words, causes are multifactorial. Truly idiopathic leukoplakia may be more at risk of malignant change. It affects males twice as frequently.

The lesions of leukoplakia are typically painless white-grey verrucoid plaques (though quite variable), mostly found in the oral cavity. There are three stages:

- Earliest – non-palpable, with white slightly translucent discolouration
- Later – slightly elevated opaque white lesions with granular texture.
- May progress to thick white lesions with induration and fissuring.
  - Ulceration is suggestive of invasive SCC.

The clinical diagnosis is one by exclusion (i.e. exclude candidiasis, lichen planus, biting/friction, lupus, etc.); it is not a specific disease entity – rather it is a keratotic white plaque that cannot be scraped off and cannot be given another specific diagnostic name. The term carries no histological definition but has classical histological features of hyperkeratosis, parakeratosis (thickened keratin layer containing nuclear remnants) and acanthosis (epidermal hyperplasia). **Dysplasia is not a feature** of simple leukoplakia but is more likely to be found in erythroplakia.

About 5%–20% undergo malignant transformation into aggressive SCCs; though some studies say that it is as low as 0.6%. The risk is closely related to the cellular appearance (see above). The highest risk seems to be associated with lesions that are long-standing, verrucous and have erosion/ulceration.

Erythroplakia has a 50% risk of transformation and can be considered as an in situ SCC. It tends to affects the 'sump' areas of the oral cavity. There are two main types:

- Uniform white plaques (homogeneous) with low malignant potential.

- Verrucous leukoplakia with more malignant potential.
  - Some are mixed white and red (speckled or erythroleukoplakia).
- 'Hairy' leukoplakia is an unusual form seen mostly in HIV-positive patients. It is associated with opportunistic Epstein–Barr virus (EBV) infection and seems to have a very low risk of malignant transformation with a tendency to spontaneous resolution, particularly when the underlying disease is treated. There are some trials with antiviral therapy, podophyllin, tretinoin and cryotherapy.

TREATMENT

Biopsy, repeated as necessary being wary of sampling error.

- Excision if precancer/dysplasia or cancer detected.
  - CO_2 laser or surgery.
- Alternatively, if there is no dysplasia, etc. or there is hyperkeratosis only, treat by avoiding precipitating factors; many may regress if the source is removed especially smoking (over half disappear within 1 year).
- **A Cochrane review (Lodi G, *Cochrane Database Syst Rev*, 2016)** assessed 14 RCTs on the subject of treating leukoplakia to avoid cancer. Treatment with beta-carotene, lycopene, vitamin A or retinoids was successful, but high rates of relapse were common. Retinoids had significant side effects. The overall quality of the evidence was poor, with little/no consideration of the effects of stopping high risk activities. The conclusion was that, to date, there are no effective treatments in preventing malignant transformation of leukoplakia.

II. STAGING

STAGING

The TMN (tumour, metastases, nodes) classification system is more useful than the overall stage in most instances as the latter is much broader, e.g. T3N0 and T1N1 are both stage III but are very different clinically.

TMN CLASSIFICATION SYSTEM

Basic staging system

Tumour
- TX – primary tumour cannot be assessed
- T0 – no evidence of primary tumour
- Tis – carcinoma in situ
- T1, T2, T3 and T4 – increasing size and extent of primary tumour

Nodes
- NX – regional nodes cannot be assessed.
- N0 – no evidence of regional lymph node involvement.
- N1 – regional lymph node involvement.

Metastasis
- MX – distant metastasis cannot be assessed.
- M0 – no evidence of distant metastases.
- M1 – distant metastases.

STAGING OF INTRA-ORAL CANCERS

This is a 'typical' system.

Tumour
- T1 – <2 cm
- T2 – 2–4 cm
- T3 – >4 cm
- T4 – extension to bone, muscle (including extrinsic muscle of tongue), skin, neck, etc.

Nodes
- N0 – no evidence of regional lymph node involvement
- N1 – mobile ipsilateral node <3 cm
- N2
  - N2a – ipsilateral node 3–6 cm
  - N2b – multiple ipsilateral nodes
  - N2c – contralateral or bilateral nodes
- N3
  - Any node >6 cm
  - Fixed nodes

Metastasis
- M0 – no evidence of distant metastases
- M1 – distant metastases

There is also the distinction between the clinical TNM (cTNM) before treatment, based on examination and investigations, and the pTNM – the pathological or post-surgical TNM, which adds information from surgery and pathological examination. This is the dual classification with cTNM guiding treatment whilst pTNM helps with prognosis; when TNM is used without a prefix, it implies the clinical classification.

- m = multiple tumours – the tumour with the highest T is classified with the multiplicity or the total number of primary tumours is indicated in parentheses, e.g. T2(m) or T2(5).
- y = following multimodal/neoadjuvant therapy.
- r = recurrent tumour when reclassified after a disease-free interval.
- a = autopsy findings.

OVERALL STAGING (ALSO 'ROMAN NUMERAL STAGING')

- Carcinoma in situ is stage 0.
- In the absence of metastasis, overall stage follows tumour stage; T1 is stage I whilst T4 is stage IV.
- Any nodal involvement is at least stage III – N1 is stage III when the tumour is not T4, and there are no distant metastases, whilst N2 or above is stage IV.
- Any distant metastasis is stage IV.

Tumours should not be restaged; if a patient without distant metastasis at presentation and before treatment then shows evidence of distant spread, then it does not change from M0 to M1.

WORK-UP OF PATIENTS WITH HEAD AND NECK CANCER

- Complete examination of head and neck – 20% have synchronous tumours especially in the larynx and nasopharynx.
- Biopsy lesion.
- Panendoscopy – DL, rigid bronchoscopy and rigid oesophagoscopy.
  - Toluidine blue said to stain malignant lesions selectively.
- Metastatic work-up – CXR/CT, basic blood tests including liver function tests and calcium. Others depending on symptoms.
- Imaging.
  - **CT for primary tumour and nodes**, chest and liver.
  - MRI has similar accuracy for nodes; useful for detecting skull base involvement or neural invasion.
  - PET can improve accuracy of staging but not yet standard of care.

III. RECONSTRUCTION

RECONSTRUCTIVE OPTIONS

- Direct closure – is rarely possible except in the smallest lesions.
- Split skin grafts can be used to resurface hard palate defects, but are not suitable for most defects.

LOCAL FLAPS

- **Mucosal flaps**
- **Tongue flaps**
- **Nasolabial flaps** are useful for reconstruction of moderate defects of the FOM, ventral surface of the tongue and oral commissure but are more difficult in the dentate. They usually require a two-stage technique with division of the pedicle after 3–4 weeks; de-epithelialising a portion of the flap in order to make it a one-stage procedure may compromise flap viability. They can be inferiorly or superiorly based, and can be used bilaterally (Varghese BT, *Br J Plast Surg*, 2001).
- **Submental flaps** (Martin D, *Plast Reconstr Surg*, 1993) are gaining popularity as an option for intra-oral reconstruction providing thin pliable tissue pedicled on the submental branch of the facial artery. There are some oncological concerns with use in cases of oral cancer; it should be avoided in those with clinically advanced neck disease.

- **Buccal fat pad** (Chakrabarti J, *Indian J Plast Surg*, 2009) lies between the buccinator and masseter and has an average thickness of 6 mm. The fat 'flap' is usually pedicled taking care to avoid excessive stretch to preserve the diffuse plexus; there are multiple feeding vessels from maxillary, transverse facial/superficial temporal and facial arteries in the subcapsular plexus. It may be an option for coverage of defects of 4–5 cm^2 of the buccal mucosa, maxilla and RMT; the fat epithelialises over 3–5 weeks with some evidence that the fat fibroses. It can be harvested via the resection defect or a superior sulcus incision around the second upper molar. It is contraindicated in large, distant defects, or in the presence of exposed bone or irradiated tissues.
- **FAMM flap** (facial artery musculomucosal flap; Pribaz J, *Plast Reconstr Surg*, 1992) is an axial flap that includes the buccinator muscle that lies between the artery and the mucosa.
  - The flap can be superiorly based (retrograde flow) or inferiorly based. The facial vein is not necessarily captured; drainage relies on a submucosal plexus and the base should be made wide enough (>2 cm).
  - It can be used for small to medium oral cavity defects; it is often used for palatal fistula, which most often occurs at the hard–soft palate junction, after repair of wide/bilateral CL/P.

PEDICLED FLAPS

- **Pectoralis major (PM) myocutaneous flap.** It is useful for large volume defects, but the donor defect is significant. Painful chest movement may promote chest infection/basal atelectasis.
- **Latissimus dorsi (LD) myocutaneous flap.** This is also a large volume flap that is reliable and safe but usually involves turning the patient at least once during surgery.

FREE FLAPS

Free flaps allow flexibility and variability in design including chimeric flaps with multiple components.

- For coverage, thin fascial flaps such as the RFF, ALT or medial sural artery perforator (MSAP) flaps are better. The RFFF is thin and reliable, but the donor usually needs skin grafting. The ALT flap may be rather bulky in some patients particularly in White patients, but can be thinned down (primarily in selected cases or secondarily). The MSAPF is a more recently described fasciocutaneous flap that is easily harvested. The lateral arm flap is similar to the RFFF but has a shorter vascular pedicle. The skin can be innervated, although for many situations, e.g. tongue reconstruction, the true effectiveness is debatable.
- For bulk, e.g. muscle, the RA, VL or chimeric ALT is particularly useful.

- In glossectomy, swallowing function seems to depend more on larynx preservation/laryngeal suspension and the amount of tongue/muscle remaining, than the actual flap used. Other than this, studies show better function in patients with protuberant bulky tongues compared to flatter depressed tongues, although this is somewhat dependent on the preoperative function.
  - Paulowski (*Head Neck*, 2004) suggests that the tongue base volume has the greatest impact on swallowing; 1:1 replacement is recommended.

RECIPIENT VESSELS

- The most commonly used recipient arteries in the head and neck are the facial and superior thyroid arteries.
- Others – lingual, superficial temporal and occipital depending on the site.

Recipient veins in the head and neck:

- Internal jugular vein (IJV) – end-to-side or end-to-end to a tributary close to the main trunk.
- External jugular vein (EJV), which is formed by the posterior auricular vein joining the posterior division of the retromandibular vein (from the superficial temporal vein and the maxillary vein) and drains into the subclavian vein. It crosses the sternomastoid (SM) muscle, and there is some concern that it may be prone to compression.
- Facial vein. The common facial vein is formed by the junction of the anterior facial vein with the anterior division of the retromandibular vein. It divides into two – one drains into the IJV whilst the other receives the anterior jugular vein before draining into the EJV.

VESSEL-DEPLETED NECK

Suitable recipient vessels can be in short supply, e.g. in the irradiated head and neck and/or after repeated surgery.

- Arteries
  - Often still available are the transverse cervical (found in the bottom lateral corner of the posterior triangle) or (branch of) the thoracoacromial vessels (which can be used even if the PM has been harvested before).
  - The external carotid artery itself can be used with a side clamp and good proximal and distal control.
  - There is some evidence that 'reverse flow' in certain arteries with significant collaterals, e.g. facial and superior thyroid, can be used – according to Batchelor, any artery with pulsatile flow can support a flap whether anterograde or retrograde. This may be useful where geometry is unfavourable, e.g. kinking more likely with using proximal portion.
- Veins
  - The IJV is usually still available in most cases; otherwise, the transverse cervical vein can be used.
  - The cephalic vein can be turned over to allow an anastomosis in the neck.

Vein grafts may be needed to reach more distant recipient vessels. The length of the vein graft does not seem to affect patency per se, but will increase the risk of kinking and thrombosis.

Hyperbaric oxygen therapy for wound complications after surgery in the irradiated head and neck (Neovius EB, *Head Neck*, 1997)

Hyperbaric oxygen therapy (HBOT) aims to increase oxygen tension in hypoxic tissues, e.g. after radiotherapy especially radionecrosis of the mandible and post-surgical, post-irradiation wounds and fistulae. Some suggest prophylactic pre-operative therapy (20 sessions), before surgery in irradiated tissues, with 10 post-operative sessions.

A session of HBOT usually consists of exposure to 2–3 bar, 100% oxygen for 75 minutes; 30–40 daily treatments may be required. Proposed benefits include

- Increased fibroplasia and angiogenesis to aid wound healing
- Facilitate oxygen-mediated phagocytic killing of pathogens to reduce infection
- Bactericidal effect on anaerobes

Complications include temporary myopia, barotrauma and oxygen toxicity and seizures. There is apparently no effect on cancer cells.

- Barotrauma to the middle ear/tympanic membrane or lung especially with repeated treatment is found in up to 15%–20% of cases. The risk can be minimised with thorough pre-treatment check-ups.
- ENT assessment – clinical screening of Eustachian tube (ET) function with active (Valsalva) and passive manoeuvres; if the results are equivocal or a failure, then formal ET testing (e.g. tympanometry) is needed. Those with sinusitis, etc. should be treated with prophylactic decongestants. Mucus plugs in the airways are more common in asthmatics and those with chronic obstructive pulmonary disease.

QUALITY OF LIFE CONSIDERATIONS IN HEAD AND NECK CANCER RECONSTRUCTION

Improvements in free flap reconstruction of advanced head and neck cancers have helped to make it a routine procedure, and simple survival is no longer an adequate goal. Whilst reconstruction should aim to maintain appearance as well as function, maximising the quality of life (QOL) is not a simple function of flap success or functional outcomes.

QOL or health-related QOL (HRQOL) has been a focus of more recent studies, in addition to survival/recurrence data, flap success, etc. The information is usually derived from patient-completed questionnaires, or patient-reported outcomes (PROs). The most common of these are the European organisation for research and treatment of cancer head and neck QOL questionnaire (EORTC-QLQ-HN35) and the University of Washington head and neck QOL

(UW-QOL), which take 18 and 5 minutes to complete, respectively.

- The greatest impact on QOL is related to radiotherapy, position and size of tumour and the age of the patient.
- The specifics of the reconstruction have little impact on the QOL scores.
- Oral function in terms of eating and speech is a major concern, and issues can lead to social isolation and psychological upset.
- Facial asymmetry is more significant than isolated scars.

IV. ORAL CANCER

Discussion of the management of oral cancer will be used to demonstrate some general points that can be applied to the majority of head and neck cancers.

This group forms 30% of all head and cancer tumours and 2%–3% of all tumours overall (in places like India, it constitutes up to 40% of all cancers). More than 90% of intra-oral tumours are SCCs.

- Other tumours include salivary gland tumours (sublingual and minor) that are likely to be high-grade malignancies including muco-epidermoid and adenoid cystic tumours. Intra-oral adenoid cystic tumours tend to excite little inflammatory response and invade the mandible without radiological change; they also show aggressive perineural spread with tendency for skip lesions.
- Less common are lentiginous melanoma (usually superficial) and sarcomas.

HISTORY

Classic risk factors include the 'S's: smoking, spirits, spices, sharps, syphilis and sunlight; 75% are most closely related to **smoking and alcohol**. In some cultures, betel nut chewing is an important factor, e.g. India and Taiwan.

- The risk in smokers is 3.43× greater than non-smokers and ex-smokers (1.4× according to Gandini S, *Int J Cancer*, 2008), and is affected by the length and frequency of smoking; the greatest risk is seen in those with more than 20 pack-years (Petti S, *Oral Oncol*, 2009). Toxins such as nitrosamines and aromatic hydrocarbons lead to mutations in tumour suppressor genes (TSGs) p53 and p16, which leads to carcinogenesis.
  - The risk of a second primary is 40% unless they give up smoking, in which case it decreases to 6%.
- Alcohol – its metabolic by-product acetaldehyde is mutagenic.
  - Smoking and drinking are synergistic.
- Erythroplakia/leukoplakia – found in up to 20%; resultant lesions tend to be more aggressive.

- Human papillomavirus (HPV) positivity is increasing; the link with tumour causation is strongest in tonsillar carcinoma – after integration into the host DNA, viral oncoproteins bind to and affect the function of p53 and pRb. HPV-positive tumours tend to present at an earlier tumour stage but a later nodal stage.
  - The most common subtype associated with head and neck cancer is HPV16 (90%).
  - HPV-negative tumours tend to have more dysplasia and are keratinising, whilst HPV-positive tumours tend to have little dysplasia and are non-keratinising.

PROGNOSIS

Overall, the 5-year survival is 50%. Mortality depends on the primary tumour (size, degree of differentiation, invasion/stromal involvement) and lymph node involvement. Patients suffering from early recurrence (within 18 months) tend to do worse.

- Age and general health.
- Smoking history, which has implications for pulmonary function but not microsurgical success.
- Alcohol history and likelihood of withdrawal symptoms.
- HPV-positive tumours have a good response to chemoradiation. Overall survival at 2 years is 94% vs. 58% in HPV-negative cancers (Fakhry C, *J Natl Cancer Inst*, 2008). HPV-positive patients tend to not have p53 gene mutations and have less cancer risk factors in general.
  - One-third of head and neck cancer deaths are due to a second primary.

RELEVANT ANATOMY

The oral cavity is the area from the lip vermillion to the junction of the hard and soft palates superiorly and circumvallate papillae inferiorly.

- The oropharynx lies from the circumvallate papillae of the tongue to the tip of the epiglottis (or hyoid bone level) and includes the soft palate, tonsils, aryepiglottic folds and valleculae.
- The hypopharynx lies from the aryepiglottic folds to the origin of the oesophagus (cricoid cartilage level). Important subsites are the postcricoid region, piriform fossa and posterior pharyngeal wall.

EXAMINATION

Assess the size (T status) and site including fixity to tongue, mandible and floor of mouth (FOM), as well as the presence of any trismus and the patient's dental status. Some patients may have had preceding erythroplakia/leukoplakia. Some countries, e.g. India, have trialled screening (visual inspection in high-risk populations) that may allow earlier detection (Subramanian S, *Bull World Health Organ*, 2009), but there is no standard routine screening test for oral cancer in most of the world.

- Synchronous tumours – detected within 6 months – up to 15%.
- Metachronous tumours – detected at >6 months – 40% in those who continue to smoke compared with 6% in those who quit.

Common sites affected in both categories include the oropharynx, lung and oesophagus.

INVESTIGATIONS

- Chest X-ray, blood tests
- MRI/CT scan of tumour and neck for staging and planning
- Panendoscopy
- Local anaesthetic (LA) biopsy of lesion for histology
- Fine needle aspiration (FNA) of any neck masses

TREATMENT

Oral lesions rarely metastasise below the level of the clavicle. T1 and T2 lesions of the oral cavity have a significant rate of **occult node metastasis;** prophylactic neck dissection (ND) can be considered especially lesions near/crossing midline, when the neck is entered for access.

- **T1N0M0 lesions may be effectively treated using either surgery or radiotherapy alone.**
- **Surgery first effectively debulks 99%+ of tumour** mass, provides a specimen and allows accurate staging; free tissue transfer facilitates post-operative radiotherapy (PORT). This is preferred for cases with bone invasion, failed prior RT, continued smoking/drinking with higher risks of recurrence or other primary. Optimal excision margins have not been rigorously tested, but it is important that excision is not compromised to preserve function:
  - Well-defined tumours should be excised with margins of at least 1 cm, preferably using Colorado needle-tip cautery.
  - Ill-defined tumours, recurrent tumours or those arising in previously irradiated tissues should be excised with margins 2 cm or more.
  - Consider perineural spread along the lingual or IANs; divide nerves as close to the skull base as possible.
  - RT is still available for salvage or a second tumour.
- **Radiotherapy** by comparison only debulks the tumour by ~25%. It also delays surgery and eliminates the possibility for further radiotherapy if surgical margins are narrow or involved. Delay for >4–6 weeks after surgery is associated with decreased local control. Late effects include (progressive) fibrosis and telangiectasia.

- Therapy for very thin/small primary, and neck.
- Adjuvant primary therapy for perineural invasion, close margins and neck disease if extracapsular spread is seen.
- RT alone may be offered to those who refuse or are not fit enough for surgery.
- There are some reported strategies to reduce the acute and chronic side effects of adjuvant therapy, e.g. amifostine (cytoprotective adjuvant) and growth factors such as granulocyte colony-stimulating factor (GCSF) (early studies showed reduction of post RT oral mucositis), granulocyte macrophage colony-stimulating factor (GM-CSF) and KGF reduce radionecrosis.
- Results show similar control rates and superior function compared with surgery.
- **Chemotherapy** can be offered as part of a controlled trial, as palliation or as neoadjuvant to reduce the tumour bulk prior to surgery.
  - Cisplatin most commonly used
  - Molecularly targeted agents, e.g. cetuximab (IgG1 chimeric antibody)
- **Chemoprevention** is not yet a reality, but the aim(s) would be to
  - Treat **premalignant conditions** such as leukoplakia. Some trials show that carotene may help in clinical resolution, but other studies show no reduction in the rate of malignant transformation (nor have studies with bleomycin or vitamin A) (see premalignant conditions).
  - **Prevent second primary** (5% risk per year) – there is evidence of reduced risk of a second primary (4% vs. 24% in placebo) or recurrence using retinoids, e.g. 13-cRA seen in early studies (Hong WK, *N Engl J Med*, 1990) but have been difficult to confirm in larger studies. Furthermore, ~1/3 need to stop due to side effects particularly with high-dose regimes.
  - **High-risk population** – there is no evidence for any benefit from taking vitamins, retinoids or carotene. In fact, β-carotene (taken during cancer prevention trials undertaken based on early 1980s epidemiology) may increase risk of lung cancer in smokers and those with asbestos exposure. A Cochrane review (2007) demonstrated 1%–8% **increased** mortality, though some dispute the methodology of these meta-analyses.

GENERAL TREATMENT BY STAGE

T1N0

- Surgery or radiotherapy only; the neck can be observed – there is a 20% risk of occult disease (Hicks WL, *Head Neck*, 1997; see below).
- T1 and low-volume/mobile T2 tumours can be reasonably treated by radiotherapy alone as long as the distance from the mandible is sufficient.

- T1N0M0 SCC tongue, 80% 5 year survival with either radiotherapy or surgery alone, compared to
- T3N0M0 SCC tongue, 30% 5 year survival with either alone

T2–3N0

- Excision and reconstruction.
- Modified radial ND (MRND). There is some debate – some would suggest ND for higher-risk areas such as tongue or FOM and where the neck would be opened for access.
- Radiotherapy is indicated for incomplete excision, extracapsular spread, perineural invasion and N2/N3 disease, i.e. multiple positive nodes (Hicks WL, *Head Neck*, 1997; see below) and also close excision margins (<5 mm).

T4N1

- Excision and reconstruction.
- Mandible.
  - Rim resection if the tumour abuts
  - Segmental resection if invading or previous radiotherapy
- Ipsilateral MRND (types 1–3) or radical therapeutic ND. Bilateral ND if the tumour crosses the midline.
- Radiotherapy. As above.

Role of radical surgery and post-operative radiotherapy in the management of intra-oral carcinoma (Robertson AG, *Br J Plast Surg*, 1985)

Two treatment modalities for FOM and tongue tumours (T2 and greater, N0–3, M0) were compared:

- Group 1 – radical surgery (including radical LND) + radical radiotherapy (4–8 weeks after).
- Group 2 – non-radical surgery (± LND) + radical radiotherapy. The 5 year survival rates (%) were given in Table 3.1.

Squamous cell carcinoma of the floor of mouth 20-year review (Hicks WL, *Head Neck*, 1997)

T1 tumours have a ~20% risk of occult nodal disease. Elective ND is often performed for reasons of access but is also warranted for occult disease. With surgery alone

- Involved margins ~40% local recurrence
- Clear margins ~10% local recurrence

Table 3.1 5 year survival rates from Robertson AG 1985

Tongue		Floor of mouth	
Group 1	Group 2	Group 1	Group 2
44	5	41	10

SPECIFIC REGIONS IN THE ORAL CAVITY

- **Tongue (30%, see below)**
- **Gingiva/alveolar mucosa**, particularly the molar area. These tumours tend to invade bone early and have a high incidence of nodal metastasis – 25% in T1 tumours. They are best treated with surgery.
- **FOM (30%).** 75% are found anterior to the lingual frenulum and lymph drainage can be bilateral; 15%–30% will have invaded the mandible at the time of presentation, i.e. T4, with nodes in 1/3.
  - More frequently involved in betel nut chewers.
  - T1 tumours can be treated with radiotherapy or surgery, but larger tumours should be resected.
  - Smaller defects of the ventral tongue/FOM can be closed with local flaps whilst larger defects will need pedicled/free flaps.
- **Buccal (10%).**
- **Retromolar trigone** (RMT) is the area between the upper and lower third molar teeth, medial to the ascending mandibular ramus and the medial pterygoid muscle.
  - Lymphatic drainage goes to the jugulodigastric and submandibular nodes; 1/3 to 2/3 of patients with RMT SCC present with nodal disease.
  - Tumours tend to spread to the FOM/tongue and to the faucial area more than to the palate or buccal mucosa.
  - Due to the thin tissues, patients almost invariably present with **bony involvement** (ascending ramus) with infiltration of the mandibular canal and IAN. Involvement of the nearby muscles (medial pterygoid, masseter and tendon of temporalis) will cause trismus.
- **Faucial tumours** may be SCC (keratinising or non-keratinising) or malignant lymphoid tumours (tonsil). They tend to spread laterally through the pterygomandibular raphe/constrictors to invade the medial pterygoid but rarely the mandible; they also invade medially to the FOM/tongue and anteriorly to the RMT.
  - T2 tumours or less have a 40% cure rate with radiotherapy alone; thus, surgery is preferred. The type of resection (of the tumour and involved bone) via mandibular split and swing depends on the degree of invasion:
    - Rim resection.
    - Rim, anterior ascending ramus, coronoid process; this includes the mandibular canal and IAN.
    - Entire ascending ramus including the condyle.

TONGUE CANCER

Tumours of the anterior 2/3 are twice as common as the posterior 1/3, which are usually more advanced at presentation and thus have a worse prognosis. The commonest presentations of a tongue cancer are

- Tongue ulcer (52%) or tongue mass (19%)
- Neck mass (4%) (69% had a clinically negative neck on presentation; Haddadin KJ, *Br J Plast Surg*, 2000)

EXAMINATION

- Tumour size (T stage) – T1 (23%), T2 (50%) and T3/4 (27%) at presentation (Haddadin KJ, *Br J Plast Surg*, 2000).
- Tumour thickness is predictive of node involvement. Elective nodal dissection has been proposed for lesions thicker than 10 mm.
- Site.
  - Does it cross the midline?
  - Is the tongue fixed to FOM?
  - Hypoglossal nerve palsy?
- Neck status – 1/3 of tongue (and FOM) tumours have nodes at the time of presentation.
  - FNAC

These are investigated similarly to other oral tumours. Examination under anaesthetic (EUA) is often necessary to establish the degree of spread within the mouth whilst pan-endoscopy excludes synchronous tumours.

- CT/MRI, including the neck, is also helpful.
  - MRI for nodal involvement, extracapsular spread
  - CT for bone involvement
- PET-CT is not part of the primary assessment but may be used under certain circumstances, e.g. exclude distant metastasis (most commonly lung and bone), before undertaking radical surgery for an advanced tumour.

TREATMENT

The tongue may be approached via

- Submandibular 'visor' incision and a pull-through technique sparing a mandibular osteotomy.
- Lip split and 'Y' incision (for synchronous ND) combined with a (paramedian) mandibular osteotomy. An *en bloc* or in continuity ND aims to remove any lymphatic pathways between the primary and superior neck nodes (I and II), but may increase complications such as fistula formation.

Excision with gross margins of 1–2 cm; frozen section control of margins should be considered, though it will be less reliable with prior irradiation. The propensity for peri-neural invasion and perivascular spread means that resection margins may be much wider than initially expected. Excisional surgery effectively 'debulks' 99%+ of the tumour; radiotherapy can be used for involved margins.

- **Radiotherapy** potentially preserves more function and can treat the neck at the same time; surgery is then the salvage option. There are significant acute and chronic side effects, particularly xerostomia and (osteo)radionecrosis (ORN).

- **Chemotherapy**
  - **Neoadjuvant** to shrink large tumours, though resection margins should still be based on the original size.
  - **Targeted therapy**, e.g. cetuximab (monoclonal EGF receptor antibody) can be combined with radiotherapy in those unfit for chemotherapy.
- **TisN0 – CO$_2$ laser**.
- **T1 tumours** can be treated with radiotherapy only or with excision with a 1 cm margin, possibly with direct closure or SSG and no ND. Surgery is often preferred for anterior lesions, whilst radiotherapy may be considered more often for posterior lesions.
- **T2 tumours usually require surgery and radiotherapy**.
  - Reconstruction with a thin free flap, e.g. RFFF. The overall function is related to the residual tongue and its mobility; it is important to avoid tethering but also to maintain volume which prevents shift of the residual tongue and allows the tongue to contact the palate for swallowing and speech. Predictors of poor post-operative function include large defect size, midline defects and PORT.
  - Ipsilateral MRND.
    - The high incidence of involved neck nodes in tongue cancer means that ND is often needed, as even stage I or II tumours have 42% occult metastases in neck nodes.
    - For tumours >5 mm invasion, 60% will have occult nodes (Fukano H, *Head Neck*, 1997; see below) and elective neck treatment is strongly indicated; upstaging of clinically negative neck occurs in 36% of patients (Haddadin KJ, *Br J Plast Surg*, 2000, see below).
    - Contralateral ND for T2 tip of the tongue tumours that are clinically N0 (35% incidence of occult nodal disease) or N2c disease.
  - Radiotherapy.
- **T3 tumours**, often involving the tip of the tongue:
  - Tumour excision and reconstruct with bulkier flaps
    - If >50% is involved, then a total glossectomy should be considered (see below).
    - Significant involvement of the base of the tongue may require a laryngectomy (see below).
    - MRND (types 1–3) is performed wherever possible, unless a RND is required.
  - Radiotherapy
- **T4 tumours** involve extrinsic muscles of the tongue.
  - As above.
  - (Re)-suspension will facilitate swallowing.

RECONSTRUCTION

Swallowing function depends less on the actual flap used and more on the amount of remaining tongue, laryngeal suspension/preservation. The mobility of the residual tongue and a well-formed sulcus are important parts of a properly reconstructed tongue.

- Direct closure/secondary healing for small areas of buccal mucosa.
- Buccal fat pad can be mobilised to cover 4 cm² defects of palate, RMT or buccal mucosa; it is left to epithelialise over 4–5 weeks. It is not reliable enough to cover exposed bone.
- Skin grafts may contract and cause tethering such that they are a little better than secondary healing.
- Local flaps, e.g. tongue, nasolabial, are often salvage options. The FAMM flap and the temporalis flaps can be useful in small defects.
- Pedicled flaps, e.g. PM, deltopectoral, etc., can provide large amounts of tissue but can be too bulky with significant donor site scarring.
- Free flaps are usually the first choice due to the wide range of tissues available, freedom of inset, etc. It is important to use robust reliable flaps; partial necrosis even of a small tip may lead to fistulae that complicates management significantly.

The value of innervated flaps, e.g. radial forearm free flap (RFFF) or anterolateral thigh (ALT), is not confirmed particularly in the long term; 90% of non-innervated flaps regain at least some sensation (probably due to axonal sprouting into the flap); innervated flaps do gain general sensation sooner, but this may not be that important for tongue function. Patients generally do not complain of a lack of taste due to taste buds being almost ubiquitous in the oral cavity.

TOTAL GLOSSECTOMY

Total glossectomy is mainly reserved for

- T3/T4 tumours.
- Post-radiotherapy recurrence.
- Where >50% of the tongue is involved (high risk of perineural and perivascular spread) – in such cases, the contralateral lingual vessels and the lingual and hypoglossal nerve may be involved precluding hemiglossectomy.

RECONSTRUCTION AFTER TOTAL GLOSSECTOMY

- Paulowski (*Head Neck*, 2004) tongue base volume has the most impact on swallowing; aim to replace 1:1.
- Bulky flap reconstruction, e.g. rectus abdominis, PM vs. flat/funnel repair, e.g. ALT perforator flap, etc.
- Laryngeal suspension – hyoid to mandible.
- Post-operative speech therapy is needed; speech is generally regained by all patients even after total glossectomy. Ruhl (*Laryngoscope*, 1997) found that reasonable QOL was possible even after total glossectomy, and that the choice of flap was not so important. Even in those with laryngectomy, realistic expectations and adaptation reduce the impact on QOL.

Natural history and patterns of recurrence of tongue tumours (Haddadin KJ, *Br J Plast Surg*, 2000)

A retrospective study of 226 patients with tongue SCC with the following management principles:

- Surgery – complete surgical excision wherever possible, with therapeutic ND for palpable disease and elective ND for 'high-risk' tumours or where the neck is opened for access/reconstruction.
  - **36% of clinically negative necks upstaged** whilst 7.7% of clinically positive necks were downstaged.
- PORT for large and/or infiltrating tumours, narrow excision margins and positive cervical nodes.
  - The resulting 5 year survival was pT2 79%, pT2 52% and pT3/4 35%.
  - The primary site and ipsilateral neck were the most common sites for recurrence (27 and 34 patients), which is more common than contralateral neck recurrence (which is also relatively high – 19 cases).
  - Second oral primary occurs in 10%.
  - Disease-related deaths occur in about half of patients and are mostly due to advanced local disease (80%) rather than systemic spread.

Depth of invasion as a predictive factor for cervical lymph node metastasis in tongue carcinoma (Fukano H, *Head Neck*, 1997)

- Depth of invasion <5 mm – ~6% incidence of nodal disease
- Depth of invasion >5 mm – ~60% incidence of nodal disease

Overall, clinically negative necks (N0 or stage I and II) had 30% incidence of occult disease. The authors recommend tumour excision with frozen section for measurement of the depth of invasion, with an elective ND for invasion >5 mm.

In general, it is uncommon to opt for observation in clinically N0 necks due to the significant risk of occult involvement, but is an option in those with very thin tumours, e.g. <4 mm. Otherwise, a selective ND (supraomohyoid) or radiotherapy is usually advocated.

- Indian T1–2 tongue cancer study showed better (63% vs. 52%) disease-free survival in those having elective ND (END) in addition to their hemiglossectomy, compared to hemiglossectomy alone. The overall survival rates were similar.
- T1–3, N0 tumours show a 49% positive END compared to 53% developing clinically apparent nodes in those who were observed closely.

OROPHARYNX

The oropharynx lies from the circumvallate papillae of the tongue to the tip of the epiglottis (or hyoid bone level) and includes the soft palate, tongue base, tonsils, aryepiglottic folds and valleculae. Tumours here can spread into the nasopharynx and hypopharynx, particularly submucosally; thus, tumours are generally larger than they appear clinically.

- Tongue base – often painless. Palpation will help reveal the degree of infiltration.
- Soft palate – usually presents early.
- Tonsil tumours may be associated with EBV; 1% of tonsil tumours are secondaries. Note that the ICA is about 2.5 cm away from the tonsillar fossa (posterolateral).
- Posterior pharyngeal wall tumours usually present late, usually when they have spread past the midline. They need to be excised at the level of the prevertebral fascia and bilateral ND is often needed.

PRINCIPLES OF EXCISION

- A major part of the surgical morbidity is related to the impact on the structures involved in swallowing. Laryngectomy should be considered for tumours involving a significant part of the tongue base due to the high risk of aspiration; those who keep their larynx should have good pulmonary function.
- Tracheostomy is usually needed to maintain the airway.
- More than half will have nodal disease at presentation and thus ND is indicated even in N0 disease.
- Access.
  - Peroral
  - Slaughter's pull through (stripping FOM structures off the mandible by subperiosteal dissection and delivering them to the neck through a submandibular incision)
  - Lip split and mandibular osteotomy
    - Access to the posterior pharyngeal wall and the base of the tongue may be gained by a midline/paramedian mandibulotomy with or without a midline glossotomy.

MANDIBULAR OSTEOTOMY

The **lip is split** in the midline with an incision curving around the chin – this is the most aesthetic and best preserves sensation and motor control. The osteotomy site can be

- Symphyseal.
- Paramedian – split anterior to mental foramen (MF) and provides good exposure. It allows genioglossus and geniohyoid muscles to remain attached to the mandible helping to maintain tongue stability.
- Lateral – posterior to the MF. This divides the inferior alveolar (IA) neurovascular bundle.

TECHNIQUE OF OSTEOTOMY

- Vertical osteotomy, e.g. between the second incisor and the canine – look for a suitable gap between teeth; an X-ray/OPG is useful.

- Step osteotomy risks exposing the dental roots but allows good osteosynthesis with two plates.
- Sagittal split leads to inevitable exposure of the dental roots.

Preplating of the osteotomy sites allows better fixation and compression.

There is discussion regarding the use of the lip/mandible split. There are those who say that it is not necessary (Cantu G, *Oral Oncol*, 2006; Li WL, *Tumor Biol*, 2014), and without it, resection margins are not compromised (Devine JC, *Int J Oral Maxillofac Surg*, 2001), and there are those who do say it does not affect that continence (with **less** risk of lip dysfunction); and despite the scar, patient satisfaction is similarly high in both groups (Dziegielewski PT, *Oral Oncol*, 2010). However, though the relationship between QOL and body image is complex (Pruzinsky T, Cash TF, Body Image: A Handbook of Theory, Research, and Clinical Practice, 2002), disfigurement does undoubtedly impact QOL in head and neck cancer patients (Arunachalam D, *Indian J Plast Surg*, 2011), particularly women.

RECONSTRUCTION

- Allow small defects of the posterior pharyngeal wall to granulate or close primarily if possible.
- Flap closure.
  - Free flap, e.g. RFF or ALT
  - PM flap
  - Temporalis muscle flap or TPF flap

Inadequate reconstruction of the soft palate may lead to VPI and hypernasality; thus, it is usually preferable to have a bulky flap (with or without a pharyngoplasty) if static, or to have a thinner dynamic flap, which is attached to working muscle.

V. MANDIBLE RECONSTRUCTION

MANDIBLE IN ORAL CANCER

The main blood supply to the mandible comes from the **periosteum**, which originates from the buccal and submandibular branches of the facial arteries (especially with advanced age) – the IA artery supplies the teeth and alveolar part of the mandible only.

- Alveolar resorption results in loss of alveolar height and approximation of gingival mucosa to the floor of the mouth at the mylohyoid line.
- After dental extraction, the cancellous bone is in contact with the mucosa overlying it.
- Ameloblastomas are benign but locally aggressive odontogenic tumours that usually present as hard painless masses around the angle of the mandible. Local curettage/enucleation is associated with a high rate of recurrence; wide local excision (>1 cm margin) gives better local control but usually requires bony reconstruction.
- Adenocystic carcinoma can invade bone with few radiological signs.

Routes of entry of squamous cell carcinoma to the mandible (McGregor AD, *Head Neck*, 1988)
Direct infiltration.

- Dentate mandible – via the periodontal membrane at the occlusal surface; **invasion is heralded by loosening of teeth.**
- Edentulous mandible – via the alveolar surface at tooth gaps; following dental extraction, the cortical bone does not regenerate so that cancellous bone is in contact with the overlying mucosa. The periosteum is resistant to tumour invasion but fails to protect the edentulous occlusal surface (where bone gaps ossify incompletely).
- Post-irradiation mandible may be invaded at several sites.

The mandibular periosteum does not need to be excised unless it is directly involved. Tumour can spread within the mandible either through the medulla or permeative spread along the mandibular canal. Trismus (suggestive of pterygoid involvement) and pain radiating to the ear or temple (auriculotemporal nerve) or lower lip (mental nerve) are poor prognostic signs.

IMAGING OF MANDIBLE IN ORAL CANCER

OPG, CT or MRI may show changes suggestive of bone involvement such as new bone formation (except on the occlusal surface) and loss of haemopoietic marrow. However, changes secondary to radiotherapy can be difficult to distinguish from tumour.

PRINCIPLES OF MANDIBULAR EXCISION

The main factors affecting mandibular involvement are dental status and irradiation, which leads to the loss of haematopoietic marrow and replacement by fibrous tissue. Tumour spread is direct and not metastatic; it spreads with a fibrotic reaction in the medulla along trabeculae and along the IAN. It can be difficult to determine the degree of tumour invasion (see above), but generally, bony excision should be limited to what is required for adequate margins.

- Approximately 1 cm controlled by frozen section
- In the non-irradiated mandible,
  - There is usually little cortical spread; thus, bone excision can be based on the mucosal spread on the alveolus.
  - If haematopoietic marrow is seen, then the resection is usually adequate.

The degree of involvement and the vertical height of the mandible determine the choice between either rim resection or segmental resection – a shorter vertical height brings the occlusal ridge closer to FOM, theoretically allows earlier tumour involvement and thus increases the need for segmental resection.

- **Rim resection** is generally only feasible in the **non-irradiated** mandible with early tumour spread (T1–2, with minimal/no involvement of the periosteum, periodontal ligaments or cortex) or because stripping of overlying densely adherent mucosa is difficult/impossible. In the former scenario, the resection level should be below the mandibular canal such that the entire canal from mandibular foramen to MF is resected, preventing tumour permeation along the IAN.
  - >1 cm of bone should remain. It is not considered to be safe in irradiated bone where clearance is less predictable along increased risk of complications including poor healing at the osteotomy site.
- **Segmental resection** for short vertical height, larger tumours (T3/4, with macroscopic involvement of the mandible) and prior mandible irradiation.

Rogers (*Head Neck*, 2004) found that QOL advantages of rim resection were lost when the segment is >4 cm long, and/or if post-operative radiotherapy is required.

Immediate reconstruction and PORT are the general management after resection; virtually all patients undergoing mandibular resections should have synchronous ND irrespective of the presence of palpable node disease.

CLASSIFICATION OF DEFECTS

- Urken: C-R-B-S (SH), i.e. condyle, ramus, body, symphysis (half).
- C-L-H: C, complete central/canine to canine segment; L, lateral defect of any length minus condyle; and H, same as L but with condyle. Thus, the possible types of defects are C, L, H, CL, CH, LCL, HCL and HCH. Optional parameters are m, mucosa; s, skin; or ms, both.

Jewer classification of mandibular defects (modified by Soutar):
Defects of different portions have different types of stress.

- **Central segment** – the anterior mandible from MF to MF includes the first point of contact and involves great stresses; thus, reconstructions of this region have a higher failure rate. Vascularised bone is recommended; recreating this curved segment requires an osteotomy.
- **Lateral segment** – from MF to lingula preserving the posterior ascending ramus and the condyle. The lower stresses mean that plate-only methods have been used, but these still have significantly high failure rates (see below) and thus not suited in younger patients with normal life expectancy. A single straight piece of bone is adequate for MF to lingula.
- **Ascending ramus** – bone or alloplasts can be used for the posterior mandible. The end can be contoured to fit the glenoid fossa if needed or the native condyle can be attached to the bone flap. Where a small segment of condyle remains, it is better to remove it and fix it to

the bone flap rather than try to plate it in situ. Titanium condylar prostheses have been used, but there is the risk of extrusion, exposure and migration.

RECONSTRUCTION OF THE MANDIBLE

Aims

- Enable normal chewing and swallowing; maintain oral competence.

- Denture rehabilitation and aesthetics.
    - An anterior mandibulectomy may cause an 'Andy Gump' deformity. **Andy Gump** was a cartoon character created by Sidney Smith, supposedly based on David Hoag who had resection of his anterior mandible and anterior FOM for lower lip cancer in 1915 and lived in the New York suburbs. The character was extremely popular in the 1920s to the 1950s, and there was legal case over the (lack of) attribution.

- Segmental loss is best treated with **vascularised bone graft** (VBG) as it allows relatively rapid union and additional tissue can be imported.
    - Non-VBGs are appropriate for **small structural defects (<5 cm)** with rigid fixation in well-vascularised non-irradiated sites providing good soft tissue cover. This size limit is related to the speed of 'creeping substitution' in non-VBG – bone deposition begins at the graft recipient interface, but at the centre, bone is replaced by fibrous tissue. Other complications include
        - Resorption – Calvarial bone is supposedly better than other bone grafts, and this may be related to the differences between intramembranous vs. endochondral ossification.
        - Poor take due to hostile recipient bed (including previous radiotherapy – hypovascular, hypocellular and hypoxic tissues).
    - Longer sections of segmental loss fixed with metalwork only are associated with a higher complication rate – 7% if <5 cm vs. 81% if >5 cm (Arden RL, *Arch Otolaryngo Head Neck Surg*, 1999).

The choice of reconstruction in a particular individual depends on many factors, but in general,

- VBGs may be needed particularly for more complex defects and when PORT is anticipated.
- Young patients with non-malignant process: rigid fixation and non-VBGs are an option for short defects (see bone healing), whilst **distraction osteogenesis** (DO) is particularly useful for developmental abnormalities (and also after trauma or to revise previous VBGs).
    - Bone segment from iliac crest or rib grafts. There is vessel ingrowth and removal of dead bone cells

and repopulation of the existing Haversian canal network.

- Particulate bone and cancellous marrow (PBCM) can be harvested from the ilium and provides marrow mesenchymal cells and endosteal osteoblasts. It still undergoes the same resorption–replacement cycle but with a lesser degree of resorption.

- Grafts must have adequate vascular soft tissue cover; pre- and post-operative hyperbaric oxygen may improve vascularisation from 30% to 80% of normal tissue levels.

- Elderly patients with poor premorbid health, poor prognosis – soft-tissue-only reconstruction with or without a reconstruction plate can be considered. There is a very significant risk of plate complications such as extrusion. Allografts such as freeze-dried bone or non-vascularised autografts may be combined with vascular soft tissue flaps in selected patients.

Reconstruction of posterior mandibular defects with soft tissue using a rectus abdominis free flap (Kroll SS, *Br J Plast Surg*, 1998)
VBG is the gold standard treatment for larger (>9 cm) or complex (soft tissue) defects and in irradiated areas. A 'simpler' soft tissue-only flap may be used in patients with poor tumour prognosis or poor general health, particularly if the TMJ has been excised as it would be very difficult to reconstruct. Posterior defects cause less morbidity than anterior defects; good aesthetics and functional outcome have been reported. Overall, we have the following:

- **No reconstruction** – may be considered for lateral defects or defects of the ascending ramus. The chin will be deviated to the deficient side, but speech and swallowing are usually satisfactory.
- **Reconstruction plates** may be appropriate for those with poor prognosis/low demand (extrusion and fracture are almost inevitable) but should be limited to lateral defects as anterior defects reconstructed in this way have an extremely high extrusion rate. You would not expect them to last beyond 18 months.
- **Non-VBG** can be used for smaller defects (<6 cm) except in cancer patients who are likely to need radiotherapy (which will lead to an extrusion/infection/resorption rate of 50%–80%).

VASCULARISED BONE

See also: 'Individual flaps'

Osteomyocutaneous flaps

- **Lateral trapezius with spine of scapula** – the flap is based on transverse cervical vessels, which should be preserved during ipsilateral ND (but not always); it incorporates bone from the spine of the scapula and a skin paddle over the acromioclavicular joint, which can be orientated horizontally or vertically. It is important to preserve the suprascapular nerve during dissection – it supplies supraspinatus, which initiates shoulder abduction.

- **Pectoralis major with fifth rib** or edge of sternum (Ariyan S, *Surg Oncol Clin N Am*, 1997) – this is based on pectoral branch of thoracoacromial artery (50% of PM blood supply); the muscle is also supplied by lateral thoracic and superior thoracic arteries, 40% and 10%, respectively.
- **SM with medial segment of clavicle** (up to 8 cm) – it is based on the occipital vessels (with some supply from the superior thyroid artery and the thyrocervical trunk) with the skin paddle overlying the clavicle, which has a 35% viability but may be increased if the middle vessel is preserved. The arc of rotation is determined by point of entry of the XIth nerve. It is contraindicated in cases with cervical nodal disease that requires RND, although the flap may be used where there is a single level I node treated by suprahyoid dissection. It is thus usually indicated for benign defects in the mandible, dysplasia or primary mandibular tumours. A bilateral flap incorporating the intervening manubrium has been described.

Osseous flaps – The 'gold standard' particularly in osteoradionecrosis (ORN)

IMF can be used to maintain the occlusion during inset particularly for lateral defects (anterior defects usually cannot be fixed this way due to lack of dentition).

- **Miniplates** (at least two sets per osteotomy) are used to fix the contoured fibula; they are cheap, low profile and easy to mould.
- Some prefer **reconstruction plates** as they are stronger and thus less likely to fracture, though being bulkier and a higher profile may make exposure more likely. There may be increased 'stress shielding' and disuse atrophy/osteoporosis and (slightly) higher complication (particularly ORN) and removal rates. In practice, using a reconstruction plate means that the demands on the bone flap are reduced.

Free flaps

- **Fibula** – this flap provides the longest length of bone available (~25 cm) that also readily accepts osseointegrated implants; the bone is straight and thus usually requires multiple osteotomies for mandibular reconstruction. The overlying skin paddle is useful for FOM reconstruction but may be unavailable in up to 10% due to the vascular configuration. This flap is probably the most common choice for mandibular reconstruction.
- **Radial forearm flap** – its use in mandibular reconstruction was originally described by Soutar (*Br J Plast Surg*, 1983). It is a reasonably good option for lateral and central segmental defects, but the low bone volume makes it less suitable when osseointegrated

implants are planned. The bone segment (~12 cm) lies between the insertion of pronator teres proximally and brachioradialis distally, and one should remove <1/3 of the cross-sectional area to avoid fracture. The periosteal supply comes from perforators in the lateral intermuscular septum and vessels, which pass through FPL. The thin pliable skin island is suited for mucosal and skin reconstruction, but the thin weak bone functions more or less as a simple spacer, and is usually combined with a reconstruction plate for strength.

- **Deep circumflex iliac artery (DCIA)** – the bone segment (15 × 6 cm, both cortical and cancellous) can accommodate osseointegrated implants, is naturally curved and thus requires no osteotomy, making it an almost ideal bone flap particularly for hemimandible reconstruction, but has a precarious skin paddle (10% risk of failure) and is often too bulky. The donor site can be quite painful with a risk of hernia developing (it is important to close the external oblique meticulously). A portion of the internal oblique muscle based on the ascending branch of the DCIA can also be harvested for intra-oral lining.
- **Scapula flap** – a thin, straight 12 × 3 cm bone segment is available from the lateral border of the scapula along with a reliable skin paddle based on the subscapular artery. It is suitable for central (symphyseal) defects, but the thin bone cannot accommodate osseointegrated implants. The patient also has to be turned during the operation.

ALLOPLASTIC MATERIALS

- **Metal plates** including reconstruction plates (three screws either side) may be used, usually as temporary support as the metal will fatigue eventually. They have been used as definitive reconstruction in selected cases where functional demands are low.
  - Salvatori (*Acta Otorhinilaryngol*, 2007) found a 22% exposure rate (early exposure is due to wound breakdown because of infection/necrosis; late exposure is due to fracture). Plates require good soft tissue cover. When used for anterior defects, there is often lip ptosis due to muscle detachment and denervation combined with gravitation effects. The main patient complaints are dentally related; there is little scope for dental rehabilitation.
- **High failure rate with anterior defects** (particularly in combination with a PM flap instead of free flaps).
  - 40% failure (Papazian MR, *J Oral Maxillofac Surg*, 1991).
  - 52% (Kim MR, *J Oral Maxillofac Surg*, 1992).
  - 35%. Patients require another 35 days of hospital stay for secondary procedures compared to VBG (Boyd JB, *Plast Reconstr Surg*, 1995).
- Free flaps, e.g. RFFF, provide more reliable coverage than PM flaps (Cordeiro P, *Head Neck*, 1994),

and the combination of free skin flaps with reconstruction plates is a reasonable option in the elderly or those with a poor prognosis, particularly with lateral defects (5% vs. 21% overall failure rate). However, Wei (*Plast Reconstr Surg*, 2003) has found unacceptably low success rates even for well-covered lateral defects – 46% exposure in cases using ALT flaps with plates, with 31% needing salvage.

- **Bone substitutes** are rigid, do not remodel and cannot support dental prostheses.
  - **Medpor** (porous polyethylene) has the risk of extrusion and infection especially in irradiated tissues. Medpor implants are more useful for reconstruction of the craniofacial skeleton rather than the mandible. The porosity offers better stabilisation but in turn may make removal more difficult.
  - **Hydroxyapatite** and tricalcium phosphates are classed together as calcium phosphate ceramics; they are osteoconductive but brittle, have low tensile strength and can be difficult to fixate. Hydroxyapatite is rigid and cannot support osteointegration.
    - PBCM (iliac) can be packed into allografts after burring out holes.

Secondary lengthening of the reconstructed mandible by distraction osteogenesis (Yonehara Y, *Br J Plast Surg*, 1998)

Mandibular DO was originally described by McCarthy (*Plast Reconstr Surg*, 1992). This paper reports two cases where the mandible was reconstructed with free fibula flaps that were initially inadequate in length. Lengthening was achieved by a midline osteotomy with gradual distraction.

Dental restoration is usually delayed. Osteointegrated implants can be placed in fibula or DCIA flaps where there is more than 6 mm bone height; other favourable features are provision of well-vascularised bone and soft tissue cover particularly a **thin** intra-oral lining.

- DO has had very mixed results in the context of reconstruction, possibly related to use of radiation therapy (no new bone formation is seen). Apart from lenghtening short flaps, vertical DO can augment bone height to facilitate osseointegration.

VI. HYPOPHARYNX

The hypopharynx is the region from the aryepiglottic folds to the origin of the oesophagus (cricoid cartilage level). Important subsites for tumours are postcricoid region (10%), piriform fossa (70%) and posterior pharyngeal wall (20%).

T STAGING

- T1 – One subsite and less than 2 cm wide
- T2 – More than one subsite or 2–4 cm without hypopharynx fixation
- T3 – More than 4 cm or with hypopharynx fixation
- T4a – Invades mid-line thyroid/cricoid, hyoid, oesophagus, strap muscles
- T4b – Invades prevertebral fascia, mediastinum or encases carotid

Hypopharyngeal tumours have a tendency to spread sub-mucosally and have skip lesions. The majority of patients (80%) present with advanced disease (stage III/IV) and 17% have distant metastases. T1 tumours can be treated with radiotherapy alone, but few patients present at this early stage; more advanced stages require surgery – resection with laryngectomy (usually), reconstruction and PORT.

- If there is adequate mucosa, then primary closure is an option as long as a **34F catheter** can be passed; at least 3 cm of mucosa is required.
- If there is inadequate mucosa, then reconstruction requires either a free jejunum or a tubed fasciocutaneous flap, e.g. RFFF or ALT, or a tubed pectoralis major. Tubed flaps are said to have a higher incidence of fistulae compared with the jejunal flap supposedly due to the extra longitudinal suture line; the bulk of the PM can hinder tubularisation of the skin island. Preservation of a strip of pharyngeal mucosa, e.g. back wall, is generally associated with better functional results compared with complete circumferential reconstructions.

JEJUNUM

Pharyngeal reconstruction using free jejunal flaps was first reported by Seidenberg in 1959. Using the jejunum has the advantages of a flexible and self-lubricating tubed reconstruction with near-normal swallowing. The flap has average donor vessel diameters of 1.2 mm (artery) and 3.0 mm (thin veins) – a 10 cm pedicle allows perfusion of a segment up to 40 cm in length (Huang JL, *Ann Plast Surg*, 1999). However, a laparotomy is required with its attendant possible complications and contraindications, e.g. in those with previous abdominal surgery, but Uchiyama (*Head Neck*, 2002) demonstrated no difference in harvesting or in post-operative abdominal complications.

- Mucus production, though it settles to a lower level after ~2 weeks, can still give a 'wet' quality to voice; there is also a risk of aspiration in patients who retain their larynx.
  - 4–5 cm loop produces 100 mL of secretions per day, decreasing to 10 mL/day after 2 weeks.
- Short ischaemic time tolerance (90 min); thus, preparation is important and some perform the vessel anastomosis before the bowel anastomoses. Intraoperative cooling has not been useful and excessive cooling can cause vessel spasm. The high metabolic rate also contributes to its susceptibility to RT effects.
- The bowel can be opened out along anti-mesenteric border as a 'patch' for the reconstruction of mucosal

defects, whilst a segment with its mucosa removed can be skin-grafted to reconstruct skin tissue defects if needed (Carlson GW, *Plast Reconstr Surg*, 1996).

TECHNIQUE

- Open or laparoscopic approach (Gherardini G, *Plast Reconstr Surg*, 1998). No bowel preparation is usually required.
- Isolate the second or third jejunal loop (or 40 cm) beyond the ligament of Treitz on a 'V'-shaped mesentery containing an artery and a vein. Gentle dissection is necessary to avoid mesenteric haematomas. The proximal should be identified with a stitch or ink. The cut small bowel ends can be repaired whilst leaving the raised jejunal flap in situ until ready to transfer (to shorten ischaemic time).
- When ready (i.e. recipient vessels prepared), divide the jejunal flap pedicle and inset the flap in an isoperistaltic direction with the mesenteric border posterior. It is conventional to complete the upper anastomosis first.
  - The upper end may be too narrow to anastomose to the wider distal pharyngeal stump – a reverse L end-side anastomosis, double-lumen J-pouch or jejunal expansion with a patch flap may be considered (Yoshida T, *Br J Plast Surg*, 1998). Place a few holding sutures at the lower end before the definitive repair.
  - Tack the posterior surface to the prevertebral fascia.
- Microanastomosis of the vessels is usually performed before the distal bowel anastomosis to reduce the ischaemic time as well as to take account of the flap lengthening that occurs after revascularisation. There will be mucus production and peristalsis at this point. The neck should be thoroughly irrigated with drains inserted. A feeding tube is passed through the anastomosis; some surgeons prefer a long tube that also goes past the jejunal anastomosis.
  - Excessive redundancy may lead to swallowing problems and should be avoided by careful tailoring of the length of the flap, and insetting with the neck in a near-neutral position (being hyperextended for tumour resection).
- Some prefer to use double-layer closure (inner 3-0 vicryl and outer serosal Lembert suture) for the superior anastomosis to reduce fistula rates and a single-layer interrupted vicryl for the inferior suture line with 1.5 cm 'V' spatulation into the anterior oesophagus to reduce stricturing.

For hypopharyngeal reconstruction, the distal margin should not be more than 2 cm below the inferior cricoid border to avoid a low anastomosis that is almost in the chest; in such a situation, a pull-up may be preferable, though an alternative is to use a jejunal flap with a stapled anastomosis.

Monitoring of the (buried) flap can be a problem and options include

- Anterior neck window to expose the serosa of the underlying flap, which is tacked to the skin, possibly covered with a thin SSG (Bafitis H, *Plast Reconstr Surg*, 1989) or closed after the third day.
- Daily endoscopic inspection (beginning on the fifth day).
- Sentinel loop – exteriorising a minor segment of the flap (~2 cm) to observe colour, secretion and peristalsis (Katsaros J, *Br J Plast Surg*, 1985). This segment is excised ~5 days under LA.
  - A similar method can be used for tubed fasciocutaneous flaps, e.g. ALT with multiple perforators.
- Alternative methods include
  - Handheld Doppler – mark position of the anastomosis on skin at the end of surgery; the pedicle always runs in an 'unnatural' course and usually more superficial. Venous hum is said to be a more specific feature.
  - Colour duplex Doppler.
  - Implantable Doppler probe – a standard of sorts but still not wholly reliable as it may detect other vessels.
    - Christian Doppler (1803–1853) was an Austrian physicist.
  - Angiography.

POST-OPERATIVE CARE

- NPO: tube feeding is commenced on the fifth day or so (when bowel sounds return).
- Vancomycin or other antibiotic swallows.
- Gastrograffin swallow on the 10th day, and gradual oral diet if the anastomosis is satisfactory (note that contrast swallow tests do not provide information on the viability of the flap). In the uncomplicated case, PORT can be commenced ~5 weeks post-reconstruction.

One review (Cordeiro P, *Plast Reconstr Surg*, 1999) on the use of routine barium swallows (average 12–17 days) found that they could be difficult to interpret. Water-soluble swallows are potentially safer but less sensitive. A normal swallow test does not ensure an uneventful clinical course with some leaks being delayed whilst radiological leaks do not imply clinical fistula (more than half do not develop overt fistula). Thus, clinical judgement is needed when deciding to restart oral intake. Some surgeons suggest refeeding at 7 days as a standard (later if irradiated) without a routine contrast swallow if progressing well, on the assumption that swallowing saliva and the presence of a feeding tube is potentially more irritating than refeeding.

COMPLICATIONS

More common complications include the following:

- Abdominal, e.g. adhesions.
- Anastomosis failure – the lower anastomosis tends to have more problems.

- Fistula: most cases will close spontaneously with conservative treatment, but this may take up to 2 months. If it occurs on the side of the vascular anastomosis, diversion may be considered.
  - Early minor leakage should be exteriorised.
  - For significant dehiscence, a controlled pharyngostome is advised to allow the tissues to recover, with the defect covered later by another flap.
- Dysphagia is a common delayed complication: early problems are possibly due to oedema or a functional problem, such as redundancy. Late dysphagia may be due to stenosis.
- If one flap fails, another can be harvested, but avoid leaving a segment of jejunum between two **donor** sites as denervation of this segment leads to motility disorders.

More recently, the tubed ALT flap is becoming popular; a 9–10 cm wide flap is needed for a 3 cm diameter tube (approximately $2\pi r$). According to studies,

- Fistula rate is slightly higher and ascribed to the additional vertical suture line (8% vs. 3%) but manifesting itself later at 4–5 weeks vs. 2 weeks, and more likely to heal with conservative treatment. Proximal leaks are less common as the ALT may cope better with the wide oropharyngeal defect.
- Stricture rates were slightly less (12% in circumferential reconstructions).
- Better return to a complete oral diet and fluent speech.

SPEECH RESTORATION

- Artificial larynx – electronic external mechanical sound source usually placed on the neck skin; sometimes intraoral devices are used. A hands-free version using EMG transducers on the strap muscles has been described (Goldstein EA, *J Speech Lang Hear Res*, 2007).
- Pneumatic artificial larynx. Popular in Hong Kong.
- Oesophageal speech – no additional surgery/equipment but needs significant training, ~50% success.
- Tracheo-oesophageal fistula (TOF) and valve, e.g. Provox, Blom-Singer.
- Autologous valve free flap, e.g. ileocaecal flap as reconstruction, free appendix for TOF, additional 'voice tube' segment with free jejunum.
- Laryngeal transplant – first case in Cleveland, 1988. Probably more suited to trauma patients.
- Speech-generating device – words/sentences input into the device are electronically spoken, e.g. from phone/tablet to dedicated devices.

Quality of life and disease-specific functional status following microvascular reconstruction for advanced (T3 and T4) oropharyngeal cancers (Netscher DT, *Plast Reconstr Surg*, 2000)

General and disease-specific QOL is decreased after surgery and RT. Most returned to baseline levels at 6 months, whilst some were better than pre-treatment after 1 year.

VII. TUMOURS OF THE NASAL CAVITY AND PARANASAL SINUSES

NASAL POLYPS

These are relatively common, occurring in about 1% of the population (up to half of cystic fibrosis sufferers – suspect this disease if nasal polyps occur in children). The risk of malignant change is thought to be very low, and nasal polyposis is not regarded as being a premalignant condition. There is no reliable way to distinguish benign from malignant clinically, although unilateral solitary polyps are more likely to be malignant.

Biopsies prior to definitive treatment are not routine for simple polyps, but should a biopsy demonstrate a malignant lesion, then a wide local excision via lateral rhinotomy or FESS and PORT is needed. Ethmoidectomy is usually achieved by piecemeal excision. Post-operative epiphora due to blocked nasolacrimal ducts is not uncommon.

NASAL CAVITY TUMOURS

These tumours usually present with epistaxis, obstruction or rhinorrhoea. Radiotherapy is a common treatment option in order to avoid potentially mutilating surgery; 15% will develop a second primary, approximately half in the head and neck.

NASOPHARYNGEAL CARCINOMA (NPC)

The nasopharynx is the region behind the posterior choanae up to the palatal plane (soft palate to posterior pharyngeal wall). NPC is common in Chinese and also North and sub-Saharan Africans. In other populations, it comprises 0.25% of all carcinomas. Risk factors apart from ethnicity (HLA linkage) include EBV and dietary nitrosamines, whilst smoking and alcohol do not seem to be major aetiological factors.

- The vast majority are SCCs – keratinising (I), non-keratinising (II) or undifferentiated (III).
- Early-stage symptoms may be trivial; common methods of presentation are cervical lymphadenopathy (70%, usually upper jugular or level V), otitis media, obstruction or epistaxis. Thus, tumours are relatively advanced at presentation. In rare cases, patients may have skull base symptoms, i.e. cranial nerve palsies or distant metastases. There are attempts to find disease at an earlier stage, i.e. screening with EBV IgA.

T STAGING

- T1 – Nasopharynx
- T2a – Extension to oropharynx, nasal cavity without parapharyngeal extension
- T2b – Tumour with parapharyngeal extension

- T3 – Bony structures or paranasal sinuses
- T4 – Intracranial extension, cranial nerve involvement, infratemporal fossa, hypopharynx, orbit, masticator space

INVESTIGATIONS

- Endoscopic exam and biopsy – may be predominantly submucosal
- Neck node FNAC
- Imaging – CT/MRI with contrast (especially for parapharyngeal involvement)

Accurate staging is important for determining the neck status and RT planning. The tumour is typically very radiosensitive and even extensive disease may regress completely; IMRT may allow better shielding of normal tissues and allow higher doses to be used. Therefore, most cases are treated with RT with or without concomitant chemotherapy depending on their state of health. Salvage surgery is usually offered for recurrences; most recurrences occur in the first 2 years.

- Stage I – radiotherapy to primary and neck
- Stages II–IV – radiotherapy or chemoirradiation

Hypothyroidism is a common complication of irradiation; 20%–60% will develop distant disease. Post-irradiation skin and soft tissues changes in the neck are a common source of morbidity.

PARANASAL SINUS TUMOURS

These are rare tumours (~$1/10^5$) in the United States, comprising 3% of all head and neck malignancies; most are SCC (80%) with adenocarcinoma making up most of the remainder. Sinus tumours are more common in Japan and Uganda, most frequently affecting males in the over 60 years age group.

- 60% occur in the maxillary antrum.
- 3% nasal cavity.
- 9% ethmoid sinuses, 1% sphenoid and frontal sinuses.

These patients usually present with late disease (T3/4). Possible risk factors include smoking and alcohol (synergy seems to exist), occupational causes such as wood dust, chromium and nickel, cyanide chemicals as well as radiation and possibly HPV.

INVESTIGATIONS

- EUA and biopsy – biopsy can be performed directly through the medial wall of the maxillary sinus for example, or via a Caldwell–Luc approach.
- Facial X-rays, OPG.
- Staging with MRI or CT for definition of soft tissue and bony involvement, respectively.

Most of these tumours are treated by surgery followed with post-operative (brachy)radiotherapy, notable exceptions being

- Sarcomas – chemotherapy then surgery
- Lymphomas – chemotherapy and radiotherapy

MAXILLARY SINUS TUMOURS

Differential diagnosis of facial/cheek swellings:

- Benign, e.g. epidermoid cyst, lipoma, ossifying fibroma
- Malignant, e.g. SCC, adenocarcinoma, lymphoma

The maxillary sinus may be affected by primary tumours or may be invaded from neighbouring regions, e.g. palatal tumours. The orbit, in particular, is an important consideration.

- The periosteum of the orbital floor is a good barrier to invasion (although the lamina papyracea may be destroyed quite quickly), and the orbital contents may be preserved with close observation (Suarez C, *Head Neck*, 2007).
- Exenteration is required once the periorbitum has been breached. Tumour types with aggressive behaviour such as adenocarcinoma or SCC compared to esthesioneuroblastomas should have a lower threshold for exenteration.
- Orbital wall reconstruction is needed if two or more orbital walls are involved to prevent displacement.

PRESENTATION

There is usually advanced disease at the time of presentation.

- Facial symptoms – swelling, pain and infraorbital/cheek paraesthesia
- Dental symptoms – gingival or palatal mass, dental pain (especially first and second premolars) or unhealed extraction socket, fistula
- Nasal symptoms – epistaxis, discharge, obstruction, pain
- Ocular symptoms – proptosis, epiphora, eyelid swelling, impaired vision, pain

STAGING

Tumour staging

- T1 – mucosal involvement only
- T2 – bony involvement including inferomedial spread (hard palate, nasal cavity) but not posterior wall extension including pterygoid plates
- T3 – bony involvement superolaterally (orbit, anterior ethmoidal sinuses) or the posterior wall of maxillary sinus, subcutaneous tissue involvement
- T4a – anterior orbit, skin of cheek, pterygoid plates, infratemporal fossa, cribiform plate, sphenoid or frontal sinuses
- T4b – orbital apex, dura, brain, cranial nerves other than maxillary division, nasopharynx or clivus

Nodes (N) and metastases (M) staging as for oral cavity. Or based on symptoms related to the degree of spread:

- Stage 1 – symptoms due to swelling itself – swelling, numbness and pain
- Stage 2 – symptoms related to inferomedial spread – tooth pain/numbness/loosening, nasal bleeding/discharge/obstruction
- Stage 3 – symptoms related to superolateral spread above Ohngren's line – ocular pain, ophthalmoplegia or impaired vision.

Ohngren's line is a plane that lies diagonally connecting the inner canthus with the angle of the mandible. Maxillary sinus tumours invading above this line i.e. high tumours carry a worse prognosis. Overall, there is local recurrence rate of 45% especially in the first year.

Malignant tumours of maxillary complex: 18-year review (Stavrianos SD, *Br J Plast Surg*, 1998)
Treatment with the combination of surgery with PORT results in 68% and 64% 5 year control and survival. This is better than

- Radiotherapy alone, 39% and 40%, respectively.
- Surgery alone – survival 30%

CLASSIFICATION OF MAXILLECTOMY DEFECTS

Class III/IV defects are complex and often require multiple components/flaps (Figure 3.6):

- Skeletal support for globe, nasal base, cheek contour and alveolus
- Obliteration of soft tissue defect
- Skin and mucosal defects

TREATMENT

In general, most maxillary sinus tumours are best treated by surgery then radiotherapy (necessitating pre-operative dental evaluation). Other factors include nutritional support as well as encouraging the patient to stop smoking.

- Resect as much maxilla as is required for tumour clearance. Maxillectomy is usually carried out via a Weber–Fergusson lateral rhinotomy approach ± subciliary Dieffenbach extension or craniofacial bicoronal approach. Tumours affecting the inferior half of the maxilla may be assessed via a lip split, whereas facial degloving is usually needed for superomedial tumours. Selected cases may need orbital or transcranial approaches.
  - Extensive maxillectomy requires ipsilateral insertion of grommets to prevent secretory otitis media.
  - Reduce post-operative trismus by excision of the coronoid process.
- Prefabrication of an obturator to close oronasal fistula (preferably with preoperative dental assessment) or reconstruct (immediate or delayed) palate using a free flap with bone or soft tissue only.
  - The orbital floor may require reconstruction with bone graft, e.g. rib or iliac crest, or with titanium mesh. Frank orbital involvement is more problematic particularly at the apex – the dural seal, the cavernous sinus and the ophthalmic artery need to be considered.
    - In general, accurate setting of the level of the visual axis is best done with a mesh repair, whilst vascularised bone is desirable when any healing issues are anticipated.
  - Skin of the cheek may need to be replaced – flaps such as the RFFF are usually a poor colour match, so some suggest a second step of **dermal overgrafting** with a scalp SSG for improved colour match.
- Lymph node metastases are rare (except for tumours of the maxillary sinus that also involve buccal mucosa) as the region is poorly supplied by lymphatics.

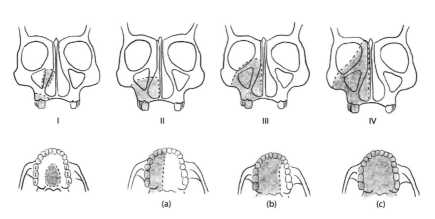

Figure 3.6 Brown classification of maxillectomy defects, considered from the vertical and horizontal components. (a) Unilateral, (b) bilateral incomplete and (c) complete.

Health-Related quality of life after maxillectomy: A comparison between prosthetic obturation and free flap (Rogers SN, *J Oral Maxillofac Surg*, 2003)

The size of the defect is associated with physical functioning, and the activity and recreation QOL domains. Otherwise, there were **no significant differences** between obturator and flap groups. Some borderline trends for obturator patients were

- More concerned about appearance, more self-conscious, including awareness of upper teeth
- More oral pain and discomfort
- Less satisfied with function

VIII. SALIVARY GLANDS

The salivary glands can be described as being serous or mucous in nature:

- Parotid gland is mainly serous (P-S).
- Submandibular gland is a mixture.
- Sublingual gland is mainly mucous.
- Minor salivary glands are almost entirely mucous.

PAROTID GLAND

The gland is ectodermal in origin and is enveloped by the parotid fascia that is derived from the investing fascia of the neck. The deep and superficial lobes (25% vs. 75% of the gland volumes, respectively) are split by the facial nerve; there may be an accessory gland that is anterior and superficial to the masseter. The following structures pass through, from superficial to deep:

- Facial nerve, its upper and lower divisions and the *pes anserinus*
- Retromandibular vein (posterior and anterior branches to post-auricular/external jugular and anterior/common facial veins, respectively)
- ECA and its two terminal branches
- Other structures in the gland include
  - Pre-auricular lymph nodes
  - Fibres of the auriculotemporal nerve

The parotid duct (of Stensen, 5 cm long) arcs around the anterior border of the masseter to pierce buccinator opposite the third upper molar and travels obliquely forward to open into the oral cavity opposite the second upper molar.

- Niles Steensen was a Danish Scientist (1638–1686) who then became a Catholic Bishop (of Titopolis) and as of 1998 is on the third of four steps to becoming a saint.

NERVE SUPPLY TO THE PAROTID:

- Sensation – the auriculotemporal nerve, which is a branch of the mandibular nerve (V3), emerges anterior to the tragus. It also supplies the upper part of the pinna (lower half is supplied by the great auricular nerve; the posterior auricular nerve is a preparotid branch of the VIIth nerve and is motor to occipitalis).
- Sensation to the parotid fascia – great auricular nerve (C2, 3).
- Secretomotor – preganglionic fibres from the inferior salivary nucleus (glossopharyngeal nerve – tympanic branch of IX – lesser petrosal nerve – otic ganglion – postganglionic fibres in the auriculotemporal nerve). The otic ganglion is closely applied to the mandibular nerve beneath the foramen ovale in the infratemporal fossa.

The posterior belly of digastric (PBD) is on the deep inferior surface of the gland and is a guide to the location of the facial nerve as it emerges from the stylomastoid foramen. The PBD is one of the **Residents' friends**; it lies superficial to ECA and its branches, ICA, IJV, XI, XII; the only significant thing above it is VII (marginal mandibular). The other Residents' friend is the omohyoid muscle.

SUBMANDIBULAR GLAND

The gland is composed of superficial and deep parts, which are separated by the free border of mylohyoid. The submandibular lymph nodes lie in contact with or within the gland.

- Superficial part is grooved posteriorly by the facial artery, but no actual structures pass through the gland.
- Deep part lies between the lingual nerve above and the hypoglossal nerve below.

The thin-walled duct (of Wharton) emerges from the anterior part of the deep lobe. It is 5 cm long and passes deep to mylohyoid and geniohyoid to open in the mouth next to the frenulum. The preganglionic fibres in the superior salivary nucleus/nervus intermedius/facial nerve/chorda tympani/via petrotympanic fissure and then go to the lingual nerve/submandibular ganglion and post-ganglionic fibres then pass directly to the gland.

- Thomas Wharton of the jelly fame (1614–1673) was an English anatomist/physician.

PAROTID TUMOURS

Eighty percent of all salivary gland tumours are found in the parotid (80% are benign):

- 75% are pleomorphic adenomas (PAs, roughly 80% for **the 80–80–80 rule**). Some people would say that the 80% rule is 80% true.
- 10% are adenolymphomas (proportions vary depending on ethnicity – much more common in Chinese) (Chung YFA. *Brit J Surg*, 1999) and may be related to smoking and EBV.
- 3% are mucoepidermoid carcinomas (most common malignant tumour of parotid and of salivary glands overall).
- 3% are adenoid cystic carcinomas (ACCs, most common non-parotid malignant tumour).
- 9% other carcinoma including carcinoma ex-PA.

Salivary malignancies comprise 3% of all head and neck tumours, and all pre-auricular masses in adults should be regarded as a parotid mass until proven otherwise. Haemangiomas are the most common parotid tumour in children.

OTHER SALIVARY GLANDS

- 10%–15% of all salivary gland tumours are found in the submandibular gland: half of the tumours in the submandibular glands are malignant.
- 10% are found in the sublingual glands (70% malignant) or the minor salivary glands – especially of the hard palate; 80% of parotid tumours are benign, whilst 80% of minor salivary gland tumours are malignant.
- The smaller the salivary gland is, the more likely that a tumour is malignant and the more likely that a malignant tumour will behave aggressively.
- Mucocoeles are uncommon in the upper lip; canalicular adenomas affect the upper lip most frequently.

Salivary gland tumours usually present as localised painless nodules ± fixity. Differential diagnoses (for a parotid lump) include sebaceous cyst (punctum and discharge), sialolithiasis (the whole gland is swollen and is related to meals) and autoimmune conditions, e.g. Sjögren's or lymphoma (examine nodes). Overall, the **clinical picture is only about 30% predictive** with regards to benign vs. malignant; often the diagnosis is made after surgery. Features suggestive of malignancy include

- **Pain** – however, it is rather subjective/nonspecific and may be due to non-neoplastic reasons such as infection/inflammation.
- Short history – steady gradual growth followed by rapid growth of a localised portion suggests carcinoma ex-PA.
- Parotid tumours may involve the facial nerve, and facial weakness is a strong indicator of malignancy (though sarcoidosis of the parotid may also present with nerve palsy).
  - Trismus from TMJ involvement
  - Duct involvement causing obstruction or bleeding (another strong sign)
- Lymphadenopathy and fixity (deep and skin) are other features strongly suggestive of malignancy.
- Tumours in children and the elderly are more likely to be malignant.

Biopsy is largely contraindicated in the major salivary glands unless the features of the lump and history are strongly suggestive of pathology *other than* PA. In contrast, biopsy of the minor salivary glands is indicated because it is less likely that the lump will be a PA – more likely to be a carcinoma for which treatment will be based on the results of the biopsy.

Examination should include

- Lump including intra-oral and bimanual
- Full head and neck examination including

- Facial nerve function
- Lymph nodes and other possible draining areas, e.g. EAM and scalp

CLASSIFICATION OF SALIVARY GLAND TUMOURS

There are many different types. **Metastatic tumours** (up to one-third of parotid malignancies) have most commonly spread from SCCs of the scalp or ears, but prostate and kidney metastases have also been described. In Chinese patients, metastases from NPC are not uncommon. It is almost mandatory to perform FNAC of parotid lumps in patients with other known malignancies including lymphomas.

Malignancies are generally divided into low (mucoepidermoid, acinic cell) or high grade (mucoepidermoid again, ACC, SCC, AC and anaplastic/undifferentiated).

ADENOMA

- **Monomorphic** (adenolymphoma, Warthin's tumour) is a benign tumour (of the parotid tail in particular) accounting for 10% or more of parotid tumours. These are most commonly found in older male patients, particularly smokers. Tumours are typically soft and cystic and composed of uniform epithelial tissue, with lymphoid stroma. They may be multifocal or bilateral (10%–15%), and there is a 10% recurrence rate after surgery, though some say the recurrence rate is closer to 2% if one excludes missed multifocal lesions, hence the 10% rule, which is not that useful due to its lack of accuracy.
  - It is much more common in East Asians and in some series is more common than PA.
- **PA** is composed of different types of epithelial tissue and different types of stroma – chondroid, myxoid, mucoid, hence the name. It is usually found in middle-aged women. It typically exhibits slow painless growth. The 2%–5% risk of malignant change is the main reason for surgery.
  - **Pleomorphism** refers to the histological features – variability in size, shape and staining of the cells.
  - There is a delicate often incomplete **pseudocapsule** composed of compressed normal glandular tissue with tumour pseudopodia that may project beyond the capsule.
  - Enucleation leads to significant risk of recurrence ~25%; excision with a margin reduces this to 1%–5%. Recurrences may be multifocal and the chance of cure is then <25%.
- **Myoepithelioma** is a tumour of minor salivary glands that is similar to PA, though much less common (1% of all salivary gland neoplasms) usually presenting as a large intra-oral swelling with a characteristic slow growth over many years. It is usually said that biopsy should be avoided; MRI defines tissue planes and

resectability. Treatment may not be required, though secondary middle ear obstruction and effusion may require grommet insertion.

- **Mucoepidermoid tumour** displays squamous and mucous metaplasia within ductal epithelium and exhibits variable behaviour according to grade/differentiation. Tumours in major glands tend to be low grade like PAs, whilst in the minor glands, they behave more like ACCs. There is rarely a discrete capsule, and recurrence after excision is fairly common. It is the commonest primary parotid malignancy (30%); the most common parotid malignancy is a metastasis. 5 year survival of low-grade lesions is 74% vs. 5% in high grade.

CARCINOMAS (EPITHELIAL TUMOURS)

Most malignant salivary gland tumours still arise from the parotid, though the risk that a particular lesion is malignant is higher in the smaller glands.

- Adenocarcinoma.
- Squamous carcinoma.
- Anaplastic carcinoma.
- **Carcinoma in PA** (carcinoma ex-PA). The diagnosis is suggested by a sudden increase in the rate of growth with the development of fixity in a previously mobile swelling that has been present for many years (typically over 10 years). There may be facial nerve weakness or bleeding from the duct. The tumour behaves like anaplastic carcinoma with a poor prognosis (30% 5 year survival) but can be unpredictable at times.
- ACC.

Lymphoid tumours (malignant lymphomas) have a typical history of a diffuse rapidly enlarging swelling with no facial nerve involvement in a previously normal gland. It may occur in a gland affected by Sjogren's syndrome. The diagnosis is made by biopsy, and the treatment is chemotherapy rather than surgery.

ADENOID CYSTIC CARCINOMAS

The smaller the gland, the more likely that a tumour arising within it might be an ACC; they are rare in the parotid. These tumours have a Swiss cheese pattern histologically with no capsule; the tendency for marked **perineural spread**, perivascular invasion and infiltration of tissue planes without a lymphocytic response and the occurrence of skip lesions mean that excision is followed by 'inevitable' recurrence.

There are several histological subtypes: solid (10%, worst prognosis), cribriform ('classic' presentation seen in more than half) and tubular (best prognosis).

ACCs present most commonly in the fifth decade, with a slow rate of growth and typically have a protracted disease course, being prone to incomplete resection (>1/2), local recurrence (20%) and late metastatic potential especially to lungs.

Overall survival after **combined surgery and radiotherapy** at 5 years was 65% (Chummun S, *Br J Plast Surg,* 2001).

- Embolic spread to lymph nodes is very rare, but nodes may be involved due to direct invasion.
- Haematogenous spread to the lungs and bones is more common (36%) than nodal spread.
- High-grade lesions may need nerve sacrifice.

Facial nerve sacrifice and radiotherapy in parotid adenoid cystic carcinoma (Iseli TA, *Laryngoscope*, 2008)

This retrospective review of 52 cases showed that selective nerve sacrifice (for pre-operative nerve dysfunction or encased nerve at surgery) improved local control and survival (not statistically significant) but worse QOL. Cummings (*Ann Otol Rhinol Laryngol,* 1977) was one of the first to advocate nerve preservation with PORT (as long as the pre-operative nerve function is intact); thus, an alternative is to accept a higher recurrence rate but with improved QOL. These issues need to be carefully discussed with patients. Patients who had radiotherapy after surgery had better local control. N0 patients rarely went on to develop lymphadenopathy. In contrast to SCCs, ACCs cannot be considered cured even after 5 years of disease-free survival.

INVESTIGATIONS IN PRIMARY PAROTID MALIGNANCY

The role of investigations is commonly debated – some would say that it is not necessary except if there are suspicions of malignancy or deep/parapharyngeal involvement. In simple terms, the aim is to answer the following:

- Is the lump parotid tissue or not, e.g. NPC nodes?
- Is the lump neoplastic or non-neoplastic?
- Is the lump malignant or benign?
- If the lump is thought to be separate from the parotid gland (e.g. sebaceous cyst), use ultrasonography (USG) to confirm. USG cannot image the deep lobe.
  - Sialography if thought to be sialolithiasis.
- If the lump is truly a parotid swelling, then FNA can be used to obtain a tissue diagnosis – FNA can diagnose PA in 95% or more of cases; it can also diagnose malignancy accurately, just not the type. It is somewhat operator-dependent and requires experienced cyto-pathologists. Core biopsies have a greater risk of facial nerve damage. Open biopsy is generally contraindicated due to the possible risk of tumour seeding.
- Sensitivity 93%–95%; **only positive results should be accepted**.
- Specificity 98%–100%.
  - Sensitivity reflects the ability of a test to find those with the condition, whilst specificity reflects the ability to find those without the condition.
- 70%–75% concordance with pathology for tumour type.

- Having a tissue diagnosis facilitates informed decisions regarding management. UK guidelines (Sood S, *J Laryngol Otol*, 2016) recommend USG-guided FNAC for all salivary tumours with an experienced pathologist.
- MRI with contrast is capable of diagnosing malignant parotid disease (poorly defined tumour boundary with radiological evidence of local tumour invasion) with up to 93% sensitivity (Raine C, *Br J Plast Surg*, 2003). It can determine the location and extent of the tumour – particularly useful for larger tumours and where there is a question of deep lobe involvement; it can assess the neck nodes and the relationship of the tumour to the facial nerve.
  - PA is usually homogeneously hyperintense on T2W, whilst presence of a mass with low-to-intermediate intensity on T2W images is more indicative of a malignant lesion. Warthin's tumour is an exception appearing hypointense on T2W images. Oncocytoma is isointense to the glandular parenchyma on fat-suppressed T2W and postcontrast T1W images (Patel ND, *Am J Neuroradiol*, 2011).
- CT with contrast shows less soft tissue detail but is still a reasonable option unless detail around the nerve is a priority. Both CT and MRI can facilitate staging. Overall, CT provides useful information in 14%.

Some surgeons argue that there is little/no need for FNAC, that a superficial parotidectomy with frozen sections is the 'biopsy' that is therapeutic in most cases. Detractors of FNAC say that it provides little information that will change management as all parotid tumours (except lymphomas) should be removed, but it is cheap, simple and quickly available and, very importantly, it helps with discussions with patients.

However, there are also valid arguments for pre-operative investigations that allow **better planning particularly for malignant tumours** that may require radical surgery with ND, facial nerve grafting or flap reconstruction.

T STAGING

- T1   <2 cm
- T2   2–4 cm
- T3   >4 cm
- T4   >6 cm or invasion
  - a – skin, mandible, ear canal or facial nerve
  - b – skull base, pterygoid plate or encasing carotid

MANAGEMENT

Note that even where there is an extensive ACC or muco-epidermoid tumour for which surgery (with or without reconstruction) would only be palliative in effect, surgery may still be worthwhile because recurrent disease may take many months or years to become apparent and is often painless.

- Parotid
  - Benign or low-grade tumours:
    - Superficial lobe – **superficial parotidectomy** (lobectomy), e.g. PA, mucoepidermoid.
    - Deep lobe – **facial nerve-sparing total parotidectomy**
  - High-grade malignancy:
    - **Radical parotidectomy** sacrificing the facial nerve and surrounding involved structures including masseter, medial pterygoid, styloid process and associated muscles and the PBD. Overlying skin may also need to be sacrificed. Immediate nerve grafting and temporary lateral tarsorrhaphy are recommended under such circumstances.
- Submandibular
  - Benign or low-grade tumours – submandibular gland excision.
  - High-grade tumours – excision of gland plus excision of surrounding structures including platysma, mylohyoid and hyoglossus muscles, hypoglossal and/or lingual nerves
- Minor gland tumours – radical local excision

RADIOTHERAPY

Salivary gland tumours tend to respond poorly to radiotherapy; therefore, one should assume that **surgical resection is the only chance of cure**. Radiotherapy has no place in the management of PAs, which should be adequately excised; radiotherapy actually may increase risk of malignant change. Adjuvant radiotherapy may be indicated in cases of high-grade or advanced (T3/4) malignancies (Mahmood U, *Arch Otolaryngol Head Neck Surg*, 2011).

- Neutron therapy may be of some benefit with ACC.

PAROTIDECTOMY

The superficial parotidectomy will provide **adequate management in 80%** of all parotid lumps (benign and low-grade malignant tumours). In malignant lesions, PORT may be needed.

- Typically, a Blair incision is used (some have described limited incisions or face-lift incisions for selected lesions); the skin-SMAS flaps are raised off the parotid.
- Then the parotid tail is separated from its adjoining muscles – SCM and PBD. The great auricular nerve (6 cm below tragus lying on the SCM) is preserved if at all possible (~70%).
- **Identification of the facial nerve** – if a nerve stimulator is to be used, then no muscle relaxant is given. Sometimes the tumour size/position makes retrograde nerve dissection necessary.
  - At the stylomastoid foramen. The styloid process is deep to the nerve and thus not a useful clinical landmark.
  - **PBD**, which can be followed back to the digastric groove. Mastoid origin of SCM.

- **Tympanomastoid suture** – the nerve is 6–8 mm deep to the inferior end of this.
- Triangular projection of the **tragal cartilage points** to the nerve, which is classically 1 cm deep (but usually 2–2.5 cm deep) and anterior inferior.
- The buccal branches run alongside the parotid duct.
- The inferior trunk/marginal mandibular branch accompanies the retromandibular vein as it emerges from the inferior surface of the gland.
- Marginal branch runs below the inferior border of the mandible and over the facial artery.
- There is often a small branch of the occipital artery just superficial to the nerve and often leads to profuse bleeding that heralds the presence of the nerve nearby.

MANAGEMENT OF THE FACIAL NERVE

Some feel that the facial nerve should be resected only when *invaded* by malignant disease.

- If the tumour is close, carefully dissect out and consider PORT to clear 'contamination'. Long-term follow-up is mandatory.
- If the nerve is involved/invaded (suggested by preoperative palsy)
  - If the patient is under 60, then reconstruct the nerve (interpositional/cross facial with great auricular/ sural/medial cutaneous nerve of the forearm).
  - If the patient is over 60, then consider instead a temporalis transfer with fascia lata extensions, gold weights or endobrow lift/mid-face lift.

After a standard superficial parotidectomy, facial palsy is usually temporary (20%, usually recovering over 2 months); it is permanent in a very small number (1% or less).

NECK DISSECTION

The parotid is a relatively common site for regional metastases – lymph nodes are incorporated into the gland due to the delay (embryologically) in the formation of the capsule. These nodes receive lymphatic drainage from wide areas of skin as well as the orbit, external ear and posterior oro/pharynx.

- If N0 (clinically/MRI) then observe.
- Positive neck (either clinical or MRI) or highly aggressive/ recurrent tumour – synchronous lymphadenectomy.
- If the parotid tumour is a metastasis from a face/scalp primary – lymphadenectomy.
- Extensive involvement of the deep lobe of the parotid with a malignant tumour.

COMPLICATIONS

- Intra-operative – facial nerve palsy, retromandibular vein damage

- Early
  - Skin flap necrosis, infection, haematoma.
  - Sialocoele – aspiration and a pressure dressing are useful in most; the use of botulinum toxin A has been described.
  - Salivary fistula.
- Late
  - **Frey's syndrome**, i.e. gustatory sweating occurs because post-ganglionic parasympathetic secretomotor fibres destined for the parotid and hitch-hiking in the auriculotemporal nerve (sensory nerve to the ear and temple) are divided by surgery. Nerves degenerate to the level of the cell bodies in the otic ganglion and then regenerate along the auriculotemporal nerve and link up with sweat glands, so that subsequent eating induces sweating in the distribution of the auriculotemporal nerve. The reported incidence varies considerably (10%–40%, many cases may be subclinical). It can be treated with antiperspirants or botulinum toxin. The latter has largely meant that more invasive treatments have become much less common, such as interposition of dermofat or ADMs like Alloderm, superiorly based SM flap supplied by occipital artery or tympanic neurectomy.
    - **Lucja Frey** (1889–1942) was a Polish neurologist who described gustatory sweating in a patient who had drainage of a facial abscess.
    - De Bree (*Head Neck*, 2007) reviewed 10 trials on the use of botulinum toxin for Frey's syndrome, which showed good consistent results, though longevity varied from 3 to 24 months.

PAROTID FISTULA

The classical conservative treatment is to restrict the patient's oral intake, administering IV fluids, probanthine or atropine, along with repeated aspirations and compression. If the fistula fails to heal in 5 days, parenteral nutrition may be needed. Radiotherapy if needed for the disease will often help.

- Exploration can be fraught with difficulties and luckily is only needed in the minority that fails conservative treatment and for suspected/known ductal injuries. Options include duct ligation/excision and tympanic neurectomy to section the auriculotemporal or Jacobsen's nerve. Techniques of local duct treatment with cautery or sclerosants (including contrast material) tend to have a high recurrence rate.
- In contrast to techniques that aim to stop the flow, others aim to divert the secretions into the mouth, e.g. controlled internal drainage/fistulisation; by T-tube or catheter, duct repair or reconstruction; saphenous vein graft, mucosa flap, or marsupialisation of duct to buccal mucosa.

Malignant tumours of the parotid gland: A 2-year review (Malata CM, *Br J Plast Surg*, 1997)

Parotid malignancies are relatively uncommon, affecting 1–4 in 100,000 in the United Kingdom. This study included 51 patients with just over one-half having T3 or T4 disease on presentation. Carcinoma exPA constituted a significant proportion (transformation in up to 10% reported).

- FNA had an 88% sensitivity in diagnosing malignancy.
- MRI is more useful than CT (especially for imaging neck nodes).

Generally, **fixed** tumours without facial nerve palsy are treated by either

- Total parotidectomy (sparing all or part of the nerve) and PORT or
- Radical parotidectomy and facial nerve reconstruction (five patients)

Overall, 3/4 received PORT (including all patients with ACC); some of these had had immediate nerve grafting after radical parotidectomy.

ND was reserved for palpable disease or positive MRI findings or where the neck is entered for access purposes. **Immediate temporary tarsorrhaphy** was performed for palsied patients to prevent exposure keratitis.

Poor prognostic factors included

- Males
- Incomplete excision
- Pre-operative facial palsy

Free flap coverage of a fungating tumour was regarded as an acceptable option for palliation.

Malignant tumours of the submandibular salivary gland: 15-year review (Camilleri IG, *Br J Plast Surg*, 1998)

Submandibular gland malignancy accounts for 8% of all salivary gland malignancy. In this review of 70 patients (mean age 64 years), the main presenting symptom was a painless enlarged gland. Sometimes malignancy was an incidental finding, diagnosed after removal of an enlarged gland previously assumed to be due to duct obstruction. The commonest tumour in this series was ACC followed by carcinoma exPA. FNA was 90% sensitive. The standard treatment was surgery with PORT. The overall prognosis was related to TMN status at presentation.

Current treatment of parotid hemangioma (Weiss I, *Laryngoscope*, 2011)

These are the most common salivary gland tumours in children. In this retrospective review of 56 patients, females were affected more frequently (2.3:1). Most had combined skin and parotid involvement; a minority required treatment for complications including narrowing/obstruction of the auditory canal.

- Systemic steroids were used in 22, with an initial response but followed by rebound in 2/3 after cessation.
- Newer modalities such as oral propranolol were promising; most patients had significant shrinkage within 1 month without side effects. Another development was the use of bleomycin for sclerotherapy instead of agents such as NBCA (a cyanoacrylate). **Interferons were no longer an option.**
- Surgery for a proliferating parotid haemangioma risks excessive blood loss and facial nerve injury. Surgery was performed in 16 with good results; approximately half had sclerotherapy 24–48 hours before surgery.
- Patients with larger lesions were more likely to require surgery during the involutional phase later in childhood; typically fibrofatty tissue was resected through a facelift-type mobilisation.

The successful use of directly injected Bleomycin with or without dexamethasone has been reported by Chinese doctors.

IX. ORBITAL TUMOURS

Most orbital tumours (89%) are **secondary** tumours (from breast, lung, prostate and melanoma) or due to local invasion, e.g. from the paranasal sinuses. Primary malignant tumours are uncommon, but include

- Lymphosarcoma and rhabdomyosarcoma
- Meningioma and glioma
- Orbital malignant melanoma (MM), which can have several origins:
  - Extrascleral extension of posterior uveal MM, e.g. from choroid or ciliary body
  - Extension of adnexal MM, e.g. from eyelid or conjunctiva
  - Primary orbital MM – melanocytosis of the meninges of the optic nerve
  - Metastatic melanoma, i.e. haematogenous spread from a skin primary

Other orbital conditions include

- Inflammatory – thyroid, autoimmune, orbital pseudotumour, mucocoeles.
- Vascular – haemangioma.
- In children, the most common lesion is a dermoid cyst, whilst the most common malignancy is a rhabdomyosarcoma. Others include
  - Haemangioma
  - Optic nerve glioma
  - Teratoma

Proptosis is a common symptom; it can be defined as protrusion of the corneal apex >21 mm beyond the lateral orbital rim or >2 mm relative to the other side measured with a Exophthalmometer. The direction of displacement is important, e.g. lacrimal tumours tend to displace the globe inferior and medially.

- Inadequate eye protection can lead to exposure keratopathy.
- Severe stretching may compromise the optic nerve.
- Proptosis secondary to a mass/tumour can cause compressive optic neuropathy.

INVESTIGATIONS

Full ophthalmological examination should be part of the assessment.

- Plain X-ray, CT, MRI.
- Biopsy (division of lateral canthal ligament allows access behind the globe).

SURGICAL APPROACHES TO THE ORBIT

In general, anteriorly placed lesions are best treated via transorbital approaches, whilst lesions of the posterior 1/3 are best treated via extraorbital routes, though this is not absolute.

- The medial wall can be approached via a Lynch incision, transcaruncular incision or endoscopic endonasal approach.
- The orbital floor can be approached via subciliary, transconjunctival or transantral approach (via a buccal gingival sulcus incision).
- The **lateral orbit** approaches include the following:
  - **Upper eyelid skin crease incision** (Harris added an extension past the lateral canthus) allows access to the orbital apex and upper 2/3. When using this route, it is important to avoid damaging the levator aponeurosis (LA) by going superiorly when the orbital septum is reached.
  - **Lateral canthotomy** (straight incision introduced by Berke) allows lateral wall access and is especially useful in children.
    - Lateral triangle flap joining an upper lid skin crease and lateral canthotomy raised as a medially based flap allows access to the lateral orbit.
    - Lateral orbitotomy may be needed for apical/large masses.
  - **Lower lid swinging** (on a **medial pivot** after lateral canthotomy and cantholysis) – allows access to the lower 2/3 of the apex. The lid may need to be shortened (transversely) when closing to reduce the risk of lid retraction/ectropion. The flap can be subclassified as low (for floor access) or high (lateral orbitomy access).

TYPES OF EXCISION

- **Evisceration** – removal of the contents within the scleral shell (e.g. with an evisceration spoon). This is not suitable for tumour surgery and may provoke sympathetic ophthalmia.

- **Enucleation** – **removal of the globe** from the orbit preserving muscles and eyelids; prostheses can be inserted with muscle reattachment. It is suitable for treatment of intra-ocular malignancy, e.g. uveal tract melanoma without extrascleral spread.
- **Total exenteration** – removal of the entire contents of the orbit; eyelid sparing may be possible in selected cases. This is multilating and is primarily reserved for situations where such resection is needed to achieve clear margins with life-threatening malignancies.
  - **Extended exenteration** – some use this term to define a total exenteration with removal of adjacent bone, e.g. in cases of extensive orbital involvement by paranasal tumours.
  - **Subtotal exenteration** – excision that removes the globe, conjunctiva and extraocular muscles without a subperiosteal dissection, i.e. leaving some periorbital and part or all of the skin of the eyelids. It may allow better functional and aesthetic results.

RECONSTRUCTION OF THE ORBIT

Surgical effects may be compounded by radiotherapy, if any.

RECONSTRUCTION OF SOFT TISSUE

Spinelli (Atlas of Aesthetic Eyelid and Periocular Surgery, 2004) suggests that orbital reconstruction should be guided by the likelihood of tumour recurrence: coverage by skin grafts allows observation for recurrence in malignant disease, but if the surgery is regarded as definitive, i.e. with curative intent, and there is no specific need for close observation, then immediate reconstructive surgery can be performed. Whether or not the eyelids can be preserved makes a big difference to the quality of the reconstruction.

- **Split skin grafts** – may be used to cover exposed tissues following subtotal exenteration or to line the bony orbit following total exenteration. Mucosal grafts and dermal/dermal fat have been discussed as alternatives.
  - Healing by secondary intention is a 'classic option' but takes weeks to months and is not practical in irradiated tissues.
- **Pedicled myocutaneous flaps**
  - **Temporalis** muscle can be tunnelled through a window created in the lateral orbital wall to line the orbit after total exenteration; the socket is able to accommodate a prosthesis, but there is a temporal hollow. Other regional flaps include the frontalis/forehead flap and the TPF flap based on the superficial temporal vessels.
  - **Pectoralis major**. Some have tunnelled this myocutaneous flap to resurface an exenterated orbit (Aryan S, *Plast Reconstr Surg*, 1983), but there is a significant risk of tip necrosis due to the long

excursion and thus some suggest a two-stage method with an exteriorised pedicle.

- **Free flaps** bring in vascularised tissues and are particularly useful in irradiated beds, or dealing with dural leaks or small areas of necrosis.
  - LD, RA can provide skin and muscle bulk to fill the orbital defect.
  - Thinner flaps such as the RFFF or ALT are alternatives.
  - Flaps can be split and lined to accommodate a prosthesis, whilst hair transplants can be used for lashes. However, results are usually not that gratifying.

BONY RECONSTRUCTION

- Free split calvarial bone grafts
- Bone composite free flaps
- Alloplastic materials, e.g. titanium plates; should be avoided in irradiated fields

CONSIDERATIONS FOR ORBIT RECONSTRUCTION IN CHILDREN

The orbit is almost adult-sized by 2 years and fully adult-sized by 7 years. Children do not have fully formed sinuses, and the roots of the maxillary teeth abut the infraorbital rim (thus at risk). **Microphthalmos** is the commonest congenital problem; the lack of expansile stimulus leads to a hypoplastic bony orbit. The original disease process may also contribute. Options for the bony orbit reconstruction include the following:

- **Expanders**. Port tube can be passed through a hole in the lateral orbital wall to lie under the scalp of the infratemporal fossa (Dunaway DJ, *Br J Plast Surg*, 1996). Complication rates can be high; infections and rupture scar/stiffen the tissue making subsequent surgery more difficult.
  - Releasing osteotomies helps reduce the resistance to expansion when planning expansion over a shorter time. When planning expansion over a prolonged period, osteotomies are generally not necessary.
- **Implants** (regularly changed, e.g. 6 monthly) are usually the preferred option. The implants can be made of silicone, Medpor (porosity may actually be problematic due to tissue integration making removal difficult) or hydroxyapatite, wrapped with fascia lata, temporalis fascia or pericranium.
- **Bone defects** resulting from expansion or due to disease/surgery can be filled by autologous bone, though the cranium is thin and more cancellous, and thus splitting should not be attempted until >9 years of age. The iliac crest and ribs are alternatives.
  - Alloplastic materials should not be used in children wherever possible.

PROSTHESIS

To facilitate wearing of a prosthesis, the infraorbital rim should be built up to provide a bony shelf, whilst the posterior cavity should be filled so that a thinner, lighter implant can be used. Heavy implants lead to more fatigue and tend to stretch out the soft tissues particularly the lower eyelid.

- None – simply use an eye patch.
- Adhesive, with or without glasses.
- Obturator prosthesis when eyelids have been preserved.
- Osseointegration of an orbital prosthesis is an option if the eyelids have been resected; abutments are placed on the inner aspect of the orbital rim.

C. RECONSTRUCTION OF OTHER FACIAL REGIONS

I. EAR RECONSTRUCTION

EAR ANATOMY (FIGURE 3.7)

The Frankfurt plane (sometimes Frankfort, established at an Anthropology congress in that city in 1884) runs from the inferior margin of the orbit (orbitale) to the upper margin of the external ear meatus (EAM, porion), is regarded as the anatomical position of the human skull and is close to the horizontal plane of the head in the living subject.

- Distance from lateral brow to ear ~ height of ear
- Axis of ear to vertical: 20°
- Distance of helical rim to scalp: 1.5–2 cm

The arterial supply comes from the branches of the external carotid: postauricular, superficial temporal and occipital arteries.

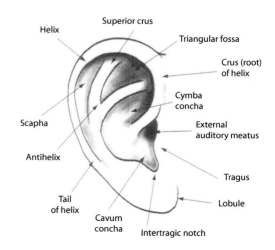

Figure 3.7 External ear anatomy.

SENSATION

- Great auricular (C2–3) – lower half of ear
- Auriculotemporal (trigeminal V2) – lateral part of upper ear, anterosuperior parts of EAM
- Lesser occipital – medial part of upper ear
- Auditory nerve of VII to EAM
- Arnolds nerve (X) – concha and EAM
- Jacobsens nerve (IX)

A ring block will probably not sufficiently numb the concha (CN X); additional local infiltration may be required.

EMBRYOLOGICALLY

- Three anterior hillocks from the first arch give rise to tragus, helix and root of helix; three posterior hillocks from the second arch give risk to antitragus, antihelix and lobule. The external ear forms lower in the neck and **migrates upwards** with the development of the mandible. Thus, any arrested growth results in a low and anterior ear.
- The malleus and incus arise from the first arch; stapes from the second arch.
- EAM and tympanic membrane from the first cleft/groove.
- Eustachian tube/mastoid air cells from the first pouch.

RECONSTRUCTION OF THE EAR

Seventy percent of tumours of the external ear are related to actinic damage and are more common in men; supposedly women's ears are protected by their longer hair. Tumours tend to spread locally fairly rapidly.

- Most tumours are SCC with a higher metastatic potential when compared with other facial SCC and tend to spread to internal jugular and parotid nodes.
- BCCs are uncommon outside the conchal fossa, but may also be found on the posterior surface and lobe.

Other tumours include melanoma and adnexal tumours (adenocarcinoma, adenoid cystic), but these are rare; they generally require amputation of the pinna and possibly ND.

CLINICAL CLASSIFICATION OF AURICULAR DEFECTS (TANZER)

This is not that useful from a management point of view.

- Anotia 1 in 6000 in whites; 1 in 4000 in Japanese
- Complete hypoplasia (microtia)
  - With atresia of the EAM
  - Without atresia of the EAM
- Hypoplasia of the middle third of the auricle
- Hypoplasia of the superior third of the auricle
- Constricted (cup or lop) ear
- Cryptotia (1 in 400 Japanese)
- Hypoplasia of the entire superior third of the auricle
- Prominent ears

MICROTIA

Microtia occurs 1 in 10,000, being more common in the Japanese and Navajo Indians (0.1%); it is twice as common in **males**. The proportion of **right**, left and bilateral microtia is 6:3:1. There is low concordance in twins.

- Causes include teratogens (thalidomide, retinoic acid) or some intrauterine ischaemic insult (stapedial artery).
- Microtia is often sporadic and isolated but is sometimes a feature of some syndromes, e.g. Treacher Collins and hemifacial macrosomia (HMF)/Goldenhars that may be detected on careful examination.
  - Some regard microtia as 'microform' HMF.
- Associated features include
  - Hearing loss – sensorineural loss is less common (10%–15%) than conductive (80%–90%). The severity of external deformity does not correlate well with middle ear function.
  - Patients with microtia are more likely to have problems at school, which may be partly due to the hearing loss, as well as self-esteem issues.
    – BAHAs vs. middle ear implants (Vibrant Soundbridge®)
    – Jahrsdoerfer grading system (1992) based on external ear appearance and CT findings especially stapes, correlates with outcome of surgery
  - Others include facial clefts, micro-/anophthalmia, limb defects, etc.
  - Whilst the auricle may be normal with middle ear anomalies, when there is microtia, there are almost always abnormalities of the middle ear.

Auricular dystopia is an ear that is displaced secondary to deformity of the facial skeleton, particularly the temporal portion; it is a common feature of HMF. The remnant is often anterior and inferior to the proposed/optimal position for reconstruction (see above). The presence of a formed EAM actually complicates the surgery, and the facial nerve is at greater risk. The question is where to situate the reconstructed ear – at the remnant or the best match for contralateral side.

CLASSIFICATION

There is a spectrum of deformities:

- Lobular vs. conchal – Nagata method, etc.
- Classic vs. atypical – used by Brent.
- Firmin classification (1–3) based on the incisions needed – 1 corresponds roughly to lobular type, 2 to large conchal remnant and 3 to small conchal remnant, etc.
- Grading – I–IV (I is small but normal features; others, see below).

NAGATA CLASSIFICATION

- Anotia (grade IV)
- Lobular type (most common) – sausage-shaped lobule remnant and helix (grade III)

- Conchal type – lobule remnant, concha, EAM and tragus; looks more ear-like but is more likely to be displaced (grade II)
- Small conchal type – lobule with small concha
- Atypical microtia – types that do not fit into the above categories

TECHNIQUES OF AUTOLOGOUS RECONSTRUCTION

Brent had a 30% complication rate when his operating time was 6–8 hours, and this reduced to 1% when the operating time was cut down to 3 hours. Whilst the results in the best hands may provide reasonably good symmetry in placement and shape that passes a 'glance test', the fine details are far from normal. Expectations must be managed.

AGE

- The ears are 85% of their final size by 3–4 years of age (close to adult size by 11 years); in unilateral cases, the normal ear can be used as a reasonable template. The reconstructed ear continues to grow, albeit at a reduced pace.
- The second constraint is the amount of costal cartilage available – at ~6 years of age, there is enough for an adult-sized ear.
  - Undeveloped X-ray film is used to make a template from the other ear; taking care to match the angle and position, particularly the position of lobe and the distance from the eye.

Initially, Tanzer and Brent operated when patients were 6–7 years old; Nagata 9–10 years (with X-ray to confirm chest circumference >60 cm). Overall, there has been a tendency to wait longer; there is more cartilage and it is easier to retain the inner perichondrium. Balanced against this are the facts that calcified cartilages are more brittle and difficult to carve, as well as psychological considerations.

- **Costal cartilage framework** is constructed and placed into position.
  - Ear shape is carved out from the contralateral 6th to 8th costal cartilages: fused (synchondrotic) 6th and 7th for the body, 8th (free floating) for the helix and held together either with wires or sutures (such as clear nylon). It is thinned

out whilst preserving as much perichondrium as possible with an **exaggerated rim and a pronounced antihelix being most important**. The Nagata technique uses ipsilateral 6th–9th rib cartilage.
  - A segment of cartilage for framework elevation can be banked in the lateral part of the donor wound; smaller fragments can often be sutured together and buried, and will coalesce to useful larger masses by the next stage.
- The **template should be slightly smaller** by a few millimetres to allow for thickness of soft tissue that will be draped over it; the lobe usually does not need a cartilage framework.
- A **pocket ~1 cm wider** than the framework is dissected out; excessive dissection should be avoided to prevent subsequent displacement. Ear contours can be improved with mattress quilting sutures, with or without bolsters. In addition, suction drains, conforming dressings and an ear bandage worn may be used, taking care to avoid too much pressure.
- The results depend more on the quality of the overlying skin rather than the intricacy of carving; details will inevitably be blunted. The main aim is to have the framework in the correct size and position so that it passes a 'glance test' at a moderate distance.
- **Scaffold elevation** – Generally, one waits 4–6 months or more to allow blood supply to be re-established and for oedema to settle. The scaffold is elevated from the side of the head through an incision 5 mm superior and posterior to the framework. This exposes a bare postauricular sulcus; part of the elevated skin will drape over the cartilage rim whilst the remainder may be covered with fascia (temporoparietal or postauricular) and a skin graft with a bolster. There may be reconstruction of the lobule and tragus at this point (Brent) or with the first stage, and depending on the exact technique, contralateral ear tissue may be utilised. See Table 3.2.
- **Definitive reconstruction of the tragus and lobule**; costal cartilage for tragus (or a composite graft) and excavate cartilage to reconstruct depression of concha.
  - Hair removal with standard methods

Table 3.2 Comparison of Brent and Nagata techniques

Brent	Nagata
	Fewer stages
Multiple stages	Thicker looking ear
Lack of definition around conchal bowl	High flap necrosis rate 14%
Loss of postauricular sulcus due to SSG contraction	More cartilage needed, more noticeable donor defect
	Need for TPF (alopecia)
	Use of wires associated with higher extrusion rate

TEMPOROPARIETAL FASICA FLAP

The temporoparietal fasica (TPF) covers the deep temporal fascia over the temporalis muscle (with an intervening loose areolar layer) and is on the same anatomical plane as the galea and superficial musculoaponeurotic system (SMAS). The TPF lies just below the dermis at the level of the scalp hair follicles with fibrous attachments to the scalp without a true anatomic plane in between; thus, meticulous haemostasis is needed.

The TPF flap (TPFF) has supply from the superficial temporal artery (STA) and posterior auricular artery but **can usually be raised on the STA alone** – 8 × 8 cm can be harvested as free flap, e.g. for dorsum of hand. The posterior auricular fascial flap (based on the posterior auricular and occipital arteries) is continuous with the TPFF and can be used as an alternative.

- In microtia surgery, the TPFF is used to resurface the postauricular area after framework elevation. The flap needs to be at least twice the size of the framework. The superficial temporal vessels need to be carefully visualised; the path can be identified with a Doppler hand-held probe. A Y- or T-shaped scalp incision allows good access; the plane lies just deep to subcutaneous fat/hair follicles. The perimeter of the flap is incised and the deep layer is raised to isolate the vascular pedicle as far as the tragus.
- A 'primary' fascial flap can be considered if more than half of the framework will be covered by hair or if the skin pocket is predicted to be tight.
- It can be used to facilitate autologous reconstruction in moderately compromised recipient sites, and to salvage significant framework exposure.

RECONSTRUCTION IN MICROTIA

Patients are often referred soon after birth; they should be screened for other anomalies. They should be seen annually until ready for surgery.

- Family history.
- Hearing test and CT imaging including temporal bones – decide which ear benefits the most from hearing restoration surgery in bilateral cases. Hearing tests include
  - Brainstem evoked response after birth.
  - Behavioural: needs a cooperative child; distraction testing requires strong neck muscles and coordination.
- MRI for facial nerve if indicated.

Auricular reconstruction generally precedes any ear surgery to ensure that the tissues are virgin. BAHAs are usually OK if placed well away from the mastoid pocket, whilst prior osteointegrated implants are a contraindication for autologous reconstruction.

Auricular reconstruction for microtia (Walton RL, *Plast Reconstr Surg*, 2002)

TANZER TECHNIQUE

- Stage one – transverse re-orientation of lobular remnant
- Stage two – framework carved from **contralateral 6th–8th costal cartilages** and buried beneath mastoid skin
- Stage three – elevation of framework to create retroauricular sulcus with FTG to sulcus
- Stage four: reconstruction of tragus by composite graft from normal ear

BRENT TECHNIQUE

It is based on the Tanzer technique but with a modified sequence; patients are aged 4–6 years.

- Stage one – high-profile cartilaginous framework as above and placed into a mastoid pocket
  - The pocket is made from an incision in the hairy temple; it should be 10%–20% bigger than the framework to take account of the thickness/profile.
  - Microdrains for closed suction.
  - At this stage, the ear can look very odd with the remnant superimposed on the framework.
- Stage two – transposition of the lobule (occasionally combined with stage three).
- Stage three – elevation of the construct as above with placement of a banked piece of cartilage behind the ear to increase projection.
- Stage four – tragus reconstruction (trend to reconstruct tragus with the framework), excavation of conchal bowl, symmetry adjustment.
  - Initially, Tanzer rotated the ear remnant as a separate first stage but later combined this with the inset of the framework. Others, such as Brent, have generally performed lobe rotation after the inset of the framework to minimise scarring of soft tissues before this crucial stage.

NAGATA TECHNIQUE

Patients are usually ~10 years old. There is a theoretically greater vascular risk to the skin from the increased dissection, and more cartilage is needed leading to significant donor site deformity (supposedly this can be minimised by leaving perichondrium intact to allow cartilage regeneration).

- Stage one – formation and placement of an ipsilateral cartilaginous framework (6th–9th ribs) **with transposition of the lobule** to include **tragal reconstruction.**
  - A pocket is fashioned through a modified W-incision over the mastoid and rudimentary lobule (maintaining the subcutaneous pedicle) with a small circular excision (2 mm) at the end for the incisura; the remnant cartilage is removed. This modification to the classic V-shaped incision aimed to avoid wasting skin behind the ear that usually meant there was insufficient skin to cover the concha.

- The contour is maintained with bolster dressings.
- Stage two – after 6 months, elevation of the construct with placement of a further crescent of costal cartilage in the postauricular sulcus to increase projection. TPF flap and SSG from occipital scalp are used to resurface the sulcus (or advance retroauricular skin and graft the remainder).

Park described a single-stage two-flap reconstruction; a thin skin flap is used for anterior coverage, and an arterialised mastoid fascial flap for posterior coverage of a cartilage framework.

The Nagata technique has its advantages, but has a significant skin necrosis rate as well as greater donor morbidity (chest wall and TPF). Thus, some prefer the Brent approach, which also tends to produce a more natural-looking lobule.

Note that there is a reasonably steep learning curve before operating times and complications decrease, and aesthetics improve. What you see in journals and books are the best results after a long practice.

COMPLICATIONS

- Infections – rare (<0.5%). Prophylactic antibiotics are routinely used; the ear should be regularly inspected for erythema and collections/haematomas. Salvage with antibiotic irrigation has been described.
- Skin necrosis with exposure of cartilage (generally due to a tight pocket or post-operative compression from dressings/bolsters); small areas of necrosis can be dressed, but larger areas should be debrided and covered with skin or fascial flaps.
- Hairy ear resulting from placement in hair-bearing skin – standard depilation techniques including laser can be used. Some have replaced the hairy skin with skin grafts, e.g. from the other ear.
- Donor site complications, e.g. pneumothorax, atelectasis, chest wall scar (some suggest an IMF scar in females) and deformity (more likely with older patients), pain.
  - Pneumothorax is rare. If it is noticed intraoperatively, the defect can be repaired over a suction catheter that is pulled out when the lung re-expands, with a CXR to check.
  - TPF harvest causing alopecia/visible scar and numbness.

Tissue expansion as an adjunct to reconstruction of congenital and acquired auricular deformities (Chana JS, _Br J Plast Surg_, 1997)

Tissue expansion can be used to generate additional skin in difficult or salvage situations when large amounts of unscarred skin are not available. If excessive scarring prevents the use of expansion, then a thin flap such as the TPF may be required, but this will further reduce the shape definition that can be achieved with the cartilage framework.

- Retroauricular rectangular expander placed via a remote incision in the temporal hairline

- Slow expansion commenced after 2 weeks and maintained for 2 weeks before removal
- Capsulectomy performed and cartilage framework inserted; suction drains used to facilitate skin draping

There is a complication rate of 30% including extrusion, infection and haematoma.

ALLOPLASTIC TECHNIQUES

- **Silicone framework** – good initial result, but permanent risk of implant exposure/failure with relatively minor trauma. Largely abandoned.
- **Medpor framework** – TPF is needed to cover framework, which tends to lead to loss of definition. Risk of late exposure/implant failure somewhat reduced, supposedly due to some tissue integration.

PROSTHESIS

Osseointegration was FDA-approved in 1995 for extra-oral use. The Branemark technique uses osseointegration to fix a tailored silicone ear prosthesis. It arguably offers the best aesthetics – better than nose/orbital prostheses that are centrally positioned and reflect light differently, making the observer aware of a difference. Meticulous hygiene is required; the patient is constantly reminded of the deformity. The prosthesis needs to be replaced every few years. It effectively precludes autologous reconstruction later; the main indications are

- Scarred recipient site, e.g. burns/trauma/failed reconstruction.
  - Especially with lack of TPF
- Severe tissue hypoplasia.
- Very low hairline that would cover the upper pole of a framework. However, the lower pole is more important for aesthetics.

There is an element of local preference. Whilst autologous reconstruction is common in many countries such as Japan, the United States and United Kingdom, prosthetics are used more frequently in Sweden (home of Branemark).

RECONSTRUCTION FOLLOWING ACQUIRED LOSS

Acquired loss is usually due to tumour surgery (60% SCC, 35% BCC and 5% melanoma), occasionally due to trauma or burns (ears are involved in 90% of facial burns). The reconstruction can be considered in terms of the anatomical part(s) affected:

- **Conchal/antihelical defects** reconstructed by
  - Full thickness skin graft
  - Trap-door flap
  - Islanded retroauricular flap
- **EAM** defects tend to heal by stenosis; acrylic moulds, typically used for 6/12, have variable results, as does surgery in the form of FTSG or local flaps.

UPPER THIRD DEFECTS

- **Helical advancement** (Antia Buch) generally recommended for defects of 3 cm or less. The helical rim is detached from the anterior skin and cartilage, pedicled on the posterior skin. The superior segment can also be advanced in a VY manner.
- **Banner flap** – from the posterior sulcus based at the root of the helical rim, along with contralateral conchal cartilage graft for support.
  - **Bilobed flap** using skin from postauricular sulcus
- Local flaps can be tubed and **bipedicled**, e.g. tubed preauricular skin for upper helical rim defects, or neck skin for lower defects. It is a three-stage procedure. The donor scarring can be very significant.
- **Chondrocutaneous composite flap** based on the skin pedicle from the root of helix (Davis J, *Symp Reconstr Auricle*, 1974) or on the outer border (Orticochea). The donor is covered with a transposition flap with skin grafting to this donor.

MIDDLE THIRD DEFECTS RECONSTRUCTED WITH

- **Composite grafts** of contralateral helical rim.
- **Ipsilateral conchal cartilage graft** covered both posteriorly and anteriorly by a transposition flap from retroauricular skin.
- **Direct closure** using either wedge excision or helical advancement (Antia and Buch). Small wedges can be excised with direct closure of a V wedge with excision of accessory triangles ('star') to facilitate closure.
- **Tubed bipedicled flaps**.
- **Converse tunnel technique** – a tailored piece of cartilage is tunnelled under the mastoid/postauricular skin and joined to the edges of the helical defect. The ear is then separated from the mastoid area in a second stage after 3 weeks with the graft attached, and the defect covered with FTSG.
- **Revolving door** flaps for conchal defects.

LOWER THIRD DEFECTS

Lobe reconstruction can be complex:

- Two-stage approach – inset free edge into adjacent skin then release with an adjacent local flap
- Contralateral composite graft
- One-stage approach
  - Alconchel technique (below)
  - Gavello procedure – a horizontal bilobed flap from the postauricular mastoid skin, supposedly based on the postauricular artery
  - Limberg/rhomboid flap technique – better for rather low/small defects (Figure 3.8)

SPLIT/CLEFT EAR LOBE

Many different techniques have been described. Pardue describes a technique of reconstructing the hole with a small flap from the cleft; it may be easier to simply pierce the ear again after a complete repair that obliterates the hole. Some suggest using Z-plasties to reduce notching from scar contraction. Although there is no cartilage in the lobe, a graft may be placed for additional contour/support.

A combined flap technique for earlobe reconstruction in one stage (Alconchel MD, *Br J Plast Surg*, 1996)
This technique avoids the classic two-stage approach and the donor defects often close directly (FTSG can be used if necessary).

- Reflect anterior skin of healed inferior edge inferiorly to form the upper part of the posterior surface.

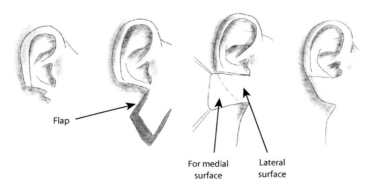

Flap

For medial surface   Lateral surface

Figure 3.8 Earlobe reconstruction. An adjacent rhomboid flap is elevated and inset into defect. The inferior portion is used to cover the medial surface of the ear.

- A vertically orientated islanded skin flap with a narrow pedicle at the postauricular sulcus is raised from the postauricular skin. It is brought forwards with the longer superior portion making the anterior surface and the lower part folded up backwards to make the posterior surface.

CAULIFLOWER EAR

It is usually preceded by a condition sometimes known as 'auricular haematoma', though the 'haematoma' is usually more of a serosanguinous collection that forms on the anterior aspect after trauma. Separation of the cartilage from its source of nutrition causes necrosis.

A 'cauliflower ear' develops from the formation of fibroneocartilage by chondrocytes over the 'haematoma' after 7–10 days (demonstrated by Skoog in 1972 with injections of blood subcutaneously and subperichondrially). The haematoma may be treated by

- Needling: often used in sport injuries but the effect is often incomplete; it may require repeating and still leads to distortion.
- Compression dressings: buttons (slightly higher risk of infection) or dental rolls, etc. after open evacuation through a small incision.
- If these fail, formal excision of the fibroneocartilage is usually necessary. Vogelin (*Br J Plast Surg*, 1998) suggest a bat-ear like posterior approach, resecting calcified haematoma and the posterior leaf of cartilage whilst the anterior leaf is resculpted by anterior scoring.

RECONSTRUCTION OF THE AMPUTATED EAR

- **Banking of cartilage beneath retroauricular skin** but it tends to flatten out (Sexton).
- **Pocket technique** (Mladick RA, *Plast Reconstr Surg*, 1971) is a reasonable salvage procedure that requires two stages. First, the avulsed segment is dermabraded (but leaving perichondrium) and reattached to the auricle in its appropriate anatomical location but buried in a postauricular pocket. At the second stage after 4 weeks or so (originally 2 weeks), the ear is released by elevating the skin off the ear and returning it to the retroauricular bed; the denuded ear is left to re-epithelialise or is grafted.
  - Dermabrasion of anterior skin and draping with a retroauricular flap (Pribaz JJ, *Plast Reconstr Surg*, 1997).
- **Banking of cartilage** subcutaneously as a prefabricated flap, e.g. forearm for later transfer as a composite free flap (Schiavon M, *Plast Reconstr Surg*, 1995). However, flap bulk often obscures definition; therefore, an option is to transfer as a fascial/cartilage flap with SSG.

- **TPF flap** coverage of denuded cartilage.
- **Baudet** technique – excision of posterior skin and cartilage fenestration to facilitate revascularisation of the lateral skin. Reconstruct sulcus 3 months later with skin graft. Survival is unpredictable, but when successful, it potentially has less flattening of the cartilage compared to pocket techniques.
- **Microvascular replantation** to available vessels, usually the superficial temporal or the posterior auricular vessels (see below). Technically difficult; small segments can survive with an arterial-only anastomosis. Leeches may help to tide the replant over until veins grow (7–14 days); topical heparinisation may be used as a chemical 'leech'.

Microvascular ear replantation (Kind GM, *Clin Plast Surg*, Apr 2002)

Pennington performed the first successful microvascular replantation of an amputated ear in 1980. Since then, dozens of successful cases of microvascular replantation of an amputated or avulsed ear have been reported in the literature.

Finding recipient vessels is a challenge. In a total amputation, the distal superficial temporal vessels can be dissected and reflected back into the operative field for length and better size match (however, this precludes later use of a TPF). Alternatively, the postauricular vessels can be used.

- Vein grafts may be needed. The skin is closed loosely.

MANAGEMENT OF THE BURNED EAR

- Padding and avoidance of pillow friction/compression.
- Topical antibiotics (sulfamylon – good penetration but painful, with risk of hyperchloraemic acidosis).
- Early debridement reduces the risk of infection and chondritis.
- **Exposed cartilage will not spontaneously re-epithelialise**, whilst non-viable areas may separate spontaneously; areas of chondritis should be aggressively debrided and covered (FTSG or fascial flaps).

An operation for Stahl's ear (Ono I, *Br J Plast Surg*, 1996)

Stahl's bar is a 'third crus' projecting from the antihelix with flattening of the helical rim. Options include

- Anterior stepped wedge excision of skin and cartilage; closure with helical advancement and a small cartilage graft (from conchal fossa) inset behind the approximated cartilage edges
- Turnover/rotation techniques
- Splinting within the neonatal period (similar to prominent ears, see below)

Posterior Z-plasty and J-Y antihelix-plasty for correction of Stahl's ear deformity (El Kollali R, *J Plast Reconstr Aesthet Surg*, 2009)

The Z-plasty is used to lengthen the skin on the posterior surface of the affected ear – the short vertical length tends to cause a bow-stringing effect. Posterior scoring and suturing are used to reconstruct the superior crus.

PROMINENT EARS

Prominent ears occur in up to 5% of the population; different cultures have different levels of acceptance and thus the rates of surgery vary greatly. This is inherited as an AD trait in some. The main features to look for are

- Poorly defined/absent antihelical fold. A small amount of the superior helical rim should be visible from the AP view.
- Conchal excess, e.g. wall height >1.5 cm, usually 7–10 mm.
- Conchoscaphal angle >90°.
- Also
  - Prominence of lobe – uncommon cause of prominence, but may be accentuated after correction of the upper and middle thirds
  - Wide angle between auricle and mastoid (males 25°, females 20°)

NON-SURGICAL TREATMENT

Neonatal cartilage is malleable supposedly due to maternal oestrogens/high hyaluronic acid levels, and moulding within this early window (1–2 weeks after birth) may be successful (Matsuo K, *Clin Plast Surg*, 1990), but does entail a significant undertaking for up to 6–8 weeks. Effectiveness is variable.

SURGICAL TECHNIQUES

History of treatment

- The use of sutures to recreate the antihelical fold described by Mustardé (*Plast Reconstr Surg*, 1967)
- Open anterior scoring to recreate an antihelical fold described by Chongchet (*Br J Plast Surg*, 1963)
- Transcartilaginous incision originally described by Lucket in 1910

Options

Some prefer to operate before the child starts school, whilst others wait until the child is able to actively participate in the decision, so that they will be more cooperative (usually around 6–7 years of age). In compliant adults, the surgery can be performed under LA ('ring block' of ear).

- **Excisional**
  - Cartilage – conchal reduction (Davis), antihelix (Luckett)
  - Skin – postauricular skin – dumbbell, fishtail, etc.

- **Suture techniques** – conchoscaphal sutures (recreate antihelical fold with mattress sutures placed from postauricular approach; Mustardé), conchomastoid sutures (along with excision of postauricular soft tissue, to reduce conchal projection but may distort meatus; Furnas). Suture-only techniques are probably more likely to lead to recurrence particularly in adults with stiffer cartilage.
  - Permanent sutures for 'suture-only' techniques, e.g. Ethibond vs. absorbable sutures for techniques also using cartilage shaping.
  - 'Single suture method' carefully defines a postauricular flap by de-epithelialising an ellipse, and then incising medially to form a laterally based flap that is relatively tough and can be sutured to the concha; it is often combined with Mustarde sutures, which will then be covered by this flap.
- **Cartilage moulding – Gibson's Law** (1958) states that cartilage will bend away from a scored surface due to the release of interlocked stresses. This is utilised in Stenstrom's technique (1978) that uses a rasp/otoabrader via a posterior approach and Chongchet (*Br J Plast Surg*, 1963) anterior scoring technique with a blade 1/2 to 2/3 of the cartilage thickness (Figure 3.9). Remember that auricular cartilage is **elastic cartilage**.
  - Mustarde sutures are best supplemented with some cartilage weakening to reduce failure in the long term.
  - **Access to outer/anterior cartilage surface**.
    - An otoabrader can be introduced via small posterior skin-cartilage incisions; some use anterior incisions. It is less useful for older stiffer cartilage (Weerda H, *Laryngol Rhinol Otol (Stuttg)*, 2007).
    - Scoring requires wider access – a wide posterior skin incision can either continue

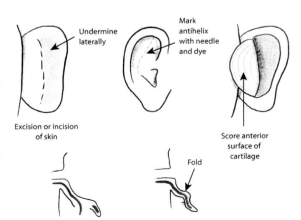

Figure 3.9 Chongchet technique of otoplasty. Some surgeons are concerned that the significant cartilage exposure may increase the risks of necrosis.

through cartilage, e.g. at the site of antihelical fold, or allow the cartilage to be degloved in a more open technique.

- **Cartilage breaking technique** – the cartilage is incised at the area of the desired antihelical fold, with (Luckett) or without some excision (Converse), and repaired with permanent mattress sutures. The fold tends to be sharp; thus, it is not a common option. Techniques that abrade the posterior surface aiming to thin down the cartilage are more cartilage-breaking than moulding.
- **Critics suggest that cartilage-shaping causes damage and degloving may lead to necrosis**.

Classically, soft conforming dressings were made with acriflavine or proflavine soaked wool, but this is not available in some localities, partly due to doubts about its antiseptic efficacy, partly due to a shortage of raw materials and partly due to the reported mutagenicity/toxicity. Alternatives are available. Avoid over-packing the concha/EAM, which may increase nausea. It is common to use a light head bandage over fluffy padding; headbands are commonly used for weeks afterwards especially at night.

COMPLICATIONS

Always be suspicious of a haematoma in patients returning early after surgery with increased pain and spotting of the dressing. Patients with wound infections tend to come back later. Both can have disastrous sequelae; therefore, there should be a low threshold for inspecting the wound.

The incidence of asymmetry can be quite high (~20%). **Dual-operator technique** is significantly more likely to give rise to asymmetry, and since young children usually have a general anaesthetic and two surgeons, this may explain the higher incidence of asymmetry in the young.

Otoplasty by percutaneous anterior scoring: Another twist to the story. (Bulstrode NW, *Br J Plast Surg*, 2003)
This is a review of patients in whom the Mustardé technique was used in combination with percutaneous anterior scoring using a hypodermic needle. Complications included a 3.5% infection rate but no haematomas. There was a 1.8% rate of hypertrophic scarring whilst 5.3% had significant residual deformity.

Otoplasty: Open anterior scoring technique and results in 500 cases (Caoutte-Laberge L, *Plast Reconstr Surg* 2000)
Anterior scoring of the antihelical cartilage was performed through a posterior skin and rather peripheral transcartilage incision; 94.8% of patients were either very satisfied or satisfied. Complications were not common but included

- Bleeding 2.6% (haematoma 0.4%)
- Wound dehiscence 0.2%, infection nil
- Keloid scars 0.4%, inclusion cysts 0.6%
- Loss of ear sensation 3.9%, tender ears 5.7%

Cryptotia is an unusual congenital deformity (more common in Asians) with an absent superior sulcus between the ear and the head so that it fails to stand out from the side of the head. In most cases, the cartilage is normal despite being buried. It is seen more often in examinations than in real life.

Surgical treatment (generally when the child is older) aims to release and reshape the cartilage and then use local flaps to recreate a superior helical sulcus. The modified trefoil technique is an alternative technique. Some have described early moulding.

CONSTRICTED EAR

In this group of deformities, the helical rim has an inadequate circumference and folds over the scapha. It is not uncommon in the mildest forms that are often 'asymptomatic' or regarded as a normal variant. Those with significant deformity form <10% of ear anomalies presenting to doctors. The appearance is sometimes described as

- Lop – downfolding of helix/scapha is the major feature.
- Cup – deep concha, short, superior fold.

Cosman classification (1978) (Cosman B, *Clin Plast Surg*, 1978)
This has many similarities to the Tanzer classification. Surgery is often delayed until ~12 years of age as the matured cartilage seems to allow more consistent results (Park C, *Plast Reconstr Surg*, 2018). Splintage in the early neonatal period may be successful in selected patients (especially Tanzer I or IIA; Tan ST, *Br J Plast Surg*, 1994); over 20 different procedures have been described.

- **Cosman A (~Tanzer I) Mild severity** – lidding, no protrusion and height difference less than 1 cm
  - Treat by excision of overhanging ('lidding') helical curl
- **Cosman B (~Tanzer IIA)** – lidding, no protrusion, height difference 1–1.5 cm
  - Treat with radial incisions of the cartilage for expansion (stabilised with a conchal strut) or to construct the helical rim with stacked double Banner flaps
- **Cosman C (~Tanzer IIA)** – lidding, protrusion, height difference 1–1.5 cm
  - Treat with **Cosman technique** – vertical expansion and correction of prominence
- **Cosman D (~Tanzer IIB)** – lidding, protrusion, height difference 1.5–2 cm
  - **Kislov technique** – unfurl margin and rotate superiorly using a middle third incision and superior rotation of the superior portion; the posterior defect is covered with a Banner flap (with cartilage graft)
- **Cosman E (~Tanzer III)** – like microtia

PREAURICULAR SINUS

This is a common congenital anomaly (US 0.25%, Taiwan 1%–2%) due to incomplete fusion of the sulci between hillocks of first and second arches. Some cases display incomplete AD inheritance, especially if bilateral (25%–50%). If unilateral, it is usually more common on the left side. Some have been described to have associations with renal malformations; however, current evidence suggests that renal ultrasound is not warranted if there are no other ear abnormalities or dysmorphia. Uncommonly, the condition may occur in the context of a syndrome, e.g. Treacher Collins and HMF.

The sinus is usually found as a narrow opening anterior to the end of the crus of helix; the sinus may fill with keratin debris and calculi can form. The sinus is of variable length and may arborise or be very tortuous. It is usually attached to cartilage especially the concha; it occasionally goes into the parotid gland, but is usually lateral and superior to the parotid and facial nerve – there is no connection to the facial nerve as it is not a true first arch syndrome. High-resolution ultrasound may be able to visualise the configuration of the sinus and its relationship to the parotid.

The majority of patients are asymptomatic, but once affected (>60% staphylococci), it tends to become recurrent and rarely settles completely. Treatment of asymptomatic patients is somewhat controversial; some believe surgery is justified as the recurrence rate after infection is much higher.

Some advocate the use of microscopes for dissection and resection. Some inject dye into the sinus 3 days beforehand (closing off orifice with a pursestring) and then use a probe and more dye intraoperatively. There is no standard surgery, but average recurrence rates are ~20% in larger series; a 4% recurrence rate has been quoted with a supra-auricular technique with a longer incision.

II. RECONSTRUCTION OF THE EYELIDS AND CORRECTION OF PTOSIS

ANATOMY

Orbital fat lies between the lamellae.

- **Anterior lamella** composed of skin and muscle, the **orbicularis oculi.**
  - Orbital fibres – contraction causes eyes to screw up tightly, e.g. to resist opening.
  - Palpebral fibres responsible for blinking gently.
  - Pretarsal for involuntary blink and tear film distribution.
  - Preseptal voluntary and involuntary assistance with blinking.
- **Posterior lamella** composed of lid retractor, conjunctiva (non-keratinising squamous epithelium) and tarsal plates. The latter are condensations of the orbital septum and are dense fibrous tissue around Meibomian glands and **are not cartilage.**
- The **orbital septum** is a dense fibrous membrane from the periosteum of the orbital rim, to the tarsal plate separating orbital from periorbital tissues. Some describe the orbital septum as the **middle lamella**; it fuses with the posterior lamella at the tarsal plate.
  - The arcus marginalis is the fusion of septum with the orbital periosteum.

Other features:

- Suspensory ligament of Lockwood forms part of the ligamentous attachments to the globe.
- Numerous apocrine glands of Moll at the lid margin.
- Lateral and medial condensations of the tarsal plates form the lateral and medial canthal ligaments.

EYELID RETRACTORS

- **Levator palpebrae superioris (LPS)**
  - **Striated muscle** (45 mm in length) attaches to the upper tarsal plate via the LA to become part of the anterior lamella. It elevates the upper eyelid (10–15 mm); it is supplied by the superior division of the oculomotor nerve. It is crossed by the superior transverse ligament (of Whitnall) in its upper part that acts as a check to levator retraction.
- **Müller's muscle** lies deep to LPS.
  - **Smooth muscle** supplied by sympathetic fibres in the oculomotor nerve. It maintains the tone of raised eyelids and effects fine adjustment on lid height; paralysis (Horner's syndrome) causes 2–3 mm of ptosis. It is involved in the sympathetically mediated startle response (eye opens wide).
- **Capsulopalpebral fascia (CPF)** of the lower lid – this is a condensation of fibrous tissue that is analogous to the LA. It is an extension from the inferior rectus muscle to the tarsus and functions to stabilise the tarsus allowing the eyelid to descend when the eyeball looks down. It splits around the inferior oblique and then reunites at Lockwood's ligament.

BLOOD SUPPLY

Marginal and peripheral arcades from lid margin.

- Upper lid – branches of ophthalmic artery (internal carotid)
- Lower lid – branches of facial artery (external carotid)

NERVE SUPPLY

Sensation comes from CN V1 and V2 for the upper and lower lid, respectively.

LACRIMAL GLAND

Secretomotor fibres come from superior salivary nucleus that travels through the pterygoid canal to relay in the pterygopalatine ganglion and travels in the zygomatic nerve (CN V2), and then joins to the lacrimal branch of CN V1. Accessory lacrimal glands include

- Meibomian glands – lubricate lid margins
- Glands of Zeiss – sebaceous glands associated with lashes
- Glands of Moll

The lacrimal apparatus consists of the following:

- **Lacrimal punctum** is located at the medial canthus – upper and lower canaliculi lead from it to the lacrimal sac, travelling beneath the upper and lower limbs of the medial canthal ligament.
- **Lacrimal sac** drains into the nasolacrimal duct, which empties into the inferior meatus of the lateral wall of the nose; the sac is pulled open during contraction of the palpebral fibres of orbicularis oculi and closes by elastic recoil. Valves in the canaliculi prevent reflux.

The LPS divides the lacrimal gland into palpebral and orbital portions. Basic secretion from the palpebral part lubricates the cornea, whilst reflex secretion from the main orbital gland responds to changes in environment or emotion. Causes of dry eyes include smoking, old age (including post-menopausal), antihistamine treatment and sicca syndrome. Functional tests (e.g. Schirmers) are recommended before eyelid surgery.

LACRIMAL GLAND TUMOURS

- PAs (50%) usually present as painless slow-growing lesions with no inflammatory signs.
  - There is a high risk of local recurrence due to tumour spillage, and generally the advice is not to biopsy, but rather to treat by total gland excision.
- ACCs (25%)
  - These spread diffusely along tissue planes and are locally aggressive; they almost always recur locally. Surgery requires total gland excision and orbital exenteration.
  - Swiss cheese appearance histologically and basaloid changes associated with very poor prognosis (20% survival at 5 years; otherwise, 70% at 5 years).
- Miscellaneous (25%) group including adenocarcinomas, malignant change in a PA or muco-epidermoid tumours. In general, these are treated by total gland excision and orbital exenteration.

EYELID TUMOURS

Consider biopsy to confirm histology before definitive excision under frozen section control and reconstruction.

- The majority of tumours are BCCs (especially lower lids); only 10% of lid tumours occur on the upper lid.
- SCC accounts for ~2% of eyelid tumours (most often the upper lid).

GENERAL PRINCIPLES

Eyebrow defects

- Hair-bearing FTSG – thickness determined by the depth of the follicle limits take
- Pedicled flap based on superficial temporal vessels
- Hair transplants

EYELID RECONSTRUCTION

Partial thickness loss

It is often worth replacing the lower lid as a unit rather than a patch; the cosmetic result is better, whilst extending past the medial and lateral canthi tends to provide more support like a hammock. Alternatively, if a lower lid patch graft is used, tightening up the lower lid by excising a wedge/pentagon before grafting over it will give better support.

- Skin – primary closure or FTSG (contralateral lid or postauricular).
- Conjunctiva – advancement for small defects, nasal/buccal mucosa for larger areas (nasal mucosa said to contract less, 20% vs. 50%), hard palate, contralateral grafts.
- Muscle defects can be closed by advancement or composite muscle-skin grafts that heal up fairly well with reasonable reinnervation and function.
- Tarsus – primary repair, palatal mucosal graft, nasal chondromucosal graft or allograft (Alloderm).

RECONSTRUCTION OF THE LOWER LID

Suggested methods include

- **Full thickness defects** between 1/4 and 1/3 of the eyelids can usually be closed directly after **wedge/pentagon excisional** (more in the elderly due to their skin laxity). Repair in layers to avoid notching: the tarsal plate should be closed with interrupted partial thickness sutures, whilst the muscles can be repaired with an interrupted or continuous suture. The conjunctiva does not need to be specifically closed if reasonably apposed (buried sutures); skin suture ends are often left long to be stuck down out of the way with tape.
  - A **lateral canthotomy and cantholysis** (inferior crus) may be required if closure is overtight, providing ~5 mm of extra advancement.

- If closure is still tight, then a **Tenzel flap** (Figure 3.10) can be elevated – it is a semicircular musculocutaneous rotation flap based high above the lateral canthus; periorbital tissue is undermined inferiorly and laterally up to the level of the brow. A Z-plasty with a superior back-cut at the end of the flap may help.
- Note that as this advances the lateral skin medially along the lid margin, the 'new' margin will not have lashes laterally. The tarsal plate is also not reconstructed laterally.
- Greater defects will require the recruitment of tissue from elsewhere:
  - **Bipedicled Tripier flap** (includes strip of orbicularis muscle). The pedicles can be incorporated into the defect or divided at 3 weeks. It can be used as a unipedicled flap up to the midpupil point.
    - These flaps tend to curl – a tie over dressing is useful to flatten it and maximise tissue contact.
    - It can be combined with the tarsoconjunctival strip flap from the other lid.
  - Hughes flap (see below).
- **Locoregional flaps** can be used when there is insufficient local tissue, but are not ideal due to the thicker skin available, which will usually need a separate lining for the inner surface.
  - Fricke flap – a flap of temporal skin above the eyebrow.
  - Glabellar or forehead flap.
  - Nasolabial flap.
  - **Cheek advancement flap**, e.g. Mustardé cheek rotation (converting the defect into an inverted triangle is helpful). The flap should be raised relatively thin (though the SMAS can be included to reduce distal edge necrosis); it should be well mobilised and anchored to the orbital margin and just above the lateral canthal ligament to reduce retraction/late ectropion, which is the commonest complication.
    - Recruit temporal skin by taking the lateral incision in a high arch.
    - Z-plasty (McGregor) allows more mobility.
  - The reconstruction of the inner lining needs to be considered:

- Conjunctiva can be advanced into lower lid defects, whilst small defects not at fornix heal reasonably well with secondary intention.
- Chondromucosal graft from the nasal septum or buccal mucosal graft. Skin grafts tend to irritate.
- Support may not be needed especially if <30% width loss. Sources of support when needed include nasal septum, palate or conchal cartilage. Alloplasts include irradiated bovine collagen (Chondroplast®) or dermal matrices (Enduragen®, porcine acellular dermis).

HUGHES FLAP

A tarsoconjunctival flap from the upper lid is advanced inferiorly to reconstruct the posterior lamellae of the lower lid; the flap is taken >4 mm away from the lid margin and includes a small portion of the upper tarsus. The flap is inset so that the upper lid tarsus in the flap is in line with the lower lid tarsal remnants.

The second stage of flap division is performed after 6 weeks. Whilst waiting for this, the eye would be occluded, though some perforate the bridge to allow some vision at the expense of vascularity. The anterior lamellar is usually reconstructed with a local skin-muscle flap or a muscle flap covered by a skin graft. The Meibomian glands in the flap tend to die, but there are few functional problems in general.

Critics such as Mustardé advised against using the upper lid to reconstruct the lower lid, as the upper lid is more important for lid function and protection. However, the Hughes flap is able to effectively reconstruct defects larger than two-thirds without distorting the canthal angles.

One-stage reconstruction of full thickness lower eyelid defects using a subcutaneous pedicle flap lined by a palatal mucosal graft (Nakajima T, _Br J Plast Surg_, 1996) A skin island from the lateral cheek is rotated 180° into the lower lid with the pedicle based on the lateral canthus and including a small portion of orbicularis. The flap is lined with palatal mucosal (leaving the periosteum of the donor area intact, and dressed with tie-over collagen sponge for 10 days), which is thicker and more durable than oral mucosa.

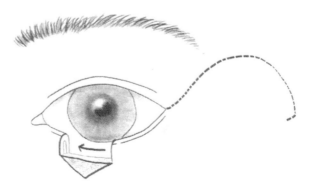

Figure 3.10 Tenzel flap for eyelid reconstruction. It is combined with lateral cantholysis.

This method enables reconstruction of the entire skin of the upper or lower lid as an aesthetic unit. A similar flap was described by Heywood (*Br J Plast Surg*, 1991).

UPPER LID RECONSTRUCTION

Direct closure of defects of up to 1/3 (more in the elderly) is possible; beyond this, local flaps are generally required.

- **Tenzel flap** (as above) for defects up to 60%. A triangular excision of skin and muscle only below the square full thickness defect facilitates advancement/ rotation.
- **Hueston lid switch** is an Abbé-like flap from the lower lid, which is most suited to defects ~50% of the upper lid. It is a technically complex two-stage technique, and the donor defect also needs reconstruction; but it may be the best option for the larger upper lid defect. It can be raised laterally or medially; the former is easier to rotate into the defect, but the vascularity is supposedly more tenuous, whilst the latter can be combined with a cheek advancement flap to help close the donor site.
- **Cutler–Beard flap** (Figure 3.11) – this is a two-stage procedure capable of reconstructing a whole upper lid. Whilst sparing the lower lid margin (5 mm), the **full thickness of the lower lid** is advanced under the margin/bridge to be sutured end to end into the upper lid defect. The pedicle is divided after 3 weeks. Support of the upper lid margin is lacking, and a cartilage graft between conjunctiva and muscle may be required.
  - Reverse Hughes flap – a lower lid flap can be raised up to the upper lid defect and covered with skin, and would be divided 5–8 weeks later. The lower lid tarsoconjunctival flap can be raised close (1.5–2 mm) to the margin and can include the whole tarsus.
- A **sliding tarsoconjunctival flap** from the remaining tarsus can be advanced to the lid margin and covered with FTSG. Shallow marginal defects with part

(>3 mm) of the vertical tarsus remaining may be repaired by advancing the remaining tarsus or by rotation of a vertical segment into a horizontal position.
- **Tripier flaps** of skin and orbicularis muscle can be combined with buccal mucosa for lining for example, though this is not strictly necessary and cartilage is not needed if the defect is <1/3.
  - Fricke flap, paramedian forehead flap
- A variety of islanded flaps have been described in the literature: supratrochlear artery (two-staged), nasojugal, paramedian forehead, lateral paraorbital and flaps based on the anterior branch of superficial temporal artery

PERIORBITAL MASSES

Dermoid cysts

Classification

- Acquired – implantation type – insect bite, minor trauma, etc.
- Congenital teratoma type.
- Congenital inclusion type – at sites of embryonic fusion plates. Orbitofacial dermoids are of the congenital inclusion type.

Most orbital dermoids are solitary masses with distinct palpable margins, and intracranial extension is rare; simple cyst excision is sufficient. However, some cysts may have intraorbital involvement – typically showing indistinct margins, and decrease in size with gentle pressure causing proptosis. CT may be required for complete assessment. Incomplete excision in such cases may lead to inflammation, abscess or sinus formation. Needle aspiration is not an effective treatment.

The management of midline transcranial nasal dermoids in the paediatric patient (Bartlett SP, *Plast Reconstr Surg*, 1993)

Most facial dermoids are subcutaneous and only a minority have deeper extension. This retrospective review of 84

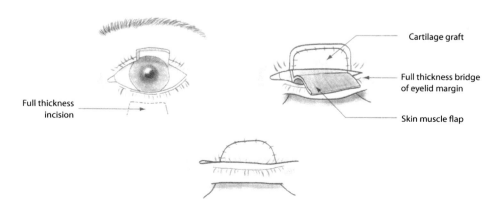

Full thickness incision

Cartilage graft

Full thickness bridge of eyelid margin

Skin muscle flap

Figure 3.11 Cutler–Beard two-stage reconstruction of upper eyelid defects.

patients demonstrated that the three commonest anatomical locations were

- **Frontotemporal** (lateral brow area) commonest at 65% and were generally soft, non-fixed and tended to be slow-growing and asymptomatic. They could be resected by splitting the orbicularis oculi and excising down to periosteum. No special work-up was needed.
- **Orbital** (25%). Females were affected twice as frequently. These dermoids could adhere to frontozygomatic or medial sutures but were usually easily dissected free with no transosseous extensions. They rarely need work-up.
- **Nasoglabellar** (10%) – often presents as a mass with or without a punctum (with fine hair growth or sebaceous debris). The nasal bones may be splayed.
  - Midline glabellar lesions had no deep extension ($n = 2$), whilst dorsal nasal lesions had occult naso-ethmoid and cranial base abnormalities on CT.
  - **Dorsal nasal dermoids need radiological work-up** and may need a bicoronal approach.

PTOSIS (BLEPHAROPTOSIS)

Normally, the upper eyelid covers 1–2 mm of the upper limbus of the cornea. Ptosis is an abnormal droopiness of the upper lid that covers more of the cornea than usual.

BEARD'S CLASSIFICATION OF PTOSIS (1981)

- Congenital
- Acquired

FRUEH CLASSIFICATION (1980)

- Neurogenic
- Myogenic
- Aponeurotic/involutional
- Mechanical

CONGENITAL PTOSIS

In most cases, there is an **absence of levator palpebrae superioris** (LPS), hence, there is a congenital myogenic ptosis; in some the ptosis is due to innervation problems. It is mostly idiopathic, but some are genetic with AD inheritance being more common. Histologically there is fibrosis and absence of striated muscle fibres in LPS with fatty infiltration, which leads to **lagophthalmos**. Muller's (smooth) muscle tends to be normal. The problem is usually noticed shortly after birth.

- Reduced palpebral aperture, with **absent or asymmetrical lid crease**.
- Reduced marginal reflex distance 1 (MRD1) – distance from the corneal light reflex to the upper lid margin.
- **Decreased, often poor, levator excursion**.

- **Lagophthalmos**, on downward gaze; ptotic eyelid is held higher due to **levator fibrosis** preventing lid descent.
- Lid lag is common.

Generally, surgery is deferred until ~5 years of age unless there is

- Severe ptosis obstructing the visual field leading to amblyopia.
- Corneal exposure risking ulceration.

Some conditions are associated with congenital ptosis:

- **Blepharophimosis syndrome** is the combination of bilateral ptosis with short palpebral fissures, epicanthus inversus and telecanthus resulting in reduced vertical and transverse dimensions of the palpebral aperture; some may also have mild hypertelorism. This can occur either in isolation or in association with other anomalies; some show AD inheritance. Treatment includes
  - Brow suspension for ptosis
  - Jumping man flap (Mustardé) for epicanthic folds or Roveda correction
  - May need craniofacial surgery for hypertelorism
- **Marcus Gunn jaw-winking syndrome** – there is synkinesis of the upper lid with chewing caused by aberrant trigeminal nerve innervation (from branch to lateral pterygoid); it is seen in about 2%–6% of patients with congenital ptosis.
  - At rest, there is ptosis, but with jaw opening, the upper lid is briefly elevated, like a 'wink'.
- **Associated anomalies**:
  - Anophthalmos/microophthalmos
  - Harmatomas/benign tumours, e.g. neurofibroma, lymphangioma and haemangioma
  - Strabismus, amblyopia

ACQUIRED PTOSIS

- Neurogenic
  - **Oculomotor nerve lesion**.
  - Horner's syndrome (effects reduced with 10% phenylephrine hydrochloride).
  - Myasthenia gravis (worse later in day). Tensilon test is diagnostic – neostigmine or edrophonium. Anti-acetylcholine receptor antibodies are 100% specific (Padua L, *Clin Neurophysiol*, 2000).
  - Demyelination, i.e. multiple sclerosis.
  - Traumatic ophthalmoplegia or ophthalmoplegic migraine.
- Myogenic
  - **Oculopharyngeal muscular dystrophy** (OPMD). Ptosis typically in middle age, with dysphagia (later), dysarthria and proximal limb weakness.
  - Steroid ptosis – localised myopathy due to chronic use of steroid eye drops, or injections for conditions such as uveitis.

- A rare cause of chronic progressive ptosis is chronic progressive external ophthalmoplegia (Kearns–Sayre syndrome – as a subset with possible risks of ataxia, deafness, diabetes and sudden cardiac death), which usually presents as adult ptosis with poor levator function with symmetrical ophthalmoplegia. It has been classed as a mitochondrial myopathy (mitochondrial DNA is transferred maternally) and can be diagnosed by electromyograph (EMG) and thigh muscle biopsy that may show ragged red fibres on Gomori trichrome staining.
  - Myotonic dystrophy.
- Aponeurotic
  - **Senile/involutional ptosis** – stretching or dehiscence of the LPS aponeurosis with age; actual levator function is usually good, and the dermal insertions are preserved, thus elevating the supratarsal fold. This is the **most common cause of ptosis** and is often categorised separately.
  - **Traumatic** (second most common).
    - **Injury to levator mechanism,** e.g. surgery including cataract surgery ~6% incidence
    - Damage/scarring of superior rectus muscle when used for insertion of a stay stitch to immobilise the eye
- Mechanical
  - Lid tumour or other masses

Pseudoptosis is the appearance of ptosis rather than true ptosis (i.e. droopy upper lid); for example,

- Globe displacement, e.g. with enophthalmos.
- Mechanical lid displacement, e.g. inflammation, oedema.
- Dermatochalasis (excess redundant skin).
- Contralateral lid retraction, e.g. thyroid eye/Grave's disease.
- Hypertropia; visual axis is higher than the fixating eye; dissociated vertical deviation.
- Blepharochalasis – rare condition in young, with recurrent lid oedema and subsequent stretching.
- Duane syndrome – absent/hypoplastic abducens nerve, and the lateral rectus is innervated by the oculomotor nerve, which leads to limitation of abduction and sometimes adduction. There may also be fibrosis of the attachments of the extraocular muscles. The globe tends to retract into the orbit.
- Blepharospasm.

ASSESSMENT

Take a history including patient concerns – functional versus aesthetic, assess general health, medications (aspirin/warfarin), smoking/diabetes, history of dry eyes.

Ascertain the cause – is the ptosis

- Congenital or acquired?
- Neurogenic or myogenic?

- Mechanical – any lid swellings?
- Trauma – history of injury or cataract surgery or blepharoplasty? A history of atopy (leading to habitual eye rubbing) or hard contact lens use?

In the absence of the above and in an elderly patient, the cause is likely to be **senile ptosis** or **pseudoptosis** due to other conditions (see above).

EXAMINATION

Look

- **Measure the degree of ptosis** in millimetres (mild 1–2 mm; moderate 3 mm; severe 4 mm or more) and compare with the other eye.
  - The distance between the mid-pupillary point to the lid margin **MRD1** is normally 4–5 mm.
  - **Asymmetric ptosis** (see below).
- Presence of lid crease – absent in congenital, high in senile ptosis.
- Dermatochalasis. **Check for brow ptosis** (brow level in relation to the supra-orbital rim).
- Assess lower lid position, e.g. scleral show, lower lid laxity.

Move

- **Levator function/excursion** (should be 15–18 mm), immobilise brow, then zero ruler over the upper lid margin on the extreme down gaze, then look upwards fully:
  - Good (10 mm or more), moderate (>5 up to 10 mm), poor (0–5 mm); normal 15 or more ('fives').
  - Levator function is the most important factor in surgical planning and also gives an indication of the likely cause of ptosis.
  - **High supratarsal fold and good levator function indicate levator dehiscence**, e.g. senile ptosis.
- **Lagophthalmos** (incomplete closure of the lids) is a sequelae of all surgeries for ptosis; avoid overcorrection in those with pre-operative lagophthalmos during downward gaze (this suggests fibrosis of LPS).
- **Bell's phenomenon**: eyeballs rotate upwards when the lids are closed. Some patients do not have this, and one should be much less aggressive with ptosis correction in these patients as over-correcting may lead to corneal exposure during sleep.

Test

- Acuity.
- Pupils.
- Extra-ocular movements.
- Dry eyes – these patients are at risk of corneal exposure with post-operative lagophthalmos.
  - History and symptoms
  - Schirmer's test I and II
  - Tear film breakup

ASYMMETRIC PTOSIS

Correction of one side may unmask ptosis in the other side. **Hering's law** states that the LPS receives equal innervation bilaterally. Severe ptosis affecting one side creates impulse for bilateral lid retraction, but after treatment of the ptosis, the impulse for lid retraction will decrease and *may reveal ptosis in the contralateral eye.*

- **Hering's test** – aims to reveal contralateral ptosis with brow immobilisation in straight gaze; elevate ptotic lid with cotton bud and check for contralateral ptosis.

SURGICAL OPTIONS

There are many options, with few controlled trials to compare them properly. The choices are largely determined by the levator function and the degree of ptosis. See Table 3.3. Many authors suggest various formulae to predict the amount of correction, but in general, every millimetre of ptosis correction requires 4 mm of **levator** excision/plication/advancement, whilst tarsal plate resection (for acquired ptosis only) is more direct – 1 mm resection for 1 mm elevation (but rim must be maintained). Surgery under IV sedation is preferred.

McCord CD Jr. Algorithm (Eyelid Surgery: Principles and Techniques, 1995)

- >10 mm levator function usually involutional – treat with levator advancement/resection
- 5–10 mm – usually congenital or myogenic – either levator surgery, aponeurotic repair or frontalis suspension
- <5 mm – usually congenital or traumatic, use frontalis suspension

Chang S. Algorithm (*Plast Reconstr Surg*, 2012) for involutional ptosis
Ptosis with good levator function (>10 mm).

- **Very mild ptosis** <2 mm (maximum 3 mm) can be treated with 'posterior' repairs, which are resections.
  - **Fasanella–Servat** procedure (see below).
    - **Putterman procedure** is F-S without tarsal resection; one criticism of the F-S is that it may cause a floppy lid due to resection of the tarsus.
  - **Mullerectomy** especially with positive PE test (see below).
  - **Mustarde split level tarsectomy.** A stepped excision centred on the level of the top of the tarsal plate. Above this, the anterior skin and muscle is excised whilst below this, the tarsus is mostly excised leaving a lower tarsal remnant that can be advanced superiorly. As a direct excision rather than a folding excision, the shortening offered by this is more precise/predictable (at least according to its proponents) but does involve an external scar.
- **Mild-to-moderate ptosis** >2 mm.
  - **Aponeurosis surgery**, e.g. resection or plication of the aponeurosis

FASANELLA–SERVAT (FIGURE 3.12)

- The upper lid is everted over a **Desmarre** retractor, and two sutures are placed through the conjunctival tarsal border. The tarsus is marked centrally and the proposed resection measured.
  - Desmarre LA was a French ophthalmologist (1810–1882).
- The tissues (**Muller's muscle and superior part of the tarsal plate**) to be resected are elevated via traction sutures and the Putterman clamp placed and secured; the original technique using two curved haemostats was rather unwieldy.
- After an imbricating 6-0 prolene is passed through the tissues just below the clamp and exteriorised through the skin, the clamped tissues are excised by 'running

Table 3.3 Surgical options for correction of ptosis

Levator function	Degree of ptosis	Procedure
Good (>10 mm)	Mild (1–2 mm)	Fasanella–Servat, Müllerectomy
Good (>10 mm)	Moderate (3–4 mm)	Aponeurosis surgery
Fair (5–10 mm)	Moderate (3–4 mm)	Levator surgery (resection/advancement)
Poor (<5 mm)	Severe (>4 mm)	Frontalis suspension surgery

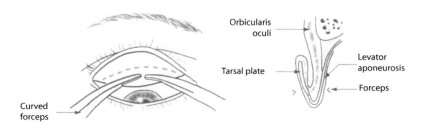

Figure 3.12 Fasanella–Servat procedure.

the blade' at 45° against the clamp. The suture is removed after 1 or 2 weeks.

- The overall success rate is about 70%. The **resection is 4:1**; thus for ptosis >2 mm, this would require excessive (tarsal) resection and levator surgery is preferred. It can also be used in patients with a positive PE test, but such patients will usually have better results with a Mullerectomy.

MULLERECTOMY AND THE PHENYLEPHRINE (PE) TEST

With a **positive PE test** (1–2 mm elevation after topical application), the Muller's muscle is deemed viable and a mullerectomy would offer 'predictable' results (more so than FS). That is if the PE elevates the eyelid to a normal position, then in theory, shortening the muscle will achieve the same result. If there is 2 mm or more of elevation with PE, then Muller's muscle (along with overlying mucosa) can be resected 4:1 to ptosis.

It is a simple procedure and patients like it. It can be performed under LA, but is painless apart from the initial injection; patient participation is not required. GA would be necessary in children. Another advantage is the lower risk of suture keratopathy as the sutures lie higher.

Mullerectomy and FS procedures are similar. The FS resection is centred lower down, closer to the lid margin. The FS can be used in patients with **negative PE** with relatively predictable results, because it is effectively a partial tarsectomy with a little Muller resection (thus, some call it a tarsoconjunctival mullerectomy). The amount of **tarsus removal** is based on the PE result in a 1:1 ratio, i.e. if lid is still 1 mm too low after PE, then remove 1 mm of tarsus (max 2 mm).

PTOSIS WITH POOR LEVATOR FUNCTION (<10 MM)

- **Moderate ptosis (>3 mm), poor levator function 4–10 mm** – treat using levator shortening (resection or plication) or advancement.

- **Levator aponeurotic repair** is the operation of choice for patients with poor levator function (which roughly equates to moderate to severe ptosis); it can also be used for mild ptosis, particularly where a concomitant blepharoplasty is needed. The main concern is that the procedure is a bigger, more painful undertaking along with a skin scar. It is best performed under LA with minimal sedation, with patient participation. The rationale is that by shortening the levator, the pulling force of the muscle is strengthened.
- Incise skin at the proposed supratarsal fold and a skin-orbicularis flap is developed to expose the orbital septum and distal levator mechanism. The orbital septum is incised higher up in its upper third to avoid damage to the underlying levator, which is then disinserted from the tarsal plate and the Müller's muscle dissected free. **A lifting suture is placed into the tarsus and levator (4: 1 ratio) with 1 mm overcorrection (i.e. 12 mm advancement for 3 mm ptosis; see below)**. Excess aponeurosis and skin-orbicularis flap, if necessary, are trimmed. Fix the crease, e.g. anchor blepharoplasty.
- A 2 mm difference may result after the operation, though with selected patients with minimal ptosis, symmetry within 0.5 mm can be achieved.
- Levator reinsertion is only indicated in true levator dehiscence, which is usually due to trauma.
- **Severe ptosis, very poor levator function <4 mm** – suspension surgery is indicated. The frontalis muscle that normally elevates the brow is used to elevate the upper lid via a sling. This is likely to cause lagophthalmos at night. In addition, the sling will cause an indent on downward gaze. In the best hands (Crawford), there is still a 10% recurrence rate over 20 years.
  - **Crawford/Fox techniques** (Figure 3.13) – frontalis is connected to the tarsal plate via a sling usually made of fascia lata, though there are alternatives (see below).

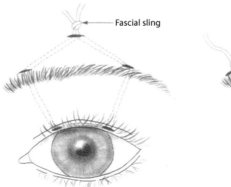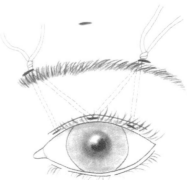

Fascial sling

Figure 3.13 Common techniques of sling repairs for ptosis include the Fox and Crawford techniques; a special 'Wright' needle is used for threading the fascia, palmaris longus or alloplastic material through.

– Harvest the fascia lata (20–25 cm) with the knee slightly flexed and rotated internally. A 5 cm transverse incision 6 cm above the knee is usually adequate.

- **Inferiorly based orbital septum flap** raised through a blepharoplasty incision (5–6 mm from lash line, at the superior border of the tarsal plate), in a trapezoidal flap that narrows superiorly. A second incision above the brow is then used to expose vertical frontalis fibres that is raised as a superiorly based flap with the medial limit 5 mm lateral to the supraorbital notch to reduce nerve damage. The septal flap is tunnelled up, sutured to the frontalis flap. A Frost stitch is kept for 48 hours. This is the modification of the frontalis-only flap, which was often too short to attach to the tarsal plate by itself.

SLING MATERIAL

Fascia lata is the classic choice, but may not always be available.

- **Silicone rods** can be used for patients with disorders that are either progressive (myogenic) or may recover. Some further adjustment of height is possible later when LA effects have worn off, but this is only practical within 24 hours; in particular, as it is easier to advance than recede, it is desirable not to overcorrect.
  - Prolene
- **Palmaris longus** (PL) is absent in 15%–30%, with a weak association with plantaris absence (7%–20%) but no association with absent FDS to little finger. It may be used in circumstances where fascia lata harvest may be difficult, e.g. in those under 3 years of age. The PL is verified with various tests including the lotus pinch and harvested via a 0.5 cm incision in wrist fold and a second 1 cm incision 7–10 cm away. The tendon can be taken partially; it can be split and it can be doubled up.
- The **plantaris tendon,** unlike the palmaris, cannot be verified clinically before surgery, though ultrasound may be useful. The tendon runs obliquely between gastrocnemius and soleus to insert into the medial posterior aspect of the calcaneus. It can be difficult to find; a 1.5 cm incision above the shoe line is made just anterior to the medial margin of Achilles tendon.

COMPLICATIONS OF PTOSIS SURGERY

The commonest complications are undercorrection or overcorrection. LA with adrenaline causes partial lid retraction through blockage of the somatic innervation of LPS and activates sympathetic innervation of Müller's muscle; hence, the final lid position should include 1–2 mm of overcorrection.

- Overcorrection can be treated by release of sutures and massage but may need ultimately reoperation.

- Undercorrection, i.e. a lid that is still too low, should probably have further surgery. Thus, after an FS procedure, the choices are either another FS procedure or a more traditional external approach. The main complaint that can be laid against the FS repair is that it is **rather imprecise** (in part due to it being a folding excision).
- Dry eyes – post-operative keratopathy may occur due to scar tissue, or loss of glands or more commonly due to the sutures and as such is often temporary (keratopathy due to scar tissue will also resolve albeit at a slower rate, after several weeks).
  - Avoid excising more than 2 mm of tarsal plate; otherwise, the potential loss of accessory lacrimal glands may exacerbate pre-existing dry eye more than other techniques.
- Correcting ptosis will cause an **apparent telecanthus** post-operatively (as ptosis gives the illusion of a narrowed intercanthal disease).
- Those with a hypoplastic tarsus, e.g. in congenital ptosis, are at risk of lid eversion after surgery.

LAGOPHTHALMOS

Patients with this condition are unable to fully close their eyelids. Common causes include

- Facial nerve palsy
- Eyelid problems – scars, proptosis/exophthalmos, enophthalmos and eyelid surgery especially excessive skin removal

Surgical treatment of lagophthalmos in facial palsy (Inigo F, *Br J Plast Surg*, 1996)

Complications of lagophthalmos include dryness leading to corneal keratitis and conjunctivitis. Treatment approaches in facial palsy include

- Artificial tears/drops/ointments, protective lenses
- Lateral tarsorrhaphy, canthoplasty/canthopexy
- Gold/platinum weights
- Cross facial nerve grafts to re-innervate orbicularis (ineffective with long-standing paralysis)
  - Platysma muscle flaps with direct neurotisation has been described (Nassif PF, IX International Facial Nerve Symposium, 2009; Leckenby JI, *J Plast Reconstr Aesthet Surg*, 2012).
- Temporalis turnover flap (but may cause involuntary closure during chewing)

In this paper, Inigo describes a technique of **levator lengthening** using autologous conchal cartilage graft sutured between the tarsal plate and LA that was successful in 11 out of 12 patients. They demonstrated that the width of graft required to reduce the palpebral fissure by 1 mm is ~4 mm.

New technique of levator lengthening for the retracted upper lid (Piggott TA, *Br J Plast Surg*, 1995)

Lid retraction may occur with Graves' disease or occasionally following an upper blepharoplasty. There are two main approaches:

- Müller's muscle division via a conjunctival incision
- Division of LA and Müller's muscle via a skin incision

The paper describes a technique of lengthening the LA by designing **'castellated' flaps** (i.e. cut in a square wave-type pattern) in the aponeurosis and suturing the resultant flaps end on end. The length of each flap should be 1 mm more than the desired correction. The authors note that this technique is not suited to skin-loss problems, e.g. burn scar contracture.

ECTROPION

Eyelid anatomy

The upper and lower tarsal plates are attached via the lateral canthal tendon (LCT) ('retinaculum') to Whitnall's tubercle inside the lateral orbital rim. The LCT is continuous with the LA in the upper lid and the suspensory ligament of Lockwood in the lower lid.

Ectropion is the outward turning of the lower eyelid margin. Other related conditions include the following:

- Blepharochalasis is laxity of eyelid skin associated with aging.
- Blepharophimosis is an abnormally narrow palpebral fissure.
- Blepharoptosis ('ptosis') is an abnormally low upper lid margin (see above).

Classification of ectropion

- **Involutional** (senile) ectropion is the most common and is characterised by **transverse lid laxity** – treat by lid shortening, e.g. wedge excision ± lower lid blepharoplasty (Kuhnt–Symanowski) or (lateral) tarsal strip procedure to counteract LCT attenuation.
- **Mechanical**, e.g. lid tumour, treat by excising the lesion.
- **Cicatricial**, e.g. burns – release scar and reconstruct, e.g. Z-plasty, FTSG or flap.
- **Paralytic**, e.g. VII nerve palsy, can treat as for involutional.

CANTHOPLASTY

The main indications for canthoplasty are as follows:

- Correction of horizontal lid laxity or ectropion from paralysis/atony
  - **Tarsal strip procedure** (Anderson RL, *Arch Ophthalmol*, 1979) is a method of horizontal lid shortening used for horizontal lid laxity, paralytic and atonic ectropion. After cutting the lower part of the LCT, a tarsal/dermis strip is raised and anchored to the superolateral orbital rim (with or without a pentagonal wedge excision) becoming the new tighter tendon.

- Prevention of cosmetic blepharoplasty lower lid retraction.
  - **Inferior retinacular lateral canthoplasty (Jelks GW, *Plast Reconstr Surg*, 1997).** The inferior limb of the LCT is suspended to the periosteum of the superolateral orbital rim at the level of the upper edge of the pupil, which can be performed via an upper eyelid (blepharoplasty) incision.
  - Less invasive variations on canthal tendon tightening (canthopexy) involve suturing the soft tissues just below the end of the tarsal plate to the tough periosteum of the orbital bone.

ENTROPION

The eyelid margin folds inwards, and the posteriorly directed lashes (trichiasis) may cause corneal irritation/infection.

- In children (uncommon), entropion can be left alone as it will usually resolve.
- In adults, **aging is the commonest cause of entropion (and ptosis and ectropion).** For transverse laxity, Kuhnt–Symanowski blepharoplasty or canthoplasty is indicated as for involutional ectropion. Vertical laxity may be treated with reattachment of the CPF to the tarsal plate.
  - **Cicatricial** – scarring in the posterior lamella; release and replace conjunctiva and tarsus with mucosa and cartilage grafts, respectively.
  - **Acute spastic entropion** may occur due to ocular irritation and overactivity of the orbicularis oculi.
    - Botulinum toxin may help.
    - Any lid laxity can be treated as above.

III. NASAL RECONSTRUCTION

(See also 'Rhinoplasty'.)

The commonest reason for nasal reconstruction is skin cancer, mainly **basal cell carcinoma** (BCC; 10 times more common than SCC). The aims after oncological clearance are good cosmesis combined with good function, primarily a patent airway. Reconstruction of nose needs to consider the different components: skin, support and lining.

SENSATION

- V1 – radix, rhinion, sidewalls (infratrochlear) and skin over dorsum to the tip (nasociliary – external nasal)
- V2 – lateral tissue over lower half of nose, columella and vestibule (infraorbital)

ARTERIAL SUPPLY

- Internal carotid – ophthalmic artery to anterior ethmoidal artery, dorsal nasal artery
- External carotid – facial artery
  - Superior labial to columellar branch.

- Angular artery to lateral nasal artery that arises 2–3 mm above the alar groove. It is the primary blood supply to the nasal tip if transcolumellar incisions are used.

SKIN

The nose is divided into thirds:

- Zone I. Proximal – over the nasal bones.
- Zone II. Middle – over upper lateral cartilages.
- Zone III. Distal – over nasal tip and alar cartilages (lower lateral cartilages, LLC). The columella is formed in part from the medial crura of the alar cartilages.

Skin over the upper 2/3 (dorsum and sidewalls) is thin and mobile, whilst skin over the lower third (tip and alar) is thick, more sebaceous and more fixed. The skin may also be divided into convex and flat units; flaps that tend to contract at the edges/trapdoor are good choices to replace convex units, whilst flat areas are better replaced by FTSG (see also 'Medial canthus').

Cosmetic subunit principle (Burget and Menick) (Figure 3.14):

- The nine subunits are the dorsum, sidewalls, alar lobules, tip, soft triangles and columella. It is suggested that when there is >50% skin defect in any one unit, total excision and reconstruction should be considered for optimal results.
- The subunit principle of reconstruction is partly based upon the observation that eyes are trained to see changes in colour, texture and contour. Scars can become raised or spread in which case they reflect a line of light, or they become depressed and cast a linear shadow. Whilst the quality of scarring cannot be controlled, the **site of scars** can be controlled, to a certain extent.
- Avoid making perpendicular (or parallel) incisions in the ala; oblique lines are preferable.

NASAL RECONSTRUCTION

Reconstruction of the skin

- Healing by secondary intention or primary closure
  - For example, small defects (<1 cm square) of the glabella/medial canthus.
- Skin grafts
  - SSGs are not a common option due to the poor appearance and tendency to contracture. However, it is simple and makes it 'easier' to monitor recurrence.
  - FTSG – an option for selected defects of zone I/II.
    - Postauricular skin is relatively thin (thinner than preauricular) and vascularises well.
    - Some suggest the use of conchal bowl skin for the tip as the concave skin will mould quite well to the convex tip.
    - **Composite grafts** of skin and cartilage (McLaughlin CR, Br J Plast Surg, 1954) can be taken from helical rim or root of helix. They are limited to <1.5 cm in size; the area of dermal contact can be maximised to optimise take. Most suggest that no part of the graft should be >0.5 cm from an edge (where the vascularity comes from). Cold compresses are suggested for 48 hours to reduce metabolic requirements.
- Local flaps are the most common method of reconstruction (Figure 3.15).
  - **Banner flap** (local transposition flap, ~single lobe of a bilobed flap) for defects <1 cm² of the dorsum/tip.
  - **Bilobed flap** (Esser JFS, *Deutsch Zschr Chir*, 1918; Zitelli JA, *Arch Dermatol*, 1989) for defects 1–2 cm². Laterally based design flaps can be used for the tip; medial for the lobule. The pivot point should be positioned away from the alar margin or lower lid to reduce distortion. Two (maximum) 50° lobes, or a maximum total of 100°.

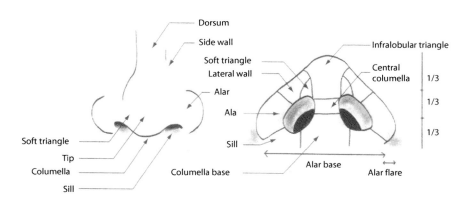

Figure 3.14 Nasal anatomy with subunits (Burget and Menick). The nasal base is often divided into thirds as well as seven subunits.

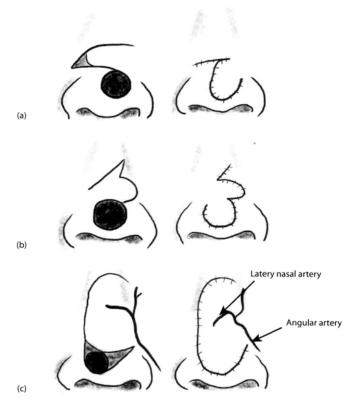

(a)

(b)

Latery nasal artery

Angular artery

(c)

Figure 3.15 Dorsal nasal flaps for coverage of increasingly larger nasal defects. (a) Banner flap, <1 cm. (b) Bilobed flap, ~1.5 cm. (c) Dorsal nasal flap, ~2 cm. Lateral nasal artery. Angular artery.

- It cannot cover the infratip lobule; it should not be used for defects within 0.5 cm of the nasal rim.
- Some degree of rim distortion is to be expected if the defect is within 1 cm of the rim.
- **Dorsal nasal/Rieger rotation flap** rotates the tissue of the whole dorsum inferiorly on a lateral pedicle with the **angular artery**. This can cover larger defects up to 2 cm²; it will not reach the columella.
- **Glabellar flap** – commonly used, often in a V-Y manner.
- **Forehead flap** (see below).
- **Nasolabial flap** especially for alar defects – superiorly or inferiorly based, one- or two-stage (for best results) or islanded (beware of tendency to trapdoor). It can be folded over rim defects; a strip of cartilage along the rim is needed; otherwise, notching is likely to occur. However, this can get quite bulky.
  - When replacing a whole ala, trapdooring/convexity can be encouraged by using a slightly larger pattern (~1 mm) to augment the contour.
- **Cheek advancement flaps** for sidewalls, e.g. V-Y cheek flaps.

- **The ala can be reconstructed with composite free flaps from the pinna** (Parkhouse N, *Br J Plast Surg*, 1985) based on the STA. Others have described a free chondrocutaneous helical flap (Shenaq SM, *J Reconstr Microsurg*, 1989).

MEDIAL CANTHUS

This is a complex anatomical region and reconstruction is potentially difficult, which is unfortunate as it is not an uncommon place for BCCs. Options include the following:

- Small partial defects will heal quite well by secondary intention particularly if the defect is symmetrically placed with respect to the MCT. It may take up to 4–6 weeks, and there is a risk of hypertrophic scarring and distortion, and thus is only suited for very small defects.
- Quilting sutures are useful to apply grafts within the concavity. FTSG can be used with a vascular bed, but there may be noticeable differences in colour and texture.
- Local flaps such as rhomboid, bilobed, glabellar. Forehead flaps tend to be a bit too bulky and create a convexity.
  - Eyelid flaps – e.g. superomedially based upper eyelid myocutaneous (hemi-Tripier)

PEDICLED FLAPS FROM THE FOREHEAD

The **forehead flap** is the reconstruction of choice for dorsum and tip defects, whilst the superiorly based nasolabial flap can be used for the alae and a superiorly based cheek rotation is used for the sidewalls. A paramedian forehead flap can cover the entire nose. Patients should be consented with a full explanation; the best result will come from a multistaged forehead flap that will require sacrifice of normal tissue and a forehead scar.

- The classic 'Indian technique' forehead flap (Sushruta) was a median flap based on two sets of vessels.
  - Supratrochlear 2 cm lateral to midline, runs towards midline
  - Supraorbital 3 cm lateral to midline
- **Paramedian forehead flap** in its current form is based on one set of supratrochlear vessels – the dissection plane starts deep (subperiosteal) up to a point 2 cm above the supra-orbital rim. The flap can be thinned 'distally' (further from the eye) as the vessels become more superficial as they near the hairline.
  - Use a handheld Doppler or palpate the pulse at the medial canthus; the stem is 1.5–2 cm wide and angled 45° upwards. The stem can be lengthened by dissecting further proximally along the pedicle.
    - Above muscle at the top of forehead, then submuscular and then subperiosteal near the orbital rim
  - The axis of the flap can be canted obliquely for extra length; due to the rich vascular anastomosis, the distal vessel does not need to be included in the flap (Shumrick KA, *Arch Otolarygngol Head Neck Surg*, 1992). The flap also can be lengthened by going into hairline.
    - A single-stage flap was described by Kishi (*Arch Facial Plast Surg*, 2012) – the origin was shifted to a lower point by making use of the connections between the angular artery and the supratrochlear, which was divided proximal to this.
    - Seagull forehead flap (Millard) is a modified midline forehead flap with a cruciate shape due to lateral extensions for the alae.
  - Pre-operative (or intra-operative) subgaleal **tissue expansion** may be useful, but critics point to (unpredictable) rebound contraction of the flap. Expansion increases vascularity (delay), thins the flap and facilitates direct closure of the donor defect; it is probably best applied to the sides of the forehead rather than the flap itself. Grafting of the donor site gives poor results and secondary healing is preferable.
    - Flap thinning is safe ~1 month post-operation; some use intradermal steroid injections to cause fat atrophy.

Alternatives to the forehead flap include the following:

- **Scalping rhinoplasty** (Converse JM, *Proc R Soc Med*, 1942) is based laterally on the STA and vein, and makes use of 60%–70% of the whole forehead, arching into the anterior scalp, which is raised on the subgaleal level. Skeletal elements can be prefabricated with cartilage grafts inset into the flap. The forehead part of the donor is grafted whilst the scalp donor is dressed; the pedicle is divided after 2–3 weeks and the unused flap returned.
- **Washio temporomastoid flap** – the **postauricular skin** (and thicker mastoid skin) is also based on the STA (and its retroauricular branch) and is transferred to the nose defect. No delay is required and there are no facial scars. Henriksson (*Scand J Plast Reconstr Surg Hand Surg*, 2005) included a portion of conchal cartilage for nostril support.

DISTANT FLAPS

- The 'Italian technique' of total nasal skin reconstruction uses a proximally based medial arm skin flap (the original description by Tagliacozzi, 1597 was distally based) with pedicle division after 3 weeks. This technique is of historical interest only.
- Free flaps – the classic choice was a radial forearm flap, but many thin small flaps are available elsewhere; however, colour and texture mismatch is always a potential issue. Using a forehead flap gives better results.

RECONSTRUCTION OF THE LINING

Unlined flaps would eventually distort from scarring and compromise the final results. Larger complex defects, in particular, often require more lining than expected after scarring is released. The lining flap can be used to support **primary** cartilage grafts; secondary grafts placed after the soft tissues that have undergone some contraction already may offer less than optimal results.

- **Intranasal flaps** can support primary cartilage grafts:
  - Septal hinge flap (De Quervains) – anteriorly based flap of mucosa and cartilage is rotated outwards about the anterior attachment to provide contralateral midvault lining (it cannot reach the nostril/rim). A fairly large septal fistula results, though refinements to the technique have minimised the donor defect.
  - Bilateral septal flaps can be used – inferiorly hinged ipsilateral mucosa for alar lining, anteriorly hinged contralateral mucosa for midvault lining, at the expense of a septal perforation.
  - Septal mucoperichondrial (pivot) flap – can provide lining and some dorsal skeletal support. The majority of the septum is pulled forward out of the nasal cavity on a narrow pedicle (septal branch of superior labial artery) pivoting near the nasal spine to be folded outward to line the dome area.
  - Bipedicled mucosal advancement flap for small vestibule defects.
- **Folded forehead flap** – it is difficult to satisfactorily place cartilage primarily in folded flaps because of their bulkiness.

- **Skin grafts** have low morbidity and are the best choice in the elderly and those with previous septal surgery. However, they cannot support primary cartilage grafts and will still **contract** to a variable degree. Flaps can be prelaminated in a staged surgery.
- **Turned-over nasal skin**, hinged on the edge, is useful when resurfacing a subunit that has some skin remaining. This is also useful to increase the contact area for composite grafts.
- **Local flaps**, e.g. nasolabial, are often bulky and require secondary thinning.
- For near total defects, a thin **free flap**, e.g. RFFF, is used to provide a lining layer for a forehead flap with skeletal elements. Some prefer to stage it, that is, to cover first with skin grafts that are removed when a cartilage framework is constructed and covered with a forehead flap.

RECONSTRUCTION OF THE SKELETON

Ideally, the skeleton should be reconstructed at the same time as skin/lining reconstruction, but the vascularity of the soft tissues (and their ability to support the skeleton) is a consideration.

- Septal cartilage is easy to carve and strong (thus good for support), but there is a limited supply and it is not a good option in children.
- Conchal cartilage (elastic cartilage) has useful curvatures for nasal tip and ala, but is often too flimsy to withstand a tight envelope. It is difficult to carve and often crumbles in the elderly.
- Rib cartilage is easy to carve and is available in decent quantities, but the potentially poor donor scar limits its wider use. It tends to warp; leaving perichondrium encourages bending on that side whilst unilateral carving/scoring often leads to curling (Gibson's principle). Costochondral junction bone is useful in children and has less tendency to warp. Calcification typically occurs after the ages of 50 or so, making it more difficult to carve but less liable to deform.

Due to the low metabolic requirements of cartilage, the take of a cartilage graft is generally high as long as it can be vascularised by surrounding tissues. Perichondrium usually needs to be excluded, as its chondrogenic potential may distort the graft.

MIDLINE SUPPORT

- 'L'-shaped costochondral strut (**Gillies**) from the nasal radix and angulated to contact the anterior nasal spine; good projection but the columella tends to be wide.
- **Cantilever bone graft** (Converse, Millard) screwed (×2) to the nasal radix with a small subjacent bone wedge to provide projection. Ideally, calvarial graft is used as it is said to be less prone to resorption and may be harvested via the skin flap incisions; rib and ilium (Tessier) are alternatives. It avoids a wide columella (Jackson IT, *Ann Plast Surg*, 1983), but often sink over time.

- **Hinged septal flap (Millard)** – similar to the 'L'-shaped strut but made from the septum in situ hinged superiorly on the caudal end of the nasal bones.
- Septal pivot flap as above, in combination with a cantilever graft for dorsal support.

Lateral support – this is inherently more difficult. Cartilage grafts are used most often.

- Anatomic grafts – supposedly provide improved alar rim correction with less nostril distortion. Autologous cartilage is shaped to resemble the lateral crura and fixed to the residual medial crura or a columellar strut.
- Non-anatomic.
  - **Alar batten grafts** (in leading edge) for alar collapse and external valve obstruction. Cartilage graft is used to bridge the collapsed area from piriform aperture to the lateral third of lateral crura.
  - Lateral crural strut graft – for retraction of the alar rim and malposition of the lateral crura. Long struts are placed between the deep surface of the lateral crus and vestibular skin and sutured, whilst the lateral end extends to the piriform aperture.
  - Alar contour grafts – cartilage buttress is inserted through an infracartilagious incision into a pocket at the rim.
  - Alar spreader grafts to treat internal nasal valve collapse or pinched tip deformity.
- Alloplasts – prolonged risk of implant exposure and infection.
  - Vitallium or titanium mesh.
  - Medpor allows tissue ingrowth, which seems to reduce infection rates but makes it more difficult to remove.

COLUMELLAR RECONSTRUCTION

- Bilateral **nasolabial flaps** – these can be tunnelled or rolled inwards to line the vestibule and create a central columellar post. Better results are possible with staged procedures.
- **Forked upper lip flaps** – transverse flaps from the upper lip (best for long-lipped patients or the elderly).
- **Chondrocutaneous composite grafts**, e.g. from auricular for small defects.
- **Free composite helical flaps** (see above).
- **Vestibular flaps** (Mavili ME, *Plast Reconstr Surg*, 2000) – use of internal vestibular skin.
- **Forehead flap**.
- **Washio flap** (Motamed S, *Br J Plast Surg*, 2003).

RECONSTRUCTION BY PROSTHESIS

This is a reasonable choice for debilitated or elderly patients.

- Branemark osseointegrated prosthesis
- Prosthesis attached to spectacles

RHINOPHYMA

This condition is characterised by sebaceous hyperplasia of the nasal skin with erythema and soft tissue enlargement. It is a severe form of acne rosacea and has no association with excessive alcohol intake. It is 12 times more common in males, typically affecting them from middle age onwards. There is said to be a risk of malignant change (typically BCC) in up to 15%–30%.

Treatment

- Non-surgical – skin hygiene, tetracyclines, isoretinoin, topical metronidazole
- Surgical – tangential excision (cold steel, dermabrasion or CO_2 laser) with secondary healing from the sebaceous elements that run very deep. An old photograph of the patient may be helpful to guide the sculpting.
  - Note that it is generally recommended that oral retinoids should be stopped 1 year before surgery due to their deleterious effects on wound healing. However, the evidence for this is not strong and it is likely that the overall risk is relatively small.

IV. SCALP RECONSTRUCTION AND HAIR RESTORATION

Scalp avulsion usually occurs in the subgaleal plane. It is usually said that due to the extensive collateral supply, a total scalp avulsion can be replanted on a single set of vascular anastomoses though in practice, it is probably advisable to have more than one pedicle.

SCALP ANATOMY

A common mnemonic is SCALP – skin, connective tissue, aponeurosis, loose areolar tissue and periosteum:

- **Skin** is thick especially in the occipital region (8 mm vs. 3 mm in temple).
  - The scalp is most mobile in the temporal regions.
  - It is a good graft donor site particularly for burns/wounds of the face.
- Vessels, nerves and lymphatics are in the **subcutaneous connective tissue** layer; supposedly, this reduces the ability of vessels to retract leading to difficulty with haemostasis.
- The scalp is supplied by both ECA and ICA branches.
  - STA has the largest territory, which is lateral.
  - Occipital artery supplies the posterior scalp above the nuchal line (the skin below is supplied by perforators from splenius capitis and trapezius muscles).
  - Other arteries, e.g. supratrochlear, supraorbital and posterior auricular, contribute less.
- The nerve distribution is analogous with slight differences, such as the supraorbital nerve supplying a large area of skin to the vertex.

- Emissary veins lie in the loose areolar layer; haematoma and infections can collect/spread here.
- The galea aponeurotica is continuous with the frontalis, occipitalis as well as the TPF (and thus also the SMAS).

SCALP SURGERY

- Incisions should be made parallel to the hair direction to minimise damage to the follicles, but at the actual hairline, a perpendicular incision may allow a softer appearance (or formal **trichophytic closure**); some have suggested immediate micrografts in the incision line. It is important to avoid excessive tension in the skin closure; this may not cause tip necrosis but can still lead to alopecia from follicle damage or anagen arrest.
- Bleeding from the edge can be a problem: use clips, adrenaline infiltration, haemostatic sutures, etc. Cautery should be used judiciously to avoid damaging follicles.
- Proper closure of the galeal reduces tension and spreading of the scar; the galea may be tacked to the periosteum with 'progressive tension sutures'.
- Galeal **does not stretch;** scoring can aid flap movement. Do not underestimate the inelasticity of the scalp.
  - Kazanjian – parallel incisions 1 cm apart gain 1.67 mm per incision.
  - Recruit from mobile parietal area where possible.
  - Multiple flaps may often be needed.
- Mattress sutures are a good way to close the scalp skin, which reduces the amount of hair you get trapped by the sutures. Staples are fast, are haemostatic in the scalp and cause a low(er) level of skin ischaemia – they do need to be removed in a timely manner, and thus a deeper layer of sutures is needed for support and good skin apposition.

PRINCIPLES

REPLACE WITH LIKE TISSUE

- Use adjacent/remaining scalp if possible; the parietal scalp is mobile and the galea can be scored to increase advancement. Flaps should incorporate at least one named vessel.
- Consider **tissue expansion** – it can be combined with flaps.

SECONDARY HEALING

Small areas granulate in about a week, and then slowly reepithelialise along with contraction; however, there is a risk of bone exposure/desiccation in the interim. A cerclage suture can be used to decrease the size of the defect.

DIRECT CLOSURE

Small defects near the hairline can be converted to A or T to preserve the hairline.

SKIN GRAFTING

As long as the grafts are thin, they can be placed on fresh bare bone without waiting for granulation (which can take weeks). Burring down the outer table to get some bleeding may improve vascularity.

- Perforating the outer table is a very old method, although what Celsus and Galen advocated was perforation or rasping of sequestrum, respectively, and not the healthy bone. Generally the skin that heals over granulation tissue is thin and can be unstable; they are prone to breakdown with minor trauma after healing, especially at the seams. They can be used as temporising measures before definitive reconstruction, e.g. tissue expansion.
  - Dermal substitutes, e.g. Integra®, Nevelia®, can be used to bridge small clean bare areas due to their low nutritional requirements.
  - NPWT can improve graft take or encourage granulation over bare bone, even irradiated bone. The role of HBOT is unproven.
- Small areas of bare bone can be covered by flaps of **pericranium** or subgaleal areolar tissue. They should be based on a major feeding artery or on a wide bipedicled base and sutured without tension.
  - **Bipedicled advancement flaps** can work well, but the incisions may compromise potential flaps in the future.
  - **Crane principle** can be used to cover small areas of bare bone. Once the flap has allowed vascularisation of the wound, the flap can be raised at a more superficial level and returned to its original donor site, leaving a vascular layer on the wound that can now be grafted.

LOCAL SCALP FLAPS

Local flaps (raised above the periosteum) are able to close areas 2–25 cm², i.e. up to 5 × 5 cm. Due to differences in body size, it is probably better to use a relative defect size; **the limit for local flaps is probably 30%.** Local flaps are limited by the amount of remaining skin available (and thus the size of defect). The galea can be scored to allow expansion (see above), taking care not to damage the vessels.

- **Rotational advancement flaps** are the most common, although the flap needs to be five to eight times the size (margin) of the defect to work well; attention is needed with the hairline and dog ears (which should be kept and left to resolve, as resecting them can reduce vascularity).
  - VY and rhomboids, particularly multiples, are useful in parietal/vertex defects.
- **Orticochea** described multi (4 and then 3) flap techniques based on known arterial territories; the central defect (up to 30%) is closed by bilateral flaps based on the STAs; the contralateral flap is usually larger and is regarded as the dominant flap. A large

posterior flap with the rest of the scalp based on one occipital vessel is moved forward by advancement and rotation. Extensive undermining and galeal scoring are needed. The results will be cosmetically inferior to tissue expansion in most cases and should be a second choice, unless single-staged reconstruction is important.

- For larger defects (>25 cm²), tissue expansion or free flaps will produce better results.
  - **The tissue expander** is filled until there is ~20% more tissue than needed to allow for recoil. A single large expander is usually preferable to several smaller expanders and reduces risk of infection, but often several expanders are placed to maximise the amount of expansion per operation.
  - **Free flaps** – Flaps allow rapid wound closure, which may be important if the patient needs adjuvant treatment such as radiotherapy. Conversely, prior irradiation makes other methods of scalp reconstruction more challenging due to fibrosis, etc.
    - **Omentum** (McLean DH, *Plast Reconstr Surg*, 1972) with SSG provides a large pliable flap that is highly vascular.
    - Muscle flaps such as the LD are 'classically' good for infected wounds. Including skin with the muscle makes the flap bulky; thus, harvesting the muscle only and covering it with an SSG is a common alternative. There is a risk of muscle atrophy/retraction with bone exposure; scalp over muscle (vest over pants for 1.5 cm) closure is recommended. The pedicled trapezius flap may reach the lateral and posterior parts.
    - The ALT is probably the new workhorse; fasciocutaneous flaps are thinner and contour well. Others include the RFFF and para/scapular flaps.

DURAL AND BONE DEFECTS

Dural defects can be patched using many materials, whilst small defects can be closed directly. Some use fibrin glue on the suture line; Tisseel® is made with pooled serum, and thus there is a theoretical infection risk. Autologous fibrin (Vivostat®) can be used, but needs a bit more advanced planning. **Calvarial reconstruction can be delayed until stable soft tissue cover is available.** Bony reconstruction is not always needed, but is often desirable particularly for the aesthetics of the forehead.

- **Rib** – using alternate ribs may reduce the contour deformity. There is a potential for regeneration (albeit unpredictably) if the periosteum is kept at the donor site. At the recipient site, ribs can be wired/sutured together and gaps smoothed/filled with bone paste, acrylic or hydroxyapatite.
- **Split clavarial bone** especially parietal bone just behind the coronal suture, because it is thicker and has fewer underlying sinuses.

- **Unicortical ilium.** Donor pain can be significant.
- **Alloplastic material** such as titanium/steel mesh or **methyl methacrylate** (MMA) (with or without mesh) can be useful to avoid a donor defect. MMA has been successfully used in cranial/frontal reconstructions and it is radiolucent, but care is needed with the exothermic reaction that may damage adjacent soft tissue. It may be complicated by late infections/ extrusions, which occurs in 4% on average but up to 40% in sites with previous infection. In most cases, vascular flap coverage of the alloplast is desirable.
  - Metal plates are being used less, as they conduct heat (cold), obscure X-rays and have a higher infection/extrusion rate.
  - Custom implants can be made by various companies based on CT data.

ALOPECIA

The average scalp has about 100,000–150,000 hairs with more in blondes and less in redheads. Rather than being in single units, hairs are arranged in **follicular units** – each with 1–4 terminal hairs, 1 vellus hair and approximately 9 sebaceous glands along with perifollicular vessels, nerves and erector pili. The follicles are subcutaneous, but the bulb is not absolutely necessary – as long as the upper two-thirds of the follicle survive, then 30% of the hairs will still grow.

HAIR GROWS IN CYCLES

There are different lengths of cycle in different parts of the body.

- **Anagen** (87%) – this is the phase of active growth that lasts about 3 years or more in men (longer in females, 5–8 years) during which follicular cells proliferate and become keratinised. This influences the length of the hair.
- **Catagen** (3%) – lasts 3 weeks during which there is degradation of the follicle; the hair base keratinises and separates from the dermal papillae.
- **Telogen** (10%) – this is the resting phase that lasts for about 3 months. Hair is shed (exogen, on average 50–100 every day) and the follicle is inactive. The telogen/anagen ratio influences the amount of hair in a region: with a prolonged telogen and a shortened anagen, hair thinning will result.

HAIR LOSS

Alopecia is hair loss and the commonest cause is **androgenic alopecia**, i.e. male pattern baldness (MPB), which is relatively common. It is X-linked dominant and related to a defect in the susceptible follicle, either excessive 5 α-reductase activity (converting testosterone to dihydrotestosterone, DHT) in susceptible (frontal scalp) follicles or excessive sensitivity to DHT. Occipital scalp follicles tend to have reduced activity and are less influenced by hormonal

factors making them good donors ('donor dominant') that will grow when transplanted to bald areas.

Other less common causes of alopecia include the following:

- **Alopecia areata** – unknown cause but involves a perifollicular lymphocytic infiltration. It affects males and females equally. The **exclamation point sign** is a pathognomonic feature. The natural history is unpredictable, and whilst spontaneous recovery is common, so are recurrences. The most common chosen options are
  - Intralesional steroids.
  - Minoxidil (5% twice daily).
  - Topical immunotherapy, unknown mechanism – weekly squaric acid dibutylester (SADBE).
  - PUVA is associated with a small risk of developing cancer and thus often regarded as a 'final' option. A 55% response rate is quoted but is generally not an effective long-term treatment.
  - Anthralin (an antipsoriatic) may be useful in children.
- **Telogen effluvium** – there is diffuse hair shedding with spontaneous recovery over several months; provoking factors include stress, hormonal upset or medication related.
- **Traumatic alopecia** – usually related to hairstyling or sometimes trichotillomania (compulsive hair pulling).
- **Cicatricial alopecia** – this subset of alopecia is characterised by the scarring and follicle destruction. It can be subdivided into secondary causes such as burns, infection, etc. or primary cicatricial alopecia (e.g. discoid **lupus erythematosus** and lichen planopilaris, both uncommon) that is characterised by inflammatory cell infiltrates and can itself be divided into neutrophil-rich, lymphocytic-rich or mixed types. A skin biopsy is usually necessary for diagnosis.
- **Female pattern baldness.** The most common cause of female baldness is probably still androgenetic, i.e. sensitivity to androgens, but with weaker inheritance and less likely to follow the typical male patterns.
  - Female baldness can be more challenging to treat; often the remaining hair is of poor quality and finasteride does not work well. Some propose high dose (5%) of minoxidil or anti-androgen therapy (spironolactone or cyproterone acetate). 5-α-Reductase inhibitors are contraindicated in pregnancy due to possible feminisation of the male foetus.

ASSESSMENT

Factors that need to be considered include

- Density of hair – affects donor availability.
- Colour of hair – lighter hair, including grey or 'salt and pepper', allows for more natural-looking results.
- Type of hair – thick or thin, straight or curly (hair with natural wave generally allows better results).

CLASSIFICATION

- **Male pattern baldness** (MPB) is most often classified by the Norwood modification of the Hamilton classification, which has types I (minimal frontotemporal recession) to VII (horseshoe shape). The McCauley classification has relevance to treatment by expanders (see 'Scalp alopecia').
- **Female alopecia** is generally classified with the Ludwig classification with grades I–III of thinning over the vertex.

MEDICAL THERAPY FOR ALOPECIA

These are often used together with surgery.

- **Minoxidil** (Rogaine® or Regaine® depending on the country) – available in 2%–5% topical solutions that need to be applied on the scalp twice daily. The main complaint is the 'messiness' whilst 5% may have skin irritation. Useful results are seen in approximately 1/3, but it needs to be used indefinitely. It is usually regarded as **first-line therapy** and there is evidence of a synergistic effect with tretinoin. The exact mechanism of action is unclear, though the original medication was intended to treat hypertension; there may be a direct mitogenic effect but it has no antiandrogenic action.
  - Oral minoxidil in low dose (off-label) a quarter of a 2.5 mg tablet a day.
- **Finasteride** (Propecia®, Proscar®) – this is a 5-α-reductase inhibitor that is effective in reducing further loss but may also increase hair growth in a proportion of patients. Side effects include 1%–2%

impotence/reduced libido; it also is rather expensive and needs to be used **indefinitely**.
  - 2011 health warning for 1 mg (propecia) and 5 mg (proscar) formulations; a small number of male breast cancer reported worldwide, though the causal relationship is not proven.
- **Spironolactone** being an androgen receptor antagonist also slows down hair loss, and is one of the most widely prescribed medications for MPB.

SURGICAL TREATMENT

Surgical options include

- **Scalp reduction** – can be considered for stable bald areas particularly at the crown/vertex <15% of the scalp; serial excision is possible. Anterior undermining should be minimised, as this would tend to elevate the brow.
- **Rotation flaps** – e.g. temporoparietal flaps can cover frontal loss but changes the hair direction.
- **Tissue expansion** – it is said that 50% defects can be resurfaced with tissue expansion without noticeable hair thinning.

TRANSPLANTATION

The aim of hair transplantation is to achieve natural-looking results, particularly at the anterior hairline, whilst minimising scalp scars. In Norwood types V–VI, there is approximately 12.5% of the scalp available as donor areas (occipital and temporal regions). A strip is harvested (and closed directly with or without **trichophytic closure** [Figure 3.16]); the hairs are then divided up into units. This

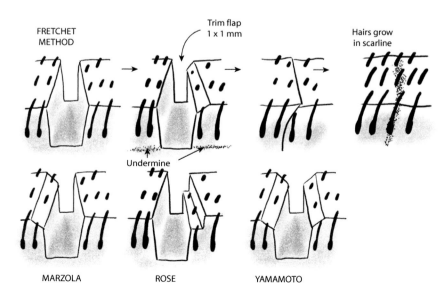

Figure 3.16 Trichophytic closure. Frechet method involves shaving a 1 × 1 mm triangle from the lower flap with closure after undermining for about 5 mm each side. Hairs will grow back in the scarline. Alternatives include the Marzola, Rose and Yamamoto methods.

is called **strip harvesting**; the transfer of follicular units is called follicular unit transfer (FUT).

- Micrografts contain 1–2 hairs.
- Minigrafts contain 3–8 hairs.

Smaller grafts are usually placed in the front of the hair-line with larger micrografts/minigrafts behind them. More than one procedure/grafting session may be needed for the most natural effect.

- In androgenic alopecia, insensitive (to DHT) occipital follicles are transplanted to the frontal region and grow (donor dominant). If there is a family history of severe MPB, i.e. Norwood VI or VII, then attempts to transplant the entire area may lead to doughnut pattern with ring of baldness. This is more likely in the younger patient where you would be less certain of the final pattern of hair loss.
  - Overall, poorer results are expected in those with low-density donor sites, thin follicles, darker hair (more contrast between hair and skin) and straighter hair. Patients are asked to stop taking anticoagulants including NSAIDs and herbal medicines such as garlic, St John's Wort and *Ginkgo biloba*, if used.
  - Field block with local anaesthesia and then tumescent infiltration to turgour (which also reduces 'collateral' damage of neighbouring follicles). Grafts should not be buried; they are better slightly above the skin level than slightly below.
- Placement
  - **Needles** 19–22 G, 'stick and place'; the needle puncture is made just before placing the graft as the hole stays open for only a few seconds. It is less traumatic and one of the favoured techniques but can be difficult to master. Some use specially designed implanters.
  - **Slit grafting** – a slit (1–2 mm long) is made with a blade, and thus transplanted units are more liable to be compressed with healing. As this does not remove alopecia, overall hair density is lower compared to needles.
- Particular attention must be paid to the direction of the follicles for a natural look:
  - Front/anterior hairline 45–60°
  - Posterior hairline 75–80°
  - Vertex/crown 90°, i.e. perpendicular
  - Posterior to crown 45–60° downwards

FOLLICULAR UNIT EXTRACTION (FUE) AND TRANSFER

A punch instrument is used to cut into the dermis around a follicular unit followed by extraction; strictly it requires an assessment of the dermal depth (level of the arrector pili muscle). The small puncture wounds heal by secondary intention. It takes longer to perform; some argue that this reduces viability of the hairs as they are exposed/out of the body for longer. Robots (ARTAS) have been used in hair transplantation since 2011 but are more expensive. FUE may be best suited for small areas in patients who prefer to wear their hair short; it causes 'pit' scarring.

- Harvests from a wider area (8×) – top of the donor area may thin out later and 'borderline' hairs may be lost later.
- Faster recovery time.
- Low total yield and more transection.

Transplantation is contraindicated in

- Diffuse female pattern baldness
- Non-donor dominant alopecia
- Alopecia areata (commonly treated by steroids, minoxidil and phototherapy)
- Active cicatricial alopecia

COMPLICATIONS

Four months or more (some say up to a year) should elapse before judging the results; transplanted hairs grow for about a month before entering telogen for 2–3 months.

- General complications include lidocaine toxicity, bleeding, infection and scarring.
- Poor growth.
- Poor appearance, e.g. unnatural hairline, dolls-head appearance.
- Cyst formation due to buried grafts.

V. LIP RECONSTRUCTION

ANATOMY

The upper lip can be subdivided into the following aesthetic subunits: lateral and median/philtrum, separated from the cheek by the nasolabial/mesolabial fold.

MUSCLES

- Orbicularis oris acts to form a whistling expression. The sphincteric activity depends on muscle continuity. The muscle also inserts into dermis and intermingles with nearby muscles.
  - Extrinsic fibres intermingle with buccinator, decussate at the modiolus.
  - Intrinsic fibres – incisive and mental slips.

ELEVATORS

- Levator labii superioris (LLS) and LLS alaeque nasi (elevates the upper lip and flares the nostrils)
- Levator anguli oris (LAO)
- Zygomaticus minor and major (elevates lips)

DEPRESSORS

- Depressor anguli oris (DAO)
- Depressor labii inferioris

- Mentalis (role in lower lip protrusion)
- Platysma (lowers the lower lip)
- Risorius – from parotid fascia to the angle of the mouth (draws the angle of the mouth laterally)

NERVES

- Motor
  - Upper lip muscles – buccal branch of VII.
  - Lower lip muscles – marginal mandibular branch of VII.
  - Orbicularis oris is supplied by both.
- Sensory
  - Upper lip – **infraorbital nerve** (ION, maxillary branch of V).
    - Block 1 cm below the inferior orbital rim in line with the medial limbus/mid pupil through skin or upper buccal sulcus.
  - Lower lip – **mental nerve** (termination of IAN, mandibular branch of V) exits the mandible at the second premolar.
    - Intra-oral infiltration in line with the lower canines; nerve may be visible by putting the lower lip on the stretch.
  - Other facial blocks.
    - **Supraorbital nerve** – approximately 2.5 cm from the midline, between the midpupillary line and the medial limbus. A notch may be palpable.
    - **Supratrochlear nerve** – exit orbit at the upper medial corner approximately 1 cm from the midline.

The blood supply comes from superior and inferior labial branches of the facial arteries with rich midline anastomoses – it is often said that a cut labial artery will bleed from both ends. The inferior labial artery branch arises from the facial artery about 2.5 cm lateral and 1.5 cm inferior to the oral commissure. The anatomy of the labial (and facial) artery is important when performing filler/injections.

- The superior labial artery runs closer to the lip edge, deep to the muscle near the wet–dry lip junction.
- The inferior labial artery travels deep to the orbicularis oris further away from the vermillion border.

Lymphatics of the upper lip tend not to cross the midline unless the lesion itself has crossed the midline, going to the preauricular/parotid, submandibular and submental nodes. The lower lip lymph drains to the submandibular and submental nodes. Lymph node metastases are uncommon (10% and 20% for the lower and upper lip, respectively) as they tend to occur late and the highly visible lesion usually leads to an early diagnosis. SCCs and melanomas have a tendency to spread along nerves, which may be suggested by symptoms of numbness or paraesthesia.

PATHOLOGY

The lack of a keratinised layer may increase susceptibility to ultraviolet radiation.

- Most upper lip lesions are BCCs (most lower eyelid tumours are BCCs).
- Most lower lip lesions are SCCs (only 5% of SCCs occur on the upper lip) and commissural/mucosal SCCs have a higher propensity for metastasis. Excision margins should be 5–10 mm for SCCs.
  - SCCs anterior to the wet–dry margin behave like cutaneous tumours, whilst those posterior to this line behave more like intraoral tumours with a higher rate of metastasis.
- Tumour size and thickness also correlate with metastatic potential.
  - 5% risk of occult metastasis in lesions under 4 cm
  - 5% risk of recurrence, 5% risk of second lip primary
- **Lip mucocoeles** are more common in the lower lip; 85%–90% are of the extravasation type due to mechanical damage to the ducts (pseudocyst) and can be associated with an inflammatory response. Retention-type mucocoeles are lined with oncocytic epithelium and are found most commonly on the buccal mucosa/FOM of older patients.
- **Avulsed lip** segments (due to bite injuries) have been successfully replanted (Walton RL, *Plast Reconstr Surg*, 1998). Regardless of venous repair, there was venous congestion in all patients, which was treated by leeches (that left visible scars) and systemic heparinisation used in 11/13.

T STAGING OF LIP SCC

As for intra-oral SCC if involving mucosa

- T1 tumour <2 cm.
- T2 tumour >2–4 cm.
- T3 tumour >4 cm.
- T4 tumour invades adjacent structures (bone, tongue, skin of neck).

LIP RECONSTRUCTION

Ideally the reconstructed lip should be competent – it should be sensate and have a complete innervated muscle ring. In addition, for the lower lip in particular, a good sulcus is needed to prevent drooling. Other considerations include speech and cosmesis (symmetry and preservation of landmarks – particularly the **vermilion border** – single 'l', derived from the French vermeil, a red dye – classically vermiculum from the insect *Kermes vermilio*, vermilion itself was mercuric sulphide/cinnabar).

- Vermilion – red lip due to rich vascularity and lack of keratinisation.
- Vermilion border – junction of skin with vermilion.

- White roll is a slight prominence next to the vermilion border that reflects light.

LOWER LIP RECONSTRUCTION

In situ cancer may be treated by lip shave and mucosal advancement (may need incisional release to convert it into a bipedicled flap) or CO_2 laser.

Losses of up to one-third of the lower lip may be closed directly (more in the elderly), whilst larger defects will require recruitment of additional tissue in the form of various flaps. Wedge excisions can be 'shield' or 'W' (skirting around the mental/labiomental crease) or a so-called 'double-barrelled excision' – the lip segment is full thickness whilst the chin segment is skin/subcutaneous tissue only.

DEFECTS ONE- TO TWO-THIRDS OF THE LOWER LIP

Most named flaps with the exception of the Abbé flap were originally designed for the lower lip, where most pathology occurs (Figure 3.17).

- **Abbé flap** – some are loathe to violate the upper lip to reconstruct the lower (see below).
- **Abbé–Estlander flap** (defects of the commissure/ lower lateral lip) – the flap is designed to be half the width of the defect, pedicled on the contralateral end of the labial artery (potentially making the vascularity more tenuous). Initial descriptions were two-staged, but currently it is most commonly used for lateral defects and can be single-staged. As the flap is rotated,

the modiolus is distorted affecting animation and the commissure is blunted (commissuroplasty may be required later). The segment is insensate.
- The commissure should not be sacrificed unnecessarily.
- **Karapandzic flap** is a neurovascular circumoral advancement flap that transfers skin, muscle and mucosa with the correct muscle orientation but requires an intact commissure. The circumoral incision is the height of the defect, and goes through skin and superficial facial muscles (with a more limited mucosal incision), but **preserves neurovascular supply** to orbicularis oris whilst dividing radial elevators or depressors. However, preserving nerves and vessels limits the advancement possible (some view it as a **modified Gillies**) and so usually needs to be applied bilaterally. The technique can also be used for upper lip defects where it may need excision of Burow's triangles.
- As it does not introduce new tissue, it will cause **microstomia**, though this will stretch out/relax to a certain extent; there is also distortion of commissures. Its use should be limited to defects less than two-thirds of the lip.
- There may still be significant sensory loss.
- **Gillies fan flap** – some regard it as being halfway between a Karapandzic flap and a McGregor flap. It is an insensate myocutaneous flap; the muscle is denervated. It is suited for upper or lower lip defects adjacent to the commissure; it can be raised bilaterally for subtotal upper lip reconstruction. There have been many modifications.
- For the lower lip, the flap is cut back to the nasolabial fold – it advances along rather than

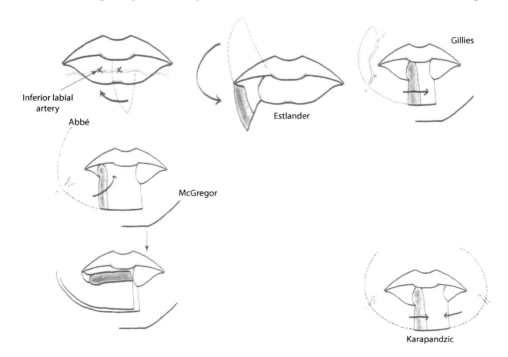

Figure 3.17 Different types of lip reconstruction: Abbé, Estlander, Gillies, Karapandzic, McGregor.

rotates into the defect and thus the commissure moves medially (and becomes rounded); again no new tissue is recruited – the lower lip is still shortened but less so than with a Karapandzic flap.

- A Z-plasty modification allows better turning around the commissure (Panje WR, *Otolaryngol Clin North Am*, 1982) and is similar to a McGregor flap.

- **McGregor flap** is a myocutaneous flap composed of three approximately equally sized squares that **rotates** around the commissure, which remains in the same place. As it introduces new tissue into the lip, **microstomia is reduced**.
  - The new lip is devoid of vermilion, which can be reconstructed by mucosal advancement or tongue flap.
  - There is a lack of a functionally complete muscle ring, but post-operative drooling is uncommon.
  - A Nakajima flap is similar but preserves the neurovascular bundle inferolaterally.

- **Johanson's step (ladder) technique** – a central defect is approximated by creating step cuts in the soft tissue of the chin, which work like a 45° W-plasty; it can close defects up to 50%–67%, though with larger defects microstomia will result.
  - Blomgren I (Scand J Plast Reconstr Surg Hand Surg, 1988) modification to preserve commissure
  - Grimm modification with curved steps (Roldan JC, *Plast Reconstr Surg*, 2007)
  - Taiwan modification with altered composition with each step: full thickness, skin to split muscle, dermis only.

(SUB)TOTAL DEFECTS

A few good options exist to reconstruct wide (sub)total lower lip defects. Much has been written about anatomical restoration and muscle reconstruction to maintain oral competence, but it may be less important in practice. Whilst conceptually attractive, the objective evidence of muscle function in reconstructed lips is rarely observed, and in most instances, the flap serves merely as a **static sling** even when the aim has been 'functional'. Likewise, sensate reconstruction is emphasised, but prospective comparative studies found no differences in terms of functional outcomes. Innervated flaps may provide earlier return of sensation, but patients with denervated flaps do not complain of loss of sensation or drooling. There may be neurotisation from adjacent tissues if there is sufficient muscle in the flap, i.e. not totally dependent on the local neurovascular pedicle.

In simple terms,

- Bilateral Karapandzic up to 70% lower lip
- Bilateral McGregor 80%
- Webster modification of Bernard-Burrow 90%
- Nasolabial flaps 100%
- Free flaps 100%

Bernard–Burow flaps/Webster modification of – advance **cheek** and chin tissue, using excisional triangles on the cheek. The vermilion is reconstructed by advancement of buccal mucosa. The **Webster** modification utilises mucosa preserving triangles adjacent and parallel to the nasolabial fold, instead of the full thickness excisions in the original technique.

- There is less microstomia than bilateral Karanpandizic/Gillies flaps, but caution is still required in defects >3/4 except in patients with substantial cheek laxity.
- There is more scarring and reduced muscle function.
- Normal tissue is sacrificed.

Nasolabial flaps. Bilateral flaps can be used for total lip defects, with the flaps pedicled inferiorly immediately superior and lateral to the defect. Donor sites for flaps 2.5–3.5 cm wide can usually be closed primarily with moderate undermining. There are many variations, e.g. Von Brun technique or Fuijmori gate flaps (larger triangular flaps rotated on the inner corner with the pedicle dissected out, and the ends staggered). Flaps are not wholly reliable due to the random blood supply and thus are not often a first choice for lower lip reconstruction.

- Innervated (motor and sensory) composite (skin, muscle and mucosa) flaps based on depressor and levator anguli oris. Bilateral full thickness flaps (up to 2.5 cm width). Labour-intensive dissection of the nerves (marginal mandibular, buccal branch and mental nerve) needed to maintain innervation.
- Steeple flap – an islanded composite cheek flap based on the facial artery.

FREE TISSUE TRANSFER

- Thin fasciocutaneous flaps, e.g. RFF with palmaris longus sling (medial cutaneous nerve of the forearm for a sensate flap) or ALT with fascia lata sling. These flaps tend to have a poor colour match (landmarks such as the vermilion border are difficult to reconstruct) and do not have functioning muscle (though a strip of vastus lateralis can be used as a chimeric ALT).
- Myocutaneous flap, e.g. gracilis with coaptation of the motor nerve.
- Constructing a sling is important for functional outcomes. Fascia lata extensions are tunnelled over orbicularis oris and sutured down to the muscle or to each other or anchored to the periosteum of the zygomatic bone with permanent sutures (Yildirim S, *Plast Reconstr Surg*, 2006).

UPPER LIP RECONSTRUCTION

Upper lip cancers are much less common; a lateral segment BCC is the commonest scenario.

- **Loss of up to 1/4** of the upper lip may be closed directly.
  - For slightly larger defects, simple advancement flaps may be combined with crescentic perialar excisions.
  - Partial thickness defects can be closed in an A-T or O-T fashion.

- **Abbé flap** (Robert Abbé 1851–1928, American surgeon and radiologist, who was a good friend of Marie Curie). Whilst midline upper lip defects can be easily closed directly, this will mean the loss of the normal philtral appearance. The Abbé flap, a lip-switch pedicled on the lateral side of the donor lip, is a useful option for central defects, especially in women, and can also be used for lateral defects up to 50% of the upper lip.
  - **A flap of the same height but half the width** of the defect along with a skin/subcutaneous only 'Burow's' triangle along the mental crease allows easy donor closure. The position of the artery is first noted on the free/unpedicled side to guide fashioning of the pedicle; there is often no recognised accompanying vein, and a muscle cuff is kept to improve venous return. The bridge is divided after 2–3 weeks.
  - It theoretically reconstructs muscle continuity. Some sensation may return after several months in the order of pain, touch and temperature. There is some evidence of reinnervation of muscle presumably via neurotisation. The segment may trapdoor and move oddly.
  - Can be combined with bilateral advancement - Websters.
- **Karapandzic flap** (see above).
- **Estlander** (see above) is similar to the Abbé flap but used for lateral defects involving the commissure.

FOR LARGER DEFECTS (GREATER THAN TWO-THIRDS)

- If there is sufficient cheek tissue for advancement, then use Bernard–Burow's technique – bilateral for central defects or ipsilateral combined with contralateral perialar advancement for lateral defects. It can be combined with an Abbé flap.
- Von Bruns nasolabial.
- Bilateral Karapandzics.
- With insufficient cheek tissue, free flaps need to be considered, e.g. RFFF.

ORAL COMMISSURE (FIGURES 3.18 AND 3.19)

Reconstruction of electrical burns of the oral commissure (Donelan MB, *Plast Reconstr Surg*, 1995)
It is very difficult to reconstruct the specialised structure of the commissure:

- Thin mobile lip segment
- Moves dynamically and symmetrically

In burns, a conservative approach is usually adopted initially with secondary reconstruction (including scar contracture release) at a later stage. The author describes the use of an anteriorly based ventral myomucosal tongue flap to reconstruct the lower lip portion of the commissure with

pedicle division at 2 weeks. It provides good volume of tissue, but the combination of awkward tongue position and significant swelling post-operatively means that a soft or liquid diet is needed for several days.

The upper lip portion of the commissure is reconstructed with a Gillies–Millard flap, which is a superiorly based flap raised from the scarred commissure and rotated upwards to lengthen the upper lip. Scar release is performed through the flap incisions.

VI. CHEEK RECONSTRUCTION

The cheek is divided into three aesthetic subunits or zones:

- Zone 1 – **suborbital** zone from the lower eyelid down to the gingival sulcus and from the nasolabial fold to the anterior sideburn
- Zone 2 – **pre-auricular** zone from the tragus to the anterior sideburn and from the junction of the helical rim with the cheek down to the mandible
- Zone 3 – **buccomandibular** – area inferior to the suborbital zone and anterior to the pre-auricular zone

Reconstructive options by zones:

SUBORBITAL ZONE (ZONE 1)

- Direct closure with a vertically orientated scar.
- FTSGs generally offer a poor cosmetic outcome (patch effect) compared to local flaps, but can be considered in those who cannot tolerate more complex procedures.
- Local flaps including
  - **Limberg, V–Y, McGregor flap** for defects <4 cm. Pay attention to the vectors – avoid pulling downwards on the lower lid.
  - **Cervicofacial flap** for larger defects (>4 cm), with wide undermining and incorporating the SMAS-platysma into the flap. To reduce the risk of ectropion, the flap should be anchored to the periosteum at the zygomatic arch and inferior orbital rim; a lateral canthopexy may be needed. This flap can be used for reconstruction of zone 1 or 3. It can be inferiorly based moving postauricular skin anteriorly onto the medial cheek or posteriorly based moving neck skin upwards onto the cheek/temple.
  - The **Mustarde flap** is inferiorly based; the skin incision is taken well laterally beyond the lateral canthus and curves upwards into the temple before curving back down to the preauricular crease.
  - **Cervicopectoral flap**.
- Tissue expansion – ideally two or more expanders.
- See also lower eyelid reconstruction.

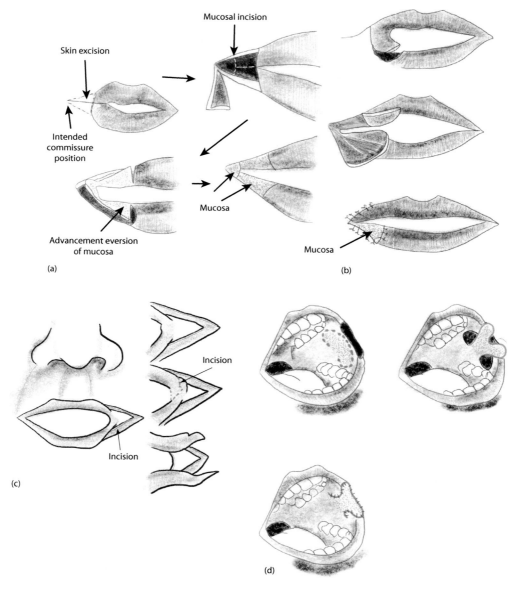

Figure 3.18 Commissuroplasty. Common techniques include (a) Converse and (b) Gillies. Mucosa is advanced out to resurface the outer lip skin. (c) The lip at the blunted commissure is split to allow lengthening. (d) The mucosal defect can be covered by a variety of means including a pedicle mucosal advancement flap.

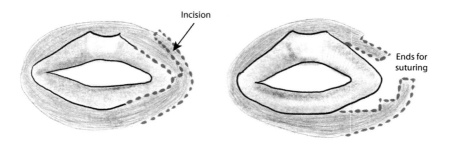

Figure 3.19 Oral sphincteroplasty. A manoeuvre to elongate the orbicularis oris when performing a commissuroplasty.

PRE-AURICULAR ZONE (ZONE 2)

- Direct closure (facelift-type undermined flap; it is said that undermining more than 4 cm does not offer additional advancement).
- Skin grafts may work quite well in the temple areas.
- Local flaps – Limberg flap, hatchet flap, anteriorly based cervicopectoral flaps.
- Distant flaps for larger defects – PM (bulky), LD myocutaneous flaps (tunnelled over or through PM), deltopectoral flaps (DP, delay may increase reliability of the tip).
- Free flaps – particularly if >10 cm – RFF, scapular flap, ALT, lateral arm.

BUCCOMANDIBULAR ZONE (CHEEK PROPER, ZONE 3)

- Skin only – direct closure, FTSG, local flaps and distant flaps as above
- Lining – tunnelled nasolabial flap, axial tongue flap (based on a lingual artery), flaps that epithelialise secondarily, e.g. buccal fat flaps
- Skin and lining – combination of procedures or **double skin paddle** PM, DP, free flaps including RFF (± bone, tendon), scapular flap, ALT

CONTOUR DEFECTS

Cheek contour defects may be part of Romberg's syndrome, HMF, facial lipodystrophy (which may be associated with AIDS/HIV treatment) or trauma. Options include

- Fillers for smaller volumes, e.g. collagen, semi-permanent (Sculptura® – poly-L-lactic acid), dermal/dermofat, fat injections
- De-epithelialised flaps, e.g. platysma, free flaps as above including omentum for larger volumes

D. MANAGEMENT OF PATIENTS REQUIRING RADICAL OR SELECTIVE ND

I. NECK ANATOMY

FASCIAL LAYERS (FIGURE 3.20)

The deep cervical fascia has four components:

- **Investing fascia.** This is the layer of deep fascia that lies beneath the subcutaneous fat and splits into superficial and deep layers as the parotid fascia surrounds the gland. A local thickening forms the stylomandibular ligament.
- **Prevertebral fascia.** This covers the muscles (splenius capitis, levator scapulae, scalenus posterior, medius and anterior) that form the floor of the posterior triangle, and forms a layer over which the pharynx and oesophagus can freely slide. It covers the brachial plexus trunks and subclavian artery but not the subclavian vein and is pierced by the four nerves of the cervical plexus.
- **Pretracheal fascia.** This separates the trachea from the overlying strap muscles to allow trachea gliding. It encloses the thyroid gland (pierced by the thyroid vessels) and blends laterally with the carotid sheath.
- **Carotid sheath.** This envelopes the carotid arteries (common and internal), the IJV (where it is thin) and vagus nerve. It is adherent to the deep surface of SM.

TRIANGLES OF THE NECK

POSTERIOR TRIANGLE

The borders are the anterior border of trapezius, the middle third of clavicle and the posterior border of SM. The posterior belly of omohyoid subdivides into an upper occipital

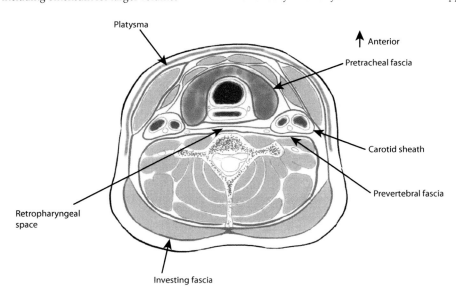

Figure 3.20 Fascial layers of the neck.

triangle and a lower supraclavicular triangle. The investing fascia forms the roof whilst the floor is composed of the pre-vertebral fascia (see above).

Contents

- Lymphatics
  - Lymph nodes: occipital, supraclavicular and lowermost deep cervical nodes.
  - Thoracic duct enters the junction of IJV and subclavian vein on the left side.
- Nerves
  - Accessory nerve (XI) crosses from the upper third SM to the lower third trapezius within the fascial roof.
  - Cutaneous branches of the cervical plexus.
    - Lesser occipital C2, greater auricular C2, 3, transverse cervical C2, 3 and supraclavicular C3, 4.
  - Muscular branches of the cervical plexus.
    - C1 travelling with XII forms the superior root of the ansa whilst C2,3 forms the inferior root of the ansa.
    - C2, 3 to SM.
    - C3, 4 to trapezius.
    - C3, 4, 5 as the phrenic nerve to the diaphragm.
  - The plexus lies on scalenus anterior beneath the prevertebral fascia and may be joined by the accessory phrenic nerve, a branch from the nerve to subclavius (from the brachial plexus).
- Vessels
  - Transverse cervical and suprascapular vessels from the thyrocervical trunk – these may be important 'stand-by' vessels in the vessel-depleted neck.
  - Subclavian artery lies low down in the triangle.
  - EJV.
- Muscle – omohyoid (the other Residents' friend)

ANTERIOR TRIANGLE

The borders are the anterior border of SM, the lower border of the mandible and the midline; note that it does not meet the posterior triangle being separated by the width of the SM mus-cle. The roof consists of the platysma and deep cervical fascia.

It can be subdivided into

- Submandibular (digastric) and submental triangles by the ABD muscle
- Carotid (jugulodigastric) and muscular triangles by the omohyoid muscle

Contents

- Lymph nodes: deep cervical nodes (which are closely adherent to the IJV), submandibular and submental nodes.
- Nerves
  - X within the carotid sheath and superior laryngeal branch.
  - Lingual branch of V3 (one of the three sensory branches from the posterior division).

- XI (at the apex of the triangle).
- XII.
- Ansa cervicalis.
- Vessels
  - Common carotid – no branches proximal to its bifurcation at C4 (upper border of thyroid cartilage). The ICA has no branches in the neck whilst the ECA has multiple branches.
  - IJV lies lateral to the ICA; the facial, lingual, superior and middle thyroid veins.
- Muscles
  - Suprahyoid muscles – digastric, stylohyoid, mylohyoid, geniohyoid and hyoglossus.
  - Infrahyoid strap muscles – sternohyoid and omohyoid superior, thyrohyoid and sternothyroid deeper.
- Other tissues
  - Hyoid bone and thyroid cartilage.
  - Thyroid and parathyroid glands.
  - Submandibular and sublingual salivary glands.
  - Trachea and oesophagus.

Branchial cysts, if present, will lie in the anterior trian-gle. The classic presentation is as a soft, cystic mass anterior to the SM that contains straw-coloured fluid with choles-terol crystals. They are usually well-encapsulated but can extend to the lateral pharyngeal wall.

SUPRAHYOID REGION

This includes the digastric (submandibular) and submental triangles between the mandible, the hyoid bone and the two PBD.

- Nodes: submental and submandibular lymph nodes.
- Nerves
  - Lingual nerve spiralling around (crossing twice) the submandibular duct of Wharton
  - Hypoglossal nerve
- Vessels – the anterior jugular veins drain into the EJV in the posterior triangle
- Muscles – supra- and infrahyoids as above
- Other soft tissue: submandibular (and duct) and sublingual salivary glands

The role of MRI scanning in the diagnosis of cervical lymphadenopathy (Wilson GR, *Br J Plast Surg*, 1994)
Clinical examination is unreliable in many patients with 30% false positive and 40% false negative, and misses nodes <2 cm in diameter, especially if deep to SM. Overall accuracy is 60%–70%.

MRI is capable of identifying all enlarged nodes >4–5 mm diameter (i.e. 100% sensitive), but it can-not reliably differentiate between benign and malig-nant lymphadenopathy (53% specific for malignant lymphadenopathy).

- Clinically negative neck but high risk – MRI scan to confirm node status
- Clinically positive neck – FNA with ND if histologically confirmed

145

On MRI:

- T1 – the **tumour signal is generally darker than normal tissues** (light – fat; darker – fluid); one limitation of the standard MRI is that it is difficult to differentiate tumour from oedema/fluid. The resolution of the MRI can be increased by special imaging, e.g. fat suppression or use of contrast such as gadolinium, a paramagnetic substance that enhances nodes making them brighter like fat.
- T2 – darker – fat, light – fluid.
- Up to 25% of clinically occult metastases are not detected radiologically.

II. TORTICOLLIS

Torticollis: *tortus* (twisted); *collum* (neck).

Causes include musculoskeletal (e.g. cervical spine abnormalities), ophthalmologic (e.g. congenital nystagmus, IVth nerve palsy), infectious (e.g. parapharyngeal abscess), neurologic (e.g. posterior fossa tumours), traumatic (e.g. brachial plexus palsy) and neoplastic conditions – may present early with only torticollis, and thus the first step in evaluation is always a careful and complete physical examination.

CONGENITAL

Torticollis in children (0.5% of births) is likely to be congenital.

- The actual cause is usually unknown; it may be due to a primary fibrosis of SM. There may be a palpable mass within the substance of the muscle in the first few weeks that gradually dissipates (8 months on average) but leaves an area of fibrosis.
  - It is loosely associated with possible birth trauma with difficult deliveries (primiparous, breech where it occurs in up to 30%, etc.), and a muscle-specific compartment syndrome either during delivery or perinatal (in utero crowding) is another theory. It may run in some families.
- In some cases, it is compensatory, e.g. **vertical orbital dystopia** (craniosynostoses especially unilateral/asymmetric coronal, craniofacial clefts, HMF). As the orbits lie on different horizontal planes, the child holds his/her head to one side to compensate attain stereoscopic vision. This is called positional torticollis as opposed to muscular torticollis.
  - Positional – no actual tightness.
  - Muscular – tightness limits ROM, concomitant mass.
  - Surgery for vertical orbital dystopia (Tan ST, *Plast Reconstr Surg*, 1996) requires orbital translocation via a bicoronal approach; it is easier to elevate the lower lying orbit. Medial canthal ligament and lacrimal apparatus are left attached if possible.
- In idiopathic cases, the initial treatment is **physiotherapy** (stretching and strengthening exercises) – home exercises may be sufficient; otherwise, patients should be referred

to physiotherapy at 6 weeks. Some may use special collars such as the TOT collar as needed.
  - Earlier treatment seems to have better results with shorter duration of treatment; 5%–10% may need surgery (best between 1 and 4 years of age).
  - **Myoplasty** can selectively denervate the muscles responsible for the abnormal movement or posture.
- Those who do not respond to 6 months of treatment, or those with additional abnormalities such as craniofacial, hip or spine anomalies, warrant referral to appropriate specialists.
  - The usual skull changes are ipsilateral craniorbital flattening with contralateral occipital flattening (i.e. **positional plagiocephaly**) that often resolves with conservative measures; cases that persist beyond 12–18 months will usually require surgery to treat the deformity.
  - Surgery produced good results in 81.8% of patients (Cheng JC, *Clin Orthop Relat Res*, 1999). Post-operative rehabilitation is also important.
  - Botulinum toxin injections are **not** recommended as first line – neutralising antibodies may develop with repeated treatments in 5%–10% of patients (though this is based on previous older formulations and higher dosage regimes).
  - Anticholinergics (50% relief but with significant side effects) and baclofen.

Efficacy of microcurrent therapy in infants with congenital muscular torticollis involving the entire sternocleidomastoid muscle (Kwon DR, *Clin Rehab*, 2014)

In a randomised placebo-controlled trial, a group of 10 infants with congenital muscular torticollis had physiotherapy/exercises along with ultrasound therapy, whilst a second group had additional microcurrent treatment. Microcurrent therapy consists of a probe placed on the skin delivering small amounts of electricity to the tissues, supposedly increasing blood flow reducing spasm. Ultrasound therapy generates deep heat supposedly decreasing inflammation. The latter group had significantly better passive range of motion, as well as a shorter treatment time (2.6 months vs. 6.3 months).

ACQUIRED TORTICOLLIS

This is torticollis presenting in a previously normal patient. This is less common than congenital torticollis; most cases are idiopathic, though a small number develop it secondarily.

In adults (25–60 years old), this is most commonly spasmodic and is a form of **focal cervical dystonia**, a chronic movement disorder. It was previously thought to be a psychiatric illness, but is now viewed as a neurological illness. The aetiology is unknown but may follow trauma. In some families, it is inherited (AD with reduced penetrance).

- 10%–20% of patients may experience remission, but nearly all patients relapse within 5 years and are left with persistent disease.

- Botulinum toxin is the most effective treatment unlike congenital torticollis.
- Anticholinergics and baclofen may also help.
- Surgery.

III. NECK DISSECTION

MANAGEMENT OF NECK NODES

Surgical education: neck dissection (Chummun S, *Br J Plast Surg*, 2004)

The occurrence of cervical node metastases in patients with head and neck cancer reduces survival by 50%. Layland (*Laryngoscope*, 2005) demonstrated that disease-specific survival drops from 67.9% for N0 disease to 39.9% for N+. The presence of any palpable lymph nodes means that the cancer becomes at least stage III. Radiotherapy reduces the risk of post-operative neck failure by >50%.

Risk factors for nodal metastases:

- Posterior tumours are more likely to metastasise compared with anteriorly located tumours.
- The highest risk of nodal metastases is associated with tongue tumours.
- T-stage and thickness (highest risk >8 mm thick, lowest <2 mm).
- Histology including perineural and perivascular invasion.

NODE LEVELS (MEMORIAL SLOAN-KETTERING)

- Level Ia submental triangle.
- Level Ib submandibular triangle.
- Level II upper deep cervical/jugulodigastric.
- Level III mid deep cervical.
- Level IVa lower deep cervical – deep to the sternal head of SM.
- Level IVb lower deep cervical – deep to the clavicular head of SM.
- Level Va posterior triangle – along the accessory nerve (XI).
- Level Vb posterior triangle – along the transverse cervical artery.
- Level VI anterior compartment.
- Level VII upper mediastinum (this is not commonly used).

PATTERNS OF SPREAD

There tend to be typical consistent patterns of lymphatic spread:

- Enlarged supraclavicular node usually indicates a primary site below the clavicle, e.g. breast, bronchus, stomach, pancreas.
- Enlarged level nodes III–V usually mean a primary site in the mid-neck, e.g. thyroid, larynx, pharynx.

- Enlarged jugulodigastric node suggests a primary in the oral cavity, face or scalp.

With multiple enlarged nodes, consider the diagnosis of lymphoma and check other node basins as well as liver and spleen.

Pattern of lymph node metastases in intra-oral squamous cell carcinoma (Sharpe DT, *Br J Plast Surg*, 1981)

Radical ND (RND) specimens from 98 patients with intra-oral SCC were examined. The important conclusions were as follows:

- There were no lymph node metastases in posterior triangle, submental triangle, salivary glands or SM muscle.
- There were **predictable patterns** of lymph node involvement:
  - Hard palate and maxilla – level I
  - Lower lip – levels I and II
  - FOM and alveolus – levels I and II
  - Tongue levels – I and II
- No lower internal jugular nodes (levels III and IV) were involved in the absence of disease higher up.
- The **more anterior the lesion, the more likely that level I** nodes would be involved first; the more posterior the lesion, the more likely that level II nodes would be involved first.

The conclusion was that functional ND, preserving XI in the posterior triangle and the SM, would be oncologically safe.

CLASSIFICATION OF ND

An ND removes lymph nodes in a block from the neck. It can be therapeutic and/or prognostic (staging). The contralateral neck is usually left alone except for tumours of the tongue tip or those crossing the midline.

MANAGEMENT OF NODAL DISEASE

- N1 – surgery (if node >3 cm) or radiotherapy (if node <3 cm)
- N2 – selective or MRND III
- N3 – RND/MRND I

It can still be considered in N0 necks (clinical examination is only two-thirds accurate at best):

- Risk of subclinical disease is high.
- Consider site – lip, sinus, glottis vs. oral cavity/pharynx.
- Tumour factors such as size, thickness, histology, e.g. patients with T3/4 N0 tongue usually undergo selective ND (SND).
- Provides surgical access to tumour or vessels for reconstruction.
- For patients who are difficult to follow up.
- Note that level V is rarely involved in clinically N0 necks.

RADICAL ND (CRILE 1906)

All nodes in levels I–V are removed along with the accessory nerve (AN), IJV and SM.

Indications:

- Recurrent tumours
- Level II node encasing XI ± extracapsular spread
- Post-irradiation field

MODIFIED RADICAL ND

The MRND spares some non-lymphatic structures in an effort to reduce the morbidity of the procedure.

- **SM** – the concerns are mostly about the contour deformity, though the muscle may offer protection for the carotid artery particularly when skin flap necrosis or fistula formation occurs. Its loss results in the least morbidity of the three non-lymphatic structures sacrificed during RND; thus, it is the one resected most often (subtypes I and II).
- **Internal jugular vein** – bilateral IJV resection is associated with serious complications such as raised ICP, oedema, stroke and death (0–3% mortality for staged RND vs. 10%–14% for simultaneous RND – Dulguerov P, *Laryngoscope*, 1998). Some clinicians believe that risks are reduced if the operative time is less than 5–6 hours, but most prefer either to stage procedures or for IJV reconstruction if bilateral IJV resection is necessary. The IJV is an important recipient vein for microvascular surgical reconstruction.
- **Spinal accessory nerve** (SAN) – nerve injury results in dysfunction of the trapezius muscle causing the shoulder to droop as the scapula is shifted laterally and rotated downward – thus patients have an asymmetric neckline, a drooping shoulder, winging of the scapula and weakness of forward elevation, but complain mostly of shoulder stiffness/discomfort with decreased range of motion, particularly abduction. Conversely, sparing the nerve reduces shoulder and neck pain and reduces the need for pain medications (Terrell JE, *Laryngoscope*, 2000). QOL studies (Shah S, *Head Neck*, 2001) show that it is the shoulder pain and neck tightness that impact the patient the most. It affects 33.3% after MRND, 20% after SOHND and 66.7% after posterolateral ND (Van Wilgen, *Head Neck*, 2004); radiotherapy did not affect this.

Suarez presented anatomical work that demonstrated that the lymphatics are generally well compartmentalised away from the non-lymphatic structures by fascial layers. Bocca proposed the term 'functional neck dissection' in 1967; different subtypes and classifications were proposed by Medina, Robbins and Byers in 1989, 1991 and 1994, respectively.

The subtypes are often referred to as 'Medina subtypes':

- Type 1 – preserves SAN only.
- Type 2 – preserves nerve and the IJV.

- Type 3: preserves nerve, vein and SM – this is equivalent to Bocca's 'functional neck dissection' (although he originally spared the submandibular gland).

The type of MRND performed depends upon clearance of the tumour and is often determined on-table. The relationship of nodal metastases to the trio of structures is evaluated using inspection and palpation, e.g. IJV thrombosis. Inability to develop a clean plane of dissection that preserves the thick reactive fibrous tissue around nodes means that the structures need to be sacrificed. Although formalised indications for MRND have not been created and clinicians vary in their preference, in general terms, MRND is indicated wherever possible without oncologic compromise.

SELECTIVE ND

The selective ND that leaves some lymph node groups based on a predictable pattern of spread was first described by Hanley in 1980. It is often performed to gain 'access'.

- **Suprahyoid dissection**: removes level I submental and submandibular nodes from the suprahyoid region.
- **Supra-omohyoid dissection** is a common option for N0 anterior tongue and FOM tumours. It can be performed *en passant* whilst gaining access to the tumour and removes nodes in levels I–III along with occipital nodes in the posterior triangle.
  - There is a 3.5% failure rate (Shah JP, *Cancer*, 1990), but the thoracic duct is not at risk, whilst the SM, SAN and IJV are spared (like type 3 MRND).
  - It is not suitable for parotid and tonsillar tumours as these all drain preferentially to levels IV and V.
- **Posterolateral ND** removes occipital nodes along with posterior triangle (V) and jugulodigastric chain (II–IV) – is an option in posterior scalp tumours.
- **Anterolateral II–IV** for oro/hypo-pharynx and larynx.

EXTENDED RADICAL ND

This is an RND along with **additional** resection (additional nodes or non-lymphatic structures).

- Paratracheal dissection (VI and VII)
- Parotidectomy

OPERATIVE TECHNIQUE – MRND

Position the patient slightly head up with the neck extended (sandbag under the shoulders) and the head turned away from the operative side. Many types of skin incisions have been described (Figure 3.21) – optimising exposure safely is the priority – most commonly a 'Y' incision (e.g. Conley, or variant) with a curved vertical limb to avoid contracture or an apron-type incision to avoid the

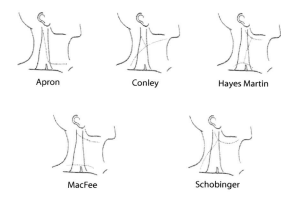

Figure 3.21 The main types of incisions for NDs. There are many subtle variations on each type, e.g. the Conley-type incisions are often called 'Y-shaped', whilst the Hayes Martin is a 'double-Y'. Apron, Conley, Hayes Martin, MacFee, Schobinger.

trifurcation. The MacFee incision is advocated if the neck has been irradiated, though some people use it as their 'default'.

- Raise the skin flaps deep to platysma to the mandible, clavicle and trapezius whilst preserving the marginal mandibular and cervical branches of VII in the upper flap and greater auricular nerve (GAN) and SAN. The EJV should be preserved for a venous anastomosis if possible.
- Clear the submental then the submandibular triangles from anterior to posterior, to the posterior border of the mylohyoid, which is then retracted to allow identification of the submandibular gland. Take care to avoid injury to the marginal mandibular nerve whilst freeing the submandibular gland; ligating the duct and the facial artery twice in the process. The lingual nerve is deep to the gland whilst the XII is deep to the **PBD (Residents' friend)** as well as Wharton's duct; the superior attachment of the SM to the mastoid can be divided.
  - **'Erb's point'** – where GAN (and other branches of cervical plexus) crosses over the posterior border of SM ~6 cm below mastoid, and 1 cm above this is the SAN, which then enters the anterior border of the trapezius 5 cm above the clavicle.
  - Strictly this is an error; Erb's point was originally described as a point 2–3 cm above the clavicle where C5 and C6 roots unite. Stimulation here will cause contraction of the upper arm, whilst pressure causes something resembling Erb's palsy.
  - Wilhelm Erb (1840–1921) was a neurologist working mostly at Heidelberg University.
- Elevate the level I contents downwards to identify the superior IJV and determine its condition. Identify the SAN and also determine how the nodes relate to it as well as the SM.
- Then define the posterior border of the posterior triangle (trapezius) taking care to leave the GAN (and SAN)

and then elevate the contents in a posterior to anterior direction. Identify the SAN and dissect it free along its course through the posterior triangle from the SM to the trapezius. Deep dissection continues on top of splenius and levator scapulae; the phrenic nerve and brachial plexus will be exposed.

- Approach level IV nodes under the SM muscle if it is to be spared; otherwise, divide it at the clavicle to expose the IJV. During exposure of the carotid sheath, the branches of the cervical plexus going into the specimen need to be divided whilst identifying and preserving the phrenic nerve. The dissection proceeds over the IJV (identifying the vagus nerve in the carotid sheath) and the carotid artery. Going upwards, divide the omohyoid from its attachment to the hyoid (absent in 10%) to elevate zones II and III. The XII is seen again at the top of the IJV.
  - **Omohyoid is another Resident's friend**; it demarcates the boundary between levels III and IV. Inferior belly lies superficial to brachial plexus, phrenic nerve and transverse cervical vessels; the superior belly lies superficial to IJV in the anterior triangle.
- The specimen can then be removed and should be marked for histology. The operative field is irrigated with sterile water before closing over drains.

COMPLICATIONS OF ND

There is a 1% mortality rate associated with the procedure.

INTRA-OPERATIVE

- **Nerve injury** – IX–XII, lingual, phrenic and sympathetic chain – manipulation of the carotid bulb may cause bradycardia/arrhythmias.
- **Inadvertent vessel injury** – especially IJV (risk of air embolus). If this happens, then
  - Anaesthetist should be informed – ask for head down.
  - Control the vein, especially distally to prevent air entering the circulation.
  - Then isolate the bleeding point and repair if possible.
  - If there is continued oozing, use the SM to plug it.
  - If air embolism has already occurred (reduced cardiac output), then the air may be aspirated with a central line or directly through the skin.

EARLY POST-OPERATIVE

- Airway problems.
- Infection.
- Seroma/haematoma.
- Carotid blow-out (salivary fistula, previous radiation therapy).

- Skin flap necrosis (especially posterior flap), wound dehiscence (up to 1/4) with the risk of vessel exposure. Previously irradiated vessels are at a greater risk of blow-out; protection with a muscle flap should be considered.
- **Lymphatic fistula** (1%–2% of NDs) chyle leak:
  - Repair if recognised intra-operatively.
  - Significant drainage is usually taken arbitrarily as >500 mL/day.
  - Low-fat diet/medium-chain fatty acids; control protein levels and electrolytes.
    - TPN dries up the drainage quickly but has potential complications of infection, metabolic derangements and cost.
  - Octreotide – 100 µg SC every 8 hours stopped low output leaks in 5 days, high output leaks in 7 days (Jain A, *Laryngoscope*, 2015). Failure of octreotide therapy is a common indicator for surgical treatment.
    - Ligate thoracic duct if possible.
    - Cover with muscle, glue (cyanoacrylate or fibrin), vicryl mesh.
    - Suction drain is vital.

LATE

- Scar hypertrophic or contracture
- SAN injury – shoulder pain and weakness
- Glossopharyngeal nerve injury – difficulty swallowing
- Neuroma
  - Trigger point sensitivity at the site of division of branches of the cervical plexus
  - Shoulder pain syndrome
- Oedema – facial, cerebral

POST-OPERATIVE RADIOTHERAPY

PORT to the **primary** may be considered for close/positive margins, invasion of adjacent soft tissues, etc.; ~20% of tumours overall will recur despite clear margins, whilst 60% of tumours recur if margins are involved. Adverse prognostic factors include

- Poorly differentiated primary tumour
- Thick tumour (>4 or 5 mm)
- Lymph node
  - Numbers (and multiple levels, especially lower levels).
  - **Extracapsular spread.** Whilst the number of nodes changes the stage, the presence of extracapsular spread will determine biologic behaviour.
- Perineural or perivascular invascular invasion
- Invasion of carotid artery, other vessels
- Poor response to radiotherapy or chemotherapy
- Increased angiogenesis, apoptosis index, non-cohesion

The most common indications for PORT after **ND** are

- Positive NDs
- Single large involved node (>3 cm)

- Extracapsular spread

If radiotherapy is planned, then a **dental check-up** is important; any caries should be dealt with prior to radiotherapy as subsequent dental infections/extractions may cause ORN.

- Brachytherapy is an alternative to external beam radiotherapy; facilitated by the insertion of selectron rods at the time of surgery.
- Irradiated tissues lose natural planes making dissection difficult; furthermore, frozen section histology is unreliable in previously irradiated tissues.
- **Field change** in oral mucosa may lead to a high second primary rate especially hypopharyngeal tumours.
- Recurrences after a full course of radiotherapy cannot be given further radiotherapy.

Complications of head and neck radiotherapy include

- Eyes (cataracts and dry eyes)
- Hearing (sensorineural loss)
- Salivary glands (xerostomia)
- Hypopituitarism
- Growth disturbances of the craniofacial skeleton in children, e.g. retinoblastomas and orbital hypoplasia; fibrosis of facial soft tissues
- Injury to dental roots and TMJ ankylosis

MANAGEMENT OF THE OCCULT PRIMARY

Clinically palpable node – T0N1+

- Full history of age, occupation, smoking, drinking, dental health, drugs, allergies, past medical history, systems review
- Thorough head and neck examination including intra-oral examination

It is important to try and differentiate it from a lymphoma (examine other node basins) or primary carcinoma in a branchial cyst.

INVESTIGATIONS

- Blood tests including EBV, IgA
- FNA (excision if suspicious of lymphoma or if FNA equivocal)
- CXR and OPG
- Panendoscopy
  - EUA upper aerodigestive tract, e.g. nose, pharynx, oesophagus, bronchus
  - Biopsy – nasopharynx, tonsil, piriform fossa, base of tongue and FOM
- MRI scan
  - Use the information from the above investigations to direct the MRI scan.
  - T2-weighted images detect peri-tumour oedema and so may overestimate size.
    - Sinister features for lymph nodes include
      - Size >1.5 cm
      - Loss of capsule definition

- Multiple nodes
- Central necrosis
- CT/PET.

SURGICAL TREATMENT

- If N1, consider MRND or primary radiotherapy (to neck and likely primary sites)
- If >N1, proceed to MRND with PORT particularly if there is extracapsular spread

SENTINEL LYMPH NODE BIOPSY IN HEAD AND NECK CANCER

Although the practice of sentinel lymph node biopsy (SLNB) is well established in melanoma (Morton DL, *Arch Surg*, 1992) and breast cancer (Krag DN, *Surg Oncol*, 1993), for head and neck cancer, it is primarily a research tool and is not commonly performed outside validation trials (Calabrese L, *Acta Otorrhinol Ital*, 2006; Kuriakose MA, *Curr Op Otol Head Neck Surg*, 2009). SLNB has been most widely studied in early oral cavity tumours – it is only of value in N0 necks; in N1 necks, the **disease may make lymphatic drainage unpredictable**.

A multicentre trial (Ross GL, *Ann Surg Oncol*, 2004) with 134 patients with T1/2 tumours found sentinel nodes in 93%. The sensitivity was 90% (lower in FOM tumours) and it upstaged the disease in 48% of anterior tongue and 33% of FOM tumours. The authors concluded that this supported the view that SLNB can be used as a staging tool in T1/T2 tumours of the oral cavity/oropharynx.

The treatment of N0 neck is somewhat controversial; ELND has been recommended when risk of lymphatic spread over 15%–20%. This means that the majority will have ELND with its associated morbidity when there is no tumour.

Diagnostic value of sentinel lymph node biopsy in head and neck cancer: a meta-analysis (Thompson CF, *Eur Arch Otorhinolaryngol*, 2013
This is a meta-analysis with 26 studies, including 766 patients with SCC of the head and neck who underwent SLNB followed by immediate ELND. Metastases were found in 31%. Overall sensitivity was 95% with a negative predictive value of 96%.

- ELND has significant morbidity; SLNB is much less traumatic particularly with regards to nerve injury and lymphoedema.
- Potential avoidance of radiotherapy in N0 neck has been advocated for N0 necks not proceeding to ELND (Shasha D, Otolaryngol Clin North Am, 1998) – five papers showed 11 recurrences in 200 cases that did not have ELND after negative SLNB. Comparable to 6% node recurrence rate after ELND in T1/2 N0 oral tongue SCC (Yuen AP, *Head Neck*, 2009).

I. THE PATIENT WITH FACIAL PALSY

The facial nerve has the following components:

- Somatic motor – muscles of facial expression, stapedius (nerve from second genu of geniculate ganglion), PBD
- Somatic sensory – EAM with vagus (Horton's nerve)
- Visceral sensory – taste to anterior 2/3 of the tongue (chorda tympani)
- Visceral motor – V1 to oculomotor–lacrimal gland (greater superficial petrosal nerve at first genu), V2 to pterygopalatine ganglion to nose and V3 to submandibular ganglion.

CONGENITAL OR ACQUIRED FACIAL PALSY

Acquired facial palsy is much more common. Up to 90% of neonatal facial palsy is due to birth trauma (forceps delivery).

- 'Spontaneous' palsy 80%
  - Bell's palsy is the most common cause of unilateral facial palsy (rarely bilateral) in adults, but it is a diagnosis of exclusion, i.e. not
    - Simultaneous bilateral palsy (central cause)
    - Progressive over >3 weeks (tumour)
- Post-traumatic (facial laceration, head injury)
  - Exploration of the facial nerve medial to the lateral canthus tends to be fruitless; in addition, the distal end can only be stimulated for up to 72 hours.
- Secondary to tumour excision (parotid, acoustic neuroma, glioma)

AETIOLOGY RELATED TO COMMON SITES

- Facial nerve nucleus
  - Usually infarction (stroke), upper motor neurone signs with contralateral weakness **sparing the brow** (cross-innervation), i.e. no brow ptosis
- Pons and cerebellopontine angle
  - Vascular abnormalities
  - CNS degenerative diseases including motor neurone disease
  - Tumours: acoustic neuroma, glioma
  - Congenital abnormalities and agenesis including Möebius syndrome
  - Trauma
- Within the petrous temporal bone
  - Tumours (including cholesteatoma)
  - Trauma (including iatrogenic)
  - Bacterial and viral infections
    - **Bell's palsy** (Charles Bell, 1812) – presumed viral infection causing swelling of the facial nerve within the petrous temporal bone.

It causes a palsy of abrupt onset, often appearing overnight. Overall, there is 70% functional recovery, mostly within 3 months – a longer delay to recovery is associated with more contracture and synkinesia; 15% have permanent palsy.

- **Ramsay–Hunt syndrome** – herpes zoster infection of the geniculate ganglion (chorda tympani).
- Extracranial
  - Tumours (parotid tumours)
  - Trauma (including iatrogenic)

MÖEBIUS SYNDROME (1888)

This is a rare (1 in 50,000 live births in the United States) congenital anomaly with multiple cranial nerve palsies – most commonly, **abducens (50%) and facial nerve**, which may be bilateral but usually asymmetrical, resulting in 'mask-like' facies. There may be secondary changes in the facial vessels and bones, e.g. flat cheeks, long face and retrognathia. There are **pectoral** and limb anomalies such as clubfoot in 1/3, whilst 10% have **mild mental retardation**. There is a high incidence of congenital cardiac disease, spinal anomalies, peripheral neuropathies and microglossia/micrognathia. The aetiology and pathogenesis of the condition are unknown; there is a 2% risk in a second child. It is present at birth and not progressive.

Patients would usually need free muscle transfer and nerve grafting to gain some useful facial movement as well as jaw surgery in the form of a Le Fort I, sagittal split mandibulectomy or genioplasty. The results are never normal and take ~2 years for peak effect; a smile may be learnt but spontaneous smiles are rare.

- Möebius PG (1853–1907) was a German neurologist who described the condition as 'nuclear atrophy' in 1888. He also wrote a pamphlet called 'On the physiological idiocy of women' that went through eight editions during his lifetime.

II. FACIAL REANIMATION

AIMS

- Symmetry at rest and with voluntary and involuntary motion
- Control of the ocular, oral and nasal sphincters (may need temporary tarsorrhaphy)

SMILE RESTORATION

There are different types of smile that vary according to vector, strength, etc. (Rubin LR, *Plast Reconstr Surg*, 1974):

- Commissure/transverse (Jennifer Aniston) ~zygomaticus major (ZM) smile (67%)
- Canine/oblique (Tom Cruise) 31%
- Complex/full denture (Julia Roberts) 2%

TECHNIQUES OF FACIAL REANIMATION

Direct nerve repair

This is usually possible for traumatic or iatrogenic injury to the nerve; repairing intracranial injuries is a little more difficult.

Facial nerve grafting

This is best performed within 3 weeks to 1 year of injury, e.g. immediate grafting after ablative surgery (up to 95% response). There is a >6 month interval to the return of facial movement.

- Common donors include branches of the cervical plexus or sural nerve (35 cm); GAN provides up to 10 cm.
- Expect 20% shrinkage of the graft; therefore, there should be no tension in the repair, which should not be dependent on positioning.
- Epineural repair is comparable if not superior to fascicular repair.

CROSS-FACIAL NERVE GRAFTING (SCARAMELLA)

When direct nerve repair or interpositional graft is not possible, CFNG aims to provide cross-innervation from the non-paralysed side to the damaged recipient nerve distal to the level of injury, with potential coordination of contraction.

- Axonal regeneration occurs at a rate of 1–3 mm/day, and it takes 9–12 months to reach the other side. Only 20%–50% of axons actually cross the nerve graft, i.e. axonal escape, which may be reduced by reversal of the sural nerve graft.
- CFNG depends upon overlap, e.g. in the zygomatic and buccal territories, allowing donor nerves to be 'spare'. Less success (~15%) is expected with the 'outer' nerves, i.e. temporal and mandibular grafts.
- There are a variety of 'wiring' patterns (Figure 3.22), e.g. Scaramella preferred to connect up the main trunks with a single graft, whilst at the other end of the spectrum, Anderl used four grafts to connect the smaller distal branches, and Fisch crossed a buccal branch to the opposite zygomatic and marginal mandibular.

Recovery of facial palsy after cross-facial nerve grafts (Inigo F, *Br J Plast Surg*, 1994)

In this study, the CFNG was coapted to facial muscle (neurotisation) with excellent results. Alternatively, the graft was coapted to the distal stump of the contralateral facial nerve.

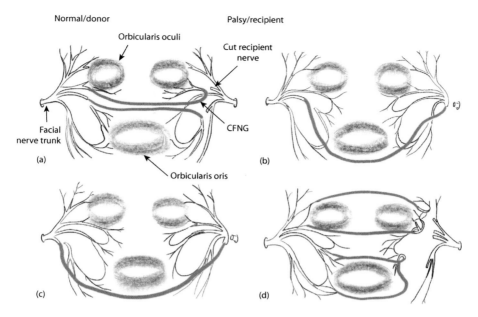

Figure 3.22 Cross-facial nerve grafts (CFNG) of various patterns. (a) Fisch, (b) Scaramella, (c) Conley and (d) Anderl. Connecting up the temporal and marginal branches is least useful with useful function in ~15%.

Patients referred within 1 year of onset of palsy are suitable CFNG; worst results are in patients undergoing surgery 4–10 years later.

SURAL NERVE HARVEST

The sural nerve is the most frequently used source of graft due to the available length (30–40 cm), being easily accessible and having a reasonable (final) donor deficit – loss of sensation on the dorsolateral foot.

- The sural nerve (S1,2) supplies sensation to the lateral and posterior third of the lower leg and the lateral ankle/foot/heel (little toe). The sensory loss improves over time (continuing for up to 5 years) due to collateral sprouting/regeneration from surrounding nerves and cortical remapping.
- The nerve is almost completely sensory except for a few autonomic nerve fibres and a small number of motor fibres according to some studies; it has a high connective tissue-to-nerve ratio.
- According to classic description, it is formed from the medial sural cutaneous nerve (MSCN) from the tibial nerve as it emerges between the bellies of gastrocnemius after being joined by the peroneal communicating (called lateral SCN by some) branch from the common peroneal nerve. The variable site of union is often quite low; more than 90% will be below the mid-distance of the calf. In approximately 20% of cases, the sural nerve is a direct continuation of the MSCN.

The most predictable position of the nerve lies behind the lateral malleolus, 2 cm posterior and 2 cm proximal (it is more posterior than one thinks) and close to the short saphenous vein. A continuous longitudinal incision may be preferable to multiple stabs, but endoscopic harvest through a 2 cm longitudinal incision behind the lateral malleolus is probably better. There is (variable) branching distal to the malleolus that can be useful if trying to reconstruct the branching of the facial nerve.

The average patient satisfaction according to one study was 90%. Its use is relatively contraindicated in those who require a functioning nerve for sports or employment and in those with pre-existing neuropathies or compromised sensation.

OTHER SOURCES OF NERVE GRAFT

- **The great auricular nerve** (GAN, C345) is a source for short (6–8 cm) segments of the nerve. It can be found along a line halfway between the angle of the mandible and the mastoid tip and the posterior border of the midpoint of the SM.
- **Cutaneous nerves of forearm**
  - Medial nerve (alongside the basilic vein, 10 cm) is found in the groove between triceps and biceps and splits into anterior and posterior divisions. The anterior is preferred because loss of sensation is then in the anterior forearm rather than the elbow and in the position of rest of the forearm; the medial arm scar may be more acceptable.
  - Lateral nerve (alongside cephalic vein, 6–8 cm) negligible sensory loss, but worse scar over volar forearm compared to the medial nerve.
- **Lateral and posterior cutaneous nerves of thigh**

- **Thoracodorsal nerve** – Biglioli (*Plast Reconstr Surg*, 2012); apparently the branching pattern allows it to reconstruct up to seven distal branches.

EXAMINATION

- Temporal/'frontal' branch – **'raise eyebrows'**. Brow ptosis, lack of wrinkling
- Zygomatic branch (orbicularis oculi) – **'squeeze eyes shut tight'**. Lagophthalmos, corneal exposure
- Buccal branch – **'smile'**. Lip weakness, lack of a smile
- Marginal mandibular branch – **'smile', 'purse lips'**. Drooling, asymmetric – lack of lower lip depression
- Cervical branch – **'grimace'**. Platysmal contraction absent

The palsy is common graded according to the **House Brackmann system** (I is normal, VI complete palsy), but it is not sensitive enough to detect the small changes seen in recovery, and does not take account of synkinesis (which is a form of cross-wiring, with motor nerves going to different parts of different muscles than intended). Alternative grading schemes include the Burres–Fisch and Sunnybrook systems.

For non-Bell's palsy, investigations include

- Imaging – CT/MRI
- Serology – syphilis, Lymes

Electrical tests **tend to underestimate** the function of nerve and muscles.

- **Electroneurography (ENoG)** stimulates facial nerve percutaneously/transcutaneously at the stylomastoid foramen (SMF) and measures the compound muscle action potential (CMAP) at the NLF. It provides an accurate evaluation of nerve degeneration and is the **most useful predictor** of prognosis, but is expensive and time consuming.
  - **Nerve excitability test (NET)**. Transcutaneous stimulation over SMF starting at the lowest current until there is contraction. There is a level of subjectivity and operator dependency.
  - **Maximal stimulation test (MST)**. Supra-maximal stimulation is used; serial testing provides more information.
- **Electromyography (EMG,** patients dislike having needles inserted into muscle), only worthwhile **after 2–3 weeks** – performing it too early whilst the motor end plates can still respond to direct stimulation will give false positive/normal results. For paralyses of more than 1 year, an EMG may be the most useful test.
  - **Fibrillations** indicates denervation and a poor prognosis.
  - Early (polyphasic) reinnervation potentials indicate axonal regeneration and a good prognosis.
  - Negative tests are generally not that useful – 30% false negative in cubital tunnel syndrome, 6%–8% in carpal tunnel syndrome.
  - Where positive, it can give the location and extent of compression.

BASIC PRINCIPLES OF TREATMENT

Important to determine

- Level of the palsy
- Duration of the palsy

In simple terms, for intracranial and intratemporal problems (no proximal stump available):

- Less than 1 year: may still have functional muscle – the aim is to **aggressively save muscle function**. Use CFNG to distal nerve stump or directly into muscle (neurotisation).
  - **Muscle atrophy can be rapid** (70% at 2 months); some fibres will die in 6–12 months.
  - **Motor end plates** remain open for ~1 year before fibrosis, which then means reinnervation is not possible.
- More than 1 year, i.e. no functional muscle.
  - In younger patients (better nerve regeneration and overall health), use free muscle flap with CFNG.
  - In older patients, consider
    - Muscle transfer – temporalis turnover
    - Nerve transfer – IX, XI, XII

Other supplementary procedures:

- Static suspension – facelift, fascia lata sling
- Correction of drooling
- Gold weight into the upper lid

For extratemporal division, proximal and distal stumps are usually available.

- Less than 1 year – direct repair or primary nerve graft.
- More than 1 year – muscle flap, coapted to ipsilateral nerve stump.

NERVE CROSSOVERS

Glossopharyngeal, accessory, phrenic and hypoglossal nerves can be used as donors to the distal facial nerve stump. The anastomosis can be made end-to-end or end-to-side.

- **Hypoglossal crossover is the most common.** Compared to CFNG, it involves only one suture line at the expense of a possibly significant donor defect: using the hypoglossal nerve will lead to moderate tongue atrophy in >50% of the patients, and severe atrophy in up to 25%. This may lead to detectable difficulties with speech and handling of the food bolus, but most patients do not complain.
  - Although the results can be rather unpredictable, 80% have good results with intensive physiotherapy and training. There is a tendency for **synkinesis** or, occasionally, hypertonia. As such, crossovers are generally reserved for those not suitable for CFNG, e.g. for older patients.
  - Crossovers can be used to 'babysit' the facial musculature awaiting the regeneration of fibres along a CFNG, or in some cases, whilst waiting for

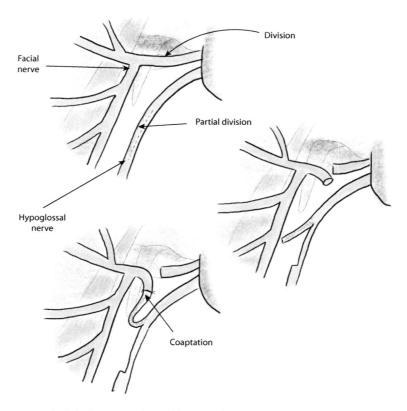

Figure 3.23 Nerve crossover. Ipsilateral nerves can be used for coaptation to the palsied nerve. A partial/subtotal crossover that reduces donor morbidity is an option, particularly when 'babysitting' during a CFNG.

uncertain nerve recovery. In these cases, usually only 1/3 of the nerve is used so that the donor deficit is less pronounced (Figure 3.23).

MUSCLE TRANSFERS

Local muscle transfers

- **Temporalis** – a turnover flap of the middle third with fascial extensions was originally described by Gillies (*J Roy Soc Med*, 1934) and Rubin (*Plast Reconstr Surg*, 1986). Alternatively, the tendinous insertion is detached by osteotomising the mandibular coronoid process (McLaughlin intraoral coronoidectomy, 1953), using fascia lata to anchor to nasolabial fold and upper/lower lips. The muscle is used here in an orthodromic manner in contrast to Gillies. The impulse for movement originates in the trigeminal nerve and is therefore not physiological; 'emotional' smiling is unlikely without extensive retraining (in the young).
  - The coronoid process can be accessed externally, with division of the zygomatic arch (Breidahl AF, *Br J Plast Surg*, 1996).
  - **Labbe** (*Plast Reconstr Surg*, 2000;105:1289) described a lengthening myoplasty without fascial

strips. It requires wide access and dissection to free the temporalis from its origin; the muscle is repositioned at the anterior part of its origin allowing it to drop inferiorly.
- **Masseter**. The vector of contraction is more lateral than superior compared with the temporalis; thus, the best choice will be determined in part by the patient's normal smile (see above). The external approach via a parotidectomy-type incision produces better results than the intraoral approach.
- **Others, less commonly used**:
  - SM – too bulky, pull in wrong direction
  - Platysma – too delicate, not enough power
  - Anterior belly of digastric (ABD) looped over the mandible to restore depressor function

Free muscle transfer

The action of **zygomaticus major** (ZM) alone nearly produces a normal smile; thus, surgical efforts are generally directed at reproducing this action. The transferred muscle should receive impulses from the uninjured facial nerve if a natural smiling response is to be provided. Normal facial muscles have ~25 muscle fibres innervated by one axon, whereas gracilis and pectoralis minor muscles have ~150–200 muscle fibres to each axon; ~50% loss of motor power is expected following transfer.

GENERAL PRINCIPLES

- A short donor nerve reduces re-innervation time.
- Fascicular nerve stimulation of the donor muscle allows determination of which fascicle supplies which strips of muscle.
- Muscle ends are plicated with mattress sutures/staples to allow sutures to hold.
- Key sutures above, below and at commissure. Test smile and NLF with traction.
- **Two-stage procedure** – this is preferred by most, particularly if the paralysis has already been of long duration.
  - A reversed sural nerve is used as a CNFG, anastomosed to the buccal branch with its end banked in the ipsilateral tragus via the upper lip. Alternatives to CFNG include a **masseteric motor branch** of V3. 'Vascularised' nerve transfers are of uncertain benefit.
  - After demonstrable regeneration, usually after 6–9 months (using an advancing Tinel's sign, which indicates that 20%–50% of axons have reached the other side or histologically), free muscle is inset with its nerve coapted to the CFNG stump. Muscle activity is seen after 4–5 months and continues to improve over the next 2 years.
- **Single-stage procedure** – the muscle is transferred and the motor nerve sutured to a (contralateral) facial nerve branch.
  - Free LD with a 'vascularised' thoracodorsal nerve allows reinnervation by 6 months. The nerve is lengthened by dissecting it out of the muscle and taking it high up to the brachial plexus. It is anastomosed via an upper lip tunnel to the contralateral buccal branches.
  - Only a single suture line, no need for nerve graft.
  - With a contralateral donor nerve, the transferred muscle will atrophy, lose motor end plates and fibrose due to prolonged denervation. Thus, some also coapt the medial motor branch of the LD to the ipsilateral masseteric nerve (i.e. regenerating nerves travel retrograde), i.e. dual innervation.
    - Some innervate the gracilis muscle flap with the ipsilateral masseteric nerve, giving a variation on the 'classic' single-stage technique.

Most commonly used muscles:

- **Pectoralis minor** (described by Manktelow).
  - Harvest by incising along anterior axillary fold, cut origin from coracoid process, medial and lateral pectoral nerves and choose the largest vessels (lateral thoracic or the pectoral branch of the thoracoacromial trunk).
  - The muscle is inserted with the pedicle orientated superficial to aid microsurgery.

- **Gracilis** (**described by Harii,** first successful transfer in humans in 1976).
  - Single-stage free tissue transfer is made possible by coaptation of the nerve to gracilis (anterior division of the **obturator nerve**) across the philtrum to the contralateral buccal branch and avoids the need for a CFNG (Kumar PA, *Br J Plast Surg*, 1995).
    - Axis – pubic bone to medial femoral condyle.
    - As the pedicle lies on the deep surface of the muscle, some thinning is possible.
    - Long pedicle (8–10 cm) but muscle is rather bulky.
  - For children, age 5–6 seems optimal in terms of muscle and vessel size.
- **Latissimus dorsi** (see above)
  - Muscle trimming is facilitated by the pedicle being on the deep surface.
- **Serratus anterior, rectus abdominis and platysma** have also been used.

Comparative objective and subjective analysis of temporalis tendon and microneurovascular transfer for facial reanimation. (Erni D, *Br J Plast Surg*, 1999)

This study compared McLaughlin's technique for temporalis tendon transfer to a two-stage free tissue transfer using LD, gracilis and pectoralis minor (only offered to patients under 50 years of age). The technique for temporalis transfer was as follows:

- Through a facelift incision, the masseter is split to approach the coronoid process, which is detached with an osteotome. A 6 mm drill hole is made through detached segment and threaded with a strip of fascia lata that is re-routed to the corner of the mouth and anchored to previously inserted conchal cartilage grafts.

The authors found that microsurgical reanimations resulted in the following:

- Significantly better excursion during smiling whilst static symmetry was similar to temporalis transfer.
- Swelling of the cheek soft tissues and skin tethering was more problematic.

STATIC PROCEDURES

These are often considered in the elderly or ill.

- **Canthal/eyelid repair.** The operation can be performed under LA and anaesthetic eye drops: after a full thickness canthotomy of 15 mm and lysis of the inferior limb of LCT, redundant tissue is trimmed and the tarsus is resuspended from the inner aspect of the lateral orbital rim (above the normal tendon). The skin-muscle flap is suspended from the periosteum of zygoma. Alternatives to canthopexy include wedge resection or temporalis sling.
  - **Gold weight** to the upper lids, placed just lateral of midline. When supine, the weight may cause

the upper lip to drop back and taping is usually required at night. Positioning the weight as low as possible in the upper lid may reduce the tendency for the upper lid to fall back when supine.

- Palpebral spring made from stainless steel and looks somewhat like a safety pin. Some have a Dacron sleeve over the inferior limb that sits on the superior tarsus. They aim to improve blink closure but have significant risk of complications including corneal damage.
- **Facelift/brow lifts**. Soft tissue can be repositioned to correct an overhanging brow with either a forehead or brow lift; both should be done cautiously as eye closure may be compromised. A **direct brow** incision lift is often useful. The frontalis muscle can be attached to the periosteum (not usually done in conventional lifts as it limits muscle movement, but it is actually useful in facial palsy). Endoscopic methods are less useful in facial palsy and the effects are mild.
  - Botulinum toxin (off-label) to weaken the contralateral (normal) side – effect lasts up to 6 months.

MARGINAL MANDIBULAR NERVE PALSY

The marginal mandibular nerve is vulnerable to trauma in the submandibular fossa, lying deep to platysma below the body of the mandible in 20%, and injury causes paralysis of **DAO and** depressor labii inferioris **(DLI),** resulting in

- Inability to form a natural smile
- Drooling with elevation of the lower lip at rest, unable to move downwards or evert

Microsurgical strategies in 74 patients for restoration of the dynamic depressor mechanism. (Terzis JK, *Plast Reconstr Surg*, 2000)
Reanimation options:

- If the palsy duration is <12 months (with EMG evidence of depressor activity), then **directly neurotise** depressors using CFNG.

- If the palsy has lasted 12–24 months (EMG still shows some depressor activity) or failure of the above, then a mini XII-to-VII **crossover** or direct neurotisation (incorporates 20%–30% of the nerve trunk).
- With long-standing palsy: transfer of platysma (if functional) or **anterior belly of digastric (ABD)**, which is supplied by the trigeminal nerve. The tendon is divided and mobilised to the corner of the mouth whilst the insertion on the mandible is then divided and inset to reproduce the smile vector. There is a scar in the submandibular fossa.
- In young patients, re-education is usually successful in reproducing a physiological smile, but older patients require coaptation to a CFNG.

Paralysis of the marginal mandibular branch of the facial nerve. (Tulley P, *Br J Plast Surg*, 2000)
Treatment options include:

- ABD transfer
  - Simple and very effective one-stage procedure.
  - ABD is sometimes absent.
- Two-stage microsurgical transfer of extensor digitorum brevis
  - Complex microsurgical procedure with greater donor and recipient site scarring
- **Balancing myectomy** – improvements in appearance, oral continence and lip biting reported
  - Botulinum toxin injection of contralateral depressors produces temporary symmetry (Hussain G, *Br J Plast Surg*, 2004). Determine surface marking of DLI on the unparalysed side by palpation of the vermilion border whilst the patient attempts to show the lower teeth.
  - Intramuscular injection of LA can be used to simulate the effect of myectomy. The muscle is exposed using an intra-oral incision 0.5 cm above the buccal sulcus, retracting the orbicularis oris fibres, and a segment of muscle is then resected across its entire width.

4

Clefts and craniofacial

A. PRINCIPLES OF MANAGEMENT OF CLEFT LIP AND PALATE

I. EMBRYOLOGY AND ANATOMY

EMBRYOLOGICAL DEVELOPMENT OF THE MAXILLOFACIAL SKELETON

During the fourth to fifth weeks of development, the **pharyngeal arches** form as ridges in the cranial mesenchyme and are separated by **pharyngeal clefts**, whilst internally out-pouchings of the foregut are formed called pharyngeal pouches. Skeletal components are formed by inward migration of neural crest cells.

The **stomodeum** is the cranial opening of the foregut (mouth and nasal apertures), and five swellings are formed ventrally:

- Paired mandibular swellings (from the first pharyngeal arch)
- Paired maxillary swellings (also from the first pharyngeal arch)
- Fronto-nasal prominence (downgrowth from primitive forebrain)

Each arch has

- Cartilage – it gives rise to skeletal structures, though not all bones arise from endochondral ossification of this arch cartilage.
- Artery.
- Nerve – both motor and sensory. The nerve has a role in muscle development, e.g. Moebius syndrome.
- Muscle – note that muscles may migrate significant distances but always keep the nerve of origin.

FIRST PHARYNGEAL ARCH

The first pharyngeal arch is the most important, from a cleft perspective.

- The arch artery is the maxillary artery from the external carotid, whilst the nerve is the trigeminal: motor from mandibular branch and sensory from all three divisions.
- Muscles – muscles of mastication as well as tensor palati, tensor tympani, ABD and mylohyoid. The mesenchyme of the first arch forms the dermis of the face.
- Cartilaginous components include
  - Maxillary process – the mesenchyme undergoes intramembranous ossification to form the premaxilla, maxilla, zygoma and part of the temporal bone.
  - Mandibular process – Meckel's cartilage forms in the mesenchyme of the mandibular process, and most of it eventually regresses to leave only the parts that form the incus and malleus, anterior ligament of malleus and sphenomandibular ligament. The mandible forms by intramembranous ossification using Meckel's cartilage as a template rather than by direct ossification of the cartilage.

FIRST ARCH SYNDROMES

Treacher Collins syndrome (TCS)

This was described by Edward Treacher Collins (1862–1932, English ophthalmologist) in 1900; Berry had described it in 1889. The condition is due to sporadic mutation in up to 60%, whilst AD inheritance with variable penetrance is

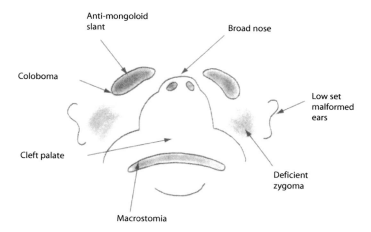

Figure 4.1 Schematic representation of the main features associated with TCS. CP is found in one-third of the patients.

demonstrated in some. The responsible gene (TCOF1) is on chromosome 5 (5q31–33, same chromosome as cri du chat). Consistent aetiological factors have not been found, though advanced paternal age and maternal isotretinoin use have been implicated. Mental retardation is unusual (10%), though deafness may contribute to some developmental delay (Figure 4.1).

It affects males and females equally, with an incidence of 1 in 25,000–50,000. TCS is otherwise known as mandibulofacial dysostosis; there is bilateral failure of the first arch neural crest. The deformities in TCS are said to be non-progressive with age, and some represent a consortium of facial clefts 6, 7, 8 centred around the zygoma. **There is significant variation in severity.** Some unkindly describe the facies as a 'sad fish' – characteristic features include the following:

- **Mid-face hypoplasia** is a key feature leading to the typical mid-facial convexity – zygomatic a-/hypoplasia with absent arches, the inferolateral orbital wall deficient with downward slant of the supra-orbital ridge, the maxilla is narrowed. Hypoplastic temporalis muscle.
- **Mandibular hypoplasia** – micrognathia and anterior open bite (type II), long chin.
  - Airway compromise at birth/sleep apnoea is not uncommon.
- **Defects of lower eyelid** – loss of medial lashes, **coloboma** (6 cleft), **antimongoloid slant** due to lack of support from the hypoplastic lateral orbital wall (8 cleft).
  - Hypertelorism.
- Macrostomia (7 cleft).
- Abnormalities of the external, middle and inner ear – low set ears/**microtia**/skin tags; >95% have moderate conductive hearing loss due to stenosis of the EAM or ankylosis of the inner ear ossicles, and sensorineural hearing impairment.
- Broad prominent nasal bridge, choanal atresia or stenosis.

- **Cleft palate** (CP) or high arched palate.
- Long sideburns.

Bilateral hemifacial macrosomia (HFM) has similarities but has

- No mid-face clefting
- No limb anomalies

Treacher Collins treatment

Patients should be treated by a multidisciplinary team, e.g. speech therapist, audiologist, orthodontist, etc. The variable expression demands that treatment be tailored to the individual patient. The combination of micrognathia and choanal atresia, in particular, means that the airway is a source of concern in neonates. 'Secondary' issues include vision, feeding and hearing.

- 0 months – tracheostomy if needed
- CP surgery at 6 months
- Zygoma surgery at 3–5 years
  - The zygoma and orbital floor is usually grafted with (split) calvarial bone. Continued differential growth of the mid-face and zygoma means that the deformity usually 'relapses' necessitating further surgery; thus Posnick advises against reconstruction before 5 years of age.
    - Flaps may be used to augment or cover the bone, e.g. pericranial flaps or temporal/temporoparietal, but the amount of muscle available is small and the donor depression is often noticeable.
    - Use of vascularised bone has not been promising, and with local flaps in particular, it is difficult to maintain the blood supply whilst optimising fit.
    - Alloplastic reconstruction is also usually disappointing.

- Mandible surgery for mandibular retrognathia and malocclusion treated at 4–5 years; augmentation by vertical sagittal osteotomy and bone grafts or distraction.
  - Classification as per Mulliken modification of Prusansky.
- 6 years – soft tissue correction:
  - Ear reconstruction, 7–8 years onwards, depending on the technique chosen. There is usually no value in middle ear surgery; BAHA should be fitted early.
  - Commissuroplasty for macrostomia (reposition muscle).
  - Sideburns set back, treat abnormal hairline.
  - The **coloboma** can often be treated once zygomas have been reconstructed. Options include a laterally based hemi-Tripier upper lid flap and lateral canthopexy, but aesthetic results are usually disappointing. Earlier surgery may be indicated under certain circumstances.
- 6–12 years – orthodontics and jaw surgery: cephalometric assessment.
  - Le Fort III maxillary advancement.
- 12–18 years – Le Fort I advancement to finalise bite, sliding genioplasty.
- 18 years – open rhinoplasty to broad nasal bridge.

Other conditions show similar features to TCS with additional limb anomalies:

- **Nager's syndrome** (acrofacial dysostosis) – preaxial anomalies especially the **thumbs** that tend to be asymmetrically affected. Colobomas are less common but almost all have **CPs**. The mandible is typically very small causing airway problems. The facial features are similar to TCS, and are also associated with defects of the extremities, usually with short stature. It is a much less common first and second arch syndrome of unknown cause; most cases are sporadic but may show AR inheritance.
- **Miller** – postaxial anomalies affecting the little finger/toe of all limbs in a symmetrical manner.

BRANCHIAL CLEFT ANOMALIES

Otherwise known as branchial cysts, these are found in the anterior triangle and probably represent entrapped remnants of the branch clefts that may manifest as cysts, sinuses or fistulae. Cysts tend to be soft and non-tender but may form abscesses if infected.

- First brachial cleft cysts
  - Type I – duplication of EAM – a fistula close to the lower part of the parotid with tracts that may terminate in the ear canal (external or middle ear)
  - Type II – usually in the anterior triangle just inferior to the angle of the mandible, with a tract through the parotid (thus closely associated to the facial nerve) to the EAM

- Second branchial cleft cysts – deep to platysma with a tract running between the internal and external carotid arteries up to the tonsillar fossae.

DEVELOPMENT OF THE TONGUE

The tongue precursors appear at ~4 weeks of development: two lateral plus one median (tuberculum impar) lingual swellings from the first arch mesenchyme form the anterior 2/3 of the tongue. Behind this, a median swelling (copula or hypobranchial eminence) of second, third and fourth arch mesenchyme forms the posterior tongue.

- Sensory innervation to anterior 2/3 by the mandibular division of V; posterior third innervation from IX and X.
- Motor innervation mainly XII – the musculature is derived from occipital somites, and all are supplied by XII except palatoglossus, which is innervated by the X nerve.

DEVELOPMENT OF THE NOSE AND UPPER LIP

The maxillary swellings lie above the stomodeum, whilst the mandibular swellings lie caudal; they are present by the fifth week of development. The frontal process lies in the midline, above the maxillary swellings.

- On each side of the frontal process just above the stomodeum, the ectoderm thickens to form two nasal placodes. Swellings develop lateral and medial to each nasal placode, which deepens to form the nasal pit.
- By week 7, the maxillary swellings advance into the midline, pushing the medial nasal swellings together to form the upper lip.

DEVELOPMENT OF THE PALATE

The undersurface of the fused maxillary and medial nasal swellings forms the intermaxillary segment, which contributes to

- Philtrum of the upper lip
- Part of the maxillary alveolus bearing the upper incisors
- Triangular primary palate

During week 6, the palatal shelves grow out from the maxillary swellings to lie lateral to the tongue. These shelves then ascend with hydration of glycosaminoglycans and fuse in the midline to form the secondary palate; the vertical movement takes place very rapidly (less than 1 second in rat embryos). The secondary palate fuses anteriorly with the primary palate with the junction marked by the incisive foramen.

- Epstein's pearls are cystic epithelial remnants of the zone of apoptosis between the fusing palatal shelves.

DEVELOPMENTAL ABNORMALITIES LEADING TO CLEFT LIP AND PALATE

Clefts can be divided into clefts of the primary palate and clefts of the secondary palate (posterior to the incisive foramen).

- **Primary palate** consists of the lip, alveolus and hard palate anterior to the incisive foramen, and clefts represent failure of mesenchymal penetration between medial and lateral palatine processes and failure of fusion of maxillary and medial nasal processes (cleft of lip and alveolus between incisors and canines extending to incisive foramen).
- **Secondary palate** consists of the hard palate behind the incisive foramen and soft palate, and clefts represent failure of the lateral palatine processes to fuse with each other and the nasal septum/vomer.
- **Rare clefts** include failure of fusion of medial nasal swellings, which gives rise to the very rare median cleft, whilst failure of fusion of maxillary and lateral nasal swellings causes an oblique facial cleft.

ANATOMY OF THE PALATE

The hard palate includes the palatal processes of the maxilla and the horizontal plate of the palatine bone with an adherent mucoperiosteum (attached to bone by Sharpey's fibres).

- Blood supply via the greater palatine artery from the maxillary artery; venous drainage occurs via venae comitantes mostly. Lymphatic drainage goes to the retropharyngeal and deep cervical nodes.
- Sensory innervation via the pterygopalatine ganglion (branches of the maxillary nerve) – nasopalatine nerves to the premaxillary area and by the greater palatine nerve posteriorly.

SOFT PALATE

- The blood supply to the soft palate comes mostly from the lesser palatine arteries, the ascending palatine branch of the facial artery and the palatine branches of the ascending pharyngeal artery.
- All muscles of the palate are supplied by the pharyngeal plexus (cranial accessory nerve and the pharyngeal branch of X) except tensor palati (nerve to medial pterygoid – branch of the mandibular nerve).

There are five paired muscles:

- **Tensor palati** from the scaphoid fossa of the medial pterygoid plate, the lateral part of the cartilaginous auditory tube and the spine of the sphenoid. It passes around the pterygoid hamulus as a tendon and inserts as a concave triangular aponeurosis to the crest of the palatine bone, blending in the midline with that of the opposite side. It acts to **tense the soft palate to form a platform** that the other muscles may elevate or depress. It also opens the auditory tube during swallowing.

- **Levator palati** arises from the quadrate area of the petrous bone and the medial part of the auditory tube and inserts into the nasal surface of the palatine aponeurosis. The paired muscles form a 'V'-shaped sling pulling the soft palate upwards and backwards to close the nasopharynx. It also opens the auditory tube.
- **Palatoglossus** arises from the under surface of the aponeurosis and passes downwards to interdigitate with styloglossus. It forms the anterior fold of the tonsillar fossa and acts as a sphincter to raise the tongue and narrow the transverse diameter of the oropharyngeal isthmus.
- **Palatopharyngeus** has two heads that clasp the levator palati muscle insertion. They form the posterior pillar of the tonsillar fossa and the innermost muscle of the pharynx, blending with the inferior constrictor. The anterior head (arising from bone) acts to raise the pharynx/larynx, whilst the posterior head (arising from aponeurosis) depresses the tensed soft palate. Some fibres, along with fibres from the superior constrictor, contribute to the palatopharyngeal sphincter (which forms Passavant's ridge when the soft palate is elevated; this is hypertrophied in CP patients and in 25%–30% of normal individuals).
- **Muscle of the uvula.**

PHARYNX

The pharynx is a 12 cm long muscular tube that extends from the skull base and becomes the oesophagus at the level of C6.

- Muscles consist of overlapping superior, middle and inferior constrictors with paired stylo-, palato- and salpingo-pharyngeus muscles. The inferior constrictor has two parts, thyropharyngeus and cricopharyngeus, with a weak area in between called Killian's dehiscence.
  - Gustav Killian (1860–1921) was an otolaryngologist who is regarded as the founder of bronchoscopy.
- Blood supply comes from the superior and inferior laryngeal arteries, ascending pharyngeal artery and also the vessels supplying the palate.
- All muscles are supplied by the pharyngeal plexus (motor fibres in pharyngeal branch of X, IX fibres are purely afferent) except stylopharyngeus (IX) and cricopharyngeus (recurrent laryngeal branch of X).

II. GENETICS

GENERAL CONSIDERATIONS

Definitions

Cleft lip is a congenital abnormality of the primary palate and may be complete/incomplete/microform or unilateral/bilateral, and may coexist with a CP. CL alone or in combination with a CP is the same entity but represents different points along the morphological **spectrum**.

CP is a congenital abnormality of the secondary palate, which may be unilateral/bilateral or a submucous cleft.

INCIDENCE AND AETIOLOGY OF CLEFT LIP WITH OR WITHOUT PALATE (CL/P)

- ~1.5 in 1000 in Europe
- 1 in 500 in Asia
- 1 in 1000 or less in Africa

CL/P is more common than CP alone (CPO), which is a distinct entity. Cleft lip and palate is the commonest (approximately 50%), whilst CPO occurs in 30% and CL alone occurs in 20%.

- CL/P is more common in boys, whilst CPO is more common in girls.
- The left lip is affected twice as often as the right – left/right/bilateral 6:3:1 (cleft-left).

Non-syndromic clefts, in general, display **multifactorial inheritance**, which may include a genetic predisposition plus one or more of the following risk factors. There is a higher incidence in the offspring of parents of advanced age (especially paternal) and smoking mothers, and there is a possible link with maternal drug ingestion including anti-epileptics (Dilantin 10× risk), salicylates, tretinoin (retinoids), benzodiazepines and cortisone. There is a 60% concordance in identical twins.

GENETIC PREDISPOSITION

Genetic counselling is an important part of the overall management of patients and their families. The inheritance of clefts may be chromosomal, Mendelian or sporadic. There are over 150 syndromes associated with CL/P; however, most (85%) cases are sporadic.

- Chromosomal inheritance includes syndromes such as trisomy 13 (Patau) and 21 (Down).
- Mendelian inheritance includes syndromes due to single gene defects that will be passed on within families – these may be AD (e.g. **van der Woude syndrome**, which is the most common CLP syndrome– CL/P, missing teeth and lip pits) and TCS (recessive or X-linked).
- Sporadic cases may be associated with developmental abnormalities (e.g. Pierre Robin sequence [PRS]) with a low risk of further affected children.

GENETIC COUNSELLING AND GENETICS OF CLEFT LIP AND CP

Non-syndromic **cleft lip (85%)**:

- With normal parents, the risk of a child with cleft lip is 1 in 750–1000.
  - **Second and third affected children – risk 4% and 10%, respectively**
- **If one parent has cleft lip, the risk of having a child with cleft lip is 4%.**
  - Second affected child – risk 17%.
- **With both parents affected, the risk is 1/3 to 1/2.**
- If a child is born with CPO, the risk of CL/P is still 1 in 750.

For non-syndromic **CPO (over 50%)**:

- Normal parents – risk of affected child is general risk, i.e. 1 in 2000.
- Second affected child – 3%.
- One affected parent – risk of first affected child is 3%.

The majority of syndromes are diagnosed clinically. Chromosomal testing may be indicated when the cleft occurs with other malformations, growth deficiency or developmental delay. Molecular (DNA) testing is available for few very specific conditions. Stickler syndrome is common enough in CPO that evaluation of the eye is recommended.

Prenatal counselling for cleft lip and palate. (Matthews MS, *Plast Reconstr Surg*, 1998)

Although no parents included in this study of nine families of patients with prenatal diagnosis felt that termination would be an option for an isolated cleft, 30% were against having a further pregnancy. There was a high incidence of associated abnormalities, and karyotyping is advised. The majority of parents felt prenatal counselling with the cleft team was helpful.

Having some photographs to show the parents is often useful. Currently, CL/P can be visualised at 13–15 weeks depending on maternal obesity and foetal position; transvaginal ultrasound can detect clefts earlier by ~12 weeks. Clefts of secondary palate are the most difficult to diagnose; the foetal palate is best seen in the axial plane, whilst the lips are best visualised in the coronal view.

Cleft lip and palate: Association with other congenital malformations. (Beriaghi S, *J Clin Ped Dentistry*, 2009)

Patients with CPO are more likely to have congenital malformations (38.7%) vs. CL/P (26.4%). These associated malformations were usually found in the orofacial region, followed by the cardiovascular and central nervous systems.

INITIAL ASSESSMENT OF THE BABY WITH A CLEFT LIP

- Breathing – if dyspnoeic, then nurse prone to allow the tongue to fall away from the airway. Insert a nasopharyngeal airway and apply tongue stitch if necessary. Continuous positive airway pressure (CPAP) may need to be considered.
- Feeding – a trial of breastfeeding is always worthwhile; using a soft teat and a squeezy bottle may be considered. Education of the parents is very important. **CP babies have more feeding** problems than CL babies.
- Patients should be referred to a multidisciplinary cleft clinic for further assessment, planning and treatment.

CLASSIFICATION

The Veau classification is descriptive:

- Soft palate
- Soft palate and hard palate

- Soft palate and hard palate and unilateral prepalatal cleft
- Soft palate and hard palate and bilateral prepalatal cleft

THE UNILATERAL CL/P DEFORMITY

- Cleft across sill (complete or incomplete)
- Alveolar cleft at canine (which is often deformed and malpositioned), leading to an open nasal floor
- Nasal tip displacement
- Flattening and hooding of alar rims
- Abnormal muscle attachment to nose; muscles run parallel to the edge of the cleft
- Cleft side columellar shortening
- Splayed medial crura with flattened nasal dome
- LLCs hypoplastic and displaced laterally
- Deviation of posterior septum to the cleft side
- Labial frenulum displacement
- Maxillary retrusion

THE BILATERAL CL/P DEFORMITY

- Short or absent columella
- Complete or incomplete cleft lip
- Nasal tip flattening with splayed medial crura
- LLCs displaced laterally
- Flattening and hooding of alar rims
- Protuding premaxilla
- Poorly formed or absent nasal spine
- Prolabium/premaxilla distortion

III. SURGERY

TIMING OF REPAIR

Classically, the **'rule of tens'** proposed surgery when the patient was 10 weeks old and 10 pounds in weight, and the haemoglobin had reached 10 mg/dL.

There is currently no evidence that points to a 'best' timing. The variety of protocols (201 teams used 194 different protocols according to Shaw WC, *J Oral Maxillofac Surg*, 2001), the lack of agreed objective outcomes and the long lag times involved make it difficult to assess.

The **Scandcleft study** looking at unilateral CL/P was initiated in 1997 and is expected to run until 2024; the UK joined the initial centres in Denmark, Finland, Sweden and Norway. Patients are being randomised to having surgery according to either a common technique or the local protocols. With the 10 centres, there were 3 local protocols, making a total of 4 different treatment groups.

- Lip and SP closure at 2–4 months, hard palate closure at 12 months (the newly defined **common protocol** taken to be the base, arm A)
- Lip and SP closure at 2–4 months, hard palate closure at 36 months (arm B)

- Lip repair at 3–4 months, hard and soft palate closure at 12 months (arm C)
- Lip and hard palate repaired at 3–4 months, soft palate repaired at 12 months (arm D)

The primary outcomes were speech and dentofacial development, some of which were reported in a series of articles in February 2017 (*J Plast Surg Hand Surg*); some conclusions included the following:

- Surgeons at each centre did have some problems familiarising themselves with the common protocol.
- There is still no statistically significant evidence that any technique is better than the others in terms of bleeding, infection, anaesthetic complications or length of hospital stay (Rautio J, *J Plast Surg Hand Surg*, 2017).
- There were no differences in VPC and hypernasality at 5 years (Lohmander A, *J Plast Surg Hand Surg*, 2017).
- Arm A vs. arm B showed higher Percent Consonants Correct (PCC) scores (Willasden E, *J Plast Surg Hand Surg*, 2017).
- There are no differences in dental arch relationships (Heliovaara A, *J Plast Surg Hand Surg*, 2017) or occlusion (Karsten A, *J Plast Surg Hand Surg*, 2017) at 5 years.
- Use of the Millard technique with or without McComb nose correction was the commonest and showed significant differences in the nose and lip areas compared to the Tennison Randall technique (Molsted K, *J Plast Surg Hand Surg*, 2017).

SURGICAL SEQUENCE

Currently, a common sequence is as follows:

6 weeks–3 months.
- **Lip (Millard rotation–advancement for unilateral cleft lip) and primary nose correction (McComb).**
- **Vomerine flap to anterior hard palate for alveolar cleft.**
- **Synchronous soft palate repair** in wide clefts may make subsequent hard palate repair easier (see below).

3–6 months.
- **Palate repair** (von Langenbeck technique including intravelar veloplasty, vomerine flap to close nasal layer at the level of the hard palate).
- **Grommets** if required (~95%). Distraction tests can be used to screen hearing from 6 months onwards.

5 years.
- **Pharyngoplasty** for velopharyngeal incompetence (VPI) (superior pharyngeal flap preferred except where there is significant lateral wall immobility – then Orticochoea).
- **Nasal correction** – Tajima, if required.
- **Lengthen columella** – bilateral forked flaps.

3–4 years: Speech therapy commenced if required.
6 years: Orthodontics – early dental management.

9 years: Orthodontics – alveolar bone graft, when the canine teeth first appear radiologically to prevent their root from collapsing into the cleft.

11 years: Orthodontics – management of permanent dentition.

16 years.

- **Rhinoplasty**.
- **Orthognathic surgery**. Le Fort I advancement to correct class III malocclusion if required. Mid-facial growth is largely undisturbed in the presence of an unrepaired cleft; deficiency is typically observed in patients having repair.

Residual lip deformity is less common with current management, but a lip revision if needed can be performed at 5–6 years. However, nasal deformity is seen in almost all, and tip revision or simple septal surgery can be performed at 5–6 years; but formal septoplasty or osteotomies should be delayed until the mid to late teens.

DELAIRE APPROACH

Delaire was a maxillofacial surgeon in Nantes who proposed a so-called 'functional' lip repair at 6 months involving more muscle dissection, and part of the rationale for operating at this time was that the muscle was better developed.

- 6 months – lip and soft palate repair
- 18 months – hard palate repair with medial relaxing incisions possible because palate has been narrowed by previous soft palate closure

Treatment of cleft lip and palate in the UK. (Boorman JG, *Br J Plast Surg*, 1998)

Seventeen of 57 units providing cleft lip and palate care in the United Kingdom were assessed, and of the 457 patients reviewed, only 2 units were judged to be of a good standard overall. The conclusion was based on numerous criteria: the unit itself (multidisciplinary team, use of protocols, data collection, experience of team members) and assessment of children treated aged 5–6 and 12–13 years at the time of the survey (appearance, speech, hearing, growth, jaw relationships and patient/parent satisfaction).

- There were no significant differences demonstrated in treatment outcomes between plastic and maxillofacial surgeons.
- There are very few high volume operators – only 7 of the 99 surgeons performed ~30 new repairs annually, whilst the others performed fewer than 10 new repairs per year. However, the only demonstrable benefit of high volume surgery was in **speech outcome**.
- The skill and experience of the surgeon were more important than the actual technique used.

The recommendations of the group were to reduce the number of units to 8–15 with each surgeon treating 40–50 new patients annually; reducing the number of units would also enable better data analysis and facilitate treatment advances. The CSAG study is often quoted as recommending centralisation of services; this is not that low volumes necessarily mean poor results, but rather that it allows a minimum number of cases for meaningful outcome measurement.

CLEFT LIP REPAIR

Unilateral cleft lip classification

- Incomplete (variable vertical lip shortness, nasal sill intact – Simonart's band)
- Complete (complete separation of the lip, nasal sill and alveolus)
- Microform ('forme fruste' – vertical furrow or scar, notch in the vermilion and white roll, variable vertical lip shortness)

AIMS OF REPAIR

- A cupid's bow and philtral dimple (rearrange tissues and lengthen the medial lip)
- Pouting of the lower portion of the upper lip (avoiding whistle deformity)
- Reconstruct orbicularis oris (re-approximation of muscle)
- Symmetrical alae (reposition displaced atrophic alar cartilages and alar base)
- A straight columella

Millard originally described the **C flap** as a medial superior rotation flap that crossed the nasal sill to inset into the lateral lip element as a lateral rotation advancement flap (type I). He refined the technique to use the C flap to inset into the medial lip element, augmenting the columellar height and creating a more natural flare at the base of the medial footplate (type II). However, there is a series of incisions/scars at the base of the columella that may be associated with poor healing if not planned properly. The C flap can be used in either position as requirements dictate (Figure 4.2).

MANAGEMENT OF THE PROTRUDING PREMAXILLA

- **Premaxillary setback** (but sacrifices incisors and compromises growth, thus now condemned).
- **Lip adhesion.** Temporarily closing the cleft lip under tension aims to reduce the size of the alveolar cleft. The adhesion is a straight line repair >3 mm away from the incision lines for definitive surgery, supposedly without compromising it, although some contend otherwise. It was first described in 1961 as a prior step before bone grafting, and in 1964 by Millard before definitive lip closure. It has been largely superseded by pre-surgical orthopaedics (PSO) but can still be offered as a substitute under certain circumstances, e.g. lack of PSO. It is a relatively crude procedure with an 18% dehiscence rate; the forces are less controlled.

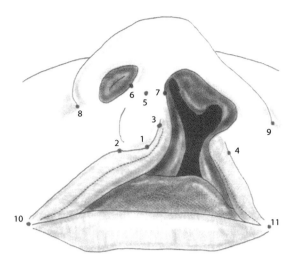

Figure 4.2 Common anatomical landmarks for cleft lip surgery.

- Some suggest that **lip taping** by reliable parents may achieve similar results.
- **Pre-surgical orthopaedics** (PSO) was pioneered by McNeil (1950), when a maxillary obturator was used to reduce alveolar and palatal clefts. It pretty much supplants lip adhesion.
  - **Nasoalveolar moulding** is the preferred form of (**passive**) PSO; it aims to take advantage of early malleability in the nasal cartilages as with ear cartilage. Within 2 weeks, a custom soft acrylic denture is worn 24 hours a day, removed only for cleaning. This also acts to separate the nasal and oral cavities to **facilitate feeding**. Subsequently, a nasal extension lifts the nose into place. It is combined with taping, and the mould is adjusted weekly to reshape the alveolus until segments are in passive contact, whilst the nose is moulded into a better shape more with more tip projection and alar cartilage symmetry. A 'tissue expansion' type effect may help to **lengthen tissues especially the columella** and the intranasal lining. Outpatient treatment takes place over 3–6 months.
    - Chang. (*Plast Reconstr Surg*, 2014): 30 patients were randomised to either the Grayson or Figueroa techniques of nasoalveolar moulding. There were some subtle differences noted by the time of surgery, but nothing significant.
  - The aims are to bring the tissues into **better alignment**, reduce the magnitude of the surgical procedure, **allow tension-free soft tissue repair** (thus a better scar) and hopefully reduce the number of revision procedures. Results are encouraging, but truly long-term improvements, i.e. into adulthood, have not yet been demonstrated. Orthodontic benefits are limited. Initial concerns about deleterious effects on growth and dental

health have not been borne out. Offering PSO requires a significant amount of time and money.
- **Active** technique, e.g. Latham device, that is adjusted daily. Some say that active devices restrict maxillary growth more than passive devices. They are said to be preferred in bilateral clefts for more premaxillary retrusion and palatal expansion; however, they require a general anaesthesia for fitting (with a 1% risk of it falling out).
- Studies have shown that **neonatal lip repair (within 48 hours)** is safe provided patients are mature with no illness, no opioids are administered and experienced nursing is available with vigilant apnoea detection. It is not scarless. There are supposed psychological benefits, and parents certainly prefer earlier repair. However, in the end, no significant overall advantage has been demonstrated.

Cleft palate closure in the neonate: preliminary report. (Denk MJ, *Cleft Palate Craniofacial J*, 1996)

Against

- Anaesthetic risk and technical difficulty.
- Implications for facial growth.
- Chance of missing undiagnosed anomalies.
- Hypoglycaemia and jaundice may result.

For

- Improved speech and easier feeding
- Psychologically better for parents
- Can perform synchronous palate (Furlow's) and lip closure under one anaesthetic

The authors report on their experience with 21 patients operated within 28 days of birth; they conclude that it is safe but do not recommend it as a standard.

REPAIR TECHNIQUES – BRIEF PRINCIPLES

As the muscle repair is theoretically the same, the differences are only 'skin deep'. The cleft side is 'shorter' and thus needs to be 'lengthened'. Although there are many techniques/protocols, good results can still be had when surgery is meticulous – results are somewhat surgeon dependent. In general, the greater the vertical deficient, the more difficult the lip repair, whilst the greater the horizontal deficit, the more difficult the nasal repair.

UNILATERAL CLEFT LIP – STENCIL METHOD

This was described by Tennison (*Plast Reconstr Surg*, 1952) and modified by Randall and Skoog. It avoids a straight line scar by fashioning a Z-plasty on each side of the cleft. This method is said to be more suited to wide unilateral clefts and very short lips, but leaves a transverse scar low down on the philtral column.

ROTATION–ADVANCEMENT REPAIR

This was described by Millard (*Plast Reconstr Surg*, 1960). The name comes from the fact that it relies upon rotation of a flap (A flap) in the philtrum (non-cleft side) downwards and advancement of a flap from the cleft side (B flap) to meet the A flap. As the A flap rotates downwards, a small triangular flap above it, the C flap, can cross the midline and be inset between the B flap and the nostril sill (Figure 4.3).

- C flap for columella
- L flap for (nasal) lining
- M flap for mucosa

The Millard technique was used by 84% of US surgeons in 2008, but over half have modifications, some of which had not been described (until then); 86% of surgeons also tend to stick to the same technique all the time.

- **Noordhoff modification**: red line – triangle inset into the junction of wet and dry vermilion and Noordhoff point (vanishing point of white roll on the cleft lip segment, at the thickest segment of vermilion and where there is a robust white roll) – position of peak of cupids bow. Additional backcut-triangular notch at philtrum to level cupids bow.
- **Fisher subunit repair** (Fisher DM, *Plast Reconstr Surg*, 2005) has similar markings to Millard, but the closure lines are placed along anatomic subunits and stress the importance of Cupid's bow levelling.

SECONDARY DEFORMITIES

- **Short lip** – some asymmetry (due to unilateral short lip) is generally expected, peaking at about 2 months after surgery and maturation/softening of the scar will usually return the lip to its immediate post-operative position. If a lip is short at the end of surgery, it will always be short. If the short lip deformity follows a Millard operation, then the usual causes are inadequate muscle repair or inadequate rotation – in that case, revision will usually help.
- **Tight upper lip** – more common after triangular repair. If a Z-plasty does not help, then an Abbé flap needs to be considered.
- **Long upper lip** – more common after triangular repair or bilateral CLs.
- **Whistle deformity** is largely due to inadequate red margin/vermilion and options include
  - Mucosal advancement from the buccal sulcus including mucosal V–Y advancement (Kapetansky DI, *Plast Reconstr Surg*, 1971)
  - Free graft from lower lip
  - Abbé flap

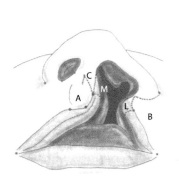

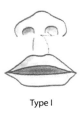

Type I

Type II

Figure 4.3 Millard advancement-rotation flap is a common choice. A – rotation flap, B – advancement flap, C – columellar base, M – medial mucosal flap, L – lateral mucosal flap. Depending on how the C flap is used, there are subtypes I and II.

BILATERAL CLEFT LIP

It can be asymmetric; more severe forms have a fly-away premaxilla and collapsed lateral segments.

- The prolabium is deficient of white roll and vermilion and lacks muscle, whilst the columella is short/almost absent. The protruding premaxillary segment is suspended from the nasal septum.
- Poorly formed or absent anterior nasal spine with retruded area under the base of the septal cartilage.
- Broad, flat nose with recession of the foot plates of the medial crura.
- The maxilla is usually underdeveloped and Le Fort I or II procedures are needed.

Surgery becomes more difficult with age as the central segment becomes more deformed. It is often said that surgery for bilateral clefts is twice as difficult, with results half as good as in unilateral clefts. There is a wider variation in techniques, each with their own set of pros and cons.

Additional considerations include the following:

- PSO for the protruding premaxilla; lip adhesion is relatively contraindicated as it uses up too much tissue and works poorly.
- Columellar length.

Common issues with bilateral cleft lip repair are

- Short columella
- Widened prolabium/philtrum
- Poorly projecting tubercle (Abbe flap after maxillary growth/Le Fort I)

Secondary (open) rhinoplasty is often performed when skeletal maturity has been reached, often requiring non-anatomic and anatomic cartilage grafts.

Closure of bilateral cleft clip and elongation of the columella by two operations in infancy. (Millard DR, *Plast Reconstr Surg*, 1971)
PSO was used for the premaxilla, and lip repair was performed at 1 month of age with banking of forked flaps. Columellar lengthening was performed at a second stage at 3 months.

- The muscle from the lateral lip segments is sutured together in the midline. The prolabial vermilion/mucosa is turned down and is used for lining behind the muscle repair, which adds bulk and helps prevent a whistle deformity. The lateral lip segment vermilion and white roll are advanced and **joined in the midline**.
- **Bilateral fork flaps** are derived from the lateral edges of the prolabium, and each flap is sutured end-on to the alar base to form a standing cone/pyramid. At a second stage, an inverted 'V' incision is made in the columella to join the bases of the two fork flaps, and the incision is closed as a V–Y to gain columellar length.

This technique combines **columellar lengthening** with advancement of the alar base.

- Some would argue that prolabial skin should be used in the lip, not the nose (Adams WM, *Plast Reconstr Surg*, 1953); otherwise, there is a difficult to correct long lip deformity.
- The subsequently modified Millard technique does **not** bank the lateral segments of the prolabium.

The Manchester repair (1965, historical interest only) preserved the vermillion and white roll from the prolabium for reconstruction of the tubercle – this results in a dry chapped patch as the prolabial vermilion does not have minor salivary glands. It preserves full prolabial width in anticipation of forked flaps for columella. The muscle is repaired to prolabial soft tissue, the thinking being that the lip would be overtight otherwise. The **straight line repairs** mean a wider philtrum with irregular peaks, and more whistle deformity. The Broadbent and Woolf modification (1984) cut the prolabium to the desired width, and parings were mostly discarded, some used to line nasal floor.

Byrd repair (2008) combines aspects of Millard and Manchester (and Cronin).

CARTILAGE TECHNIQUES

The older Millard and Manchester techniques are sometimes called **skin-only techniques** as they are focused on the 'skin problems' especially the short columella. Subsequent growth of the deranged nose would lead to a bulbous tip that could be very difficult to correct.

More recent techniques from Mulliken (1988) and McComb (see below) integrate nasal correction (not addressed by Millard or Manchester techniques) with lip repair to give adequate tip projection as well as **primary columellar lengthening**. McComb has described a staged approach (*Plast Reconstr Surg*, 1990).

- Prolabial white roll and vermillion are discarded; mucosa is rolled in for buccal lining/sulcus.
- Cupids bow and tubercle are constructed from lateral segments. Muscle is advanced medially below the elevated philtral flap, which is wider inferiorly.
- **Alar cinch sutures** to reposition alar bases.

BILATERAL INCOMPLETE CLEFT LIP

These are typically clefts involving only the lip with a near-normal nose with Simonart's bands across the nasal floors, and a normally positioned premaxilla. They can be repaired using the rotation–advancement technique as for unilateral repair in two stages, one side at a time.

CLEFT PALATE

Failure of fusion of the palatal shelves (~7–12 weeks) leads to a cleft of the secondary palate, the hard palate posterior to the incisive foramen. By comparison, the critical time for clefts lips is 4–6 weeks.

Patients with CPs will have **speech (see below) and feeding problems**. The goal of CP surgery is to close the palate with a technique and timing that produces optimal speech whilst minimising facial growth disturbances.

FEEDING

CP patients have greater problems with feeding than CL patients.

- Breast feeding is always worth trying, though supplements are often needed.
- Haberman feeder: slit valve (control flow by orientation), reservoir in teat that can be squeezed to deliver milk, valve between teat and bottle.

CPO, which involves only the secondary palate:

- 1 in 2000 with fewer racial and gender differences
- Often syndromic (~50%)
  - DiGeorge/Shprintzen (chromosome 22q deletion, cardiac defects) most common (15%–25%)
  - Stickler (AD, mutation in type 2 collagen) 25% of syndromic clefts
  - Van der Woude (20%)
  - Crouzon, Aperts
- Multifactorial environmental factors
  - Folic acid supplements may help, but the evidence is not wholly conclusive

CLASSIFICATIONS

- **Veau classification (see above).**
- **Kernahan's** striped Y, further modified by Millard and Jackson, allows the cleft to be located anatomically: 1–3 on the right, 3–6 on the left, from lip anteriorly to the incisive foramen, 7, 8 hard palate and 9 soft palate.
- **LAHSAL** classification that is used by the national database on clefts with the capital indicating complete clefts of lip, alveolus, hard palate, soft palate, alveolus, lip.

SUBMUCOUS CP (SCP)

This occurs in ~1 in 1000 (Kaplan EN, *Cleft Palate J*, 1975) to 1 in 600 (Nasser M, *Cochrance Database Syst Rev*, 2008). Signs sometimes called the Calnan triad (1954) include

- **Bifid uvula** (occurs in general population ~1%–2%; 10% will have SCP and thus it is not an accurate predictor).
- Shortened soft palate with muscle diastasis.
- Palpable notch in hard palate.

Some have a blue line/translucency aka 'zona pellucida' indicating a separation of the palatal musculature. Most patients have normal speech, though about **15% have VPI**,

which can be the presenting complaint. Others can present with feeding or hearing problems, or else simply found on routine paediatric examination. The severity of the VPI is not directly correlated to the physical signs. If speech and ENT assessment are acceptable, then palatal or pharyngeal surgery can be avoided; otherwise, the traditional surgical option is pharyngoplasty. Other options include palatoplasty (Furlows, intravelar veloplasty).

Interventions for the management of submucous cleft palate. (Nasser M, *Cochrane Database Syst Rev*, 2008) A literature review of RCTs found one methodologically satisfactory trial (Ysunza A, *Plast Reconstr Surg*, 2001) comparing 72 patients randomised to minimal incision palatopharyngoplasty (MIPP, uncommonly used), pharyngeal flap or sphincter pharyngoplasty. They conclude that there is some weak and unreliable evidence that there is no significant difference between MIPP and other methods.

CP SURGERY

Aims of CP correction include

- Closing the oronasal fistula whilst minimising maxillary growth retardation
- Allowing normal development of speech whilst facilitating velopharyngeal closure

STAGED OR DELAYED SURGERY

Some stage the palatal surgery, repairing the soft palate earlier with the aim of improving speech development whilst reducing growth disturbance by performing the hard palate repair later. The early lip and soft palate repair is said to have a constraining effect on the remaining palatal cleft, making it easier to repair later. The benefits of early surgery on speech development need to be weighed against the increased technical difficulty with early surgery and deleterious effects on dentofacial development. Simply put, it is more difficult to correct disordered speech than facial growth issues. In addition, babies are obligate nasal breathers until about 6 months; the nasal airway can be compromised by early palatal surgery.

Some techniques proposed an even longer gap: **Schweckendiek** (*Cleft Palate J*, 1978) repaired the soft palate at 6–8 months and the hard palate at 12–15 years, which tended to give good facial growth but with a 50% VPI rate and worse speech (Marburg study), as well as having to use an obturator until the hard palate repair. Perko (*J Maxillofac Surg*, 1979) repaired the soft and hard palate at 18 months and 5–8 years, respectively, and long-term follow-up confirms good facial growth but poor soft palate length/mobility and VPI. The global concept of a 'functional repair' (proposed by Delaire based on the premise that normal growth is possible and that there should be restoration of structures particularly muscles; see above) is attractive in principle, but long-term results have not been fully assessed.

Currently, the arbitrary definitions are as follows:

- Early – 6 months (best speech outcomes; Dorf DS, *Plast Reconstr Surg*, 1982)
- Traditional – 12–18 months (acceptable facial growth; Semb, *Cleft Palate Craniofac J*, 1991)
- Staged – soft palate at 3–6 months (or with lip repair), hard palate at 15–24 months (Byrd)

TECHNIQUES

General anaesthesia with a south-facing endotracheal tube, and a Dingman gag.

VOMERINE FLAP

This is used to close the anterior hard palate/alveolus at the time of lip repair; it decreases the frequency of alveolar nasal fistulae but may exacerbate the maxillary growth retardation.

FLAP-LESS REPAIR

This relies upon movement of the mucoperiosteum off the arched palate to lie horizontally to gain enough length for primary closure in the midline without lateral releasing incisions and is only suited for narrow clefts. The closure is under some tension; thus, a higher fistula rate is expected.

SOFT PALATE LENGTHENING (VEAU–WARDILL–KILNER)

The mucoperiosteum of the hard palate is pushed posteriorly whilst transposing myomucosal flaps based on the greater palatine neurovascular bundles towards the midline. New bone is formed under the transposed periosteum. The relatively large anterolateral donor defects are usually packed with a haemostatic material such as Surgicel; there are concerns that the extensive denudation of bone may inhibit maxillary growth. Original descriptions included

fracture of the hamulus to release tensor palate, but it is no longer commonly done.

- Although palatal musculature is detached from the hard palate, fibres still course anteriorly rather than transversely. It is known as the **'push-back'**, but the effect on the soft palate alone is often insufficient to correct significant VPI without a formal veloplasty (Figure 4.4).

Effect of Veau–Wardill–Kilner type of cleft palate repair on long-term mid-facial growth. (Choudhary S, *Plast Reconstr Surg*, 2003)

There are concerns that this type of CP repair causes inhibition of maxillary growth due to the extensive denudation of the palate. The author presents experience with 25 nonsyndromic complete unilateral cleft lip and palate patients with an average of 12 years of follow-up. Mid-facial growth was analysed using 12 year dental models and lateral cephalograms taken before definitive orthodontic treatment; 72% of patients had a good or satisfactory outcome, whilst 28% obtained a poor score of 4 or 5.

The results suggest that satisfactory long-term midfacial growth can be obtained, but did not compare it with other techniques.

VON LAGENBECK TECHNIQUE

This is the oldest technique and is still being used. The palatal tissues are moved towards the midline using lateral releasing incisions that lie lateral to the greater palatine artery. By avoiding disturbing the anterior palate, it is hoped that there is less disturbance to the nearby maxillary growth centres (Figure 4.5).

- As part of the technique, the muscle is dissected out from nasal and oral mucosa and swept backwards off the hard palate mobilised to the midline, and then closed. There is no increase in length of the soft palate.
- Delaire used more medially placed incisions/flaps with the aim of reducing maxillary growth inhibition, but it was associated with a higher fistula rate due to higher tension as well as the essentially random pattern flap perfusion.

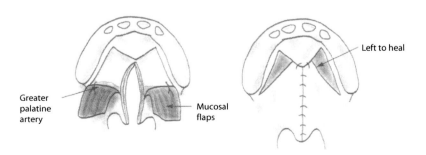

Figure 4.4 Veau–Wardill–Kilner. Mucosal periosteal flaps are raised and sutured together medially leaving areas that are left to heal secondarily. There is retropositioning of the posterior border of the soft back, hence the alternative term 'push-back repair'.

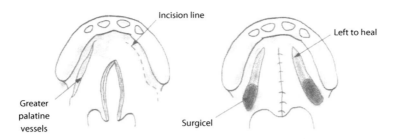

Incision line
Left to heal
Greater palatine vessels
Surgicel

Figure 4.5 von Langenbeck repair. A bipedicled mucoperiosteal flap is raised by incising behind the alveolus, and mobilised medially whilst preserving the greater palatine vessels.

- The **Bardach two-flap palatoplasty** (1967) was conceived as a modification of the von Langenbeck with the incisions extended anteriorly to allow elevation of two large posteriorly based mucoperiosteal flaps that have good mobility. It is one of the most common repairs used; studies report low fistula rates (2.4%) and good speech (Murthy, *Indian J Plast Surg,* 2009). It is worth repeating that there is little to choose between the common techniques; surgical expertise in applying a particular technique is probably more important.
  - It is often combined with an intravelar veloplasty.

VELOPLASTY – REALIGNMENT OF THE PALATAL MUSCLE

Intravelar veloplasty was popularised by Sommerlad and involved radical muscle dissection under an operating microscope. Dissection included taking the tensor muscle back to the pterygoid hamulus and repositioning to lie more posteriorly and transversely, and then reconstructing the sling.

Kriens (*Plast Reconstr Surg,* 1969) provided a detailed description of the abnormal muscle insertions and directions of pull as well as guidance to the dissection of individual muscles at operation to restore them as near to normal anatomy as possible.

A technique for cleft palate repair. (Sommerlad B, *Plast Reconstr Surg,* 2003)
Four hundred forty-two primary palate repairs were performed using an operating microscope, and were followed up for >10 years; 80% had hard palate repair with minimal dissection, combined with radical veloplasty. Secondary velopharyngeal surgery rates decreased from 10.2% to 4.6% over 10 years during which the muscle dissection became more radical. The conclusion was that radical muscle dissection improves velar function.

Cleft palate repair by double opposing Z-plasty. (Furlow LT, *Plast Reconstr Surg,* 1986)
The author described his technique of soft palate repair using double opposing Z-plasty flaps to create a muscle sling across the cleft. In the author's view, this also allows the soft palate to be lengthened without using tissue from the hard palate. It is combined with a von Langenbeck hard palate repair.

- The nasal Z-plasty is a mirror image of the oral Z-plasty with the central limb formed by incising the cleft edges. Anteriorly based flaps are composed of mucosa; the posteriorly based flaps are myomucosal to incorporate palatal musculature. The nasal flaps are transposed before the oral flaps and create an overlapping sling of palatal muscle.
- The suture lines are at the right angles to each other on the nasal and oral layers, reducing the chance of fistulae.
- It is reported to produce superior speech and less VPI compared with historical controls.

However, subsequent reports suggest that if there is any lengthening with a Furlow's technique, it does in fact do so at the expense of tissue that would be used for closure around the hard–soft palate junction. The Furlow technique is often regarded as an exaggerated muscle repair.

With the various repairs, the degree of muscle retroposition and palatal lengthening **does not directly correlate** with the effect on speech.

Arm restraints in children with cleft lip/palate. (Sommerlad BC, *Plast Reconstr Surg,* 2003)
This randomised trial demonstrated that there was no benefit in using any form of arm restraint.

IV. COMPLICATIONS

Of most concern are the airway obstruction and bleeding.

- **Airway obstruction** occurs especially with pharyngoplasty, push-back, and combined procedures, particularly in patients with Pierre Robin. Significant obstruction is rare in the absence of excessive bleeding.
  - **Nasal airway obstruction** occurs at two time periods: early due to post-operative swelling and late due to altered nasal morphology (25% decrease in pressure flow through the nasal airway).
- **Fistulae** (0%–34%) may present as a deterioration in speech intelligibility. There may actually be

an increasing incidence with the trend for less undermining to avoid growth issues; some combine primary surgery with buccal fat pads (BFPs; see below).

- Assess by examining and enlisting an experienced speech therapist; listening for hypernasality, nasal regurgitation and nasal air emission ('p's or 's's) and articulation errors. The intraoral appearance of a fistula does not reflect the complexity of its shape/course to the nasal side. The effect of the fistula may be tested by occluding it; nasal inflammation may also modify speech.
- Timing is controversial, but there is no evidence that spontaneous closure will occur once the wound itself has healed. The usual treatment is to excise the fistula, raise large palatal flaps and close in tension-free manner; some also use bone graft (or cartilage or Alloderm). Fistula closure is prone to recurrence (25%; Cohen, *Plast Reconstr Surg*, 1991) and may adversely affect growth.
  - BFP or FAMM flaps are gaining in popularity.
- Obturators (temporarily or permanently) may be used in selected patients.
- **Maxillary growth retardation** may be less pronounced in later repair but at the expense of delaying speech development due to late correction of VPI. Growth retardation (Semb G, *Cleft Palate Craniofac J*, 1991) is related to age at surgery; the seniority of surgeon, the type of lip repair and pharyngoplasty are not prognostic. Facial growth may be inherently impaired in some CP patients

The use of buccal fat pad (BFP) as a pedicled graft in cleft palate surgery. (Grobe A, *Int J Oral Maxillofac Surg*, 2011)

This is a retrospective study of 24 patients who had a pedicled BFP (7 × 4 × 3 mm) to cover the area at the posterior end of the hard palate where there would be high tension, with the aim of preventing fistulae (Pittsburgh type III). Without skin grafts for coverage, epithelialisation takes about 4 weeks; there were no donor site complications.

PIERRE ROBIN SEQUENCE

- **A sequence** is a single developmental defect that results in a chain of secondary defects; for example, in PRS, mandibular hypoplasia causes posterior tongue displacement, which leads to airway obstruction and hinders closure of the palatal arches, leading to a cleft of the secondary palate. The entire cascade of events is the sequence.
- **A syndrome** is a group of anomalies that contain multiple malformations and/or sequences. A given anomaly may be incompletely expressed or absent; the

pathogenic relationship of the group of anomalies is frequently not well understood.

The PRS sequence is theorised to start with hindrance of the neck to come of flexion, e.g. oligohydramnios; subsequent retrogenia and glossoptosis limit tongue descent, which prevents fusion of the palatal shelves.

PRS was first described in 1822 and affects 1 in every 8000 live births or just under 50 babies per year in the United Kingdom. The risk of further children being affected is 1%–5%. It is part of a larger syndrome in >50%, the most common of which are **Stickler syndrome** (see below), van der Woude and VCF.

- Glossoptosis and airway obstruction.
- Retro-genia/gnathia (also some micro-genia/gnathia): in milder cases, the mandible will gradually grow to more normal proportions to acquire a normal profile by 6 years of age, and mandibular advancement is rarely required.
- CP (60%–90%) that tends to be wide and U-shaped – usually closed surgically at 12–18 months.
- Defects of ear and eye.

AIRWAY MANAGEMENT IN PRS

The affected neonate suffers from airway obstruction during sleep and will become exhausted if the problem is not corrected.

- Try nursing **prone** first – this is adequate in 80%.
- Nasopharyngeal airway aiming to end just above the epiglottis – adequate in another 18%.

Surgery may be needed in a very small number: in particular, if the neonate desaturates during sleep, requires prolonged nasal CPAP, etc.:

- **Emergency management** – pull **tongue forward** with stitch/towel clip, nasotracheal airway/intubation.
  - Longer-term techniques for managing the tongue include suturing the tip to the inner surface of the lower lip, i.e. **labioglossopexy** (Routledge) Figure 4.6, or passing a K-wire through the mandible to skewer the base of the tongue in a forward position.
- A definitive airway in the form of a tracheostomy is rarely required (<1%), and the decannulation process can be prolonged.
- Mandibular advancement by **distraction osteogenesis (DO)** has been described but should not be used without trying other methods first; in addition, there is a risk of permanent dental in those under 2 years of age, whose bones are too soft anyway. Distraction has the advantage of also stretching the soft tissues (distraction histiogenesis).
  - Traditional osteotomies have become less commonplace.

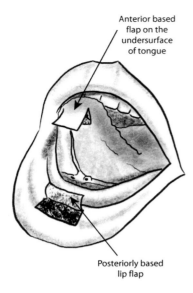

Anterior based flap on the undersurface of tongue

Posteriorly based lip flap

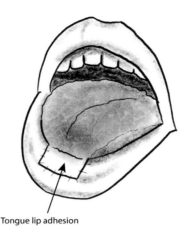

Tongue lip adhesion

Figure 4.6 Lip tongue adhesion. Complementary flaps are raised on the tongue tip and the lower lip, and then sutured together.

STICKLER'S SYNDROME (HEREDITARY PROGRESSIVE ARTHRO-OPHTHALMOPATHY)

This is a connective tissue disorder first described in 1960 by Gunnar Stickler from the Mayo Clinic. It is a progressive condition with AD inheritance – there are several subtypes: COL2A1 (75% of cases, defect on chromosome 12), type XI COL11A1 and 2 (chromosome 6) and type IX COL9A1 (also chromosome 6, recessive variant). Characteristic features include

- **Severe progressive myopia**, retinal detachment, vitreal degeneration, glaucoma, cataracts
- Progressive sensorineural hearing loss
- Valvular prolapse, e.g. mitral valve prolapse
- Scoliosis
- **PRS features** – **CP** and mandibular hypoplasia – flat face with small nose that tends to improve with age
- Hyper- and hypomobility of joints, leading to osteo-arthritis in later life; variable epiphyseal dysplasia causing joint pain, dislocation or degeneration
  - It should be considered in any infant with congenitally enlarged wrists, knees or ankles, particularly when associated with PRS (30%–40% of those with PRS have Stickler's). It should also be suspected in those with features of the Marfan syndrome with hearing loss, degenerative arthritis or retinal detachment.

Influence of surgical technique on early post-operative hypoxaemia in children undergoing elective palato-plasty. (Xue FS, *Br J Anaesth*, 1998)
Post-operative hypoxaemia is potentiated by oedema of palate, pharynx or tongue along with the inability to clear pulmonary and oral secretions and low elastic recoil of the thorax and lungs. Children also have comparatively higher oxygen consumption.

Three treatment groups studied 312 patients altogether:

- von Langenbeck palatoplasty
- Push-back palatoplasty
- Push-back plus superior pharyngeal flap pharyngoplasty

Oxygen saturation dips to <85% were recorded most frequently in patients with combined procedures, whilst von Langenbeck repairs were significantly less likely to cause hypoxaemia than the others. Desaturation was most profound within the first 30 minutes of arrival in the recovery room but depended somewhat on the technique used:

- von Langenbeck palatoplasty – within the first 15 minutes
- Push-back palatoplasty – the first 40 minutes
- Push-back plus superior pharyngeal flap pharyngoplasty – 120 minutes

Cleft palate fistulas: A multivariate statistical analysis of prevalence, aetiology, and surgical management. (Cohen SR, *Plast Reconstr Surg*, 1991)
This is a retrospective review of 129 non-syndromic CL/P patients with an overall fistula rate of 23%. The fistulae were mostly small (1–2 mm) and located in the anterior part of the hard palate.

Multivariate analysis showed that causative risk factors were **push-back** palatoplasty (43% developed fistulae), Veau classifications 3 and 4 and the operating surgeon. Factors that did not seem to contribute included intravelar velo-plasty and age and gender of the patient, although recurrent fistulae (37%) were more common in females.

Surgical options include total revision of the palate repair, local mucoperiosteal flaps, vomerine flaps, bone grafting plus soft tissue closure and tongue flaps.

- 16% large fistulae (>5 mm), repaired early due to speech problems
- 47% small fistulae (1–2 mm), repaired at the time of lip revision, nasal surgery or bone grafting, i.e. delayed

V. CLEFT LIP NOSE

UNILATERAL CLEFT LIP NOSE DEFORMITY

- Mild – wide alar base, but with normal alar contour and dome projection
- Moderate – wide alar base, depressed dome or alar crease (minimal alar hypoplasia)
- Severe
  - Wide alar base, deep alar crease, under-projecting alar dome (alar hypoplasia) with caudal rotation (downwards) of the alar cartilage (loss of overlap) so that the dome is retroposed and the nose is lengthened on the cleft side.
  - Cleft lip nose (CLN) is caudally rotated – normal columellar angle ~60°.
  - Base of the septum is deviated away from the cleft side – the pull of normal muscles is not counterbalanced.

BILATERAL CLN DEFORMITY

- Short columella
- Broad, depressed nasal tip

In general, primary nasal correction is carried out at the time of lip correction (McComb) or age 5–6 years (Tajima) with definitive rhinoplasty at ~16–17 years. Asymmetry and nasal obstruction are common problems (Figure 4.7).

PRIMARY REPAIR OF THE UNILATERAL CLN

Primary repair of the unilateral cleft lip nasal deformity. (McComb H, *Plast Reconstr Surg*, 1985)
Surgery for the CLN aims to correct caudal rotation of the alar cartilage at the time of lip repair and shorten the nose on the cleft side. The skin is mobilised off cartilage framework and the alar lift achieved with mattress sutures passing from within the vestibule of the cleft nostril and tied over a bolster at the level of the nasion.

Reverse 'U' incision for secondary repair of cleft lip nose. (Tajima S, *Plast Reconstr Surg*, 1977)
This technique uses an inverted 'U'-shaped incision in the nasal vestibule to mobilise the dorsal nasal skin and allow suturing of the displaced alar cartilage (cleft side) to the normal side, but significant undermining is required. As the normal anatomical correction of the alar cartilage is achieved, the mobilised dorsal skin is in slight excess and closure gives rise to a natural in-rolling effect.

The use of this technique has been reported in primary repairs also (Byrd HS, *Plast Reconstr Surg*, 2000).

Primary repair of the bilateral cleft lip nose. (McComb H, *Plast Reconstr Surg*, 1990)
Following primary correction of the bilateral CLN by elevation of the alar cartilages and columellar lengthening with forked flaps, three undesirable features become apparent at adolescence:

- Nostrils are larger than normal.
- Broadening of the nasal tip due to separation of alar domes.
- Downward drift of the columella base.

Supposedly, it makes more embryological sense for the columella to be reconstructed from nasal tissue rather than from the prolabium, and the use of forked flaps is questioned. The lip repair is performed at a second stage 1 month later, so that the blood supply to the prolabium is thus not compromised by concurrent nasal tip dissection and undermining, as it is elevated off the premaxilla.

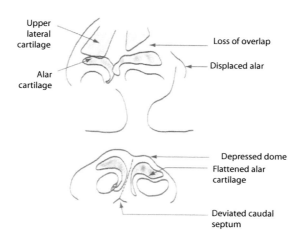

Upper lateral cartilage — Loss of overlap — Displaced alar
Alar cartilage
Depressed dome — Flattened alar cartilage
Deviated caudal septum

Figure 4.7 The CLN deformity is complex. Nasal bones are flattened. There is loss of overlap between the upper lateral and lower lateral (alar) cartilages, and the cleft side alar base is displaced laterally (up and back). The cleft side alar cartilage is flattened, buckled and hypoplastic contributing to a depressed, bifid dome. In addition, the nasal spine and causal septal cartilage are deviated to the opposite side; there is also maxillary hypoplasia.

PSO helps to reduce the soft tissue cleft before operation.

- Stage 1 – Repair of nostril floor and **lip adhesion** of prolabial segment to adjacent lip
- Stage 2 (1 month later):
  - **Open rhinoplasty approach** – internal incisions above each alar rim meeting in the midline and mobilise alar domes with wide undermining.
  - Lip adhesions taken down and a **formal lip repair** performed using lateral mucomuscular flaps to the undermined prolabium.
  - Suture the displaced alar domes (now under less tension) together.
  - Close skin incisions as a V–Y to a length of 5 mm as the vertical limb in the columella.

VI. ORTHODONTICS

TOOTH DEVELOPMENT AND CLEFT ORTHODONTICS

The alveolar cleft is usually located between the lateral incisor and the canine. The lateral incisor tooth bud may develop two incisors on either side of the cleft, may erupt into the cleft space or may be absent (10%–40% of patients).

The permanent lateral incisor normally erupts at 7–8 years of age, whilst the canine erupts at 11–12 years of age. Permanent teeth are generally slower to erupt around a cleft than non-cleft teeth, and adjacent teeth usually have poorly formed enamel.

STAGES OF ORTHODONTIC TREATMENT

- PSO (see above) can be useful in assisting the closure of wide alveolar clefts. A prosthetic plate may also aid feeding.
- Early dental management from age 6 onwards consists of extraction of troublesome displaced deciduous teeth and correction of malocclusion of erupting permanent teeth.
- Management of permanent dentition from age 11 onwards includes orthodontic treatment aimed at realigning teeth and correcting cross-bite. Some patients may need Le Fort I osteotomy and maxillary advancement or distraction.
- Orthodontics relies upon bone resorption along the pressure side of a tooth and growth on the tension side.

OCCLUSION (ANGLE CLASSIFICATION)

- Class I – Normal occlusion. The mesiobuccal cusp of the permanent maxillary first molar occludes in the buccal groove of the permanent mandibular molar. **Essentially each upper molar tooth should sit half a tooth *in front* of the corresponding lower tooth**.
- Class II – lower incisor contacts posterior to class I, e.g. TCS, PRS, HMF.

- Class III – lower incisor contacts anterior to class I, e.g. Crouzon's syndrome.
  - Edward Hartley Angle (1855–1930) – 'Father of American Orthodontics'

BONE–BASE RELATIONSHIP

- Class I – maxilla slightly over-projects mandible (normal).
- Class II – maxilla excessively over-projects.
- Class III – mandible over-projects maxilla.

The occlusion may be normal in some cleft patients, but there is often class III occlusion. There are also variable degrees of cross-bite in the posterior teeth, some uppers biting inside the lowers – unilateral clefts tend to be associated with unilateral areas of cross-bite, bilateral clefts with bilateral cross-bite. Some teeth may be significantly displaced and need to be extracted.

AIMS OF ALVEOLAR CLEFT CLOSURE

Alveolar deformity in complete clefts can be either narrow or wide, with or without collapse. The aims of cleft closure are

- To stabilise the maxillary arch (especially in bilateral clefts) and close oronasal fistulas and anterior palatal cleft
- To provide periodontal support for teeth to the cleft and provide a matrix into which permanent teeth may erupt

Alveolar bone grafting (ABG) involves raising flaps of gingiva, packing cancellous iliac crest bone into the cleft and then closing the gingival flaps. In contrast, gingivo-periosteoplasty (closure of the alveolar cleft using periosteal flaps – Skoog) does **not** achieve all of these aims.

Movement of the premaxilla and maxillary segments is impossible after bone grafting; thus, it is necessary to establish good arch alignment **before grafting**. The eruption of permanent dentition may be needed to facilitate orthodontic treatment before bone grafting, particularly in bilateral clefts.

There is some debate regarding the optimal timing – early (5–6 years) versus late (9–11 years), or when 25%–50% of the canine tooth is visible on the OPG. Early grafting may reduce maxillary growth, and the bone graft resorbs in the absence of an erupting tooth. Late grafting deprives erupting permanent dentition of periodontal support.

COMPLICATIONS:

- Wound dehiscence and graft exposure
- Resorption of graft

VII. EAR DISEASE

EUSTACHIAN TUBE DYSFUNCTION

The abnormal attachments of tensor palati and levator palati onto the Eustachian tube lead to dysfunction during swallowing. This leads to generation of negative pressure within the middle ear and collection of serous or mucoid (glue ear) effusion in the middle ear. There is usually a conductive hearing loss of 40 dB that exacerbates speech problems.

- Hearing can be tested at an early age by evoked response audiometry.
- The natural history is for the dysfunction to improve by ~8 years of age: as mid-face grows, the Eustachian tube begins to drain by gravity.
- Repair of the palate alone does not improve otitis media; palatoplasty often helps but does not always correct the dysfunction. Adenoidectomy may improve Eustachian tube patency.
- Some patients may need treatment by myringotomy and insertion of grommets before or at the time of palate repair. Grommets fall out after 6–9 months and thus benefit may be temporary; there are also known complications such as damage to the tympanic membrane (4.8%), displacement into middle ear, tymanosclerosis, etc.

B. INVESTIGATION AND MANAGEMENT OF VPI

I. NORMAL SPEECH

In the English language, there are 24 consonants, 15 short vowel sounds and 9 long vowel sounds.

CLASSIFICATION OF CONSONANTS:

- Voicing of sounds
  - Vocal folds vibrating – all vowels and B, G, D, Z
  - Vocal folds held apart – mainly plosive sounds P, T, K, S
- Place of articulation
  - Lips – M, P, B
  - Labiodental – F, V (lower lip and upper incisors)
  - Dental – TH (tongue plus teeth)
  - Alveolar – T, D (tongue plus alveolar ridge)
  - Palato-alveolar – SH (air passes beneath the palate)
  - Palatal – Y
  - Velar
  - Glottal

During normal speech, the soft palate ascends to close off the nasopharynx, and inadequate closure causes VPI. Symptoms include

- Lack of voice projection and articulation.
- Hypernasality (rhinolalia).
- Audible nasal escape – **only the sounds M, N and NG normally allow nasal escape** in the English language.
- **Maladaptive**/compensatory substitutions, e.g. glottal stops and pharyngeal fricatives.

SECONDARY SYMPTOMS OF VPI

- There is an inability to generate enough air pressure to pronounce explosive sounds **(stop plosives) such as P, T, K, B, D and G**, which are substituted for by **glottal stop** sounds (compensatory articulatory method characterised by forceful adduction of vocal cords – the build-up and release of air pressure underneath the glottis results in a grunt-type sound).
- **Consonants such as S, Z, SH** and occasionally CH are substituted by **pharyngeal fricative sounds** (making the sound in the throat instead of the mouth).
- Unintelligible vocalisation, nasal grimacing (attempting to close anterior nasal aperture), snorts (attempting to close posterior aperture) and breathlessness.

About 20% of patients require pharyngoplasty after palatoplasty, which seems to be independent of the type of surgery. VPI may result from anatomic factors (e.g. abnormal dentition), neuromuscular, mental disability, behavioural or a combination of disorders.

- Furlow 87% normal speech (Kirschner, 2001)
- Von Lagenbeck 86% (Marrinan, 1998)
- Veau–Wardill–Kilner 85% (Marrinan, *Cleft Palate Craniofac J*, 1998)

II. SURGERY FOR VPI

INDICATIONS FOR SURGERY

Nasal escape is a prominent feature and hampers the development of normal speech.

- VPI, despite adequate correction of a palatal cleft, is found in approximately 20% of patients (see above).
- CP patients with mid-face hypoplasia having maxillary advancement of more than 1 cm.

Investigation of VPI aims to define the site and size of the gap:

- Speech and hearing assessment.
- **Multiview videofluoroscopy** (VF, asked to say 'EE') – allows definition of the level of closure. Palatal plane ~C1 tubercle.
- **Nasendoscopy** – allows visualisation of closure mechanism. Closure patterns include coronal (most common, >50%), circular (20%), circular with Passavant's ridge (20%) and sagittal (10%).
  - Passavant's ridge is usually 1 cm below the usual level of closure.
- MRI.

Surgery may lead to obstructive sleep apnoea (OSA) in some patients; 1% of patients may need intubation postoperatively. Other complications include bleeding, wound dehiscence and inadequate correction.

TIMING OF SURGERY

After 5 years but before 12 years; after 12 years, there is a decline in the rate of learning of new speech sounds.

CHOICE OF PROCEDURE

The most commonly used procedures are pharyngeal flap, sphincter pharyngoplasty or posterior wall augmentation. There are those who suggest that the **pharyngeal flap** provides superior results in almost all situations and that seems to be the trend (Collins, *J Plast Reconstr Aesthet Surg*, 2012).

- Speech assessment/therapy may be sufficient for minor VPI.
- Palatal procedures:
  - Lengthening the palate with push-back procedures, Furlow's
  - Improving palatal movement – intravelar veloplasty (redirection of muscles)
- Narrowing the nasopharyngeal isthmus (exclude velocardiofacial syndrome [VCF], e.g. using FISH cq22). Procedures can be partly tailored to the problem:
  - Immobile soft palate (sufficient lateral wall motion) – flap pharyngoplasty/pharyngeal flap
  - Mobile soft palate but inadequate lateral wall closure – sphincteroplasty
  - Nasal escape following adenoidectomy: implant (Teflon, cartilage)
    - Posterior wall augmentation had been largely abandoned due to the unpredictable results; however, more recently, submucosal fat grafting has become an alternative.
    - **Wardill technique (*Br J Surg*, 1928)**: similar to a pyloroplasty, a horizontal incision is made in the posterior pharyngeal wall at the level of Passavant's ridge and sutured vertically, creating a ledge of tissue to act as a 'valve seating for the upper surface of the soft palate'. The closure is under some tension.
    - A palatal obturator may be considered in those with very wide clefts with little movement, and with little prospect of a good surgical outcome.

Alternatively, a suggested algorithm is

- Minimal circular gap – Furlow or intravelar veloplasty
- Moderate circular gap or sagittal gap – pharyngeal flap
- Large circular gap, coronal or bowtie gap – sphincter pharyngoplasty

SPHINCTEROPLASTY/SPHINCTER PHARYNGOPLASTY

The modern muscle sphincteroplasty was originally described by Hynes (*Br J Plast Surg*, 1951) and then modified by Orticochea (*Plast Reconstr Surg*, 1968) and Jackson (*Clin Plast Surg*, 1985). It is indicated when there is **poor**

medial excursion of the lateral pharyngeal walls and a short anteroposterior diameter. Creating a central posterior mound will narrow the central port and shorten the AP distance. Sphincter pharyngoplasties are effectively combinations of dynamic and static repairs, but the dynamic part may not be evident for 6 months until the muscles recover.

Pharyngoplasty by muscle transplantation. (Hynes W, *Br J Plast Surg*, 1951)

According to the author, a drawback of using Wardill's technique (see above) was that the ridge was too low for velopharyngeal closure particularly if the repaired palate is short. To be effective, a pharyngoplasty must

- Reduce the transverse diameter of the pharynx and reduce the AP diameter of the pharynx at a level higher than Passavant's ridge
- Allow normal superior constrictor function; maintain functional muscle around the nasopharyngeal isthmus rather than create an inert scar

Thus, Hynes suggested using **superiorly based mucosal flaps** from the posterior tonsillar pillars including the underlying **salpingopharyngeus**, taking care to preserve branches of the vagus nerve entering the muscle at the level of the soft palate. Flaps should be 3–4 cm long and ~1.5 cm wide and then inset in the midline into a horizontal incision in the posterior pharyngeal wall, one above the other to form a bulky ridge. This reportedly provides static and dynamic closure of the velopharynx. The donor is closed directly (Figure 4.8).

Construction of a dynamic muscle sphincter in cleft palates. (Orticochea M, *Plast Reconstr Surg*, 1968)

The author describes the transposition of **palatopharyngeus** myomucosal flaps towards the midline and inset into an **inferiorly based posterior pharyngeal flap**. The donor defects are left to heal by secondary intention with cicatrisation, which gradually closes off the lateral pharyngeal apertures.

In adults or where there is a very short palate, there is increased risk of dehiscence of these palatopharyngeus flaps – it is often preferable to perform the surgery in two stages, one flap at a time.

Sphincter pharyngoplasty. (Jackson IT, *Clin Plast Surg*, 1985)

The palatopharyngeus flaps are sutured **end–end** when inset into a transverse incision on the posterior pharyngeal wall level with the upper margin of the tonsillar fossa, under a **superiorly based mucosal flap**.

The preferred level of inset is determined by the results of videofluoroscopy, although in practice, it is placed as high as possible above C1 arch and Passavant's ridge. Only 1/3 retain significant levels of muscle contraction, i.e. in most cases, it is **not dynamic**.

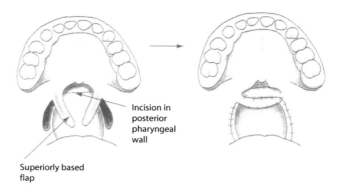

Incision in posterior pharyngeal wall

Superiorly based flap

Figure 4.8 Sphincter pharyngoplasty. Better results seem to be associated with higher level of inset.

Complications of sphincter pharyngoplasty include OSA/snoring and airway obstruction but less than with pharyngeal flaps; there is a higher rate of hypernasality.

PHARYNGEAL FLAPS

These are **superiorly or inferiorly based** single flaps that provide **static closure** of velopharynx. The aim is to allow less air through by acting as a central obturator; the lateral ports – aiming for a diameter of ~0.5 cm – are partly closed off by the medial movement of the lateral walls. Overcorrection will lead to mouth breathing, hyponasality and OSA (2%–10%). Judging the correct flap width is the biggest challenge.

The flap is raised in the plane of prevertebral fascia, i.e. full thickness, and inset into reflected flaps from the soft palate or nasal mucosa. The donor defect is partially closed or allowed to heal by secondary intention. **Superiorly based flaps are usually preferred** as they avoid having to inset into friable adenoidal tissue, and scarring will tend to pull the soft palate upwards (Figure 4.9).

Posterior pharyngeal flap for VPI patients: A new technique for flap inset. (Emara TA, *Laryngoscope*, 2012)

A high but relatively short and narrow superiorly based posterior pharyngeal wall flap is inset through a 1 cm wide transverse full thickness buttonhole in the soft palate, coming through into the oral surface. Several levels of

sutures make it relatively secure. Lateral pharyngeal ports were determined by 45° nasoendoscopy.

Pharyngeal flaps vs sphincter pharyngoplasty for the treatment of VPI. (Collins J, *J Plast Reconstr Aesthet Surg*, 2012)

There were only two RCTs comparing the two types of surgery. The analysis seems to suggest a trend towards performing pharyngeal flaps.

Velocardiofacial (Shprintzen's) syndrome. (Shprintzen RJ, *Cleft Palate J*, 1978)

VCF is the most common syndrome associated with clefts (5%–8% of all CP). There is inadequate development of the facial neural crest tissues, resulting in defective organogenesis of pharyngeal pouch derivatives. There is a **22q11.2 deletion** that can be diagnosed by fluorescent in situ hybridisation (FISH test) for the gene. These patients generally do badly as a group; associated abnormalities include CATCH (22):

- Cardiac anomalies – **medially displaced anomalous carotid arteries** – 25% have median carotid artery (preoperative MRI angiography is advised), congenital heart problems, e.g. tetralogy of Fallot, coarctation, pulmonary stenosis and ventricular septal defect (VSD) (most commonly).
- Abnormal facies (**flat expressionless face**), vertical maxillary excess, epicanthic folds, anti-Mongoloid

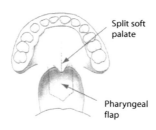

Split soft palate

Pharyngeal flap

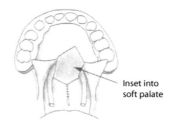

Inset into soft palate

Figure 4.9 Superiorly based pharyngeal flap.

slant, malar flattening, class II malocclusion, abundant scalp hair.

- **T**hymic aplasia (overlaps with Di George syndrome).
- **C**left palate (more commonly submucous) and **VPI** (poor lateral wall movement). Magnetic resonance angiography (MRA) is recommended before VPI surgery (usually a high wide pharyngeal flap).
- **H**ypocalcaemia.

Also

- Small stature
- Abnormal dermatoglyphics
- Mild hypotonia in early childhood
- Spindly fingers
- Learning difficulties and psychotic illness in adult life

Surgical management of VPI in velo-cardiofacial syndrome. (Mehendale FV, *Cleft Palate Craniofacial J*, 2004)

The pre-surgical assessment included pre-operative intra-oral examination and lateral VF with or without nasendoscopy, and intra-operative assessment of velar muscular anatomy.

Surgical options were based upon assessment. They preferred a staged approach, opting to maximise palatal function first.

- Radical dissection and retropositioning of velar muscles (submucous CP repair) followed by
- Hynes pharyngoplasty

Outcomes were assessed by evaluation of resonance and nasal airflow and repeating lateral VF and nasendoscopy. There was improvement in hypernasality in all groups.

- Staged approach showed significant improvement in nasal emission.
- Submucous CP repair resulted in increased velar length and increased velocity of closure.

Velopharyngeal surgery: A prospective randomized study of pharyngeal flaps and sphincter pharyngoplasties. (Ysunza A, *Plast Reconstr Surg*, 2002)

This is a study of 50 patients with residual VPI after palate repair. They were evaluated by videonasendoscopy and multi-view VF and equal numbers were randomised to undergo 'customised' pharyngeal flap repair or 'customised' sphincter pharyngoplasty ('customised' means according to the operative findings). Results were similar in each group.

Velopharyngeal insufficiency managed by autologous fat grafting in patients with aberrant courses of internal carotid arteries. (Bois E, *Int J Pediatr Otorhinolaryngol*, 2017)

The authors describe a retrospective review of nine patients (eight with 22q11 microdeletion) who had autologous fat grafting in addition to speech therapy. All had improved VPI at 11 months (BMS and intelligibility) that was stable at 3 years without reports of severe complications.

C. CRANIOFACIAL ANOMALIES

I. CRANIOFACIAL ANATOMY

EMBRYOLOGY

The face is recognisably human by the end of week 8. The majority of craniofacial anomalies arise during the first 12 weeks of embryological development.

The face is derived from five facial prominences – the frontonasal process and paired maxillary and mandibular processes, which fuse around days 46–47, and failure of which leads to facial clefting. The **mesodermal penetration theory** postulates that clefting occurs due to failure of migration of mesoderm into a bilaminar ectodermal membrane resulting in the loss of support to the overlying epithelial seam.

CRANIOFACIAL ABNORMALITIES

Potential factors contributing to craniofacial anomalies include

- Genetic (e.g. FGF receptor mutations)
- Radiation (associated with microcephaly)
- Maternal infection (toxoplasmosis, rubella, CMV) or other health problems (phenylketonuria, DM, vitamin deficiency, smoking)

Some useful definitions:

- Malformation – intrinsic inborn error of the foetal development process.
- Dysplasia – abnormal organisation of cells into tissue, e.g. Stickler's.
- Disruption – initially normal foetus subjected to tissue injury/breakdown, e.g. vascular, infection, metabolic, mechanical causes, e.g. thalidomide.
- Deformation – foetus with no intrinsic problem, but abnormal external forces cause secondary distortion/deformity, e.g. amniotic band.
- Syndrome – dysplasia affecting two or more sites not linked embryologically.

American Society of Cleft Lip and Palate classification of craniofacial deformities:

- Clefts and encephalocoeles
- Synostosis – syndromal and non-syndromal
- Hypoplastic conditions – hemifacial microsomia (HFM), hemifacial atrophy
- Hyperplastic conditions – fibrous dysplasia

Van der Meulen classification (most recent, European and uses 'dysplasia'):

- Cerebral craniofacial dysplasia – poor brain development usually means that these foetuses are non-viable.
- Craniofacial dysplasia – clefts and synostoses.

- Craniofacial dysplasia of other origin – i.e. miscellany, neurofibromatosis, vascular anomalies and fibrous dysplasia.

ENCEPHALOCOELES

These have a worldwide incidence of 1 in 5000 births and are herniations of cranial contents through a defect in the skull:

- Meninges (meningocoele)
- Meninges and brain (meningoencephalocoele/ encephalomeningocoele)
- Meninges, brain and ventricle (meningoencephalocystocoele)

ENCEPHALOMENINGOCOELE

These are congenital midline swellings that consist of the herniation of meninges and brain tissue from the anterior cranial fossa via the foramen caecum. It is a form of neural tube defect and may be associated with metopic synostosis and hypertelorism. They can occur in occipital (most common 80%), parietal, frontal, nasal and nasopharyngeal sites. Occipital encephalocoeles are usually large and the outcome is poor; 75% die or are severely disabled.

Frontoethmoidal lesions are said to arise due to failure of regression of a dural diverticulum projecting through the developing nasal and frontal bones (subtypes: nasofrontal, nasoethmoidal and naso-orbital).

Common craniofacial anomalies: Facial clefts and encephalocoeles. (Hunt JA, *Plast Reconstr Surg*, 2003)
Encephalocoeles can be investigated using skull X-ray and CT/MRI. The surgery can be performed by intra-/ extracranial approach via a bicoronal incision with the assistance of a neurosurgeon. In rare cases, only the meninges protrude, i.e. meningocoele; if the herniation involves only glial tissue, it can be safely excised.

- Urgent closure of open skin defects
- Incision of sac and amputation of excess tissue beyond the limits of the skull
- Dural closure, then reconstruction of soft tissue and bone (diploic bone graft)

Prenatal sonographic diagnosis of major craniofacial anomalies. (Wong GB, *Plast Reconstr Surg*, 2001)
Craniosynostosis – ultrasound imaging of cranial sutures is possible from week 13, though detection of single or multiple suture fusions is only possible from week 16; hence, an early normal scan does not exclude later synostosis. Ultrasound findings should be combined with available genetic/molecular information.

- Head measurements may indicate pattern of suture fusion (e.g. scaphocephaly vs. brachycephaly).

- Measurement of interorbital distance to diagnose hypertelorism.
- Imaging of hydrocephalus, encephalocoele and spinal defects.
- Syndromic synostoses identifiable from associated limb abnormalities; transvaginal ultrasound is useful for demonstrating hand abnormalities.

Pharyngeal and oromandibular abnormalities – imaging of the foetal maxillofacial skeleton possible from week 10.

- Craniofacial abnormalities of HMF can be diagnosed from week 29.

  TCS can be diagnosed from 15 weeks onwards.

- Canted palpebrae, microphthalmia and hypertelorism
- Microtia and micrognathia (also found in PRS and Stickler's syndrome)
- Nager syndrome (TCS phenotype with preaxial limb abnormalities)
  - Proximal radioulnar synostosis, thumb hypoplasia or aplasia

3D ultrasound complements traditional ultrasound and may allow earlier diagnosis of conditions such as Aperts (wide metopic suture, absent coronal suture; Esser T, *Am J Obs Gynecol*, 2006). MRI may be useful particularly for its negative predictive value when the ultrasound is suspicious (Fjortoft MI, *Neuroradiology*, 2007). 3D CT can also provide useful information but is limited by the issue of foetal irradiation. Overall, routine ultrasound may be able to reliably detect craniosynostoses in the second or third trimester.

II. CRANIOFACIAL CLEFTS

FACIAL CLEFTS

The commonest facial cleft is cleft lip/palate followed by isolated CP; other facial clefts are **actually relatively rare** by comparison (up to 5 cases per 100,000 live births). These other clefts exhibit a mixture of tissue deficiency and tissue excess. Environmental factors thought to contribute to facial clefts include influenza A2 virus and toxoplasmosis infection, and also drugs such as anticonvulsants, steroids and tranquillisers. See mesodermal penetration theory above.

- The Tessier classification, the most commonly used, is anatomical, whilst the Van der Meulen classification is embryological. The classification is 'oculocentric'.

AIMS AND PRINCIPLES OF RECONSTRUCTION

Functional and aesthetic correction of deformities with particular attention to

- Eyelids (to prevent corneal exposure)
- Macrostomia
- Separation of confluent oral, nasal and orbital cavities

SURGICAL TECHNIQUE

- Excision of cleft scar tissue and abnormal elements.
- Layered soft tissue closure: provide skin cover with local skin flaps and reattach soft tissue in the correct position, e.g. muscles of facial expression to reanimate the face and stimulate growth.
- Delay skeletal reconstruction until the child is older. Remove abnormal bone elements and reconstruct the defect with transposition of neighbouring bone or bone grafts.

CRANIOFACIAL CLEFTS

Anatomical classification of facial, craniofacial and laterofacial clefts. (Tessier P, *J Maxillofac Surg*, 1976)

These are numbered 0–14; facial clefts (from orbit downwards) extend to cranial clefts (orbit upwards). The numbers relate to their position relative to the midline with cleft 8 forming the equator at the lateral angle of the eye. The facial cleft number plus cranial cleft number = 14, e.g. 0–14, 1–13, 2–12, 3–11, etc. In general,

- Lateral clefts tend to have more severe bony abnormalities.
- Medial clefts have more severe soft tissue abnormalities.

Clefts **do not** pass through bony foraminae, which are the site of neurovascular structures. Each can be considered in terms of bony and soft tissue characteristics (Figure 4.10).

- Bilateral clefts do not have to be equally severe.
- Facial clefts may coexist with craniosynostoses.

Cleft 0 (0–3 are sometimes referred to as the oronasal clefts)

- Midline facial cleft.
- Median cleft lip (absent prolabium), bifid nose, bifid tongue, maxillary midline cleft.

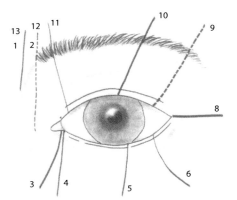

Figure 4.10 Craniofacial clefts in relation to the eye.

- Extends to cleft 14 – holoprosencephaly deformities (including cyclopia) and frontonasal encephalocoele may be present, though the deformity is very variable. The crista galli is bifid.

Cleft 1

- Soft tissue cleft from Cupid's bow through alar dome and bony cleft passes between central and lateral incisors. The septum is intact, but the alar dome is notched, the columella broad, with absent nasal bones. The prognosis is related to the degree of brain development.
- It extends to cleft 13 that passes medial to the inner limit of the eyebrow, producing hypertelorism; encephalocoeles may be present. The cribriform plate is widened, and the ethmoid cells are hypertrophied.

Cleft 2

- This is a rare cleft, a soft tissue cleft from Cupid's bow but lateral to the alar dome, which is hypoplastic and drawn upwards. Lacrimal drainage is usually normal.
- Maxillary alveolar cleft lateral to the lateral incisor.
- The cleft 12 passes through the medial third of the eyebrow; there is hypertelorism and telecanthus. The frontal and sphenoid sinuses are enlarged.

Cleft 3

- **This is one of the most common Tessier clefts**. It is an oblique facial cleft (oronasoocular cleft) from the Cupid's bow to the lacrimal punctum, with MCT agenesis and colobomata. The nasolacrimal duct is disrupted.
- Bony cleft begins between the lateral incisor and canine, and passes along the nasomaxillary groove into the orbit. Absence of the medial wall of the maxillary sinus produces a confluent cavity of mouth, nose, maxillary sinus and orbit. It involves the secondary hard palate.
- Surgery is directed at the cleft lip and palate repair, nasal correction, bony reconstruction of orbital floor and maxilla and transnasal medial canthopexy.
- Cleft 11 passes through the medial third of the upper lid and eyebrow; the bony cleft lies lateral to the ethmoid, producing hypertelorism.

Cleft 4

Cleft 4 (4–6 are oral ocular clefts that pass through the cheek without the disrupting nose, i.e. classic meloschisis)

- Similar to a number 3 cleft but begins just lateral to Cupid's bow and passes more towards the eye, to the lower lid just lateral to the punctum. There is deficiency of the medial/inferior orbital wall that may cause secondary nasal deformities. **It is the most disruptive and complicated cleft.**

- The bony cleft passes medial to the infra-orbital foramen, and there may be microphthalmos or anophthalmia.
- Cleft 10 continues through the middle third of the supra-orbital rim; a fronto-orbital encephalocoele displaces the eye inferolaterally causing hypertelorism.

Cleft 5

- This is one of the rarest. The soft tissue cleft runs from around the lateral commissure to the middle third of the lower lid that draws the lip and lid together.
- Bony cleft from the premolars passing lateral to the infraorbital foramen to involve the orbit in its middle third, and the eye can herniate into maxillary sinus.
- **Cleft 9 is the rarest cleft** and passes from the supra-orbital rim into the forehead as the continuation of a number 5 cleft, with an association with encephalocoeles, facial nerve palsy and cranial base abnormalities.

Cleft 6

- Soft tissue abnormality includes lower lateral lid colobomas, hypertelorism and anti-Mongoloid slant.
- Bony cleft centred on the zygomaticomaxillary suture and lateral third of the infraorbital rim, with loss of malar prominence.
- Cleft numbers **6, 7 and 8 – Treacher Collins syndrome**.
- Cleft number 8 with disruption of the lateral canthus (incomplete closure) is a component of the Goldenhar syndrome. Isolated cleft 8 is rare; there is a cleft at the frontozygomatic suture.

Cleft 7 (7–9 are lateral facial clefts)

- **Cleft number 7 is HFM** and may be bilateral in 10%; it is the **commonest cleft** at 1 in 3000 and more common in males. Cases are usually sporadic; supposedly secondary to the disruption of the stapedial artery.
- It is centred on the line between the oral commissure and the ear and affects structures around this line.
- Soft tissue structures – **macrostomia**, ear defects (**microtia**), facial and trigeminal nerve, parotid.
- Bony structures – ascending ramus of mandible, maxilla, etc. There is an open bite on the affected side.

Clefts 10–14

Clefts 10–14 are called **cranial clefts**. Number 30 cleft: midline cleft involving the mandible, the hyoid bone and sternum.

Amniotic band syndrome – The association between rare facial clefts and limb ring constrictions. (Coady MS, *Plast Reconstr Surg*, 1998)
Facial clefts that occur with limb ring constrictions are of paramedian type (2–12, 3–11, 4–10), and these patients may also have truncal defects. Theories for this rate association include

- Mechanical disruption due to amniotic bands
- Disorders of foetal blood supply

- Genetic programming error
- Disorder of tissue morphogenesis

Down syndrome: Identification and surgical management of obstructive sleep apnoea. (Lefaivre JF, *Plast Reconstr Surg*, 1997)
In Down syndrome, OSA may be caused by craniofacial issues:

- Mandibular and maxillary hypoplasia
- Macroglossia or disproportionately sized tongue (small oral cavity)
- As well as
  - Increased upper airway secretions and infections
  - Tonsillar and adenoid hyperplasia
  - Hypotonia

Treatment options include

- CPAP at night
- Tonsillectomy and adenoidectomy
- Uvulopalatopharyngoplasty (UPPP)
- Septal surgery to correct deviation and inferior turbinectomy
- Maxillary advancement (Le Fort I or III) or distraction but over-advancement may precipitate VPI
- Genioplasty
- Central tongue reduction

JLH Down (1828–1896) followed his father into chemistry and was Faraday's research assistant. When his father died, he entered medical school at age 25 and became interested in treating the mentally ill particularly children with 'mongolism'. It is better to refer to Down syndrome instead of Down's syndrome as the latter connotes ownership or possession. Dr Down did not have the syndrome – he described it.

III. CRANIOSYNOSTOSIS

Virchow's law relates to growth retardation in the direction perpendicular to the prematurely fused suture, with compensatory growth parallel to the suture (Figure 4.11).

AETIOLOGY

Theories of Suture Closure

- Cranial base – exerts abnormal tension.
- Intrinsic suture biology – secondary to the osteo-inductive properties of dura mater (Cohen, 2000). Dura mater communicates with the overlying cranial suture via paracrine activity of growth factors to regulate suture fusion.
- Extrinsic factors – in utero compression, hydrocephalus decompression (e.g. after VP shunt), abnormal brain growth (e.g. microcephaly) or systemic pathology (e.g. hypothyroidism or rickets).

Virchow stated that primary suture fusion caused secondary deformation of the cranial base; others suggest the opposite (Van der Klaauw and Moss), that a cranial base problem causes secondary growth deformities at the sutures with **brain**

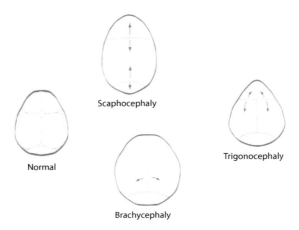

Figure 4.11 Typical skull shapes resulting from premature synostosis of cranial sutures: scaphocephaly (sagittal synostosis), trigonocephaly (metopic synostosis) and brachycephaly (bilateral coronal synostosis [BCS]).

enlargement being the primary stimulus for skull growth (functional matrix theory), whilst some say that a mesenchymal defect causes malformation of both. Though the primary event in craniosynostosis (CS) is still unclear, current evidence points mostly to a primary suture/skull vault problem.

- Many forms of CS are associated with mutations in FGFR genes that encode tyrosine kinase receptors.
  - FGFR1 – Pfeiffer
  - FGFR2 – Pfeiffer, Apert, Crouzon
- Elevated FGFR2 levels have been found in dura just prior to suture closure in rats (Mehara BJ. *Plast Reconstr Surg*, 1998).

CS can be classified as

- **Simple vs. complex** (two or more sutures involved)
- **Primary vs. secondary**
  - Premature fusion due to other diseases (see above); these patients are less likely to have raised intracranial pressure (ICP).
- **Syndromic vs. non-syndromic** (much more common)
  - Syndromic synostosis accounts for ~10%–20% of all synostoses; 50% are hereditary. It is often associated with other anomalies; the commonest syndromes are Crouzon, Apert and Pfeiffer. Regular CT scans and monitoring of ICP, e.g. visual evoked potentials, are recommended. Coronal synostosis is most likely to be syndromic.
  - Non-syndromic synostosis occur 0.6 in 1000 and tend to be of single suture type. They are usually sporadic and not inherited; they may be due to
    - Gestational influences
    - Toxic influences

TYPES OF CRANIOSYNOSTOSES

Sagittal synostosis is more common in males, whilst unilateral coronal synostosis is more common in females. Differences are less noticeable with the remainder.

- Metopic (between the frontal bones) synostosis – trigonocephaly
- Sagittal synostosis (M>F) – scaphocephaly
- Unilateral coronal synostosis (F>M) – plagiocephaly
- BCS – brachycephaly
- Unilateral lambdoidal synostosis – plagiocephaly

Positional (deformational) plagiocephaly of the occiput is a non-synostotic deformity, otherwise known as self-correcting 'plagiocephaly without synostosis' (PWS). PWS is the commonest cause of skull deformity.

RAISED ICP

Disparity between brain growth and remodelling of overlying bone due to premature fusion of sutures may lead to raised ICP (often defined as >15–20 mmHg under unstressed conditions), though the relationship is not so straightforward and may be related to venous hypertension. Raised ICP is more common in those with **multiple fused sutures** and is uncommon when only one suture is fused (42% vs. 13%, Marchac). Clinical signs include the following:

- **Examination** – papilloedema that may lead to optic atrophy, fontanelle bulging.
- **Headaches, irritability and other neurological symptoms** – fits, seizures.
- **Imaging shows thumb printing, copper beating or a Wormian appearance as well as the absence of suture lines at synostoses.** Clinical and radiological signs are usually only seen in late stages.
  - Although CT appearance is not predictive of which patients will develop ICP, progressive ventricle enlargement is an indication for shunt placement.
- **ICP and hydrocephalus is commoner in syndromic CS especially Crouzon** (66%) and uncommon in non-syndromic CS. Apert patients may have ventriculomegaly without hydrocephalus.

- **Developmental delay.** Very generally, the higher the ICP is, the lower the IQ tends to be; mental disability is more common when ICP is raised (multiple suture synostosis) and with hydrocephalus (syndromic synostosis). However, the relationship is not simple/ direct as mental retardation may also be related to prematurity or primary brain abnormalities. Although favoured by Marchac, the effect of early surgery in CS and mental development remains controversial, particularly in single suture synostosis. Single synostosis patients with significant mental retardation are probably more likely to have a primary brain problem.
  - Kapp-Simon (*Cleft Palate Craniofac J*, 1998). Children with unilateral coronal synostosis are two to three times more likely to suffer from learning disabilities than the general population.
  - Low self-esteem may affect social interaction and learning.

ASSESSMENT OF PATIENT WITH CS

History

- Family history of CS
- Problems during pregnancy (including maternal drug history) or delivery, and condition at birth (Apgar scores)

Investigations

- Skull X-ray
- CT, with or without 3D CT reconstruction
- Paediatric consultation

The general aim is to determine whether the patient has a deformational synostosis or true CS – and if the latter, which one? Possible diagnoses may be suggested by specific features, e.g. turribrachycephaly plus

- No hand abnormality – Crouzon
- Spade, mitten or hoof hand – Apert
- Broad thumbs ± ankylosis of elbow – Pfeiffer
- Low forehead, ptosis, short stature – Saethre–Chotzen
- Dry frizzy hair, grooved nails, bifid nasal tip – craniofrontonasal dysplasia
- Scaphocephaly – Carpenter

Patients with CS are best treated within a **multidisciplinary set-up**. Surgical treatment aims to treat the deformity (create aesthetic head shape) or to prevent deformity and to provide adequate volume for the growing brain.

MODERN PRINCIPLES OF TREATMENT OF CRANIOFACIAL SURGERY

Principles include

- Good access
- Rigid fixation
  - Beware of using titanium mini-plates during infancy as bone resorption may lead to intracranial

migration; as such, absorbable plates may be preferable (also to avoid potential growth restriction). Absorbable plates can be made from Vicryl® (polyglactic acid) or Dexon® (polyglycolic acid), with variable degradation rates, but generally lose strength at 9–15 months by hydrolysis. They are thicker than metallic plates and thus more likely to be palpable, and screw holes need to be tapped.

- Bone graft
  - Autologous – split calvarial (parietal), split rib (hard to mould, more resorption).
  - Methylmethacrylate, hydroxyapatite – calcium phosphate, Medpor®, demineralised bone.
    - Replamineform is a process to create hard porous implant material similar to coral.
- Pericranial/galeal flap.

TYPES OF SURGERY

Good comparative studies looking at optimal timing and techniques do not exist.

- **Treatment of CS**
  - Cranial vault remodelling ~3–6 months
  - Fronto-orbital advancement ~1 year
- **Treatment of mid-face hypoplasia**
  - Le Fort III with advancement vs. distraction
    - ~5–7 years of age when features 85% of adult size, or
    - 12 years of age, waiting for permanent dentition
- **Treatment of malocclusion**
  - Orthognathic – Le Fort I/BSSO/distraction

TREATMENT OF CS

Strip craniectomy may be needed in the first few months of life; it is best viewed as a **temporary decompression** until the patient is old enough for frontal advancement (which is part of the definitive treatment). Simple suture removal tends to be inadequate – the cranial shape is not immediately corrected, and many have secondary deformities due to re-closure of the suture before adequate remodelling.

Cranial vault remodelling is usually performed at **6 months**, sooner if raised ICP supervenes, e.g. pan-sutural involvement. At this age, the skull bones are malleable and heal better, and large bony defects can be reconstituted with new bone formation from the dura (in children <2 years); the surgery tends to be less radical/quicker and involves less blood loss. On the other hand, operating later may reduce the need for revisional surgery. Malleability and re-ossification potential are largely minimal after 3 years of age. Overall, there is a 5% re-operation rate.

- Transcoronal incision and subperiosteal dissection.
- Cut barrel staves and out-fracture as needed.
- Use split bone grafts as needed, moulding bone by burring, scoring or radial osteotomies.

Patients are usually kept in ICU for 24–48 hours; the haematocrit should be monitored and transfused as required.

Whilst cosmesis is important, mental development is paramount. Although the ICP may not be raised in Apert syndrome (wide open fontanelles), **frontal advancement** in these patients in Marchac's series (see below) may have allowed better intellectual development (other surgeons have said that earlier surgery does not affect intellectual development). Parents are often reluctant to accept craniofacial surgery, and **objective measurements** such as a raised ICP help to provide stronger arguments for surgery.

The effects of whole vault cranioplasty versus strip craniectomy on long term neuropsychological outcomes in sagittal craniosynostosis. (Hashim P, *Plast Reconstr Surg*, 2014)

This was a multicentre retrospective study of 70 patients with isolated sagittal synostosis. They found that those who had cranial vault remodelling before the age of 6 months performed better at a host of neuropsychological tests than those who had strip craniectomy before 6 months or before 3 months.

A criticism is that remodelling is often performed at 6–12 months but a comparison was not made; there was also no comment on the severity of the deformity. There were quite a few comments on this article; the small patient numbers from individual centres and the potential for bias were the main criticisms.

Neurodevelopment outcomes in infants and children with single-suture craniosynostosis. (Knight SJ, *Developm Neuropsychol*, 2014)

This review of 33 articles had contrary conclusions to Hashim; they found little evidence of factors affecting outcome. The review suggests that children with single suture CS have an increased risk of developmental problems, though they emphasise that individual patients will have very different trajectories.

Timing of treatment for craniosynostosis and faciocraniosynostosis: A 20-year experience. (Marchac D, *Br J Plast Surg*, 1994)

For patients with brachycephaly, **frontal advancement** (1.5–2.5 cm) is performed at age 2–4 months; for other CS, correction can be performed later, between **6 and 9 months**. Note that the authors suggest that there are increased reoperation rates compared with surgery performed after 9 months. This view is supported by Wall (*Br J Plast Surg*, 1994) who go further to suggest that unless there is raised ICP or severe exorbitism, surgery should be delayed until after 12 months.

Frontofacial **monobloc** advancement is only indicated for severe exorbitism in infancy as there is

- Infection risk due to dead space and intracranial communication with the nasal airway (see below; Fearon JA, *Plast Reconstr Surg*, 1997).
- Major surgery with risk of blood loss.

- If performed too early, e.g. <5 years of age, the deformity may return.
- Between 2 and 5 years, supra-orbital bar advancement is complicated by the development of the frontal sinus, although in these patients, the frontal sinus will usually redevelop after it has been cranialised.

Thus, in most cases of CS with mid-face hypoplasia (Apert, Crouzon), **a two- (or three-) stage approach** is preferred:

- **Frontal advancement** first before 1 year of age, then facial advancement 6–12 years (Le Fort III). The eyes can be protected in the interim with corneal lubrication, temporary tarsorrhaphies.
- Le Fort I advancement may ultimately be required for final correction of the bite at 12–18 years if the mandible outgrows the maxilla.

Another option is for DO including **monobloc distraction** (Bradley JP, *Plast Reconstr Surg*, 2006). Facial bipartition surgery can be performed to correct the hypertelorism associated with Apert, and accompanies facial advancement.

PROTECTION OF THE BRAIN DURING AND AFTER INTRACRANIAL SURGERY

- Pre-operative antibiotics and dexamethasone (4 mg 6 hourly).
- Post-induction drainage of 100–120 mL CSF leads to relaxation of the brain, and less retraction is needed during the operation.
- Controlled hyperventilation to decrease $PaCO_2$ leading to cerebral vasoconstriction and decreased brain volume.
- IV infusion of mannitol to decrease ICP.

COMPLICATIONS OF SURGERY

Death (1%–2%) due to

- Uncontrolled intra-operative haemorrhage (disruption of dural sinuses, large areas of raw bone)
- Air embolus
- Cerebral oedema
- Respiratory infection or obstruction
- CSF leak (check with intra-operative Valsava), which may lead to meningitis – use antibiotics which cross the blood–brain barrier

Other complications:

- Optic nerve injury if bicoronal flap is reflected over the eyes for too long.
- Persistent CSF leak.
- Seizures.
- Plate migration.
- Recurrence: further surgery was needed in 27% of syndromic cases, 6% for isolated synostoses.
- Infection.

Infections in craniofacial surgery. (Fearon JA, *Plast Reconstr Surg*, 1997)

The authors reported a 2.5% infection rate in 567 intracranial procedures. Interestingly, no patients younger than 13 months developed an infection, and they suggested that this may be due to rapid brain growth quickly obliterating the dead space. Half of all infections were related to frontofacial **monobloc surgery**. The infection rates were higher in secondary surgery, possibly related to

- Longer operating times
- Scarring with decreased tissue vascularity
- Older patients with more sinus development

Shaving hair did not influence infection rates. Cephalosporin prophylaxis of meningitis may have contributed to incidence of *Candida* and *Pseudomonas* infection.

METOPIC SYNOSTOSIS (10%)

The metopic suture normally fuses ~2 years of age. Metopic synostosis leads to **trigonocephaly** with flattening of the frontal bones, a midline forehead ridge and **bitemporal narrowing** with flaring of the parietal bones.

- Comprises <10% of non-syndromic synostoses.
- Most occur spontaneously; AD inheritance has been reported.
- ~4% have raised ICP and mental disability; there is an association with abnormalities of the corpus callosum.

There is also a Mongoloid slant (surgery can correct orbital rim hypoplasia) and **hypotelorism**. Note that with the notable exceptions of Down and Binder syndromes, most other craniofacial syndromes have hypertelorism.

- Frontoparietal advancement and remodelling with radial barrel stave osteotomies
- Supra-orbital bar advancement
  - The hypotelorism is then self-correcting without the need for orbital translocation and interorbital bone grafts.

SAGITTAL SYNOSTOSIS (50%)

This is **the most common CS** (50%) and results in a long and narrow skull, i.e. scaphocephaly, supposedly keel-shaped. There are reduced biparietal width and increased AP measurement with frontal and occipital bossing, which may affect anterior or posterior areas unequally. Cases are usually sporadic, though 2% have a genetic inheritance. It is four times more common in males.

Surgery aims to reduce AP length and increase skull width.

- Sagittal strip craniectomy (sagittal sinus injury is a risk)
- Frontal, parietal and orbital bone remodelling (barrel stave).

Correction of scaphocephaly secondary to ventricular shunting. (Shuster BA, *Plast Reconstr Surg*, 1995)

In some cases, premature fusion of the sagittal suture may be precipitated by the insertion of a VP shunt (secondary synostosis) possibly due to acute reduction in intracranial volume with overriding of the sutures. However, the synostosis may also be related to the primary pathology that caused the hydrocephalus.

This affects mainly children <6 months of age. It can be treated by excision of the fused suture (sagittal strip craniectomy) and occipital remodelling ± frontal remodelling.

UNILATERAL CORONAL SYNOSTOSIS (20%)

This is rather uncommon (1 in 10,000, 79% being female) and results in **anterior plagiocephaly** (Greek for oblique skull). It needs to be distinguished from secondary moulding deformities that may be associated with torticollis or Klippel–Feil syndrome (fusion of cervical vertebrae, a fairly rare association).

There is retarded growth in an AP direction on the affected side – the anterior cranial fossa becomes shorter with ipsilateral frontal flattening and contralateral parietal bossing (due to increased bone deposition directed away from the fused suture). Elsewhere, there is **altered growth:**

- Upwards – causing a long flat forehead. The supraorbital rim is raised but recessed and the orbit is shallow. **Proptosis** may lead to corneal exposure and ultimately blindness.
- Downwards – distorting the sphenoid with a loss of height of the lateral wall of the orbit; this is seen as the **'harlequin orbit'** on X-ray that is **pathognomonic** of coronal synostosis – the 'devil's eye' is slanted upwards. The eyebrow is elevated on the affected side, whilst the face tends to be C-shaped with chin and nose deviation away from the affected side.

Surgery restores the supra-orbital rim by advancing this segment (bilateral fronto-orbital advancement) along with frontal remodelling as above.

- Unilateral frontal craniotomy and supra-orbital bar advancement may give unsatisfactory results, and bilateral surgery has been shown to give a superior appearance (Sgouros S, *J Craniofac Surg*, 1996).
- Supra-orbital bar advancement may inhibit growth of the frontal sinus, which then affects the projection of the glabellar region, but this a theoretical complication not borne out in practice (Marchac DA, *Plast Reconstr Surg*, 1995).

BILATERAL CORONAL SYNOSTOSIS (20%)

Growth retardation in an AP direction leads to **brachycephaly**, which is a shortened skull, or turribrachycephaly, which is a shortened and **tower-shaped** skull due to compensatory growth upwards and laterally (thus tall forehead and bitemporal widening). X-rays may also demonstrate frontal flattening and hypoplasia of the supra-orbital rims, which are recessed below a bulging forehead; bilateral harlequin orbits.

- This type of deformity is a feature of syndromic CSs especially Apert or Crouzon; patients with BCS should have genetic testing.
- The commonest treatment is frontal advancement within the first year – 'floating' advancement of the frontal bone releases the synostosed suture and advances the supra-orbital bar to protect the globe.
- This is followed by mid-face advancement by Le Fort III osteotomy at ~9–12 years of age at which time mid-face growth is complete and the patient is less likely to require secondary surgery.

Alternatively, the whole frontal advancement and Le Fort III advancement can be done as a **monobloc** (Monasterio), but bone grafting is needed and the communications between nasal and cranial cavities lead to a high infection risk.

Secondary **Le Fort I osteotomy** may be required later to correct occlusal problems; less commonly mandibular osteotomy (~18 years of age) may be needed, with risk of causing VPI.

Multiple synostoses cause a variety of skull abnormalities including the following:

- **Turribrachycephaly due to BCS.**
- **Oxycephaly** – a pointed head with recessed forehead that is tilted backwards (parallel to the plane of the nasal dorsum), is due to fusion of the coronal and lambdoidal sutures, sometimes described as a postnatal 'pansynostosis'. There is usual raised ICP and the optic nerve is at risk.
- **Kleeblattschädel** is prenatal 'pansynostosis'.

Kleeblattschädel – a clover leaf skull that results from synostosis of coronal, lambdoidal and metopic sutures with compensatory bulging at the sagittal and squamosal sutures,

leading to a trilobe-shaped skull (and brain). Sutures are often re-opened due to the elevated ICP, and there is bone erosion. It is usually regarded as a type II Pfeiffer syndrome (Cohen, *Am J Med Genet*, 1993).

- Exorbitism and exophthalmos, eyelids may retract behind the globe.
- Marked hydrocephalus and raised ICP.
- Variable degree of mid-face hypoplasia.

Patients with profound mental disability often have a poor prognosis. Treatment consists of urgent cranial vault expansion (within days), and repeat/revisional procedures are usually needed.

LAMBDOID SYNOSTOSIS

This is the **least common synostosis** and leads to synostotic posterior plagiocephaly:

- There is occipital flattening and mastoid bossing on the affected side but no ipsilateral frontal bossing.
- The ear is displaced inferiorly and posteriorly (**skull is trapezoidal in shape**).
- The foramen magnum deviated towards the fused suture on X-ray.

It is a severe progressive deformity, and surgery to remodel occiput (occipital bandeau with barrel staving, or spiral osteotomy) is usually advocated.

DEFORMATIONAL/POSITIONAL PLAGIOCEPHALY (PWS)

Ninety-eight percent of posterior plagiocephaly is due to deformation. It occurs in up to 1 in 300 births including those with very minor plagiocephaly. In simple terms, the deformity is a **'parallelogram head'** ('p' for 'positional' and 'parallelogram') – occipital flattening with ipsilateral frontal bossing; contralateral frontal flattening and occipital bossing (Figure 4.12) (Table 4.1). There is no radiographic

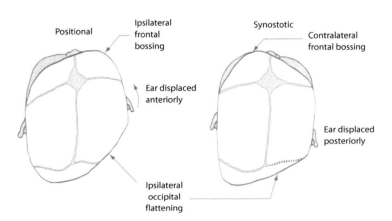

Figure 4.12 Comparison of the features of positional plagiocephaly (parallelogram head) and plagiocephaly due to unilateral lambdoid synostosis. Pushed forward vs. pulled back.

Table 4.1 Features of true synostosis compared to plagiocephaly without synostosis (PWS)

	True synostosis	PWS
Position of ear	Posteroinferior	Anterior
Shape of occiput	Flattened	Flattened
Shape of frontal area	No bossing	Bossing
Overall cranial shape	Trapezoid	Parallelogram

synostosis and the foramen magnum is in the midline (in contrast to lambdoidal synostosis; see above). The ear is positioned anteriorly on the side of occipital flattening; 5% have mental disability. It may be related to

- Restricted movement in utero.
- Moulding in the birth canal. Premature infants have softer skulls.
- Decubitis position/supine sleeping in those with normal shaped skulls at birth. This may be exacerbated by the infant's preference for lying on the flattened side.
- Vertebral abnormalities, **congenital torticollis** or abnormal vision (ocular torticollis).

The deformity is usually **self-correcting** and can be managed by conservative means, but it must be distinguished from plagiocephaly due to unilateral coronal or lambdoidal synostosis – 3D CT reconstruction may be helpful. Once the diagnosis of PWS is established

- Correct underlying factors.
- **Head positioning** of baby at sleep, supervised 'tummy' time. Improvement often comes as the baby sits up more.
- Physiotherapy for the two-thirds with torticollis (see 'Torticollis'). Early treatment gives better results.
- Shaping helmets, e.g. dynamic orthotic cranioplasty – an acrylic head mould with a space into which the head can grow whilst applying mild pressure to prominences.
  - More effective when used early (before 18 months of age).

True lambdoidal synostosis (or PWS failing to respond to conservative treatment) requires operative intervention to release (resect) the fused suture – resected sutures usually show sclerosis rather than true fusion histologically, i.e. true synostosis at this suture is rare.

ACROCEPHALOSYNDACTYLY (ACS) SYNDROMES

Most of these conditions have AD ± variable penetrance except for Carpenter syndrome, which is AR. Some are associated with mutations in the FGF receptor genes. There is some evidence that tyrosine for cysteine substitution in the FGFR2 gene results in uncontrolled signalling. Apert and Pfeiffer syndromes are both AD craniosynostoses with FGFR2 mutations, mid-face hypoplasia and exorbitism,

but can be distinguished by their hands with severe syndactyly, normal hands and broad thumbs and toes, respectively. **Turribrachycephaly** (turret-like) due to BCS is an associated feature.

TEMTAMY AND MCKUSICK CLASSIFICATION (1978)

- Type 1 – Apert syndrome – both Crouzon and Apert have FGFR2 gene mutations on chromosome 10.
- Type 2 – Carpenter syndrome: AR.
- Type 3 – Saethre–Chotzen syndrome. TWIST1 gene mutation; AD. Normal intelligence.
- Type 4 – Goodman syndrome, later removed due to its identification as a variant of type 2.
- Type 5 – Pfeiffer syndrome – FGF2R mutation with AD inheritance; broad thumbs and toes (compared to acrosyndactyly in Apert and normal hand in Crouzon).

There have been several revisions of the classification, and it is generally best to avoid referring to the type/number and use the eponymous syndrome instead. Note that there is another list of acrocephalopolysyndactyly (ACPS) syndromes with different numbers.

CROUZON SYNDROME

Octave Crouzon (1874–1938), a French neurologist, described this in 1912. It is the commonest of the syndromic craniosynostoses; it occurs in 1 in 25,000 live births. It is associated with FGFR2 mutation. It is usually sporadic – the risk of a second affected child is less than 1%; some cases show AD inheritance with variable penetrance. It is sometimes referred to as the Apert–Crouzon syndrome, and some regard it as a variant of Apert but it is more common and there is no syndactyly. There is raised ICP in two-thirds of patients that often have normal intelligence and development (<5% learning disabled compared with Apert patients who are rarely normal).

- Usually there are no digital abnormalities.
- **Mid-face hypoplasia**
  - **Class III malocclusion**. The mandible is short with a distinctive ramus/body ratio (ramus is normal or longer, but the body is significantly shorter) producing the **relative prognathia**.
    - There may be airway problems just after birth.
- High arched palate.
- **Parrot beak nose**.

- Shallow orbits – along with the maxillary hypoplasia leads to ocular proptosis, **exorbitism** that may lead to keratitis.
  - Visual disturbance may be due to nystagmus, strabismus, hypotelorism.
- Conductive hearing impairment due to cranial base abnormalities.
  - Generally less severe than Apert syndrome (Reitsma JH, *Cleft Palate Craniofac J*, 2012), but shows more variability and may show progression with growth.

APERT SYNDROME

Eugene Apert (1868–1940) was a French paediatrician who described the syndrome in 1906 (it had been described by Wheaton in 1894); he was a founding member of the French Eugenics society (not named after him; *eu* good, *genos* birth). It occurs in 1 in 100,000–160,000 live births (four times less common than Crouzon) with most cases being sporadic – advanced paternal age is a risk factor; AD inheritance has been reported. A FGFR2 mutation on chromosome 10q26 has been described. Out of the ACS syndromes (type I), it usually has the most **severe hand deformities** – there is a complex symmetrical **syndactyly** of hands and feet:

- Type I – 'spade hand' – mid-digital hand mass composed of second to fourth digits. The thumb may be broad and have clinodactyly.
- Type II – 'mitten' or 'spoon' hand – thumb joined to mid-digital mass by a simple syndactyly.
- Type III – 'hoof' or 'rosebud' hand – complete osseous fusion between the thumb and ring fingers with simple syndactyly in the fourth web space. Nail synaechia.

Types I–III will also have a short radially deviated thumb and symphalangism. The atypical type of Apert does not have a mid-digital hand mass.

The cranial deformity is most commonly **turribrachycephaly** due to BCS. There is **raised ICP in ~43%**; however, **mental disability** is common (~50%) even in the absence of raised ICP, presumably due to primary brain abnormality, and surgery does little to affect the mental disability. Ventriculoperitoneal shunting is often needed. Other associated features are as follows:

- Paronychial infections during infancy.
- **Acne** especially over forearms.
- Vertebral fusions C5–6, hemivertebrae, butterfly vertebrae.
- Dysplasia of shoulder and elbow.
- Polycystic kidneys and cardiopulmonary abnormalities.
- **Mid-face hypoplasia** (more severe than Crouzon). The craniofacial features are more asymmetric than Crouzon (Turvey TA, 1996).
- Class III malocclusion with prominent mandible, high narrow arched palate; 30% have **CP**.
  - Unusual speech associated with a long soft palate

- Orbital proptosis (exorbitism), **anti-Mongoloid slant** and **hypertelorism**.
  - Some extraocular muscle palsies
- Flat face and short parrot beak nose.
- Low set ears and conductive hearing loss.
- Hydrocephalus 30%.
- Agenesis of the corpus callosum.

Although it shares some features with Crouzon syndrome, the development is different and distinct. The overall craniofacial features may often be more severe in Apert, but the **exorbitism/proptosis** in particular is often more severe in Crouzon. Other differences include

- Normal hands in Crouzon
- Mental retardation more common in Apert
- Conductive hearing loss in Apert

PFEIFFER SYNDROME

This was first described in a family by Rudolf Pfeiffer, a German geneticist in 1964; the family had also been studied by Noack in 1959 but had been classified as Apert. It affects approximately 1 in 100,000. Inheritance is AD, but many arise due to sporadic mutations; FGFR1 and FGFR2 mutations on chromosomes 8 and 10, respectively, have been described. It is also known as ACS type 5. Raised ICP is common, though many have normal intelligence. Some call it 'lower Apert' as opposed to Saethre–Chotzen being 'upper Apert'.

- **Type I 'Classic Pfeiffer'**
  - CS and turribrachycephaly.
  - **Broad thumbs and halluces**, incomplete syndactyly of second web space.
  - **Severe mid-face hypoplasia**, shallow orbits/exorbitism, hypertelorism/anti-mongoloid slant.
  - Cervical fusion 30%.
  - Intelligence and lifespan more likely to be normal.
- **Type II**
  - As above but with ankylosis of elbows and Kleeblattschädel and mental disability.
- **Type III**
  - Ankylosis of elbows but no Kleeblattschädel and mental disability. Types II and III are associated with FGFR2 gene mutations only.

DISTRACTION OSTEOGENESIS

Le Fort III advancement with gradual distraction using internal devices. (Chin M, *Plast Reconstr Surg*, 1997)
The authors describe results of gradual distraction in CS patients (Crouzon, Apert and Pfeiffer) between 4 and 13 years of age.

- Advancement gap of ~10 mm created by Le Fort III osteotomy before distraction was tolerated well with no non-union and increased advancement compared with bone–plate fixation alone.

- Nasal–frontal osteotomies were grafted with cancellous bone.

The distraction devices were custom-made based on cephalometric assessment and were left in place for 6 months. Conventional advancement occurs at 1 mm of advancement per day, whilst the authors describe a technique of **accelerated distraction** with the rate guided by the resistance created in the soft tissues and use of a torque wrench. This increased advancement to ~2 mm/day for ~5 days.

Their results show improvements in exorbitism, class III malocclusion and OSA post-operatively.

- Britto, (*Br J Plast Surg*, 1998) described cases that were advanced at a rate of 1 mm/day initially, and then increased to 2 mm/day after the first week – the aim of this gradual advancement was to reduce the formation of a dead space with the resultant danger of infection.
- Higuera (*J Plast Aesthet Surg*, 2009). Although some surgeons believe that a latent period allows formation of a 'bone haematoma' as a foundation for bone regeneration, the authors demonstrated the successful use of DO in seven paediatric maxillae after a 24-hour latent period, followed by a distraction rate of 2 mm/day. They suggest that Ilizarov's 'ideal' protocol of 3–5 days of latency and distraction at a rate of 2 mm/day does not apply to the paediatric facial skeleton.

SAETHRE–CHOTZEN SYNDROME

This ACS type III was described by Saethre in 1931 and Chotzen in 1932. It occurs in 1 in 25,000–50,000. There is AD inheritance with incomplete penetrance and that has been associated with deletion or mutation of the **TWIST gene on chromosome 7**. Mild mental disability and schizophrenia have been reported.

- Short stature and incomplete syndactyly, mainly second web space
- CS, mainly turribrachycephaly due to **BCS** but may be asymmetric
- Mid-face hypoplasia including CP
- **Low set hairline**, flattened forehead and **ptosis** of the eyelids
- Facial asymmetry with deviation of the nasal septum

CARPENTER SYNDROME

This was described by George Carpenter, a British physician, in 1909 and is distinct from the others by exhibiting **autosomal recessive** pattern inheritance. The diagnosis is made clinically, though it is **often confused for Apert**. It is one of the **least common** of the CS syndromes and affects 1 in 1 million live births in the United States (Table 4.2).

- **CS** – sagittal synostosis, BCS and also lambdoid synostosis in some cases. There may also be acrocephaly or turribrachycephaly depending on the combination of sutures involved, which is often asymmetric.
- Short hands, symbrachydactyly and **preaxial polydactyly of the feet**.
- **Congenital heart defects** in 1/3, VSD/atrial septal defect (ASD).

Patients have short stature, **moderate obesity**, umbilical herniae, cryptorchidism and decreased hip mobility; many have **mental disability**. Treatment aims to treat/prevent raised ICP as well as the airway and eyes.

Table 4.2 Summary of the features of the common types of craniosynostosis

Abnormality	Calvarial deformity	Main operation	Other operations
Bicoronal synostosis Most syndromal synostoses including Crouzon's, Apert's, Pfeiffer's	Turribrachycephaly	Floating frontoparietal advancement and remodelling with supraorbital bar advancement: if raised ICP/exorbitism, perform early (3 months). Alternative is monobloc advancement.	Palatal cleft surgery ~6 months. Surgery to hands <2 years. Le Fort III advancement ages 6–12 years. Le Fort I advancement 12–18 years.
Unilateral coronal synostosis	Plagiocephaly	Bilateral supraorbital bar advancement with frontoparietal remodelling aged 6–9 months.	
Sagittal synostosis Carpenter's syndrome	Scaphocephaly	Sagittal strip craniectomy and frontoparietal remodelling aged 6–9 months.	
Unilateral lambdoidal synostosis	Plagiocephaly	Occipital remodelling aged 6–9 months.	
Metopic synostosis	Trigonocephaly	Supraorbital bar advancement and frontal remodelling aged 6–9 months.	Hypotelorism does not need correction.

PATAU SYNDROME

Klaus Patau, a geneticist, identified the cytogenetic basis of the disease in 1960. The clinical picture had been described in 1656 by Thomas Bartholin (1616–1680), a Danish physician and father of Caspar Bartholin (of the eponymous gland/duct).

Patients with the syndrome have **trisomy 13** (mostly nondisjunction). Prechordal mesoderm midline fusion defects during the first 3 weeks leads to multiple morphological defects of the mid-face, eyes and forebrain. Patients have severe mental disability and a very poor prognosis with almost half dying by 1 month and three-quarters by 1 year. Only six cases have been described as surviving beyond 10 years. For the purposes of genetic counselling, the recurrence rate depends on the genotype.

There is microcephaly with a sloping forehead, wide sagittal sutures and fontanelles and aplasia cutis congenita. There may also be holoprosencephaly (lack of septation of the forebrain – lack of a corpus callosum).

Facial features:

- Eyes – micro/anophthalmia, coloboma and retinal dysplasia
- Mouth – **midline cleft lip (60%–80%)/palate**
- Ears – low set ears with abnormal helices, deafness (sensorineural, conductive), recurrent otitis media
- Hands – camptodactyly and polydactyly of hands/feet, rocker-bottom feet

Other features:

- Coarctation, ASD, patent ductus arteriosus (PDA), VSD, dextroposition
- Males – cryptorchidism, abnormal scrotum, ambiguous genitalia
- Females – bicornuate uterus
- Polycystic kidneys

IV. CRANIOFACIAL ASYMMETRY

Congenital:

- HFM (unilateral or bilateral – still asymmetrical)
- Unilateral coronal synostosis
- Beckwith–Wiedemann syndrome

Acquired:

- Hemifacial atrophy
- Lipodystrophy
- Differential growth due to radiotherapy/surgery for childhood malignancy
- Hypoplasia

PARRY–ROMBERG DISEASE (HEMIFACIAL ATROPHY)

This was described by Parry in 1825 and Henoch and Romberg in 1846. It is characterised by a slowly **progressive atrophy** of the soft tissues of one-half the face that begins before age 20 (5–15) and eventually 'burns' itself out (2–10 years).

- On average, it appears at 9 years of age and lasts 9 years.
- Saxton-Daniels (*Arch Dermatol*, 2010) followed up 27 patients for a mean of 30 years; 89% had some disease activity into adulthood and 56% had permanent sequelae.

The inheritance pattern is unclear; most are sporadic, with some suggestions of AD with variable penetrance. It is more common in females (1.5×) and is unilateral in 95% (R > L).

The presentation is quite variable. The main feature is the slowly progressive hemifacial soft tissue atrophy affecting **skin and subcutaneous tissues** (including tongue and salivary glands) early on, then later muscle and bone. Atrophic tissues show **chronic inflammation** and scarring. The aetiology is poorly understood – some believe that it may be a form of localised scleroderma, possibly viral or due to an abnormal sympathetic system.

- ***En coup de sabre*** deformity – distinctive subcutaneous atrophy in a line from the chin to the malar area, eyebrow and forehead.
- **In the upper face**, soft tissue changes predominate, whilst in the lower face, which is usually involved afterwards, bony changes are more common.

Other features:

- Neurological – seizures, contralateral Jacksonian epilepsy, trigeminal neuralgia and migraine-like headaches
- Skin – **hyperpigmentation** and vitiligo
- Hair – blanching and alopecia
- Teeth – delayed dental eruption and malocclusion
- Eyes (1/3) – enophthalmos, refractive error and heterochromia iridis

There is no cure, and no treatment has been shown to change/halt disease progression. Some have tried immunosuppression such as methotrexate, but RCTs are lacking. Reconstruction is conventionally delayed until the disease is stable for at least 6 months. Choices include

- Fat/dermofat grafts.
  - Some suggest using ADSCs.
  - Hunstad (*Ann Plast Surg*, 2011) injected autologous fat into the face of a 9 year old during the 'active' phase of the disease with good results; in fact, there was some hypertrophy of the treated area as the patient gained weight.
- Onlay grafts or implants for skeletal abnormalities.
  - Stacked Integra and fat grafts with PRP for cheek volume (Ortega VG, *J Craniofac Surg*, 2015).
- TPF, temporalis transfer.
- Free tissue transfer, e.g. ALT, scapular/parascapular – some suggest a degree of overcorrection to allow for (unpredictable) post-operative atrophy, waiting at least 6 months before revising.

- The use of the omentum-free flap for this condition was popularised by Wallace JG (*Br J Plast Surg*, 1979).

Microvascular free flap correction of severe hemifacial atrophy. (Longaker MT, *Plast Reconstr Surg*, 1995)

The average duration of disease in this series was 6.7 years.

The authors used superficial inferior epigastric and parascapular free flaps. Advantages of the latter included a long pedicle with good vessel diameter and a good donor site scar. In addition, the fascia could be extended beyond the de-epithelialised skin paddle whilst achieving primary closure – this can be used to 'feather' the edge of the contour augmentation.

Two-thirds of patients required revision, e.g. debulking/augmentation/recontouring, but only after 6 months.

HEMIFACIAL MACROSOMIA

HFM patients may have a variety of functional problems, e.g. airway, feeding, speech, eyes and facial growth. A multidisciplinary team is important.

The OMENS classification of hemifacial microsomia. (Vento AR, *Cleft Palate Craniofac J*, 1991)

A grading system of structures involved in HFM:

- **Orbital** dystopia (includes maxilla, zygomatic bone hypoplasia, etc.)
- Mandibular hypoplasia, cleft lip and/or CP
- **Ear** defects – abnormalities of ear bones, external ear and tympanic membrane, preauricular skin tags
- **Nerve** – facial nerve deficits (muscles of facial expression with variable agenesis)
- **Soft tissue** abnormalities – hypoplastic muscles of mastication, hypoplastic parotid, macrostomia

The incidence of HFM is ~1 in 5600 births; it is the commonest craniofacial anomaly (cleft lip and palate is the commonest facial anomaly). It is usually unilateral (~90%). It must be distinguished from TCS, which has the following:

- Loss of the medial lower eyelashes.
- **Deformity is symmetrical**, whereas in bilateral HFM, it is usually asymmetrical.
- Well-defined pattern of inheritance (AD) with a genetic basis on chromosome 5, but bilateral HFM has no inheritance pattern, being mostly sporadic (possibly due to stapedial artery thrombosis). The risk of an affected parent having an affected child is 3%.
- TCS is a consortium of abnormalities associated with clefts 6, 7 and 8, whereas HFM is the result of a **Tessier number 7 facial cleft**.

AETIOLOGY – THEORIES

- 'Mesodermal insufficiency' (Stark RB, *Plast Reconstr Surg*, 1962).

- Vascular insult to the arches (**stapedial artery**) – evidence from haemorrhage and haematoma (Poswillo D, *Oral Surg Oral Med Oral Pathol*, 1973) and thalidomide-induced hemifacial-like defects in **monkeys**. This is currently the most favoured; it helps to explain how the deformity does not fit exactly the pattern of the **first and second arches**.

Goldenhar syndrome is essentially (some but not necessarily all the features of) HFM with certain additional features such as epibulbar dermoids, (cervical) vertebral anomalies, colobomata as well as renal and cardiac problems. Most cases of Goldenhar are sporadic with variable severity.

Less than 5% of HFM patients have the other features of Goldenhar, and thus it is probably better to view **HFM as a feature of the syndrome**. A slightly different take is that HFM and Goldenhar are moderately severe and most severe forms of a broader condition called oculo-auriculo-vertebral spectrum (OAVS) – the mildest form is called OAV disorder.

MANDIBULAR HYPOPLASIA

This is the cornerstone of HFM and, in general, the severity of this reflects the severity of other associated abnormalities.

PROZANSKY CLASSIFICATION OF MANDIBULAR HYPOPLASIA

- Type 1 — All parts present but hypoplastic
- Type 2a — Condyle articulates as hinge
- Type 2b — No condyle
- Type 3 — Mandible ramus absent

The a and b subtypes are part of the Kaban modification. Types 1 and 2a can be treated with distraction, whilst the others need a costochondral graft – transfer of a growth centre is useful. However, sometimes the cartilage side grows more rapidly causing asymmetry the other way. In 2b, the condyle is malformed and not in the plane of the contralateral side, the TMJ is not functional and there is restricted hinge-like movement only.

Isolated microtia as a marker for unsuspected hemifacial microsomia. (Keogh IJ, *Arch Otolaryngol Head Neck Surg*, 2007)

The authors examined 100 patients with isolated microtia who had further examination to determine their OMENS score. They found that 40 patients fit into the diagnosis of HFM (cranial nerve deficits, mandibular asymmetry and hearing loss were the commonest) and suggested that isolated microtia is a marker for HMF, that they represent different points on a spectrum of expression of the same phenomenon.

Surgical options during childhood include cleft lip/palate surgery (CPO is most common) and

- O – see 'Skeletal surgery'.
- M – mandibular advancement/distraction or reconstruction (if severely hypoplastic).

- E – hearing device; excision of accessory auricles; microtia reconstruction.
- N – need to import muscle and nerve with two-stage facial reanimation.
- S – commissuroplasty.

There is a dilemma of sorts in that early corrective surgery may cause disordered growth in the future – there is growth of the globe/eye until about 5 years of age, and growth of the mandible and maxilla continues until approximately 18 years of age and is driven primarily by the secondary dentition. Multiple surgeries increase the risks of complications. The aim is to encourage growth whilst preventing functional deformities, and to ideally correct deformities when growth is complete ~16–18 years of age.

- **Infancy** – treatment during this time usually consists of crisis intervention, e.g. eye, airway, feeding and speech. Early correction of deformity may be needed or possible – e.g. remove auricular appendages, correction of cleft or orbits.
- **Childhood** (time of mixed dentition).
  - Prevent secondary deformity, e.g. **distraction,** orthodontics or costochondral grafts in Prozanky 3 (overgrowth may occur later)
  - Deformity correction, e.g. distraction, orthodontics
- **Adolescence/maturity** – definitive correction of deformity (both soft tissues and skeleton) delayed until skeletal maturity.
  - Osteotomy, e.g. zygomatic
  - Distraction, e.g. Le Fort I
  - Soft tissue augmentation – fat transfer, seems most effective in the younger age group
  - Onlay grafts – autologous (costochondral, calvarial) or alloplastics (Medpor®, MMA, hydroxyapatite) for non-load bearing areas

SKELETAL SURGERY

Surgery is usually delayed until skeletal maturity; early surgery does not seem to reduce teasing significantly due to the other deformities.

- Fronto-orbital advancement for frontal flattening
- Correction of orbital dystopia
- Le Fort III osteotomy used to correct exorbitism
- Le Fort I maxillary advancement osteotomy and/or sagittal split osteotomy to correct cant and restore bite.

Skeletal surgery has significant complications:

- Airway compromise, haemorrhage
- Nerve injury
- Non-/mal-union
- Trauma to tooth roots
- VPI
- Malocclusion

Skeletal surgery should be allowed to settle before soft tissue reconstruction is contemplated. **DO** techniques are being increasingly used instead of vascularised bone reconstruction (as long as the condyle is present). The phases include corticotomy/osteotomy, **latency** (5–7 days, for callus), **distraction**/activation (1–2 mm per day vs. 0.25 mm four times a day) and **consolidation** (8 weeks, for bone mineralisation). There is also **distraction histiogenesis** – soft tissue elongates and there is less tendency for it to shrink back. It is a major undertaking but is the only technique that offers lengthening whilst also dealing with soft tissue contractures and misalignments. Distractors may be internal or external, depending on the space available for the device as well as the vectors of pull required. Motorised distractors offer 'continuous' distraction. Although complications are not uncommon (30%), most are relatively minor. Pin tract problems are almost inevitable.

Optimising the rate of distraction is important as

- Too slow leads to premature fusion.
- Too fast leads to non-union – eradicate any infection, then options include recompression or bone transport.
- The rate is adjusted according to the bone formation radiologically, or to symptoms such as nerve palsies.
- Some question the need for the latent period; waiting too long leads to consolidation.

It is very reliable in the craniofacial skeleton but should be used cautiously before the age of 18 months as the bones may be too soft. Some suggest that mandibular distraction should be timed to coincide with time of rapid maxillary growth ~6 years of age (Cousley RR, *Br J Plast Surg,* 1997).

ZONES IN DISTRACTION OSTEOGENESIS

- Zone I – fibrous tissue or fibrous interzone in the centre, highly organised parallel collagen strands with fibroblasts
- Zone II – extending bone formation or primary mineralisation front or transitional zone, either side of zone I, with osteoblasts on bone spicules
- Zone III – remodelling zone, with osteoclasts
- Zone IV – mature bone, thicker spicules

The fibrovascular bridge becomes ossified by tension forces into new bone by intramembranous ossification. If there is excessive motion, chondrocytes form and fibrocartilage non-union occurs. It takes about 8 months for the new bone to be close to (90%) mature bone in structure.

HYPERPLASTIC CONDITIONS

Fibrous Dysplasia

This condition is characterised by accumulation of immature woven type bone; it was described by von Recklinghausen in 1891. There are monostotic (70%–80%) or polyostotic forms (generally more severe and presents earlier). The aetiology is unknown. von Recklinghausen (1833–1910) was a German pathologist who studied under Virchow, and had many achievements; he famously disagreed with Koch's theory that the mycobacterium *Bacillus* was the cause of tuberculosis.

It is related to Gs protein mutation (of α-subunit) causing osteoblast and osteoclast activity; there is fibrous formation in the medulla of bones particularly the mandible and maxilla. The disease presents as bony swellings in the under 30 year age group with some pain.

- Disfigurement.
- Local symptoms due to bony overgrowth.
  - Neurological symptoms including compression of optic, facial, trigeminal nerves, etc.
  - Deafness and blindness
  - Dental problems
- Pathological fractures may occur.

In addition,

- Active fibrous dysplasia may show elevated serum alkaline phosphatase and urine hydroxyproline (indicating bone turnover). The X-ray appearance is usually distinctive enough to make the diagnosis – ground glass appearance, expansion/deformity; MRI may provide additional information including malignant change.
- **(McCune)–Albright's disease** is fibrous dysplasia combined with patchy skin pigmentation and precocious puberty (due to pituitary tumours). Inheritance is AD. Patients also have short neck and short metacarpals/metatarsals due to early epiphyseal closure.
- **Cherubism** is a familial form (AD) of polyostotic fibrous dysplasia that presents early and affects the maxilla and mandible. It may regress (after puberty), but some form of corrective surgery especially for dental or aesthetic considerations is appropriate in certain cases. Some view it as a giant cell granuloma rather than fibrous dysplasia. There is an association with mutation of the SH3BP2 gene that activates osteoclasts. It is rare with about 300 cases described in the literature.
  - A family with several affected members was described by Jones WA in 1933.
- There is a 0.5% incidence of **osteosarcoma**, which may be increased by radiotherapy.

It is self-limiting (by about the patient's 30s) but will not regress. The main options in treatment include curettage (20%–30% recurrence) or, preferably, total excision and reconstruction. Bone grafts placed in areas of disease tend to become replaced by fibrous dysplasia. Nerve decompression may be needed.

Medical treatment includes IV bisphosphonates (pamidronate), with calcium and phosphate supplements, and vitamin D. This reduces bone pain and may reduce bony fibrosis, but the use of bisphosphonates is associated with severe complication of osteonecrosis.

BECKWITH–WIEDEMANN SYNDROME

This overgrowth disorder with unknown aetiology was described by Beckwith (US paediatric pathologist) in 1963 and Wiedemann (German geneticist) in 1964; 85% of cases are sporadic (slightly increased in assisted reproduction); other cases are familial but with mixed patterns of inheritance. Mutations of chromosome 11p15.5 have been described. It affects about 1 in 15,000. It features variable combinations of

- Metopic synostosis, microcephaly and large prominent eyes, **pits/grooves in earlobe**.
- **Macroglossia** (90%), gaping mouth, prognathism – it often becomes less noticeable with age; some perform reduction surgery but the optimal time is unknown.
- **Large body size** (which may affect one side of the body only) and visceromegaly, hemihypertrophy of the face may require surgery.
- **Midline abdominal wall defects** – omphalocoele, umbilical hernia or diastasis recti.
- **Neonatal hypoglycaemia**, which may be profound, leading to brain damage if untreated.

Most patients do not have all these features; some recommend that two of the five common features (in bold font above) suggest the diagnosis (DeBaun MR, *Am J Hum Genet*, 2002).

Patients do have an **increased risk of cancer**; ~10% develop cancer with Wilm's tumour being the most common. Screening with ultrasound every 3–4 months is suggested. Other than this, the prognosis is very good.

Other causes of hyperplastic lesions:

- **Neurofibromatosis** – 1 in 2500; sporadic or AD with variable penetrance. Type 1 is related to a mutation on chromosome 17, whilst type 2 has a mutation on chromosome 22.
- **Gorlin's syndrome** – affects 1 in 100,000 demonstrating AD inheritance. There are multiple BCCs with cysts of the jaw and pits of the palm and soles. Typically these patients have hypertelorism, widened nose, frontal bossing and calcification of the falx cerebri.

HYPERTELORISM

Tessier introduced the term **orbital hypertelorism** (true lateralisation of the whole orbit, i.e. medial and lateral wall, which is usually due to failure of medialisation). See Table 4.3. Telecanthus is the increased intercanthal distance (where the orbit may be normal). It is a physical finding and not a disease/syndrome by itself.

- Pseudohypertelorism is the increased distance between the medial walls but normally spaced lateral walls – this may occur with midline

Table 4.3 Tessier classification of orbital hypertelorism

Degree	Interocular distance (mm)	Standard deviations more than normal
1	30–34	2–4
2	35–40	4–8
3	>40	>8

tumours or encephalocoeles. Otherwise known as interorbital hypertelorism (van der Meulen) or bony telecanthus.

- Pseudotelecanthus is the illusion of telecanthus due to a flat nasal bridge or medial epicanthal folds.

Tan and Mulliken classification of hypertelorism (*Plast Reconstr Surg*, 1997) based on cause and anatomy.

- **Frontonasal malformation** (median cleft syndrome) is most common.
  - Widow's peak, short broad nose and short upper lip.
  - Symmetrical hypertelorism/telecanthus (interorbital).
  - Amblyopia and encephalocoele.
- **Craniofrontonasal dysplasia** (Cohen syndrome), the second most common, is a combination of coronal synostosis with frontonasal dysplasia, hypertelorism, bifid nasal tip and a broad nasal bridge.
  - EFNB1 gene (ephrin-B1 protein) mutation on X chromosome; affecting females more frequently and more severely affected (unusual for an X-linked disorder).
  - Mid-face hypoplasia with high arched palate (scaphomaxillism) and/or V median CP.
  - Patients have unilateral coronal synostosis with plagiocephaly, corpus callosum dysgenesis and **characteristic frizzy hair**.
  - Extremity deformities, e.g. Sprengel deformity, syndactyly and **nail pitting** – disordered deposition of large keratin filaments.
- **Craniofacial clefts** – especially paramedian Tessier (3–11, 2–12) – asymmetric orbital hypertelorism.
- **Encephalocoeles** – interorbital (usually) hypertelorism.
- **Miscellaneous groups,** e.g. syndromic CS (Apert, Pfeiffer).
  - Noonan (1 in 1000–2500) with hypertelorism, chest deformities, short stature and cardiac disease in 50%.

MANAGEMENT

Medialisation of orbit by surgery:

- **Facial bipartition** (removal of central bony segment) for less severe problems; it narrows the entire mid-face and rotates orbits, affects upper dental arch. In syndromic cases such as Apert, this approach also allows mid-face advancement.
- **Box osteotomy** (rectangular osteotomy around each orbit, then remove/add bone around as needed) – allows a greater degree of medialisation and can correct vertical and horizontal problems, i.e. good for asymmetric anomalies. It does not affect dentition.

The ideal timing is said to be about 9–11 years, after eruption of the permanent incisors and canines. This is affected by functional issues such as management of airway, eyes, clefts/encephalocoeles.

Craniofrontonasal dysplasia. (Orr DJA, *Br J Plast Surg*, **1997)**

The article describes 10 patients treated at the Oxford craniofacial unit (all females) with forehead advancement and remodelling for synostosis within the first year. Hypertelorism was treated by facial bipartition and excision of paramedian bone and ethmoid sinuses between 4 and 9 years of age – it is a cosmetic procedure in principle, thus not urgent, and at this age, the patient may understand the deformity and the need for surgery.

The skin is allowed to re-drape, and a medial canthoplasty is performed a year later to remove any residual excess skin/epicanthal folds (Mustardé canthoplasty – jumping man). There was no subsequent impairment of mid-facial growth in these cases.

MISCELLANEOUS CONDITIONS AFFECTING THE HEAD AND NECK

Binder syndrome

This was described by Binder in 1962 as dysostosis maxillonasalis in the original German paper. This has an unknown aetiology but is familial in 15%. Patients have normal intelligence; there is maxillonasal dysostosis with mid-face hypoplasia, i.e. the structures around the nose are poorly formed.

- Decreased vertical height of maxilla, absent anterior nasal spine, class III malocclusion
- Short, flat nose and **short columella**, acute nasolabial angle, perialar flatness
- Convex upper lip with wide but shallow philtrum
- Vertebral abnormalities in 50%

Treatment can be difficult but usually includes nasal augmentation and Le Fort II advancement osteotomy.

Klippel–Feil sequence

Maurice Klippel (1858–1942) and Andre Feil were French neurologists who co-authored a publication (1912) describing a French tailor who appeared to have no neck. Feil's thesis (1919) was important in moving public opinion away from regarding congenital deformities or 'monstrous births' as being the result of a moral failing or regression.

This condition occurs with an incidence of about 1 in 40,000 and is due to a mutation on chromosome 8q, inherited in an AD manner with variable penetrance. It is characterised by the failure of segmentation of the cervical spine, causing **cervical fusion** (most commonly C2–3), a short neck with limited movement, congenital scoliosis, Sprengel's deformity and a low hairline in 40%. It can be a feature of syndromes such as Goldenhar; ~1/3 have hearing loss whilst 1/5 have CP. AR inheritance has been reported with C5–6 fusion.

Classification

There is a contraindication to contact sports in Feil types I and II (Samartzis DD, *Spine*, 2006).

- Type I – a single congenitally fused cervical segment

- Type II – multiple non-contiguous, congenitally fused segments
- Type III – multiple contiguous, congenitally fused cervical segments

Aplasia cutis congenita

The cause is unknown, though some have a familial component. It is usually an isolated defect, though it may be multifocal in 25%. It may be associated with anomalies of lip/palate, fingers, trunk as well as the nervous system, e.g. hydrocephalus and myelomeningocele. It usually affects the scalp, but may affect the limbs or other regions.

Typically there is an absence of the midline vertex tissues to a variable depth, presenting as a sharply demarcated patch usually <2 cm in diameter. At birth, it may already have healed with scarring (atrophic, paper-like scar with alopecia) or remain eroded to a variable depth and occasionally involves the dura or meninges with exposed brain. In certain cases, it may lead to haemorrhage from sagittal sinus bleeding or even death, but in the majority, it is simple and heals spontaneously with dressings, e.g. SSD, to prevent desiccation. There is usually no rush to operate.

Hurler syndrome (gargoylism)

Gertrude Hurler (1889–1965), a paediatrician from the then East Prussia, described this syndrome whilst training in 1919. This is a mucopolysaccharidosis (type 1H) with a build-up of dermatan and heparan sulphate due to deficiency of α-L-iduronidase, which is a **lysosomal enzyme** that degrades mucopolysaccharides. There is a defective IDUA gene on chromosome and inheritance is AR.

Patients are apparently healthy at birth (may have herniae) but develop typical signs and symptoms (coarse features/prominent forehead – **gargoylism**, skeletal deformities, hepatosplenomegaly, corneal clouding, short stature, progressive mental disability) by 6–24 months and are usually dead by 10 years (due to obstructive airway disease or respiratory infections).

Laronidase (recombinant enzyme replacement, IV once a week) may help to reduce pain and non-neurological symptoms. Haematopoietic stem cell transplantation (HSCT) and umbilical cord blood transplantation before deterioration are among the best treatments and may halt degeneration, but these are high-risk procedures and do not offer an actual cure. Gene therapy is one for the future.

V. GENIOPLASTY

ASSESSMENT

- Medical history.
- Previous orthodontic history.
- Dentition – unerupted teeth, e.g. in those under 15 years of age may be at risk during osteotomies. The elderly will have relatively poor bone stock and are also poor candidates for osteotomy.

- Occlusion – orthognathic surgery should be considered for those with abnormalities of occlusion.
- Rickett's E line – a line between soft tissue pogonion (most anterior point of chin) and nose tip should lie just anterior to the lips with the upper lip approximately twice as far from the line compared with the lower lip.
- Chin–nose relationship.
- Soft tissue.

IMAGING

- Orthopantomogram
- Cephalogram

CEPHALOMETRICS

Cephalometry is the measurement of the human head by imaging (Broadbent, 1931) and is used to evaluate dentofacial properties and clarify the anatomic basis for problems such as malocclusion. For example, if there is significant maxillary retrusion, then formal orthognathics are indicated rather than genioplasty.

Cephalometric radiographs use a cephalostat – a device that keeps the head in a stable horizontal position whilst the images are being acquired. Cephalometric landmarks of relevance include

- Frankfurt plane – porion (highest part of EAM) and suborbitale (lowest part of orbit).
- Pogonion – the most forward projecting part of the chin.
- Menton – the lowest part of mandibular symphysis.
- Subspinale – the deepest point on the premaxillary outer contour between the anterior nasal spine and central incisor.
- Supramentale – the deepest point between pogonion and incisor.
- Radix is the area where the nose meets the brow.
  - Nasion is the deepest part of the radix and lies at the apex of the nasofrontal angle, the nasofrontal junction or the anterior point on the frontonasal suture. The vertical level of the nasion is the take-off and should be 6 mm above the medial canthus or at the level of the supratarsal fold.

OSSEOUS GENIOPLASTY/CHIN OSTEOTOMY

Preserving soft tissue attachments helps to reduce resorption (Figure 4.13).

- **Sliding** – for sagittal projection deficiency. Genioglossus and geniohyoid are still attached to the inferior segment. More extensive advancement may need a stepladder genioplasty, which is a two-tiered advancement.
- **Jumping** – the fragment is placed anterior to the symphysis as an onlay similar to an implant; it improves the sagittal projection whilst decreasing the height of the lower third.

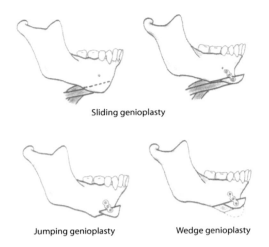

Sliding genioplasty

Jumping genioplasty   Wedge genioplasty

Figure 4.13 Common types of genioplasty. Sliding genioplasty, jumping genioplasty and wedge genioplasty.

- **Interpositional** – with bone graft (or hydroxyapatite) to advance chin as well as increase lower face height.
- **Wedge** – for height reduction, which will result in a degree of soft tissue **ptosis**. The segment between two parallel osteotomies is resected.
- **Reduction** – for sagittal and vertical excess.
- **Centralising** or asymmetric genioplasty – to correct asymmetry.

The average satisfaction rating for osteotomy (90%–95%) is slightly higher than for implant genioplasty (85%–90%).

IMPLANT GENIOPLASTY

Implants cannot usually correct deficiencies of vertical height as they are generally placed over the pogonion for mild/moderate deficiencies of projection. Materials such as ivory, acrylic and precious metals are of historical interest only. In general, implants are only suitable for augmenting **<5 mm**; greater degrees of augmentation are best treated with osteotomy. The ratio of soft tissue response to skeletal change is 0.66, i.e. a 1 cm thick implant will usually result in 0.66 cm soft tissue projection.

- Synthetic – **silicone is the most popular**, Medpor® (porous high-density polyethylene that allows a degree of tissue ingrowth, which seems to reduce infection rates and reduces capsule formation). Materials such as nylon mesh or expanded PTFE (both soft) or hydroxyapatite (hard) are not commonly used.
- Biological – autologous bone, e.g. calvarial, rib or chondral cartilage or allogenic – irradiated cartilage, etc.

According to Pitanguy (1968), the principles for implant augmentation are to position the implant at the lowest point of the mandible and that it must be immobilised. Implants can be fixed with screws, Mitek or sutures, though some say that fixation can be avoided if the pocket is precisely made and closed. Implants can be positioned via

- Submental exposure (extra-oral), which allows precise placement with less risk to the mental nerve but leaves an external scar.
- Intra-oral route (incision 1 cm above gingivolabial sulcus) leaves no scar and supposedly has similar infection rates to extra-oral placement. However, it is more difficult to place implants accurately in this way; often they end up being too high.

The choice between supraperiosteal or subperiosteal dissection is controversial; most agree that supraperiosteal positioning reduces bone resorption under the implant.

COMPLICATIONS

- Haematoma (rare).
- Infection – uncommon, <3% for osteotomies, <5% for implants but may need to be removed.
  - If an implant is removed and not replaced, then either the soft tissue needs to be repositioned to reduce chin pad ptosis or an osseous genioplasty is needed to advance the bone to fill the tissue void.
- Nerve injury ~5% – usually a neuropraxia of the mental nerve leading to lower lip paraesthesia (and possible drooling). It can be caused by an implant that is too large. Permanent damage is rare.

5

Breast

A. BREAST AUGMENTATION

I. RELEVANT ANATOMY AND EMBRYOLOGY

EMBRYOLOGICAL ASPECTS

- Breast tissue comes from the mammary ('milk') ridge from the axilla to the groin, which develops from the ectoderm during the fifth week. Most parts of this ridge disappear, except for the small portion around the fourth intercostal space that persists and penetrates the underlying mesenchyme (10 to 14 weeks). Accessory nipples (2%) can lie anywhere along the ridge but are most commonly inframammary. No further development occurs until puberty.
- As a result of its ectodermal origin and its invagination into the underlying mesenchyme, the breast tissue is contained within a fascial envelope, the superficial and deep layers of the superficial fascia.
  - Thelarche – oestrogens stimulate duct and stromal growth whilst progesterone stimulates lobular growth.
- The breast parenchyma is penetrated by fibrous attachments – suspensory ligaments of Cooper – which join the two layers of the superficial fascia and extend to the dermis of the overlying skin and the deep pectoral fascia.
  - Sir Astley Paston Cooper (1768–1841) was an English surgeon and anatomist. He once stole his neighbours' corpses for dissection.

TANNER STAGE

Tanner staging is most commonly used; they do not correspond to chronological ages but rather are maturity stages.

- Stage 1 – nipple only – there is no glandular tissue and the skin follows the breast.
- Stage 2 – nipple and small breast bud form with some glandular tissue and areolar widening.

- Stage 3 – further enlargement and **breast develops beyond borders of the areola**.
- Stage 4 – enlargement of areola and increased pigment, **double mound** appearance.
- Stage 5 – final adolescent development and smooth contour.

Breast development occurs mainly at puberty at ~10–12 years of age, as a result of hypothalamic gonadotrophin releasing hormones (GRHs) stimulating the anterior pituitary to release LH and FSH:

- FSH stimulates the ovaries to produce oestrogens that causes proliferation of breast ductal epithelium.
- Ovarian follicle maturation – production and release of oestrogen and progesterone that completes breast development.

PREGNANCY

There are various hormones involved – oestrogen, progesterone, placental lactogen, prolactin, chorionic gonadotrophin – that cause breast ductal, lobular and alveolar growth.

- First trimester – oestrogen causes ductal sprouting and lobular growth (thus the breast enlarges) and the nipple areolar complex darkens.
- Second trimester – progestins cause lobular colostrum production/accumulation.
- Third trimester – at the time of delivery, the breast may be up to three times the normal size due to a combination of vascular engorgement, epithelial proliferation and colostrum accumulation.
- Delivery – withdrawal of placental lactogen and breast is now predominantly influenced by prolactin.

After delivery, the nursing infant stimulates production of pituitary hormones.

- Prolactin (anterior pituitary) causes milk production and secretion.
- Oxytocin (posterior pituitary) causes breast contraction and milk ejection.

Involution will begin about 3 months after breastfeeding ceases with regression of extralobular stroma.

AGEING

With menopause, there is loss of glandular tissue that is largely replaced by fat.

BREAST SURGICAL ANATOMY

The breast gland is formed by a collection of lobules (functional units each with hundreds of acini) draining into 16–24 lactiferous ducts to the nipple via a central collecting duct. The breast is supported by a fascial layer, and the ligaments of Cooper that penetrate from the deeper layers of this fascia into breast parenchyma and attenuation/degeneration will lead to ptosis.

- **Montgomery glands** (12–15) are sebaceous-type glands, and their openings on the periphery of the areola form Montgomery tubercles (also called Morgagni tubercles – Giovanni Battista Morgagni was the first to describe the surface feature). William Featherstone Montgomery (1779–1859) was an Irish obstetrician.
- **Wuringer's septum** (1998) is a horizontal septum from medial to lateral at the level of the fifth rib. It is well vascularised and has been used to support breast reduction pedicles (Hamdi M, *Plast Reconstr Surg*, 2009).

The nerve supply to the nipple comes from the T4 intercostal nerves; the lateral cutaneous branch pierces the deep fascia at about the midaxillary level to lie in the pectoral fascia up to the midclavicular line where it runs forwards to the nipple via the parenchyma. The breast on the whole is supplied by T3–5 dermatomes, whilst the lower fibres of the cervical plexus/supraclavicular nerves supply the upper and lateral breast.

BLOOD SUPPLY

- Internal thoracic – 60% – the largest perforator is usually the second.
- Lateral thoracic – 30%.
- Intercostal vessels – 10%.

The nipple gets its blood supply from the subdermal plexus as well as the parenchyma.

VENOUS DRAINAGE

The main venous drainage does not accompany the arteries – it is mostly provided by the superficial system.

- Internal mammary veins
- Axillary vein
- Intercostal veins
- Superficial veins draining upwards to communicate with neck veins and medially to communicate with internal mammary veins

LYMPHATIC DRAINAGE

- Predominantly to the axilla (breast–central node–apical node–supraclavicular), but 3%–20% to the internal mammary chain
  - Level I – lateral to pectoralis minor, which arises from the third to sixth ribs to insert to coracoid process. The pectoralis minor is innervated by the medial pectoral nerve, which is more lateral than the lateral pectoral nerve on the chest wall.
  - Level II – beneath the pectoralis minor.
  - Level III – medial to the pectoralis minor (III–II–I from superior to inferior).
  - Rotter's nodes – interpectoral nodes between the pectoralis major and minor, often regarded as level II. The clinical significance is uncertain; they are not routinely removed but may be the site of tumour spread.
  - Josef Rotter (1857–1924) was a German surgeon.

Rotter's node metastases. (Cody HS, *Ann Surg*, 1984)
Interpectoral nodes were sampled at the end of 500 consecutive modified radical mastectomies (MRMs) for early-stage breast cancer. Nodes were found in 73% and tumour metastasis in 2.6% of all (patients/4% of all with nodes sampled) 8.2% and 0.5% of axillary node positive and negative patients, respectively, had interpectoral metastasis.

Analysis of metastatic involvement of interpectoral (Rotter's) lymph nodes related to tumor location, size, grade, and hormone receptor status in breast cancer. (Vrdoljak DV, *Tumori*, 2005)
A total of 172 breast cancer patients had their Rotter's nodes removed as part of their surgery; 77% had identifiable Rotter's nodes, with tumour in 20% of these; 30% of T3 tumours had positive Rotter's nodes; 35% and 4% of axillary node positive and negative patients, respectively, had interpectoral metastasis. The authors suggest that these nodes should be routinely removed.

II. BREAST IMPLANTS

- 1895 – first breast augmentation procedure carried out in Germany by Vincent Czerny (1842–1916) – a giant lipoma from the back was transferred into a breast that required surgery. Apparently it was smaller and firmer but seemed to have been otherwise successful at 6 months.
- 1945 – Japanese prostitutes inject liquid silicone into breasts to satisfy American servicemen clients.
- 1962 – Frank Gerow and Thomas Cronin were the first to implant what became Dow Corning's silastic mammary prosthesis. The first patient was Timmie Jean Lindsey, who still has her original implants. She agreed to have the operation in exchange for free otoplasties.
- 1992 – Moratorium.
- 2006 – Final re-approval.

GENERAL CONSIDERATIONS

The silicone used in implants is polydimethyl siloxane, a polymer of silicon that is not the same as elemental silicon (Si). Silicone is also found in heart valves, joint prostheses, IV cannulae/syringes and baby bottle nipples. The foreign body reaction to implants is not immune-mediated; no specific antibodies have been detected yet.

About 100,000–150,000 women in the United Kingdom and ~1–2 million women in the United States (~1%) are estimated currently to have breast implants. It is the second most common cosmetic surgical procedure in the United States after liposuction. Ten year PMA data show a 15%–24% reoperation rate (saline and silicone).

The choice of implant depends on many factors:

- Preference of patient and surgeon
- Breast characteristics – skin quality, volume required, etc.

Breast milk contamination and silicone implants. (Semple JL, *Plast Reconstr Surg*, 1998)

There have been reports of abnormal oesophageal motility in children breastfed by women with implants (Levine JJ, *JAMA*, 1994). This study measured elemental silicon (used as proxy measure for silicone) in the breast milk of patients with and without implants and found them to be the same. In fact, silicon was 10 times higher in cows' milk and even higher in infant formula. Grain, rice and beer also have high levels of silicon.

Kjoller (*Pediatrics*, 1998) conducted a register-based follow-up study and found higher rates of oesophageal disorders in the children of mothers with breast implants (939), but the same excess was found in those born before the implant surgery as those who were born afterwards.

SILICONE IMPLANT CONTROVERSY

- 1982 – van Nunen (*Arthritis Rheum*, 1982) links silicone breast implants with connective tissue disease (CTD) for the first time, in three patients, but the data are largely anecdotal.
- 1984 – Stern vs. Dow Corning. Patient Maria Stern's claim that her autoimmune disease is caused by her implants is upheld by the court.
- 1988 – US Food and Drug Administration (FDA) classifies implants as Class III, i.e. manufacturers need to show that they are safe and effective to keep them on the market.
- 1991 – Hopkins vs. Dow Corning. Marianne Hopkins awarded US$7.34 million for mixed CTD that the court believed was related to her ruptured implants.
  - Ramasastry (*Plast Reconstr Surg*, 1991). Administering a chemical carcinogen caused a high cancer incidence in rats; placing an unexpanded tissue expander reduced the cancer incidence, whilst expanding the expander led to an even lower cancer incidence.

- 1992 – FDA ban on silicone implants with onus on manufacturers to prove safety despite lack of evidence that implants cause CTD. The argument was that as implants offered cosmetic advantages only, no risks would be tolerated. Only women undergoing breast reconstruction are allowed to receive silicone implants, and as part of a scientific study.
  - Dow Corning leaves silicone breast implant business along with Bristol-Myers-Squibb and Bioplasty.
  - Hennekens (*JAMA*, 1996). The relative risk of CTD in patients with breast implants was said to be 1.24. The cohort was big (395, 543), but a major flaw in methodology was **self-reporting**.
- 1994 – 30,000 lawsuits filed against Dow Corning and 440,000 women register for class action settlement. Manufacturers agree to pay US$4.25 billion to women with breast implants as part of a class action settlement. Those entitled to compensation were those who had, or developed within 30 years, any of 10 CTDs providing the symptoms began or worsened after the implants were placed. These ranged from scleroderma to non-specific aches and pains; even husbands were entitled to compensation for emotional suffering.
  - Medical devices agency (DoH) concludes no reason for a ban.
  - Mayo Clinic study (Gabriel SE, *N Engl J Med*, 1994) found the rates of CTD were comparable to control, but was criticised for accepting funding from the American Society of Plastic and Reconstructive Surgery/Plastic Surgery Educational Foundation, which receive contributions from Dow Corning and other implant manufacturers.
- 1995 – Dow Corning files for bankruptcy protection; Dow Chemical ordered to pay US$14.1 million to one patient by a jury in Nevada.
  - FDA recognises body of evidence against a link to mixed CTD but maintains ban due to potential local complications.
  - Nurses' health study – no increased risk (Sanchez-Guerrero J, *N Engl J Med*, 1995).
  - Su (*Plast Reconstr Surg*, 1995). Placing a silicone implant and administering a chemical carcinogen in rat led to a 17% cancer incidence; without an implant, the carcinogen alone caused a 50% cancer incidence.
- 1998 – UK Independent Review Group on Silicone Gel Breast Implants (Sturrock R) publishes review and finds no link.
  - Nyren (*Br Med J*, 1998) found no difference in 7442 augmentation vs. 3353 breast reduction patients.
  - Miller (*Plast Reconstr Surg*, 1998). Rheumatological markers such as RF, ANA as well as CRP and ASO titres did not increase after implants (up to 13 years).
- 2006 – the restriction for the United States was lifted by the FDA in November, but patients had to be carefully monitored.
  - Post-approval Core studies.

The moratorium imposed additional studies that showed that implants were medically safe but that there was a high reoperation rate – 17% for saline implants, higher for silicone implants. **The FDA estimated in 2011 that 20% of patients with implants would need to have them removed within 10 years; up to 50% in those for reconstruction.** They advised patients with silicone implants to get MRI for silent ruptures 3 years after, then every 2 years (this is being reviewed). The FDA also recommends that silicone implants be used in patients **22 years of age or over**; it is not 'illegal' to use them in younger women but it is 'off label', and manufacturers may not offer their standard warranty.

Long-term health status of Danish women with silicone breast implants. (Breiting VB, *Plast Reconstr Surg*, 2004) This is a retrospective study comparing three cohorts of women: breast augmentation, breast reduction and population controls. The data indicated no difference between any cohort in

- Incidence of breast cancer
- Seropositivity for ANA, RF and IgM Ab recorded in 5%–10% of women in each group

The implant cohort was compared with the non-implant patients:

- Breast pain reported more commonly (three times) – 18% of patients reported severe pain associated with Baker IV capsular contracture.
- Higher self-reported use of antidepressant and anxiolytic drugs; increased risk of suicide amongst augmentation mammoplasty patients reported elsewhere (Koot VCM, *Br Med J*, 2003).
- Fatigue and Raynaud-like symptoms were similar in implant and reduction cohorts, but reported more frequently than in the population control group.

ASSESSMENT

The aims of the procedure seem simple enough, but the patient's motivations and expectations may be very complex. The evaluation should include the psychological and relationship status – there is an excess of suicides in breast-augmentation patients. Full informed consent is mandatory (more than ever).

- Lipworth (*Ann Plast Surg*, 2007) – 175 deaths vs. 133.4 expected in general population; there were increases in deaths from alcohol and drug abuse.

EXAMINATION

It is vital to plan the surgery based on the patient's tissues. In general, get the patient reclined for breast cancer examination and sat up for aesthetic examination – symmetry, ptosis, etc.

- Skin quality – tone, elasticity and striae.
- Soft tissue thickness.

- Asymmetry – chest wall, scoliosis, inframammary fold (IMF) and nipple and areola complex (NAC). Although all breasts are asymmetric, significant breast and chest wall asymmetry is a very difficult problem to overcome.
- Ptosis – severity – a degree of ptosis may be improved by augmentation (this can be gauged by asking patients to lift their arms behind their head), but moderately severe ptosis will need a formal mastopexy.
- Breast examination – as per oncological examination, assess nipple sensation.

MEASUREMENTS

Remember to take account of **skin fold thicknesses** – in simple terms, choose an implant narrower than the breast base, and profile less than the skin stretch.

- **Implant relevant**
  - **Breast width** (BW) – from medial edge/cleavage (designate a safe zone of 2–3 cm in the middle to reduce symmastia and spare the IMA perforators) to the anterior axillary fold (or obvious lateral edge of breast). Implants should not be wider than the breast base width (BBW), which is BW minus soft tissue thickness.
    - Going more medial does not improve cleavage; it just makes the edge of the implant more obvious; the best way to increase cleavage is a push-up bra.
  - **Height** from IMF to crease that forms when you push up (for anatomical implants).
- **Symmetry**
  - Sternal notch to nipple.
  - Internipple and intermammary.
  - Midclavicular line to nipple.
  - NAC diameter.
- **Tissues**
  - **Pinch test** – superior and inferior pole.
  - IMF to NAC, under stretch.
  - Anterior pull skin stretch (APSS).

TEBBETTS HIGH FIVE (2005)

In order, the important practical considerations are

- Optimal soft tissue – coverage and thus pocket for implant – otherwise visible/palpable
- Implant volume relative to breast envelope, i.e. fill volume required
- Effects on tissue, e.g. skin thinning, gland atrophy

Desired/optimal fill volume – it is important to take note of tissue limitations – placing an implant larger than suggested will come with trade-offs, including visibility or thinning of tissues, and give unnatural results:

- Wide breast base with loose skin – small implant will look like a 'rock in a sock'.
- Narrow breast with tight skin – large implant like a basketball, excessive stretching/thinness, etc.

He describes five important measurements in his **High Five® measurement sheet:**

- BBW
- APSS on nipple (>3 cm, need to fill lower pole volume)
- Nipple to IMF distance (>9.5 cm, need to fill lower pole volume)
- Soft tissue pinch upper pole (STPUP; <2 cm, muscle coverage advised)
- Soft tissue pinch at IMF (STPIMF; <4 mm, implant not advisable)

EXPECTATIONS

It is important to manage patient expectations particularly during the consultation/consent process. Patients should be told that

- If the ribs can be felt beneath or to the side of the breast, then the implant will be palpable beneath or lateral to the breast.
- The larger the implant, the worse it will look over time due to stretching and tissue thinning. **Big implants mean big troubles**.

The important messages to deliver are as follows:

- If patients do not accept **palpable** implants, they should not have an augmentation.
- If patients want a totally 'natural' breast, they should not have an augmentation.

There are many different ways to estimate the volume of augmentation required; 1 cup size is approximately 125–150 mL (see below), but there are many variables involved. When consenting, it is important to explain that one cannot guarantee shape, size, nipple direction, IMF or height. **The ONLY predictable effect is an increase in size but not any specific shape**.

PROBLEMS WITH PREGNANCY, LACTATION AND BREASTFEEDING

All are unaffected by implants; early concerns about oesophageal motility were unproven (see above).

- Patients may experience lactorrhoea post-augmentation.
- Nipple sensation is altered in ~20%.

TYPES

- **Textured vs. smooth** – a textured shell decreases the rate and degree of capsular contracture, though the effect is less pronounced than initially thought particularly when compared to smooth saline implants. Texturing reduces implant movement and is required for anatomical implants to maintain orientation. Textured implants may cause traction rippling when placed subglandularly and may be more palpable due to their thicker shell. They are also more expensive.
  - **BIA-ALCL** (see below) seems to be associated with macrotexturing.
- **Motiva** silicone implants have a novel 'nanotextured' shell. In the process of getting FDA approval in August 2017.
- **Silicone vs. saline** – silicone implants tend to feel more breast-like than saline implants, but the latter can be used for limited incision surgery including endoscopically assisted. Some patients may feel that saline implants are 'safer' and associated with a lower contracture rate. Underfilling will cause more rippling, and earlier rupture whilst overfilling (to reduce rippling, increase projection) will make it firm.
- Some implants had a **polyurethane coating** around the silicone shell that reduces capsule formation, but the material was shown to induce sarcomas in rats (breakdown to toluene-diamine [TDA] dimers); however, studies used extreme in vitro conditions. Though TDAs have been detected in the urine of patients, the estimated risk is about 1 in 1 million lifetime risk (Hester TR, *Plast Reconstr Surg*, 1997); although there have been no reports of associated sarcoma in humans, the manufacturers withdrew them from the US market. FDA recommendations are that existing implants need not be removed.
  - Although **polyurethane implants** such as Silimed are not FDA approved, they are used in some European countries (CE marked), Latin America and Australia. They were withdrawn in the United Kingdom in 1991 and then reintroduced by one manufacturer (Polytech Silimed) in 2005.
  - **PIP implants** used a non-approved industrial-grade silicone and were more prone to ruptures and leakage. Recommendations for removal vary between countries; in the United Kingdom, prophylactic removal was not mandated. PIP folded in 2010.
  - **Hydrogel** (PIP hydrogel and Novagold) and **triglyceride** soya oil (Trilucent) implants were removed from the UK market in 2000 and 1999, respectively.
- **Cohesive gel vs. liquid gel** – there is a range of cohesiveness, and this has varied with different generations of implants; currently favoured implants have a thicker type of cohesive gel that does not 'run' when cut; 410 or CPG are terms used by manufacturers; patients call them 'gummy bears'.
- **Anatomical vs. round** – anatomical implants avoid too much upper pole fullness and provide ~25% more projection than with equivalent round implants. They contain a cohesive gel to maintain their shape and need to be textured to reduce rotation. The pocket cannot be overdissected.
- **For a long time, there were only two choices for implants (in the United States) – Mentor (J&J) and Allergan (formerly Inamed and McGhan)/Natrelle.** Sientra silicone implants gained FDA approval in 2012. In 2015, Sientra put a voluntary hold on the implants to investigate potential issues with implants made by their Brazilian manufacturer, Silimed, after German

inspectors found (sterile) particle contamination in some devices. Such particles are found in all implants; thus, after the investigation, Sientra implants were available again in March 2016.

- There is **no 'best implant'**.
- Sientra, unlike the other two manufacturers, will only sell implants to board-certified plastic surgeons.

PLACEMENT

Subglandular vs. submuscular

- **Subglandular placement** is suited to most cosmetic situations as long as the skin envelope is sufficient (>2 cm). A natural breast shape is possible by filling out redundant skin envelope in the ptotic breast. However, the edges of the implant may be palpable/visible particularly at the upper pole, there is a higher contracture rate and there is more interference with mammography.
- **Subfascial plane** – some surgeons have described placing implants behind the pectoralis fascia, which is physically quite thin. Reports of benefit are largely anecdotal.
- **Subpectoral placement** is primarily indicated in very thin patients with insufficient soft tissue to **cover the superior pole of the implant**. In addition, there is less **capsular contracture** and less alteration of nipple sensation, but there may be a **higher rate of implant displacement and asymmetry**, due to contraction of the overlying pectoralis major muscle.
  - The lower pole shape/IMF definition tends to be less attractive; a double bubble deformity may develop in the very ptotic breast (consider augmentation – mastopexy in these patients). It is more difficult to place large implants in this plane, due to the limited space and greater spasm.
    - Senior (*Plast Reconstr Surg*, 2000) used Botox to reduce spasm. Similarly, Schwartz (*Mov Disord*, 1998) and Van Dam (*Plast Reconstr Surg*, 2004) treated spasmodic LD and TRAM flaps, respectively, with BTX.
  - In the 'traditional' subpectoral position, the muscle is not cut; this will increase displacement with muscle contraction and will also lead to dead spaces under the muscle, which will fill with fluid and fibrose up, further displacing the implant. Thus, it is common to release the lower rib attachments to allow the implants to sit better. However, the muscle should not be cut less than 1.5 cm from the midline; the medial attachment is never cut.
  - The inferior 1/3 is uncovered, but with modern (saline) implants, the capsular contracture rate is similar to the total submuscular positioning. The 'benefit' in terms of reducing contracture is seen in both smooth and textured implants.

- **Submuscular placement** usually refers to having the whole implant being covered by muscle, and this usually involves dissection of the serratus anterior (SA) also.
  - Tebbetts advises against this in primary augmentation – it is difficult to dissect the SA without tearing due to the lack of a natural plane, and it often atrophies later anyway.
- **Dual plane** (Tebbetts, see below) aims to combine the advantages of subglandular and submuscular methods. In addition to a subpectoral dissection, a second plane of dissection is between the breast and the muscle (up to the upper level of the areola) to allow soft tissue redraping, to avoid pseudoptosis/'double bubble (A)'.
  - **Double bubble A** – can happen with the (total) submuscular placement when the implant is held high on the chest wall whilst the parenchyma slides downwards over it – sometimes called 'waterfall deformity' or Snoopy appearance.
  - **Type B double bubble** occurs when the lower border of the implant is visible below the breast mound, creating two 'IMFs'. It may be due to 'bottoming out' or a capsular contracture under the breast parenchyma.

Whilst there are many different options and surgeons have their own preferences, many choose a **subglandular silicone implant** as 'default' as long as the soft tissue cover is sufficient (>2 cm) because of the following reasons:

- More natural feel compared with a saline implant.
- Subglandular placement takes up skin envelope better.
- Avoids issues with muscle contraction.

In thin patients, this may not be advisable due to the incidence of wrinkling and one may need to consider either

- Submuscular placement to reduce wrinkling (and capsule formation) or
- Change to a smooth saline implant for subglandular placement (at the cost of slightly more capsular contracture)

INCISIONS FOR ACCESS

Incisions are/should not be the primary focus. Overall, avoid trying too hard to shorten the scar as it will increase skin trauma – usually 5–5.5 cm is sufficient for implants <300. **Asymmetry of nipple** position is common pre-operatively and is often magnified by augmentation mammoplasty, but the implants should still be placed in symmetrical pockets.

- **Periareolar incisions are the most versatile**, being compatible with all planes and types of implant. They provide good access for capsulectomy and a submuscular pocket.
  - Also a good option in the tubular breast where concurrent circumareolar mastopexy is indicated.

- **Avoid in the small (<3 cm) or lightly pigmented areola**. There may be more trauma and potential bacterial exposure, and higher risk of reduced nipple sensation and reduced ability to breastfeed.
  - Put the incision just inside the pigmented border; some use an irregular line. Avoid a straight vertical dissection through the parenchyma; use stair step.
- **Inframammary fold (IMF) incisions** are the simplest to use and almost as versatile as the periareolar. It is easier to change planes with this incision and allows accurate subpectoral placement particularly for those with less experience. It is less useful for secondary cases requiring capsulectomy as it is at the periphery of the pocket. They are ideal in those with significant breast volume beforehand and have significant ptosis. Conversely, they should be **avoided in patients with a poorly defined IMF**.
- **Axillary incision placement** is more accurate when endoscopy is used but is not really suited for subglandular positioning, though it can, in theory, be used for all pockets/types of implants. There is less control and a greater chance of malposition. It is a reasonable choice in patients with low pre-operative breast volume and high breast position, as well as small areola and no IMF crease (thus precluding the above two choices). It precludes the use of larger implants, particularly anatomical and gel types.
- **Transumbilical** – this is a difficult route especially to access the subpectoral plane or for gel implants. It is not FDA-approved and thus is regarded as off-label.

Dual plane breast augmentation. (Tebbets JB, *Plast Reconstr Surg*, 2001)

This is a paper with a great deal of detail on this technique.

Patients with a **pinch thickness** of <2 cm in the upper pole are not suitable for subglandular implants and require muscle coverage to avoid rippling. Essentially, the dual plane controls the position of the inferior PM border by dissecting the muscle from the overlying parenchyma to allow redraping. The dual plane pocket is created through the following:

- Releasing the inferior insertion of PM parallel to and 1 cm above the IMF, which allows the muscle to retract 2–4 cm upwards. It is important not to divide the muscle medially along the sternum to avoid visible retraction and a palpable implant edge. This is type 1 and is used in patients where the entire breast parenchyma is above the IMF and the muscle is tightly attached to the parenchyma, and a short nipple–inframammary fold (NAC-IMF) distance of 4–6 cm under stretch, i.e. **nonptotic breast**, e.g. in nulliparous.
  - Muscle division reduces implant distortion and lateral displacement at the expense of a widened cleavage gap.
  - Do not divide PM if the IMF pinch thickness is <0.5 cm; it is important to maximise soft tissue cover over the lower pole.

- Division of muscle–breast parenchyma attachments to a point level with the inferior edge of the NAC (type 2) is used in patients where most of the breast is above the IMF, and there are looser attachments of breast to muscle and the NAC-IMF is 5–6.5 cm under stretch. **DP2 for ptotic breasts**.
- The attachments may be divided to the superior edge of the NAC (type 3) in patients with glandular ptosis, very loose attachments between the gland and muscle and markedly stretched NAC–IMF 7–8 cm. It is also suited for constricted lower pole, i.e. tuberous breast deformity, combined with radial parenchyma scoring.
  - Be conservative when separating the gland from the muscle – release 1 cm at a time.

BREAST AUGMENTATION AND BREAST CANCER

The recommendations for **patients at high risk of developing breast cancer** (e.g. positive family history) are as follows:

- Inform them that having breast implants may delay diagnosis of breast cancer but does not affect overall survival.
- Suggest mammogram/USG before augmentation if >30 years old (some say 35).
- Recommend submuscular placement for better post-operative visualisation – see later.
- Regular screening afterwards – the recommendations are no different for augmented patients (Jakubietz MG, *Plast Reconstr Surg*, 2004).

Early reports (Silverstein MJ, *Arch Surg*, 1988) suggested that breast tumours in augmented patients were more advanced, but this has not been confirmed (including Silverstein's own follow-up paper). Other evidence followed to suggest that the risk of breast cancer is actually reduced (Berkel H, *N Engl J Med*, 1992; Deapen DM, *Plast Reconstr Surg*, 1992). Hypotheses include smaller amounts of breast tissue or that detected cancers may be smaller possibly due to increased body consciousness. Studies in rats suggest an increased immune response, which may be related to tissue expander effects on blood flow, and blood from implant patients has been shown to kill cancer cells in vitro.

- Shons (*Plast Reconstr Surg*, 2002) – no evidence of increased incidence of breast cancer in those with implants. Those who develop cancer have the same survival as the general population; tumours are detected at a similar stage and are not any more aggressive.
- Berkel (Birdsell DC, *Plast Reconstr Surg*, 1993) reanalysed the data and found 13,246 women with breast cancer, and that those with breast augmentation had the same 5 year survival and same incidence of lymph node disease as non-augmented women with breast cancer. Although there was no difference in the pathological stage at diagnosis, the tumours in

augmented patients were smaller, and augmented patients were ~12 years younger at diagnosis.

- Bryant (*N Engl J Med*, 1995) performed their own reanalysis of Berkel (12,569 patients) and found no difference in 5 and 10 year breast cancer incidence in patients with or without implants.

Breast cancer diagnosis and prognosis in women augmented with silicone gel-filled implant. (Silverstein MJ, *Cancer*, 1990)

Patients with implants are more likely to require open biopsy for histological diagnosis than percutaneous needle techniques, but the presence of an implant does not preclude radiotherapy or FNA/Trucut biopsy.

According to this paper, augmented patients with breast cancer present with a higher percentage of invasive lesions and involved lymph nodes.

DETECTION OF BREAST CANCER IN AUGMENTED BREASTS

The fear is that delayed diagnosis may occur due to **a high false-negative mammography rate**. Saline implants are slightly more radiolucent than silicone, but both are fairly radio-opaque; thus, a higher dose of radiation is needed. In addition, microcalcification within the capsule may theoretically obscure microcalcification associated with malignancy. Overall, studies have shown no significant difference in the mammographic detection of breast cancer.

In augmented breasts, compression and displacement techniques visualise ~60% of breast if subglandular and ~80% if submuscular (**Eklund views**); they should be interpreted by experienced radiologists. Capsular contracture makes Eklund techniques more difficult.

TREATMENT OF BREAST CANCER IN AUGMENTED PATIENTS

Patients with implants are more likely to undergo mastectomy rather than lumpectomy. Small breast volume and distortion of tissue due to the presence of the implant capsule may make wide local excision of the tumour difficult.

Breast conservation therapy (BCT) may still be possible depending on the size of the residual breast, but there will be increased risk of complications such as contractures (up to ~2/3). Those who choose explantation may need a mastopexy, which should be delayed, if possible, to reduce the risk of nipple necrosis.

- Sentinel lymph node biopsy is less reliable in patients who have undergone axillary placement of their implant.

Surgical treatment of breast cancer in previously augmented patients. (Karanas YL, *Plast Reconstr Surg*, 2003)

Half of the 58 breast cancer patients with previous implants were treated with an MRM with implant removal, whilst the other half underwent BCT – lumpectomy, axillary lymph node dissection and radiotherapy.

- One-third initially retained their implants, but half of these ultimately required complete mastectomies with implant removal (local recurrence, residual disease and implant complications).

INJECTABLES FOR BREAST AUGMENTATION

Liquid silicone was actually developed by Dow Corning during World War II, when it was commissioned to do so by the US government. It is well documented that Japanese prostitutes hoping to attract more American soldiers had their breasts injected with materials such as paraffin and liquid silicone (with olive/cottonseed oil to stop migration by deliberately causing scarring). The latter was initially called the **Sakurai formula**, after the first physician to perform the procedure, who eventually opened a practice in California. It was noticed that large quantities of transformer coolant made of silicone were disappearing from Yokohama docks. This 'doctored' non-medical-grade silicone was being injected directly into breasts.

The practice of injecting silicone passed back to the United States and the complications were so severe that the state of Nevada had to pass emergency legislation to make the injections a felony. The FDA finally banned the practice in 1965. With these events in the background, Thomas Cronin and Frank Gerow developed the first breast implants with Dow Corning in 1962.

- Robert Gersuny (1844–1924), an Austrian doctor, injected paraffin into breasts in 1890, which has largely overshadowed his other achievements – he was resident to Bilroth and he improved intestinal anastomotic and abdominal closure techniques.
- Symmer (*Br Med J*, 1968) – a surgeon who reported on 31 cases of breasts filled with 'paraffin waxes, beeswax, silicone wax, silicone fluid, shellac, shredded oiled-silk fabric, silk tangle, glazier's putty, spun glass and epoxy resin'.

MACROLANE VRF® ('LUNCHTIME BOOB JOB')

NASHA injections for breast enhancement were popular especially in Japan, for a while (2008–2012) – it was 'voluntarily' withdrawn by QMed in 17th April 2012 but only for breast augmentation; the other indications remain. It was never approved by the FDA; it was banned for breast augmentation in France in 2011 and in the United Kingdom in 2012.

- There were concerns that it could impede radiological screening 'rather than safety concerns with product itself'. There is a consensus that radiologists have the techniques to properly assess women treated with Macrolane, though some challenges come from the variability in placement (it was supposed to be injected between the gland and the muscle), appearance and longevity.
- Encapsulation was found in some patients.

- Ishii (*Plast Surg*, 2014) reported <10% local adverse effects in 274 (out of >4000 total) who returned for retreatment or complications. Events included gel migration, nodules and infection (rare, 0.08%).
  - There were far fewer problems compared to polyacrylamide gel.

FAT INJECTION TO THE BREAST

(See also 'Fat injection')

The ASPS did a complete 180° on the issue, from discouraging it in 1987 to its current position (see below). Fat injection seems safe; it is useful for filling in contour defects, softening scars and improving the implant–soft tissue interface. Some surgeons like to expand the soft tissue envelop to enhance results; Khouri is a great proponent of pre-injection use of the Brava® system for 3 weeks or so; Yoshimura has described use of a breast implant for its tissue-expanding effect before removing it prior to fat injection. Similarly, Del Vecchio (*Plast Reconstr Surg*, 2012) uses fat injection before and after a prosthesis – simultaneous implant exchange with fat (SIEF) technique.

- Coleman (*Plast Reconstr Surg*, 2007). Post-operative mammograms in 17 patients who received fat injections to the breast for a variety of indications identified changes expected after breast surgery.
- Rubin (*Plast Reconstr Surg*, 2012) found that fat grafting (average 526.5 mL) produced fewer radiologic abnormalities than breast reduction.
- Hyakusoku (*Plast Reconstr Surg*, 2009) discussed general complications after fat injections to the breast such as induration, pain, infection and discharge. The author made it clear that fat grafting should only be performed by trained and skilled surgeons.
- The Brava® system was initially marketed to increase breast volume by applying suction pressure (200 mmHg) for 12 hours a day for 10 weeks. One study showed modest increases in volume (~100 mL) with early recoil; after about half a year, about 55% of this remained.

Current applications and safety of autologous fat grafts: A report of the ASPS fat graft task force. (Gutowski KA, *Plast Reconstr Surg*, 2009)

It was only in 1987 that the ASPS Ad-hoc Committee on New Procedures had previously stated that 'the committee is unanimous in deploring the use of autologous fat injection in breast augmentation'.

The new task force had the following recommendations:

- Fat grafting may be considered for breast augmentation and correction of defects associated with medical conditions and previous surgeries, with the proviso that results are quite **operator-dependent** and additional treatments may be needed.
- Fat grafting can be considered a safe method of augmentation and correction of defects. A sterile technique is necessary. Patients should be made aware of **potential complications**.
- **Caution should be exercised in high-risk patients** – those with risk factors for breast cancer: BRCA, personal or family history of breast cancer. Baseline imaging is recommended.
  - There was no increase in local recurrence after fat grafting seen in a multicentre study (Myckatyn, *Plast Reconstr Surg*, 2017).

2012 POST-MASTECTOMY FAT GRAFT/FAT TRANSFER ASPS GUIDING PRINCIPLES (REAFFIRMED 2015)

The existing evidence suggests autologous fat grafting as an effective option in breast reconstruction following mastectomy (with no remaining native breast tissue) and yields aesthetic improvement and significant patient satisfaction. In addition, the available evidence also cites autologous fat grafting as a useful modality for alleviating post mastectomy pain syndrome and a viable option for improving the quality of irradiated skin present in the setting of breast reconstruction with no increased risk of complications.

- Based on available literature, complication rates are relatively low and include bleeding, calcification, fat embolism, fat necrosis, infection, oil cysts and graft volume loss. Cases of severe complications and death appear to be extremely rare.
- Fat grafting to the post-mastectomy reconstructed breast does not delay breast cancer detection or increase breast cancer recurrence. When reviewed by experienced radiologists, the presence of oil cysts and fat necrosis on mammography, ultrasound and MRI imaging is distinguishable from suspicious lesions. Surveillance should continue to be rigorous.
- The safety, efficacy and final outcome are dependent on the technique used; many variants have been described. The majority of patients require more than one fat grafting session to achieve adequate aesthetic results, and that each additional session will contribute to gradual improvement of the overall outcome.

RADIOLOGICAL CHANGES AFTER FAT INJECTION

Radiological studies have demonstrated that suspicious lesions could be differentiated from the sequelae of fat grafting using current imaging:

- Combination of targeted ultrasound and mammography.
- MRI – benign changes have reduced uptake of contrast and will have a fatty signal intensity (often with fat-fluid levels).
- A study of 30 fat-grafted patients monitored with multimodality imaging a year after surgery found that four had benign calcifications, one had biopsy of a suspicious area that turned out to be a granuloma, whilst the rest had normal imaging (Pierrefeu-Lagrange AC, *Ann Chir Plast Esthet*, 2006).

- A literature review (Claro F, *Br J Surg*, 2012) with 60 studies found an overall complication rate of 3.9% – most commonly, induration and palpable nodules with radiological abnormalities in 13% (mostly cysts).

Furthermore, similar changes are seen in up to 13% of breast reconstructed with flaps as well as other forms of breast surgery such as reduction mammoplasty. Although fat can be injected into various planes, e.g. subcutaneous, subglandular, submuscular and intramuscular, most do not inject into the breast parenchyma, whilst others have done so 'safely' (Illouz, *Aesthet Plast Surg*, 2009).

Fat grafting: Evidence-based review on autologous fat harvesting, processing, reinjection, and storage. (Gir P, *Plast Reconstr Surg*, 2012)

This is a systematic review of many procedural variables in fat grafting, and the main conclusions were as follows:

- **Infiltration before harvest** – no significant difference with lignocaine or adrenaline.
- **Liposuction technique** – there was insufficient evidence, but studies seem to support the use of lower suction pressures (cell damage >10% with vacuum of 700 mmHg) and larger diameter cannulas to increase adipocyte viability.
- **Fat processing** – no significant differences between centrifugation and using sieves or gauzes, but that centrifugation at higher RPM (>3000) caused more damage.
- **Fat storage** – fat should generally be used immediately; some studies suggest that cryopreservation is possible but should include strict methodology.

Outcomes of prosthetic reconstruction of irradiated and non-irradiated breasts with fat grafting. (Komorowska-Timek E, *Plast Reconstr Surg*, 2017)

This is a retrospective review of a single surgeon's outcomes in 75 patients who had fat grafting for soft tissue deficiencies at the time of exchange of the tissue expander for permanent implants. The average volume injected was 151 mL.

The most common complications were fat necrosis and oil cysts – most resolved without treatment except in three patients who required drainage. There was a 22% capsular contracture rate in this series. Previous irradiation did not increase the complication rate. Fat grafting of irradiated skin can increase pliability and improve implant outcomes.

III. COMPLICATIONS

COMPLICATIONS

The reoperation rate due to implant complications is 1/4–1/3 over 5 years.

GENERAL

- Scars – Medicines and Healthcare Products Regulatory Agency (MHRA) says that 1 in 20 get 'bad scars'.
- Temporary change in nipple sensation reported in 15%.

- Thromboembolic disorders (TEDs; deep venous thrombosis [DVT]/pulmonary embolism [PE]). Assess risk and manage as per local protocols; promote early mobility.
- Very rarely, pneumothoraces have occurred, presumably from inadvertently penetrating the intercostal muscles.

Local complications are the primary issue with breast implants; they occur with significant frequency that accumulates over time. It has been estimated that one in four patients with implants will need a second operation within 5 years (one in three for reconstructive and one in eight for augmentation). Some studies quote 15%–20% at 3 years, which is also high, although it includes **any** surgical procedure to the same breast, e.g. biopsies, scar revisions or even a staged, i.e. planned, mastopexy, in addition to implant-related problems (which perhaps are better defined as 'revisions'), and also includes a mixed population.

- The **2000 FDA prospective study** demonstrated that removal rates for saline implants used for cosmetic augmentation were 8% and 12%–14% at 3 and 5 years, respectively, whilst the corresponding rates for reconstructive implants were approximately two to three times higher (confirming the **Mayo 1997 study** with 5 year complication rates of 12% and 34% in cosmetic and reconstructive patients, respectively). However, these are higher than more recent prospective studies.
- Irradiation increases the risk of most complications associated with implants.

AESTHETIC COMPLICATIONS

The final result may be too big or too small.

- **Asymmetry**. Always check the intraoperative appearance of the breasts properly – with the patient sitting up.
- Rippling, palpable edge.
- Symmastia is due to violation of the midline and is difficult to treat. Risk factors include multiple operations, large implants and excessive medial dissection.

LOCAL COMPLICATIONS

Capsular contracture is most common (see below).

- **Infection. ~2% (usually *Staphylococcus aureus*)**. Management needs to be individualised. Infected implants are best treated by removal; some may be salvageable with an 'aggressive' regime of thorough irrigation, IV/instilled antibiotics and possibly replacement with slowly inflated expander-implant. Salvage takes a long time (months), and generally this means more scarring and risk of permanent deformities.
  - It is common to cover the nipple with an adhesive dressing to reduce contamination.

- **Exposure** is uncommon (2%) but increases in those with thin skin envelopes as well as smokers. Salvage by conservative means is more successful (up to 50%) in those **without overt signs of infection**; removal of the implant and delayed replacement (particularly under muscle) produces the most predictable results. A trial of conservative salvage even when ultimately unsuccessful does not seem to affect the final results, *as long as there is no infection.*
- **Haematomas (3%). Haematomas of a significant size should be evacuated** to avoid infection and late deformation.
- **Lymphoma.** In January 2011, the FDA released a report on the occurrence of breast implant–related **anaplastic large cell lymphoma** (BIA-ALCL) in patients with implants (34 cases from 1997 to 2010), with an association with late onset (average 8 years), persistent peri-implant seroma.
- As of September 2017, the FDA received 414 reports of BIA-ALCL including 9 deaths; 242 of 272 were textured and 234 of 413 were silicone gel. Loch-Wilkinson (*Plast Reconstr Surg*, 2017;140;645) This Australian and New Zealand study found that Biocell salt loss textured implants (Allergan, McGhan and Inamed) accounted for 58.7% of the ALCL, and had a 14.11 times higher chance than Siltex textured implants.
  - As of March 2018, there have been 16 confirmed deaths globally.
- The Australian Therapeutic Goods Administration estimates the risk of BIA-ALCL after breast implants to be between 1 in 1000 and 1 in 10,000. The risk for smooth implants is zero.
- It is rare, but it should be considered in those who develop a late seroma (>6 months after). Symptoms include pain, swelling or lumps. Aspirated fluid should be sent for histological examination and CD30 immunohistochemistry, advising the pathologist of the potential diagnosis.
  - Capsule may be sent – anaplastic lymphoma kinase (ALK).
- It seems to run a more benign course compared to other forms of ALCL.
  - Explantation with capsulectomy is usually sufficient; chemotherapy is rarely indicated and usually reserved for those with unresectable disease or metastasis.
  - Better prognosis if ALK negative.
  - FDA does not suggest prophylactic removal or additional screening in the asymptomatic.
- **Others**
  - **Skin numbness** is usually temporary but may be persistent in 10%–15% of patients. Nipple numbness is more likely when implants are placed subglandularly or via the periareolar route.

- **Breast pain** of varying degrees is experienced by 10%–20%; 5% of patients may experience intense nipple sensations.
  - Mondor's disease (Henri Mondor, 1939) – tender venous thrombosis, which fades to a fibrotic cord that may cause contracture. It is usually benign and may follow local trauma but has been associated with breast cancer.
- **Galactorrhoea** (1–2 weeks after surgery) is rare and may be related to prolactin release due to nerve irritation. Bromocriptine or intercostal blocks may help.

Breast implants and the risk of anaplastic large cell lymphoma in the breast. (De Boer M, *JAMA Oncol*, 2018)
This is currently the largest population-based study based on the Dutch registry (1990–2016). They found that the relative risk was 421.8. Associated implants were usually macrotextured (23 out of 28 known types, out of a total of 43 patients with BIA-ALCL). The number of women with implants required to cause 1 BIA-ALCL case before age 75 years was 6920.

CAPSULAR CONTRACTURE

All implants will have a surrounding capsule of some sort; capsular **contracture** is the problem.

- **Capsular calcification** – may be mistaken for malignant disease and make MMG interpretation difficult: 0% under 10 years, 100% over 23 years; of little significance and can be removed with capsulectomy.

Baker classification of capsular contracture (1975):

- Class I – no contracture
- Class II – palpable contracture
- Class III – visible contracture
- Class IV – painful contracture

The assessment is still rather subjective: there are no universally accepted objective measures, although some use callipers or tonometry. Most cases occur within 3–6 months after surgery, and there is low risk after 1 year.

INCIDENCE

How you define the condition, as well as the time span studied, affects the incidence; also consider the fact that implant designs have changed over time. New implants seem to be less prone to capsular contracture.

- The MHRA (2010) states that 1 in 10 patients will develop capsular contracture (without a specific time).
  - Mentor Core Study (2005) and Allergan (formerly Inamed) Core Study (2003) – studies for primary augmentation show a capsular contracture rate of 8.0% for silicone and 9% for saline.
  - Allergan/Mentor pre-market approval studies in 2007/8, grade III/IV contracture at 4 years:
    - 15% augmentation
    - 15%–30% reconstruction

PATHOGENESIS OF CAPSULAR CONTRACTURE

There are some theories regarding the following:

- **Subclinical infection** especially *Staphylococcus epidermidis* – biofilms have been implicated; betadine washout has been shown to reduce colonisation rates but is banned by FDA.
  - Pajkos (*Plast Reconstr Surg*, 2003). Samples were obtained during explantation from 27 breast implants. There were 17 positive cultures in the 19 patients with significant capsules; 14 of these yielded *S. epidermidis*.
  - Tamboto (*Plast Reconstr Surg*, 2010). *S. epidermidis* was inoculated into submammary pockets made in pigs to form biofilms (72%). After 13 weeks, there were 80.6% capsular contractures vs. 47% in the non-inoculated.
- Fibroblastic foreign-body type reaction.

Strategies for reducing capsular contracture:

The incidence of capsule formation may also be related to surgical technique and patient factors.

- **Submuscular**/pectoral placement is the most predictable way to reduce contracture.
  - Benefit is most pronounced for smooth (saline) implants.
- **Use of textured implants**; Malata, *Br J Plast Surg*, 1997; Hakelius, *Plast Reconstr Surg*, 1997.
  - Texturing makes less difference when placed submuscularly.
- **Antibiotics** – Gylbert (*Plast Reconstr Surg*, 1990). A randomised blinded series of 76 patients undergoing subglandular augmentation with half receiving perioperative antibiotic prophylaxis found that there was no significant effect on the incidence of contracture.
  - In contrast, pocket irrigation with **betadine has a consistent beneficial effect** (capsule contracture rate of 12% vs. 28% using saline irrigation) that is independent of the effect of texturing. However, this practice is banned by the FDA. The concern came from reports of implant deflation possibly due to **valve patch delamination** by affecting the adhesive; most cases of failure came from one surgeon who was using betadine intraluminally. In vitro studies confirmed that intraluminal betadine does indeed cause deflation, but soaking in betadine even for 4–7 weeks does not. Clinical studies have shown no increase in deflation rates with the use of betadine externally. Despite the evidence, surgeons who continue to use betadine leave themselves open to litigation. Currently, many have turned either to combination regimes (e.g. soak in bacitracin 50,000 U, cefazolin 1 g, gentamicin 80 mg in 500 mL saline for 5 minutes) or to continue to use betadine solutions for pocket

irrigation only, and then thoroughly rinsing with saline before placing the implant (and thus avoiding the 'contact' between the implant and betadine).

- **Other strategies** such as strict asepsis, meticulous haemostasis and use of lint-free gauze and powder-free gloves are fairly standard. The use of steroids and vitamin E has no value according to most studies.
  - **Keller funnel** 'no touch' technique (bought out by Allergan in 2017). Flugstad NA (*Aesthet Surg J*, 2016) showed that the rate of reoperation (within 12 months) due to capsular contracture was reduced from 1.49% to 0.68% when a funnel was used.
- **Exercises/massage** – moving the implant within the pocket is also controversial; early massage (2–3 days) may be better than later (2 weeks) for up to 3 months. Whilst there are psychological benefits, the effect on capsule formation is largely unproven.

Treatment of capsular contracture:

- Closed capsulotomy – this is not recommended as the forces involved exceed the breaking strength of the implant, and several studies have demonstrated that increase in MRI detected ruptures in those with previously closed capsulotomies.
- Open capsulotomy.
- Open capsulectomy – this reduces breast parenchymal volume, and there is no guarantee that recurrent capsule formation will not occur. Patients with one episode of capsular contracture are more likely to develop capsules with further operations.

Textured or smooth implants for breast augmentation? A prospective controlled trial. (Coleman DJ, *Br J Plast Surg*, 1991)

Fifty-three patients in this prospective randomised double-blind study (usually referred to as the **'Bradford study'**) had subglandular smooth or textured implants and were assessed at 12 months. There was adverse capsular contracture (Baker grades III/IV) in 58% of breasts augmented with smooth implants compared with 8% in the textured surface implant group.

- Malata (*Br J Plast Surg*, 1997) reviewed the study after a total of 3 years (data on 49 of the 53 patients), and adverse capsular contracture was 59% for subglandular smooth implants and 11% for textured ones.

Capsular contracture in subglandular breast augmentation with textured versus smooth breast implants: A systematic review. (Wong CH, *Plast Reconstr Surg*, 2006)

This review identified six RCTs comparing textured and smooth implants and found that smooth implants were associated with more contracture (III/IV) at 1 and 7 years, with relative risks of 4.16 and 2.98, respectively.

The effect of Biocell texturing and povidone–iodine irrigation on capsular contracture around saline-inflatable breast implants. (Burkhardt BR, *Plast Reconstr Surg*, 1995)

This is a prospective, controlled, blinded 4 year trial with 60 volunteers, testing the effect of two independent variables (texturisation and betadine irrigation) on the incidence of capsular contracture around subglandular saline implants.

- Textured devices irrigated with betadine – 4% contracture
- Smooth devices irrigated with saline solution – 50% contracture

RUPTURE

Older silicone implants have a reported silent rupture rate of 15%–30% (most are intracapsular); but newer cohesive gel implants are more durable with **6 year rupture rates of less than 1%**, whilst prospective FDA studies for modern saline implants show rupture rates of 3% at 3 years and 10% at 5 years.

Rupture is easily detected in saline implants, but cohesive silicone implants do not extrude and ruptures are usually asymptomatic/diagnosed inadvertently; thus, published rates are likely to be underestimated.

- The accuracy of clinical detection is poor; **MMG cannot detect intracapsular rupture reliably**, and conventional MMG (more than Eklund) may actually cause rupture. Blood silicone levels are not helpful. Endoscopic examination has been suggested but is obviously impractical for outpatient screening.
- **MRI** ('linguine' sign on T2 with increased sensitivity with breast coils/step-ladder/salad oil sign, 99% positive predictive value) then **USG** (requires an experienced ultrasonographer, 80% sensitivity and specificity) are the best radiological techniques for diagnosing rupture (Ahn C, *Plast Reconstr Surg*, 1994). Most ruptures are intracapsular (with little change in size/shape), and though it may not be dangerous, the FDA recommends removal. There have been reports of silicone granulomas/nodes with extracapsular rupture (Austad ED, see below).
- Some have suggested an algorithm for investigation based on symptoms and the age of implants.
  - Asymptomatic (6.5% rate of rupture) – screen with USG
  - Symptomatic and age less than 10 years (31% risk)
  - Symptomatic and age more than 10 years (64% risk) – use MRI as those with negative USGs still have 37% rate/risk

- The FDA recommends (i.e. not mandatory) routine MRI screening for rupture 5 years after insertion, and then after every 2 years, but not many countries have adopted this policy.
- **Microscopic gel bleed** (leakage of silicone oil) may occur, and elevated tissue silicone levels can be detected around **intact implants** (silicone > saline > controls). Scar tissue that forms quickly around implants means that silicone is usually not detectable more than 2 mm beyond the implant and asymptomatic in the majority. Newer implants with much thicker shells are supposedly 'low bleed'.

Mentor contour profile gel implants: Clinical outcomes at 6 years. (Hammond DC, *Plast Reconstr Surg*, 2012)

According to this review of a specific implant, the rupture rate at 6 years is 2.1% and the capsular contracture rate is 2.4% (III/IV) for primary augmentation.

Breast implant-related silicone granulomas: The literature and the litigation. (Austad ED, *Plast Reconstr Surg*, 2002)

A silicone granuloma is a foreign-body type reaction to the presence of silicone formed by aggregates of macrophages and polymorphs. There is no evidence to suggest that they bear any relationship to any form of systemic disease; most are excised simply to exclude malignancy.

- Granulomas are relatively rare; though the exact incidence is unknown, it is probably between 0.1% and 0.5%. It may not always be associated with implant rupture; in some cases, it may be associated with low-grade *S. epidermidis* infection. Thus, excised granulomas should be submitted for culture.
- Fragments of silicone were found in the capsules of 46 of 54 textured implants in one study. Silicone lymphadenopathy has been reported many years after the placement of an implant or MCP joint prosthesis.

IV. TUBEROUS BREASTS

Tuberous breast deformity: Classification and treatment. (von Heimburg D, *Br J Plast Surg*, 1996)

Tuberous breast deformity was first described in 1976 by Rees and Aston (due to its similarity in shape to 'tubers'). Sometimes called 'tubular' or 'constricted' breasts. Developmentally, the superficial layer of the superficial fascia is absent in the area underneath the areola. There is also a constricting fibrous ring at the level of the periphery of the NAC that inhibits the normal development of the breast. This results in

- Deficient horizontal and vertical development of the breast, especially lower pole – **deficiency of parenchyma and skin envelop with a high IMF**
- **Herniation** of the breast parenchyma towards the **widened areolar**

CLASSIFICATION

von Heimburg Classification (1996, modified by the author in 2000)

- Type 1 – hypoplasia of the inferior medial quadrant
- Type 2 – hypoplasia of both inferior quadrants, sufficient subareolar skin
- Type 3 – hypoplasia of both inferior quadrants, sub-areolar skin shortage
- Type 4 – severely constricted breast, minimal breast base

GROLLEAU CLASSIFICATION

- Type I (deficiency of the lower medial quadrant)
- Type II (deficiency of both lower quadrants)
- Type III (deficiency of all four quadrants)

The problem may be unilateral or bilateral; asymmetry is common. The true incidence is unknown – whilst severe forms tend to present early at or after breast development, mild degrees of deformity may go unnoticed, and some studies suggest that many who present with asymmetric/hypoplastic breast have previously unrecognised tuberous breast deformity (Figure 5.1).

SURGICAL OPTIONS

The important features that need to be addressed are as follows:

- Constricted breast base needs to be expanded – enlarge skin envelope and augment volume where appropriate, e.g. rigottomies and expander/implants. A short IMF to NAC distance makes it difficult to place an implant.
- Breast herniation into areola – **release constriction** at the edge of the areola to allow breast tissue to reduce and then **reduce the areola**.
- High IMF – needs to be lowered.

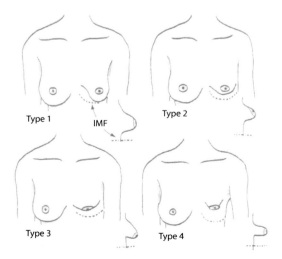

Figure 5.1 Schematic representation of the classification of tuberose breast deformity. The dotted lines represent the level of the IMF.

The subglandular approach is the best for remodelling but may leave inadequate tissue cover.

- **Type 1 – augmentation** with a subglandular implant via inframammary or infra-areolar incision, taking care to avoid a 'double bubble' deformity.
- **Type 2 – augmentation plus internal flap** by 'unfurling' of breast tissue on the posterior aspect of the gland, turned downward to augment the lower half of the breast (Puckett CL, *Aesth Plast Surg*, 1990). This can be performed through a circumareolar incision.
- **Types 3 and 4 – augmentation plus internal flap plus skin importation** to break up the constricted base at the abnormal IMF, which would tend to cause a 'double bubble' deformity.
  - Z-plasty across the IMF – modified Millard technique.
  - De-epithelialised thoracoepigastric flap.
  - Tissue expansion (Scheepers JH, *Br J Plast Surg*, 1992) followed by circumareolar mastopexy.
    - Becker expander-implants can be replaced gradually by serial fat injections.
  - Contralateral breast reduction may be considered if adequately sized.

Aesthetic reconstruction of the tuberous breast deformity. (Mandrekas AD, *Plast Reconstr Surg*, 2003)
The authors describe their surgical approach in 11 patients, which uses a periareolar incision:

- The inferior skin flap is dissected to the chest wall and to **the new IMF**, and also behind the breast leaving only the superior parenchyma attached to the chest wall.
- The constricted lower parenchyma is exteriorised through the periareolar opening and is divided vertically down the middle, creating two breast pillars that can redrape. The breast is flatter and wider at the expense of projection.
- In cases of volume deficiency, a silicone breast implant is placed in a subglandular pocket.
- Doughnut mastopexy addresses the wide NAC.

The tuberous breast revisited. (Pacifico MD, *J Plast Reconstr Aesthetic Surg*, 2007)
The authors suggest that herniation of breast tissue through the NAC is the only major deformity in tuberous breast and that there is **no significant actual skin shortage**. They place a subglandular implant before NAC reduction if necessary, preferring an IMF approach over the periareolar. The new NAC size is agreed beforehand with the patient, and the position is determined by several parameters:

- Inferior NAC to IMF no more than 6 cm
- Medial NAC to midline 8–10 cm

The areolar is de-epithelialised around the 'new' areolar margin up to its margin with further subdermal undermining outwards for 2 cm. Deep tension sutures that double-breast the dermis are then placed during wound closure.

Management of tuberous breast deformity with anatomic cohesive silicone gel breast implants. (Panchapakesan V, *Aesth Plast Surg*, 2009)

This paper presents results in 50 cases of tuberous breast deformity with single-stage surgery using **anatomic implants**. For cases requiring areolar reduction, a periareolar approach is used for the implants, whilst for cases with small areola/minimal herniation, the incision is at the site of the planned IMF. A **subglandular** position is preferred for the full or extra-projection implants; for those with insufficient superior pole tissue, a dual plane procedure is performed. If further release of constricted tissues is required, then **radial scoring** with electrocautery is used up to the dermal level if necessary. After the implant is in place, **areolar reduction** or mastopexy is performed as needed.

Those with severe deformities may benefit from a staged procedure. Scoring and expanding with a tissue expander of the lower pole is done first, followed by implant exchange and a periareolar mastopexy.

B. BREAST REDUCTION

I. INDICATIONS FOR BREAST REDUCTION

The aim of breast reduction surgery is to achieve smaller breasts with aesthetic shape and volume symmetry. Reduction mammoplasty is commonly performed for bilateral macromastia, but can also address asymmetry (congenital and acquired).

INDICATIONS IN MACROMASTIA

The top three of the following list are most common. Older women tend to complain of physical symptoms, whilst younger women tend to have more psychological symptoms. **Size does not correlate well with symptoms**.

- Secondary back, shoulder and neck pain; poor posture
- Difficulty with exercise
- Low self-esteem/other psychological symptoms
- Mastalgia
- Difficulty with finding clothing
- Submammary maceration, intertrigo

Although patients commonly refer to bra sizes for reduction and augmentations, it is close to meaningless as it does not accurately correspond to volumes. Patients (as well as surgeons) may have very different perceptions of what constitutes a 'full C cup', for example.

- Bra band size is generally not affected by surgery unless the thorax is liposuctioned to reduce girth.
- The cup size is relative to the band size – for a 32–34 inch chest, each cup size ~100 g, whilst for a >36 inch chest, one cup size ~ 180–200 g.

Symptoms and related severity experienced by women with breast hypertrophy. (Sigurdson L, *Plast Reconstr Surg*, 2007)

Patients should be warned about the change in breast shape with weight gain/loss, and bottoming out and ptosis with time (especially with the inferior pedicle technique).

- 93% report improvement in symptoms and 62% increased their activity levels (Miller AP, *Plast Reconstr Surg*, 1995).
- 87% overall satisfaction (Davis GM, *Plast Reconstr Surg*, 1995) despite minor complications; 93% would have the surgery again and 94% would recommend it for others.
- There is only weak correlation between the volume excised and symptom relief.

EXAMINATION

- Cancer examination (lie back) – lumps, nodes, scars, etc.
- Aesthetic examination (sit up) – size/shape/symmetry, degree of ptosis, sternal notch–nipple distance, NAC-IMF distance, general body habitus

II. BREAST REDUCTION SURGERY

Operative techniques are usually classified according to the type of **pedicle used** for the nipple and the type of **skin markings**/resection. These are independent of each other and can be combined in various ways. For example, Khan (*Aesth Plast Surg*, 2007) combined a vertical scar with a vertical bipedicle McKissock technique, and Blondeel (*Br J Plast Surg*, 2003) combined a latero-central pedicle with a Wise pattern. However, the most common variations in use are the inferior pedicle with an inverted T scar (ITIP) and vertical scar mammoplasty (VSM, with variety of pedicles).

Skin incisions:

- Inverted T.
- Vertical scar – requires healthy skin elasticity for remodelling, high revision rate for dog ears/scar.
- B-shaped (Regnault) – less commonly used.
- Circumareolar – generally not a useful option in breast reduction, or for >2 cm of ptosis. Excessive disparity between the NAC and the defect in the flap will result in flattening of the breast and puckering of the scar.

PEDICLE TECHNIQUES

Excess tissue is debulked around the pedicle that carries the NAC and allows it to be transposed safely to its new position. It turns out that most pedicles are fairly reliable axial pattern flaps rather than the random pattern perfusion they were initially thought to have. It is the resection not the pedicle that directly determines the aesthetic result. Glandular rearrangement is the key to long-lasting results; skin alone cannot be used for support.

- **No pedicle** (Thorek M, *NY Med J Rec*, 1922) breast amputation and **free nipple graft**. This was conceived as a more reliable means of preventing nipple loss when previous pedicle techniques were insufficiently reliable.
  - It can still be considered in the elderly, those with poor anaesthetic risk, the very obese and those requiring a resection of more than 1.5 kg per breast. Some return of sensation after grafting is not uncommon.
- **Central mound** (Balch CR, *Plast Reconstr Surg*, 1981).

- **Dermoglandular pedicle**. The dermal portion was meant to improve venous return, but it has not been shown to have major effects in practice.
  - **Horizontal pedicle**
    - Horizontal bipedicle, with inverted T scar (Strombeck JO, *Br J Plast Surg*, 1960).
    - Horizontal single pedicle, with inverted T scar (Skoog T, *Acta Chir Scand*, 1963).
  - **Lateral pedicle**
    - Lateral pedicle and lateral scar (Duformentel C, *Ann Chir Plast*, 1965).
    - Hamdi described the septum-based mammoplasty (**Wuringer septum** – a horizontal septum from the chest wall at the level of the fifth rib, carrying neurovascular bundle to the nipple).
  - **Vertical pedicle**
    - **Bipedicle**, with inverted T scar (McKissock PK, *Plast Reconstr Surg*, 1972). There is often superior fullness pushing the nipple to point downwards. When it was realised that the 'additional' superior pedicle could be safely dispensed with, several inferior pedicle techniques were developed and remain widely used.
    - **Superior pedicle** (Weiner D, *Plast Reconstr Surg*, 1973). Superior pedicles tend to have limited arcs of rotation; they should be ~2 cm thick to include the axial vessels.
    - **Superior vertical pedicle, vertical scar only** (Lejour M, *Ann Chir Plast Esthet*, 1990).
    - **Inferior pedicle with inverted T scar** (Robbins TH, *Plast Reconstr Surg*, 1977). Some have suggested that the longer the nipple to the IMF distance, the wider the pedicle base should be, e.g. 3:1 ratio; however, extra wide pedicles may actually impede circulation by increasing skin tension during closure. They adversely impact on the aesthetic results whilst contributing little to perfusion. Most use a maximum pedicle width of ~10 cm.
    - **Glanduloplasty technique**, inferolateral resection, B-shaped scar (Regnault P, *Plast Reconstr Surg*, 1980).

There are a wide variety of safe techniques. Different countries/regions seem to favour one over the other, e.g. the United States and United Kingdom commonly use ITIP, whilst vertical techniques are more common in Europe.

INFERIOR PEDICLE WITH INVERTED T SCAR

This technique, often called the **'Wise' pattern** (although this strictly refers to the skin incision), is popular as the results are predictable, and is suited for larger reductions, as it allows excision in both horizontal and vertical directions (Figure 5.2). The skin incision can be marked according to a template or performed 'free hand' – the nipple position is not precut, allowing more flexibility in positioning to increase symmetry, etc. The **measurements are primarily aimed to ensure nipple symmetry** rather than to design a certain breast shape. Important landmarks/measurements are as follows:

- NAC diameter 38–45 mm
- Nipple to the IMF distance 6–8 cm. Note that this is not the same as NAC/areolar to IMF distance; you need to account for the areolar radius.
  - **Nipple/breast meridian** – from the midclavicular line to the nipple at IMF
  - **Sternal notch to nipple distance** ~ 21 cm, depending on the stature/body size.
    - The basic pattern (Penn J, *Plast Reconstr Surg*, 1955) is a triangle with sides 18–22 cm long and corners at the sternal notch and new nipple positions. It forms a good starting point but should only be used as a guide; in particular, some degree of nipple medialisation may be necessary.
  - **Nipple position at Pitanguy's point**, i.e. IMF of breast along the meridian. Some suggest that the nipple height should be slightly lower in mature breasts and higher in firmer young breasts, although high nipples are very difficult to correct.
    - Placing the nipple too high, particularly in those with inadequate upper pole fullness, would lead to a **ski-jump type** breast with the nipple pointing upwards.

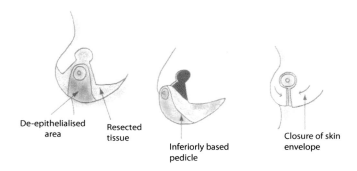

De-epithelialised area   Resected tissue   Inferiorly based pedicle   Closure of skin envelope

Figure 5.2 ITIP technique. The perfusion of the NAC is maintained by an inferiorly based parenchymal pedicle. The method largely relies on the skin envelope to maintain its shape.

A longer sternal notch to nipple distance (>40 cm) is usually associated with IMF to nipple distance (>20 cm), which means that the inferior pedicle will need to be folded, and the risks of complications increases.

- **Central vertical limbs** should be limited to less than 8 cm long (the NAC radius accounts for 2 cm of this) to reduce bottoming out (although this reduces projection).
- **Central angle.** A pinch/displacement test can be used to roughly assess the scale of the reduction possible. An excessively wide angle will make closure more difficult and will result in a flat boxy base; keeping it <60° reduces T-junction tension/ischaemia. A small triangular wedge at the T-junction may reduce tension.
- **The pedicle base should be 8–10 cm wide.**
- **Drains may not be necessary.**
  - Wrye (*Plast Reconstr Surg*, 2003). This was an RCT with 49 patients with ITIP reductions, with patients randomised to having a drain in either their left or right sides, and none in the other side. There was no difference in the incidence of haematomas or complications, whilst patients reported that they preferred the early post-operative comfort in the side with no drain.
  - Collis (*Br J Plast Surg*, 2005). This RCT with 150 patients did not show any difference in the rates of haematoma formation with or without the use of drains. The rate of wound infection was also not affected.
- Post-operatively, patients are usually advised to wear sports bras for 24 hours a day for up to 6 weeks.

When to use drains in breast reduction surgery? (Ngan PG, *Ann Plast Surg*, 2009)

This retrospective review of 182 patients with breast reductions identified age >50 years and reductions >500 g as risk factors for higher output states where drains should be considered.

VERTICAL SCAR MAMMOPLASTY

The superior pedicle in early techniques was difficult to inset and prevented wider acceptance; the pedicle needed to be thinned to allow folding without compression/kinking, but this also reduced sensation and the capacity for subsequent breastfeeding (Figure 5.3).

- **Patient selection is important**, as always; VSM techniques are most suited for small–medium volume reductions, and best avoided in those with excessive amounts of ptosis or redundant skin. The risk of nipple numbness is higher, but otherwise, the incidence of other complications is comparable. There is a learning curve that adds to the inertia involved in changing from a reliable and well-tested technique such as the ITIP despite its shortcomings.
- **The IMF and the nipple tend to end up higher** than the ITIP and thus should be marked somewhat lower at the beginning.
- **The puckering and shape may take weeks to months to settle,** and it may be difficult to reassure patients

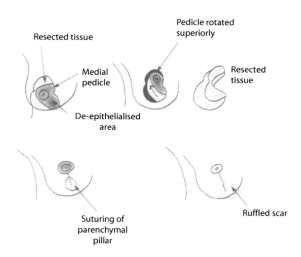

Figure 5.3 Simplified VSM technique based on a medial pedicle. Bringing together the parenchymal pillars cones the breast tissue and achieves a longer-lasting shape.

particularly if the surgeons themselves have little experience with the technique. The bottom line is that if a surgeon is performing a large number of reductions, then a VSM has the potential to produce better long-term results; however, for those with a lower volume of cases, a 'reliable' method like the ITIP is a reasonable choice.

A 30-year experience with vertical mammaplasty. (Lassus C, *Plast Reconstr Surg*, 1996)

Lassus first described his technique in 1970, and this paper presented his cumulative experience.

- Initial markings indicate the position to which the nipple must move, and a second point 2–4 cm above the IMF defines the inferior limit of skin resection.
- Vertical lines are marked to connect these points after medial and lateral displacement of the breast, and a keyhole pattern is incorporated to mark the inset of the NAC.
- The **superior dermal pedicle** used must be thin but with adequate tissue above the nipple to avoid venous congestion. Central breast parenchymal excision is then undertaken. There is **no skin undermining** in this technique.
- The nipple is inset temporarily, and tacking ('framing') sutures are used to generate the desired breast shape and guide secondary resection. The vertical scar is closed and pleated to ensure that the scar does not descend below the IMF.

Vertical mammaplasty and liposuction of the breast. (Lejour M, *Plast Reconstr Surg*, 1994 [The original paper in 1990 was in French.])

Several significant differences from the Lassus technique include the following:

- Fairly aggressive liposuction to model and shape the breast; the area behind the areola is not suctioned.

- Pillar plication. It relies upon substantial post-operative skin contraction and inferior breast remodelling. The contour is overcorrected to create a high, projected, narrow-based breast ('**upside-down breast**') that will improve after several months for a more aesthetic final result.

Nipple numbness is not uncommon due to use of the superior pedicle (nerves enter inferolaterally). In about 10% of patients, particularly those with larger ptotic breasts, a second procedure was needed to excise skin redundancy from the lower part of the scar. Lejour suggests that this is useful for reductions of up to 1000 g, but most other surgeons would be more comfortable with a limit of 400–500 g.

'I' becomes 'L': Modification of vertical mammaplasty. (Pallua N, *Plast Reconstr Surg*, 2003)

The authors propose a **lateral** IMF incision to reduce the problems with the bunched-up wound of the classic Lejour, whilst sparing the medial side for a 'scar-free cleavage'. They combined this with a superior pedicle in 45 patients and reported good results.

Other strategies to deal with the vertical skin excess include a caudal extension to the IMF, medially or medio-laterally (mini-inverted T). Excessive bunching up to avoid these extensions does not seem to result in a better scar in the long term (Hall Findlay, 2010).

Vertical versus Wise-pattern breast reduction: Patient satisfaction, revision rates, and complications. (Cruz-Korchin N, *Plast Reconstr Surg*, 2003)

This is a prospective, randomised study that compared the outcomes of ITIP reduction with medial pedicle VSM reduction.

- Complication rates and overall patient satisfaction were not significantly different.
- However,
  - VSM was ranked significantly higher by patients with regard to scars and overall aesthetic results.
  - VSM for moderate macromastia has a significantly higher revision rate.

The vertical mammaplasty: A reappraisal of the technique and its complications. (Berthe JV, *Plast Reconstr Surg*, 2003)

Criticisms of the Lejour vertical mammoplasty are as follows:

- **Delayed healing of the vertical scar**
- Risk of seromas, haematomas, glandular necrosis and increased need for **secondary corrections**

In this study, the results of 170 consecutive vertical mammoplasty procedures (330 breasts) were reviewed:

- Minor complications observed in 30% (minor skin edge necrosis)
- Major complications in 15% (glandular necrosis and severe infection)

- Surgical revision for scar or volume correction necessary in 28%

The original technique was modified, decreasing the skin undermining, avoiding liposuction and primary skin excision performed in the submammary fold at the end of the operation for redundant skin. This resulted in much fewer minor and major complications but no significant change in the rate of revisional surgery for secondary scar and volume corrections.

Lassus wrote a discussion piece for the article above (Lassus, *Plast Reconstr Surg*, 2003). He stresses that what are lumped together as 'vertical techniques' can be very different procedures; in particular, he compares his technique with the Lejour:

- Liposuction is part of Lejour but not Lassus.
- Skin undermining is part of Lejour but not Lassus, where the skin remains attached to the breast reducing dead-space formation.
- Lejour sutures the lateral pillars; Lassus does not.
- Lejour relies on skin contraction for the scar; Lassus does not.

He comments that the modifications described by Berthe actually make it closer to a Lassus. Several authors have modified the Lejour technique in a similar manner (Hall Findlay, *Plast Reconstr Surg*, 1999; Hidalgo, *Plast Reconstr Surg*, 2005; Serra, *Ann Plast Surg*, 2010 – see below).

Benefits and pitfalls of vertical mammaplasty. (Beer GM, *Br J Plast Surg*, 2004)

This survey shows that VSM is more popular in Europe than in the United States (12% according to a survey in 1999). Complication rates are similar to ITIP breast reduction. From their review of a **modified Lassus reduction** technique in 153 patients:

- Early complications in 21.6% including
  - Haematoma 4% and infection 4%.
  - Wound dehiscence 12% especially infra-areolar area.
  - Nipple necrosis 0.7%.
- Late complications in 26%:
  - Problems with the vertical scar including scar below the new IMF.
  - Major late complications required reoperation in 11.1%.

The authors suggested that the benefits over the ITIP technique, including the long-lasting and enhanced projection and reduced scarring, justify its use as a standard technique.

Vertical mammaplasty. (Hidalgo DA, *Plast Reconstr Surg*, 2005)

The author reviews the evolution of VSM and in particular points to several key issues that improve outcomes:

- **Not using liposuction** as a major part of the procedure.
- **Not suturing** the gland to the pectoralis major (as this tends to cause distortion).

- **Not undermining** the lower pole skin and leaving it attached to the gland.
- **Creating additional pillars of adequate size** and careful approximation to avoid flattening or notching. The significant parenchymal resection means that drains are more important than in ITIP methods.
- **Avoiding tight closure**/excessive skin resection, both of which distort the lower pole significantly.
- Positioning of nipple after tacking and sitting up, rather than using a predetermined position – in addition, it should be no higher than the IMF as it will be pushed up by closure of the pillars.
- **Restricting purse stringing** of the vertical incision to the lower portion only.

The author suggests that surgeons taking up VSM should start with small volumes and minor ptosis. Not all cases are suited for this technique, particularly those with extreme problems of size and/or ptosis.

Breast reduction with a superomedial pedicle and a vertical scar. (Hall-Findlay's technique; Serra MP, *Ann Plast Surg*, 2010)

The authors present their results in 210 consecutive patients using a set of modifications as described by Hall-Findlay (*Plast Reconstr Surg*, 1999) with no skin undermining, no routine liposuction and no pectoralis suspension sutures in association with a superomedial pedicle.

- The IMF is marked 2 cm below Pitanguy's point to accommodate the increased projection with this procedure.
- The lateral and medial limbs are marked by displacing the breast in, out and up; these lines are joined up in a U shape 2–6 cm above the IMF.

Most complications involved the vertical scar, particularly in larger-volume reductions – the authors suggest a short horizontal component to the scar.

Other techniques are less commonly used:

- **Regnault B technique** has an oblique scar extending laterally that avoids a large medial component. It offers an aesthetic roundness and can also be used to manage moderate ptosis.
- **Periareolar techniques** (concentric/eccentric) have the advantages of reduced scarring but tend to produce a flatter, poorly projecting breast and the areolar tends to stretch out. They are not recommended for larger volume resections.
- **Some have described endoscopic techniques for piecemeal resections,** which are only suited for young women with no/minimal ptosis and good elasticity.
- **The use of liposuction alone for reduction is controversial;** only 20% of the breast volume can be extracted by liposuction. It does not remove the parenchymal tissue, and thus the risk of unknowingly removing the malignant tissue is small.

- It may be useful in those with moderate-sized fatty breasts and good skin tone (as it can increase ptosis) with normally located NACs. It can be used as an adjunct particularly mid-line, IMF and subaxillary areas, or to make minor adjustments after surgery.
- The concern that it may cause microcalcification that obscures tumour detection does not seem to have been borne out by studies.

- **Free nipple graft** (for massive reductions >2500 g or nipple IMF distance 20–25 cm or more).
- **Modified Robertson technique** for large ptotic breasts. The initial description (1967) involved leaving a large inferior flap for coning the breast shape, and covered by the upper skin flap coming down to meet a bell-shaped flap of inferior skin. The NAC was grafted, and there was a transverse scar running through it. The Hurst modification (1983) eliminated the nipple grafting, but the visible transverse scar remained. The Boston modification (Movassaghi K, *Aesthet Surg J*, 2006) involved raising a longer superior flap to extend 5 cm below the new NAC position; the NAC based on a broad de-epithelialised inferior pedicle would come out through the superior flap, like the umbilicus in an abdominoplasty flap.
- **Transverse resection** (Piza-Katzer H, *Br J Plast Surg*, 2003). Although this is not a new technique contrary to what the authors say, it may be useful particularly when performing a 'balancing' reduction on the contralateral breast for those with reconstructed breasts after MRM.

SPAIR TECHNIQUE

The short scar periareolar inferior pedicle reduction (SPAIR) was described by Hammond (*Plast Reconstr Surg*, 1999). There is a fairly steep learning curve with extensive intra-operative design:

- Design of skin excision pattern by breast displacement, so as to allow tension-free NAC inset.
- After de-epithelialising around the new NAC shape, the inferior pedicle is developed. The skin flaps are elevated, and the parenchyma is resected. A significant amount of gland suturing is needed to obtain the desired shape.
- With the patient sat up, the lower pole skin redundancy is fixed temporarily with staples before definitive resection. The NAC is inset and with a CV3 Gore-Tex purse-string suture.

COMPLICATIONS OF BREAST REDUCTION SURGERY

General

- Infection
  - A single dose of perioperative antibiotics is sufficient.

- Haematoma
  - Infiltration of **adrenaline solutions** can reduce blood loss and does not seem to increase the risk of haematoma (Kerrigan, *Plast Reconstr Surg*, 2013; Wilmink H, *Plast Reconstr Surg*, 1998).
  - Drains are generally unnecessary though may be considered in patients with looser skin and larger resections.
- Dehiscence (particularly at T-junction)
  - Fat necrosis is probably more common than thought.
- DVT/PE

Specific

- **Nipple numbness** occurs in around 5%–15% of patients and is more frequent with more radical reductions (in one study, >440 g was a threshold value). Empirical numbness is more pronounced with superior pedicle techniques compared to inferior pedicle techniques. Canting pedicles medially or laterally has also been suggested to improve sensation.
- **Nipple position** – the biggest aesthetic mistake to make is to position the nipple too high; one measure (that is often temporary) is to excise some tissue below the nipple; otherwise, a VY-plasty or skin grafting is needed but will leave obvious scars on the upper half of the breast.
  - ITIP methods tend to lower the IMF, whilst VSM tends to raise it.
- **Shape** – **asymmetry**, 'bottoming out' of the vertical scar or 'dog ears' may require subsequent revision. The IMF–nipple distance may increase post-operatively by up to 30% especially in inferior pedicle techniques, which will reduce projection.
- **Scar hypertrophy** is not uncommon but can be reduced with standard treatments such as silicone and steroid therapy.
  - Some studies suggest that a 5 day course of antibiotics reduce the incidence of hypertrophic scarring and wound dehiscence.
- **Nipple loss** – partial/complete 4%–7%. Free nipple grafting is suggested for large reductions (>1500 g) with potentially long nipple translocations (>25 cm), in smokers/diabetics or revisional reductions where the first pedicle used is not known. Hypopigmentation is fairly common.
  - Laser Doppler (LD), fluorescein flowmetry or ICG may be useful in predicting loss/guide timing of grafting, particularly in darker-skinned patients where clinical judgement may be more difficult.
  - Grafts will survive better than bordeline nipples on pedicles due to reduced metabolic demands. Questionable nipples should be converted to free grafts as soon as possible, certainly within 24 hours.
- **Lactation** and breastfeeding compromised but ~75% can still lactate following inferior pedicle technique (Schlenz I, *Plast Reconstr Surg*, 2005).

- Thibaudeau (*J Plast Reconstr Aesthet Surg*, 2010). This systematic review of 26 articles found no difference in breastfeeding capacity during the first month after delivery. With the exception of Strombeck's horizontal bipedicle technique, the majority of studies show that lactation is possible with the variety of pedicles, with the limiting factor being the connection of the nipple to a significant portion of ducts and lobules – recanalisation is rare. They state that difficulties appear to be mostly explained by psychosocial issues such as inadequate/inappropriate advice and coaching as well as other considerations. They recommend that these patients should all be encouraged to breastfeed.
- Problems are more likely with dermal pedicles, e.g. superior pedicle, compared to dermoglandular, e.g. inferior pedicle.

III. BREAST CANCER AND BREAST REDUCTION

PATHOLOGICAL FINDINGS IN BREAST REDUCTION SURGERY

Incidence of breast cancer in women <28 years of age is ~8 in 100,000; in patients <30 years of age, there is no absolute need to send tissue for histology unless there is a strong family history or the tissue appears macroscopically abnormal.

- ~25% of all breast reductions show abnormal pathology, mostly fibroadenosis (Titley OG, *Br J Plast Surg*, 1996).
- Analysis of 5008 breast reductions by Snyderman RK (*Plast Reconstr Surg*, 1960) demonstrated nine cancers **(0.38%)**.
- 1998 survey of plastic surgeons in New Orleans revealed four cancers after 2576 reductions **(0.16%)** (Jansen DA, *Plast Reconstr Surg*, 1998).
- Tang (*Plast Reconstr Surg*, 1999) documented invasive carcinoma in **0.06%** of 27,500 breast reductions from the **Ontario registry**.
- Colwell (*Plast Reconstr Surg*, 2004) reported six cases **(0.8%)** of breast cancer in 800 breast reductions; half were invasive, and the other half were ductal carcinoma in situ (DCIS). The **pre-operative mammography was negative in all cases**.

The surgeon must indicate the areas from which separate blocks of tissue have been removed – 60% of breast cancer occurs in the upper outer quadrant. It is a challenge for the pathologist to find a small clinically undetectable cancer in a large mass of breast parenchyma and fat – often the specimens are evaluated by thin slicing and selectively sending blocks for histology. Some have used specimen radiography to aid detection (Ozmen S, *Aesth Plast Surg*, 2001).

The role of pre-operative investigations is controversial. In the United States, it is common to

- Recommend a baseline mammogram. Perras (*Aesthetic Plast Surg,* 1990) found 34 cancers by mammography in 1149 patients undergoing cosmetic breast surgery who were over 35 or had a positive family history.
  - Campbell (*Am J Surg,* 2010). This study involved 207 patients (average age 49) considering reduction mammoplasty who had recent screening mammograms; 16% had abnormal radiographs, but all were **false positives**.
- Send all specimens.
- Obtain baseline mammogram at 6 months after surgery; there will be typical changes that do not hinder screening (see below).
  - Palmieri (*Breast Cancer Res Treat,* 2005). A 20 year literature review concluded that breast reduction decreases the risk of breast cancer and is related to the amount of tissue resected.
  - Tarone (*Plast Reconstr Surg,* 2004). Five studies concluded that the risk of breast cancer was less in the breast reduction patients than in the controls (relative risk, 0.2–0.7).
    - The possible mechanism(s) may be the removal of microscopic disease or simply the reduction of the mass of breast tissue.
  - Bilateral prophylactic mastectomy reduces the risk of breast cancer by 90% compared with 95% reduction of risk for prophylactic contralateral mastectomy after cancer in one side.

BREAST REDUCTION SURGERY AND BREAST CANCER RISK

Screening for breast cancer post reduction mammaplasty. (Muir TM, *Clin Radiol,* 2010)

This study reviewed 4743 women who had breast screening **after** breast reduction; 51 cancers were detected (4.28 per 1000 screens), which was less than the controls without breast reduction (5.99 per 1000) with a relative risk of 0.71. There were no significant differences in the pathological types or anatomical location of the tumours. The authors conclude that the post-operative changes of breast reduction (skin thickening, non-anatomical retro-areolar bands that may become fibrose, fat necrosis with oil cyst calcification or calcification along suture lines) do not hinder screening.

SECONDARY BREAST REDUCTION

It is uncommon for patients to present for repeated reduction surgery as the overall patient satisfaction is high. The general advice is to use the same pedicle as before. There have been mixed outcomes with transecting pedicles.

- Hudson (*Plast Reconstr Surg,* 1999) recommends using the same pedicle or free nipple grafting if the previous pedicle/technique is unknown. There is

an increase in complications such as delayed wound healing and loss of NAC with repeat reductions.
- Losee (*Plast Reconstr Surg,* 2000) – three of four patients with complications (out of a total of 10) had transected pedicles (average time from first surgery 15 years), but these complications all healed conservatively.

IV. MASTOPEXY

REGNAULT CLASSIFICATION OF BREAST PTOSIS

Ptosis is Greek for the act of 'falling'. The underlying reason is usually volume loss due to post-pregnancy, significant weight loss, larger cup size/BMI or aging-related changes. Breast feeding itself was not found to be a factor (Rinker B, *Ann Plast Surg,* 2010) (Figure 5.4).

- First degree – the nipple descends to the level of the IMF.
- Second degree – the nipple falls below fold but remains above the lowest contour of the breast.
- Third degree – the nipple reaches the lowest contour of the breast.
- Pseudoptosis – loose, lax breast but the nipple remains at/above IMF whilst the majority of parenchyma falls below the level of the fold. There is an increase in the NAC–IMF distance.

ASSESSMENT

- Evaluate the patient's concerns and expectations.
- Breast history and relevant past medical history.

EXAMINATION

- **Skin and parenchymal quality**
  - The amount of skin stretch is an important factor in deciding what procedures will produce the best results.
- **Areolar size and shape**
- **Degree of ptosis**
- **Measurements – sternal notch to NAC, NAC to IMF**

The basic aims are similar to breast reduction, i.e. to produce a pleasing breast shape whilst ensuring reliable NAC transposition and optimisation of the scar. However, often reduction is not desirable; instead, volume maintenance or

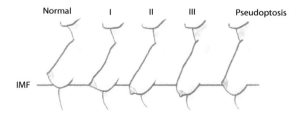

Figure 5.4 Classification of breast ptosis. Normal, I, II, III and pseudoptosis.

some sort **of volume replacement is required**, which sets up a set of conflicting stresses. Many different techniques for mastopexy have been described in the literature, which usually suggests the absence of a single ideal technique.

Mastopexy preferences: A survey of board-certified plastic surgeons. (Rohrich RJ, *Plast Reconstr Surg*, 2006) According to this survey with 487 responses, the traditional inverted T scar technique is the most popular technique. Satisfaction was highest with short-scar techniques, e.g. SPAIR and Hall-Findlay techniques, but physician satisfaction was lowest with periareolar techniques with a higher rate of revision surgery. Overall, the complications were similar to breast reduction, with the most common being suture splitting, excess scarring and bottoming out (ITIP).

BASIC TECHNIQUES

- **Periareolar** – this is suited for mild to moderate ptosis. At its simplest, it is a periareolar incision with concentric de-epithelialisation and closure (Bartels RJ, *Plast Reconstr Surg*, 1976), but this tends to enlarge and flatten the areola/breast when used too aggressively (e.g. the outer diameter more than twice the inner diameter). Many other variants involve parenchymal reshaping, whilst use of permanent purse-string sutures has reduces areolar/scar widening. Contraindications include sternal notch to NAC distance of >24 cm, ptosis grade of 2 or more or implants being removed or downsized.
  - **Benelli round block technique** incorporates some parenchymal moulding. The nipple is kept on a superior pedicle whilst the gland is undermined; medial and lateral parenchymal flaps are coned. The periareolar incision is closed with nylon, i.e. permanent sutures (Figure 5.5).
  - **Goes technique** with mesh support (*Aesthet Surg J*, 2003).
- **Vertical/short scar techniques** – based on the VSM techniques, are useful for moderately severe forms of ptosis. They have increased in popularity as they tend to incorporate parenchymal rearrangement and do not rely on the skin for long-term support.
  - Hall-Findlay (*Clin Plastic Surg*, 2002) prefers to use a lateral pedicle for the nipple and a medial pedicle for the inferolateral breast tissue that is mobilised and rotated up as an autoaugmentation.
  - SPAIR technique (Hammond DC).
- An inferior dermoglandular flap is tunnelled superiorly under a loop of PM muscle – this is usually referred to as the Graf/Biggs flap (**Graf** R, *Aesth Plast Surg*, 2000).
- **Flowers. 'Flip-flap' mastopexy** (*Aesth Plast Surg*, 1998). The inferior parenchyma is folded under the superior pedicle and sutured to the pectoralis fascia.
- **Inverted T inferior pedicle** – these may be considered in severe ptosis and severe skin excess, but the main criticisms are the scarring and the bottoming out over the long term. The inferior parenchyma can be repositioned and sutured to the pectoralis fascia to restore some upper pole fullness.
  - **Double flap technique** (Foustanos A, *Plast Reconstr Surg*, 2007). The authors use a Pitanguy skin pattern (similar to Wise, resulting in an inverted T); the nipple is carried on a superior pedicle (first flap), whilst an inferior pedicle is developed and sutured to the superior chest wall (second flap). This has been likened to a form of 'auto-augmentation'; something similar was described by Honig (*Aesth Plast Surg*, 2009).

AUGMENTATION MASTOPEXY

Augmentation mastopexy is the **most frequently litigated operation** in plastic surgery in the United States.

Volume replacement in the form of implants is more likely to be needed in those with relatively poor skin quality and deficient parenchyma particularly in the upper pole. Whilst augmentation alone will restore breast volume, **some skin excision** will be required for more severe degrees of ptosis.

Most cases needing more than 3 cm of nipple elevation usually require a mastopexy **and** augmentation preferably in two stages (usually augmenting before mastopexy),

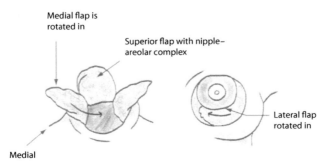

Figure 5.5 Benelli mastopexy. The NAC is supported by a superior flap; medial and lateral glandular flaps are developed. The medial flap is rotated in under the superior flap and sutured in; the lateral flap is rotated medially over the medial flap. The NAC complex is sutured in with a round-block permanent purse-string suture.

though some suggest a one-stage procedure, which has a greater risk of complications (see Spear, *Plast Reconstr Surg*, 2003). In such cases, the implant is usually placed subglandularly (if soft tissues allow this) as this will fill the skin envelope better.

When making the decision, it is important to ask the patient many questions, particularly **how large do they want to be?** The larger the augmentation/implant, the less lift required, etc. Many variables need to be considered:

- Choose one- or two-stage (4–6 months apart)
  - If staged
    - Augmentation or mastopexy first.
    - Augmenting first means shorter final scars but the patient will need to live with sagging before the second stage.
    - With severe ptosis, it is better to excise skin first via inverted T (with or without autoaugmentation).
    - Staging halves the risk of revision from 20% to 10%.
  - When performed together, it is preferable to only mark the new nipple position tentatively and to confirm the position after the implants are in place and the skin is tailor-tacked with the patient sitting up.
- Best plane for implant
  - **Subglandular** – reasonable choice in mild–moderate ptosis with good soft tissue envelope.
  - **Subpectoral preferred** with thinner skin envelope. It adds less weight to breast, but the breast will continue to descend over the muscle (ptotic breast likely to have deficient Coopers ligaments) causing a double bubble deformity.
- Type of implant. Silicone is much preferred; if the patient insists on saline implants, then it should be placed subpectorally.
  - Avoid large implants due to weight as well as risk to vascularity.

Key points in mastopexy. (De Benito J, *Aesth Plast Surg*, 2010)

This author prefers anatomical implants because when the implant is placed 60% below the NAC, the NAC tends to move up whilst a round implant would tend to move the NAC down. Silicone gel implants have less tendency to expand or atrophy the lower pole than saline implants (Tebbetts JB, *Clin Plast Surg*, 2001). The authors prefer to use a subpectoral or subfascial plane.

Augmentation/mastopexy: 'Surgeon beware'. (Spear SL, *Plast Reconstr Surg*, 2003)

The author explains his viewpoint on combining augmentation with mastopexy. He states that individually they are simple procedures with relatively few complications; however, **in combination, they increase the likelihood of complications of the other**. Where a mastopexy tends to reshape the breast and reduce the skin, an augmentation enlarges the breast volume and expands the skin, setting up a set of competing factors that may lead to insufficient soft tissue cover, with the implant also creating tension and reduced vascularity.

- There is an increased risk of infection and implant exposure due to the overlying soft tissue rearrangement.
- There is an increased risk of loss of nipple sensation or malposition as the mastopexy after augmentation will reposition the breast.

A follow-up by the same author (*Plast Reconstr Surg*, 2006) found that combined procedures had 5× the reoperation rate of primary augmentation and 10× the complication rate.

Conservative augmentation with periareolar mastopexy reduces complications and treats a variety of breast types. (Cannon CL, *Ann Plast Surg*, 2010)

This paper emphasises the combination of a small/moderate implant and a periareolar mastopexy to reduce the incidence of complications. The authors suggest that favourable factors are implant size 360 mL or less, flaccid empty breasts, nipple elevation 4 cm or less, light skin tones and absence of stretch marks.

Aesthetic management of the breast following explantation: Evaluation and mastopexy options. (Rohrich RJ, *Plast Reconstr Surg*, 1998)

This is a retrospective review of 282 patients who had their implants explanted. Almost 50% chose not to replace the implants. Other options include the following:

- Capsulectomy alone. The presence of microcalcification or silicone granulomas makes detection of breast cancers more difficult if the capsule is left behind.
- Re-implantation. If the plan is to replace the implant with a saline implant, then submuscular placement is preferred to avoid rippling.
- Mastopexy – grade I periareolar/vertical, grade II Wise pattern.
- Pseudoptosis – inframammary wedge excision.

A follow-up study (Rohrich RJ, *Plast Reconstr Surg*, 2007) found that the commonest choices were now implant exchange (usually a subpectoral smooth saline implant) with or without mastopexy.

V. GYNAECOMASTIA

Gynaecomastia (Galen) is abnormal breast development in the male that can be due to a wide variety of causes. It has an incidence of 32%–65% in the male population; this range is partly due to a lack of a standard definition. Most cases are due to a variety of subtle hormonal factors and may be reversible; sometimes it is caused by a serious underlying disease particularly of the pituitary or testes. Very rarely, male breast cancer may masquerade as gynaecomastia; a hard eccentric mass should raise suspicions.

AETIOLOGY

The aetiology is multifactorial, but in many cases, a clear identifiable cause is missing. The age of onset is an important clue to the most likely cause of the enlargement; up to two-thirds of patients will be labelled as 'pubertal' gynaecomastia.

PHYSIOLOGICAL

- Neonatal (up to 60%, lasts 2 weeks), pubertal and senile (up to 60%) gynaecomastia that may be due to some **androgen–oestrogen imbalance**.
- **It affects up to 75% of pubertal males** (can almost be considered 'normal' – 75% resolve within 2 years, and by 17 years of age, the incidence is less than 10%). It is possibly due to increased androgen to oestrogen conversion in the tissues and/or increased tissue hypersensitivity. It is typically asymmetric and possibly tender.
- In the elderly, it may be due to testicular failure or increased fat levels/aromatase activity.

PATHOLOGICAL

Pathological gynaecomastia (40% overall) is more common in non-pubertal patients.

- **Hormone-producing tumours**
  - Seminomas, teratomas and choriocarcinomas of testis that produce human chorionic gonadotrophin (HCG).
  - Leydig, Sertoli and granulosa theca cell of testis producing oestrogen.
  - Lung, liver and kidney tumours producing GRH.
- **Systemic disease**
  - Liver disease (e.g. cirrhosis, reduced oestrogen clearance) and hyperthyroidism increase serum hormone binding globulin, which decreases free androgens.
  - Renal disease increases luteinising hormone (LH) and oestrogens.
  - General debility that interferes with the pituitary–hypothalamic axis, e.g. burns.
- **Hypogonadism/testicular failure**
  - Pituitary disorders (decreased GRH).
  - Androgen insensitivity syndrome (5-α-reductase deficiency).
  - Klinefelter's syndrome. These patients have 20–60× increased risk of breast cancer; patients with other forms of gynaecomastia do not have an increased risk.

PHARMACOLOGICAL (10%–20%)

Drugs are the most common cause of gynaecomastia in men over 40 years of age.

- Spironolactone, cimetidine (blocks androgen action), digoxin, metoclopramide, tricyclics, methyldopa, marijuana, steroids (adrenal suppression)

- Drugs used in the treatment of prostate cancer
  - LH releasing hormone (LHRH) analogues (e.g. Zoladex used in the treatment of prostate cancer) increases testosterone and then decreases it due to negative feedback.
    - There is increasing use in transgender patients – primarily as puberty blockers but also in adults; here, increasing breast size is a welcome side effect.
  - Anti-androgens (cyproterone acetate) and oestrogens (stilboestrol).

ASSESSMENT

History

- Age of onset and rate of growth.
  - Gynaecomastia of less than 1 year duration may still respond to medical therapy.
- Psychological effects.
- Symptoms such as pain, nipple discharge, etc.
  - Gynaecomastia with **visual disturbance and headache** is a pituitary tumour until proven otherwise.
- General state of health and **drug history**.
- Family history – familial forms have been described.

Examination

This should include the thyroid, abdomen (liver, kidneys) and genitalia/testes.

- Testicular asymmetry may be due to tumours (steroid producing or paraneoplastic HCG); 5% of testicular tumours present with gynaecomastia.
- Small testes may be associated with Klinefelter's syndrome (patients have low testosterone).

Investigations

Routine tests are usually not required; extensive work-up is rarely indicated, but in certain groups, selected investigations may be useful, e.g. **prepubertal gynaecomastia** (infants) – testicular examination/ultrasound may yield a significant number of functional endocrine tumours. Other clues include small testicles, decreased libido/fertility, lack of male hair or eunuchoid body.

Adult gynaecomastia is usually due to excess fat rather than glandular hypertrophy. The common identifiable causes are drugs, liver dysfunction and hyperthyroidism. Routine endocrine screening is not fruitful.

Other significant features include tenderness, rapid enlargement, eccentric hard/irregular mass or lesion >4 cm in diameter.

- FNA of simple gynaecomastia is to be avoided.
- Liver function test.
- Hormone screen – reduced testosterone and/or elevated oestrogen.
  - Serum testosterone, LH/FSH for hypogonadism

- HCG, oestradiol (consider CT to exclude adrenal tumour – increased substrate for oestrogen production by peripheral aromatase) and DHEA
  - TSH/free T4 in selected patients
- Chest X-ray (CXR).
- Karyotyping can be considered if the testosterone is low, or features of feminisation with Marfanoid characteristics (to exclude Klinefelter's).

CLINICAL CLASSIFICATION

Pseudo-gynaecomastia is sometimes used to describe purely fatty enlargement.

(Simon BE, *Plast Reconstr Surg*, 1973)
- Grade I – Subareolar 'button'
- Grade II
  - a – Moderate enlargement, no skin excess
  - b – Moderate enlargement with extra skin
- Grade III – Marked enlargement with extra skin

A new classification system based on the amount and character of breast hypertrophy as well as the degree of ptosis was proposed by Rohrich (*Plast Reconstr Surg*, 2003, see below).

- Grade I – minimal hypertrophy (<250 g of breast tissue) without ptosis
  - IA primarily glandular
  - IB primarily fibrous
- Grade II – moderate hypertrophy (between 250 and 500 g of breast tissue) without ptosis
  - IIA primarily glandular
  - IIB primarily fibrous
- Grade III – moderate–severe hypertrophy (>500 g of breast tissue) and grade I ptosis
- Grade IV – severe hypertrophy (>500 g of breast tissue) and grade II/III ptosis

Cordova classification. (Cordova A, *J Plast Reconstr Aesthet Surg*, 2008)
- Grade I – swelling limited to the areolar region; no IMF. Adenectomy via semicircular periareolar incision.
- Grade II – NAC above IMF. Ultrasound-assisted liposuction (UAL) with skin-sparing adenectomy.
- Grade III – NAC at the same height or less than 1 cm below IMF. UAL followed by periareolar skin removal. Scar wrinkling usually improves spontaneously.
- Grade IV – NAC more than 1 cm below IMF. Breast reduction with nipple repositioning usually a central pedicle.

HISTOLOGICAL CLASSIFICATION

The enlargement is due largely to ductal tissue with some fat, without true gland development. The histologic appearance changes with time from hypervascular ductal tissue to acellular fibrosis with few ducts. This gives rise to three histological patterns with varying degrees of stromal and ductal proliferation:

- **Florid pattern** – increased numbers of budding ducts in a highly cellular fibroblastic stroma. This pattern is more common in the first 4 months.
- **Intermediate type** – overlapping.
- **Fibrous type** – extensive stromal fibrosis with minimal ductal proliferation. The hypertrophic breast tissue becomes **irreversibly fibrotic** after about 12 months.

MANAGEMENT

Non-surgical

Medical management has had limited success overall. It is more effective during the active proliferative phase, with very little effect after fibrosis occurs.

- Correction of underlying causes.
- Pharmacological treatment of hormonal imbalances.
- Medication – The level of evidence is generally low.
  - Danazol. 60% and 35% show intermediate and moderate response respectively to this drug. It inhibits oestrogen production with androgenic side effect; there may be significant weight gain.
  - Tamoxifen is useful to reduce pain but seems less useful in reducing the size. Its long-term effects on males are not clear.
  - Clomiphene (oestrogen receptor modulator, often used to treat female infertility), testolactone (aromatase inhibitor that was discontinued in 2008).
- Obesity is often associated with large fatty breasts but the effectiveness of weight loss is very variable.

Surgical treatment

Pubertal gynaecomastia is less likely to resolve when it has reached moderate sizes (4 cm or more) or in particularly obese patients. Overall, ~15% of patients have surgery; classically, the type of surgery depends on the grade as follows:

- Grade I – circumareolar/inferior semicircular **areolar incision**, excise 'button' taking care to leave some soft tissue under the areola to reduce the dish deformity. Take care to place the incision exactly at the edge; some use an irregular incision to disguise it further.
- Grade II.
  - A – Liposuction alone or in combination with excision of a disc of breast tissue via a **circumareolar incision**.
  - B – Excision of skin using doughnut mastopexy technique, bevelled excision of the breast disc and liposuction to feather the edges.
- Grade III – 'breast reduction' - some non-areolar skin will need to be excised leaving chest scars. A wide range of techniques have been described and no single technique is suitable for all.
  - **Circumareolar concentric** skin reduction with subcutaneous mastectomy can be successfully treat severe gynaecomastia (Tashkandi M, *Ann Plast Surg*, 2004). The authors suggest free nipple

grafting in some cases due to massive weight loss or tuberose breasts.

- Horizontal skin ellipse with nipple–areolar vertical bipedicle leaving transverse scar
- Letterman technique – nipple transposition on superomedial pedicle
- Inferior pedicle markings
- Lejour-type vertical short-scar type technique

Complications

- Early
  - Haematoma/seroma – fairly common. Drains may be needed in more extensive resections; pressure dressings are commonly used.
  - Infection.
- Late
  - **Dish deformity** and having nipple stuck to the chest wall – keep at least 1 cm of soft tissue behind the areola.
  - Inadequate correction of gland volume or skin excess.
  - Problem scarring.

LIPOSUCTION FOR GYNAECOMASTIA

Currently, there is a trend for more liposuction especially UAL, with excision reserved for severe (glandular) gynae-comastia or for significant skin excess after UAL.

- Grades IA and IIA. Liposuction, but the firm breast bud is fairly resistant to standard liposuction.
- UAL (e.g. Vaser®) is effective in (almost) all grades of gynaecomastia; it is more effective for fibrotic tissue and also promotes skin tightening, and thus reducing the need for skin excision. Removal of redundant skin should be delayed for 6 to 9 months.

Classification and management of gynecomastia: Defining the role of ultrasound-assisted liposuction. (Rohrich RJ, *Plast Reconstr Surg,* 2003)
In UAL, piezoelectric crystals produce ultrasonic energy that 'liquefies' fat through cavitation whilst preserving adja-cent nervous, vascular and connective tissue elements, i.e. it is (somewhat) selective (see 'Liposuction').

- Subcutaneous infiltration of a wetting/tumescent solution.
- Tunnelling with the UAL probe to treat the fat.
- Releasing the IMF is important.
- Evacuation and final contouring by suction-assisted lipectomy.
- The endpoints for UAL (time and loss of resistance) differ from those for standard suction-assisted lipectomy (pinch and contour).

This review of 61 patients demonstrated that UAL is effective in treating most grades of gynaecomastia and is better than conventional liposuction in addressing dense, fibrous lipodystrophy. Excision is reserved for skin excess after liposuction, after approximately 6–9 months.

Some surgeons, e.g. Mladick RA in his discussion of the article above, prefer to address skin excess in the same operation rather than wait for retraction.

Laser-assisted lipolysis in the treatment of gynaecomastia. (Trelles MA, *Lasers Med Sci,* 2013)
In a prospective study of the use of a 980 nm diode laser, 18 of 28 patients graded their results as very good, 6 as good. There were no reported complications. The same author described a second slightly expanded study ($n = 32$) in 2013 (Trelles MA, *Rev Col Bras Cir,* 2013).

Yoo (*Dermatol,* 2015) reported success with a 1444 nm Nd:YAG laser in 13 patients.

C. BREAST RECONSTRUCTION

I. BREAST CANCER AND SCREENING

EPIDEMIOLOGY

The lifetime risk of developing breast cancer is estimated to be 12% (ACS data) with a median age at diagnosis of approximately 60.

About 30,000 new cases of breast cancer are diagnosed annually in the United Kingdom, and half of those in the <65 year age group require mastectomy, making around 7500 breast reconstructions per year in the country.

BREAST CANCER GENES

- 25% of women who develop breast cancer before age 42 have a definable hereditary component.
- **BRCA1 and BRCA2** genes (mutated tumour supp-ressor genes) account for 2%–3% of breast cancer cases; there are other as yet unidentified genes that may also contribute to the risk. When more than four cases of breast cancer at <60 years of age occur within one family, there is likely to be a genetic cause; with two to three cases per family, it may be due to chance only.
  - Patients with the genes (0.1% of women with either) are likely to develop breast cancer before 50 years of age. From the age 25 onwards there is an 85% lifetime risk of developing breast cancer (60% ovarian cancer).
  - These patients may elect to undergo prophylactic (subcutaneous) mastectomy and reconstruction; 50% of BRCA1 carriers treated by lumpectomy and radiotherapy recur or develop a second cancer in the same breast.
  - Tamoxifen has been shown to decrease the risk among BRCA1/2 mutation carriers by 50%–62%.

OTHER FACTORS

- Hormonal factors – increased number of menstrual cycles (i.e. early menarche, late first pregnancy, nulliparity, late menopause), which increases oestrogen exposure, oestrogen HRT.

- Women with an increased BMI tend to have more fatty tissue and elevated peripheral oestrogen. This is associated with increased breast cancer risk in postmenopausal (though not premenopausal) women.
- Prophylactic mastectomy is shown to decrease cancer risk by 90%–100%.
- Bilateral oophorectomy before menopause reduces risk by 25%–53%.

SCREENING

Identifies approximately 6 cancers for every 1000 women screened.

- Screening is currently offered every 3 years after 50 years in the United Kingdom. An extension for ages 47–73 is (still) being phased in – it was meant to have been completed by 2012. The ACS (2015) recommends that women of average risk aged 45–54 should get annual mammograms. Younger patients (40–44) have the choice to start screening whilst those 55 or older should switch to a mammogram every 2 years.
    - The benefit of screening in terms of lives saved is greater than the harm in terms of over-diagnosis; 2–2.5 lives are saved for every over-diagnosed case (Duffy SW, *J Med Screen*, 2010).
    - BRCA1-related tumours tend to be cellular rather than scirrhous, with less microcalcification, and are more difficult to differentiate from benign lesions on mammography, particularly in the typically younger patients.
- MRI is a sensitive investigation in the premenopausal breast (which would be difficult to screen with MMG). A Canadian study (Warner E, *JAMA*, 2004) demonstrated clear superiority over MMG or ultrasound in BRCA patients, whilst combining all three offered the highest rate of detection (95%). A follow-up study (Bigenwald RZ, *Cancer Epidemiol Biomarkers Prev*, 2008) demonstrated that MRI was still far better than MMG for older BRCA patients with less dense breasts.
- Ultrasound is good for differentiating between solid and cystic lesions and for guiding biopsies. High-resolution ultrasound can pick up some cancers and can be used to monitor tumour response to chemotherapy or radiotherapy.

EXAMINATION

- Oncological examination – site, size, chest wall fixation, skin involvement, nodes and thorough examination of the contralateral breast
- Donor sites, e.g. abdominal/back scars, rectus diastasis, skin and soft tissue laxity

PATHOLOGY

- 75% of breast tumours are invasive ductal carcinomas – DCIS presents as microcalcification on MMG.

- 10% invasive lobular carcinomas – lobular carcinoma in situ (LCIS) has no mammographic changes and is a 'coincidental' finding on biopsy; it is a **marker** of invasive disease rather than a precursor, and tumours in such cases have the tendency to bilaterality (40%) and multifocality (60%).
- Special types generally have a better prognosis:
    - Medullary (numerous lymphocytes) <5%
    - Mucinous (bulky mucin-forming tumours) <5%
    - Tubular (well-differentiated adenocarcinoma)
    - Phyllodes (mixed connective tissue and epithelial tumour, with a fern-like cellular pattern)

STAGING

TNM classification – main landmarks (approximate 5 year survival %)

- Stage I – tumour <2 cm confined to the breast (T1) (85%)
- Stage II – mobile axillary nodes (N1) (65%)
- Stage IIIa – fixed axillary nodes (N2) (40%)
- Stage IIIb – chest wall or skin involvement (T4) 25%
- Stage IIIb – internal mammary nodes (N3)
- Stage IV – distant metastases (M1) (10%)

TUMOUR

- Tis – carcinoma in situ or Paget's disease of the nipple with no associated tumour
- T1 – ≤2 cm
- T2 – 2–5 cm
- T3 – >5 cm
- T4 – extension to the chest wall or skin

LYMPH NODES

- N0 – no regional lymph node metastasis
- N1 – mobile ipsilateral axillary lymph nodes
- N2a – fixed ipsilateral axillary nodes
- N2b – internal mammary nodes without evidence of axillary nodes
- N3a – axillary and infraclavicular nodes
- N3b – axillary and internal mammary nodes
- N3c – supraclavicular lymph node

METASTASIS

- M0 – no distant metastasis
- M1 – distant metastasis

II. MASTECTOMY AND ADJUVANT THERAPY

TUMOUR EXCISION

Modified radical mastectomy (MRM) includes an in-continuity axillary clearance but leaves the pectoralis major.

Large tumours may also require neo-/-adjuvant chemotherapy, e.g. cyclophosphamide, methotrexate and 5-fluorouracil (CMF). Most patients receive tamoxifen. The NAC is usually excised; nipple-sparing mastectomy (NSM) is still rather controversial.

- Skin-sparing mastectomy (SSM) the 'traditional' option for extensive DCIS; no node surgery/radiotherapy
- **Breast conservation therapy** (see also 'Oncoplastic surgery')
  - Small lump – lumpectomy (1 cm margin) + **radiotherapy** + node sampling/clearance, adjuvant radiotherapy. RT is a mandatory part of BCT; it reduces recurrence from 40% to 8%.
- Axillary nodes
  - Node dissection – standard level I and II clearance will identify 98% of metastasis; level III only indicated in those with gross nodal involvement.
    - Intercostobrachial nerve injury 70%–80%
  - Sentinel node lymph biopsy (SLNB) with radioisotope and blue dye in those with clinically negative axilla. Some surgeons are using indocyanine green (ICG).

NEO-ADJUVANT THERAPY

- Neo-adjuvant chemotherapy treats systemic disease and downstages tumour size but with a significant morbidity. The overall response rate is about 80% with complete response in 30%, but there is **no evidence of a survival advantage.**
- Radiotherapy is usually used post-operatively but neo-adjuvant radiotherapy may also be used, with the exception when local tissues are required for flap closure. Radiation has unpredictable effects on reconstructions and usually precludes the use of expander/implants.

Angiosarcoma of the breast: A review of 70 cases. (Hodgson NC, *Am J Clin Oncol*, 2007)
Although angiosarcoma is a very rare complication of breast irradiation, it is being reported in increased numbers with the increase in BCT. These 'secondary' types of breast angiosarcomas tend to present with more advanced disease and in an older age group (~30 years older).

Wide local resection may be curative; the most common site of recurrence is the contralateral breast, possibly due to lymphatic spread.

Angiosarcoma of the breast. (Georgiannos SN, *Br J Plast Surg*, 2003)
All 4 patients in this study were alive and disease free 3–7 years post-mastectomy. Prognosis is generally related to histological grade and excision margins; with high-grade tumours, the median disease-free survival is 15 months.

Primary and secondary angiosarcoma of the breast. (Arora TK, *Gland Surg*, 2014;3:28)
There is little consensus in the management of AS of the breast. Deep margins are most likely to be positive after wide local excision and some advocate muscle resection. Some suggest excision of all irradiated skin.

Skin-Sparing Mastectomy. (Toth B, *Plast Reconstr Surg*, 1991; Kroll SS, *Surg Gynecol Obstet*, 1991; Slavin SA, *Plast Reconstr Surg*, 1998)
An SSM removes breast, nipple–areolar complex and biopsy scar, and it aims to produce a **superior aesthetic result** because

- It preserves native breast skin except for skin close to a superficial tumour.
- It preserves the IMF.
- It is only appropriate when immediate reconstruction is planned.
- A separate incision may also be needed for axillary sampling/clearance (some choose to use the same incision) and/or for microsurgery.

Classification of SSM (Carlson GW, *Ann Surg*, 1997)

- Type I – NAC only excised (prophylactic) surgery
- Type II – NAC + separate scar excision
- Type III – NAC + in-continuity scar excision
- Type IV – NAC excision within a breast reduction pattern (large breast, unsuitable for TRAM flap and contralateral reduction planned)

Common indications include

- Prophylactic mastectomy.
- Stages 1 and 2 invasive breast cancer – BCT is an alternative.
- DCIS – usually combined with SLNB.
- Multicentric tumours.
- Phyllodes tumours.
- Where immediate reconstruction is planned.

SSM aims to remove all breast tissue, but in practice, this is difficult to achieve, i.e. **cancer reducing not cancer preventing**. Most agree that it seems to be a safe treatment for early invasive cancer that does not compromise local control.

- A **nipple-sparing mastectomy** (NSM) is an SSM that preserves the NAC along with its ductal epithelium, which is a theoretical oncological risk. Although the nipple may be flattened, dyspigmented and insensate, it offers better aesthetic results than NAC reconstruction. It may be an option in **prophylactic mastectomies** (strong family history, BRCA genes, atypia/precancerous changes) or in cases of very small tumours far away from the nipple.
  - Some would argue that higher risk patients should have a standard mastectomy that removes the maximal amount of breast tissue (although deposits of breast tissue will **still** remain on the skin flaps and the pectoralis muscle) without formal axillary dissection (there should be complete removal of the axillary tail of Spence, obliging removal of some low axillary lymph nodes).

- Others say that the oncological risks of preserving the NAC seem to have been overestimated (Simmons RM, *Ann Plast Surg*, 2003), and it may be safe as long as the tumour is not close to the nipple and frozen section assessment of the subareolar tissue is performed. A variation on this is to remove the nipple but preserve the areolar (areolar-sparing mastectomy [ASM]).
- The term *subcutaneous mastectomy* (preserves significant breast tissue) is rather defunct.
- **Radiotherapy** is not a contraindication to SSM per se but will affect the final cosmetic outcome.

Local recurrence is a marker for disseminated disease; most patients with local recurrence after total mastectomy eventually die of metastatic disease. In the end, **all forms of mastectomy leave behind some breast tissue**, and the local recurrence rate is related more to the stage of disease and tumour biology rather than the type of surgery. The flaps should be of the same thickness as a standard mastectomy; the risk of residual tumour in the skin flaps increases when the flaps are >5 mm (Torresan RZ, *Ann Surg Oncol*, 2005); 60% of skin flaps contained residual breast tissue. Skin flap necrosis is a recognised complication of SSM (11%), though it does not seem to be much higher than for other types of mastectomy and can be minimised with careful patient selection (avoiding smokers, diabetics, obese patients, etc.).

III. BREAST RECONSTRUCTION

Once it had been demonstrated that immediate breast reconstruction was oncologically safe, it became the preferred option as the aesthetic results are superior with more superior fullness and better ptosis.

Adjuvant therapy is not affected by (immediate) reconstruction; general wound complications are similar to a standard mastectomy, though transfusion requirements may increase (a 3 unit threshold may be significant in terms of the immunosuppression). On the other hand, some argue that the additional surgical trauma of a second surgery may cause a degree of relative immunosuppression allowing dormant tumour cells to flourish.

However, adjuvant treatment may affect the quality of reconstruction – most often, there is a variable/unpredictable volume loss.

- With **delayed reconstruction**, there is a loss of the (3D) native skin envelope, a new IMF is required, surgery involves exploration/dissection of previously operated/irradiated tissues and, overall, the outcome is less aesthetic.
  - Need to wait at least 6 weeks after last chemotherapy dose (and blood tests have normalised) and 3–6 months after radiotherapy (when skin has regained most of its softness).
  - Delayed reconstruction costs up to 70% more.
  - More psychological trauma.

- **Delayed immediate (MD Anderson)** – submuscular expander is placed to preserve skin envelope whilst awaiting definitive pathology, avoiding the problems associated with RT after immediate reconstruction (Kronowitz SJ, *Plast Reconstr Surg*, 2010). This is a common scenario in countries with variable levels of funding for reconstruction.
  - If RT is required, then delayed reconstruction after 4–6 months.
  - If RT is not needed, then immediate reconstruction can proceed.

It is important to appreciate that **breast reconstruction is a process**, involving several procedures, rather than a one-off operation, and this needs to be clearly conveyed to patients. Mimicking natural ptosis and achieving a good IMF are often the most difficult parts to get right. Reconstruction can either be

- Designed to match the contralateral breast, and/or
- Contralateral breast can be modified to match the reconstruction.

Routine histological examination of the mastectomy scar at the time of breast reconstruction: Important oncological surveillance? (Soldin MG, *Br J Plast Surg*, 2004)

This is a review of the histology of 48 mastectomy scars in patients who had delayed breast reconstruction; there was no evidence of malignancy in any of the scars, whilst six patients had a local recurrence at the time of presentation for reconstruction (1 was clinically 'occult').

Up to 90% of local recurrence following mastectomy occurs within 3 years, and since local recurrence is detectable clinically, routine histological evaluation of the mastectomy scar at the time of reconstruction is **unnecessary**, especially after 3 years.

This was confirmed by Munir (*Ann Plast Surg*, 2006) and Woerderman (*Plast Reconstr Surg*, 2006), a study with 728 scars.

Positive impact of delayed reconstruction on breast-cancer treatment-related arm lymphedema. (Blanchard M et al., *J Plast Reconstr Aesth Surg*, 2012)

Twenty consecutive patients with secondary lymphoedema related to the breast cancer treatment requested delayed breast reconstruction that was achieved through a variety of means (3 TRAM, 5 LD with implants and 12 implants alone) after a median period of 30 months. The mean lymphoedema volume (truncated cone method with 5 cm segments) at 22 months after surgery was 235 mL compared to 378 mL before surgery ($p < 0.02$). Patients continued with their previous specific therapy, e.g. MLD, pressure garments, etc. Numbers were too small to investigate the effect of different reconstructive methods.

RECONSTRUCTION OF A SMALL BREAST

Implants

Implant-based reconstruction is the commonest type of reconstruction in the United States and the United Kingdom.

Implant-based reconstructions basically compromise **long-term** aesthetics for the sake of a simpler procedure, but may be (one of the) best options for a particular patient and his/her circumstances. The lower initial cost, simpler surgery and shorter inpatient stay are significant advantages but need to be balanced against the need for revisional surgery for complications, and poor late appearance. The increasing use of fat graft in combination with implants may improve results.

- **Implants alone** may be considered if sufficient skin remains, e.g. SSM/NSM in those not needing radiotherapy; patients will need to accept a breast of smaller size. **Skin compromise is the major concern**; thus, subcutaneous implants are contraindicated, and implants are usually positioned (wholly) submuscularly or within an **ADM pocket**. ADMs supposedly allow bigger fill volumes but at the expense of more complications – seromas and infections are 4 and 5 times more common respectively.
  - Implants suffer a gradual loss of cosmesis – patient satisfaction with saline implants is 86% at 2 years, reduced to 54% at 5 years.
  - Fifteen percent of those having implant reconstruction after NSM have nipple malposition.
  - **'Red breast syndrome'** – some (5%–10%) patients with Alloderm® develop a delayed (weeks) erythema that is attributed to a poorly characterised tissue reaction. There are no signs of systemic upset or local induration, and the condition resolves as the ADM becomes incorporated (months).
- **Tissue expander followed by implant**. With some skin deficiency, e.g. after MRM, skin/tissue expansion is usually required to accommodate an implant. Most often, a tissue expander is followed by an implant, but an alternative is that a combined expander–implant is used (see below).
  - **Longer overall treatment**. The process is relatively simple with a few serious complications, but numerous visits are involved. The expander is inflated weekly until it is 'over-expanded' (approximately 25%–30%) **compared to the opposite side**. It is then left for about 3–6 months with continual massage for the capsule to 'mature'.
  - **Expanders can be held/deflated as needed for radiotherapy, followed by autologous tissue reconstruction.** If radiotherapy is not required, then the expander can be exchanged for an implant after six months to avoid the inflammatory phase (MSK protocol) (Cordeiro PG, *Plast Reconstr Surg*, 2015); using a smaller prosthesis will recreate a degree of ptosis.
  - **The normal sized port (20 expansions vs. 10 expansions for miniports) is often a better choice,** particularly for fatter patients to facilitate palpation. It is usually preferable to remove the filling port early, e.g. within 6 months; otherwise, there is an increased risk of leakage. This is often seen in patients who are lost to follow-up and return several years later with leakage/deflation of implants.

- Implants are oncologically 'safe', but they are foreign bodies and can cause problems such as infection, extrusion, leakage and capsule formation. Capsular contracture risk is increased when implants are used for reconstruction, compared to primary augmentation.
- **Expander implants**. Hilton Becker (1984) described a 'permanent' expander with textured silicone around saline that could be placed immediately and then expanded gradually until the desired volume is reached. There are products available in various silicone to saline ratios, from 25:75 to 50:50. The filling port may be distant (connected by e.g. Allergan Natrelle 133 tubing) and usually placed in the midaxillary area or integrated; however, the latter type is licensed for temporary use only with integrated ports, a magnet is used to locate the port and its metal backing plate; when the expander is underfilled, the shell can fold over the port and be inadvertently punctured. The metal in the expander implant is not MRI safe.
  - The use of expander/implants is relatively contraindicated **after** irradiation of the chest wall because the skin and the muscle may not be capable of stretching sufficiently; thus, implants are generally not an option in BCT.
  - Use of expander implants does not affect adjuvant therapy; however, radiotherapy (given to ~20%–30% of patients after mastectomy) increases the chance of capsular contracture. Half of patients with expanders treated with irradiation will subsequently need flap salvage.
  - Adjustable implants make matching the other side easier and thus are particularly useful for treating asymmetries or for bilateral reconstructions.

Becker (*Plast Reconstr Surg Global Open*, 2017;6:e1541) described the use of air to Mentor Spectrum expander implants in a small series.

RECONSTRUCTION OF A MODERATE-SIZED BREAST

- Expander implant
- LD and implant
- Pedicled TRAM (pTRAM) or free TRAM (fTRAM)
  - Contralateral pedicle is generally preferred as the ipsilateral pedicle usually involves a more acute angle and may compromise venous flow, but either is possible.
- Free deep inferior epigastric perforator (DIEP) flap where only zones 1 and 2 are needed

RECONSTRUCTION OF THE LARGE BREAST

A contralateral breast reduction can be considered in combination with a smaller reconstruction.

- Bipedicled TRAM. The donor defect is significant, but it can still be used in patients with a midline scar.

- Free TRAM utilising zones 1–3/4.
  - Anastomosing end–end to the circumflex scapular vessels saves LD as a lifeboat.
  - Anastomosing end–end to the thoracodorsal artery (TDA) proximal to the serratus branch also preserves LD (retrograde flow from intercostal supply to serratus).
- Bipedicled DIEP.

RECONSTRUCTION OF BILATERAL BREASTS

- Bilateral pedicled TRAM flaps
- Bilateral free TRAM/DIEP flaps
- Bilateral LD and implants

AUTOLOGOUS FLAPS FOR BREAST RECONSTRUCTION

Studies have demonstrated that the long-term cost of implants is actually greater than for autologous reconstruction. Patients should stop smoking, preferably weeks before surgery.

- Vertical flaps orientation provides better infraclavicular fill. The inferior tissue can be folded underneath for more projection.
- Transverse flap orientation is better for large broad breasts but with less infraclavicular fill.
- Flaps can be coned for projection, taking care with vascularity.
- In delayed reconstruction, an upward backcut at the lateral end of the inset releases the pocket for a better shape.

LATISSIMUS DORSI RECONSTRUCTION (SEE 'INDIVIDUAL FLAPS')

The LD flap (Schneider, *Br J Plast Surg*, 1977; Bostwick, *Clin Plast Surg*, 1979) is reliable with a necrosis rate of <1% (less than pTRAM). The LD flap improves aesthetics (and durability) of the expander/implant alone, and the difference becomes greater with time, especially if radiotherapy has been given.

For delayed reconstructions, the flap should be inset into the new IMF, rather than into the reopened mastectomy scar. The skin of the LD flap is thicker and darker than the front of the chest, thus creating a **patch effect**. The donor scar on the back can be large and seromas are not uncommon, although the incidence may be reduced by the use of quilting sutures.

The need for changing patient position limits its wider use somewhat. In addition, it has traditionally been regarded as being too small to reconstruct anything other than small breasts; thus, it is **usually combined with an implant**. If possible, aim for a breast 15%–30% larger than the other side to allow for shrinkage.

- According to some, the skin paddle is best taken diagonally along the RSTLs that run downwards and laterally (perpendicularly to the direction of the muscle fibres) with less hypertrophic scarring and dog ears compared with laterally placed diagonal and horizontal flaps (to hide the scar in the bra band line). However, recent studies show that the **greatest patient satisfaction** is with bra band or low oblique scars.
- The tunnel should be made high to avoid disrupting the lateral breast border. Secure muscle to the chest wall, and define the IMF. If an implant is also used, then the LD border overlaps the PM, pants over vest fashion.
- The practice regarding the tendon is variable. The tendon is often cut through 90% on the posterior surface to improve advancement whilst protecting the pedicle from excessive traction; but in delayed reconstruction, total detachment may be needed for better movement. Reattaching the tendon may allow reconstruction of the anterior axillary fold.

The size of an LD reconstruction can be maximised by

- **Fleur-de-lis skin** paddle (McCraw) or **boomerang** incisions (a transverse ellipse with an upward curve at the axilla – which is partly random as it extends beyond the muscle – and a downward curve at the middle of the back) also allow for bigger flaps, but then poor scar is often criticised.
- **Extended LD** – leave more fat on the muscle and/or take more of the adjacent soft tissue particularly the pockets of fat near the scapular tip and posterior iliac crest, which require careful dissection to preserve the fragile blood supply. The emphasis is not on widening the skin flap; this manoeuvre does not significantly increase the bulk of the reconstructed breast but makes closure much more difficult. There may be a greater risk of seroma.
- Primary fat injection to LD muscle (see below); similarly, others have proposed fat filling the PM muscle.

Latissimus dorsi flap for total autologous immediate breast reconstruction without implants. (Santanelli di Pompeo F et al., *Plast Reconstr Surg*, 2014)
Twenty-three patients underwent breast reconstruction with primary fat augmented LD flaps. Fat was harvested using the Coleman technique with 10 mL syringes and injected into the adipose layer and under the muscle fascia of the LD flap skin paddle with 1 mL syringes. Mean injected fat volume was 101 mL. No fat grafting–related complications were observed.

THORACODORSAL ARTERY (TDA, 1.5–3 MM)

The artery gives off one to two branches to the SA before entering the LD muscle. The pedicle (average 8–10 cm) can be lengthened through the following:

- Dividing the tendon – the anterior fold of the axilla can be reconstructed by reattaching the tendon.

- Dividing the SA branch (not before the TDA is identified).
- A couple of centimetres is gained by taking it back to the subscapular artery (thus sacrificing the circumflex scapular), although this may make the artery too wide for microanastomoses at 6 mm.

The **thoracodorsal nerve** arises from the posterior cord of the brachial plexus and lies deeper and more posteriorly. The nerve is often cut to reduce unwanted contraction, though there is no consensus – some choose to preserve it to maintain bulk as it atrophies unpredictably, dividing later if necessary as the contractions stop spontaneously in most. However, MRI studies have not shown any consistent benefit in maintaining bulk. The nerve also has a proprioceptive component, and some have suggested using nerve grafts in an attempt to keep protective sensation in the muscle, e.g. for walking on muscle.

VARIANTS

- **Endoscopic (assisted) harvest** – the incisions are smaller with less pain and allow earlier movement (though not statistically significant) with no differences in complications (bleeding, haematoma/seroma and infection). Others have described balloon-assisted harvest techniques.
- **Divided TDA** – the flap can still be raised after division of the main TDA, as there is reversal in flow of blood from the intercostal arteries to the SA branch to the LD branch. The collateral vessels will increase in size with time (seen in primate studies). However, the arc of rotation is reduced.
  - Parents who have had axillary dissections should be **assumed** to have transected thoracodorsal vessels unless specifically mentioned. The function of the muscle can be tested by asking the patients to put their hands on their hips and to press in; palpate the muscle. This is an indirect indicator of the integrity of the pedicle, so there will be false positives and negatives.
- **Mini-LD flaps** have been used for larger partial breast defects following BCT/oncoplastic surgery. To preserve muscle function and chest contour, the upper part of the LD can be harvested based on the transverse branch of the TDA; the descending branch is ligated and the vascularity to the rest of the muscle is maintained through the secondary supply.
  - Bittar (*Plast Reconstr Surg*, 2012) described the harvest of a partial LD muscle flap from within the SSM incision with the patient supine. The flap was used to cover the lower part of a submuscular implant, reaching to the sternum and creating an IMF.

TRANSVERSE RECTUS ABDOMINIS MYOCUTANEOUS (TRAM) RECONSTRUCTION

For a unilateral breast reconstruction, the procedure of choice is usually a free flap; if the reconstruction is delayed, the internal mammary arteries (IMAs) are often the best choice as recipient vessels.

- The rectus abdominis (RA) muscle is responsible for the first 30° of flexion and also for raising the intra-abdominal pressure. Sacrificing the muscle also adversely affects the function of the internal obliques as they need resistance against which to contract, and this leads to a decrease in rotational strength.
  - The incidence of post-operative bulges is about 5%–20% with true hernias in 1%–2%. Despite this and though objective testing will reveal measurable weakness, most are asymptomatic except for athletes/labourers, those with pre-existing problems such as lower back pain and those with bilateral harvest. However, others have found that 10%–20% of patients **do not return to their jobs and hobbies afterwards**.
  - Use of a mesh if required for donor site repair does not interfere with subsequent pregnancy. The trend is to use the mesh in the retromuscular position when appropriate, where the abdominal pressures hold it against the deep surface of the muscle.

PEDICLED TRAM (SUPERIOR EPIGASTRIC ARTERY)

The pTRAM is a commonly used flap.

- The flap tends to migrate more, with **less a distinct IMF** compared to the LD flap. The medial IMF in particular may be distorted by the muscle bulge, but this may be reduced by cutting the nerves particularly up to T8.
- The flap is based on soft tissue that is supplied by a set of choke vessels (the anastomosis between the superior and inferior epigastrics). The flap has low vascularity to tissue volume ratio.
  - There is an increased risk of fat necrosis (12% in some series) and is relatively contraindicated in the obese (>20% overweight), diabetics and smokers.
  - Consider **surgical delay** in cases with higher risk of fat necrosis (see above) as well as those requiring a large proportion of the whole TRAM tissue. It can be performed either open or endoscopically, 2 weeks before the definitive flap procedure. In the work of Codner (*Plast Reconstr Surg*, 1995), found that delay increased the 'flap perfusion pressure' from 13.3 to 40.3 mmHg.
  - The superior epigastric vein usually flows towards the umbilicus; thus, a pTRAM may be prone to venous congestion until the valves become incompetent allowing reverse flow. Even though gross congestion may resolve, there may be more fibrosis and fat necrosis. It can **be 'super-drained'** by anastomosing the DIEV/SIEV to available recipient veins or 'supercharged' by anastomosing DIEA.
- A pinch test can be used to 'eyeball' whether the (half) abdomen can provide sufficient tissue – for larger breasts, the pTRAM can be combined with

an implant or used as a bipedicled flap (though the better option is a free TRAM). For delayed reconstruction, the flap should be inset into the new IMF, angling up the axillary tail, to avoid creating an 'eyeball'. Close the abdomen before flap inset as the latter will change the IMF level and the shape of the breast.

- Moon K (*Plast Reconstr Surg*, 1998) conducted radiological studies in 64 fresh cadavers:
    - 29% type 1 with single superior and inferior epigastric.
    - 57% type 2 with double vessels.
    - 14% type 3 with three or more.
    - Only 2% have symmetrical pattern.
- There are no perforators below the arcuate line; thus, there is no need to include the muscle below this. The rectus sheath is repaired along with the contralateral rectus plication for balance, which creates a more defined waistline.
- **Contralateral vs. ipsilateral**.
    - **Contralateral flaps** where the umbo area ends up being inferior, supposedly have fewer problems with venous drainage due to less acute folding and have been popular. The contralateral pedicle is less likely to be in the 'RT field'. The tunnel should be more medial but should not cross the midline.
    - There has been a 'revival' somewhat for the **ipsilateral pTRAM** with the pedicle draped in a curve rather than folded on itself as described by Hartrampf. For this design described by Olding M in 1998, the flap tunnel is in the central portion of the IMF, and the flap height is the BW, rotated so that thicker medial edge is now at the IMF. There is less epigastric fullness.

BIPEDICLED TRAM

Indications

- Midline lower abdominal scar
- A large tissue requirement
- High-risk patient

Supposedly there is no increase in complications compared to unipedicled TRAM flaps (Paige, *Plast Reconstr Surg*, 1998). However, Hartrampf reported that patients had problems with doing 'sit-ups' in 17% after a single pTRAM, compared to 64% bipedicled pTRAM. Overall, it seems that single pTRAM leaves a mild problem that is usually well tolerated, but harvesting a bilateral pTRAM is much more debilitating, and it would be better to use free TRAM in those situations.

Breast reconstruction with a transverse abdominal island flap. (Hartrampf CR, *Plast Reconstr Surg*, 1982)
This paper presented a variety of cases using a horizontal skin island. (Holmstrom H, *Scand J Plast Reconstr Surg*,

1979 was the first to report on a **'free abdominoplasty' flap**.) The first case was a high ipsilateral flap from the epigastrium to just below the umbilicus. The muscle was transected below the flap and detached superiorly from the ribs – two costochondral cartilages were removed to allow the vessel to be traced back to the internal mammaries. The authors also described a low infraumbilical horizontal flap, with the first three patients undergoing flap delay by ligating the DIEA/V 2 weeks beforehand.

ADVANTAGES OF FREE FLAPS COMPARED WITH PEDICLED TRAM

A better-shaped breast mound can be achieved without the epigastric fullness that results from the tunnelled pedicle, and shaping and insetting are not limited by tethering at the pedicle.

- The inferior pedicle (DIEA) is sturdier than the superior epigastric artery and does not involve choke vessels, contributing to better vascularity and less fat necrosis (<5%). It can thus be used where a pedicled flap is relatively contraindicated, e.g. in the overweight, in smokers as well as in cases where the superior pedicle is unavailable due to previous surgery.
- It can reliably supply larger volumes of tissue, allowing for better breast shape/ptosis.
    - The amount of (abdominal) tissue required determines the choice of the flap – SIEA is able to support 50% of 'flap area', DIEP up to 70%, whilst fTRAM provides the largest amount of tissue – some (zone IV) needs to be discarded. To harvest the whole area, bilateral inferior pedicles are required – using either two separate recipient sites or an intra-flap anastomosis, to join one system to the other.
- Easier insetting/shaping.
- Less muscle is usually sacrificed, reducing the degree of abdominal wall dysfunction.

FREE TRAM/MSTRAM/DIEP FLAPS

Although there are many advantages over the pTRAM (see above), free flaps require microsurgical experience and special equipment. There is also the potential for complete flap loss (1%–6%); in addition, the longer operating times/greater anaesthetic risk means that it may not be suited to those with medical problems.

The DIEP flap was first described by Allen (*Ann Plast Surg*, 1994); perforator flaps have the advantage of leaving the muscle mass and fascia behind, with potentially less donor site morbidity, specifically in terms of strength of the trunk flexion on the hip and incidence of bulging/hernias, although the difference may be less pronounced with time and specific training. Blondeel (*Br J Plast Surg*, 1999) was one of the first to promote the functional benefits of the DIEP over the fTRAM; however, dissecting the vessel out of the muscle takes more time and may damage the vessels.

- The main perforators lie close to the umbilicus, usually just below it. On average, one to three perforators can be harvested with a longer pedicle (~10 cm) than the fTRAM. More than half the time, one perforator is sufficient (Blondeel PN, *Br J Plast Surg*, 1999).
- It is important **to preserve the segmental nerves** to the muscle; the nerves usually pass superficial to the inferior pedicle. If the muscle is denervated, there is little point in preserving it. More denervation is likely with use of the lateral row. Zone III of (contralateral medial) lateral row dominant flaps may need to be discarded to reduce fat necrosis (Bozikov K, *Ann Plast Surg*, 2009).
- Man (*Plast Reconstr Surg*, 2009) found that DIEP patients had double the risk of flap necrosis and flap loss, but half the risk of abdominal bulge or hernia.
- The incidence of fat necrosis is slightly higher (10%); changes may be difficult to distinguish from tumour recurrence. Interestingly, the fat necrosis rates increase with the number of perforators, implying perhaps that more perforators are usually included due to small individual sizes. If a large flap volume is required, medial row perforators may support contralateral tissue better but tend to have a longer intramuscular course; otherwise, using the lateral row perforators is usually easier.
- Muscle-sparing TRAM (msTRAM) takes the lateral and medial rows with a variable amount of muscle down to ~**2 inches** below the umbilicus. Nahabedian (*Plast Reconstr Surg*, 2002) described the subtypes:
  - MS0 – full width of rectus
  - MS1 – preserved lateral segment
  - MS2 – preserved lateral and medial segments
  - MS3 – preserved entire muscle, i.e. DIEP
- The use of mesh is debated; prolene is probably as good as any. Luijendijk (*N Engl J Med*, 2000) found that mesh repair was superior to suture repair in incisional herniae repair. There is also discussion of inlay, onlay vs. sublay techniques; sublay/underlay theoretically pushes the mesh against the abdominal wall.
  - The long-term success of mesh repair depends on whether the fascial layer can be closed or if there is a defect that needs to be **bridged** (8% vs. 50% failure).

Some suggest that the difference in abdominal wall morbidity between DIEP and msTRAM flaps may not be that great (Nahabedian MY, *Plast Reconstr Surg*, 2005; Bajack AK, *Plast Reconstr Surg*, 2006).

It should be appreciated that **what different surgeons report as a DIEP may involve very different levels of muscle damage** and denervation, making controlled comparisons with TRAM (muscle-sparing or otherwise) difficult.

Preoperative imaging of perforators

Where possible, image the perforators with the patient in the operative position.

- Duplex ultrasound.
- Handheld Doppler.
- CTA (99.6% positive predictive value for perforators >1 mm, allows 3D visualisation of the course of the perforators with better resolution than MRA. Studies have shown that use of CTA shortens the operating time, but any effect on outcomes is unproven.
- Thermal cameras.
- Indocyanine green (ICG) fluoroscopy.

Gynaecological Pfannenstiel incisions usually do not affect flap harvest as the recti are spread apart, but a general surgical Pfannenstiel approach may cut the muscle (and the artery). A preoperative CTA may be helpful

- Mark the patient standing up – mark the extent of the breast using the contralateral side as a guide, noting BBW, height from take-off to the IMF, projection and the level of the IMF.

An experienced anaesthetist will help. Paralysis will help to reduce avulsion of the fine vessels when dissecting the perforators and allow easier abdominal closure (may need to 'break' the table). Controlled ventilation will facilitate IMA anastomosis.

One suggested strategy is as follows:

- Exploration of the SIEA/V system.
  - **SIEA** >1–1.5 mm makes a SIEA flap feasible. If small, proceed to explore the DIEA perforators.
  - **Large SIEV** (>1.5 mm) may mean that a DIEP/TRAM needs superdraining. Try to harvest a good length for this eventually.
- Elevate the lateral row of perforators and release the fascial collars to allow vessel expansion. If the (arterial) perforator is <1.5 mm, then explore the medial row. If these perforators are also small (<1.5 mm), then a **muscle-sparing TRAM (msTRAM)** is preferable to a DIEP, but if the medial row vessels are larger, then a DIEP is possible:
  - If the size of the medial row vessel is 1.5–3 mm, then a DIEP should be raised on more than one perforator.
  - If the size of the medial row vessel is >3 mm, then a single perforator DIEP is feasible.
  - Check for the presence of a **good artery and vein** in the perforator 'bundles'.
- Zone III/IV (i.e. contralateral zones) will be less reliable if the flap is raised on the lateral row of perforators.

If possible, the contralateral flap is usually used and rotated 90° to have the pedicle orientated medially to go to the IMA. The best perfused regions (zones I and II) are thus placed superomedially to avoid fat necrosis in this region, which would otherwise lie over the anastomosis and be more difficult to deal with than lateral necrosis.

- **Recipient vessels**:
  - **Axillary vessels** can be used in immediate reconstruction, but the fibrosis that follows means that the IMA (second/third space) is preferred in delayed reconstructions (see below). Some worry about the theoretical risk of avulsion with arm/shoulder motion.
  - Using the ipsilateral IMA allows for a shorter pedicle length.
  - A contralateral flap is required if anastomosing to the axilla.
  - **Lifeboats**:
    - **Contralateral** IMA/V.
    - Vein – EJV, cephalic.
    - Artery – TDA, thoracoacromial and circumflex scapular.
- The manner of inset depends partly on the defect:
  - **Vertical inset** is the best option for reconstructing a ptotic breast; it gives the best infraclavicular fill. The width of the breast base should correspond roughly to the height of the flap.
  - **Transverse flap orientation** is more suited for a broader breast by providing more central tissue, but less infraclavicular fill. A triangular wedge (including umbilicus) can be de-epithelialised and closed for projection, but unipedicled flaps may not tolerate this.
  - **Tacking** may be helpful to optimise shaping – one suggestion is to attach the superomedial aspect first, followed by the sternal border and then the superolateral border to the soft tissue in front of the axillary fold, to avoid an unattractive gap that often appears at the lateral breast.

INTERNAL MAMMARY VESSELS

IMA at the third rib provides good size match for the flap artery; the vein is usually single but at this point often thin walled. Arnez (*Br J Plast Surg*, 1995) found (in an anatomical study with 34 fresh human cadavers) that the most common configuration was (type I) having a vein medial to the artery, dividing at the level of the fourth intercostal space into the medial (2.7 mm mean) and the lateral (1.8 mm).

- Incise perichondrium as an 'H'; peel off carefully to expose the cartilage that is resected as needed. Some may be banked for nipple reconstruction.
- Use blade to incise the posterior/deeper layer of the perichondrium **lateral** to the vessels, and use a cotton bud to push vessels off the perichondrium before splitting it with scissors. The vessels can be raised up, e.g. on pledgets to facilitate anastomosis.

Internal mammary vessels: A reliable recipient system for free flaps in breast reconstruction. (Ninkovic M, *Br J Plast Surg*, 1995)
The IMA lies 1.5 cm lateral to the lateral border of the sternum; pre-operative Doppler may allow more precise localisation. The third or fourth costal cartilage (a 2 cm segment 2.5 cm from the sternal edge) is removed subperichondrially to facilitate recipient vessel dissection in the third or fourth spaces. Magnification is advisable for vessel dissection.

Advantages of using the IMA:

- A **shorter pedicle is needed** vs. 9–10 cm to reach the axilla. The vessels are a good size match for the DIEP vessels at 1.5 mm.
- Allows for flexible positioning of the flap on the chest wall.
- Avoids further dissection of the axilla, which may be difficult (with risk to vessels and brachial plexus) and worsen lymphoedema. It spares latissimus dorsi as a lifeboat.
  - Crosby (*Plast Reconstr Surg*, 2012) found that lymphoedema after immediate breast reconstruction was related to BMI, axillary interventions and high number of positive nodes, but not the reconstructive method.
- Zone IV lies lateral rather than medial; >80% of TRAM flaps were ipsilateral.

Disadvantages:

- Veins in particular can be very fragile. This, the depth and respiratory movement may make microanastomosis difficult.
- Potentially compromises blood supply to sternum and removes an option for future bypass grafting.
- Risk of iatrogenic pneumothorax.
- Removal of cartilage leads to visible contour deformity.

REDUCING DONOR DEFORMITY

- Taking less than 1.5 cm of cartilage.
- Shaving the costal cartridges above and below to widen the space instead.
- If the pectoralis muscle is incised as an 'L' shape from the second rib to the top of the fourth, it can be redraped and sutured to the sternal cuff to disguise the defect. Leave a 1 cm gap for the pedicle to come through.
- IMA perforators in the second and third spaces may be usable in ~39%, defined as >1.5 mm and good flow on release of clamps. Haywood (*Br J Plast Surg*, 2003) used these vessels for DIEP, S-GAP and SIEA flaps.

A call for clarity in TRAM/DIEP zones. (Henry SL, *Plast Reconstr Surg*, 2010)
The zones of the transverse abdominal flap are generally numbered according to their perfusion. It is commonly accepted that zone 1 is the zone overlying the pedicle and zone 4 is the contralateral lateral zone, but there is confusion over what constitutes zones 2 and 3 of the TRAM/DIEP flap. Initially, Scheflan (*Ann Plast Surg*, 1983) and Dinner (*Ann Plast Surg*, 1983) described the **contralateral** medial as zone 2. Despite this, these are often referred to as **Hartrampf zones**. It became clear that if one was

considering the perfusion, then it was incorrect – ironically, this had been picked up by Dinner et al. (1983) later that year, but the nomenclature persisted.

- Holm (*Plast Reconstr Surg*, 2006) performed a perfusion study with ICG that confirmed the **modified** Dinner scheme. Others suggested renaming for 'clarity' by combining II and III as 'II' making IV now 'III', but this did not catch on.
- Henry (*Plast Reconstr Surg*, 2010) suggested a descriptive classification – contralateral as C, medial as M and lateral as L; thus, the zones would be CL, CM, IM and IL with IM as zone I, etc., which seems clear and sensible enough.

Perforasomes of the DIEP were described by Wong and Saint-Cyr (*Plast Reconstr Surg*, 2010). They found that medial row perforators contribute more to the CM zone than lateral row perforators, which contribute more to the IL zone.

TRAM flaps in patients with abdominal scars. (Takeishi M, *Plast Reconstr Surg*, 1997)

The authors present their experience with 46 TRAM breast reconstruction patients who had pre-existing abdominal scars. Free TRAM flaps were preferred and performed wherever possible; vessel exploration was an important part of the assessment process.

- Patients with **low transverse scars** (Pfannenstiel) were explored, and if the DIEA was not intact, then an ipsilateral pedicled TRAM flap or free contralateral TRAM flap was raised.
- All patients with **lower paramedian scars** had divided ipsilateral vessels.
- In patients with **lower midline scars**, the **flap was designed higher** up on the abdomen so that 5–7 cm of unscarred skin formed a bridge above the umbilicus. This leaves a high, mid-abdominal, transverse scar.
- **Subcostal incisions** usually meant that an ipsilateral flap had to be a free flap due to division of the superior pedicle.
- Appendectomy scars do not compromise the TRAM flap.

Broyles (*Plast Reconstr Surg*, 2012) harvested a DIEP flap in a patient having had **a prior abdominoplasty** and laparotomy – he used a superiorly positioned flap after CTA visualised a suitable perforator. Liposuction is another (relative) contraindication to the use of abdominal flaps, and although UAL may be 'gentler', it is probably wise to have a preoperative CTA, as well as a lifeboat.

A 10-year retrospective review of 758 DIEP flaps for breast reconstruction. (Gill PS, *Plast Reconstr Surg*, 2004)

This review of 758 DIEP flaps for breast reconstruction demonstrated complication rates comparable to pedicled and free TRAM flaps. Breast or abdominal complications had

a significant association with smoking, hypertension and post-operative radiotherapy.

- 0.5% total flap loss, 2.5% partial flap loss and 12.9% developed fat necrosis, which **increased** with the number of perforators.
- 5.9% returned to the operating theatre, 3.8% because of venous congestion (which was unrelated to the number of venous anastomoses).
- Post-operative abdominal hernia or bulge occurred in only five (0.7%).

A systematic review of abdominal wall function following abdominal flaps for postmastectomy breast reconstruction. (Atisha D, *Ann Plast Surg*, 2009)

A meta-analysis of 20 studies found demonstrable objective differences:

- Isometric dynamometry – pTRAM patients had an average of 23% deficit in trunk flexion vs. 18% in fTRAM; DIEP patients had less flexion deficit than free TRAM patients.
- Physiotherapy measures – pTRAM patients had the greatest deficit in rectus and oblique muscle function (53%), whilst free TRAM had minimal deficit and DIEP returned to baseline.

However, with the exception of bilateral flaps (pedicled or free TRAM), this **did not translate to any decrease in their ability to perform ADL**.

SIEA FLAP

The SIEA is a direct cutaneous vessel from the common femoral artery 2–3 cm below the inguinal ligament, either by itself (17%) or from a common trunk with the superficial circumflex iliac (48%). It crosses the midpoint of the inguinal ligament deep to Scarpa's fascia, then runs towards the umbilicus piercing Scarpa's to lie in the superficial subcutaneous tissue and may anastomose with periumbilical perforating arteries. **The SIEA flap is an axial pattern fasciocutaneous flap, not a perforator flap**.

The use of the SIEA flap in breast reconstruction was first described by Grotting (*Ann Plast Surg*, 1991) and potentially has minimal **donor site morbidity** as the fascia and musculature are not disturbed. However, it is not a common choice as the vessels are generally short and small (average 7 mm long and 1.6 mm wide at the inguinal ligament) and need to be dissected further down into the groin; it cannot adequately supply tissue across the midline. The vessels are absent or hypoplastic in 65%–70%.

- These vessels may have been cut in Pfannenstiel incisions.
- They are cut along with the DIEA/DIEV when delaying a pedicled TRAM.
- There is an increased seroma rate related to the inguinal dissection.

Breast reconstruction with superficial inferior epigastric artery flaps. (Chevray PM, *Plast Reconstr Surg*, 2004)
The author successfully used the SIEA flap in 30% (14 of 47) of consecutive cases of breast reconstruction; the remainder were either absent or too small (a limit of 1.5 mm is used to increase reliability). The author prefers using the IMAP to reduce size mismatch and to allow the flap to be positioned more medially.

OTHER FLAPS

On average, **the TRAM (and related) flaps are not available** in 25% due to previous surgery, e.g. abdominoplasty, or inadequate bulk.

SUPERIOR GLUTEAL ARTERY PERFORATOR FLAP

The use of the superior gluteal artery perforator (S-GAP) flap in breast reconstruction was first described by Allen (*Plast Reconstr Surg*, 1995). It can be regarded as a descendant of the traditional gluteus maximus myocutaneous flap but has less donor site pain. The skin paddle is relatively small, but the **stiff fat** provides good projection. The learning curve is significant (Boyd JB, *Plast Reconstr Surg*, 2009); haemostasis may be difficult, and there is a moderately high risk of developing seroma. The patient needs to be repositioned after harvest in the prone or lateral decubitus position.

- **Superior gluteal artery (SGA) flaps** are commonly harvested as a horizontal ellipse on the upper buttock centred on the pedicle (approximately 1/3 from the posterior superior iliac spine [PSIS] to the greater trochanter). A **handheld Doppler** is useful to localise perforators. Dissection begins laterally to expose the lateral edge of the gluteus maximus and then in continues the plane between this and the gluteus medius to find the superior gluteal vessels between the gluteus medius and piriformis about 5 cm lateral to the edge of the sacrum.
  - The **perforator flap** has a longer pedicle due to utilisation of the intramuscular portion – **lateral perforators will provide a longer pedicle but involves more intramuscular dissection.**
  - It results in an element of buttock lift. Although the scar may be hidden, the contour deformity may be obvious; the other side may need surgery to improve symmetry.
- **Inferior gluteal artery (IGA) flaps** have longer pedicles that pass below the piriformis, and courses close to the sciatic nerve. The dissection begins inferiorly at the gluteal crease, lateral to medial, exposing the hamstrings; the sciatic nerve does not actually need to be exposed during the dissection, but it is still at risk from the effects of post-operative scarring and there is an additional variable functional

loss associated with division of the inferior gluteal nerve. Inclusion of the posterior cutaneous nerve of the thigh allows for a sensate flap, where needed. It is less commonly used than the SGA flap.
- **Lumbar artery perforator (LAP) flap** is a fasciocutaneous flap (12 × 24 cm, potentially sensate) harvested usually on the fourth or second perforator (6–7 cm from the midline). The patient needs to be prone/lateral decubitis. The perforators pierce the psoas and run between the erector spinae and the quadratus lumborum. The short pedicle with small vessels means that it usually requires an interpositional pedicle – it is a useful option in those who have had a TRAM/DIEP previously and thus contralateral DIEA/V pedicle is available and 'dispensible'.
- **PAP flap** – the perforator can be lower down the thigh, ~10 cm, which would mean a lower skin island/scar. Harvest in a supine position has been described, but the closure of the posterior donor site can be a problem in this position, having to hold the leg up whilst suturing.

The sensate free superior gluteal artery perforator (S-GAP) flap: A valuable alternative in autologous breast reconstructions. (Blondeel PN, *Br J Plast Surg*, 1999)
The authors present experience with 20 free S-GAP free flaps vascularised by a single perforator from the S-GAP identified pre-operatively by Doppler. The flaps were anastomosed to the IMA/V in the third intercostal space. The author proposes it as a second choice to the DIEP flap when the latter is not available, e.g. due to scars or lack of tissue. It can be made sensate by coaption of sensory nerves entering the flap from above (dorsal branches of lumbar segmental nerves) to the fourth intercostal nerve. The authors state that this provides early sensory recovery.

- It provides a skin paddle 25–35 × 9–13 cm with a fat layer of up to 8 cm and flap volume of up to 800 mL. The pedicle length is short at 3 cm, but the vessels are a good size with a diameter of 2–3 mm, and can be anastomosed to IMA or axilla (vein grafts may be needed).

GRACILIS FLAP (TRANSVERSE UPPER GRACILIS FLAP)

This is a type II **myocutaneous free flap** and the pedicle comes from the ascending branch of the **medial circumflex femoral artery** (from the profunda femoris artery) that is only 5–6 cm long and 1.6 mm in diameter. Thus the IMA/V is the preferred site of anastomosis. The pedicle enters the proximal third of the muscle 10 cm below the inguinal ligament; skin vessels run transverse to the muscle.

- Line – adductor longus origin to medial tibial condyle; gracilis is two to three fingers breath behind this.
- Doppler may be used to identify skin perforators, ~**6 cm below the inguinal crease.**

- The skin paddle is orientated transversely over the upper part of the muscle in the proximal third of the medial thigh; the anterior extent ends before the long saphenous vein whilst posteriorly it can go to the middle of the gluteal crease.
  - Start anteriorly.
- The maximum width is 10–12 cm and in selected patients provides a moderate amount of tissue for autologous breast reconstruction. The donor–site morbidity is similar to that of a classic medial thigh lift – Wechselberger (*Plast Reconstr Surg*, 2004) found no functional deficits.
  - Lack of volume is the main disadvantage.

It is a valuable alternative for immediate autologous breast reconstruction (Arnez ZM, *Br J Plast Surg*, 2004) after SSM in patients with small- and medium-sized breasts, and who cannot have/want flaps from the lower abdomen and the gluteal region. Donor site wound problems may be more common.

Transverse myocutaneous gracilis flap: Technical refinements. (Fattah A, *J Reconstr Aesthet Surg*, 2010)
The authors describe their experience with 19 flaps and their improved technique including recruitment of inferior fat and sparing of the long saphenous vein. The flap is usually raised as an ellipse (with the muscle more anteriorly based, and the upper border 1 cm below the actual thigh groin sulcus) that is shaped by coning. The most common complication was minor wound dehiscence at the donor site.

YET OTHER FLAPS

Unilateral flaps may need balancing procedures.

- **Rubens flap** – this relatively small flap composed of the soft tissue around the iliac crest is based on the deep circumflex iliac artery (DCIA) flap and has a moderately long consistent pedicle (5–6 cm long, 2–3 mm artery and 2.5–4 mm vein). However, the abdominal wall muscles must be meticulously sutured back to the iliac crest. Post-operative pain is common, and there may be paraesthesia due to injury to the lateral cutaneous nerve of the thigh. It is not a commonly used option.
- **Thoracodorsal artery perforator (TAP or TDAP) flap**. Compared with the LD, there is sparing of the muscle and **less risk of seroma**; however, the size is limited and involves a small amount of intramuscular dissection.
  - The flap is based over the anterior edge of the LD, but can be orientated in various directions as long as it captures a perforator that tends to be 8 cm below the axillary crease and within 5 cm of the anterior muscle edge.
  - The perforator position can be checked preoperatively with handheld Doppler probes (**in surgical position**). The donor is closed directly or a bilobed design can be used.

- **Lateral transverse thigh flap** (Elliott LF, *Plast Reconstr Surg*, 1990) – this uses the TFL muscle based on the lateral circumflex femoral vessels but leaves a significant contour defect and a risk to the femoral nerve.

RECONSTRUCTION AND THE IRRADIATED BREAST

Radiation is detrimental to reconstruction; it adversely affects the cosmetic results due to **unpredictable** contractures and is more likely to lead to complications, particularly with implants due to poor wound healing, increased wound dehiscence, risk of implant exposure and less effective tissue expansion. In addition, it is difficult to predict individual reactions as there are variable dosage/regimens between institutions as well as genuine variable patient responses.

- **Implants** have high complication with radiotherapy; half require autologous tissue in the end.
  - **LD with an implant in an irradiated patient** may produce results similar to an implant alone in non-irradiated patients.
- **Autologous reconstruction** is preferable in those with prior irradiation or considering radiation; delayed breast reconstruction is performed after >3 months when the redness has subsided and the soft tissue suppleness has been restored.

IV. MALE BREAST CANCER

Male breast carcinoma constitutes 1% of all breast cancers; the mean age at diagnosis is ~60 years, approximately 10 years later than females. It affects about 240 men a year in the United Kingdom (Agrawal A, *Breast Cancer Res Treat*, 2007).

- Patients with Klinefelter's syndrome and Klinefelter's related gynaecomastia have up to a 60× greater risk of developing breast cancer (incidence 1:400 to 1:1000).
- There is **no increased risk** for breast cancer in other patients with **gynaecomastia** compared with the normal male population, and surgical treatments (liposuction and excision) do not impair detection of male breast cancer.
- Some risk factors include BRCA2 mutation, family history and irradiation.

Carcinoma of the male breast: An underestimated killer. (Di Benedetto G, *Plast Reconstr Surg*, 1998)
The tumours are hormone dependent and the aetiology often relates to hyperoestrogenic states. The pathological types and relative incidences are the same as for female breast cancer except that invasive lobular cancer is only seen in association with Klinefelter's syndrome.

They present as painless masses that are subareolar in 68%–90%. The tumours tend to be aggressive; there is a higher incidence of positive internal mammary nodes at presentation. Reconstructive options depend on the disease stage at diagnosis, but most will need flap coverage, e.g. local thoraco-epigastric fasciocutaneous flap or LD flap.

Adjuvant therapies are similar to disease in women – tamoxifen is the mainstay for metastatic disease in oestrogen receptor-positive tumours (80%), though it is poorly tolerated – there is weight gain and loss of libido. Doxorubicin is used in receptor-negative tumours. Orchidectomy is reserved for those refractory to other medical treatments.

- Relative stage-matched survival does not seem significantly different from women. Axillary node status is the major predictor.

V. NIPPLE RECONSTRUCTION AND INVERTED NIPPLE CORRECTION

NIPPLE RECONSTRUCTION

In general, a period of at least 3 months after breast reconstruction is recommended to allow the breast mound to achieve its stable shape. Where the breasts remain asymmetric, symmetry of absolute nipple position is more important than the relationship to each mound.

NIPPLE SHARING

Either the superficial half is shaved off (donor defect is purse-stringed down) or the inferior half is removed (donor defect is closed directly). Zenn (*Plast Reconstr Surg*, 2009) reported high patient satisfaction. Although it is a relatively simple procedure, there are problems including scar distortion, reduced height and sensation of the donor that make it a less popular choice except perhaps in those with overly large nipples.

LOCAL FLAPS

Many different flaps have been described, and the main challenge is always to reduce scarring and to achieve longevity of projection – one should expect 50% reduction with most techniques. Some propose inserting materials such as cartilage, dermis, Alloderm or calcium hydroxyapatite to augment the nipple, but results have been inconsistent.

- **Skate flap** – the designed height is approximately twice the desired nipple height to allow for loss; the lateral wings are raised on a subdermal level, whilst the central portion includes a core of fat. **Typically an FTSG** is needed; attempting to close with tension will cause flattening. This technique is the most popular for large nipples (Figure 5.6).
  - The **Twin flap** is a variant of the skate with square flaps and islanded central flap (Figure 5.7).
  - **Star flap** – this is similar in design to the skate flap but is designed with direct closure in mind and thus is more limited in its dimensions. It is a good alternative for small-/medium-sized nipples.
  - In general, reconstruction of a sizeable nipple will leave a donor site that requires grafting; techniques that avoid grafting represent a compromise and will provide less projection.

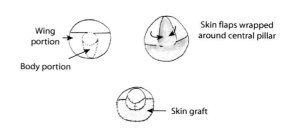

Figure 5.6 Skate flap for nipple reconstruction. The base of the flap is three times the diameter of the desired/contralateral nipple. The lateral 'wing' flaps are elevated in the subdermal level, whilst the body includes some subcutaneous flap. Some variants dispense with the skin graft, but this will limit the projection.

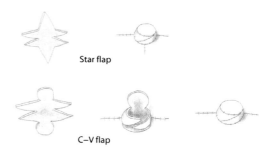

Figure 5.7 Twin flap technique. Suitable for cases where the reconstructed nipple would lie over a scar line. The areolar can be reconstructed with a skin graft.

- Other techniques described in the literature include the following:
  - **C–V flaps** – C for the top of the nipple cylinder, whilst two Vs interlock to provide the sidewall (Figure 5.8).
  - **S flap** – also known as the 'double opposing tab' flap after Cronin (*Plast Reconstr Surg*, 1988). The flaps **(diameter ~3× the nipple height)** are raised on the subdermal level with about 10 mm of fat; they come together in a 'hands in prayer' configuration. Proponents of this technique say that there is less loss of projection.
    - Kroll (*Plast Reconstr Surg*, 1989) double opposing flap (18 mm base, original backcuts eliminated) is similar.
    - These are said to be useful in the vicinity of scars; another alternative in such situations is the Twin flap (Ramakrishnan VV, *Ann Plast Surg*, 1997).

Complications are relatively uncommon except for flattening out, which is almost to be expected: tissue necrosis is a concern, and surgery should probably be avoided in smokers.

AREOLAR RECONSTRUCTION

Areolar sharing provides the best match; however, there can be a significant donor site morbidity (except if the patient is also undergoing a reduction/mastopexy to the

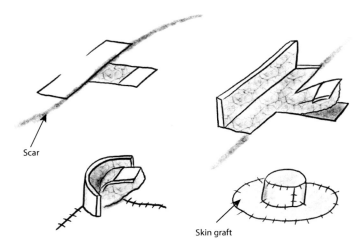

Scar

Skin graft

Figure 5.8 The star and C–V flaps are similar to the skate flap but do not require skin grafts.

contralateral side). Use of an interlocking CV3 Gore-Tex suture in a wagon spoke configuration to control the areolar diameter was popularised by Hammond; the breast flaps are undermined subdermally for 1–2 cm, whilst a 5 mm rim of dermis on the areolar is preserved for suture holding and covered vest over pants by the breast flap.

- **Skin grafts** – other sites available as skin donors include labial FTSG, inguinal or perineal skin (the donor site is easily hidden but can sometimes be inconvenient) and upper inner thigh. The selection of skin graft solely on the basis of pigmentation is largely obsolete.
  - **'Returned skin grafts'** – skin is elevated from the same site as the 'recipient', i.e. around the reconstruction nipple. Gruber used ultraviolet light to enhance graft pigmentation, but the results were not permanent.
  - Dermabrasion has also been used to induce hyperpigmentary changes, and again, the long-term results are unclear.
- **Tattoo** – it is common to wait 6–12 weeks after nipple reconstruction to allow for tissue recovery; however, some suggest tattooing **before** nipple reconstruction on the premise that it results in a more uniform colour. Tattooing is generally safe; allergic reactions are rare but have been described. Some **fading is normal** and to be expected – tattooing can always be repeated.
- **The surface texture of Montgomery glands has been reproduced by placing diced cartilage under the skin.**
- **Seasoned tattoo artists can 'draw' in the glands.**

PRESERVING THE NIPPLE

Instead of reconstructing the nipple after resection during mastectomy, could it actually be preserved?

- In the past, some surgeons had described **NAC banking**, e.g. in the groin, etc.; however, this practice was stopped due to several cases of cancer spread to the inguinal nodes (Cucin RL, *CA Cancer J Clin*, 1981), and other studies demonstrated NAC involvement in invasive and non-invasive breast cancers. Some have attempted to modify the nipple to reduce the chances of 'preserving' tumour cells, e.g. keep in a fridge/cryopreservation until final histology is available; however, these methods are inevitably less effective at preserving the nipple, which would lose pigment and projection. Long-term results have generally been disappointing.
- **Nipple sparing.** Several groups have reported their experiences with NSM with low local recurrence rates ranging from 0% at 52 months to 1 nipple recurrence in 61 patients (Sakamoto N, *Ann Surg Oncol*, 2009; Gerber B, *Ann Surg*, 2003). Patients with non-central tumours (at least 2 cm away from the nipple–areolar complex) were chosen, with intra-operative frozen sections for confirmation. Nipple necrosis occurred in 18% in the first study; some authors noted that the nipple may be insensate/non-erectile after nipple-sparing surgery.

Analysis of nipple/areolar involvement with mastectomy: Can the areola be preserved? (Simmons RM, *Ann Surg Oncol*, 2002)

This article presents data from histological evaluation of the NAC from 217 mastectomy patients between 1990 and 1998.

- 10.6% of patients overall had involvement of the nipple that increased to 27.3% if the tumour was central but decreased with non-central locations to 6.4%.
- Less than 1% had involvement of the areola (large tumours >5 cm and lymphadenopathy, located centrally below the areola).

As areolar skin does not contain ductal cells or breast parenchymal tissue, areola-sparing mastectomy may be considered in selected patients **but not the preservation of the nipple**. The author followed this up with an article in 2003 reporting on areola-sparing mastectomy with immediate reconstruction in 17 breasts (12 patients) (*Ann Plast Surg*, 2003).

INVERTED NIPPLE

This is a relatively common condition affecting up to 10% of women by some estimates. As well as the cosmetic issues, it may interfere with breastfeeding.

The aetiology is not fully understood; congenital deficiencies may be important in most cases, whilst postmastitis fibrosis may be responsible in some other. There is a reduction in the subareolar soft tissue, the lactiferous ducts are shortened and fibrotic and there may be bands tethering the nipple. There are many different techniques described; a problem is that extensive dissection/manipulation can cause more fibrosis leading to recurrence of the inversion.

Non-surgical management with suction devices such as the **Niplette** (McGeorge DD, *Br J Plast Surg*, 1993) is of limited use, particularly for those with established fibrosis.

CLASSIFICATION

Han (*Plast Reconstr Surg*, 1999) described a classification scheme that guided clinical management.

- Grade I – minimal fibrosis. Easily correctable manually and position can be maintained without traction. Treatment with a purse-string suture is usually sufficient.
- Grade II – moderate fibrosis and mildly retracted ducts. Correctable manually but position is not maintained after release of the traction. Fibrosis needs to be released with blunt dissection whilst sparing the ducts, before the purse-string.
- Grade III – severe fibrosis, severely retracted ducts and insufficient soft tissue. Difficult to correct manually. Sharp release of fibrosis and ducts is required; **dermal flaps** of many variations have been described. They create scars on the areolar skin.
  - Two thin de-epithelialised flaps are raised pedicled at the nipple base and threaded through tunnels in the nipple (Ritz M, *Aesth Plast Surg*, 2005).
  - Two triangles of areolar dermis are de-epithelialised and tunnelled through the nipple (Kim DY, *Ann Plast Surg*, 2003). The tunnel is created **by blunt dissection in grade II or sharp division in grade III**.

Little (*Plast Reconstr Surg*, 1999) commented on the article in the same issue and suggested an alternative to dermal flaps in grade III inversion – that is to divide the fibrosis at a deeper level to avoid the 'empty cylinder' defect that comes from division closer to the dermis. A purse-string with suture is then applied.

The repair is protected from compression post-operatively; some have described tethering the nipple to an inverted medicine cup with a suture for 2–5 days.

Minimally invasive correction of inverted nipples. (Kolker AR, *Ann Plast Surg*, 2009)

The authors presented their experience with surgery for 58 'congenitally' inverted nipples. The nipple is everted with a temporary traction suture, and an 18G needle inserted in the 6 o'clock position is used to divide the tissue (below the skin level) to allow the nipple to sit everted without traction. A monofilament purse-string suture (nylon or PDS) is inserted through the same needle hole, looping around the nipple circumference coming out every 3–5 mm and then tied with moderate tension. Two additional 5'0 catgut sutures are placed at the junction of the nipple and areola to reduce dead space and provide stability. Antibiotic ointment is applied, and the patient is advised not to compress them with tight clothing or otherwise for 2 weeks.

They report no recurrences in grade I nipples; there was 22% and 50% recurrence in grades II and III respectively. They suggest repeating the procedure for recurrences.

ONCOPLASTIC SURGERY

Oncoplastic surgery as a concept is uniting the resection and reconstruction at least as a philosophy between two closely cooperating surgeons (breast and plastic) if not in a 'single' surgeon.

Clear margins and radiotherapy are essential. The effect of the resection margin on survival and local recurrence is unknown; however, involved margins will predictably increase recurrence. More attention is paid towards planning skin incisions and tissue excision so that in addition to oncological clearance, aesthetic closure is facilitated in terms of restoring skin continuity, overall shape and nipple position. It may be viewed in simple terms as 'partial mastectomy with reconstruction' with the latter being achieved through a variety of techniques that basically aim to fill the skin and volume void by shifting the remaining breast tissue, or in larger defects, bringing in other tissue. The exact techniques available depend on the relative size and position of the defect (the upper outer quadrant is most commonly affected). **Breast conserving treatment (BCT) is often breast distorting treatment**; without using oncoplastic techniques, the breast would probably be severely deformed. In general,

- There should be a lower threshold for balancing the contralateral breast.
- Surgery is best performed before irradiation, but radiation can still destroy otherwise good results.
- According to Clough (*Ann Surg Oncol*, 2010),
  - Level I – maximum 20% volume excision – does not require skin excision or mammoplasty for reshaping
  - Level II – 20%–50% volume excision – requires mammoplasty techniques.

CLASSIFICATION OF TECHNIQUES

The basic distinction is between **volume displacement and volume replacement**.

- **Volume rearrangement/displacement works well for smaller defects for up to 10%–20%**. This is sometimes described as a 'therapeutic reduction mammaplasty' as the breast will become smaller; obviously it will be most intuitive for defects that lie in excision areas for standard breast reduction patterns, e.g. scenario A of the Nottingham approach (McCulley SJ, *Br J Plast Surg*, 2005). Periareolar Benelli-type incisions (so-called 'doughnut mastopexy lumpectomy') work well for upper or lateral tumours, whilst the Wise pattern incision can be used to access most of the breast with different pedicles – the inverted T can be rotated or angled to a certain degree. Defects that fall outside of normal patterns (scenario B) require different strategies that may be classified in various ways:
  - **Extended pedicles** (extensions of the pedicle carrying the nipple providing tissue that can be transposed into the defect) vs. **secondary pedicles** (a separate pedicle).
  - **Parenchymal flaps** without overlying skin (e.g. the lunate or Grisotti flaps, which are generally safe if the breast is glandular) vs. **full thickness (of breast) local flaps** with basic designs such as rotations and advancement flaps with Burrows triangles, e.g. 'batwing' for lesions near the NAC (Silverstein).
  - The **'cosmetic quadrantectomy'** is effectively a parenchymal quadrantectomy with flap advancement that may work well for a segmental tumour in the lateral part of the breast with an elongated incision radially orientated to the NAC.
    - Radial ellipses are versatile and will not alter the NAC position much.
    - Incision lines that may otherwise cross the NAC can be 'fishtailed'.
  - **For larger defects in larger breasts** (20%–50%), a **contralateral procedure may be needed**. Bilateral breast reduction is a worthwhile consideration for breast cancer patients with macromastia to reduce complications from radiation by reducing the dosage.
- **Volume replacement** – importation of local or distant tissue to restore volume particularly if >20%; it is generally preferred if there has been previous RT. Flaps have a higher complication rate than rearrangement; replacement is better delayed or 'immediately delayed' until definitive margins are available. Surgical clips can be used to mark the tumour bed to guide post-operative radiotherapy if necessary. Critics say that some options such as the partial LD may 'burn bridges', i.e. should a mastectomy (and 'full' reconstruction) be necessary in the future.
  - Inferior – IMAP, inverted T pattern superior pedicle (Clough)
  - Lower medial/inferior – IMAP, thoracoepigastric, ITIP
  - Lateral – LD (partial), lateral intercostal artery perforator (LICAP), TDAP, inferior pedicle
  - Superior – ITIP (except for very high tumours), periareolar, omega/batwing
    - The superomedial quadrant is most difficult to restore and may necessitate free flaps. Fortunately it is also the least commonly affected area.
- Other considerations:
  - The nipple may need to be 'recentralised' and the contralateral breast may need 'balancing' (which is best delayed until after radiotherapy). Due to tissue rearrangement, close co-operation with the radiation oncologist regarding the position of the target is needed; post-operative irradiation will adversely affect the aesthetic result.
  - **Fat grafting** is becoming an option; there is also a softening effect, though the late effects/longevity are largely unknown.

Fat necrosis occurs in >10% and 5%–10% will have complications involving the NAC. Overall, 20%–30% will have unfavourable outcomes, with two-thirds requesting further surgery. **Unfavourable outcomes are more likely with >20% volume change**. Being too ambitious/overextensive resection will likely lead to poor cosmesis. Avoid in

- Stage III/IV, >5 cm. Some say that 2 cm size is significant with reference to recurrences (Rietjens M, *Breast*, 2007).
- Multifocal/multicentric disease
- Recurrence.
- Previous irradiation.
- Patients with BRCAs.

The psychological impact of such surgery is difficult to quantify, although most patients seem satisfied; there are factors that can modify this, e.g. complications following balancing procedures on the contralateral breast that can cause significant distress (average 5%, skin necrosis, infection and dehiscence). Careful patient selection is obviously a key; patients need to have realistic expectations. Survival rates are similar, but the risk of recurrence is higher in BCT.

CLOUGH CLASSIFICATION

- I (mild) volume deformity with asymmetry – best left alone and treated with contralateral reduction
- II (moderate) contour deformity
- III (severe) significant volume and contour deformity

II and III are best treated with flaps, though irradiated skin will tend to shrink around the flap. Whilst patient satisfaction tends to be ~80% after I, it can be as low as 20% after II and III.

6

Hands

A. TRAUMA

I. EXAMINATION

LOOK

Start with the dorsum of the hand – **skin/swellings/ shrinkage/shape**

- Skin – sudomotor changes, benign lesions (Garrod's pads, Heberden's nodes), malignant lesions (actinic keratoses, SCCs), pigment changes, scars, etc.
- Swellings – dorsal wrist ganglia, exostoses.
- Shrinkage, i.e. wasting – particularly dorsal interossei.
- 'Shape', i.e. position of the hand – e.g. ulnar claw, rheumatoid deformities; measure angles with a goniometer for greatest accuracy.

Turn the hand over to look at the volar surface.

- Skin – sudomotor changes, scars, palmar nodules of Dupuytren's
- Swellings – volar wrist ganglion, palmar lipomata, etc.
- Shrinkage/wasting – thenar and hypothenar muscles

FEEL

- Test for sensation in each of the nerve territories. It should be routine to check nerves before operating on any part of the hand, e.g. Dupuytren's, where digital nerves may be injured.
- Feel the relevant feature to complete examination of texture, tenderness, mobility, etc. If a joint is the relevant feature, then 'feel' stability. Do not elicit pain!

MOVE

- Passive range of movement.
- Active range of movement – global and movement in an area of special interest:
  - Flexor tendon division – test flexor digitorum profundus (FDP) and flexor digitorum superficialis (FDS) tendons.
    - FDS has less power but more independent function; 15% have conjoint ring and little finger slips.
    - Note that FDP has dual innervation: the median nerve supplies index and middle finger bellies; the ulnar nerve supplies the ulnar two.
    - Having a common belly increases the power of FDP, at the cost of less independent movement. The index has most independence (about 30°), being the first belly to separate off.
  - Basal joint osteoarthritis (OA) – ask the patient to circumduct the thumb.
  - Rheumatoid arthritis (RA) – look at active wrist pronation/supination, flex/extend meta-carpophalangeal joints (MCPJs).
  - Test the motor nerves to the whole hand.

EXAMINATION FOR SPECIFIC NERVES

MEDIAN NERVE

Look: wasting of the thenar musculature and sudomotor changes in the nerve distribution.

Motor:

- Median nerve at the elbow – palpate tendon of flexor carpi radialis (FCR) with resisted wrist flexion.

- Anterior interosseous nerve (AION) sign – inability to make an 'O' sign due to denervation of FDP to the index finger and flexor pollicis longus (FPL).
- Pronation of the forearm (quadratus) with the elbow extended to neutralise the pronator teres (PT).
- Motor branch of the median nerve:
  - Weakness in abduction of the thumb (abductor pollicis brevis [APB])
  - Opposition to the little finger (true pulp to pulp – opponens pollicis)

Sensory: Pulp of the index

- Moving two-point discrimination (2pd)
- Sharp/blunt sensation

ULNAR NERVE

Look:

- Interosseous guttering and first dorsal interosseous (DO) wasting
- Hypothenar wasting
- Ulnar claw hand
- Sudomotor skin changes

Motor:

- **Froment's test** – tests adductor pollicis (**last muscle innervated by the ulnar nerve**); can perform individual Froment's tests to the fingers – palmar interossei.
- Resisted abduction of the index finger (first DO) and the little finger (abductor digiti minimi [ADM]).
- Flex the MCPJ of the little finger with the proximal interphalangeal joint (PIPJ) straight – flexor digiti minimi (FDM).
- Absent flexion at the distal interphalangeal joint (DIPJ) of the ulnar two fingers (ulnar-innervated FDPs).

  Sensory: little finger – as above.

RADIAL NERVE

Look:

- Sudomotor changes in the superficial branch of radial nerve (RN) distribution
- Wasting of triceps, brachioradialis (BR) and extensor compartment
- Wrist drop

Motor:

- Above the elbow – elbow extension (triceps)
- At the elbow:
  - Elbow flexion, arm in mid-pronation to neutralise biceps (BR).
  - Wrist extension and radial deviation, fist clenched (extensor carpi radialis longus [ECRL] and extensor carpi radialis brevis [ECRB] tendons).

- Below the elbow – posterior interosseous nerve (PIN):
  - Supination with the elbow extended to neutralise the biceps (supinator).
  - Thumb extension with the palm flat (extensor pollicis longus [EPL]). Screen with 'thumbs up'.

  Sensory: first web space – as above.

SPECIFIC PROVOCATION TESTS FOR NERVE COMPRESSION

Provocation tests aim to reproduce the symptoms of compression neuropathy.

MEDIAN NERVE

- **Pronator syndrome** – pain with resisted pronation of the flexed forearm, which pinches the median nerve between the two heads of PT
- **Anterior interosseous syndrome** – resisted FDS flexion of the middle finger
- **Carpal tunnel syndrome** (CTS) – paraesthesia with Tinel's and Phalen's tests
  - **Tinel's** – 60% sensitivity and specificity
  - **Phalen's** – more sensitive but less specific

ULNAR NERVE

- **Cubital tunnel syndrome**
  - Paraesthesia with flexion of the elbow; Tinel's test is less reliable.
  - Note – reduced/lack of clawing due to denervation of ulnar FDP.
- **Ulnar tunnel syndrome** (Guyon's canal) – paraesthesia with pressure over Guyon's canal

RADIAL NERVE

- **Radial tunnel syndrome.**
  - Pain with middle finger test (resisted extension of the middle finger).
  - The RN may be compressed by multiple structures – the medial tendinous edge of the ECRB, proximal border of supinator (arcade of Frohse) or radial recurrent vessels (leash of Henry).
- **Wartenberg's syndrome** – there is dysaesthesia with compression of the superficial branch of the RN beneath the tendon of the BR. Finkelstein test (positive in de Quervain's) may give a false positive.

LOCAL ANAESTHETICS

Local anaesthetics (LA) **are mostly weak bases** (pKa 7.7–9.1 – at pH equivalent to the pKa, the non-ionic and ionised forms are in equal proportions). Most preparations come at pH 5–6 (without adrenaline) or 2–3 (with adrenaline, because it is unstable at alkaline pH; these solutions tend to sting more). Therefore, after injection, they will need to be 'buffered up' closer to their pKa first, leading to a short delay in the onset of action before a significant amount of the non-ionised base is formed. They work by preventing membrane depolarisation and blocking the generation of action potentials by binding to the **inner portion of sodium channels**. They work quicker in smaller unmyelinated nerve fibres, e.g. pain C fibres.

- **Non-ionic form** can cross plasma membranes, whilst it is the ionic form that binds to the target. Thus, by affecting the equilibrium, the pKa will influence the **speed of onset.**
  - A compound with pKa closer to body pH will act quicker.
  - Inflammation lowers pH (i.e. even further away from the typical pKa), pushing more into ionic form, inhibiting its effect.
  - Addition of bicarbonate will raise the pH closer to the slightly basic pKa and thus speed the onset of action.
- **Potency** is related to **lipid solubility** (a property of the aromatic ring), allowing more to enter nerves (they **act from the inside of the membrane**). More potent LAs work at a lower concentration.
- **Adrenaline** counters the vasodilatory effects of most LAs (cocaine is an exception in that it causes vasoconstriction) – allows faster onset of and longer duration of action.

Procaine (Novocain®, 1905) was a synthetic analogue of cocaine that did not have the same issues with addiction but had other significant problems of its own; it had a weak action, took a long time to work and was short acting. Furthermore, there was a high frequency of allergic reactions (up to 33%), and as such, it is no longer in common use.

Lignocaine/Lidocaine is an amide (see Table 6.1) and was developed in 1943. It is the most commonly used LA and also a type Ib anti-arrhythmic, but can cause arrhythmias by itself.

Bupivacaine is slower but longer acting, and can be combined with lignocaine. Out of the commonly used LAs, it is one of the most cardiotoxic (including a direct effect on Purkinje fibres) and is thus usually contraindicated in Biers blocks. It is a racemic mixture, and the left isomers (levobupivacaine and ropivacaine) have lower cardiotoxicity; the latter is said to be less potent and has less motor blockade.

ADRENALINE AND LOCAL ANAESTHESIA

Many use adrenaline in hand surgery to reduce bleeding, decreasing the need for tourniquets and GA. Adrenaline also increases the duration of action and effectiveness of LA (by reducing systemic absorption) and thus increases the maximum safe dose.

- Time of onset of action –5–7 minutes (peak ~20 minutes; Lalonde D, *J Am Acad Orthop Surg*, 2013).
- Concentrations of 1 in 10^6 are sufficient, and no additional benefit is seen in going above 1 in 10^5.
- Adrenaline does not actually abolish blood flow to skin/bleeding; no cases of tissue necrosis have been reported with injections of lignocaine and adrenaline (accidental injection of 1 in 1000 is not that uncommon).
- It is safe for use in local flaps, fingers (Thomson CJ, *Plast Reconstr Surg*, 2007), toes, penis, nose and ears.

The use of adrenaline has been shown to increase infection rates in contaminated wounds in vitro; reduced blood flow decreases leukocyte numbers and hypoxia reduces their function, especially killing. However, the in vivo effect on infections is unclear. Adrenaline may cause arrhythmias and should not be used in those with severe hypertension, severe PVD, Raynaud's disease or phaeochromocytoma.

ISSUES WITH LA

- **Severe pain** may occur if the needle directly hits a nerve – withdraw and avoid injecting in that area. There may be some numbness that lasts weeks/months. Nerve damage is more common when infiltrating **after** a previous block.
- **Ischaemia.** Inadvertent injection of LA with adrenaline (or Epipen) may cause blanching and pain. The half-life of adrenaline is only 2 minutes, but the vasoconstriction will last longer. Thus, permanent damage is rare, but signs of ischaemia can be treated with phentolamine.
- **(True) allergies to LA** are generally rare (<1% of LA adverse reactions), though it is more common in esters than amides (see Table 6.1). In most cases, it may be due to **methylparaben**, a preservative/bacteriostatic found in multidose vials.
- **Methaemoglobinaemia** may occur due to oxidation of ferric iron to the ferrous form, which most commonly

Table 6.1 Comparison of amide and ester local anaesthetics

Amide	Ester
Lidocaine	Cocaine
Bupivacaine	Benzocaine
Prilocaine	Procaine
Degraded in liver	Hydrolysed in plasma by pseudocholinesterase to para-aminobenzoic acid (PABA), which can trigger antibody formation and lymphocyte stimulation

241

occurs with prilocaine/benzocaine, and leads to cyanosis. Treat with **methylene blue**.

- **Tourniquets.** Post-operative neuritis may occur with tourniquet use and may be related to high pressures (>250 mmHg), long duration (>2 hours) or poor limb positioning/pressure protection, e.g. the ulnar nerve is particularly vulnerable at the elbow.
- **Toxicity.** There is a dose-dependent relationship with toxicity; peak blood concentrations are also related to the rate of absorption, which is related to the vascularity. **The commonest cause of toxicity is inadvertent injection into a vessel. See below.**
  - Reports of localised eyebrow (Patrizi A, *J Clin Pharmacol*, 2009) and chin necrosis (Torrente-Castells E, *JADA*, 2008) near but distant to an injection of lignocaine (2% plain) were attributed to thromboembolic phenomenon and vasospasm, respectively.
- **Pain** – injection pain may be reduced by the following:
  - **Distraction** – applying pressure or vibration stimulus nearby excites A fibres; chatting with the patient also helps.
  - **Topical anaesthetics** – EMLA, 'freeze sprays'.
  - **Warm LA and add sodium bicarbonate** (0.1 mL of 1.26% bicarbonate per mL of LA).
  - **Use small gauge needle** to inject slowly and use the smallest amount required.
  - **If you need to give another injection, go through previously anaesthetised areas**.

TOXICITY

1 mL of 1% has 10 mg.

- Lignocaine. Maximum dose is 3.5 mg/kg (7 mg/kg with adrenaline). The effects last ~2 hours; using adrenaline approximately doubles this.
- Bupivacaine. Maximum dose is 2.5 mg/kg (3 mg/kg with adrenaline). It takes longer to work (2–10 minutes) but lasts longer (up to 4 hours).

CNS disturbance is usually the first sign of toxicity – excitation before depression. At higher levels. there are cardiac effects due to direct binding to muscle cells; 10% exhibit ventricular fibrillation or other arrhythmias (dose dependent).

- **Adrenaline toxicity** – hypertension, tachycardia or arrhythmias. It should be used cautiously in those with cardiac disease or thyrotoxicosis, those taking β-blockers or MAO inhibitors.
- **LA toxicity** – note that the seizure threshold is lowered by hypoxia/hypercarbia and acidosis.
  - **Central nervous system** (CNS) – dizziness, tinnitus, **circumoral numbness/tingling** (usually the first symptom), then excitation (due to blockade of inhibitory pathways, leading to tremor, confusion, agitation and fits), before depression (respiratory, cardiorespiratory).
  - **Cardiovascular** – sodium channel blockage with decreased Purkinje discharge and prolonged conduction times, lowers threshold for ventricular arrhythmias (re-entrant). Classically CNS toxicity precedes cardiovascular, but it can be quite variable.

If toxicity is suspected, stop the injection.

- Give oxygen and commence conventional treatment of hypotension and **arrhythmias, which can be quite refractory** – resuscitation should be continued for at least 60 minutes.
- Benzodiazepines may be useful for seizures. Reversal with **Intralipid®** (works by sequestration mechanism; optimal regime has yet to be determined) may be worth trying if available.

Evidence-based recommendations on the use of intravenous lipid emulsion therapy in poisoning. (Gosselin S, *Clin Toxicol [Phila]*, 2016)

A systematic review of the literature was used to reach a consensus. In the end, recommendations were based on very low quality of evidence. The workgroup recommended dose-finding and controlled studies reflecting human poisoning scenarios.

Intravenous lipid emulsion is recommended for the management of cardiac arrest with **bupivacaine** toxicity, whilst recommendations are neutral for all other toxins. Intralipid® 20% is most often reported, but there is no evidence for a best formulation; there was no consensus on dosing and infusion duration.

TOPICAL ANAESTHETICS

- EMLA (eutectic mixture of LA) 2.5% lignocaine and 2.5% prilocaine that takes 60 minutes for effect (maximal 2–3 hours) and lasts for 1–2 hours after removal. Eutectic means a mixture with a melting point lower than either component alone; being partly solidified makes it more convenient for topical application. Use of an occlusive dressing over a generous application improves absorption; it is a vasoconstrictor.
  - Prilocaine is regarded as one of the least toxic LAs but can cause methaemoglinaemia in the susceptible.
- Ametop® (4% Amethocaine) works quicker in ~30 minutes, lasts longer and has a vasodilatory property that facilitates intravenous cannulation, and unlike EMLA is not contraindicated in the young.
  - It is a potentially toxic ester that is only used topically.
- Tetracaine.
- ELA-Max, LMX4 – 4% liposomal lidocaine.
- Betacaine – often used in OTC pain-relieving gels.

Such preparations should be used cautiously – there have been severe complications including coma and death in patients overdosing on topical LA – in one case, Laser Gel 10-10 (10% lidocaine and 10% tetracaine) was applied to reduce the pain of laser hair removal; in others, a 6%:6% preparation was made by a pharmacy.

II. HAND INFECTIONS

The most common organisms involved in human hand infections are *Staphylococcus aureus* (up to 80%) and Streptococci, with increased risk in diabetics, the immunosuppressed and malnourished.

- Staphylococci tend to produce a purulent infection 3–5 days later with nonsmelly pus.
- Streptococci tend to lead to cellulitis with lymphangitis.
- Gram negatives can give rise to either a cellulitic picture or **pus, which is smelly**.
- Anaerobes include *Eikenella* and *Pasteurella*.

Most common infections will be covered by empirical treatment with penicillin or antistaphyloccal cloxacillin or first-generation cephalosporin, or a third-generation cephalosporin alone.

COMMON MANIFESTATIONS

- **Cellulitis** – group A Streptococci (β-haemolytic), sometimes Staphylococci (usually less severe). Treat with dicloxacillin or cephalexin (erythromycin if penicillin-allergic). Diabetic patients may have higher risk of Gram-negative/polymicrobial infections.
- **Paronychia** is the commonest hand infection and is often associated with nail biting or other minor trauma. There is a high density of dermal lymphatics and lymphocytes in the hyponychium.
  - **Acute** – *S. aureus*, occasionally anaerobes from oral contamination. Treat with drainage and dressings three to four times a day; nail plate removal may not always be needed but should be considered in cases that fail to improve as the nail will then act as a foreign body.
  - **Chronic** paronychia is usually fungal (*Candida albicans*) or atypical mycobacteria. It may be more common in the immunosuppressed, diabetic patients or those with vascular insufficiency. Treat initially with topical/systemic antifungals; some success has been described with the use of topical steroids or tacrolimus. Those who do not respond can be treated by marsupialisation of the eponychium (avoid damaging the germinal matrix) via a crescentic excision that is left to heal by secondary intention. Alternatives include en bloc excision of the proximal nail fold or the 'Swiss roll technique' (Pabari A, *Tech Hand Surg*, 2011).
- **Felon** is an abscess of the pulp space commonly due to *S. aureus*, and is often secondary to a puncture – an X-ray to check for a foreign body may be prudent. The pulp space is quite unique with 15–20 septae anchoring the skin of the pulp/tip to the distal phalanx (DP) and will tend to compartmentalise an infection.

Early infections may respond to antibiotics; but in general, a felon should be drained where it points or is most tender by midvolar or high lateral incisions (avoid fishmouth-type incisions that can compromise the vascularity of the pad, and avoid crossing joint crease). Care should be taken to ensure that all pockets are released.

- **Herpetic whitlow** – this is a herpes simplex virus (HSV) vesicular eruption in the fingertip that is typically preceded by burning-type pain the day before. It may resemble a felon, but the pulp itself should not be tense and the vesicles are filled with clear fluid (sometimes cloudy, may coalesce). These should only be incised if a secondary bacterial abscess has developed; otherwise, the open wound is at risk of super-infection. A vesicle may be deroofed for viral culture or a Tzanck smear (quicker and cheaper). It is usually self-limiting (7–10 days), but topical 5% acyclovir may be used in severe infections to shorten the disease course. There is a 20% risk of reactivation usually resulting in milder disease; oral acyclovir taken during the prodrome may abort recurrence. It is infectious until epithelialisation is complete.
  - Adolescents with genital herpes comprise the largest group – usually HSV2.
  - Children with stomatitis usually HSV1.
  - Health care professionals usually HSV1.

FASCIAL SPACES OF THE HAND

Deep space infections of the hand constitute ~10% of all hand infections and usually follow penetrating trauma, or are spread from elsewhere. It may be difficult to differentiate clinically from flexor tenosynovitis. Infections should be treated aggressively with wide incisions for good access (avoiding incisions in web spaces); wounds should be packed, re-inspected and closed secondarily.

Hand bursae – there are two bursae consisting of the synovial sheaths that project into the hand from just proximal to the flexor retinaculum (FR) where they may communicate.

- Radial bursa – encloses the FPL tendon, and continuous with the flexor sheath to the DP.
- Ulnar bursa – also called the common flexor sheath; it is larger and encloses the long tendons to the little–index fingers as they pass under the FR (and is continuous with the flexor sheath to the little finger).
- Over the second to fourth digits, the bursa stops at the midpalm level, and these digits have their own separate flexor sheaths.

Palmar spaces – thenar, adductor (deep or dorsal to the adductor pollicis), hypothenar, mid-palmar. The deep spaces are potential spaces and include the thenar, mid-palmar, subtendinous (Parona), dorsal subaponeurotic and subfascial web.

- Thenar space infection – painful thumb movements. Classically, infection will cause an abducted thumb.

- Mid-palmar space infection – painful flexion of the three ulnar fingers.
- Web space infection – abducted fingers. It may have dorsal and volar components – a collar stud abscess.

Dorsal spaces – dorsal subaponeurotic (deep to extensor tendons) and dorsal subcutaneous.

FLEXOR SHEATH INFECTIONS

This is usually due to *S. aureus* from penetrating injuries, less commonly due to gonococci (haematogenous spread).

Kanavel's four cardinal signs of flexor sheath infection are as follows:

- **Pain with passive extension.** This is the most sensitive sign that appears early.
- **Fusiform digital swelling** (not in original description).
- **Stiffness in a semiflexed position**.
- **Tenderness along the flexor sheath into the palm**.

Not all signs may be present in individual cases, particularly at an early stage. Diagnosis is largely clinically, though USG may show tendon swelling with surrounding fluid. Delayed treatment will lead to stiffness, tendon rupture or **rupture of infection into other spaces**.

Some have summarised the principles of hand infections as **AIDED**: antibiotics, immobilisation, debridement, elevation and drainage; alternatively, HER: heat (to enhance local circulation), elevation (to reduce oedema) and rest (for comfort and to reduce the spread of infection). Early infection may respond to 'closed drainage' with limited palmar and distal digital incisions to allow a catheter to be inserted for drainage and irrigation; otherwise, open drainage is required taking care to spare the A2 and A4 pulleys.

- Very early injections may respond to elevation/splintage and IVAB but treatment should proceed to surgery if there is no significant improvement after 24 hours.
- Older patients with comorbidities such as diabetes tend to do worse; there is an 8% amputation rate if there is subcutaneous pus, which rises to 80% if there are signs of digital ischaemia.

ANIMAL BITES

All respond to Augmentin (to a certain extent), and this is a good first-line treatment; doxycycline and metronidazole can be used in penicillin-allergic patients. The commonest organisms in bites are streptococci and staphylococci. Tetanus prophylaxis should be administered if needed; follow local guidelines for rabies.

Human bites (2%–23%) – *Staphylococcus*, *Streptococcus viridans* (α-haemolytic), *Streptobacillus*, **Eikenella corrodens** (found in one-third), anaerobes, e.g. *Bacteroides*. There is a risk of septic arthritis or osteomyelitis.

- Human 'bites' (often due to punching someone in the face, i.e. 'fight bites') may have penetrating MCPJ injuries. Septic arthritis, in general, can be due to haematogenous spread (suspect gonococcal infection) or penetrating injury; gouty arthritis can mimic a septic arthritis. Examine in the clenched fist position; more superficial layers will become more proximal relative to deeper levels of injury as the hand is flattened out.
- HIV transmission after human bites has been described, though this is very rare – some recommend a 28 day course of antiretroviral therapy if either the biter or the bitten are HIV positive.
- Dangers are often underestimated.
  - Acute non-infected injuries that potentially involve joints or tendons should be properly explored and irrigated, then splinted, elevated and treated with antibiotics. Hard evidence is lacking, but these injuries should probably be left open/loose, with secondary closure if necessary.
  - Infected wounds should be explored (debridement and drainage/irrigation systems may be necessary).

ANIMAL BITES

The role of antibiotic prophylaxis is unclear, but empirically it can be given to those with puncture wounds, hand/foot/face wounds, wounds that have been closed primarily and in compromised patients, e.g. diabetic, asplenic or otherwise immunosuppressed (Monteiro JA, *Eur J Int Med*, 1995).

- **Dog** (69%–90%) – *Pasteurella multocida*, *Streptobacillus*, *Staphylococcus*, anaerobes. Bites have high force and there may be significant tissue shearing/devitalisation particularly with bigger dogs. *Pasteurella* infection typically causes a discharging wound after 24 hours. Wounds can usually be closed loosely after irrigation; infection in dog bites is an uncommon occurrence (4%) compared to cat bites (50%).
  - *Capnocytophaga canimorsus* may cause severe sepsis after contact with dog saliva, especially in post-splenectomy patients (Bulter T, *Eur J Clin Microbiol Infect Dis*, 2015). Penicillin is the drug of choice.
- **Cat** (5%–18%) – mainly *P. multocida*. Cats tend to have sharper, thinner, longer teeth and that cause deep punctures with less tissue damage. Irrigation and suture are possible in most cases.
  - **Cat-scratch fever** is caused by *Bartonella* and not *Pasteurella*. Classically there are papules at the initial site of infection (1–2 weeks prior) along with regional lymphadenopathy and mild systemic upset. Generally, it has a good prognosis and is self-limited but responds well to ciproxin and doxycycline. The skin test is rarely used now as enzyme immune assay (EIA) antibody tests are available.

OSTEOMYELITIS

Osteomyelitis of the hand is uncommon. It is usually due to *Staphylococcus aureus*, *Streptococcus pyogenes* and possibly Gram-negative anaerobes. Necrotic bone should be debrided followed by antibiotics for 4–6 weeks; there is a 39% amputation rate.

OTHER INFECTIONS

Onychomycosis – nail fungal infection that leads to a thickened, discoloured and flaking nail. Dermatophytes such as *Trichophyton rubrum* are the most common cause in temperate countries, whilst *Candida* is more common in the tropics and in diabetics, and those that frequently immerse their hands in water. Laboratory confirmation is recommended before treatment: direct smear (potassium hydroxide) with histological examination and periodic acid–Schiff (PAS) staining of the biopsy of the nail plate.

- Debridement of nail combined with oral terbinafine (a newer antifungal that is better tolerated) is better than taking the drug alone (Potter LP, *J Dermatolog Treat*, 2007). Nail avulsion can reduce the duration of oral therapy needed (Jennings MB, *J Am Podiatr Med Assoc*, 2006).
- Combining oral terbinafine with amorolfine nail paint is more effective than the oral drug alone (Baran R, *Brit J Dermatol*, 2007).
- Some laser-based treatments have been described.

Sporotrichosis is a fungal (*Sporothrix schenckii*) infection of the skin and subcutaneous tissues, most commonly due to puncture wounds sustained during gardening, particularly rose thorns – hence 'Rose gardener's disease'. It is a chronic disease that begins as a plaque/nodule at the puncture point that then tends to ulcerate if untreated. Rarely it may spread to the lungs or become disseminated. Definitive diagnosis requires fungal culture. It is usually treated with antifungals – itraconazole, terbinafine or fluconazole – for 3–6 months (at least a month after symptoms clear). Oral saturated solution of potassium iodide (SSKI) has also been used with some efficacy in the past, though its exact mechanism of action is unclear; it is cheap but poorly tolerated by most.

Atypical mycobacterial infections are relatively rare; the most common is probably *Mycobacterium marinum*, which can be contracted from either fresh or salt water (except swimming pools as chlorination kills the organism). It grows optimally at 31°C and thus is seen mostly on the cooler extremities. It should be suspected in those with a chronic sinus/ulcer with a compatible history; the diagnosis can be made by culturing for 8 weeks at 31°C in a Lowenstein–Jensen medium, Ziehl–Nielson staining. Skin lesions generally do not need surgical debridement and will respond to specific antibiotics, e.g. doxycycline/minocycline, ciproxin as well as the combination of rifampicin and ethambutol, which should be used where possible for 2–6 months (empiric duration but most recommend at least 1 month further after resolution of lesions).

- Other water-borne infections include *Aeromonas hydrophilia* (fresh water, may be found in leeches).
- *Vibrio vulnificus* (coastal sea water) may cause a form of necrotising fasciitis.

III. FLEXOR TENDON INJURY

ANATOMY

- Tendons are mostly made of collagen type I, with ground substance and specialised fibroblasts called tenocytes.
  - Endotenon is the fine covering around tendon fibres that binds them together; blood vessels, nerves and lymphatics are carried in this layer. It is continuous with the epimysium.
  - Epitenon is the fibrous outer layer of the tendon within synovial sheaths.
  - Paratenon is the loose adventitial layer where there is no true synovial sheath.

TENDON NUTRITION

In the past, there was much debate regarding the source of nutrition for the tendons of the hand.

- **Perfusion** (direct vascularity) – Blood supply to the tendons comes primarily from the **vincula** (from the Latin *vincio*, meaning to bind) that have segmental branches from the digital arteries forming a vascular territory. Vessels also enter the tendon at bony insertions and musculocutaneous junctions; extrasynovial tendons have supply from random small vessels from the surrounding tissue. The vascularity is concentrated mainly on the dorsum of the tendon and remains quite superficial in the endotenon septae. There is no overlap in the flow between the territories of the vincula, and the supply to the tendons over the PP, in particular, is poor. Presumably these areas are sustained by diffusion (Figure 6.1).
  - Short – vinculum in the angle between the tendon and insertions, FDP to the neck of the middle phalanx (MP).
  - Long – from the periosteum of phalanges to the dorsum of the flexor tendon, FDP to the neck of the proximal phalanx (PP).
  - The FDS also has long and short vincula both attaching to the PP.
- Nutrients from the **synovial fluid** can reach the tendon by diffusion; some propose that finger movements pump fluid into the narrow canaliculi that pass through the tendon. Current thinking is that diffusion plays an important role; in particular, the FDP tendon is more dependent on diffusion than the FDS.

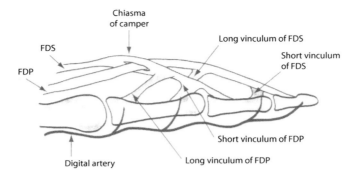

Figure 6.1 Schematic diagram of the flexor tendon arrangement of the fingers along with the vincula derived from branches of the digital artery. There may be a slip to the FPL from the index FDP (Linburg–Comstock anomaly 1979).

PULLEYS

The synovial fluid within the tendon sheath allows smooth gliding of the FDS and FDP tendons within it. There are thickened areas along the sheath that are called pulleys. In the fingers, there are five annular pulleys and four cruciate pulleys. The **crucial pulleys are A2 (proximal PP) and A4 (middle MP).** The closer the tendon is to the bone, the less tendon excursion needed to bend the joint, i.e. pulleys **maximise mechanical efficiency**.

- A1 – overlying MCPJ, attached to the base of PP
- A2 – overlying shaft of PP – proximal part of PP
- A3 – overlying PIPJ, attached to the base of MP
- A4 – overlying shaft of MP – middle of MP
- A5 – overlying DIPJ
- C1–4 – between annular pulleys, except A1 and A2

In the **thumb**, there are two annular pulleys and one oblique pulley. The tendon of the adductor pollicis is attached to A1 and oblique pulleys.

- A1 – overlying MCPJ, attached to the volar plate.
- A2 – overlying IPJ, attached to the head of PP.
- Oblique – overlying shaft of PP (analogous to A2 in the finger – the thumb A2 and oblique pulleys are most important).

FLEXOR TENDON INJURIES

Mechanism of tendon healing

Tendons contain few cells: tenocytes, fibroblasts and synovial cells. The paucity of cells and the presence of avascular zones within the synovial areas led to the impression that tendons would not heal well intrinsically and needed extrinsic cells; however, whilst the collagen bundles are dense, tendons are still metabolically active. Theories on the mechanism(s) of healing are as follows:

- **Extrinsic** – it was initially thought that healing comes from fibroblasts producing peritendinous adhesions that act as pathways for cell migration and revascularisation,

and this theory was the basis for the immobilisation regimes of the past. By this mechanism, the tendon heals 'typically' with inflammation, proliferation and remodelling.
- **Intrinsic** – tendons bathed in synovial fluid were found to heal well with minimal inflammation; collagen is produced by tenocytes (in epitenon) that act like fibroblasts and can bridge a tendon gap. This type of healing is increased by tendon motion.

There is a similar sequence to cutaneous wound healing:

- **Haemostasis** – it occurs by platelet and fibrin deposition, vasoconstriction.
- **Inflammation** – there is an accumulation of inflammatory cells and cytokines that attract fibroblasts to the injury and lasts up to a week.
- **Proliferation** – (from days 2–3 up to 1 month) fibroblast proliferation close to the cut tendon end leads to deposition of disorganised collagen fibres with subsequent vascular ingrowth. There is also proliferation of epitenon cells that covers the injury to restore a smooth surface in a fashion analogous to a fracture callus. Adhesions are a by-product.
- **Remodelling** – it begins at about 3 weeks with a parallel reorientation of collagen fibres that increases the strength of repair, and thus increased mobilisation can start at this stage. Movement limits adhesion formation and thus promotes intrinsic healing at the expense of extrinsic.

VERDAN'S ZONES

The zone of tendon injury is described as the position of the injury when the fingers and thumb are extended, rather than the site of the surface laceration.

- Fingers extended at the time of injury – distal ends lie in the wound
- Fingers flexed at the time of injury – distal ends distal to the skin wound

FINGERS

- Zone 1 – Insertion of the FDP to the insertion of FDS/distal to FDS insertion.
- Zone 2 – Between the insertion of FDS and the A1 pulley (distal palmar crease) – 'No man's land' (Bunnell, largely historical term); 'critical zone' (Boyes). The FDS divides at the level of the distal palmar crease. Digital nerve injury is common in zone 2 tendon injuries.
- Zone 3 – From the A1 pulley to the distal border of the carpal tunnel (CT).
- Zone 4 – CT.
- Zone 5 – CT to musculotendinous junctions of muscles.

THUMB

- Zone 1 – From the A2 pulley to the insertion of FPL (distal to IPJ)
- Zone 2 – A1–2 pulley (MCPJ to IPJ)
- Zone 3 – A1 pulley to CT; then as above (MCPJ to CT)
- Zone 4 – CT
- Zone 5 – Proximal to CT

BOYES' CLASSIFICATION OF FLEXOR TENDON INJURIES

- Injury to tendon only
- Tendon and soft tissue
- Associated with joint contracture
- Associated with neurovascular damage
- Multiple digits or combinations of II–IV

CLOSED AVULSIONS OF THE FDP

Seventy-five per cent of the cases involve the ring finger. This is the classic 'rugby jersey finger' – typically the tendon is avulsed from the DP whilst attempting to hold onto an opponent's collar as he is running away at speed.

LEDDY AND PACKER CLASSIFICATION (1977)

- **Type I**. The FDP tendon ruptures along with both vincula but with no fracture; hence, the tendon retracts into the palm and presents as a tender lump. Early repair (within 10 days) is needed as the vincular and synovial supplies have been disrupted. It is the **most severe type** of avulsion injury.
- **Type II**. The FDP ruptures but the long vinculum remains intact and holds the distal tendon end at the PIPJ level. There may be a small fracture fragment. Repair within 3 months is recommended. This is the **commonest type** of avulsion injury.
- **Type III**. There is a large fracture fragment that will become caught at the A4 pulley; the tendon is unable to retract further and hence both vinculae are protected. There is no specific deadline for repair and it has the best prognosis.

FLEXOR TENDON REPAIR

History

- Age, hand dominance
- Occupation (complex reconstruction vs. pragmatic lesser option) and hobbies
  - Patients should be made aware that they will not regain full use of their hand for **up to 3 months** after a tendon injury.
- Pre-existing hand problems
- Mechanism of injury – laceration, crush, avulsion, etc.
- Time of injury (if long-standing may need two-stage reconstruction)
- General questions relating to factors relevant to fitness for surgery and wound healing (drugs, medical history including diabetes, smoker, etc.) and tetanus status

EXAMINATION

In general, expose the whole upper limb and examine systematically:

- **Look** – perfusion, old scars, swellings, sudomotor changes, wasting, finger cascade, identify zone of injury
- **Feel** – sensation especially distal to the injury, feel for tender mass in the palm – Leddy and Packer type I
- **Move** – passive and active movement distal to the injury plus full neurological examination of the three nerves
  - Specific examination of FDP and FDS (see below)

SPECIFIC TISSUES

- **Soft tissue** – lacerations and tissue loss.
- **Circulation** – bleeding from a pinprick is not wholly reliable as bleeding can occur several hours after arterial occlusion (though the colour of blood may help) and may cause infection. Allen's test will show that the superficial palmar arch is incomplete in 10%–15%. Pulse oximetry is useful.
  - Arterial insufficiency – pale cold part with loss of turgor and delayed refill.
  - Venous insufficiency – congested part with brisk refill.
- **Sensation** – it is useful to note that denervated fingers will be dry and smooth, and will not wrinkle in when dipped in water >5 minutes. This may be useful in children or otherwise uncooperative patients. Neurovascular injuries are not uncommon in flexor tendon injuries. For quick screening, test sensation of the index fingertip, little fingertip and dorsal first web, which are supplied by the median, ulnar and radial nerves, respectively.
  - **Two-point discrimination** (2pd) relates to innervation density and is dependent on cortical integration. It is potentially more objective than threshold tests; furthermore, moving 2pd (>3 mm) is a more sensitive indicator of nerve dysfunction than static 2pd (>6 mm).

- Vibration and pressure thresholds (Semmes–Weinstein monofilament) are more sensitive but are less practical to use.
- **Bone** – fractures should be described according to location, type (oblique, transverse, comminuted, etc.) and deformity (angulation by direction of apex and rotational by distal segment relative to proximal). Rotational deformities can be detected by looking for an **overlap of the** finger cascade (and comparing with the other side). AP and oblique X-rays of the hands are needed as normal examination does not rule out fractures (see below).
- **Joints** – passive range of motion (ROM)
- **Muscles** – active movements, active ROM and strength testing (MRC). Look at the resting posture and the tenodesis effect to passive wrist flexion/extension.

SPECIFIC EXAMINATION OF FDP AND FDS

- **FDS** – With the patient's hand palm up and other fingers fixed in extension by the examiner, the patient is asked to flex the finger at the PIPJ. The finger will bend at that joint **and** the DIPJ will become lax. For the index finger, this test is less reliable and the test can be performed keeping the DIPJ extended. The ulnar three digits have a common FDP muscle belly, and any flexion of the finger with the others in extension demonstrates intact FDS to that finger.
  - **DIPJ extension test** – the inability to hyperextend the DIPJ with the finger and thumb in a precision pinch suggests isolated FDS injury (can quickly check for all fingers by asking the patient to press finger pulps onto the palm).
  - **Little finger**. When there is no active PIPJ joint flexion of the little finger, and considering the possibility of FDS injury:
    - 15% have a non-functioning FDS to the little finger.
    - Some have adhesions between FDS to the ring finger and little finger preventing independent movement.
- **FDP** – with the hand dorsum flat on the table, hold MP down and ask the patient to flex the DIPJ.

RADIOLOGY

It is important to exclude other injured structures especially nerves and bones, as well as to exclude foreign bodies.

- Hand – posteroanterior (PA), frontal, oblique (for MCPJ) and lateral (progressive finger flexion with thumb as frontal).
- Fingers – lateral, PA views only if injuries definitely limited to MP and DPs.
- Wrist – PA, lateral and oblique. Special views include scaphoid projection that makes the bone appear elongated allowing better views of the cortex and trabeculae of wrist, oblique hamate view or CT view.

GENERAL PRINCIPLES

Timing

The urgency/severity of limb injuries can be classified as requiring

- **Immediate treatment**, e.g. severe haemorrhage with risk of exsanguination (life threatening), ischaemia (limb threatening – warm ischaemia time of muscle is short).
  - Blind clamping or tourniquets are not recommended as they can cause damage; instead limb elevation and direct pressure are preferred.
- **Early treatments**, e.g. **flexor tendons**, open fractures/joint injuries.
  - Less severe, e.g. minor injuries including extensor and nerve injuries. Note that tendons with independent muscle units, e.g. EPL, will shorten quickly and thus need earlier treatment.

TENDON REPAIR

Timing

- **Repairing early,** e.g. within 6 hours has been the conventional teaching, but repair even after 24 hours (see below) is also acceptable if antibiotics are used. In general, there has been a tendency to move away from regarding tendon repair as an 'emergency'; results are better when performed during the day by an experienced surgeon, rather than in the middle of the night. **A good repair within 1 week gives results similar to repair within 1 day.**
- **Primary repair within 24 hours.**
- **Delayed primary** – more than 24 hours but less than 2 weeks. The patient may present late or have ongoing infections that need to be treated first. This will still provide good results.
- **Secondary repair**. Satisfactory results are still possible with early secondary repair, but more adhesions are likely.

  - Early secondary (2–5 weeks), before **significant muscle contracture** occurs, and thus results are similar to delayed primary. Note that independent muscles contract quicker.
  - Late secondary – after 5 weeks, the gap between muscle and tendon means that a tendon graft is required for continuity, or a transfer to restore the 'action'.

Antibiotics and tetanus booster immunisation are administered as indicated.

- **Anaesthesia**
  - GA or Wrist block.
  - Brachial plexus block – effective but often incomplete and risk of pneumothorax (less with ultrasound guidance).
  - Biers block (intravenous block) – tourniquet failure is rare but potentially lethal.

- **Adequate visualisation**
  - Tendons are repaired under **tourniquet control** (100 mmHg above systolic, or 250 mmHg adults, 150 mmHg children, placed high on the arm and limited to 2 hours at a time, with 15 minute breaks if required). Exsanguination is contraindicated in tumours and active infection – elevation is preferred. Tourniquets should be removed completely when not needed to reduce venous congestion. Complications are usually related to direct pressure rather than length of time, and include nerve injuries or ischaemia particularly of muscle.
  - **Incisions** aim to maximise exposure of injured parts – extend lacerations as necessary remembering that **all incisions heal with a scar, and all scars contract** and thus incisions should not cross flexor joints perpendicularly. Use either **Bruners** (Bruner JM 1967 volar zigzag), Bunnell (non-dominant mid-lateral incision, involves significant elevation of soft tissue) or volar midline oblique, taking care to avoid injury to neurovascular bundles (NVBs). Incisions on the contact areas, i.e. the ulnar side of the little finger or the radial side of the index finger, should be avoided (Figure 6.2).
    - Dissection begins from uninjured areas towards the injury.
    - The midaxial is not true midlateral (where vessels are) but a dorsal lateral, joining the dorsal points of the flexed finger creases (Figure 6.3).
    - Longitudinal lacerations crossing joints should be converted to Z-plasties.
- **Tendon retrieval**
  - 'Milking' the tendon and flexing proximal joints; fix tendon with 22 G needle.
  - Make an incision in the distal palmar crease (just proximal to A1), feed a cannula down and pull back after attaching the tendon. Other incisions can be made as needed as long as the A2 and A4 pulleys are left intact.
  - Other methods – reverse Esmarch tourniquet or endoscope; avoid 'blind' grabbing if possible.
- **Tendon repair**
  - Handle tendons carefully – avoid handling uninjured areas and grasp only the end of the tendon, as injuring

 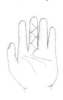

Bruner   Modified Bruner   V-Y flaps

Figure 6.2 Some common incisions used for exploring volar finger injuries or disease such as Dupuytren's contracture – Bruner (midaxial to midaxial), modified Bruner and V-Y flaps. The modified Bruner incision was described by Hettiaratchy (*Plast Reconstr Surg*, 2003).

the epitenon will increase the risk of adhesions. The aim is to repair the tendon without a gap (strongly associated with rupture) or bunching (which would shorten as well as increase bulk).

- **Avoid shortening** tendons by excessive excision/debridement, as this can result in a **quadriga effect** (incomplete flexion due to shortened FDP tendons reaching maximum flexion too early); a **loss of >1 cm** of tendon will severely limit excursion.
- The **A2 and A4** pulleys are important but can be vented (~25%, Tomaino M, *J Hand Surg Br*, 1998) without compromising function. The A2 pulley is often damaged by trauma and should be repaired, e.g. by double-wrapped palmaris longus (PL) tendon or extensor retinaculum. There is no advantage to repairing flexor sheaths, and it may actually increase friction.
- Avoid narrowing Camper's chiasm; some advocate repairing only one slip of FDS.

TWO- OR FOUR-STRAND TECHNIQUES

The common choice is a non-absorbable monofilament (e.g. Prolene®, easier to use but in vitro tests have shown stretching under tension leading to a tendon gap) or non-absorbable braided (Ticron®, braided sutures have a tendency to cause deformation and need greater attention to detail in their placement and tightening). Absorbable sutures (PDS, Maxon®) are not commonly used but can also be satisfactory since the metabolic rate of the tendon tissue is low, and suture material is retained long enough to maintain tensile strength during healing.

The **modified Kessler** 4′0 (or **Tajima** modification, quadrilateral suture with small grasping bites at each corner) **plus epitendinous suture** (5′0 Prolene) is as good as most other techniques. The epitendinous suture was introduced by Kleinert and contributes 20% to the strength of the repair; some use sutures as fine as 7′0. Placing the back wall epitendinous suture first may facilitate a 'no touch' technique.

- A cadaver study (Taras JS, *J Hand Surg (Am)*, 2001) showed that a 4′0 suture is 66% stronger than a 5′0; a 3′0 suture is 52% stronger than 4′0. Suture failure includes pull-through, unravelled knots or breakage at knots.
- Take a 0.5–1 cm bite of the tendon; 5 mm is sufficient for zone 1 injuries.
- To maximise tendon vascularity, keep sutures volar to preserve vinculae during repair; some studies have shown that dorsally placed Kessler sutures are stronger (Komanduri M, *J Hand Surg Am*, 1996; Soejima O, *J Hand Surg Am*, 1999).
  - Stein et al. (*J Hand Surg Am*, 1998) found that volarly placed sutures were as strong as dorsal using the Becker technique.

There are a variety of **four-strand** techniques based on the finding that the strength of the core suture is most important and is related to the number of strands crossing

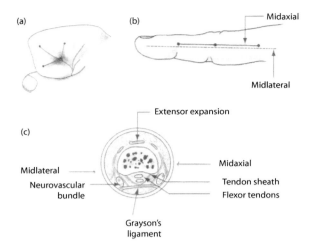

Figure 6.3 (a) The ends of the interphalangeal creases are marked with the digit fully flexed, and joining them up forms the 'midaxial' line. (b) This lies slightly dorsal to the midlateral axial and the NVB. (c) A Bruner incision should touch the midaxial line.

the tendon, e.g. four-strand cruciate, MGH criss-crossing locking stitch/augmented, Becker technique (two external knots). Six- and eight-strand techniques have also been described; adding strands **increases complexity, handling and bulk**, and the possibility makes unevenness and adhesions more likely (Figure 6.4).

- **For partial tendon division** up to 50% (or even 60%; Bishop AT, *J Trauma*, 1986; Chow SP, *J Hand Surg*, 1984), repair with an epitendinous stitch alone to improve gliding may be adequate. A tendon may be lacerated up to 90% but still functional (but not for long).
  - Without repair, there may be delayed rupture, triggering or entrapment.
- A second single horizontal mattress core suture can be placed where possible, slightly dorsal (this is where most gapping occurs) to the centre to make a four-strand Kessler.
  - Try to bury any external knots within longitudinal slits.

- **Zone 1 injuries** lead to loss of DIPJ flexion. FDP repairs may demand a reinsertion technique (Mitek anchors) as 5 mm of distal stump is usually needed for suture repair. Studies have shown that direct anchoring of tendon to the bone is stronger than suturing tendons together; the FDP tendon can be advanced up to a maximum of 1 cm for direct anchoring.
- **Zone 2 injuries** – repair both the FDS and FDP except in replants where the FDP only may be repaired. Not repairing the FDS may lead to increased risk of FDP repair rupture, loss of grip strength and dexterity and late swan neck deformity.
- **Tendon loss** – consider primary graft or insertion of a Hunter rod, but good-quality soft tissue cover muscle must be available.

POST-OPERATIVE PROTOCOL

The tensile strength of the repair is weakest at 7–10 days, just as collagen is beginning to be laid down. Strength gradually increases through collagen deposition and then

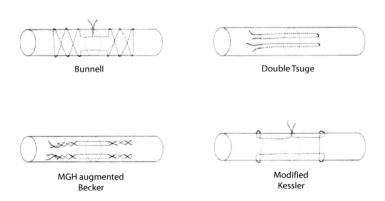

Figure 6.4 Some methods of flexor tendon repair.

remodelling; maximum strength is attained after ~3 months whilst further remodelling continues.

- **Dressings in layers** – optional tulle dressing, fluffy gauze and crepe with diminishing compression from distal to proximal.
- **Safe or protective position.** Extension block splint (dorsal slab). MCPJ flexed to 50–70° and IPJ extended (to keep ligaments taut to avoid shortening), thumb abduction (to maintain web space), 30° wrist flexion. Some prefer splintage in MCPJ 70–90°, IPJ in full extension and wrist in neutral. The amount of MCPJ flexion is variable, but the IPJs should always be fully extended; trying too hard to bend the MCPJs may cause some IPJ flexion.
  - Wrist extension (to reduce tenodesis effect – wrist flexion would cause digital flexion and pull on the extensors) is not strictly necessary with adequate support from the dressings.
  - 70° MCPJ flexion and full IPJ extension, also known as intrinsic-plus position, was originally described by James (*Acta Ortho Scand*, 1962).
- **Elevation above the level of the heart.**

Most **rehabilitation protocols** involve **early motion** that progresses to full active flexion. This increases the speed and strength of tendon repair with fewer adhesions, but this needs to be balanced against the greater risk of tendon rupture. For zones 1–3, early mobilisation is recommended except for unreliable patients, children, poor quality tendons, e.g. crush injuries, and those with additional damage. **Tendons move 1 mm for every 10° of isolated DIPJ or PIPJ flexion.**

- **Belfast protocol** of controlled active movement for 6 weeks under the supervision of the physiotherapists.
  - From day 2 to 6 weeks, every 2 hours:
    - Active flexion (IPJ movement) – to limit adhesions and increase the strength of repair/intrinsic healing. PIPJ 30°, DIPJ 10°, then mass movement of all fingers to gentle fist twice.
    - Passive flexion (for joint mobility and to reduce contractures) – complete flexion, apply gentle fingernail pressure to push fingers into the palm twice after each set; there should be active extension to touch splint with nails.
    - Passive flexion and hold – isometric force on muscle bellies helps to maintain function.
  - 6 weeks – remove splint and use active flexion exercises. The hand can be used but avoid heavy work.
  - 8 weeks – slow increase in activity, fine work.
  - 10 to 12 weeks – heavier work including driving.
  - After 12 weeks – normal activities allowed but only 60% strength at 16 weeks.
- Early active extension and passive flexion – **Kleinert;** not 'early active motion'. A dorsal splint prevents over-extension, whilst **elastic bands** in a pulley system maintain finger flexion – it allows active extension and then passive flexion by elastic recoil. The patient fully needs to understand the treatment;

otherwise, there is risk of causing flexion contracture especially of PIPJ. There is less risk of tendon rupture.

- Active ROM excursion exercises begin at 4 weeks, blocking at 5 weeks, passive ROM in extension at 6 weeks and graded excursion strengthening at 8 weeks.
- Early passive mobilisation – Duran.
- Immobilisation, e.g. in a cast, may be more appropriate for children and non-compliant adults, e.g. those with learning difficulties.
  - Tuzuner (*J Pediatr Orthop*, 2004) used botulinum toxin A to temporarily paralyse the muscles in children under 6 to reduce the risk of rupture.

COMPLICATIONS

Overall, better results are expected if the injury is outside zone 2 (85%, compared to 80% in zone 2), and poorer results are expected if there are other injuries such as fracture or nerve transection. The most common complication is adhesion, causing stiffness that may lead to flexion contractures unless discovered early and the protocol modified.

- **5% rupture rate** (more with FPL repair) – most commonly on post-operative days 7–10 but can be as late as 6 weeks. Patient education is vital as rupture commonly follows inadvertent strong gripping/lifting. Acute ruptures should be explored; MRI or ultrasound may be useful if the diagnosis is uncertain.
  - Starting active motion rehabilitation later than day 5 increases the risk of rupture. Between 5 and 21 days, the repair strength is dependent on the suture.
- **Adhesions causing pain and stiffness** may be more common after
  - Trauma to tendon or sheath, e.g. crush injuries or poor intraoperative handling.
  - Prolonged immobilisation.
  - **Tenolysis** is indicated if active flexion is still limited despite normal passive ROM >3 months after. Timing and indications are individualised; it depends on age, pain tolerance, motivation and occupational needs. Although there is no consensus, it is best to wait at least 6 months before embarking on surgical tenolysis, after a full course of hand therapy to **maximise passive ROM** and to allow maturation of soft tissue.
    - Requires wide exposure.
    - Although the dissection can be quite difficult, an effort must be made to free ALL adhesions; some can be quite distant from the site of injury. ADCON-L® (absorbable porcine gelatin and glycosaminoglycan) gel may inhibit further adhesion formation. Steroids do not help. Extensor tendon tenolysis is usually easier but may need to plan for elective skin cover. Balloon 'angioplasty' technique to expand pulleys has been described.

- Pulley reconstruction may be needed – two-stage reconstruction should be considered.
- Early post-operative mobilisation is essential and a brachial plexus block may help. The tenolysed tendon is weak and **may rupture** (8%) at up to 2 months post-operation; it is important to avoid resisted movement.
- Failed tenolysis (no improvement in up to 1/3, worse in 8%) – consider two-stage tendon grafting, arthrodesis or amputation.
- **Contractures**. Flexion contractures occur in up to 17% of flexor tendon repairs. Severe cases require release with or without capsulotomy.
- **Injury to NVB and other tourniquet-related injuries.**
- **Infection is rare** – the role of prophylactic antibiotics is unclear; irrigation and debridement are most important.
- **Reflex sympathetic dystrophy/CRPS** (see below).
- **Excessive shortening with quadrigia effect.**

The effect of partial excision of the A2 and A4 pulleys on the biomechanics of finger flexion. (Tomaino M, *J Hand Surg*, 1998)
Disruption/loss of the A2 and A4 pulleys will weaken the grip and reduce the function.

This fresh-cadaver study quantified angular rotation at finger joints and the energy required for digital flexion. **Venting** pulleys facilities repair in zones 1 and 2 and reduces tendon impingement on intact pulleys without significant functional sequelae. Venting may be performed without compromising the pulley function up to

- 25% A2 pulleys alone (greatest effect at the DIPJ)
- 75% A4 pulley alone
- 25% of the A2 and 25% of the A4 pulleys (greatest effect at the MCPJ)

A2 and A4 pulleys may need reconstruction:

- Encircling graft of the extensor retinaculum of the wrist (Lister)
- Encircling tendon graft (two to four wraps if possible)
- Tail of superficialis

An evidence-based approach to flexor tendon laceration repair. (Lalonde DH, *Plast Reconstr Surg*, 2011)
This literature review had some useful conclusions:

- There is still no consensus on what to do with the superficialis tendon in zone 2; at best, there is level V evidence. Some suggest repairing both but adhesions may increase, though total active movement (TAM) achieved was no different; others suggest repairing only one slip of the FDS.
- There is a move towards more strands in the core suture, though there is no high-level evidence to justify this.
  - A six-strand Lim/Tsai repair obtained better TAM and grip strength results compared to a two-strand Kessler, but the former group also had additional place-and-hold in the rehabilitation regime (Hoffman GL, *J Hand Eur Vol*, 2008).

- The use of topical agents, e.g. ADCON-T/N or 5-FU, is still largely experimental.
- Cochrane review (Thien TB, *Cochrane Database Syst Rev*, 2004) found insufficient evidence to define the best rehabilitation regime, but there was a trend towards early active movement protocols (level II evidence).

FLEXOR TENDON GRAFTING

The indications for tendon grafting as opposed to primary repair include the following:

- Primary repair not possible, e.g. tendon loss or muscle contracture
- Failed primary repair
- Need for good soft tissue cover over potential repair site

However, the following must be satisfied:

- Full range of passive movement with stable joints
- Hospitable tissue planes and sensate soft tissue cover
- Patient compliance with surgery and rehabilitation

TENDON GRAFTING IN ZONE 2

A one-stage procedure is suitable for selected cases such as tendon avulsion injury with good soft tissue cover and tendon sheath and pulleys are preserved. There are a variety of autologous graft options (see Table 6.2); tendon allografts are available but less commonly used.

- Suture distally first:
  - To the FDP stump
  - Into the bone (Bunnell)
  - To the pulp/nail bed (Pulvertaft)
- Connect proximally after checking appropriate tension by tenodesis effect and matching up the cascade.
  - **Pulvertaft weave**.
    - The ends can be woven into each other for extra strength due to the extra length available. **Guy Pulvertaft** (1907–1986) was a renowned hand surgeon who was an inaugural member of the Hand Club
  - **Bunnell criss-cross.**
    - Sterling Bunnell (1882–1957) was an American general surgeon with great expertise in hand reconstruction. He played a lead role in Army hand surgery during World War II.
- Kessler suture.

Table 6.2 Sources of autologous tendon grafts

Source	Length cm
Palmaris longus (PL)	13–16
Plantaris (found anterior and medial to Achilles tendon)	31–35
Extensor digiti minimi	16
Extensor indicis proprius	13
Toe extensor (usually second)	30–35

COMPLICATIONS

- **Tendon adhesion** is the most common complication.
- **Rupture of graft**.
- **Quadriga effect** limiting full flexion:
  - This results because the FDP has a common belly for each tendon. Thus, if one tendon is tethered distally (e.g. to an amputation stump through adhesions or sutured to FDS, or over-advance when repairing or using a graft that is too short), then the ability of the other tendons to achieve full flexion is affected, i.e. an **active flexion deficit in uninjured fingers**, whilst there is still a normal passive ROM.
  - It leads to a weak grasp.
- **Lumbrical plus** if the tendon graft is too long.
  - It represents the opposite of quadriga. If the FDP tendon is left too loose, it acts via its lumbrical insertion, causing MCPJ flexion and IPJ extension. Thus, there is **paradoxical PIPJ extension with attempted finger flexion**, and an intrinsic plus position. It may also occur if the FDP is lacerated distal to the lumbrical origin.
  - Treat by dividing the lumbrical.

Two-stage repair is indicated for

- Loss/damage to sheath and pulleys
- Late tendon reconstruction
- Accompanying fracture or overlying skin loss
- Nerve injury requiring nerve grafting

  Stage 1 – excise old tendon remnants, reconstruct pulley and insert Hunter (silicone) rod, which is fixed distally only.

  Stage 2 – (at least 6 months later, though a pseudosheath is evident by 8 weeks): harvest and insert tendon graft to replace the silicone rod – fix the distal part first before pushing through the pseudosheath for the proximal repair, e.g. Pulvertaft weave for zone III or V. Slight over-correction of the normal cascade is aimed for.

The choice of repair depends in part on whether the FDS is intact, which digit is involved and patient factors (occupation, compliance, etc.).

- Thumb with FPL loss (Mannerfelt lesion) – arthrodese the IPJ (usually does well) and reconstruct FPL with a two-stage tendon graft. Follow with FDS transfer from the ring finger.
- Digit with loss of both FDS and FDP – two-stage FDP graft.
- Digit with FDS intact – most patients benefit from DIPJ arthrodesis. Other options include tenodesis of a long distal end to FDS or FDP reconstruction. The latter can be considered particularly in children and young patients; Sakellarides (*J Hand Surg*, 1996;21:63) found improved pinch and improved power.

COMPLICATIONS

- Intra-operative – neurovascular injury
- Early
  - Synovitis, infection and buckling of the implant
  - Implant extrusion or migration
  - Pulley breakdown
  - Skin flap necrosis
- Late
  - Chronic flexion deformity
  - Complex regional pain syndrome (CRPS) type 1

IV. EXTENSOR TENDON INJURY

VERDAN'S ZONES

- Odd numbers overlie joints starting at zone 1 – DIPJ. Injuries in these zones tend to be more difficult to treat.
  - Zone III is the most complex.
- Even numbers overlie intervening segments finishing at zone 8 – distal forearm.

WRIST COMPARTMENTS

There are six synovial-lined compartments at the extensor surface of the wrist. Over the wrist, the tendons are separated into six compartments; the individual extensor tendons are divided into several longitudinal zones. The extensor tendons are not uncommonly injured, being superficial and covered by thin skin.

1 Abductor pollicis longus (APL; multiple strips to the base of the thumb metacarpal). Extensor pollicis brevis (EPB) – the base of the thumb PP.
2 ECRL – the base of the index metacarpal. ECRB – the base of the middle metacarpal.
3 EPL – the base of the thumb DP.
4 Extensor digitorum communis (EDC) – occasionally has two slips to the ring finger; 56% have no slip to the little finger. Extensor indicis (EI) – is ulnar to EDC.
5 Extensor digiti minimi (EDM) – there are two slips in 80%; also ulnar to EDC – both EI and EDM have no juncture.
6 Extensor carpi ulnaris (ECU).

Extensor digitorum brevis manus is an anomalous muscle found in approximately 3% (bilateral in 1/3 of these) that may cause pain and a mass between the finger extensors especially at the fourth compartment at the wrist (often misdiagnosed as a ganglion/tumour). It has variable origins from the dorsum of the radial wrist and inserts into the extensor apparatus of the fingers. It can be diagnosed preoperatively by MRI or ultrasound, and can be excised without functional deficit (although in some cases, it can be the only independent index extensor in the absence of EIP).

Extensor tendon: Anatomy, injury, and reconstruction. (Rockwell WB, *Plast Reconstr Surg*, 2000)

The anatomy and function of the extensor mechanism of the hand are more complex than the flexors. The **extensor apparatus is a linkage system** created by

- RN-innervated extrinsic system
- Ulnar nerve and median nerve-innervated intrinsic system

These interconnecting components **can compensate** for certain deficits in function.

- IPJ extension occurs due to intrinsic action when the MCPJ is in extension.
- IPJ extension is due to extrinsic action when the MCPJ is flexed.

EXTRINSIC TENDONS

The muscle bellies of the extrinsic extensors arise in the forearm and enter the hand through six compartments formed by the extensor retinaculum, a fibrous band that prevents bowstringing of the tendons (see above). **The extrinsics act mostly at the MCPJ**.

- At the wrist, the tendons are covered by a synovial sheath, but not over the dorsal hand or fingers.
- At the wrist, the extensor tendons are rounder and have sufficient bulk to hold a suture; in contrast, the thin and flat tendons over the dorsum do not hold sutures well.

The four EDC tendons originate from a common muscle belly and have limited independent action. In contrast, the extensor indicis proprius (EIP) and EDM have independent muscle bellies and are common donor tendons for transfer; they are usually ulnar ('horn hand') and deep to the EDC at the level of the MCPJ.

- The EDC to the little finger is present <50% of the time, and when absent, it is almost always replaced by a juncturae tendinae from the ring finger to the extensor apparatus of the little finger.
- A variety of mechanisms keep the tendons centralised over the MCPJ.
- The **extrinsic extensor tendons** contribute the **central slip** to the extensor mechanism; they also contribute the lateral bands that join the lateral slips from the intrinsics to make the conjoint lateral band, over the distal MP. They extend:
  - The MCPJ primarily
  - The IPJ secondarily
- The extrinsic extensor tendons have **four insertions**. At the MCPJ level, they are held in place by the intrinsic tendons and the sagittal band that arises from the palmar plate and the deep intermetacarpal ligament. At the PIPJ, the transverse retinacular ligament (TRL) maintains the position of the extensor mechanism and limits its dorsal–palmar excursion (Figure 6.5).

- A tenuous insertion on the PP and strong insertions on the middle and distal phalanges.
- Over the distal portion of the PP, the central slip trifurcates as the central slip and lateral bands (sharing fibres).
  - The **central slip** inserts on the base of the MP.
  - The **lateral band** component continues to insert on the base of the DP.

INTRINSIC MUSCLES

The intrinsic muscles

- Flex the MCPJ
- Extend the proximal and distal IPJ

The **intrinsic tendons** are composed of

- Three palmar **interossei** (adductors, PAD) and four dorsal interossei (abductors, DAB) that originate from the sides of the metacarpals and run distally on both sides of the fingers except the ulnar side of the little finger. The tendons enter the finger dorsal to the intermetacarpal ligament. The tendons split into two – the superficial slip inserts onto the PP, whilst the deep tendon becomes part of the lateral slip.
- Four **lumbrical** muscles arise from the radial side of the FDP tendon and pass palmar to the intermetacarpal ligament.

The intrinsic tendons join to form the **lateral slips** (that join the lateral bands to form the conjoint lateral bands); the bands join the extrinsic extensor mechanism proximal to the middle of the PP and then continue distally dorsal to the axes of the IPJs. Distal to the PIPJ, the conjoint lateral bands fuse to form a conjoint tendon that inserts into the base of the DP.

Other important structures are as follows:

- The **sagittal bands** are transverse ligamentous structures passing from the extensor tendon to the MCPJ volar plate – they **centralise** the extensor tendon over the metacarpal head at the MCPJ as contraction of the extensor muscle pulls on the PP to flex the MCPJ. They roll proximally and distally with MCPJ extension and flexion, respectively, somewhat like the visor on a motorcycle helmet. Laceration to one side of the sagittal bands causes subluxation of the extensor tendon to the other side.
- The **intermetacarpal ligament** separates the lumbrical tendons that are palmar from the interossei tendons that are dorsal.
- The **transverse retinacular ligament** stabilises the extensor tendon at the PIPJ. It arises from the volar aspect of the flexor sheath and PP to inset into the lateral bands and triangular ligament dorsal to the PIPJ axis.
- The **oblique retinacular ligament** (ORL; Landsmeer) is a component of the linkage system that helps to stabilise the lateral bands and is said to coordinate

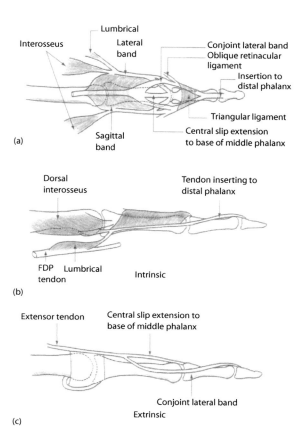

Figure 6.5 Diagram of the extensor mechanism (a) with intrinsic (b) and extrinsic (c) components isolated for clarity.

flexion and extension in the finger joints. The ligament arises from the proximal PP and the A2 pulley and inserts into the conjoint lateral band; it spirals to pass volar to the axis of the PIPJ and dorsal to the axis at the DIPJ. It is shortened in Boutonniere deformities and is said to be a reason why you cannot voluntarily flex the DIPJ with the PIPJ extended.

- The **triangular ligament** connects the conjoint lateral bands over the dorsum of the MP, keeping them in close proximity and preventing them from shifting volarly and so become an IPJ flexor.

The **excursion of the extensor tendons over the finger is less** than the flexor tendons; excursion may vary from 2 to 8 mm at the PIPJ.

- The preservation of relative tendon length between the central slip and lateral bands is important, and disturbance causes deformities that are progressive, making restoration of normal balance difficult.
- Overlapping **linkage systems** also contribute to this balance; the components of the linkage system pass palmar to one joint and dorsal to the next:
    - The intrinsic tendons create the linkage at the MCPJ and PIPJ.
    - The ORL function at the PIPJ and DIPJ.

- Thus, **deformity at one joint may cause a reciprocal deformity at an adjacent joint.**

GENERAL PRINCIPLES

The structure and interconnections of extensor tendons mean that they tend not to retract. Loss of tendon continuity will lead to extensor lag but may be disguised by juncturae.

- Repair with interrupted over-over sutures (Prolene® or Ticron®) in zones 1–6 and Kessler/core suture in zones 7 and 8. Independent tendons, e.g. EPL, may retract quickly and should be repaired early.
- Gutter splint for injuries in zones 2–4, outrigger for zones 5–8 injuries plus night gutter splint.
- If there is loss of tendon tissue, then either graft if adequate skin cover or reconstruct with a distally based tendon flap.
- Central slip rupture/loss – reconstruct with medial portions of lateral bands.
- Repair sagittal band injuries in zones 4/5; otherwise, tendon will sublux into the metacarpal gutter on the intact side.
- Partial lacerations proximal to the MCPJ may not need open repair due to the intertendinous connections.

ZONE I INJURIES (MALLET FINGER)

This deformity is due to forced flexion of the extended digit that leads to disruption of continuity of the extensor tendon over the DIPJ; it can be open or closed. If left untreated, hyperextension of the PIPJ (**swan neck deformity**) may also develop because of proximal retraction of the central band. It has been postulated that there is a zone of relatively poor vascularity at the site of mallet ruptures.

Doyle Classification. (Doyle JR, *Operative Hand Surgery*, 3rd Edn, 1993)

- Type 1 – closed, with or without small avulsion fracture. This is the most common.
- Type 2 – open laceration at or proximal to the DIPJ with loss of tendon continuity.
- Type 3 – open, deep laceration with loss of skin, subcutaneous cover and tendon substance.
- Type 4 – avulsion fractures, mostly treated with splintage unless there is significant subluxation of the fragment.
  - A – transepiphyseal plate fracture in children
  - B – fracture involving 20%–50% of the articular surface (hyperflexion)
  - C – hyperextension injury with fracture >50% of the articular surface, with early or late volar subluxation of the DP.

MANAGEMENT

The management of the mallet finger is still a topic for debate. In the vast majority of cases, splinting alone is sufficient as the tendons do not retract much. Operative treatment of a mallet injury can be demanding and may **downgrade active flexion**, so it is preferable to treat conservatively if possible – the primary indications for surgery are large fragments that are rotated or persistent DIPJ subluxation.

- The **PIPJ is of utmost importance, and it should be kept active**/free to move to avoid a boutonnière deformity.
- Neglecting a mallet finger injury will lead to DIPJ dysfunction – 1 mm lengthening will cause 25° extension lag (Schweitzer TP, *J Hand Surg Am*, 2004).

- A Cochrane review (Handoll HHG, *Cochrane Database Syst Rev*, 2004) showed little evidence of any difference between the various types of splints used (standard Stack, custom made, Zimmer padded, etc.), though they did recommend that splints be hardy enough to tolerate daily use and be easy to use; proper fit is essential (avoid skin blanching).
- Perforated splints may be better tolerated than solid stack splints (Kinninmonth AW, *J Hand Surg Br*, 1986).

TYPE 1 (MOST COMMON)

- **Stack splint – continuous full time** (i.e. 24 hours a day, even when washing [Figure 6.6]) splinting of the DIPJ in extension (some propose slight hyperextension but no more than 5°, avoid skin blanching and inspect skin regularly) for 6 weeks, followed by 2 weeks of night splinting unless there is an occupational need for early return to work or poor patient compliance, in which case consider a buried K-wire. Poor skin condition is also an indication for K-wiring instead of splintage.
  - 6 weeks needs to be restarted if the patient inadvertently flexes the finger.
  - Although splintage is still considered for <6 months after the injury and will give good results in the majority, it is said to be less effective if initiated >3 months after.
  - For chronic injuries/failed splintage, then tenodermodesis (Iselin F, *J Hand Surg Am*, 1977) may be considered. An ellipse of skin and scar is excised to produce full extension, which is supported by K-wires.

OTHER TYPES

- **Type 2**
  - Suture of tendon (simple figure-of-eight suture) and skin either separately or together (roll-type suture; tenodermodesis/dermatotenodesis).
  - Stack splint 6 weeks.

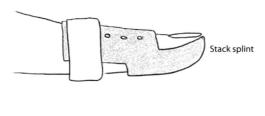

Stack splint

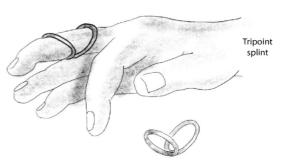

Tripoint splint

Figure 6.6 Finger splints. Stack splint for mallet finger. Tripoint splint for swan-neck deformity.

- **Type 3**
  - Primary tendon reconstruction with immediate soft tissue coverage (distally based EDC flap) plus oblique K-wire to DIPJ or
  - Secondary tendon reconstruction with tendon graft.
- **Type 4**
  - A – the extensor mechanism is attached to the basal epiphysis, so closed reduction (MUSA) results in correction of the deformity, followed by a Stack splint for 4 weeks.
  - B–C (fracture of DP base >25% of the articular surface) – open or closed reduction and K-wiring of the DIPJ, maintaining reduction with the pull-out suture over button on pulp; miniscrew fixation.

OTHER OPTIONS

- Arthrodesis – comminuted intra-articular fracture, elderly
- Amputation – severe soft tissue injury, devascularisation

Zone 2 injury (MP) – if <50% of the tendon width is cut, routine wound care and splinting for 7 to 10 days can be followed by active motion. Injuries involving >50% (or tender swollen dorsal capsule with slight extension lag at the PIPJ) should be repaired primarily and splinted in extension for 6–8 weeks.

Zone 3 injury – open or closed, with or without avulsion

- The **boutonnière deformity** is caused by disruption of the central slip at the PIPJ, which results in loss of extension at the PIPJ (often, weak PIPJ flexion is still possible with intact lateral bands) and hyperextension at the DIPJ.
- **The deformity usually appears 10–14 days** after the initial injury, especially after closed rupture as the TRLs stretch and the lateral bands move anterior to the PIPJ axis, becoming a PIPJ flexor and DIPJ hyperextensor. The initial treatment for closed injury should be splinting with the PIPJ in extension. The surgical indications for a closed boutonnière deformity are as follows:
  - Displaced avulsion fracture at the base of the MP.
  - Instability of the PIPJ associated with loss of active or passive extension of the joint.
  - Failed non-operative treatment.
  - Tendon can be repaired with simple mattress.

THREE STAGES OF BOUTONNIÈRE DEFORMITY HAVE BEEN DESCRIBED:

- **Stage 1** – the finger is supple and passive extension at the PIPJ corrects the deformity. It may be treated by splinting the PIPJ in extension with the DIPJ free to flex actively; this allows dorsal migration of the lateral bands to re-establish the normal relationship.
- **Stage 2** – passive extension at the PIPJ is still possible, but the deformity does not correct, implying that the volar TRL is shortened holding the lateral bands adherent to the volar aspect of the joint, whilst the triangular ligaments that normally hold the lateral bands dorsal are stretched.
- **Stage 3** – involves secondary joint changes at the PIPJ.

TESTS FOR TRAUMATIC BOUTONNIERE

- **Elson** – with the finger over the edge of the table and the PIPJ flexed to 90%, the patient is asked to extend the PIPJ against resistance; weakness of this with DIPJ hyperextension (due to lateral band recruitment) suggests **central slip rupture** and can be performed in the acute situation.
- **Passive** – flex wrist and MCPJ; poor passive resistance to pressure over the MP suggests weak extensor mechanism.
- **Boyes** – with the PIPJ held passively in extension, the patient should be able to flex the DIPJ unless the central slip has ruptured.

Zone 4 injuries usually involve the broad extensor mechanism but are usually partial, sparing the lateral bands, so that splinting the PIPJ in extension for 3–4 weeks is equivalent to repair. However, for complete lacerations, primary repair should be performed.

- Open sagittal band lacerations should be repaired to prevent extensor tendon subluxation.
- Closed sagittal band injury is suggested by pain with inability to extend the MCPJ actively, though the patient can hold the finger extended if positioned passively. There is subluxation of the extensor tendon. Acute cases presenting within 2 weeks can be treated with splintage of the MCPJ in extension for 6 weeks whilst older injuries need repair.

Zone 5 injury (MCPJ) – injuries over the MCPJ are almost always open**; human bites,** for example due to a punch injury, need an X-ray to exclude foreign bodies including fragments of teeth. In a 'fight bite', the joint is in flexion at the time, so the actual tendon injury will be proximal to the level of the overlying skin wound when the hand is flat. Primary tendon repair (Kessler core suture or similar) is indicated after thorough irrigation; broad spectrum antibiotics are often given. Splint for 3–4 weeks, but some begin early active motion.

Zone 6 injuries (dorsum of hand) – such injuries may be masked by adjacent extensor tendons through the juncturae tendinae, and the diagnosis would only be made at exploration. In this zone, the tendons are thicker and more oval, so repair should be performed with stronger, core-type sutures. Juncturae are found on the ulnar fingers, acting mostly to limit independent extension.

Zone 7 injuries (wrist) – partial release of the retinaculum is required in most cases to gain exposure to the lacerated tendons, which tend to retract significantly. Part of the retinaculum should be preserved to prevent extensor bowstringing.

Zone 8 injuries (forearm) – often multiple tendons may be injured, potentially making it difficult to identify individual units correctly. With injuries at the musculo-tendinous junction, the fibrous septa tend to retract into the substance of the muscles hindering repair.

DYNAMIC SPLINTING FOR EXTENSOR INJURIES

Post-operatively, the involved joints are kept in extension, with the wrist in 45° extension and the MCPJ in slight hyperextension. Injuries to zone 5 and above do not need splinting, whilst joints distal to the MCPJ do. It can take several months for extensor tendons to recover to full strength.

There are a variety of rehabilitation protocols – most propose 3–4 weeks of rest followed by active controlled motion. Early controlled motion with a dynamic extensor splint has been found to decrease adhesions and subsequent contractures, especially with more proximal injuries.

THUMB EXTENSOR TENDONS

The extensor mechanism of the thumb is different from that of the fingers.

- Each joint has an independent tendon for extension – the EPL extends the IPJ, the EPB extends the MCPJ and the APL extends the carpometacarpal joint (CMCJ).
- The APL almost always has multiple tendon slips, whereas EPB usually has one.

The intrinsic muscles of the thumb primarily provide rotational control whilst also contributing to MCPJ flexion and IPJ extension.

- On the radial side, the APB tendon continues to insert on the EPL.
- On the ulnar side, fibres of the adductor pollicis also insert on the EPL.
  - Thus, these two muscles can extend the IPJ to neutral, significantly **masking an EPL laceration**.

THUMB EXTENSOR INJURIES

The terminal extensor tendon of the thumb is much thicker; therefore, mallet thumbs are rare (closed – splint for 6 weeks; open – repair and splint).

- Zone 3 – repair EPL and EPB and splint for 3 weeks.
- In zones 6 and 7, the APL retracts significantly when divided and usually requires first compartment release for successful repair.

V. REPLANTATION AND RING AVULSION

REPLANTATION

Replantation of parts offers a result that is usually superior to any other type of reconstruction. There are pros and cons to replantation. A thorough assessment of the patient and their injury is needed to ensure that the right choice is being made. The overall success rate is 80%, but a viable replant does not equate to a valuable digit.

The first successful replantation of a severed limb was undertaken by Malt RA in Boston in 1964 (replanted the arm of a 12-year-old boy, Everett Knowles, who despite needing additional surgeries regained the use of his arm enough to drive trucks); revascularisation of incompletely severed digits was performed by Kleinert and Kasdan in 1965. The first successful digital replantation was performed by Komatsu and Tamai in Japan in 1968.

- Ronald Malt (1931–2002) was the chief surgical resident at MGH when he and his colleagues performed the replant. He was once arrested in China for inadvertently photographing a military facility.

ANATOMY OF DIGITAL ARTERIES

Dominant supply:

- Ulnar digital artery – thumb, index, middle finger (radial digits)
- Radial digital artery – ring finger, little finger (ulnar digits)

The **ulnar artery** gives rise to the **superficial palmar arch**, which gives off all the digital arteries. The radial artery gives rise to deep palmar arch about 1 cm proximal to the superficial arch and palmar to the flexors. There are some anastomoses over the dorsal carpal arch.

- In the palm, arteries are volar/palmar to nerves (P-A-N).
- In the digits, arteries are dorsal to nerves (D-A-N).

RELEVANT HISTORY AND EXAMINATION

General

- Age, occupation, hand dominance, hobbies
- Pre-existing hand problems
- General health including drugs, alcohol and smoking.
- Tetanus status

GENERAL PRINCIPLES

Specific

- **Mechanism of injury – sharp amputations** do better than avulsions or crush injuries. **Avulsions** are suggested by the red streak sign along the lateral aspect of the digit or coiled/'corkscrew' vessels – arteries (unlike nerve and tendons, which tend to remain as long dangly segments) tend to break off quite proximally and grafts are often needed (see below). Electron microscopy has shown damage up to 4 cm from the transection site compared to 1 cm when examined under a light microscope.

- Artery grafts can be harvested from the posterior interosseous or subscapular vessels. Arterial grafts may be needed for
  - Long revascularisations (e.g. thumb replants are best revascularised using grafts where necessary, to the radial artery).
  - Significant size discrepancy between proximal and distal ends.
- **Ischaemic time** – ideally under 6 hours for a digit; cold ischaemia >24 hours or warm ischaemia time of >12 hours is usually not salvageable, though cases have been described of up to 33 hours warm and 94 hours cold ischaemia.
  - In more proximal amputations, the ischaemic tolerance is significantly shorter due to the sensitivity of muscle to ischaemia – irreversible histological changes have been seen after 2.5 hours tourniquet time. Forearm amputations have a maximal tolerable warm ischaemia time of 4–6 hours.
  - The part should be wrapped in saline gauze after gentle cleansing, then placed in a plastic bag on ice for transport; the digit should not be placed directly on ice. Marginal benefit has been demonstrated with specialised storage solutions such as the University of Wisconsin solution.
- Full examination to identify other pathologies, e.g. crush injuries more proximally. X-ray the hand and the amputated part.

INDICATIONS

- **The thumb** is almost always replanted; it contributes 40% of hand function according to most analyses. Replantation probably offers the best functional return even with poor motion and sensation; the thumb will still be useful to the patient as a post for opposition. The larger vessels and nerves mean that the surgical results are generally better even if IPJ fusion is sometimes needed. With more distal amputations or unsuitable stumps, alternatives include
  - **Phalangisation** of metacarpal by deepening web space (which still tends to be short and has poor cosmesis).
  - **Distraction** of phalanx or metacarpal (long overall process) or both.
  - **Toe-to-thumb transfers** in amputations at the level of the MCPJ (potential problems with cosmesis and donor deficit).
  - **Pollicisation** of the index finger.
  - See 'Thumb reconstruction'.
- Replantation should be attempted with **almost any part in a child** including replantation and revascularisation of the foot or lower leg.
- **Multiple digits amputations** present reconstructive difficulties that may be difficult to correct without replantation of one or all of the amputated digits. Chinese surgeons in particular push the limits with multisegment multidigit replantations.

- **The finger with the highest chance of success is replanted first**, and not necessarily to the original finger, e.g. with MF and IF amputations; if the MF is not salvageable, then the IF can be replanted onto the MF stump to avoid a gap in the rays.
- **Partial or whole hand**. Any hand amputation offers the chance of reasonable function after replantation, and is usually superior to available prostheses.

ABSOLUTE CONTRAINDICATIONS

- Life-threatening concomitant injuries
- Multi-level injury
- Severe premorbid chronic illness

RELATIVE CONTRAINDICATIONS

- The wisdom of **single digit replants in adults** is open to debate; there is functionally little to gain, though most will tend to replant if conditions are favourable.
  - **PP replantation**, proximal to the PIPJ – even with good viability, has a **high risk of poor movement** and results due to adhesions in zone 2. With a functional thumb, a replanted index is often 'ignored', and the patient automatically 'replaces' the index with the middle finger. To allow early motion, the joints should not be transfixed except in cases of PIPJ injury in which case the joints should be arthrodesed 20°, 30°, 40° and 50° from the index to the little finger. Those that share a common tendon (III–V) may interfere with the other tendons.
  - **Through MP**, distal to FDS (zone 1), replantation has good motion and sensory return.
    - Single digit proximal to FDS insertion may impact on the remaining digits.
  - **DP replants** – may have problems with finding adequate veins, but if they survive, have a good outcome. Technical difficulty with venous repair increases distal to an arbitrary line 4 mm proximal to the nail fold. A systematic review by Sebastin (*Plast Reconstr Surg*, 2011) found that high success rates and good functional outcomes were possible with distal amputations.
  - **Other specific considerations** – children, thumbs, young women, cosmetic or specific occupational needs, e.g. musicians, certain cultures, e.g. Japanese, where missing digits may be regarded as a stigmata of criminals. Chinese culture in particular values an 'intact' body.
- Parts of fingers that have been completely **degloved; avulsion** of tendons, nerves and vessels. Extreme **contamination** or widespread **crush**.
- **Lengthy warm ischaemia time**. For major limb replants, reperfusion shunts/temporary anastomosis can be used.
- **Elderly** with micro-arterial disease (poor tendon/ nerve recovery expected – in the very young, the small vessels are prone to vasospasm, though this is not a contraindication per se).

- **Heavy smokers**.
- **Patients with severe systemic disease or trauma, severe mental disease** – self-harm/psychosis, intractable substance abuse, unwilling/uncooperative.
- **Although usually indicated, the replantation of any hand or arm proximal to the level of the mid-forearm must be carefully considered**. The risk of complications increases, and the chance of functional return decreases with amputations above the elbow.
- The corollary is that **non-thumb injuries, those proximal to the FDS insertion or due to avulsion, generally do not do well**.

SURGICAL SEQUENCE

Patients should be stabilised and concomitant life-threatening injury excluded/managed. Consent for graft harvest (vessels, tendon and skin) and terminalisation should be specifically sought.

- **General anaesthesia**; a brachial plexus or axillary block may provide useful vasodilatation and post-operative analgesia.
- **Examination of the part** in the operating room before/whilst the patient is anaesthetised allows time for appropriate decision-making. Vessels must be examined under the **microscope**; if in doubt, cut back to 'normal'-looking vessel as it is better to use grafts than unhealthy vessels. Suitable nerves and vessels need to be tagged with fine sutures. The 'spurt test' can be used roughly assess pressure in stump.
  - Corkscrew appearance suggests avulsion/traction.
  - 'Red line sign' bruising along the course of the digit where the NVB runs suggests a severe avulsion injury with disruption of side branches of the digital artery.
  - A 'cobweb' sign describes the appearance with multiple laceration-like patterns on the vessel wall.
  - Measles sign – pinpoint petechiae along the vessel adventitia after anastomosis due to micro thrombosis.
- **Stabilise bones** (K-wires, wires, etc.); first, shortening may be needed (maximum 5–10 mm) and should be anticipated particularly for more proximal injuries; slight shortening may be beneficial to reduce tension.
- **Repair extensor tendons first**, then muscles if any, then flexor tendons. The A2 and A4 pulleys should be kept intact/repaired.
- **Coapt nerves**, using grafts if needed; alternatively use conduits or vein grafts.
- **Anastomose two veins per artery and two arteries per digit** if possible, though one good artery is enough. When ischaemia has been prolonged (>2 hours), arteries can be repaired first to reduce reperfusion injury particularly for more proximal injuries, then (dorsal) veins will fill up and can be spotted more easily and allow metabolites to be flushed out. Beware of reperfusion; more proximal replants particularly involving muscle should have **prophylactic fasciotomies**, along with release of the nerve tunnel and intrinsic compartments. Monitor for hyperkalaemia and myoglobinuria.
  - Vein grafts can be harvested from the dorsum of the hand, other limbs. The proximal anastomosis is usually performed first; the second anastomosis can be performed with blood in the graft or flushed out with heparin–saline.
  - 80% of failed replants fail due to a venous problem.
  - With DP replants, veins may not always be available in which case venous bleeding can be encouraged by leeches, nail bed bleeding etc.
- **Cover with soft tissue but avoid overtight skin closure** as it may lead to venous compression. Some skin overlying the vein graft may be taken with the vein graft as a small flow-through venous flap.

DRUGS

- **Aspirin** – acetylates cyclooxygenase to reduce arachidonic acids, thromboxanes and prostaglandins to reduce platelet aggregation and vasoconstriction.
- **Dextran 40** – a polysaccharide. Some suggest a test dose due to risk of allergies including anaphylaxis, but this is not often performed. It has antiplatelet (negative charge decreases platelet activation and inactivates vWF) and antifibrin functions, and also provides volume expansion.
- **Heparin** – activates serum antithrombotic III and lowers blood viscosity. Systemic heparin is not absolutely necessary; heparin-soaked pledgets can be used on the nail bed after nail plate removal ('chemical leech'), if the venous repair is tenuous.

REPLANTATION (PEDERSON WC, *PLAST RECONSTR SURG*, 2001)

Post-operative care

- Splint in a position of function and elevate the limb.
- Monitor perfusion – capillary refill, temperature and turgor. Others include Doppler signal, transcutaneous oxygen, temperature probes and fluorimetry.
- Avoid vasoconstrictors including caffeine and nicotine; control pain well.
  - Keep the patient warm, wet (hydrated) and well (pain free).
  - Consider drugs (see above) also.
  - Antibiotics, e.g. first-generation cephalosporin.
  - Axillary infusion of marcaine may be given to provide both pain relief and a chemical sympathectomy.
  - Chlorpromazine orally (25 mg 8 hourly) is a potent peripheral vasodilator and sedative.

WHITE FINGER POST-REPLANTATION

- Ensure that the patient is warm, wet and well.
- Loosen dressings and remove sutures as needed.
- Re-explore.

BLUE FINGER POST-REPLANTATION

- Elevate the limb.
- Loosen dressings (remove the venous tourniquet) and remove sutures.
- Encourage venous bleeding, e.g. leeches, fish-mouth incision in the nail bed or heparin injections/soaks ('chemical leech').
- Re-explore.

FUNCTIONAL OUTCOMES

Overall success with guillotine-type amputation is 77% compared with 49% in crush injuries.

- 70% achieve <15 mm 2pd.
- 50% achieve TAM, 50% grip strength.
- Poor movement may be due to stiffness. With flexor tenolysis, TAM can improve by 43%.
- Zone I – regain 82° of motion at the PIPJ vs. 35° in zone II.

COMPLICATIONS

- Secondary amputation.
- **60% require secondary surgery** especially replants proximal to the FDS (93%) vs. 11% of thumb replants.
- **Stiffness** due to tendon adhesions and joint contracture.
- 22% require open reduction and internal fixation (ORIF) for non-union.
- Cold intolerance that improves over 3 years (at least 2 years, possibly life-long).
- CRPS, chronic pain.

The PNB classification for treatment of fingertip injuries. (Muneuchi G, *Ann Plast Surg*, 2005)

PULP, NAIL, BONE (PNB) CLASSIFICATION

- Zone I – distal to lunula. Volar veins can be used for repair; otherwise, consider arteriovenous (AV) shunting, nail-bed bleed, leech/heparin 'chemical leech'.
- Zone II – DIPJ to lunula. Digital arteries and dorsal veins can be used.

Other commonly used classifications include Tamai, Chung, Hirase and Allen.

AMPUTATIONS/TERMINALISATION

Sometimes the part cannot be reattached, or that it may not be in the patients' best interest to reattach (though they may not know it). Patients are often quite sceptical about the need for bone shortening. Cases must be judged individually; in particular, multiply injured patients should aim to avoid amputation if possible, salvaging as much function as possible from damaged parts. There are well-described

levels for elective amputation; however, in trauma, the basic rule is to save as much length as possible provided there is good soft tissue cover, even if it requires the use of distant flaps.

Patients need to be warned of the following:

- **Unrealistic expectations** of results and recovery time and effort/rehabilitation time/need for revision involved
  - Possible need for vein/nerve/skin grafts and flaps, i.e. additional donor sites/scars.
  - Fasciotomies in proximal amputations may be needed due to tissue swelling.
  - Replanted parts may have poor movement may be due to tendon adhesions, stiff joints, muscle contractures and reduced sensation (average final 2pd is 11 mm).
  - Late complications such as CRPS and cold intolerance are common complaints but may improve by 2 years.
- **Possible need for eventual amputation**

Disbelief (denial) is followed by recognition with turmoil and anxiety, with the final phase being acceptance of the loss.

- Yim (*Plast Reconstr Surg*, 2004) suggested 'primary' toe transfer (within 7 days) in non-transferrable replants.
- Transplants – immunosuppression is the key issue and is generally well tolerated but increases the risk of diabetes, infections and malignancies, whilst the long-term results are unclear; most organ transplants have a half-life of less than 10 years.

VERTICAL AMPUTATIONS

- Radial amputations (thumb/index).
- Ulnar amputations – the little and ring fingers are important parts of the power grasp and require length and good flexion particularly at IPJs.
- Central amputations – ring, middle finger defects can be troublesome; small objects may fall out of the hand, and the gap can be aesthetically unattractive (prostheses may be fitted if there is 12–15 mm beyond the web, or the index may be transposed to replace a middle finger loss).

TRANSVERSE AMPUTATIONS

Middle Phalanx

If the FDS insertion into the base of the MP can be preserved, some function of the PIPJ may be preserved; however, if the tendon insertion is no longer intact, there is little reason to preserve the MP, and disarticulation through the PIPJ may be considered though preservation of length is generally preferred with joint fusion as needed. To fashion an amputation stump, bone may need to be trimmed to allow primary closure with a volar flap.

- Condyles, etc. should be smoothed down with rongeurs, though the need for cartilage removal is no longer absolute as the risk of chondritis is much reduced in modern practice.
- Suturing flexor and extensors together will limit movements and is to be avoided; shortening and tethering of FDP tendons may lead to quadriga effects, meaning the patient cannot properly make a fist.

PROXIMAL PHALANX

These frequently need dorsal skin flaps for closure. **Lasso (Zancolli) procedure:** a flexor tendon (preferably FDS) is kept long enough to pass around the A2 pulley over the proximal PP and then sutured back to itself, adjusting tension to allow full extension of the remnant. Amputations close to the MCPJ or involving metacarpals/carpals may be best treated with a **ray amputation** as stumps and gaps in the fingers may interfere with function, and the overall appearance is better.

MORE PROXIMAL AMPUTATIONS

- **Metacarpal hand** – the thumb is often preserved. Digit reconstruction to provide a post for the thumb may work well but can be rather unattractive and means that a prosthesis (good appearance and reasonable function) cannot be fitted.
- **Arm/forearm** – 90% of ADL can be performed easily with one good hand. Children born without one limb/hand do not experience the same sense of impairment as those who acquire an amputation after establishing functional patterns; often it is the parents who need guidance and support, and prostheses are delayed until the child requests them.
  - With prostheses, it is important to accurately identify and prioritise the needs of the patient and to target these.
- **Elbow/wrist** – length preservation is very important – at least 6–8 cm of forearm with a functioning elbow joint, and the wrist with at least the radial styloid flare; both make very significant differences to the potential function.

PROSTHESES

Prostheses can be active or passive. It is inaccurate to say that one is better than the other; they perform different functions better.

- **Active** – with clamping devices, e.g. shoulder harness/cable arrangement (shrugging shoulders opens the clamp, whilst relaxing allows the clamp to close under elastic forces), or externally powered (slow and lack feedback – thus trial–error movements, bulky and noisy). Modern-powered prostheses are mostly myoelectric – electrodes on the skin pick up activity from underlying muscles, and process and feed them to motors. The feedback is solely visual; patients do not know what the prosthesis is doing when they shut their eyes. When used for above elbow amputations, the prosthesis is likely to be very bulky and heavy, and generally not worthwhile.
- **Passive** prostheses have no mechanical parts but are able to hold light objects such as a wine glass, and are most useful to restore appearance. Partial hand/finger prostheses can enhance function significantly, particularly by acting as a post for other parts to work against; digital prostheses, in particular, can provide some position and pressure sense.

RING AVULSION

Microvascular management of ring avulsion injuries. (Urbaniak JR, *J Hand Surg Am*, 1981)

Urbaniak classification

- Class I – soft tissue injury without vascular compromise, i.e. circulation adequate and best treated by standard techniques.
- Class II – soft tissue injury with vascular compromise, i.e. circulation inadequate and microvascular repair required in addition to soft tissue cover:
  - A – digital arteries only
  - B – arteries plus tendon or bone
  - C – digital veins only
- Class III – complete degloving/amputation, circumferential laceration. Type III injuries are unlikely to regain adequate function, and amputation is usually recommended.

The authors suggest that apart from wishes of the patient for replant in view of need to return to work, complications, etc. (see below), surgeons should consider the status of the amputated part (sharp amputation vs. crush) and the patient (healthy vs. systemic illnesses) and assess the potential for long-term function.

THUMB RECONSTRUCTION

The history should include general health, co-morbidities and willingness of the patient to comply with rehabilitation and tolerate an average of 6–7 months off work. The aim is to improve the function of the hand/limb by replantation compared to simple closure/amputation with or without a prosthesis. At least 1 cm beyond the MCPJ can offer potentially good function.

DISTAL ONE-THIRD

Amputation, i.e. at the level of the IPJ, is compensated fairly well leaving minimal functional impairment. For more distal amputations, and where thumb replantation is

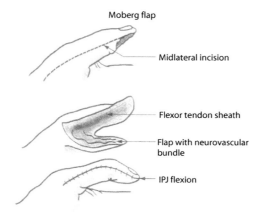

Figure 6.7 The raised volar flap should include both NVBs. Advancement to the tip of the defect requires IPJ flexion.

impossible, there are options for reconstruction. The general aims are as follows:

- Restore skeletal stability
- Provide well-padded sensory soft tissue as coverage

THUMB PULP

Local options are often sufficient.

- Homodigital – **Moberg** volar advancement flap raised at the level of the tendon sheath can resurface pulp defects up to 1.5–2 cm and has good sensation (Figure 6.7). Flexion contracture or stiffness may occur at the IPJ. It can be applied to other digits but is most suited for the thumb with its dual circulation as the flap takes both digital bundles – in digits, the dorsal circulation in these is less reliable.
- Heterodigital.
  - **Cross finger flaps** (Figures 6.8 and 6.9).
  - **Neurovascular flaps – cortical reintegration** may be an issue.
  - **Littler flap**, using the ulnar pad of the middle finger or the radial pad of the ring finger,

which is tunnelled across the palm, i.e. involves significant dissection. Flap transfer usually requires division of the radial digital artery of the ring finger, which becomes solely dependent on the ulnar digital artery; thus, checking with a Doppler or Allens test is advisable. Venous congestion is not uncommon. Problems with cortical reintegration and cold intolerance post-operatively have reduced its use. The donor site requires a skin graft.

- **Kite flap** – first dorsal metacarpal artery flap – a neurovascular flap from the radial artery just distal to the EPL. The donor area needs to be grafted.
- Free pulp transfer (medial aspect of the hallux) can restore a near-normal pulp and nail and offers the best functional results.

MIDDLE THIRD

For amputations involving the middle third (PP), the functional impairment is related to the length of the PP left but there is generally

- Loss of fine pinch and grasp.
- Thumb index cleft is shortened/shallow.

The aim of reconstruction in this situation is to **lengthen** whilst preserving sensation, stability and mobility. Gain in actual length even of 2 cm will significantly improve the function of the thumb in proximal half amputations.

- **Phalangisation** (of thumb metacarpal). For more distal amputations, the length (1.5–2 cm) may be 'gained' by deepening the web with a Z-plasty (two- or four-flap); however, the web skin must be pliable and the first metacarpal mobile. The first interosseous is released, and the adductor pollicis insertion is transferred, which impacts on their mechanical advantage/power. It is simple but little actual functional improvement is gained whilst the resulting web looks unnatural.
- **Pollicisation** of the remaining digit, usually the index (EI becomes the new EPL). It usually provides good

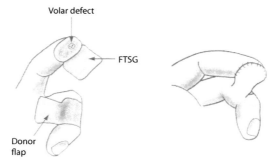

Figure 6.8 The cross finger flap can be used to cover a volar/pulp defect with exposed bone. An FTSG is first sutured along the edge nearest the donor digit (this is easier than suturing at the end). A dorsal flap is raised on the donor digit based on the side adjacent to the injury. This is sutured to the edge of the defect, whilst the FTSG is sutured to the edge of the donor.

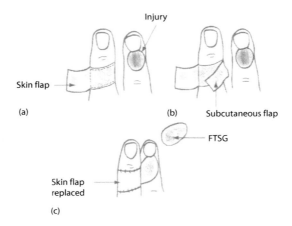

Figure 6.9 A reverse cross finger flap can be used to cover ungraftable distal dorsal defects. A skin flap (equivalent to the thickness of a thin FTSG) is elevated from the donor digit based on the edge away from the defect. A flap of subcutaneous tissue is then raised based on the other edge and is used to cover the defect (along with a thin FTSG). The donor skin flap is sutured back and a tie-over bolus dressing applied.

function and cosmesis, with minimal sacrifice, but narrows the palm. It is particularly useful if the basal CMCJ is nonfunctional.

- **Distraction osteogenesis** can lengthen the metacarpal by 3–3.5 cm over several weeks (1 mm/day plus latency) but generally needs at least 2/3 of the metacarpal remaining along with good soft tissue cover, which is also expanded to a certain extent. Complications include non-union and tissue necrosis. Bone grafting may be needed for bone gaps of more than 3 cm, particularly in older patients. Web deepening may also be needed subsequently.
- **Toe–hand transfer.** The functional results are superior to other methods as well as being the only way of replacing glabrous skin, fibrous septa and a nail.
- **Osteoplastic reconstruction** – bone graft (usually iliac crest, which may resorb significantly) plus a neurosensory (where possible) flap (e.g. reverse radial forearm, tubed groin flap or ALT). This option is usually reserved for situations where other fingers are not available and toe transfer cannot be done. It is, however, a multi-stage procedure and the results may be neither aesthetic nor functional.

PROXIMAL THIRD

When most of the metacarpal is missing, a whole thumb is needed. Options include the following:

- Pollicisation.
- Free toe–hand transfer offers the best reconstruction in a single operation, providing better sensation, stability and motor control (can expect good pinch and grasp) than the above; however, the patient's age, motivation and functional requirements also need to be taken into account. It can be performed secondarily or acutely, including a wrap-around flap for salvage of avulsion injuries with most of the skeleton still remaining. It also has good growth potential in children.

TOE–HAND TRANSFER

Toe–hand transfer is an established option, and it must be borne in mind during treatment of acute injuries. Fourteen per cent will require revisional surgery, e.g. flexor tenolysis, joint arthrodesis or web-space deepening; surgery may also be required for mal/non-union.

DONOR SITE

- The first dorsal metatarsal artery (DMTA) from the dorsalis pedis (70%, 20% from plantar metatarsal artery, 10% equal) supplies both the first and second toes and lies between the first and second metatarsals at varying levels. The EHB tendon is cut during the pedicle dissection.
- The superficial dorsal – great saphenous vein is usually used.
- Volar digital nerves from the medial plantar nerve.

The function of the thenar muscles affects the functional outcome of thumb reconstructions. Donor site complications (of the hallux) may be reduced by preserving as much skin as possible for direct closure; the metatarsal head should be preserved along with 1 cm of the PP for 'push-off'.

OPTIONS

- **Hallux transfer** – the ipsilateral toe provides the optimal mobility, stability and strength; however, on average, it is more than 20% larger than the thumb and the nail is flatter and broader. The donor site cosmesis is rather poor, but the effect on walking is slight. The hallux should not be harvested proximal to the MTPJ. For drivers, the non-driving foot is used.
- **Second toe** is thinner, has a shorter nail, and is narrower than the thumb. It is not as strong/stable as the hallux, and skin grafts are often needed. However, it offers a way of reconstructing the CMCJ in more proximal injuries when the metatarsal and metatarsal phalangeal joint (MTPJ) is harvested (first metatarsal cannot be

sacrificed without significant gait disturbance). In addition, the donor site is more aesthetic and is the preferred technique for some surgeons, e.g. Kay S.

- **Wrap-around** (Morrison) partial toe transfer – taking soft tissue and nail from the hallux, with bone from a degloved phalanx or an iliac bone graft (thus requires a second donor site). It has relatively poor mobility (no IPJ) and may resorb but does offer a sensate thumb (pulp and glabrous skin) with very good cosmesis.
- **Trimmed toe** (Wei) – hallux is trimmed to the size of the thumb, including a longitudinal osteotomy. The result is a thumb with good sensation, strength, cosmesis and function; the disadvantage is reduced IPJ function.
- **Partial toe transfer** – from the second toe – MTPJ, pulp, skin and nail.

SIMPLE ALGORITHM FOR TOE TRANSFER

- Distal to the IPJ – transfer not needed.
- PP stump with intact MCPJ – wrap-around gives best cosmesis, whilst hallux has best strength (and has growth potential and thus is preferred in children).
- Long metacarpal – hallux is the best option when harvested at the MTPJ, with thenar muscle reconstruction.
- Short metacarpal – second toe is the best option as the MTPJ along with some MT can be harvested; opponensplasty is often needed.
- Metacarpal missing (along with intrinsic muscles) – pollicisation is the best option unless this is not possible due to finger injuries, when a second toe with MTPJ is the best option. An index metacarpal remnant can be pollicised as a base for toe transfer.

VI. FRACTURES

Finger fractures, particularly the outer rays, are the commonest upper limb fractures. The most common hand bones to be fractured are the distal phalanges and the metacarpals. Middle phalangeal fractures are the least common.

- An **unstable fracture** is one that cannot be reduced closed or cannot be held reduced without fixation.
- Antibiotics – there is a 30% infection rate in open DP fractures without antibiotics compared to 3% if antibiotics are used (Sloan JP, *J Br Hand Surg*, 1987). A DP fracture underlying a subungual haematoma should be considered to be open.
- Healing time ~ 4 weeks (phalangeal fractures) – 6 weeks (metacarpal fractures); note that typically radiological healing lags behind clinical healing.

PHASES OF FRACTURE HEALING

- Inflammation (immediately to a few days) – haematoma formation and infiltration by haematopoietic cells and osteogenic precursors.
- Repair (24 hours to 3 weeks) collagen deposition and cartilaginous callus formation (it can be seen on X-ray by 3–6 months). Endochondral ossification.
- Remodelling (months to years) lamellar bone formation and repopulation of marrow. Resorption of callus.

EPIPHYSEAL FRACTURES

Salter–Harris classification for paediatric fractures – there is increasing amount of growth plate injury and potential growth disturbance:

- I – Shearing through the growth plate, transverse fracture (5%)
- II – Epiphysis and growth plate separate from the metaphysis, small metaphyseal fragment attached (75%)
- III – Intra-articular fracture of the epiphysis (10%)
- IV – Fracture passes through epiphysis, growth plate and metaphysis (10%)
- V – Growth plate crushed. Uncommon

Eighty per cent of Salter–Harris fractures are type II. Some propose a 'SALTR' mnemonic – i.e. 'slipped' through the growth plate, 'above' the growth plate, 'lower' than the growth plate, 'through' the growth plate and 'rammed' (Figure 6.10).

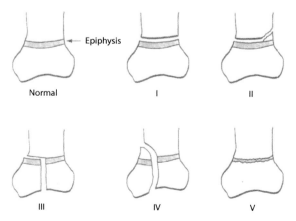

Figure 6.10 The Salter–Harris classification of paediatric fractures.

TREATMENT

The method of treatment depends on a variety of factors including age, occupation and likely compliance with the full treatment course. Other factors are related to the injury itself.

'ACCEPTABLE' HAND FRACTURES

- Tuft of DP
- AP displacement of metaphyseal fractures in children
- Metacarpal neck fractures
  - <15° angulation in the middle finger and the ring finger
  - <50° angulation in the index finger and the little finger
- Metacarpal base fractures
  - <20° in adults
  - <40° in children

Most closed hand fractures (most commonly DP and MC) can be treated without ORIF. In general, **immobilisation in a plaster** after closed reduction that is stable/minimally displaced **is 'acceptable' if there is no rotational deformity, >4 mm of shortening or angulation >10°**.

Closed fractures of MC, PP or MP can be treated either conservatively or operatively. Those without rigid fixation should have a follow-up X-ray 7–10 days later to verify the bone position.

'UNACCEPTABLE' PHALANGEAL FRACTURES

- **Open or intra-articular fractures.** The priority is soft tissue repair as secondary bony repair is almost always possible.
- **Angulation**.
  - Rotational angulation
  - Severe dorsal angulation
  - Lateral angulation
- **Rotation**/finger scissoring. Rotational deformities are not well tolerated and must be corrected. Rotation of 5° of MC will cause 1 cm of fingertip overlay.
- **Shortening** – Minor shortening is more acceptable than angulation or rotation.
- **Fractures with bone loss/comminution (usually more serious than the radiograph) or associated with neurovascular or tendon injury.**

ORIF is indicated for the 'unacceptable fractures' above and

- **Closed fractures that cannot be reduced adequately (irreducible) or cannot be maintained in reduction (unstable)**
- **Multiple fractures**

SPECIFIC FRACTURES THAT USUALLY NEED ORIF ARE

- Bennetts/Rolando
- Metacarpal fractures that are
  - Spiral/long oblique
  - Multiple transverse
- Proximal phalanx
  - Intra-articular base of the PP
  - Spiral/long oblique PP
  - Condylar fracture PP
- Fracture dislocation of the PIPJ and the base of the MP

COMPLICATIONS OF FRACTURES

- **Stiffness** – loss of motion that may be due to adhesions, capsular contracture, joint injury. **Finger stiffness is the most common complication** following **surgical treatment** of phalangeal fractures.
  - 3–4 weeks splintage is sufficient for most fractures of the hand.
- **Infection 2%–11% of open fractures**.
- **Malunion** – rotation, angulation, shortening.
- **Non-union** (which may require osteotomy and bone graft).

TECHNIQUES OF FIXATION

Fracture management represents a compromise of sorts between fracture healing and mobility. ORIF with plates/screws provides (close to) rigid fixation and permits early mobilisation, but the surgical trauma will lead to adhesions and stiffness. Closed non-rigid fixation with K-wires is associated with less trauma and adhesions, but often requires splintage for a period that encourages stiffness. Thus, the choice between ORIF and K-wire fixation is not so clear-cut. See 'Unacceptable phalangeal fractures'.

- **Lag screw fixation** – spiral fractures
- **Screw plus miniplate** (generally only metacarpal fractures)
- **Crossed K-wiring**
- **Wiring** – tension band, Lister loop, 90/90; bone tie (Sammut D, *J Hand Surg Br*, 1999)
- **External fixation** (S-QUATTRO) – comminuted open/closed fractures
  - Small intra-articular fractures
  - Combined soft tissue and bony injury
  - Segmental bone loss, pending bone graft
  - Mal/nonunions
  - Disadvantages – tethering of tendons, neurovascular damage (<1%), infection of pin sites (8%), osteomyelitis (<1%)

PHALANGEAL FRACTURES

- **Distal phalanx** – the most common hand fractures especially the MF and the thumb. Avulsion fractures associated with flexor or extensor tendon injuries (see 'Flexor tendon injuries'). Watch out for nail-bed injuries.
- **Middle phalanx**
  - Distal fractures can be pinned after closed reduction.
  - Middle fractures tend to be stable due to the action of the FDS insertion and should be pinned after closed reduction.
  - **Proximal fractures** can involve the volar plate, and intra-articular fractures can be complex – traction may be the only option and **functional outcomes tend to be rather poor**.
- **PP** – flexion forces typically result in an apex volar angulation.
  - Proximal fractures are often comminuted and involve the MCPJ.
  - Neck fractures tend to be unstable.

CLASSIFICATION

- Unicondylar/bicondylar – tend to be unstable – displaced fractures usually need open reduction.
- Neck – closed reduction and plaster of Paris (POP) for non-displaced fractures, whilst displaced fractures require an open approach and K-wiring.
- Shaft fractures – transverse or spiral fractures are usually stable and can be treated by splintage, whilst oblique fractures tend to be unstable and need fixation (closed or open). Comminuted fractures may need external fixation.
- Base – these fractures are typically impacted with **apex volar angulation** – up to 25° is reasonably well tolerated, but greater degrees should be reduced and fixed. Fractures at the base of the MP are often associated with PIPJ dislocation (usually dorsal with avulsion of the volar base of the MP).

Non-union of phalangeal fractures is uncommon (except in severe soft tissue/bone injury/loss), whilst **malunion is fairly common** and may require corrective osteotomies.

METACARPAL FRACTURES

These bones most commonly fracture at the neck (20% of all hand fractures).

METACARPAL HEAD

Like MC base fractures, these are relatively rare and are usually intra-articular. Closed fractures without joint problems (stable MCPJ on stressing) or with <20% articular surface involvement may be managed non-operatively.

- Percutaneous K-wires with or without a cerclage wire in parallel splinting to adjacent metacarpal ×2 intramedullary K-wires.
- Miniplate fixation via dorsal approach.
- External fixation if there is soft tissue loss or the PP is also fractured.
- MCPJ arthrodesis is a salvage procedure for a severe comminuted fracture.

METACARPAL NECK

This is the **commonest place for the metacarpal bones** to fracture. These fractures usually involve axial load to a clenched fist, i.e. punching a hard object (e.g. **'boxers' fifth metacarpal neck fracture**, actually rarely found in boxers). There is usually **apex dorsal angulation** (depressed knuckle and head protrudes into palm), since the intrinsics are volar and maintain a flexed MC head/MCPJ posture. The soft tissues including muscles around the metacarpal bones may help to reduce the distortion to a certain extent, but significant deformities may still result.

Treatment is required in cases with

- **Angulation >10–15°** in the (fixed) index/middle or 30–40° ring, 50–60° (some say 40–45°) little finger (which has greater mobility). Less angulation is tolerated in the index/middle fingers due to the reduced CMCJ mobility.
  - In general, proper reduction is advised as it improves cosmesis and avoids the palmar MC head deformity, which may interfere with grasping.
  - Angulations of more than 30–40° may interfere with extensor function and lead to **pseudoclawing** (MCPJ hyperextension with extension deficit/flexion contracture at the PIPJ as the patient attempts to extend the finger).
- **Rotational** deformity/scissoring – every 5° rotation causes 1.5 cm digital overlap.
  - In extension, the fingers should be in parallel, whilst in flexion, they should point towards the scaphoid tuberosity.
- **Shortening** >3 mm.

MANAGEMENT

- **Closed reduction** should be attempted in those with angulation. **Jahss manoeuvre** (*J Bone Joint Surg*, 1938) – flex the MCJP to 90° to relax the intrinsics and tighten the collateral ligaments, also flex the IPJs, then reduce the fracture with downwards (volar) pressure on the metacarpal shaft at the angulation whilst applying dorsally directed pressure at the PIPJ.
  - If it is then stable – place in the POP in the position of function (the MCPJ flexed but the IPJ extended) for 2–3 weeks followed by aggressive mobilisation.

It may be difficult to maintain reduction with the swelling.

- **If unstable, then K-wires can be used** (crossed at neck or transverse with adjacent metacarpal).
- MCPJ and CMCJ mobility can compensate for moderate amounts of residual deformity.
- **Open reduction** – dorsal approach, rarely needed.
  - Fractures with rotational deformity are often unstable and may need ORIF.

METACARPAL SHAFT

These tend to be transverse from a direct/axial force or spiral/oblique from torsion. Most are inherently stable; the border metacarpals tend to be less stable as they have less support from the intrinsics or transverse metacarpal ligament. There is usually apex dorsal angulation due to the action of interosseous muscles.

Treat if

- Angulation >10° index, middle or 20° ring or 30° little fingers
- Shortening >3 mm
- Rotational deformity/scissoring
  - Spiral fractures are commonly missed in extension, accentuated in flexion.

MANAGEMENT

- Non-operative – closed reduction and splint with wrist 30° extension, 90° MCPJ and IPJ extension
- Surgery – if unstable/irreducible, **multiple or open fractures** via a dorsal approach – K-wires, plates or lag screws
  - Fracture with segmental loss – stabilise and maintain length with external fixation, with immediate or delayed bone grafting; soft tissue cover may be needed.
  - K-wires can be technically difficult and do not provide rigid fixation, requiring supplemental external support. Longitudinal K-wiring does not prevent rotation; crossed K-wires may cause distraction of the fracture.

THUMB FRACTURES

- **Bennett's fracture – oblique intra-articular** (CMCJ) fracture of the **base** of the first metacarpal in the dorso-volar axis. It is caused by compression along a partly flexed metacarpal and is thus often sustained when punching. It is the most frequent thumb fracture and **tends to be unstable**.
  - The **metacarpal base is subluxed** dorsally, proximally and radially due to traction by the **APL tendon**. The anterior fragment of bone is attached to the ulnar collateral ligament (UCL) and the volar plate.

- **Non-operative treatment often leads to arthritis and subluxation**. The optimal treatment is AO screw fixation via a radial approach, particularly in moderately displaced fractures; an alternative is a percutaneous K-wire through the thumb metacarpal, trapezium and second metacarpal. The small fragment does not need to be pinned.
- **Reversed Bennett's fracture** is analogous to Bennett's except that it occurs in the fifth metacarpal base; hence, some call it 'baby Bennett'. Deformation occurs due to traction by the ECU tendon and hypothenar muscles. The motor branch of the ulnar nerve may be injured. It is usually treated by closed reduction and K-wire fixation to the fourth metacarpal and hamate.
- **Rolando fracture** – similar to Bennett's except that the dorsal, avulsed segment has a 'T-condylar' fracture or Y or comminuted form. Treat by K-wiring or T-plate, except for comminuted fractures (spica cast or external fixation).

VII. DISLOCATION

Dislocation joint injury is suggested by tenderness and pain that is aggravated by stressing the joint; LA/nerve blocks may aid in the diagnosis by facilitating examination. **PIPJ dislocations are the commonest dislocations in the hand.**

With many dislocations, stabilisation after reduction may be sufficient to allow healing of torn ligaments; K-wires are often used. Some notable exceptions include

- Dorsal PIPJ dislocation – torn volar plate interposed in joint cavity
- Volar PIPJ dislocation – rupture of the central slip
- UCL thumb tear – Stener lesion, i.e. interposition of the adductor pollicis tendon between ligament ends

PHALANGEAL DISLOCATIONS

Joint dislocations are named according to the **distal bone position** and can be dorsal, volar or lateral. **Dorsal dislocations resulting from forced hyperextension are the most common** and are often sports related. Alternatively, dislocations can be classified as simple, complex or fracture.

- Simple injuries can usually be reduced by traction and appropriate pressure. The adequacy of reduction should be verified radiologically and stability with movement confirmed.
  - ROM exercises are allowed after a few days of extension block splinting. PIPJ injuries (all forms) can lead to significant joint stiffness, and early active movement is important.
- Lateral dislocations are less common; they often reduce spontaneously and can be treated with buddy taping.

- Volar dislocations are rare (blow to partially flexed finger) and often involve extensor tendon central slip disruption that can lead to boutonnières if left untreated.
- Fracture dislocations are mostly stable, but a minority are unstable particularly when >40% of the MP volar articular surface has been avulsed. Most of the collateral ligaments remain with the fragment; thus, ligamentous support of the MP is lost and dorsal dislocation tends to recur. These will need fixation and possibly open treatment if closed techniques (pin for 2–3 weeks, then ROM exercises) fail.

Stability should be assessed under a block (wrist or ring) and compared to the contralateral digit.

- Passive stability – lateral stress to joint at full extension and 30° flexion, assess collaterals.
- Active stability – active ROM, any dislocation with motion indicates an unstable joint.

METACARPOPHALANGEAL DISLOCATION

The MCPJ has a shape likened to a box that can resist injury and dislocation with the support of intrinsic ligaments and surrounding structures, e.g. sagittal bands, tendons, etc. The volar plate is the floor of the joint. The shape means that with flexion there is linear stretch of the collateral ligaments, and when at >70°, the joint is laterally stable.

CLASSIFICATION OF MCPJ DISLOCATIONS

- Open or closed. For closed and stable dislocations, movement can begin with buddy strap as pain allows.
- Simple (reduces easily) or **complex** (will not reduce due to soft tissue **interposition** especially the volar plate in between the MC head and the base of the PP). In general, complex dislocations are more common in 'border' digits – thumb, index and little fingers.
- Dorsal or volar
  - Dorsal – more common and usually stable after reduction.
  - Volar – rare. The MC head protrudes into the palm between lumbrical and flexor tendons, and the volar plate is in the joint space with the flexor tendons still attached and tightened, counteracting any reduction force – thus, open reduction may be needed with A1 release to relax tension.

Collateral ligaments may be ruptured particularly on the radial side (rarely UCL) and may present late with persistent swelling and pain with localised tenderness as well as demonstrable instability. The joint can be immobilised in 30° flexion for 2 weeks and reassessed – persistent instability may respond to buddy strapping or may require repair, especially if >6 weeks.

COLLATERAL LIGAMENT SPRAIN CLASSIFICATION

- Grade I – stable with microscopic tear
- Grade II – intact ligament but with abnormal laxity on stressing
- Grade III – complete tear with instability

INTERPHALANGEAL DISLOCATION

The IPJ volar plate is confluent with the periosteum of the phalanges – it prevents hyperextension and provides some lateral stability. Due to its box-like shape/configuration, dislocation usually implies disruption of at least two parts.

- **DIPJ dislocations are less common and are usually dorsal**. They are usually easily reduced by longitudinal traction and should then be splinted.
- **PIPJ dislocations are one of the commonest ligamentous hand injuries**. They commonly result in flexion contracture and permanent fusiform enlargement of the joint.

CLASSIFICATION OF PIPJ DISLOCATION

The PIPJ has the largest arc of motion (120°) in the finger joints; 85% of the movement in grasping occurs at the PIPJ.

- **Type 1 – hyperextension injury** with volar plate damage, avulsed from the MP base with or without a bone fragment; there is partial articulation with the MP locked in hyperextension. They can be quite painful but are relatively benign, with most returning to normal function. These can usually be reduced without surgery and then immobilised for 1–2 weeks. Avoid prolonged immobilisation.
  - Untreated injury may lead to chronic PIPJ subluxation and **swan neck deformity,** which is treated by FDS tenodesis, aka sublimis sling.
- **Type 2 – dorsal dislocation, more common** – usually a complete dislocation with major ligament damage and volar plate avulsion (bayonet appearance). Often reducible; immobilise in reduction 2–3 weeks.
- **Type 3 – Fracture dislocation** – avulsion of the volar MP base with the volar plate. The hastings classification is based on the amount of the MP articular surface involved.
  - Fragments of >40% articular surface are usually unstable. Large fragments need ORIF with fixation, hemihamate autograft (Hastings) or volar plate arthroplasty. Dynamic (Suzuki) traction is an option for comminuted fractures.
  - Stable injuries usually have less than 40% injury and are usually stable after reduction due to dorsal collateral ligaments remaining intact; extension block splint.

Volar PIPJ dislocation/fracture dislocations are less common and often involve injury to the central slip and at least one collateral ligament; failure to treat may lead to boutonniere deformity.

MANAGEMENT

- Simple, closed dorsal dislocations (volar plate avulsion ± small volar fragment) may be treated conservatively (mobilise plus extension-block splint).
- Complex dislocations (unstable type 3 usually) require open reduction and volar plate removal and repair.
- **Collateral ligament fibrosis** may follow approximately a year after PIPJ dislocation – it can be reduced by rehabilitation but may ultimately require excision (taking care to preserve the lateral band).

THUMB DISLOCATIONS

The **thumb MCPJ** has proper and accessory collateral ligaments in addition to support by muscle insertions.

Thumb MCPJ dislocation injuries are more common than finger MCPJ injuries. **Dorsal MCPJ dislocation is more common** than volar in the thumb and is usually secondary to hyperextension injury. Reducible injuries can be splinted, whilst irreducible dislocations (sesamoid bone, FPL tendon or volar plate interposition) will need surgery.

- **Acute UCL injury** is often called 'ski thumb' as it is associated with fall on hand with an abducted thumb. It is much more common than RCL injury. There may be avulsion fractures of the PP – small fragments can be treated with a thumb spica, whilst large displaced fragments will need ORIF and K-wire.
  - Partial tears may be treated by splintage in POP for about 4 weeks followed by active exercises. Complete ruptures generally need repair.
  - **Stener lesion** is a completely torn UCL that lies superficial to the adductor expansion and the injury will not heal without surgery.
- **Gamekeeper's thumb** is a **chronic type of UCL injury** due to either progressive attenuation, e.g. RA, or secondary to untreated complete tears. There is a tear of the MCPJ UCL due to hyperextension injury causing volar plate disruption. There is pain and thumb weakness.
  - Reattach the ligament using an interosseous wire, suture or Mitek bone anchor and K-wire the MCPJ joint (6 weeks). Repair the UCL (may need reconstruction with PL/plantaris, FCR/APL slip), accessory ligament, volar plate and dorsal capsule as all of these will lend stability to the joint.
  - Bony Gamekeeper's thumb may be treated conservatively if the fracture fragment involves <15%–20% of the articular surface.

VIII. WRIST PAIN

DIFFERENTIAL DIAGNOSES

Radial wrist pain

- Basal joint OA (CMC axial grind test)
- Ischaemic necrosis of scaphoid
- de Quervain's tenosynovitis (first compartment) – see below
- Intersection syndrome (second compartment tenosynovitis) – see below
- Wartenberg's syndrome (superficial branch of RN entrapment)
- SL dissociation
- Synovitis

CENTRAL WRIST PAIN

- Kienbock's disease – see below.
- Ganglia/metacarpal boss – a small mass of bone usually found at the base of the second/third metacarpal bones where they meet the small bones of the wrist. Patients present with pain and lack of mobility.
- Synovitis.

ULNAR WRIST PAIN

- Ulnar impingement syndrome
- Lunotriquetral dissociation/instability (ballottement test/shuck test)
- DRUJ subluxation – piano key
- Synovitis especially flexor carpi ulnaris (FCU) tenosynovitis

TREATMENT

Treatment is tailored to the individual problem (see relevant sections).

De Quervain's disease (1895)

Musculotendinous units can become inflamed where they pass through tunnels or at a bony attachment. De Quervain's disease is a stenosing tenovaginitis of the APL tendon within the first dorsal compartment. In 20%–30% of patients, there may be two separate tunnels for each tendon (APL and EPB); EPB is absent in ~5% of people. It commonly affects middle-aged women who usually present with several months of radial wrist pain aggravated by movement and may be associated with overuse (anecdotally 'new mothers' and 'new grandmothers').

SIGNS

- Positive **Finkelstein test** (pain on ulnar deviation with the thumb clasped in the fist).
- It may co-exist with basal joint OA, and there may be a small ganglion in the first dorsal compartment.

- It can be differentiated from the intersection syndrome (see below) where the pain is more proximally located.

MANAGEMENT

- Non-operative – NSAIDs, wrist immobilisation and steroid injections.
- Operative – longitudinal release of the first compartment by incising extensor retinaculum through a 2 cm transverse incision just above the level of the radial styloid. In RA cases, synovectomy may also be required. It is important to preserve the superficial branch of the RN.

INTERSECTION SYNDROME

Pain and swelling of muscle bellies of APL and EPB at the site at which they cross (hence 'intersection') the tendons of the second dorsal compartment, ECRL and ECRB, about 4 cm proximal to the wrist. Basic pathology relates to a tenosynovitis of the second dorsal compartment. Operative treatment is by release of the second compartment in a similar fashion to De Quervain's, though most cases respond to activity modification and/or steroid injections.

KIENBOCK'S DISEASE

This is an **avascular necrosis** of the dorsal pole of the lunate (called lunatomalacia in 1910 by Keinbock) with collapse. It is usually idiopathic, possibly due to some primary vascular insufficiency or secondary to trauma (>50% have a history of wrist trauma). There is a strong association with ulnar minus/negative variant (short ulna), which is present in 23% of normal wrists but present in 78% of Kienbock's wrists – in these patients, the lunate is subjected to greater shear stress forces potentially compromising its volar blood supply.

- Fault plate hypothesis (Watson HK, *J Hand Surg (Br)*, 1997).
- Extrinsic factors, e.g. lunate loading due to differential radii of the curvature of the lunate and capitate.
- Intrinsic factors, e.g. cortical strength of the lunate, trabecular pattern, vascular anatomy – the bone has many articulations and is almost completely covered by articular cartilage, with a lack of a dominant vessel.

CLINICAL FEATURES

It usually presents as a painful, stiff, swollen wrist in young active adults (four times more common in males) with decreased grip strength, but there is a very variable symptomatology and rate of progression. The condition is usually unilateral, favouring the dominant wrist, and is more common in manual workers or those performing repetitive tasks.

PLAIN RADIOGRAPHS MAY SHOW

- Radiolucent line indicating compression fracture
- Demineralisation surrounding a fracture line (<3 months)

- Sclerosis of the dorsal pole (~3 months)
- Fragmentation and flattening
- Wrist arthrosis
- Capitate collapse (end stage)

Other methods:
- Bone scan
- MRI/CT (shows occult fractures)

STAGING

Lichtman staging (radiological)

- Stage 1 – normal except possibility of linear or compression fracture.
- Stage 2 – lunate sclerosis – density changes in lunate.
- Stage 3A – collapse of the entire lunate without fixed scaphoid rotation.
- Stage 3B – collapse of the entire lunate with fixed scaphoid rotation – in such cases, further collapse is hastened due to shifting load onto the lunate's shortened radius.
- Stage 4 – as above with generalised degenerative changes in carpus. Carpal arthritis.

MODIFIED STAHL'S CLASSIFICATION OF KIENBOCK'S DISEASE:

- Stage 1 – normal structure of the lunate, with evidence of compression fracture usually appearing as a radiodense or radiolucent line
- Stage 2 – rarification along the line of previous compression fractures, developing within the first 3 months
- Stage 3 – changes of stages 1 and 2 together with sclerosis of proximal pole, occurring at about 3 months
- Stage 4 – fragmentation or flattening of the lunate
- Stage 5 – changes of arthrosis of radial carpal and inner-carpal joints

TREATMENT

Treatment aims to prevent deformity and restore normal appearance and function.

EARLY DISEASE

- Positive bone scan, X-ray normal – treat with immobilisation and analgesia but rarely effective even in the early stages.
- Sclerotic changes on X-ray – **joint levelling** procedure, either radial shortening (about 2 mm) to restore neutral ulnar variance and redistribute load or some suggest ulnar lengthening (more difficult). This is one of the most common procedures.
- Lunate resection, fill with tendon or capito-hamate fusion to prevent capitate subluxing into proximal carpal row in the absence of the lunate (Treatment of Kienbock's disease with capitohamate arthrodesis. Oishi SN, *Plast Reconstr Surg*, 2002).

LATE DISEASE

- Intercarpal fusion/limited wrist arthrodesis
- Scaphoid–trapezium–trapezoid fusion with excision of the radial styloid
- Scaphoid capitate fusion
- Revascularisation procedures
- Pronator quadratus (PQ) turnover flap
- Pedicled DMCA buried in lunate

Other options include

- Wrist denervation
- Excision of the lunate and replacement with a silastic implant, rolled tendon graft or vascularised pisiform (Saffar P, *Ann Chir Main*, 1982)

SCAPHOID FRACTURES

The scaphoid is the most commonly fractured wrist bone (80%). Most are sustained by a fall on an outstretched hand – the wrist is dorsiflexed and radially deviated. The head of the capitate is compressed onto the concave portion of the scaphoid. There is poor blood supply to the proximal pole by retrograde intraosseous flow, which is threatened further by a fracture; healing is via the endosteal blood supply.

The **scaphoid series** is a PA wrist with ulnar deviation (to rotate the scaphoid away from the radius), lateral and oblique wrist. The scaphoid view, i.e. ulnar deviated PA with 20–30° tube angle, aims to get an en face view. Features are similar to Kienbock's: initially cystic and sclerotic and may lead to fracture or collapse of the bone. Clinically there may be pain or tenderness when palpating the anatomical snuff-box or performing a scaphoid compression test.

The fracture is visible after 10–14 days, or earlier by CT or MRI (local decrease in intensity on T1) – the latter is the most sensitive and specific assessment of post-traumatic avascular necrosis (Gaebler C, *J Trauma*, 1996). Bone scans have a high false-positive rate (Waizenegger M, *J Hand Surg [Br]*, 1994), but a negative result can generally **exclude** any occult fracture.

- **Avascular necrosis** of the proximal pole is heralded by radiological sclerosis.
- The mal-/non-united scaphoid adopts a flexed attitude (apex dorsal) leading to the so-called humpback deformity. It is most commonly associated with DISI.
- There is a fairly predictable sequence of arthritic changes in the radioscaphoid and capitolunate joints, leading to scapholunate advanced collapse (SLAC wrist), rotatory subluxation of the scaphoid and a decrease in the Huber index on the X-ray.

Primary avascular necrosis of the scaphoid (**Preiser's disease**) is rare. It may be due to repetitive microtrauma or may be drug-related, e.g. steroids or chemotherapy, in conjunction with defective proximal pole vascularity. It presents with wrist pain at rest and with movement and decreased grip strength. It is more common in the dominant hand.

TREATMENT

Uniting the fracture will increase function, reduce pain and reduce the risk of future degenerative disease. Surgery can be performed by either a volar approach (for waist and distal fractures) or dorsal approach (proximal pole including AVN).

- **No displacement** – stable fractures can be managed conservatively by immobilisation in a **scaphoid plaster** (short arm thumb spica – wrist pronated, radial deviated and moderately dorsiflexed – which should allow thumb IPJ flexion, finger MPCJ and elbow flexion); the traditional cast has its critics. Ninety-five per cent of waist fractures unite when fixed. Late presentation increases the rate of non-union and eventual degeneration.
  - Surgery is usually reserved for unstable fractures, very proximal fractures or mal-/non-united fractures.
- **Displacement** – unstable fractures (displacement and angulation) and very proximal fractures (**risk of AVN**) usually need ORIF (**Herbert screw** – double-threaded headless cannulated screw, AO screw or Acutrak screw) – with **cancellous bone graft** from the radius to correct humpback deformity. ORIF is associated with 80% union rate.
  - **Russe bone graft** made of two opposed corticocancellous grafts can be 'stuffed' into the cored-out bone in cases of non-union.
  - **Vascularised bone graft** for failed non-vascularised graft, proximal pole AVN.
- **Non-union without AVN** – non-vascular bone graft (Matte–Rewse), e.g. iliac.
- **Avascular necrosis** – vascularised bone graft, e.g. Kuhlmann procedure with volar radial bone flap from beneath the PQ on a branch from the radial artery (the volar carpal artery can be traced to the bone surface and can be raised alone with the ulnar bone graft), or scaphoid excision and rolled tendon graft; four-corner fusion (lunate to capitate to hamate to triquetral to lunate wrist arthrodesis) may be a 'salvage' option.
- **Arthritis** – radial styloid excision, radioscaphoid fusion, proximal row carpectomy or total wrist arthrodesis (SLAC wrist).

NON-UNION OF SCAPHOID

General factors

- Gap too large or separation of ends, e.g. soft tissue or dead bone interposition
- Avascularity and infection
- Excessive interfragmentary movement
- Poor internal fixation holding ends in distraction
- Adverse systemic factors (anaemia, steroids, malnutrition, etc.)

IX. NAIL-BED INJURY

ANATOMY

The fingernail grows ~3 mm a month; it takes an average of 3 months for full nail growth (there is often a 3 week delay after injury). Growth is faster in longer digits, in younger patients, in nail biters and in the summer.

- Hyponychium (*onychium*, Greek for little claw) – this is the junction between the skin of the fingertip and the sterile matrix at the distal end of the nail. It has a large number of lymphocytes as an immune barrier to deal with the heavy contamination at this site.
- Eponychium (cuticle) – the proximal part of nail fold attached to the surface of the nail.
- Nail bed – the proximal floor is the germinal matrix whilst the distal sterile matrix provides adherence.
  - The germinal matrix contributes 90% of the volume of the nail plate. The lunula is the white arc of the germinal matrix where nuclei persist in the basilar cells; as the nuclei gradually disintegrate distally, the nail plate becomes clear.
  - The smooth surface layer is derived from the tissue at the roof of the nail fold.
- Nail plate – strongly adherent to the sterile matrix, whilst it is only loosely attached to the germinal matrix. The nail acts as a counterforce to the fingertip pad to improve grip and increase sensitivity; the 2pd decreases when the nail is absent and fingerprints tend to become less obvious (Figure 6.11).

INJURY OF NAIL BED

Fifty per cent of nailbed injuries are associated with a fracture of the DP.

VAN BEEK CLASSIFICATION OF NAIL BED INJURIES

- I – small (<25%) subungual haematoma
- II – larger (>50%) subungual haematoma
- III – nail-bed laceration associated with fracture of the DP
- IV – nail-bed fragmentation
- V – nail-bed avulsion

CLASSICALLY

- Types I and II can be treated with trephination.
- Type III – remove the nail plate for exploration as there is a high risk of nail-bed injury, which should be repaired with 6'0 vicryl. Splint the nail fold (with the nail plate or other spacer) to prevent adhesions that may otherwise lead to ridging or other abnormalities.
- Types IV and V – secondary healing will tend to leave misshapen non-adherent nails.

In general, nail plates that are still adherent with intact nail folds should be left alone where possible, whilst injuries where the nail fold is disrupted or the plate is dislodged from the nail bed should be explored/repaired.

- **Acute treatment is preferred** as secondary nail-bed repair/revisions are rarely satisfactory.
  - The nail bed that has been detached can be replaced as a free graft.
  - Narrow (<2 mm) defects can be closed with bipedicled advancement after wide undermining.
  - For wider avulsions, one can use a split thickness nail-bed graft (from the same digit if <50% missing, or a toe if more) aiming to harvest a graft of 0.001 inch thickness that is then sewn in. Full thickness grafts, e.g. the lateral nail bed of hallux (close donor primarily), are an alternative.
  - Grafting the germinal matrix produces average/unpredictable results – nail bed ablation may be advisable with the other option being a free vascularised nail bed transfer.
- X-rays are advised as 50% of nail-bed injuries are associated with a fracture of the DP – most are minor/non-displaced and require no specific treatment other than repair of the nail bed.

FINGERTIP INJURIES

The fingertip can be defined as the portion distal to the extensor and FDP tendon insertions. The skin is glabrous with a thick epidermis and deep papillary ridges that form the fingerprints. Under this, the pulp is fibrofatty tissue that has a dense network of fibrous septae from dermis to periosteum, as well as bound laterally by extensions from Cleland and Grayson's ligaments.

- Digital nerve – trifurcates at the DIPJ to the nail bed, distal fingertip and volar pulp.
- Digital arteries – trifurcate to the nail fold, and two dorsal branches to the volar pulp; the branches are interconnected by two anastomoses, one parallel to the lunula and the other parallel to the free edge of the nail.
- Veins – predominantly via the dorsal veins that have valves even distally.

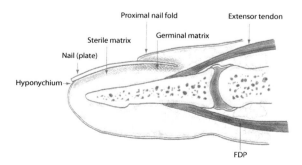

Figure 6.11 Sagittal section of a fingertip showing the structures of the nail area; the nail bed is composed of the sterile and germinal matrix.

- Cleland ligaments are dorsal to the NVB and attach the bone to the skin (B-C-D, bone-Cleland-dorsal); Grayson's ligaments are volar to the NVB and attach the flexor sheath to the skin.

FINGERTIP INJURIES AND RECONSTRUCTION

History

The patient assessment should include

- Age, gender, occupation, handedness
- Mechanism of injury and comorbidities

    Examination should concentrate on

- Size, position and orientation of defect and its components including bone
- State of flexor/extensor tendons

CLASSIFICATION OF FINGERTIP INJURIES

- Distal only soft tissue
- Middle third of the nail
- Up to the nail fold
- Up to the DIPJ

ALLEN CLASSIFICATION OF FINGERTIP INJURIES (FIGURE 6.12)

- I – **pulp involved only** – distal to the nail bed; can be treated non-operatively, e.g. dressing/Hyphecan cap or with a skin graft.
- II – **pulp and part of the nail bed** but the bone is not exposed. Treatment choices include non-operatively, composite graft, skin grafts or flap closure.
- III – **involves distal phalanx**, i.e. fractured – flap/terminalisation/Hyphecan cap.
- IV – **involves lunula as well**. Replantation may be considered; flap or amputation.

The basic requirements of a successful reconstruction are sensate, durable padding and freedom from pain whilst preserving length and cosmesis. There are many options including the following:

- **Replant** – replantation distal to the DIPJ has been increasingly reported with success (Sebastin SJ, *Plast Reconstr Surg*, 2011) especially if not crushed, contrary to conventional thinking. However, it involves a longer period of rehabilitation.
- **Dressings/secondary intention** – areas less than 1–1.5 cm^2 can heal satisfactorily by second intention over several weeks; with selected defects, often the results will be as good as local flaps. This reduces the size of insensitive skin by contraction; it is less suited for dorsal injuries that may lead to nail beaking that is difficult to fix.
- Mennen and Wise (*J Hand Surg*, 1993) looked at a series of 200 fingertip injuries treated conservatively (with Opsite). Healing took 20–30 days and good functional recovery.
  - Only the most minor of tissue loss should be closed directly; otherwise, tight closure will limit function and/or cause nail deformity.
- **Grafts**
  - Skin grafts allow immediate one stage coverage, but there is a higher incidence of cold intolerance and post-operative tenderness, and it does not seem to hasten the return to work (Holm A, *Acta Ortho Scand*, 1974). Avoid use in the index/thumb.
  - Split skin grafts (instep or hypothenar eminence provides an excellent texture match) may be considered and may be used as a temporising measure. They tend to have more reliable take, but contract more (than FTSG) and thus reduce the size of the defect.
    - One way to harvest a hypothenar graft is to shave the first layer with a Goulian knife but leave it attached, and then shave a second layer for use whilst the first layer is replaced as a dressing for the donor site.
  - Sensory return with grafts is variable; lack of reinnervation is a concern, though a review of 100 injuries (Braun M, *Can J Surg*, 1985) showed little difference in 2pd compared to local flaps (but less than secondary healing). Half report a good result compared to 90% with conservative therapy.
  - Composite grafts tend to work better in children under 6 years of age where replacing the fingertip part at the very least works as a biological dressing.
- **Revision amputations** probably offer the **quickest return to work** and should be considered in amputations proximal to the lunula or FDP/extensor tendon insertion. It is important to prevent the quadriga effect by leaving the FDP tendon untethered, though it can be secured to the A4 pulley to prevent a **lumbrical plus** deformity (which would cause PIPJ extension and MCPJ flexion with attempted flexion due to the retracting FDP pulling at the lumbrical origin).

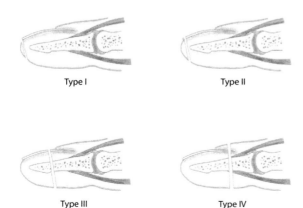

Type I   Type II

Type III   Type IV

Figure 6.12 Types of fingertip/nail-bed injuries.

Other complications include bone spicules, hook nail and neuroma.

- **Local flaps.** Defects >1/3 of the distal segment are best repaired by soft tissue/flaps particularly if the defect is not graftable or has deeper tissue loss with exposed nerves or other vital structures. There are many choices:
  - Homodigital vs. heterodigital.
  - Local, regional, distant or free.
  - Pedicled neurovascular island flap – (Foucher flap – first DMCA flap but may be of insufficient length to cover the thumb pulp), Littler (1960) – classically from the ulnar aspect of the middle finger, but also from the radial border of the ring finger. These are good choices for reconstruction of the ulnar thumb pulp, with the median nerve skin. Cortical misrepresentation can be a problem. Significant dissection is needed, along with sacrifice of the proper digital artery to the adjacent finger.

HOMODIGITAL FLAPS FOR FINGERTIP INJURIES

Homodigital flaps do not damage a normal finger and involve less immobilisation. This may mean that tissues used may be close to the zone of injury, making flap failure more likely at least in theory. In general, they can potentially provide near-normal sensation and are the method of choice for the pinch grip areas of the index and thumb.

Advancement

- **Volar V–Y advancement flap** for dorsal oblique (i.e. more dorsal loss)/transverse amputations less than 1 cm (**Atasoy** E, *J Bone Joint Surg*, 1970). The flap is advanced with blunt but meticulous dissection (Atasoy–Kleinert); defatting may be needed to facilitate closure (Figure 6.13).
- **(Bi)lateral V–Y advancement** of lateral distal skin (**Kutler** W, *J Am Med Assoc*, 1947; Geissendorfer H, *Zentralbl Chir*, 1943) (Figure 6.14). Good appearance and sensation are possible but advancement is often limited (~1 cm); the vascularity may be unreliable particularly in its original form, and a scar lies at the tip. Other **lateral flaps that are based on its own NVB** are preferred, providing larger sensate flaps that can advance ~2 cm.
  - **Segmuller** lateral flap elevated to the DIPJ or the PIPJ (Lanzetta modification). Flaps can be bilateral with their own innervation (Segmuller G, *Handchirurgie*, 1976; Biddulph SL, *Hand*, 1979).
  - **Venkataswami oblique triangular flap.** Half digit oblique volar skin advancement. The advancing edge is denervated, further from the pedicle (Venkataswami R, *Plast Reconstr Surg*, 1980).
  - **Evans** step advancement flap that exploits laxity at the base of the finger. Flaps are raised down to the

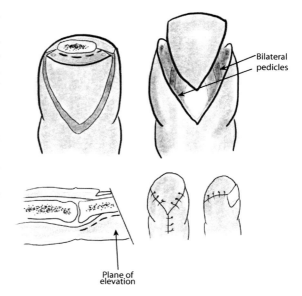

Figure 6.13 Atasoy flap. This is technically a bipedicled VY advancement flap of volar tissue of the finger used to cover a distal fingertip amputation. The expected advancement is ~1 cm. The V flap is lifted off the bone and relies on lateral attachments, which should be dissected gently. Although it avoids a midline scar, the degree of advancement is often slight. A K-wire may be needed to fix the flap.

flexor sheath and under an NVB. The angles are predrawn, getting smaller proximally – it needs more planning and is less adaptable than the others. It supposedly causes less flexion contracture than the Ventaktaswami flap (Figure 6.15; Evans DM, *Br J Plast Surg*, 1988).

- **Moberg flap** – volar digital V–Y skin advancement is the most appropriate for the thumb. Moberg described it in 1964 with incisions dorsal to the NVBs and thus are included in the flap; it also means that there is a risk of dorsal skin necrosis. The flap should be 'spread-dissected' and not cut free except at the most distal extent. The tissue movement for such a big flap/dissection is actually quite small but can be improved by islanding it and grafting the proximal defect.

TRANSPOSITION

- **Hueston volar skin transposition/rotation advancement** based laterally on the other NVB losing innervation to the leading edge (Hueston JT, *Plast Reconstr Surg*, 1966).
  - Similar to the Souquet flap, which keeps the ipsilateral bundle intact, thus limiting movement. **Sammut modification** of Souquet adds proximal flap dissection to aid mobilisation (Figure 6.16).
- **Reverse digital artery island flaps** that rely on sacrifice of one set of vessels with retrograde flow.

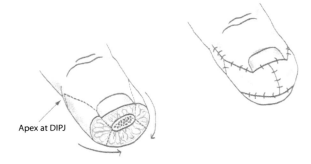

Figure 6.14 Kutler bilateral V–Y advancement flaps. The apex of the triangle reaches the level of the DIPJ; the triangles do not need to be equilateral. The flaps should be advanced with minimal disturbance of the subcutaneous tissue.

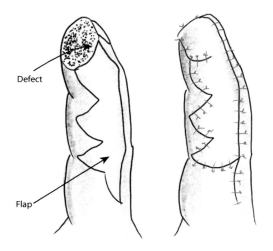

Figure 6.15 Evans step advancement flap.

Preoperative digital Allens test is required (see below; Lai CS, *Ann Plast Surg*, 1989).

- Dorsal digital defects especially over the DIPJ, can be covered by splitting proximal skin and raising an **adipofascial turnover flap** – a flap of subcutaneous tissue hinged on the proximal border of the defect (Lai CS, *Br J Plast Surg*, 1991).

Reverse digital artery island flap in the elderly. (Wilson AD, *Injury*, 2004)

This technique reconstructs the volar pulp and fingertip using an island of skin from the non-dominant border of the digit. The flap is based upon **reverse flow** in the ipsilateral digital artery via volar communicating vessels from the other side at a level 5 mm proximal to the DIP joint crease. The digital artery is ligated proximal to the flap, and a segment of the dorsal nerve can be included for coaption to the distal stump of the digital nerve on the other side to render the flap sensate. A good functional outcome is possible even in elderly patients.

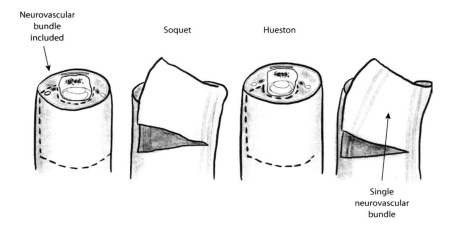

Figure 6.16 Soquet and Hueston flaps. In the latter, the ipsilateral NVB is also included to improve vascularity at the expense of advancement.

Digital artery perforator flaps for fingertip reconstructions. (Koshima I, *Plast Reconstr Surg*, 2006)
The authors describe five cases of using the small skin perforators from the digital arteries. A propeller-type flap is designed based on this perforator and rotated into the fingertip defect. Beginning proximally, the distal perforators are preserved during dissection under magnification. When no dominant perforators are found, an adipofascial base is kept for vascularity.

HETERODIGITAL FLAPS

The use of non-injured digits can provide large areas of tissue but at the expense of a normal digit and reduced sensation. Most of these are composed of dorsal skin.

- **Foucher or kite flap** (Foucher G, *Plast Reconstr Surg*, 1979) is based on the first DMCA. The distal skin paddle over the dorso-radial aspect of the PP of the index finger is a random pattern extension from the dorso-radial aspect over the distal second metacarpal. It was originally described for covering dorsal thumb defects (see above). The flap is raised with a pedicle 1–2 cm in width with fascia and epimysium using a dorsal lazy-S incision, leaving paratenon for graft take; nerves are deep to veins but superficial to arteries. In 20%, there may not be a definitive vessel, but there are several branches instead. The 'sink' branch at the level of the metacarpal head needs to be ligated. The superficial RN can be included for protective sensation. The donor site needs to be grafted.
- **Second and first DMCA flaps** (Earley MI, *Br J Plast Surg*, 1987) are based on the same principles as the Foucher flap and can cover **dorsal defects up to the**

PIPJ. There is a large anastomosing vessel between dorsal and palmar metacarpal arteries in the second web space, which needs to be ligated (this is the vessel for the Quaba flap). However, as the vein and artery lie on either side of the EC tendon, this does limit the arc of rotation. The second DMCA is larger than the first DMCA in one-third of hands and can be used as a free flap.
- **Quaba flap** (Quaba AA, *Br J Plast Surg*, 1990) is a distally based flap based on the communicating vessel between the second DMCA and the palmar vessel, which runs in the second web space. It is essentially a perforator-based propeller flap raised at the level of the paratenon, leaving the sensory nerves behind (though commonly the pedicle is not skeletonised). It is useful for full length defects of the dorsum of the finger.
- **Flag flap** (Vilain R, *Plast Reconstr Surg*, 1977) – the flag pole is the pedicle based on the dorsal vein, the dorsal branch of the digital artery and the dorsal branch of the digital nerve, which is based at a web space and can cover dorsal and palmar defects pivoted at the pedicle (Figure 6.17).
- **Cross-finger flaps** (Cronin TD, *Am Surg*, 1951) – a random dorsal skin flap (subdermal plexus) from the adjacent digit MP that is used mainly for volar defects of the digits. The flap can be based on any of the borders but most commonly laterally; it should not cross the knuckle creases. It is a relatively simple technique but is two-staged and the donor site needs a graft. Joints are immobilised in 30–40° of flexion for 10–14 days after which the flap is divided; some physiotherapy may be needed afterwards due to the stiffness.
  - The tissue is not an ideal pulp replacement as it is thin due to lack of subcutaneous tissue. The

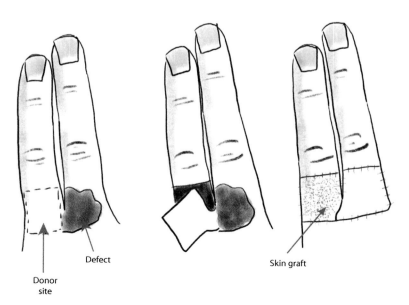

Donor site

Defect

Skin graft

Figure 6.17 Flag flap. The flap is rotated about the web space to cover adjacent defects.

average 2pd is 9 mm with recovery maximal after 1 year, and including a sensory nerve does not seem to make a functional difference – there may be some protective sensation.

- Many variations on the technique exist, including raising a skin-only flap over the definitive flap, which is a turnover de-epithelialised flap, i.e. **reverse cross-finger flap,** for dorsal defects.

- **Littler neurovascular flap** from the ulnar aspect of the middle finger classically, but can be harvested from other digits – e.g. the radial aspect of the ring finger for sensate coverage of the thumb. It is not often used due to the donor site morbidity.
- **Heterodigital venous flaps** for small defects, raised on the single vein pedicle from the dorsum over the PP for adjacent digits.

REGIONAL FLAPS

- **Thenar flap** – a reasonable choice for volar injuries of the index and middle fingers particularly in children (adults are prone to problems with contracture). Classically it is proximally based.
- **Reversed** (sacrifice of major vessel) or perforator-based radial forearm flap. Cosmesis of the donor site is the major issue with this flap.
- **Reversed ulnar artery flap** (can also be perforator based).
- **Posterior interosseous artery flap** (Zancolli EA, *Surg Radiol Anat,* 1986; Zancolli EA, *J Hand Surg,* 1988). The posterior interosseous vessels (from the ulnar artery) lie in the vertical septum radial to the ECU and ulnar to the EDM. They can support a fasciocutaneous flap with a long axis along a line joining the ulnar head to the lateral epicondyle (LE) when the arm is pronated. When distally pedicled, the ulna head is the pivot point with around three perforators.

DISTANT FLAPS

- Pedicled, e.g. groin or abdomen
- Free – first web space of the foot based on the first dorsal metatarsal artery from dorsalis pedis, dorsalis pedis flap (poor donor site), radial or ulnar flaps, lateral arm, para/scapular flaps, groin, etc.

DIGITAL NERVE INJURY

Primary repair with end-to-end repair with minimal tension with the finger extended is regarded as the gold standard. For nerve gaps 4–8 mm, a nerve graft can be regarded as the gold standard as well, but at a cost of the donor site.

What is evidence based reconstruction of digital nerves? A systematic review. (Rinkel WD, *J Plast Reconstr Aesthet Surg,* 2012)
There is not much evidence in the literature (eight RCTs), but it seems that

- There is no difference between fascicular or epineural repair.
- In sural nerve graft vs. vein conduit, there is no difference; vein conduits may have a role in emergency repair of defects up to 30 mm.
- There is very low quality evidence suggesting a role for polyglycolic conduits (Neurotube®) for defects 4–8 mm, possibly better than direct closure or autologous grafts.
- In Neurotube™ vs. vein graft, there is no difference.
- In Neurolac™ (polylactic acid) vs. end to end, there is no difference.

B. UPPER LIMB NERVE INJURIES

The commonest cause of brachial plexus injury (BPI) is high-velocity trauma particularly motorcycles (85%). Five per cent of all motorcycle injuries have BPI. The other large group are obstetric complications.

I. BRACHIAL PLEXUS ANATOMY

The brachial plexus has contributions from C5–T1; a plexus is termed pre-fixed or post-fixed if C4 or T2 contributes, respectively.

- 'Roots' – lie behind scalenus anterior
- Trunks – cross the lower part of the posterior triangle
- Divisions – lie behind the clavicle
- Cords – embrace the axillary artery behind the pectoralis minor

  - Lateral cord – musculocutaneous nerve
  - Posterior cord – radial and axillary nerves
  - Medial cord – median, ulnar and thoracodorsal nerves

The dorsal root contains sensory afferents with cell bodies (but no synapses) **outside of the spinal cord** in the dorsal root ganglion (DRG), whilst the ventral root contains motor efferents (relay in anterior horn cells). The ventral roots combine to form the spinal nerve that splits into anterior and posterior rami. It is the **anterior rami of C5–T1** that form the 'roots' of the brachial plexus (the posterior rami become the posterior intercostal nerves and supply the erector spinae muscles).

- The serratus anterior is innervated by the long thoracic nerve – from the nerve roots of C567: if there is no winging of the scapula, then the injury is more distal, i.e. in the nerve trunks.
- Erb's point marks the convergence of the C5 and C6 roots to form the upper trunk.

MILLESI CLASSIFICATION OF BPI

- I Supraganglionic.
- II Infraganglionic.
- III Trunk (or supraclavicular) – **about 75% of cases**.

- IV Cord (or infraclavicular) – e.g. shoulder dislocation. In general, it has a better prognosis than supraclavicular injuries.

LEFFERT CLASSIFICATION

- I – Open
- II – Closed
  - A Supraclavicular
    - Preganglionic
    - Postganglionic
  - B Infraclavicular
- III – Radiation induced
- IV – Obstetric
  - A Erb's (upper)
  - B Klumpke (lower)

PREGANGLIONIC VS. POSTGANGLIONIC

It is important to distinguish the **pattern of injury:** preganglionic injuries have little chance of recovery (roots avulsions are not repairable), whilst postganglionic injuries that remain in continuity have a chance of spontaneous recovery. A **preganglionic lesion** is where the disruption occurs at or proximal to the level of the DRG (e.g. root avulsion from the cord, intradural rupture of rootlets). Such lesions are within the spinal canal and hence are **not amenable to grafting** (or repair and thus usually treated by **nerve transfers**). As sensory nerves remain in continuity with their cell bodies in the DRG, sensory nerve action potentials may still be elicited. However, motor repair is not possible, as the nerves have been separated from the spinal cord (Figure 6.18).

Signs suggestive of preganglionic injury:

- **Denervation**/paralysis of paravertebral muscles – scalenus anterior, levator scapulae and rhomboids
  - Winging of the scapula (serratus anterior)
- **Horner's syndrome**
  - Partial ptosis, pupillary constriction, anhidrosis
- **Pseudomeningocoele** seen on myelography
- **Elevation of hemidiaphragm** (phrenic nerve C345, keeps the man alive)
- **Cervical spine fracture**
- **Sensory loss above shoulder/glenohumeral joint**, e.g. C34
- **Intractable pain**
- **Lack of Tinel's at the neck**
- **Sensory action potentials** in anaesthetic arm with absent motor potentials
- **Negative intra-operative somatosensory evoked potentials**

A **postganglionic lesion** is where the disruption occurs in the spinal nerve distal to the DRG. Wallerian degeneration leads to no recordable action potentials. The paracervical muscles are intact.

II. OBSTETRIC BPI

This occurs in ~1 per 1000 live births and is associated with

- Shoulder dystocia and high birth weight (maternal diabetes).
- Assisted delivery – breech presentation.
- Prolonged labour.
- Multiparity.
- It is very rare after caesarean section.

Diagnosis of injury is suggested by the lack of active movement with full passive mobility; **Horner's**

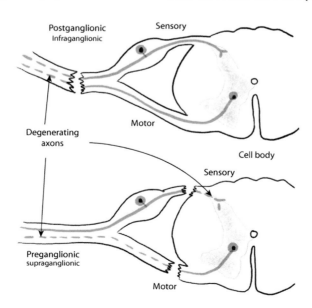

Figure 6.18 Types of brachial plexus injury. The dotted lines represent the axon segments that degenerate after the respective types of injury.

syndrome (due to interruption of sympathetic outflow via the stellate ganglion, near to C8, T1) is a strong sign; 5% are bilateral.

INVESTIGATIONS

Direct diagnostic imaging is difficult:

- CXR to check for elevation of the hemidiaphragm.
- Myelography in children (needs GA) has high false-positive rate for root avulsion.
- MRI unreliable.
- EMG can be used to select muscles for transfer; in ~20% of patients with EMG showing prolonged conduction block, good recovery is possible.

TYPES OF PALSY

- **C5, 6 (+/− 7). Erb's/Erb Duchenne palsy** due to downwards traction (or lateral flexion of the cervical spine or blow to the neck). It is the most common type of obstetric BPI (OBPI, Narakas type 1; ~75%).
  - Affects lateral and posterior cords (musculocutaneous, radial and axillary nerves).
  - Porter's or waiter's tip position – shoulder adduction and internal rotation, elbow extension, forearm pronation, wrist flexion and finger flexion.
  - If C7 is also involved, then the elbow may be slightly flexed.
  - C5–T1 – flail limb with claw hand, mottling due to vasomotor disturbance +/− Horners.
- **C7, 8, T1. Klumpke paralysis** is less common (2%–3%) and is due to traction upwards (breech delivery).
  - Affects medial cord (ulnar and median nerves).
  - Flail limb, claw hand, intrinsic muscle wasting, marbled appearance due to vasomotor changes, with or without Horner's syndrome.
- Where there is some or complete damage to all roots, is the second most common.

Note that the axillary and musculocutaneous nerves are at particular risk; there is often a second distal injury due to fixity and a superimposed traction injury at these points (quadrangular space and intramuscular, respectively).

Obstetric brachial palsy. (Kay SP, *Br J Plast Surg*, 1998)
Most cases make a full recovery (though a wide range has been reported, 30%–96%); poor recovery occurs more likely in patients with

- Lower root lesions, particularly those with Horner's syndrome
- Associated fractures of clavicle, ribs, humerus
- Avulsion injuries

Thus, it is advisable to wait at least 3 months for recovery of elbow flexion before exploring; if there is no return of **biceps**

function by 3 months of age, then exploration is warranted. Exploration is also indicated if there is failure of recovery to progress after 9 months.

- Early management consists of
  - **Physiotherapy** to maintain passive ROM whilst awaiting recovery and also allows spheroidal moulding of the humeral head and glenoid cavity
  - Indications for primary plexus exploration (repair, grafting):
    - Complete palsy with a flail arm
    - C5–6 palsy with no biceps contraction at 3 months
    - Horner's syndrome
    - Phrenic nerve involvement
- Late management – tendon transfers, etc.

III. TRAUMATIC BPI

These most commonly occur in young males (15–25) particularly motorcyclists. Most BPI are closed injuries due to traction, compression or a combination. Complete involvement of all roots is the most common pattern (75%); upper trunk only is the next most common (20%–25%), whilst lower trunk palsy is the most rare (1%–3%).

CAUSES OF NON-OBSTETRIC BPI

Rule of three's: repair within 3 days for sharp transection (nerves can still be stimulated), 3 weeks for blunt injury and 3 months for closed injury (lesions in continuity, if no clinical or electrophysiological improvement).

- **Road traffic accidents** are the most common cause (70%, and 70% of these involve motorcycles). Forceful abduction of the arm overhead injures the lower trunk, whilst violent bending of the neck tends to cause an upper trunk injury.
- **Open injuries** – it is important to exclude concomitant trauma to the axillary artery, which may cause life- or limb-threatening haemorrhage. Sharp open injuries should be explored with immediate brachial plexus repair.
  - Low-velocity bullet injuries may cause concussive effects (neuropraxia) on the plexus and transection is rare: explore after 3 months if no recovery.
- **Iatrogenic.**
  - **Post-surgery**, e.g. the lower trunk and long thoracic nerves are at risk during first rib resection in the thoracic outlet syndrome.
  - **Post-anaesthetic** BPI is usually a closed traction injury with an excellent prognosis and recovery is expected within 6 weeks. Avoiding excessive abduction of the arms or lateral neck flexion in unconscious patients may minimise these injuries. Nerve injury in the course of administering a brachial plexus block is rare but has been reported.

- **Post-radiotherapy** palsies have a poor prognosis due to the intraneural ischaemia and fibrosis. There are pain and paraesthesia that may be difficult to distinguish from tumour invasion. Any nerve grafts used should be wrapped in vascularised tissue, e.g. classically omentum (Chamorro M, *Br J Plast Surg*, 1993).

The surgical treatment of brachial plexus injuries in adults. (Terzis JK, *Plast Reconstr Surg*, 2000)

HISTORY

- **Age, occupation, hand dominance, hobbies and general health**.
- **Time**. This is the most important determinant of the final outcome; within 6 months, there is less end organ denervation, muscle atrophy, scarring, nerve retraction, etc.
- **Mechanism of injury** – open/closed, high/low velocity. **Limb position**, e.g. arm hyperabducted or neck laterally flexed?
- **Nature of injury**, e.g.
  - **Traction** – downward force with forced neck flexion (root/trunk injury), downward force on shoulder (upper trunk) and arm hyperabduction (lower trunk).
  - **Crush, direct blunt trauma to the neck and upper extremity** – plexus can be crushed between the clavicle and the first rib or compressed by haematoma or adjacent injured tissue elements.
  - Direct laceration.
  - Concomitant injuries.
- **Defect**
  - Immediate or delayed weakness in the arm?
  - Pre-existing neurological status.

EXAMINATION

- Thorough clinical examination, evaluation of vascularity of arm, specifically exclude **Horner's syndrome** and assess the function of the **phrenic** nerve
  - Use preprinted brachial plexus diagrams that include all muscle groups of the upper extremity, sensory mapping and pain threshold to document observations.

- Look – attitude of the limb (including winging of the scapula), wasting of muscles (delayed presentation), sudomotor changes, scars, swellings in the posterior triangle (subclavian artery aneurysm)
- Feel
  - Sensation of C5–T1 – pain and temperature, vibration, 2pd, touch, sweating.
  - Tinel's.
- Move
  - Test motor power (MRC, M2 is movement with gravity eliminated) at shoulder, elbow, wrist, fingers and thumb.
    - Winging of the scapula suggests a preganglionic injury (see above).
    - Test trapezius – SAN may be used for nerve transfer.
  - Nerve screening.
    - Axillary nerve (shoulder abduction).
    - RN (wrist extension – low, elbow extension – high).
    - Musculocutaneous nerve (elbow flexion).
    - Median and ulnar nerve (finger and wrist flexion).
  - Passive and active ROM of all joints.

INVESTIGATION

A priority is to classify the level of injury according to Millesi (see above). See Tables 6.3 and 6.4.

- **Radiographs** – complete radiological study of the cervical spine and the involved shoulder with special attention to the clavicle and scapula (more likely to be fractured in high-energy injuries).
  - **Fractures of the transverse processes may** be associated with avulsions of the corresponding roots, due to the attachments of the deep cervical fascia between the two.
  - Chest X-ray – hemidiaphragm elevation.
  - Rib fractures may imply concomitant damage to the plexus (first two) or potential intercostal nerve donors.
  - CT scan if there are any doubts particularly about the neck.
- **MRI** – this is less useful for (lower) root avulsions but provides good visualisation of the distal brachial plexus beyond the spinal foramen/nerve roots. It can also define shoulder anatomy.

Table 6.3 Summary of the actions used to screen for types of BPI

Levels	Action	Muscle; Nerve
Roots	Retract shoulders	Rhomboids; dorsal scapular (C5)
Trunk	Abduct shoulder to horizontal	Supraspinatus; suprascapular (C5,6)
Posterior cord	Adduct arm	LD; thoracodorsal (C7)
Medial cord	Push hands against hips	Sternal head of PM; medial pectoral (C8)
Lateral cord	Push hands together at shoulder level	Clavicular head of PM; lateral pectoral (C6)

Table 6.4 Summary of the methods used to screen for the motor functions of the main peripheral nerve branches from the brachial plexus

Peripheral nerve	Action for testing	Muscle tested
Axillary nerve (C5, 6)	Abduct shoulder above horizontal	Deltoid
Musculocutaneous (C5, 6)	Flex elbow	Biceps
Radial (C5–8)	Extend elbow	Triceps (C7)
	Extend wrist	ECRL, ECU (C7, 8)
Posterior interosseous (C8)	Extend fingers	EDC
Ulnar (C8–T1)	Cross fingers, PAD–DAB	Interossei (T1)
Median nerve (C5–T1)	Abduct thumb	Abductor pollicis (T1)
Anterior interosseous	'O' sign	

- MRA can be used as an alternative to angiography in cases with suspected vascular injury, e.g. axillary artery avulsion.
- **CT myelography** to demonstrate root avulsion particularly C8–T1; avulsion causes the dural sheath to heal with a meningocoele. The positive predictive value of combined CT myelography is more than 95% and is regarded as a '**gold standard**' investigation; however, avulsed roots can still exist despite a normal myelogram and occasionally a meningocoele occurs without nerve root avulsion i.e. the sign falls short of being pathognomonic. It is most useful to wait for >1 month after injury (for the meningocoele to form and for clot to clear).
  - MRI myelogram with T2 weighting. State-of-the-art techniques are capable of high-quality images, but MR myelography cannot replace CT myelography completely.
- **Electrophysiological studies** – Wallerian degeneration results in the emergence of spontaneous electrical discharges or **fibrillations**. Electromyography (EMG) and nerve conduction studies (NCS) should wait at least 3–6 weeks until these fibrillation potentials appear. Evoked potentials performed 4–6 weeks after the trauma/injury are more sensitive at identifying nerve continuity.
  - **Needle electromyogram** of the paraspinal muscles, innervated by the dorsal rami of the spinal roots, should also be routinely performed; denervation of the paraspinal muscles **(fibrillation potentials that appear weeks after)** provides strong evidence of avulsion of the corresponding roots. If these muscles are electrically intact, then the injury is most likely preganglionic and the root is most likely ruptured. Serial EMGs allow monitoring of any re-innervation with reduced fibrillation, nascent potentials and increased voluntary motor unit potentials (MUPs).
    - Looking for recruitment and abnormal spontaneous potentials such as positive sharp waves and **fibrillation,** which is low amplitude spontaneous activity found in denervated muscle (and is not visible through skin as compared to fasciculation).
    - MUPs will be reduced in number in denervated muscle, but the remaining MUPs will be normal; with time, however, they will increase two to three times in amplitude and become longer in duration.
    - Late responses, e.g. H reflex, F wave—may be abnormal but less useful overall.
- **Nerve conduction studies** (NCS) looking at nerve conduction velocity (NCV, m/s), which is reduced with demyelination (one of the first changes with chronic compression).
  - Most often used for main branches, e.g. median and ulnar; less commonly radial, musculocutaneous, axillary and subscapular.
  - Proximal NCS, e.g. C5–6, Erb's point, is technically possible, although difficult and can be uncomfortable.
  - **Amplitude** (related to the number of nerve fibres present, i.e. a marker of axonal degeneration) **is the key parameter**; distal latency and NCV are not that helpful.
  - Demyelinating conduction block is detectable during the first few weeks unless the axons are severed, i.e. it indicates a reasonably good prognosis.

For a closed injury, it is common to observe for 4–6 weeks before requesting electrodiagnostics.
- If some recovery is seen, then follow carefully until 3/12.
- If recovery is not appropriate or nonanatomic (e.g. hand recovery without axillary/musculocutaneous nerve function in complete BPI), then proceed to surgery. Investigate with MRI or CTM before surgery.

TREATMENT

Terzis states that the **delay** between accident and operation was prognostic for return of function but stressed the need for proper investigation rather than embarking on emergency surgery. Earlier surgery is indicated in high-velocity RTAs and in the presence of Horner's syndrome. In general,

- The best results are achieved with intervention before 6 months.
- Worse if delayed for more than a year.
- No benefit after 2 years.

Infraclavicular injuries had a better prognosis and if the injury was closed, then waiting 3–6 months for recovery before exploring was reasonable. A delay of >6 months would lead to more muscular atrophy, fibrosis and joint stiffness.

- In a **flail limb**, the priorities are elbow flexion and shoulder abduction/stability, followed by hand sensibility, wrist extension/finger flexion and then wrist flexion/finger extension.
- In a **total plexus injury**, the available donor nerves are the intercostals, SAN and phrenic (the latter two will require nerve grafts).

NON-SURGICAL TREATMENT

- Physiotherapy to maintain joint mobility.
- Functional bracing, splintage.
- Nerve stimulation of paralysed muscles to maintain motor end plates whilst awaiting recovery.
- Motor re-education and strengthening exercises.
- **Pain management.** Pain after BPI may be due to interruption of afferent signals (deafferentation), which can be intractable but may improve after nerve reconstruction. Patients with debilitating pain often have poor outcomes; **preoperative** pain relief permits patients to focus on rehabilitation. Drugs are the mainstay, e.g. narcotics, TCA, antipsychotics, sympathetic block and more recently gabapentin; involvement of a specialist pain team is useful.

SURGERY AFTER ~3 MONTHS (IMMEDIATELY IF SHARP INJURY)

- Neurolysis for neuroma in continuity
- Nerve grafts – for discontinuous injuries
- Nerve transfers if supraganglionic/root avulsion
- Muscle transfers – local or free

EXPLORATION

In general,

- Light anaesthesia without paralysing agents.
- Explore the brachial plexus through a lymphadenectomy approach in the posterior triangle – the omohyoid and the transverse cervical vessels are identified and retracted, and the phrenic nerve is identified. The incision is extended via the deltopectoral groove to the infraclavicular area.
  - Clavicle osteotomy optional – a risk of non-union or compression from callus; plating is usually avoided.

Intraoperative diagnosis: despite all the preoperative testing to assess the state of nerves, the **exact lesion (level, type and extent) can only be accurately determined at the time of surgery**. Intraoperative cortical evoked potentials can help determine whether there is supraganglionic injury.

- **Neuromas** (in continuity or at the end of a ruptured plexus segment) are usually found between the upper roots and the trunks, but may also be present distally at the cord or the peripheral nerve level. Neuromas should be excised to the level of healthy fascicles; resection and grafting provide better results than neurolysis alone.
  - Rising vital signs during resection of a neuroma indicates continuity with the spinal cord.
- **Avulsed spinal nerves** – feel empty to palpation, pale in appearance and negative to electrical stimulation. Biopsies of root with histochemistry can be useful.
- **Microneurolysis for 'hard' segments** – longitudinal epineurotomies to relieve pressure.

Nerve transfers and grafts: motor and sensory donors are matched to their corresponding distal targets. Restoration of sensation particularly of median and ulnar nerves is useful. Patient cooperation and motivation are vital to successful treatment; recovery from nerve grafting may take over 18 months, and all the while the patient has to maintain joint movement and manage deafferentation pain, etc. The availability of donors and the adequacy of graft material are the main concerns.

- **Intraplexus motor donors**, e.g. ipsilateral C5–7 roots that have escaped injury or proximal stumps of ruptured roots are preferred. Distal nerve transfers close to the target muscle would avoid the need for grafting and reduce the regeneration distances.
  - **Contralateral, e.g. C7 root.**
- **Extraplexus donors** (used in multiple-root avulsions), e.g. intercostal nerves, accessory nerve and contralateral C7 root.
- **Postganglionic injuries have the better prognosis** and are best treated with grafts between the motor donor and the distal target. Those with an isolated upper plexus injury do particularly well due to the sparing of the hand and only short grafts are needed.
  - **Nerve grafts** can be vascularised or non-vascularised (sural nerve ~ 40 cm, medial cutaneous nerve of the forearm ~ 20 cm); the former offer a faster reinnervation rate, at least in theory.

RESTORE JOINT MOVEMENT

- **Shoulder abduction** – transfer to suprascapular and axillary nerves; a 'good result' is 45° of abduction
  - Distal SAN (to suprascapular nerve).
  - Phrenic or cervical plexus (axillary).
- **Elbow flexion** – aiming to restore innervation of **biceps** and brachialis (musculocutaneous nerve)
  - Intraplexus donors, e.g. medial pectoral, thoracodorsal.
  - Extraplexus donors, e.g. distal SAN (may need a segment of nerve graft), phrenic nerve, intercostals (third to fifth, to be avoided with prior chest trauma).
    - The contralateral C7 (a good donor of large numbers of motor nerves and up to half can

be used) with a vascularised ulnar nerve to the median nerve is a useful way of restoring finger flexion (particularly in children).

- **Oberlin** (partial ulnar nerve, preferably FCU fascicles) transfer using one to two fascicles of the ulnar nerve to motor branch to biceps; recovery takes 4–6 months (faster than, e.g. the medial pectoral nerve) as the repair is close to the muscle. The success rate is also higher (97% > M3, 94% > M4) compared with nerve transfers (71% > M3, 37% > M4).
- **Hand sensation**
  - From intercostobrachial, intercostal sensory or supraclavicular nerves.
  - To the ulnar nerve in the upper arm, lateral cord to the median nerve.
  - Also transfer fourth web sensory supply to the first web.

MUSCLE TRANSFERS

- **Shoulder**
  - Trapezius transfer (to deltoid insertion) to restore abduction. Alternative is PM.
  - Advance the origins of biceps and triceps to the acromion (flexion/extension).
  - LD – taking the muscle around the humerus can restore external rotation (L'Episcopo).
  - Alternatively, particularly with severe injury, shoulder fusion to provide a stable platform for elbow transfers to work against – 30° abduction, flexion and internal rotation.
- **Elbow**
  - PM transfer – pedicled on the clavicular head into the forearm.
  - LD transfer (if the thoracodorsal nerve spared).
  - Triceps transfer to the biceps insertion to provide flexion (which is more important than extension) when the RN (posterior cord) is available but the musculocutaneous nerve (lateral cord) is not. The alternative is pectoralis minor to biceps.
  - Transfer the forearm flexor mass (medial epicondyle [ME]) higher up on the humerus so that the moment for elbow flexion is increased; it does require near-normal power in these muscles (flexor-pronator) for useful elbow flexion to occur. Steindler flexorplasty provides less power and ROM than LD transfer.

Adjunctive procedures may be considered if the injury is more than a year old.

- **Tendon transfers** should be considered in older patients (>40 years), though optimal results still require good passive ROM.
- **Arthrodeses to stabilise joints** if necessary, addressing shoulder, elbow, wrist (Sauvé–Kapandji procedure) and fingers in sequence.
- **Free functioning muscle transfers**, e.g. gracilis, contralateral LD and rectus abdominis, are a useful

option in total avulsions. They require an appropriate motor nerve for coaption and would need extra-plexus neurotisation; skin paddles can be included for soft tissue cover if needed.

In general, in terms of outcomes after BPI/surgery,

- Better outcomes in the young.
- Better prognosis with distal lesions.
- Better outcomes for infraganglionic lesions over root avulsions.
- Motor nerve transfers are usually better than nerve grafts.

Complete traumatic brachial plexus palsy. (Bentolila V, J Bone Joint Surg, 1999)

The authors state that the priorities in complete BPI are restoration of (in order)

- Elbow flexion (most important) – musculocutaneous nerve (lateral cord)
- Elbow and wrist extension – RN (posterior cord)
- Finger flexion for prehension – median nerve (medial cord), may need tendon transfers
- Shoulder abduction – axillary nerve (posterior cord)

If there is no central connection for repair

- Accessory nerve transfer to lateral cord or musculocutaneous nerve
- Grafts from intercostal, accessory and thoracodorsal nerves (if spared) to distal stumps

IV. MECHANISMS OF NERVE INJURY

CLASSIFICATION OF NERVE INJURY

Wallerian degeneration is the orthograde/anterograde degeneration in the nerve distal to the site of division, ultimately to the end receptor. This begins at 24 hours and takes ~6 weeks, being slower in the CNS compared with the peripheral nervous system (PNS).

- **Axonal degeneration** is followed by degradation of myelin sheath with macrophage infiltration to clear debris. The axonal disintegration is an active process and is dependent on ubiquitin and calpain proteases.
- The neurolemma remains as a hollow tube to provide pathways for regenerating axons that begin sprouting (growth cone and filopodia) after 4 days. The limiting step seems to be transportation of cytoskeletal elements along the axon; generally the rate is described as 1 mm/day plus 30 days with an apparent initial latent period. Pure motor or sensory nerves recover better than mixed nerves.
  - Augustus Waller observed this sequence after severing the IX/XII nerves in frogs (1850).
- **Retrograde degeneration** is the 'die-back' in the nerve **proximal** to the site of division back to the next most proximal branch and the cell body undergoes

changes that include chromatolysis. Regenerative sprouting proceeds down the original Schwann cell myelin sheath but through new endoneural tubules.
- Scar blocks sprouting axons.

CLASSIFICATION

Table 6.5 Nerve injuries and their classification; Seddon (1943) and Sunderland (1951) compared.

Sir Sydney Sunderland modified the surgical model of Sir Herbert Seddon into an anatomical one (1951). Sunderland classification relates to the conduction block (numbers are 'degrees' of nerve injury): 1–3 will recover usually without surgery; 4–5 will need surgery. The sixth degree is a combination of I–V injuries (Mackinnon), a pragmatic addition reflecting the fact that a nerve may have varying degrees of pathology at different levels. Nerve compression impairs axonal transport function of the whole nerve and increases susceptibility to a second injury, i.e. **double-crush phenomenon**. She uses the term 'neuroma in continuity'; the recovery pattern will be mixed (Table 6.5).

NCS would be expected to yield the following results in nerve injuries:

- Neuropraxia – absent conduction over the site of the block, normal above and below
- Incomplete lesion – prolonged latency, reduced amplitude
- Complete lesion – no conduction

PROGNOSIS

Regeneration occurs at a rate between 1 and 3 mm/day (advancing Tinel's sign). Muscles can potentially regain ~100% of function even after 1 year of denervation provided that enough axons reach the motor end plates.

- Younger patient age and more distal transections do better, i.e. division close to motor end plates better than proximal division.

- Sharp transection injuries usually have better recovery than avulsion injuries.

Recovery can be graded by the Medical Research Council (MRC) grading for both sensory and motor return.

SENSORY RECOVERY – MRC GRADING OF FUNCTION

- S0: no recovery
- S1: deep pain
- S1: + superficial pain
- S2: light touch
- S2: + hyperaesthesia to light touch
- S3: 2pd >15 mm
- S3: + 2pd 7–15 mm
- S4: complete recovery (2pd 3–6 mm)

Innervation density tests – moving and static 2pd. Getting 2/3 correct is deemed a pass; the normal 2pd decreases proximally from 4 mm at the tip of the finger to 8 mm at the mid-palm.

Threshold tests – Semmes–Weinstein monofilament, vibration.

Motor recovery – MRC grading of function

- M0 – no contraction
- M1 – perceptible contraction of proximal muscles/'flicker'
- M2 – perceptible contraction of proximal and distal muscles/movement with gravity eliminated
- M3 – recovery to allow contraction against gravity
- M4 – recovery of power allowing synergistic and independent movements/gravity and resistance
- M5 – complete recovery

PRINCIPLES OF REPAIR

Closed nerve injuries

The majority show signs of spontaneous recovery within 12 weeks and are managed conservatively.

- **Observe for 4–6 weeks; if there is no evidence of clinical recovery, request NCS and EMG** (except in cases where injury localises to known areas

Table 6.5 Nerve injuries and their classification; Seddon (1943) and Sunderland (1951) compared

Seddon	Sunderland	Insult	Prognosis
Neuropraxia	First degree	Segmental demyelination, interruption of axon conduction whilst anatomic continuity maintained. Recovery by remyelination, regeneration not required.	Full recovery 1–4 months
Axonotmesis	Second degree	Axon severed, endoneurium intact. Wallerian degeneration and proximal nerve regenerates. Recovery is complete unless end organ has degenerated.	Full recovery 4–18 months
Neurotmesis	Third degree	Endoneurium (and axon) disrupted. Incomplete scar block causes incomplete recovery.	Incomplete recovery
Neurotmesis	Fourth degree	Perineurium disrupted. Complete scar block with no recovery unless block removed and nerve repaired.	Incomplete recovery
Neurotmesis	Fifth degree	Epineurium disrupted, i.e. total loss of nerve continuity	No recovery

of entrapment, consider earlier investigation and intervention).

- If there is some recovery, then continue conservative therapy.
- **If there is no evidence of recovery by 3 months, consider surgical intervention.** Explore with intraoperative NCS – if there is some signal, then neurolysis; otherwise, excise and graft.

Open repair

Primary repair within 10 days if at all possible is preferred. Some define repair on the day/at the time as primary repair, up to 7 days as delayed primary repair and after 7 days as secondary repair.

- Aim for good fascicular **alignment** with superficial bites that do not go deep into the nerve tissue. Connective tissue constitutes 1/4 to 3/4 of the cross-sectional area of the nerve (quite high in the sural nerve).
- Sunderland demonstrated that nerves can move from one fascicle to another and that the longest length with a consistent pattern is about 15 mm.
  - **Epineurial suture** (most commonly used) in small purely sensory or motor nerves, e.g. digital nerves. The **vascular pattern of the vaso nervorum** and the fascicular pattern can be used for orientation. Avoid deep bites with the needle; use the minimal number of sutures to reduce the foreign body response and bulk. It is common to leave sutures long for manipulation and to use fibrin glue (or similar) at the end.
  - **Grouped fascicular repair** may be considered in larger nerves.
  - **Individual fascicular repair** offers no advantage in terms of outcomes in clinical studies; additional scarring offsets any advantage from improved alignment, meaning that superior outcomes have not been demonstrated.
  - Improved matching:
    - **Mirror image matching.**
    - **Topography**, e.g. the ulnar nerve in the forearm has three fascicles: ulnar sensory, radial volar sensory and dorsal motor, and after the dorsal sensory branch has been given off, then there are two fascicles, with the motor branch ulnar to the sensory until Guyon's canal. Similar patterns have been noted for major peripheral nerves.
    - **Histochemical staining** (initially took 24 hours, now possible within 1 hour but not always available); acetylcholinesterase, carbonic anhydrase.
    - **Awake stimulation** – within 72 hours; otherwise, remaining neurotransmitters are depleted. It also requires a cooperative patient who is able to describe the exact site and nature (motor – dull ache; sensory – sharp pain).

- For neuroma-in-continuity, do not separate out functioning fascicles (stimulators) from the neuroma as the micro/neurolysis may cause additional damage.
  - Transect the non-functioning and repair with grafts around/outside of the neuroma. Patients over 30 do poorly; those over 40 years old have minimal recovery, and early tendon transfers should be considered.
- Nerve endings should be trimmed to healthy tissue, and repairs should be covered by vascular tissues.
- Avoid excessive tension/mobilisation – **gaps >2–2.5 cm** should be grafted (reversed to reduce axonal escape).
  - **Suturing under tension** that causes >20% increase in the length of the nerve is likely to cause conduction impairment. Some length may be gained under certain circumstances by transposition, e.g. the ulnar nerve at the elbow or the intratemporal dissection of the facial nerve.
- **Nerve grafts** means that regenerating axons have to cross two sets of anastomoses; they can be harvested from
  - The sural nerve (35–40 cm) found posterior to the medial malleolus – numbness to the lateral aspect of the foot dorsum.
  - The lateral cutaneous nerve of the forearm (8 cm) next to the cephalic vein.
  - The medial cutaneous nerve of the forearm (20 cm) next to the basilic vein.
  - The PIN – short segment at the end of the nerve.
- End to side nerve transfer. The proximal end of the distal nerve segment, sutured to a side window of a normal nerve, with minimal deficit to the donor nerve.
- Autologous nerve transplantation is nearly always possible, if not **nerve conduits** (NCs) may be considered. They seem to be better for small sensory nerves. Options include the following:
  - Silicone and PTFE tubes. Early use based on biocompatibility and availability; most current NCs are made of biodegradable materials, e.g. polyglycolic acid (Neurotube™), and can be quite pricey.
  - **Vein conduit** acceptable for defects **up to 3 cm;** tendency to collapse and may actually **hinder** growth.
  - Bone, denatured skeletal muscle.
  - Nerve allograft (MacKinnon SE, *Plast Reconstr Surg*, 2000); as allograft only needed temporarily, immunosuppression can be stopped after ~6 months.
  - Fibronectin impregnated with growth factors, pseudosynovial sheaths.
  - Human nerve growth factor (NGF) and glial growth factor (GGF) may augment regeneration. Nerve conduits guide the regenerating nerves, but improved recovery may come from also providing GF delivery (Madduri S, *J Control Release*, 2012).

GENERAL PROGNOSIS

Use a tourniquet for a bloodless field; fascicular repair is feasible at the wrist where the ulnar and median nerves are well separated into fascicles.

- **Median nerve** – slow and incomplete recovery is typical. With proximal injuries, recovery of the forearm is possible but not of the distal thenar groups; wrist injuries do better with some return of thumb opposition. Sensory recovery is usually better than motor, but maximal recovery is not reached until 5 years.
- **Ulnar nerve** – results of repair at the wrist tend to be poor (in contrast to the median nerve).
- **RN** – injuries due to closed fractures of the humerus or radius tend to recover spontaneously, whilst those associated with open fractures or occurring after fracture reduction should be explored.

FUNCTIONAL RECOVERY

Muscle fibres undergo atrophy, and motor end plates decline at a rate of 1% per week. Thus, early surgery is recommended; repairing after a delay of >1.5 years is probably futile.

NEUROMA

The diagnosis of a neuroma may be suggested by

- Pain and exquisite tenderness
- Pain when moving adjacent joints
- Pressure pain
- Dysaesthesia in the distribution of the nerve

  Common sites for upper limb neuromas include

- Palmar cutaneous branch of the median nerve
- Superficial branches of the RN or the radial digital nerves
- Dorsal branch of the ulnar nerve

  The neuroma may be in-continuity or an end-neuroma:

- Neuroma-in-continuity
    - Spindle – chronic irritation in an intact nerve (e.g. entrapment of the lateral cutaneous nerve of the thigh).
    - Lateral – develops at a site of the partial nerve division or following nerve repair and is generally smaller.
- End-neuroma – often follows traumatic nerve division or amputation

MANAGEMENT

Non-surgical conservative management includes

- Desensitisation exercises especially vibration (stimulation of large Aβ-fibres to damp out smaller pain fibres)

- Transcutaneous electrical nerve stimulation (TENS)
- Drugs – carbamazepine, etc.

SURGICAL MANAGEMENT

The nerve can be identified by selective nerve blocks and examination with percussion (Tinel's). Nerves in the hands that are important functionally should be grafted if possible.

- **Resection and coagulation** – bipolar, cryotherapy, chemical (alcohol, formaldehyde), laser, etc. Surgical strategies include the following:
    - Ligation or crushing; multiple sectioning may form multiple smaller neuromas.
    - Capping (silicone, vein, Histoacryl glue®) or epineural repair over the cut end.
    - Lateral neuromas can be treated by resection and repair of the disrupted perineurium of the involved fascicles only.
- **Bury the nerve ending.**
    - In nearby muscle (of low excursion) or bone (especially for finger/hand amputations where muscles are small or have large excursions) or depending on the location, e.g. into the PP or metacarpal in palm/digits, into PQ at wrist and into the BR at the forearm.
    - Implantation into a nerve, e.g. centro-central implantation into another nerve or implantation into the same nerve.

V. NERVE COMPRESSION SYNDROMES

NERVE INTERCONNECTIONS

Nerve compression and diagnosis of the level of nerve injuries can be made more difficult by the presence of the following anatomical variations.

- **Martin–Gruber anastomosis** (Taams KO, *J Hand Surg Br*, 1997). A branch from the median nerve joins onto the ulnar nerve in the forearm, which provides all the motor fibres to the ulnar nerve. Thus, lesions to the ulnar nerve above this branch cause no motor deficit, whilst lesions to the median nerve cause a simian hand. This connection is present in ~23% of subjects.
- **Riche–Cannieu anastomosis**. This is similar to the Martin–Gruber anastomosis but occurs in the palm of the hand. It is more common and is found in up to 70% of subjects. It may allow for improved prognosis in low divisions of the median and ulnar nerves at the wrist.
- **Nerve of Henlé**. This is a branch of the ulnar nerve in the forearm that travels with the ulnar artery to supply sensation to the distal medial forearm and proximal hypothenar eminence. It is present in ~40% of subjects, and in these cases, the palmar cutaneous branch of the ulnar nerve will be absent.

PATHOGENESIS OF NERVE COMPRESSION

There are a wide variety of possible causes of compression.

- Anatomical, e.g. carpal tunnel (CT)
- Postural – which may be related to occupational factors
- Developmental – cervical rib, palmaris profundus
- Inflammatory – tennis elbow, synovitis, scleroderma, amyloid, gout
- Traumatic – lunate anterior dislocation, hand trauma, midshaft of humerus fracture (radial)
- Metabolic – pregnancy, myxoedema, diabetes
- Tumour – ganglia, neoplasms
- Iatrogenic – trapped by plate fixation devices, inappropriate positioning on operating table, tourniquet, plaster casts (e.g. peroneal)

Increased compression pressure reduces intraneural blood flow:

- 20–30 mmHg – impaired epineural venous flow
- 30 mmHg – **axonal transport halted;** there is endoneural oedema.
- 30–40 mmHg – anaesthesia.
- 50 mmHg – reduced arteriolar flow, epineural oedema.
- **>60 mmHg – perfusion stops** and complete ischaemia leads eventually to fibrosis.
  - Altered nerve physiology makes a compressed nerve susceptible to a 'double crush' from injury at a second site.

Initially, these changes are temporary and reversible, but long-term circulatory impairment may result from mechanical injury to intraneural blood vessels.

- The most common symptom of nerve compression is **pain**, even in pure motor nerves. Patient descriptions are often vague; provocation tests exacerbate/reproduce the symptoms.
- Involvement of motor nerves causes weakness and wasting.
- **Nerve conduction tests (with nerve conduction speeds NCS) are the most sensitive tests for nerve compression with demyelination.**
- **EMG is most helpful for detecting denervation** with axonal loss (fibrillation potentials after >3 weeks).

COMPRESSION NEUROPATHY OF THE MEDIAN NERVE

The median nerve (C5–T1) arises from the lateral and medial cords of the brachial plexus. It runs between the intermuscular septum and the brachialis passing medial to the brachial artery. It passes below the ligament of Struthers, the bicipital aponeurosis and between the heads of PT in the forearm, deep to the FDS arch and under PL at the CT. The nerve generally does not supply anything above the elbow, though in some cases, the branch to PT can come off just above. In the hand, it supplies the LOAF muscles. The usual sequence is as follows:

- PT, FCR, FDS, PL, AION, FDP and PL.
- There are nerve cross-overs with the ulnar nerve in 80%.

ANATOMICAL SITES OF COMPRESSION

- Pronator syndrome
- Anterior interosseous syndrome (nerve to FPL, FDS index and middle, PQ)
- CTS

PRONATOR SYNDROME

There is pain in the proximal volar forearm that increases with activity and with resisted forearm pronation. It is accompanied by decreased sensation in the median nerve territory (over PT down to the thumb and the index – including the palm) with NCS showing increased **latency** at the elbow. EMG demonstrates fibrillations in FPL and PQ but is generally not helpful. Pronator syndrome deficits are sensory and motor with loss of precision pinch. It is commonly due to compression at one of four sites:

- Beneath the **ligament of Struthers** (attaches the humeral head of PT at the supracondylar process of the humerus 5 cm above the ME to the ME – a *relatively rare* variant [1%]). Test by flexing the elbow against resistance.
  - John Struthers (1823–1899) was a professor of anatomy at Aberdeen.
- Beneath the **lacertus fibrosus** (bicipital aponeurosis) – provoke by resisted elbow flexion with forearm supination.
- Where the nerve passes between the humeral and ulnar heads of **pronator teres (most common)** – provoke with resisted pronation with extended arm.
- Under arch of the FDS – provoke by resisted flexion of the MF PIPJ.

TREATMENT

- Splint in neutral/slight pronation, wrist at 15° of dorsiflexion and elbow 90° flexion for 4–6 weeks, along with NSAIDs and activity modification. It may work in up to 50%.
- Release the nerve by dissecting it out from a point 5 cm above the elbow to below the bicipital aponeurosis, dividing the possible compressing structures above.

COMPARING CTS WITH PRONATOR SYNDROME

With pronator syndrome,

- There is less of a nocturnal pattern with symptoms.
- There is **no Tinel's sign at the wrist** (in proximal third of the forearm instead).
- Nerve conduction may be delayed but not at the wrist; NCS can be normal as the compression may be intermittent/postural.
- However, Phalen's test is positive in 50% of patients with pronator syndrome (elbow flexion may compress the nerve in its tunnel).
- Palmar cutaneous branch is affected.

AION SYNDROME

The AION is a branch of the median nerve that arises 4–6 cm below the elbow and supplies FPL, FDP (index and middle) and PQ. There may be multiple sites of compression in the distal forearm:

- **Gantzer's muscle** (accessory head FPL).
- Muscles and fascial bands at their origins, e.g. PT, FDS, FCR.
- Aberrant radial artery.
- Thrombosis of the ulnar collateral vessel, aberrant radial artery in the forearm.
- **Trauma** – fractures/penetrating injury.
- HNPP (hereditary neuropathy with liability to pressure palsies) should be considered in those with multiple nerve compressions (spontaneous recovery is common); AD inheritance, with deletion/mutation in PMP22 on chromosome 17 (genetic testing is available).

AION syndrome is relatively rare, making up less than 1% of all nerve compression syndromes. Patients tend to present with pain in the forearm and **weakness of pinch grip** – when asked to make an 'O' or 'OK' sign between the index finger and the thumb to test for the FPL and the index FDP, those with the syndrome tend to make a triangle. There is **no sensory deficit**, and the presence of a Martin–Gruber anastomosis (see above) may complicate interpretation.

- MF FDS flexion test.
- NCS indicates latency in the upper forearm.
- Rest, activity modification, NSAIDs.
- Dissect out the nerve from its origin to the lower third of the forearm (may need to detach both heads of the PT) and divide vessels that cross over it.

CARPAL TUNNEL SYNDROME

Anatomy of the CT

The transverse carpal ligament or flexor retinaculum (FR) attaches to the scaphoid tubercle and the trapezium on the radial side and to the hook of the hamate and the pisiform on the ulnar side. There are 10 structures in the CT: median nerve, FPL and eight finger flexors. FDP tendons lie side by side, whilst the FDS tendons stack up like crossing fingers (try it), MF and RF on top of IF and LF tendons.

- The **palmar cutaneous branch of the median nerve** arises 4–6 cm proximal to the FR and passes superficial to it (occasionally, this nerve may pierce it from deep to superficial and suffer from an entrapment syndrome of its own).
- The **motor branch** may follow several common variations in anatomy (Lanz U, *J Hand Surg*, 1977); other variations are rare. It arises from the radiovolar aspect of the nerve; **Kaplan's line** (apex of the first web to the hook of the hamate or the ulnar border of the

abducted thumb) intersection with the index–middle finger web provides a rough approximation to the motor branch.
- **Extraligamentous branch**, arises distal to the FR and runs in a recurrent to thenar muscles (~50%)
- **Subligamentous branch**, arises beneath the FR and emerges out of the CT distal to the FR, to run recurrent to thenar muscles (~30%)
- **Transligamentous branch**, emerging beneath the FR and piercing it to reach the thenar eminence (~20%).

CAUSES OF CTS

Causes of CTS can be either congenital or acquired, but it is **idiopathic** in the majority of cases. Literature reviews, e.g. Palmer, (*Best Pract Res Clin Rheumatol*, 2011), suggest that there is reasonable evidence that prolonged used of powered vibratory tools or prolonged repetitive flexono and extension of the risk at least doubles the risk of CTS. The evidence for keyboard/computer use is not strong.

- Congenital
  - Persistent median artery.
  - High origin of lumbrical muscles.
- Acquired
  - Inflammatory – synovitis, RA, gout.
  - Traumatic – perilunate dislocation, Colles's fracture.
  - Fluid retention – pregnancy, renal failure, cardiac failure, myxoedema, diabetes, steroid medication.
  - Space-occupying lesions – lipoma, ganglion.
  - Effort-associated CTS may be due to the lumbricals causing symptoms with repetitive gripping.

SYMPTOMS

Compression of the median nerve within the carpal canal was first described by Paget in 1854. Approximately 1% of the population is affected. It affects **females** six times more frequently; 40% have bilateral involvement. Patients present with

- Weakness/clumsiness – decrease in fine motor skills, e.g. writing, dropping things.
- Pain in the hand, occasionally referred proximally.
- **Sensory disturbance (hyperaesthesia/paraesthesia) especially at night in the radial 3 and 1/2 fingers (index and thumb). The palm is spared.**
- Morning stiffness and numbness.
- Sympathetic dysfunction in 55% (Verghese J, *Muscle Nerve*, 2000) – consisting of swelling of the fingers, dry palms, Raynaud's phenomenon and blanching of the hand. Sympathetic skin response (SSR) has a sensitivity/specificity ratio of 34/89% in CTS with autonomic symptoms. Associated with female gender but not age, duration of disease or clinical severity.

- Some suggest using skin capacitance measured with a Corneometer to aid diagnosis (Ibrahim I, *Ortop Traumatol Rehabil*, 2012).

When assessing the patient, the entire upper limb should be examined and more proximal compressions, e.g. in the neck, should be excluded. Hand examination should focus attention on

- Median nerve sudomotor changes
- Muscle wasting
- Objective assessment of sensory deficit and motor deficit

CTS is a clinical diagnosis; nerve studies can be useful to confirm the diagnosis when there is doubt, e.g. in diabetic neuropathics; dual pathologies, e.g. coexistent higher nerve compression, to determine severity, to localise level of problem and to monitor post-operative progress (improvement would be expected within 2 weeks of surgery).

- Electrophysiological testing demonstrating median nerve latency >4 ms is diagnostic, but a normal latency does not rule out CTS – 10%–15% of those with classic clinical signs of CTS have false-negative NCSs. When compression is severe, NCS may not record a sensory action potential. Electrophysiological studies are not needed in every case.
  - Sensory NCS is more sensitive than motor – 70%–90% vs. 35%–55%.
- EMG is useful in assessing nerve degeneration and differentiating CTS from root compression. It is also important to appreciate that they are snapshots of the status only at the time of testing.
  - Negative tests are generally not that useful, e.g. 30% false negative in **cubital** tunnel syndrome, 6%–8% in CTS.
  - Where positive, it can give location and extent of compression.
- Threshold tests such as Semmes–Weinstein may show reduced sensation but innervation density tests, e.g. 2pd, are often normal (unlike nerve injuries).

Diagnosis of carpal tunnel syndrome. (Gunnarsson LG, *J Hand Surg*, 1997)

Clinical examination by an experienced doctor is usually sufficient to diagnose typical CTS. However, atypical symptoms or signs, or a prior history of fracture in the limb, may warrant the use of NCS.

- Numbness in the median nerve distribution is the most sensitive symptom (95%) but is not very specific (26%).
- **Phalen's test** is more sensitive (86%) than Tinel's sign (62%) but less specific (48% vs. 57%).
  - In the former, the flexed wrist compresses the nerve between the edge of the CT and the radius (30–60 seconds), whilst the latter is direct percussion. Some have described a reversed Phalen's (2 minutes).
  - Tinel was a French neurologist. George Phalen was an American orthopaedic surgeon.

- **NCS can be used if unsure**; they are highly sensitive (85%) and specific (87%), but there is a **10% false-negative rate**.

MANAGEMENT

Non-operative treatment may be considered when entrapment of the nerve may be temporary, e.g. pregnancy.

- **Activity modification and NSAIDs**; the latter may be more effective in those with tendonitis. Avoid repetitive/prolonged wrist flexion.
- **Steroid (hydrocortisone) injections** just proximal to distal wrist crease and ulnar to PL – one-third have maintained relief of symptoms at 3 months, 10%–20% at 18 months. However, there is a risk of tendon/nerve injuries.
  - Benefit lasting <2 weeks or requiring three or more injections is an indication for surgery.
- **Futuro (wrist) splint** (stabilises wrist whilst allowing finger movements) at night and during provoking activities. Some patients benefit but not as much as with surgery. The optimal regime, including which is the best splint (OTC vs. custom, neutral or resting position), is not clear.
  - Futuro is a brand of splints designed by Jung G Jr (1917); it was sold to 3M in 2008.
- **Unclear benefit** – vitamin B6, (nerve and tendon) gliding exercises and ultrasound.

OPERATIVE

- Longitudinal release of the transverse carpal ligament (Brain WR, *Lancet*, 1947)
- Endoscopic release

OPEN PROCEDURE

Surgery provides superior results and is generally safe. The key to success is **complete release** regardless of incision type.

- LA, tourniquet.
- Incision in line with the radial border fourth ray and ulnar back-cut.
- Spread superficial palmar fascia to reveal and spare transversely orientated nerve fibres, then divide the transverse carpal ligament from proximal to distal preserving the median nerve under direct vision.
  - If concerned about the motor branch, look for this specifically.
  - If concerned about the ulnar nerve compression, then release it as well.
- Irrigate the wound and close 5/0 prolene (remove at 2 weeks).
- **Post-operative splint** for 3–4 days then change to a Futuro splint (to prevent wrist flexion but allow finger flexion) for about 2 weeks, and then used at night or whilst driving for another month. However, there is some debate over splints – they do not speed up recovery and

may cause more temporary pain/tender scars and a slower return to work (Henry SL, *Plast Reconstr Surg*, 2008).

- Formal rehabilitation accelerates recovery, but the final function and outcome are the same as home exercise programs.
- No proven benefit for epineurotomy (Borisch N, *J Hand Surg [Br]*, 2003) or tenosynovectomy (Shum C, *J Bone Joint Surg*, 2002).

Overall, there is 92% patient satisfaction, and these patients would have the same operation on the other side.

RECOVERY

- 'Immediate' relief of pins and needles
- 2pd – recovery takes about 2 weeks
- Sensory and motor nerve latencies, i.e. NCS – 3–6 months
- Pinch and grip strength – 6–9 months
  - Long-standing cases with muscle atrophy may need opponensplasty.

The more severe the symptoms and the longer the duration, the longer it takes to recover. The average time for returning to work is 3–5 weeks. Overall, 90% will improve significantly.

COMPLICATIONS

The most common complication is a sensitive palmar scar (62%). Serious complications are rare:

- Intra-operative – injury to median nerve or deep palmar arch
- Early – infection, haematoma, dehiscence
- Late – inadequate release (persistent symptoms), flexion weakness, tender scar, CRPS, nerve injury/neuroma
  - **Pillar pain** is persistent discomfort in hypo/thenar eminences that may be caused by sensory nerve damage or widening of carpal arch and is also possible after endoscopic surgery.
  - Hyperaesthesia and neurological complications, e.g. pisitriquetral pain syndrome.

ENDOSCOPIC SURGERY

With shorter incisions, it aims to reduce scar/palm tenderness to allow faster recovery but has not consistently shown significant difference in terms of outcomes, e.g. sick leave, time to ADL/work. In addition, it involves more blind dissection, which leads to a steeper learning curve and other complications especially nerve injury (motor branch, palmar branch).

- Earlier recovery of pinch and grip strength at 3/52 but **no difference at 3 months (80%)**
- **Less post-operative pain**, avoids painful hand scar especially hypertrophic scar at the distal wrist crease

There are many variants:
- The **3M Agee**/'Inside job' (now Microaire) is a single-port device that uses a composite blade and scope system.
  - Named after JM Agee, introduced in 1990 initially, withdrawn and redesigned in 1992.
- A two-portal system developed by **Dyonics** ('Chow' device) – a proximal incision starting 1 cm proximal and radial to pisiform is used to introduce a trocar into the tunnel and the palm. Inserting a device into the tight confines of the carpal tunnel risks causing damage to the median nerve. Small windows increase the risk of injury to the palmar arch and the motor branch of the median nerve (see below) as well as incomplete division.
  - Designed by orthopaedic surgeon James CY Chow.
- These were the early devices; other manufacturers such as Athrex, Brown-Instratek, Linvatek and ECTRA II have introduced newer devices on similar themes.

Complications associated with endoscopic surgery include

- Conversion to open surgery 14%
- Failure to divide completely 4%
- Guyon's canal release due to incorrect placement and possible ulnar nerve injury

Neurovascular damage should be repaired if possible; further management of delayed nerve symptoms is often deferred for several weeks if mild and incomplete but should be explored if complete. If the superficial palmar arch is accidentally cut, it can usually be safely ligated except in rare cases where there is an incomplete deep arch and the digits remain pale. Post-operative pain may be due to developing regional pain syndrome. The variety of different endoscopic techniques/modifications makes comparison difficult; there are no RCTs.

A meta-analysis of randomized controlled trials comparing endoscopic and open carpal tunnel decompression. (Thoma A, *Plast Reconstr Surg*, 2004)
This is a meta-analysis of 13 RCTs that compared endoscopic release with open release. Methodological issues reduced the number of conclusions that could be drawn. It found that endoscopic surgery was associated with the following:

- Improved post-operative pinch and grip strength in the early post-operative phase (12 weeks) and less scar tenderness
- Increased risk of reversible nerve injury (three times compared with open release) – but uncommon with either technique
- No difference in post-operative pain or time to return to work

Endoscopic release is a well-established technique that has some benefits (shorter scar, slightly faster recovery, slightly less early pain) but slightly higher complication and recurrence rates. Some (TJ Fischer) believe that the benefits do not outweigh the risk of median nerve injury (unable to view variants of motor branch, 4.3% reversible nerve injury vs. 0.9% in open surgery).

Relative contraindications for endoscopic surgery include the indications for open surgery (see below) – when the contents of the tunnel need exploration, e.g. mass lesions, synovitis, associated with an acute fracture and cases of recurrent CTS/revisional surgery.

Endoscopic versus open versus mini incisions

An **open approach** allows the surgeon to be fairly confident of complete release, reducing the risk of inadvertent damage and allowing concomitant Guyon's canal release. Patients tend to have longer off work (the evidence is not that strong), and a tender scar persists for months.

Common indications for open surgery include the following:

- Revisional surgery/recurrence
- Acute burns (see 'burns') due to direct injury, reperfusion, over-resuscitation, etc.
- Other surgery planned, e.g.
  - Opponensplasty.
  - Synovectomy – generally not needed except those with florid disease such as rheumatoid and amyloid.
  - CTS associated with acute fracture.
  - Neurolysis is of little benefit with risks of scarring and further tethering; it will usually need to be combined with other procedures to reduce adhesions, e.g. vein wrap, muscle flaps, steroids or early motion.

RECURRENT CTS

Surgical release of CTS typically has a high success rate with up to 90% returning to their old jobs. Causes of recurrent symptoms after surgery include

- Incomplete division of the FR
- Median nerve compressed by scar tissue
- Flexor tenosynovitis, i.e. wrong diagnosis

Secondary carpal tunnel surgery. (Tung TH, *Plast Reconstr Surg*, 2001)

Reasons for further surgery include the following scenarios.

- Persistent symptoms after surgery (7%–20% reported incidence) are commonly due to **inadequate release** (usually distally). However, it may also be due to additional undiagnosed proximal compression ('double crush') or misdiagnosis.
- Recurrent symptoms (i.e. previous symptoms returning after a period of initial relief).
  - Post-operative scarring compressing the median nerve
  - 'Reformation' of the transverse carpal ligament with recurrent compression
- Completely new symptoms.
  - Neurological – tender scar due to injury to multiple small cutaneous branches (one of the most

common complications), entrapment or division of the palmar cutaneous branch of the median nerve, injury to the main trunk of the median or ulnar nerves or its branches

- Vascular – haematoma following injury to the superficial palmar arch
- Wrist complaints – carpal arch alteration causing pain, pillar pain, pisotriquetral pain syndrome
- Tendon problems – increased incidence of triggering, thought to be due to transference of initial pulley-related forces from FR to A1 pulleys, bowing or adhesions of flexor tendons

Clinical evaluation is used to assess the possible underlying causes for the symptoms, and exploration is warranted for

- Positive Phalen's test.
- Night symptoms.
- Positive NCS after 3–6 months. Neurophysiological testing may help identify the level of residual or recurrent compression.

SURGERY

- 'Re-release' of ligament.
- Exploration of alternative compression sites.
- Neural surgery is controversial:
  - External neurolysis to separate the nerve from the scar tissue.
  - Internal or interfascicular neurolysis or epineurotomy has been proposed for severe CTS, but opinions differ (Curtis RM, *J Bone Joint Surg Am*, 1973)
- Interpositional nerve grafts to injured segments of the median nerve.
- Revascularisation of the nerve, e.g. PQ turnover flap for mechanical protection of the nerve, reduction of new scar tissue and improvement of local vascular support.
- Tissue interposition flaps to separate the overlying scar from the median nerve such as muscle or distally based radial forearm fascial flaps.

COMPRESSION NEUROPATHY OF THE ULNAR NERVE

The ulnar nerve is the terminal branch of the medial cord. It runs medial and posterior to the brachial artery, and then pierces the middle of the medial intermuscular septum to enter the posterior compartment and then passes behind the ME in the cubital tunnel. Distally it lies between the FDS and the FDP, then radial to the FCU tendon to **Guyon's canal**. It reliably innervates the second and third dorsal interossei, and nerve dysfunction would leave the patient unable to move the middle finger side to side with the palm flat on a table top.

- The deep branch of the ulnar nerve dives down at the level of the pisiform into the hypothenar musculature.

ANATOMICAL SITES OF COMPRESSION

- **Arcade of Struthers.** Fibrous condensation of intermuscular septum about 8 cm proximal to the ME, present in 70%.
- **Medial intermuscular septum** (between brachialis and the medial head of triceps) that is distinct from the arcade.
- **Hypertrophy of medial head triceps.**
- **Stretching caused by cubital valgus** (e.g. post-supracondylar fracture).
- **Cubital tunnel.** The roof of the cubital tunnel is formed by the fascia of the FCU and the cubital tunnel retinaculum (CTR) (also known as the arcuate ligament of Osborne). The elbow capsule and medial collateral ligaments form the floor. This is the **most common** site of ulnar nerve compression. See below.
- **Guyon's canal.** Second most common.
  - Jean Guyon, 1831–1920, was a French urologist; it is not clear why the canal is attributed to him.

The last muscle to be supplied by the ulnar nerve is the first DO – and hence it shows the earliest sign of wasting with nerve compression. It supplies all the intrinsic hand muscles except LOAF (and except the deep head of the FPB).

CUBITAL TUNNEL SYNDROME (COMPRESSION AT THE ELBOW, MOST COMMON)

- Passage of the ulnar nerve beneath the aponeurosis joining heads of the FCU.
- Trauma at the elbow; fracture, especially in children.
- Recurrent dislocation of the nerve in the ulnar groove of the medial condyle – leading to neuritis. Asymptomatic nerve dislocation is seen in 16% of volunteers.
- Humero-ulnar OA or RA.
- Ganglion at the humero-ulnar joint.
- Anconeus epitrochlearis.

Hyperflexion of the elbow usually provokes symptoms of cubital tunnel syndrome as it increases the distance the nerve has to travel and also tightens Osborne's ligament.

SYMPTOMS

- Ill-defined pain in the forearm
- Numbness in the ulnar digits especially at night
- Pain with elbow flexion
- Weakness of pinch grip (adductor pollicis)

SIGNS

- Look
  - **Wasting** of the first DO, other intrinsics and hypothenar eminence.
  - **Ulnar claw.** Lack of clawing if palsy occurs above the branch to the FDP. With palsy at the wrist, the action of long flexors causes IP flexion whilst there is a failure of lumbrical-mediated extension at the IPJs and flexion at MCPJs.
  - **Wartenberg's sign** – abducted little finger in the presence of an ulnar nerve injury at the wrist and an ulnar claw hand, due to insertion of the EDM tendon into the tendon of ADM (this is not Wartenberg's syndrome, which is a neuritis of the superficial RN).
- Feel
  - **Tinel's sign at the elbow** (can be positive in asymptomatic patients) and Phalen's analogue sign with elbow (elbow flexion test).
- Move
  - **Positive Froment's sign** (hold a piece of paper between the radial border of the index and the thumb) – patients with ulnar nerve palsy compensate for the lack of a working adductor pollicis by flexing the thumb IPJ (median innervated FPL).
  - **Test pure intrinsic function** – flex the MCPJ and abduct/adduct the fingers.

NCS will show delayed nerve conduction at the elbow in cubital tunnel syndrome; if the problem is in the neck, dysaesthesia is encountered in the C8/T1 dermatomes, i.e. the inner aspect of the forearm and the elbow. Presence of either Martin–Gruber or Riche–Cannieu anastomoses may cause confusion.

X-rays are not that helpful but some suggest:

- A–P and lateral
- Cubital tunnel view – elbow flexed

MCGOWAN CLASSIFICATION

- Mild – mild, intermittent dysaesthesia
- Intermediate – persistent dysaesthesia, early motor loss
- Severe – marked atrophy and weakness

MANAGEMENT OF CUBITAL SYNDROME

- Splintage to keep the elbow from bending during sleep, e.g. wrapping the towel around the elbow, soft sports **knee** splint.
- Medication – unclear benefits from NSAIDs, vitamin B6 and steroids.
- Surgery is often needed, but results are much less predictable compared to the CTS. Damage to the medial cutaneous nerve of the forearm during surgery may cause neuromas.
  - **Decompression** – division of aponeurosis connecting the humeral and ulnar heads of the FCU (Osborne's ligament)
  - **Ulnar nerve transposition** (with risk of nerve devascularisation)
    - Transpose the nerve anteriorly over the muscle belly of the FCU (**subcutaneous transposition**, more common)
      - Fascia wrap modification (Han HH, *Scientific World Journal*, 2014)

- **Submuscular transposition (Learmonth's technique)**: the humeral head of the FCU and the PT are divided in a step fashion and repaired after the nerve has been transposed anteriorly. This is an option for those in whom a previous decompression has failed, has severe ulnar neuritis or persistent valgus deformity. The nerve is better protected and vascularised in this way.
- The medial intermuscular septum is split above the elbow where the ulnar nerve passes through to enter the volar compartment of the forearm.
- **Medial epicondylectomy** – can be performed in association with the above.
- **Chronic clawing** with loss of thumb adduction and index abduction may necessitate a Zancolli procedure.

ULNAR TUNNEL SYNDROME (COMPRESSION WITHIN GUYON'S CANAL)

The ulnar nerve and artery lie on top of the FR and beneath the volar/palmar carpal ligament in Guyon's canal (~4cm long); nothing else traverses the canal and it does not contain any synovium; thus, compression is less common compared with the CT. Within the canal, the nerve divides into the motor branch that can be rolled over the hook of the hamate and **the palmar cutaneous branch** (dorsal branch splits off earlier in distal forearm).

There is a great deal of more variation in the causes of ulnar nerve compression in Guyon's canal (compared to CTS), which means that imaging has a greater diagnostic role. Masses are the cause in up to half of cases. The isolated occurrence of ulnar nerve compression within the canal is usually due to ganglia or lipomas; other causes include anomalous muscles (aberrant FCU or abductor digiti minim) or an **aneurysm of the ulnar artery**, which would have to be resected and restored with a graft.

- Ulnar nerve signs (see above).
  - Sensory, motor or mixed disturbance – some divide the canal in zones.
  - Typically there is dysaesthesia of the ulnar palm and ulnar one and a half fingers (palmar surface), and weakness of the intrinsics and thumb adduction.

If the **dorsal sensory branch** (arises 7 cm proximal to the pisiform) is involved (altered sensation to the dorso-ulnar hand), then the **compression cannot be in Guyon's** canal – it must be proximal to it, e.g. within the cubital tunnel. Tinel's sign is the best provocation test. EMG (first dorsal interosseous) will demonstrate slow conduction at the wrist.

TREATMENT

- Conservative.
- Surgery – release of the volar carpal ligament via a longitudinal incision radial to the FCU, isolating the ulnar nerve proximal to the wrist. The volume of

Guyon's canal increases after CT release; thus, CTR release **improves ulnar compression** symptoms in one-third of the patients.

RN COMPRESSION

The RN is the largest branch from the brachial plexus (includes all the posterior divisions) and innervates the extensors of the arm as well as overlying skin. The usual sequence of innervation is

BR, ECRL, ECRB, Supinator, EDC, ECU, EDM, APL, EPB, EPL and EIP

Sites of compression syndromes:

- Triangular space.
- Radial tunnel syndrome.
- Posterior interosseous nerve (PIN) syndrome.
- Wartenberg's syndrome.
- Compression may occur over the humerus, related to humeral fractures, use of tourniquets or external compression (**Saturday night palsy**). Most resolve within 6 months.

RADIAL TUNNEL SYNDROME

The RN passes through the **triangular space** formed by humerus laterally, triceps (long head) medially and teres major superiorly, to lie in the bicipital groove in the posterior compartment of the arm. It pierces the lateral intermuscular septum 10–12 cm above the LE and enters the **radial tunnel** (from the radial head to the distal edge of the supinator) where it may become compressed.

Within the radial tunnel, within 3 cm of the elbow, the nerve gives off the motor branch (PIN, third extensor compartment) and continues as a purely sensory nerve that stays close to the BR. All forearm extensors are supplied by the PIN (C7, 8) apart from the ECRL, ECRB and BR (RN above the elbow). A fracture of the humerus may cause injury to the RN, whilst a fracture of the radius may cause injury to the PIN.

There are three common constriction points (of the PIN) within the radial tunnel:

- Sharp tendinous medial border of the ECRB.
- Fan of vessels from the radial recurrent artery ('leash of Henry') that can compress various branches of the RN.
- **Arcade of Frohse** – the free aponeurotic margin of the supinator under which the PIN passes (thus the PIN syndrome). This is the most common site of RN compression.
- Fibrous bands around the radiohumeral joint may also cause constriction; some suggest that RTS may be a result of overuse.

SYMPTOMS AND SIGNS

This is mainly a nocturnal pain syndrome.

- **Pain in the radial tunnel** (4 cm distal to the LE, distinguishing it somewhat from lateral epicondylitis).

Relief of pain and symptoms with LA is diagnostic. Patients generally complain about the pain, not the sensory loss/weakness.

- **Sensory disturbance** radiating to the distribution of the superficial branch of the RN. This is absent with compression of the PIN, i.e. PIN syndrome.
- **Positive middle finger test** – pain over the radial tunnel upon extension against resistance (ECRB inserts into MF metacarpal and contraction causes impingement of the border onto the nerve). There may also be symptoms with resisted supination with elbow extended.
- **Tenderness over the supinator mass,** four finger-breadths distal to the LE – it can be distinguished from tennis elbow/lateral epicondylitis by the tenderness over the LE in the latter. There is no sensory disturbance or motor loss (except due to pain) in tennis elbow (golfer's elbow = medial epicondylitis).
- **Weakness and numbness are not prominent features of the RTS.** In the PIN, there is weakness of the extensors without a sensory deficit (see below).

MANAGEMENT

Electrophysiological studies are less useful for this type of nerve compression.

- Splintage, activity modification, NSAIDs. A 3 month trial is reasonable.
- Treat by nerve decompression by exploring the radial tunnel via BR muscle-splitting or anterolateral approaches that have been described. Generally, a complete release is advised (all the structures above are divided) even if no obvious evidence of compression can be seen during surgery. There is usually a good prognosis after surgery if the symptoms can be relieved by a preoperative nerve block. Motor recovery may take over a year.

PIN SYNDROME

The main features are **weakness of the wrist and finger extension** with some forearm pain without sensory disturbance. The BR, ERCB and ECRL are spared. It may be provoked by a variety of causes:

- Trauma, e.g. elbow fracture/dislocation
- Inflammation, e.g. RA in the elbow
- Swellings/masses, e.g. lipoma, ganglia
- Iatrogenic, e.g. injections for tennis elbow, etc.

Due to the above, investigations to clarify the cause are more valuable (than in the PIN syndrome), e.g. NCS, X-ray and CT/MRI.

TREATMENT

Conservative treatment as above, proceeding to surgery if the NCS is positive and there has been no recovery for 3 months.

WARTENBERG'S SYNDROME

This is neuritis of the superficial branches of the RN, which may occur due to entrapment beneath the tendinous **insertion of the BR**, anomalous fascial bands, tight jewellery and watchbands, overuse, scarring, e.g. following de Quervain's release, etc. It is a relatively rare cause of radial wrist pain and may resemble de Quervain's (Finkelstein's test may be positive).

- Tenderness 4 cm proximal to the wrist.
- Numbness or pain in the distribution of the superficial branch of the RN over the whole of dorsum/lateral hand. The symptoms are reproducible by pressure over the nerve, and worsen **with wrist movement** especially i.e. **pronation** (test for 30–60 seconds). There may be local tenderness to percussion. There is reduced 2pd on testing.
- Symptoms improve with injection of lignocaine.

Treat by surgical exploration, neurolysis and release of constricting tissues (some recommend lengthening of the BR) if conservative measures do not work.

- Robert Wartenberg (1886–1956), a Russian-born neurologist who eventually settled in California, was sometimes called the 'Rebel of Book Reviewers' due to his honest and accurate critiques.
- **Wartenberg's sign** is the inability to hold the little finger against the ring finger when the fingers are in extension and is due to the action of the EDM (radial innervation) being unopposed by weak palmar interossei (ulnar).

TRACTION NEURITIS

This may occur after open CT release or ulnar nerve transposition and is manifested as chronic pain. It may be due to

- Nerve devascularisation
- Neuroma
- Incomplete decompression

Re-explore if symptoms persist with internal/external neurolysis. Severe neuritis may require additional soft tissue coverage. For the ulnar nerve, **submuscular transposition** with or without epicondylectomy is recommended. Some cases may not improve after further intervention, and this may be related to scarring.

SUMMARY

Radial nerve (Table 6.6)

- Check for wasting of triceps, BR and extensor, wrist drop, sweating change in nerve distribution
- Motor loss:
  - Above elbow – elbow extension.
  - Elbow – elbow, BR (flex elbow in mid-pronation), wrist extension and wrist deviation (ECRL/B.)

Table 6.6 Nerve compression syndromes and their common causes

Neuropathy	Congenital/Anatomical	Acquired
Pronator syndrome	Between heads of PT Ligament of Struthers Lacertus fibrosus (biceps)	Swellings: lipoma, ganglion
Anterior interosseous syndrome	All the above plus: Fibrous bands of FDS Ganzer's muscle (accessory head of FPL)	Swellings: lipoma, ganglion
Carpal tunnel syndrome	High insertion of lumbricals Persistent median artery	Swellings: lipoma, ganglion, bony exostoses Inflammatory: RA, OA Metabolic: pregnancy, hypothyroidism, renal failure Traumatic: lunate dislocation
Cubital tunnel syndrome	Anconeus epitrochlearis Two heads of FCU	Swellings: lipoma, ganglion Inflammatory: RA, OA Traumatic: cubitus valgus, supracondylar fracture
Ulnar tunnel syndrome	Accessory PL tendon High insertion of hypothenar muscles	Swellings: lipoma, ganglion Inflammatory: RA, OA Traumatic: fracture hook of hamate
Radial tunnel syndrome	Arcade of Frohse (supinator) Leash of Henry Tendinous border of ECRB	Swellings: lipoma, ganglion Inflammatory: RA, OA Traumatic: elbow dislocation, Monteggia fracture
Posterior interosseous syndrome	As for radial tunnel syndrome	As for radial tunnel syndrome
Wartenberg's syndrome	Free edge of brachioradialis	Extrinsic compression by watchbands, etc.

- Below elbow – PIN (supinate with elbow extended), EPL (thumb extension).
- Provocation tests:
  - Radial tunnel – pain with resisted finger extension (ECRB medial edge), Wartenberg's syndrome.
  - PIN – wrist dorsiflexion causes radial deviation; BR and ECRL action due to RN without opposing ECU, which is innervated by PIN.

MEDIAN NERVE

- Check for thenar wasting, sweating change
- Motor loss:
  - Elbow – wrist flexion (FCR)
  - AION – test O-sign (FDP index and FPL), pronation with extended elbow (PQ)
  - Recurrent motor – APB, pulp-to-pulp thumb to little finger
- Sensory – moving 2pd
- Provocation tests:
  - Pronator syndrome – pain with resisted pronation of forearm
  - AIO – no sensory loss
  - CT – Tinel's and Phalen's

ULNAR NERVE

- Check for – interosseous guttering/wasting, hypothenar wasting, ulnar claw hand (paradox: less clawing with higher lesion)

- Wartenburg's – abducted little finger due to unopposed EDM.
- Motor:
  - Froment's test (adductor pollicis and palmar interossei).
  - DIPJ flexion ulnar fingers (ulnar FDP).
  - ADM (resisted abduction of the little finger) and FDM (flex MCPJ of the little finger).
  - First DIO (resisted abduction of the index) – last muscle to be supplied and thus the first to become wasted.
- Sensory – 2 pd
- Provocation:
  - Cubital tunnel – Phalen analogue, Tinel's sign is unreliable.
  - Ulnar tunnel – pressure causes paraesthesia.

MUSCLE/TENDON TRANSFERS FOR SPECIFIC NERVE LESIONS

Nerve injury is the most common indication for tendon transfer – tendon is attached to the parent muscle, but insertion is moved to another tendon or bone. Others include the following:

- Muscle/tendon injury secondary to trauma or other disease (see also 'RA')
- Spastic disorders (see also 'cerebral palsy')
- Polio – wait 6 months for any recovery
- Leprosy – disease must be under control

PRINCIPLES OF TENDON TRANSFER

The aim is to identify specific task deficits and to re-establish this function through the use of existing muscle/tendons.

Tendon transfer utilises **existing motor function** (none is created) and thus power will be **lost during transfer** – at least one MRC grade. Therefore, muscles used should have 4–5/5 power and be **expendable** and preferably synergistic. Whilst power must be adequate, over-powerful transfers may deform the joints. Transferred tendons require free passage in vascularised tissue planes with a **straight line of pull** (only change direction once) (Table 6.7).

Strength is related to the cross-sectional area of the muscle, whilst the length determines the excursion – wrist tendons have an excursion of 3 cm, whilst finger extensors and flexors have excursions of 5 and 7 cm, respectively, meaning that when wrist tendons are used to restore finger function, correction will usually be incomplete.

- One function per muscle transferred.
- **Full passive ROM** (in joints in between the origin and insertion) is required **before** transfer; contractures should be corrected.
- Joints must be stable; there should be only one joint crossed by the transfer. Active control at the wrist is paramount for tendon transfers for the fingers.
- Fractures and soft tissue **injuries have completely healed**.
- Restore function only to an area that is **sensate** (at least protective sensation). Sensory deficits limit the usefulness of tendon transfers, and every effort should be made to restore function prior to tendon transfer.
- Loss of one major nerve is amenable to tendon transfer; trying to compensate for more than one nerve will lead to more impairment.

OTHER CONSIDERATIONS

- Complete division of recipient tendon burns bridges. Attachment in-continuity compromises mechanics, but the concept of reversibility may be important ('baby-sitting' transfers in case re-innervation of paralysed muscles occurs).
- All transfers slacken with time; use the **tenodesis effect** (finger extension with wrist flexion) to get the tension right. Transfers should be within **synergistic muscle groups**, e.g. hand opening (wrist flex/finger extend) and hand closing/grip muscles (wrist extend/finger flex). Donor muscle should be independently innervated and not act in concert with other muscles (e.g. lumbricals).
- Immobilise 3–4 weeks and then begin active ROM.
- Success requires a well-motivated patient likely to be compliant with the post-operative hand therapy. Multiple transfers may be too complicated – for the patient. Thus, contraindications include
  - Advanced age (reduce recovery/re-education and reduced demands)
  - Poor motivation/compliance
  - Lack of a specific task deficit
  - Local or systemic disease affecting the surgery, e.g. RA must be controlled

TIMING

- Immediate – when chances of nerve (to muscle) recovery are low, e.g. muscle loss, advanced age or as an interim 'baby-sitting' procedure whilst waiting for **high nerve** recovery, e.g. in RN compression, or at the time of nerve repair. Classically, PT to ECRB transfer after RN palsy for some wrist extension.

Table 6.7 Nerve injuries, their symptoms and suitable transfers

Injured nerve	Active deficit	Muscle functions missing	Donor muscles/tendons available
Median nerve (elbow)	Forearm pronation	Pronator teres	Biceps
	Wrist flexion	FCR, PL	FCU split
	Finger flexion	FDS (all), FDP (median)	Tenodese to ulnar FDPs
	Thumb IP flexion	FPL	Brachioradialis
	Thumb abduction	Thenar muscles	Opponensplasty using ADM or EI
Ulnar nerve (elbow)	Wrist flexion	FCU	Split FCR
	Finger flexion	FDP (ulnar)	Tenodesis to median FDPs
	Thumb adduction	AP	Brachioradialis
Ulnar nerve (wrist)	Metacarpophalangeal flexion (hyper-extended)	Lumbricals (ulnar)	FDS to radial sagittal band
Radial nerve (elbow)	Elbow flexion	Brachioradialis	Flexor mass resisted higher on humerus
	Radial wrist extension	ECRB, ECRL	Pronator teres
	Finger extension	EC, EI, EDM	FCU
	Thumb extension	EPL	Palmaris longus

- Conventional – after muscle innervation fails to occur within expected interval.
- Delayed – if conditions (e.g. soft tissue shortage) are not ideal initially, then a delay to achieve better conditions (flap coverage) is necessary.

LOW MEDIAN NERVE PALSY

Deficit is loss of median nerve muscles (mnemonic: Lumbricals 1 and 2, Opponens pollicis, APB, Flexor pollicis brevis = LOAF muscles) and sensation. There is **thenar atrophy**; the main aim is to restore **thumb opposition**, i.e. **APB** (with contributions from opponens and FPB superficial head – deep head is usually ulnar innervated). Reliable options for **opponensplasty** include the following:

- PL (Camitz, requires strip of palmar fascia).
- EIP (Burkhalter) – probably one of the commonest; it requires no pulley or tendon graft and no loss of grasp force.
- FDS ring (Bunnell, with pulley around FCU).
- ADM (Huber) – needs intact ulnar nerve. It is the classic choice in the congenital hypoplastic thumb and also restores the bulk of the thenar eminence.
- It is important to define the functional requirements of individual patients; only 2/3 of median nerve injuries require/benefit from an opponensplasty.

HIGH MEDIAN NERVE PALSY

As above with additional loss of FPL, FDP index and middle, FDS, PQ, PT and FCR.

- **Opponensplasty** for thumb abduction and opposition.
- BR to FPL for thumb flexion, or ECRL/B.
- Suture together ulnar nerve FDPs to median nerve FDPs to achieve a finger flexion (mass action) or ECRL to FDP.
- FCU split to restore balanced wrist flexion.
- Re-route biceps to restore pronation.

LOW ULNAR NERVE PALSY (CLAW HAND)

Loss of hypothenar muscles especially ADM, ulnar lumbricals, adductor pollicis and FPB deep head (muscle usually has dual innervation, superficial head is supplied by the median nerve), interossei and sensation. There are **Froment's** and Jeanne's signs (hyperflexion of the IPJ and hyperextension of the MCPJ, respectively, with key pinch). Aims of treatment are as follows:

- **Correct clawing** (MCPJ hyperextension and inability to fully extend IPJs of ring and little fingers – Duchenne's sign, due to **absent intrinsic** function). Procedures may be divided into static (e.g. tenodesis of lateral bands) or dynamic transfers, e.g. ECRL transfer to lateral bands (see below).

- **FDS transfer** to the radial lateral band (or A1 pulley), aka FDS tenodesis (see below). Stiles–Bunnell transfer.
- **FDS slip** looped back on itself around the A1 pulley (Zancolli Lasso) providing dynamic flexion movement at the MCPJ.
- ECRL to correct claw (Stiles–Bunnell).
- Stitch down volar plate to flex the MCPJ (static Zancolli capsulodesis) but does not add power and will stretch with time.
- **Restore key pinch.**
  - BR and PL graft (Boyes, functions in both wrist flexion and extension).
  - ECRB with tendon graft (Smith), strong motor donor.
  - FDS (Littler) ring or middle finger.
  - MCPJ/IPJ arthrodesis.
- **Correct Wartenberg's sign** (inability to adduct extended little finger due to unopposed EDM, which is radially innervated) – re-route the ulnar half of the EDM to the radial aspect of the PP or A2 pulley of the little finger.
- **Enhance power grip** – some recommend no treatment (Brand).
  - ECRL to lateral bands, PP and A2 – or use BR.
  - Suture together ulnar FDPs to median FDPs to achieve a finger flexion (mass action).

HIGH ULNAR NERVE PALSY

As above with palsy of the FDP to the ring and little fingers (which reduces clawing), FCU – the functional deficit is the same, although clawing may seem less obvious.

- FCR to FCU if radial wrist deviation causes problems as ulnar deviation is important for wrist flexion.

LOW RN PALSY

Loss of ECRB, ECU, supinator and finger and thumb **extensors**. The loss of wrist extension (and stabilisation) will reduce grip strength significantly. A combination of

- **PT to ECRB** to restore wrist extension.
  - Maintains some useful pronation from the PT to the most central wrist extensor ECRB.
- **FCR to EDC** to restore finger extension (Brand); alternatively, FCU or FDS (Boyce, middle and ring finger) to EDC. The middle finger FDS with its separate muscle belly has the theoretical advantages of a straight line of pull with sufficient strength and excursion and being relatively expendable; it is usually routed through a window in the interosseous membrane of the forearm.
- **PL to EPL** to restore thumb extension, or FDS (middle) to EPL.

With **a high RN palsy**, there is additional loss of ECRL and BR, but treatment is essentially the same. Conversely with lower RN (PIN) palsy, the ECRL can be transferred to the distal ECRB.

POST-OPERATIVE CARE

- Splintage usually in the position of the function being reconstructed, for 4–5 weeks, then night splints.
- Mobilise under supervision until strength increases at 6–8 weeks. The involvement of a good hand therapist is vital to the outcome.
  - There are some studies comparing results of early active motion with passive motion or immobilisation by cast.

Complications include

- Rupture
- Adhesions
- Incorrect tension

VI. COMPLEX REGIONAL PAIN SYNDROMES

STANTON–HICKS DEFINITION

'A variety of painful conditions following injury exceeding both in magnitude and duration the expected clinical course of the inciting event'. The term 'complex regional pain syndrome (CRPS)' has been used since 1995 when it was felt that the previous terms reflex sympathetic dystrophy (RSD) and causalgia were inadequate.

It is an abnormal pain response to (typically minor) injury with multifactorial causes. It primarily affects the extremities, but sometimes the face is involved. The true incidence is unclear; estimates are roughly 5% after some causes such as Colles fracture and surgery, 2%–5% of peripheral nerve injury and 13%–70% of those with hemiplegia. It may follow burn injuries, but the incidence is unknown. Overall, 10%–30% of cases are deemed 'spontaneous'. Women are affected more frequently than men.

CRPS TYPE 1

- No predisposing **nerve** event ('primary' non-nerve related CRPS) – **reflex sympathetic dystrophy**, algodystrophy
- Follows a noxious event that may or may not be traumatic; can be an early and late complication of any hand surgery
- 90% of CRPS

CRPS TYPE 2

- **Identifiable primary nerve insult** ('secondary' CRPS) – **Causalgia** (Greek *causis* warm and *algos* pain) is usually related to nerve injury, and the effect is often seen within hours.
  - Types 1 and 2 only differ by supposed initiating factor. Some suggest that type 2 tends to be more painful and difficult to control symptomatically.

- Many are military injuries where the stress of conflict may contribute to the overall condition.
- Differential diagnosis includes Secretan's disease: brawny swelling and induration in the hand as a result of factitious tapping/rubbing of the hand.

There is some doubt over the validity of this distinction; some type 1 cases turn out to have a history of nerve injury. Some divide it into **sympathetically** maintained or independent pain syndromes. An alternate classification of RSD was based on the response to nerve blocks:

- Pain that is not limited to a nerve territory
- Pain that is associated with major nerve injury and distributed primarily in a nerve territory but may spread up or down – **causalgia**
- Pain independent of the sympathetic system, i.e. does not respond to block

The limitations of this classification are seen when patients have pain that partly responds to block or is apparently spontaneous. The **phentolamine block** (α-adrenergic inhibitor with short half-life ~19 minutes) was used as a diagnostic criterion as well as a therapeutic option; however, studies are generally of low quality. There are doubts that it is much better than placebo.

PATHOGENESIS

Little is known about the mechanism of CRPS.

- **Sympathetic system abnormality** (hair loss, sweat and oedema), hence previous name 'sympathetically maintained pain', but the situation is more complex than this as early stages of the disease may show reduced sympathetic function with increased arterial flow (thus receptor hypersensitivity is suggested by some); but phentolamine block seems to be no better than placebo.
- **Substance P** (vasoactive neuropeptides) from efferent pain receptors stimulates the inflammatory process and fibroblast activity. Their contribution is difficult to quantify.
  - **Opioid/central endorphins** block substance P release. Patient confidence and expectation of pain relief seem to be important factors; the doctor needs to be positive. Feedback methods are useful.
- **Psychological findings** – CRPS/RSD is not a psychiatric condition, but there is an excess of anxiety, depression, somatisation and interpersonal sensitivity.
  - There is often significant emotional or psychological distress, which patient is usually unaware of or denies; there is alexithymia, the inability to verbalise emotions but can be angry, desperate, sensitive and easy to feel rejected or resentful if the doctor tries to play down their problems. It is important to be compassionate – the worst thing is to belittle.

PREDISPOSING FACTORS

- Surgery or trauma (e.g. Colles' fracture) that may be relatively minor
- Increased sympathetic activity
- Smoking
- Tight dressings
- Psychological profile of the patient

DIAGNOSIS

CRPS is a clinical diagnosis that can be difficult to make. It is suggested if there are >5 of the following:

- **Pain** out of proportion
  - **Allodynia** – marked pain from a usually non-painful stimulus.
  - **Hyperpathia** – excessive perception of a painful stimulus.
  - **Hyperalgesia** – increased pain to a normally painful stimulus.
  - **Hyperaesthesia** – increased sensitivity to a stimulus, e.g. light touch.
  - **Dysaesthesia** – abnormally perceived unpleasant sensation, spontaneous or provoked.
  - **Causalgia** is usually described as a burning pain, with allodynia and hyperpathia after traumatic nerve injury.
- **Autonomic (sympathetic) dysfunction**, e.g. hyperhidrosis, (dis)colouration (white mottling/red blue), temperature (vasomotor activity), pilomotor ('goosebumps').
- **Oedema** is often the first sign. There may also be
  - Colour changes and dermographia – triple response to a light object drawn across the skin
  - Some joint swelling and decreased ROM
  - Pitting or hard/brawny particularly if well demarcated
- **Stiffness** or dystonia.
- **Changes in tissue growth** (dystrophy or atrophy), e.g. altered hair growth (first coarse and then thin), shiny skin, osteoporosis – there may be osteopaenia on plain X-ray.

There is no single diagnostic test. Functional assessments are especially important if they are able to provide simple measurements, e.g. oedema, temperature, sweating or range of movement to allow documentation of progress. Objective findings should be sought out aggressively.

- **Thermography.** Up to 80% will have a measurable temperature difference (0.6°C on thermography), which may be dynamic depending on local temperature as well as emotional stress, but can be spontaneous. However, it is of little clinical use except to demonstrate to the patient and to help to monitor progress.
- **X-rays** may show patchy osteoporotic changes in Sudecks, but these are relatively late signs; a three-phase bone scan may demonstrate earlier signs,

and whilst it is specific, it is relatively insensitive and its value is controversial. MRI features are deemed non-specific. Nevertheless, radiology can be useful when the findings are positive, but a negative result does not rule out RSD.
- **Electrodiagnostic testing** – EMG and NCS. Others include skin conductivity, quantitative sensory testing, quantitative sudomotor axon reflex test (QSART), laser Doppler flow and response to sympathetic block.

STAGING

- **Acute** (3 months) – mostly vasomotor type symptoms:
  - Inappropriate pain within 48 hours of trauma or surgery pain, swelling, warmth and sweating.
  - Hair and nail growth may be faster than normal.
  - Pain – hyperpathia, hyperalgesia with reduced mobility as a consequence.
- **Subacute or dystrophic** stage (3–12 months):
  - Some atrophy, patchy osteoporosis and myofascial trigger points.
    - Myofascial trigger points are proximal triggers causing immediate pain distally, often at muscle insertions. There may be a palpable lump or taut band. The diagnosis is clinical, and most of the time the patient is unaware of it.
  - Pain is more constant and widespread with increased sensitivity.
  - Organised oedema ('brawny').
  - Discolouration and sudomotor changes – blue, cool, dry.
  - Trophic changes – shiny/glossy skin, brittle nails.
  - Stiffness – joint contractures.
- **Chronic or atrophic stage** (after 1 year):
  - More pronounced atrophic changes to soft tissue.
  - Intractable pain – pain at rest may decrease but pain with motion persists.
  - Dry stiff atrophic skin/tissues.
  - Joint stiffness/fixed contracture.
  - Loss of bone density with increased uptake on bone scan (osteoclastic resorption). It is a late sign, whilst changes resembling disuse appear quicker than expected (1 month vs. 10 years in actual disuse).
  - Sudeck's atrophy is sometimes used as a synonym for RSD/CRPS, but often it refers to this late atrophic stage.

Some would say that the concept of staging is not useful in a disease with such an unpredictable and variable course, whilst others feel that the disease does not actually progress through these stages; rather they represent forms with differing severities.

The prognosis is generally difficult to gauge, but it is accepted that the condition is unlikely to 'burn out' as previously thought. Complete remission is rare, and the condition has the tendency to recur. Much of the published literature is low in scientific quality in terms of numbers of patients and length of follow-up (requires at least 1 year).

TREATMENT

Principles of treatment

Many treatment methods have been described, but the majority have not been that successful. The aims of treatment are to relieve pain and prevent progression.

- **Prevent** full-blown CRPS/RSD by treating early, including support, physical therapy, removing painful casts if present, avoiding external fixation and using nerve blocks for surgery. **The consensus is that early treatment is beneficial/more effective.**
  - Pain exposure physical therapy
  - Mirror box therapy, graded motor injury
- Minimise harm and individualise the treatment plan – some of the more effective treatments include reducing sympathetic symptoms with blocks, temperature feedback, steroids for inflammation, gabapentin for central symptoms, acupuncture, and treat bone disease with calcitonin or bisphosphonates.
  - Control known irritants.
  - Start with the safest, least invasive treatment (see below).
  - Be positive with the patient and communicate; rapport improves results – be honest but positive.
  - Try to use objective measurements to convey progress to the patient. Control excess pain and symptoms before surgery if contemplated.

PROCEDURES

- **TENS** for cases complaining mostly of pain but with few inflammatory, sympathetic symptoms. Better response is seen if used early.
- **Biofeedback** especially temperature.
- **Implantable stimulators** may be a reasonable option when others have failed, though symptoms may recur after initial effectiveness. It aims to replace the CRPS with a less unpleasant paraesthesia. It is possible to have a trial with temporary electrodes before implanting permanent ones.
- **Sympathectomy** is of little value except in those who experience temporary but dramatic relief with blocks.
- **Acupuncture** – the response seems to be better in Chinese patients, possibly reflecting the higher level of acceptance/'belief' in this modality.
- **Stellate ganglion blockade** is commonly used in the United States but not always successful. It is primarily used for patients with florid sympathetic signs including causalgia, but there is a 30% **placebo effect** in those without.
- **Intravascular Bier block** with guanethidine (UK), steroids or bretylium and sometimes reserpine or

phentolamine (controversial). Recent studies have cast doubts on their usefulness.
- **Brachial plexus** block to allow movement and to distinguish stiffness due to pain from fibrosis.

DRUGS

- **Sympatholytics**, e.g. clonidine (α2 agonist) as a patch or orally, phenoxybenzamine (α-1 and -2 agonists) is effective but the side effects can be severe. Calcium channel blockers such as nifedipine may help in those complaining of cool extremities.
- **Anti-inflammatory** – steroids may help for inflammatory symptoms.
- Centrally acting drugs – **gabapentin/pregabalin**, clonazepam, baclofen, **ketamine**.
  - Ketamine coma (5 days) described by Schwartzmann R in 2005 is not approved in the United States; thus, patients are sent to Germany (and Mexico). Pain returns in two-thirds after 6 months.
- **Antidepressants** – amitriptyline and diazepam have the tendency to exacerbate the condition. Some avoid the use of opioids due to theoretical concerns of reducing endogenous endorphins.
- **Calcitonin, bisphosphonates** for patients with Sudeck's or those with abnormal bone scan.
  - 88 patients were randomised to iv neridronate or placebo (Varenna M, *Rheumatology*, 2013). VAS pain scores reduced significantly within 20 days.

A sample protocol may be as follows:

EARLY

- Treat primary insult.
- Physiotherapy (splintage and mobilisation) ± brachial plexus block. Normal use of the limb without re-injury should be encouraged.
- Sequential therapy to maximal doses rather than multidrug therapy from the beginning is encouraged.
- Drugs should be tailored to the type of pain, e.g. chronic pain, pain disturbing sleep, inflammatory pain, paroxysmal pain, muscle cramps, sympathetically maintained pain.

INTERMEDIATE

- Steroids
- Sympathetic blocks

LATE (DIFFICULT AND OFTEN INTRACTABLE)

- Sympathectomy
- Clonidine epidural infusion (or transdermal patch)
- Implantable spinal cord stimulators
- Hyperbaric oxygen – 40 sessions (no evidence of long-term effect)
- Ketamine coma

EMERGING TREATMENTS

- Low dose/sub-anaesthetic ketamine
- Alpha lipoic acid (ALA) – being used in Germany, but lack of trials in CRPS
- Intravenous immunoglobulins
    - Some evidence for immune system involvement (Calder JS, *J Hand Surg Br*, 1998) including the role of cytokines and growth factors for pain and hyperalgesia.
    - Detection of antineuronal autoantibodies (Kohr D, *Pain*, 2009).
    - Goebel (*Ann Intern Med*, 2010) randomised trial IVIG vs. placebo in longstanding CRPS. At 4 weeks, patients reported a 20%–30% reduction from baseline in pain. However, IVIG is very expensive (~US$100 per gram), whilst results seem to be similar to ketamine, magnesium (downregulates NMDA receptor) and tadalafil (Cialis, for 'cold' CRPS).

C. DIAGNOSIS AND MANAGEMENT OF CONGENITAL HAND CONDITIONS

I. RELEVANT ANATOMY AND EMBRYOLOGY

About 1 in 600 children is born with a congenital upper limb deformity; 1 in 10 has significant functional or cosmetic deformity; 50% are due to unknown causes; 10% chromosomal, 20% single gene, 60% multiple gene and only 10% environmental, e.g. drugs, irradiation, anoxia or infections. Children cope surprisingly well with what they have and usually do not become self-conscious until school. Parents, on the other hand, are extremely distressed.

- Small object pinch develops at about 9 months of age. Hand dominance emerges at about 1.5–2 years and becomes consistent by 3–4 years.

The most common conditions are **syndactyly, polydactyly and camptodactyly**. Swanson's classification of congenital hand deformities is based on the work of Frantz and O'Rahilly, first described in 1976 and subsequently adopted by the American Society of Surgery of the Hand as well as the International Federation of Societies of Surgery of the Hand. It is based upon prediction of an embryonic failure leading to the clinical identifying features. However, Swanson's classification is often regarded as being inadequate for clinical use as it is phenotypic with little relevance to treatment and prognosis. The categories are not mutually exclusive, whilst ~10% like symbrachydactyly do not fit clearly into any.

- **Failure of formation of parts (15%)**
    - Transverse – amelia, brachymetacarpia.
    - Longitudinal – radial/ulnar/central deficiencies ('club/cleft hand').
    - Mixed – phocomelia, symbrachydactyly (terminal differentiation). Some lump non-transverse into 'longitudinal'.
- **Failure of differentiation of parts (35%)**
    - Camptodactyly, clinodactyly, symphalangism, syndactyly, arthrogryposis, synostosis.
- **Duplication (33%)**
    - Polydactyly.
    - Mirror hand.
- **Overgrowth**
    - Macrodactyly.
- **Undergrowth**
    - Madelung's deformity.
- **Constriction ring syndrome**
- **Generalised skeletal abnormalities**

Overview of limb development (Bates SJ, *Plast Reconstr Surg*, 2009) is a good review.

Limb buds appear by ~day 26 as swellings on the ventrolateral aspect of the embryo; these are areas of undifferentiated mesenchyme with overlying ectoderm. Components in the bud direct growth and differentiation. Apoptosis of fingers occurs on day 52; limb development is generally complete by 8 weeks with only minor changes in size and proportion thereafter.

FORMATION OF THE LIMB BUD

A **morphogenetic field** is a cluster of cells in the embryo, which undergo similar development because they lie within the same set of boundaries. Hox gene expression makes the limb field competent to respond to initiating factors such as FGF. The AP or radio-ulnar axis develops first (even before the limb bud appears), followed by dorsal/palmar with the proximodistal axis (limb elongation) being the last to develop.

- **Apical ectodermal ridge (AER).** The mesoderm of the limb bud induces the overlying **ectodermal** cells to elongate, become pseudostratified and form the AER. Both the AER and the underlying mesoderm are required for limb development – removal of the AER or loss of contact of the AER with limb bud mesoderm prevents limb development. Removing the AER early results in a severely truncated limb (e.g. formation of a humerus only).
    - AER is required for **proximo-distal outgrowth and patterning**, e.g. the interdigital apoptosis.
    - Mesenchymal cells beneath the AER proliferate rapidly to form the **progress zone (PZ)**. The AER actually prevents PZ cells from differentiating by releasing a factor that promotes proliferation, but once they have left the PZ and are no longer under its influence, thus they differentiate in a regionally specific manner.
- **Zone of polarizing activity (ZPA)** is a small block of mesoderm at the junction of the posterior part of the limb bud and the body wall. It is central to the A–P axis (the thumb-to-little finger, i.e. radio-ulnar axis) specification. According to the diffusible morphogen model (Wolpert L, *J Theor Biol*, 1969), a

soluble morphogen (Shh) is released from the ZPA creating a P–A concentration gradient, and cells exposed to high concentration of the morphogen form the posterior side and those exposed to low concentration (furthest away) form the anterior side. The ZPA also maintains the AER that, in turn, is responsible for initiating and maintaining growth and development of the limb.

- **Hox (homeobox) genes** act on the limb bud. Their expression is dependent upon FGF, Sonic Hedgehog Shh and Wnt-7a. Hox genes (A, B, C and D) coordinate the model for proximo-distal patterning in the PZ. Mutations in HoxD13 are associated with synpolydactyly.

  - **Shh** gene is a patterning gene that encodes a secreted factor that may act directly as the limb morphogen or, perhaps more likely, leads to transcriptional activation of the true morphogen. Downstream of Shh is BMP-2, which interacts with another group of patterning genes, the Hox genes.
  - **Wingless type** (WNT) is a third signalling centre in the dorsal ectoderm acting via genes Wnt-7a/LMX-1 for dorsal and En1 for ventral development.

In summary, limb development occurs in three axes. Congenital limb abnormalities involving either the absence or duplication of parts may be attributed to

- **Dorsal–palmar – centre** in non-AER dorsal ectoderm.
- **Disruptions of AP patterning** (post and preaxial/radial to ulnar), **which are normally mediated by the ZPA** on the preaxial surface acting through Shh/BMP-2/Hox, **lead to 'longitudinal disorders'**.
  - ZPA disturbances can result in mirror hand or ulnar dimelia, essentially ulnar duplication.
  - Syndactyly – failure of apoptosis in web zones.
  - Polydactyly – anterior ectopic Shh expression and disruption of Hox gene combinatorial code.
- **Proximo-distal limb outgrowth disorders, i.e. transverse deficiencies secondary to the premature failure of specification of parts by the AER via FGF.**
  - Symbrachydactyly.
  - Amelia.
- **Combination of AP and PD patterning.**
  - Intercalated deficiencies.
  - Phocomelia.

RECONSTRUCTIVE CONSIDERATIONS

- Defect
- Availability of normal proximal structures
- Assessment, investigation, planning and treatment within a multidisciplinary team environment

Patterns of hand function are established about age 4. Most surgeons will perform surgery in the subject's second year of life or before, with this 'early surgery' providing better growth potential, acceptance of the part and adaptive patterns of use, which is balanced against the greater technical difficulty and anaesthetic risk.

II. FAILURE OF FORMATION OF PARTS

LONGITUDINAL ARREST

The term 'deficiency' is preferred to 'club hand', named after the missing/deficient bone. Partial forms include radial, central and ulnar deficiency; some regard phocomelia as a complete form.

RADIAL DEFICIENCY

This was commonly called **'radial club hand'** with hypoplasia or absence of the radius with radial deviation of the hand, with an appearance resembling a golf club. It is bilateral in up to 50% or more (depending on classification) though rarely symmetrical; the right arm is affected twice as often as the left. In 'unilateral cases', the thumb is usually hypoplastic. It occurs 1 in 30,000 to 1 in 100,000; males are mostly affected.

Function tends to be poor due to associated abnormalities such as **thumb hypoplasia,** bowing from fibrosis and stiff a elbow. It is likely related to errors in the shh pathway. This usually worsens with age unless treated.

- Impaired movement in the radial digits (index and middle).
- Carpal fusion.
- **Ulna is bowed** and thickened and only 60% of its normal length; 25% have a duplicated median nerve, which replaces an absent RN. Similarly, the radial artery is often missing.
- There is fixed extension at the elbow. **Elbow stiffness** may be due to ulnar dislocation caused by the fibrous anlage restricting growth.
- The humerus is shorter and almost all muscles in the affected limb are abnormal.

FRANTZ AND O'RAHILLY CLASSIFICATION

- I – Deficient radial epiphysis – short distal radius making the radius mildly shortened, with thumb hypoplasia the prominent clinical feature requiring treatment
- II – Hypoplastic radius (rare) not requiring treatment itself like above
- III – Partial absence distally – (most common) centralisation
- IV – Total absence distally – radial agenesis, requires centralisation

It can be associated with other (mostly visceral) anomalies, i.e. syndromic radial club hand:

- **Holt–Oram syndrome** – association between the radial club hand and cardiac septal defects. AD inheritance.
- **VATER syndrome** – Vertebral abnormalities, Anal atresia, Tracheo-oesophageal fistula and Renal abnormalities, and Limb anomalies (VACTERL syndrome).
- **Fanconi syndrome** – pancytopenia, predisposition to malignancies, cardiac lesions and blood dyscrasias – the anaemia tends to develop later at

~6 years and is fatal without a marrow transplant (Fanconi's anaemia); also **TAR** (thrombocytopaenia that is present at birth but tends to improve, absent radius) but thumb is typically present. Both show AR inheritance.

- All those with radial deficiencies **should have Fanconi's excluded** (chromosomal challenge test) to allow additional time to find a suitable marrow donor.

ASSESSMENT

Those presenting with radial deficiencies should be asked about a family history of congenital hand abnormalities with focused investigations relating to suspected associated syndromal anomalies (see above).

In addition to development in general, the child should be observed particularly to assess the way the hand and elbow are used, e.g. can the hand be put to the mouth? Straightening the wrist in those with inadequate elbow flexion would make feeding of themselves impossible. Similarly adults with established functional patterns should probably not have surgery.

MANAGEMENT

Types I and II usually do not require specific treatment.

- **Restore elbow flexion** with stretching, physiotherapy and splints, then
- **Centralisation (Bayne's classification)** at 6–12 months
  - Centralisation of carpus on ulna (excising lunate to create space), **if there is good elbow movement**.
  - Ulnar transfer of radial wrist deviators – FCR, ECRB, ECRL.
  - Closing wedge osteotomy of ulna and ulnar carpus.
  - Release of radial soft tissues – Z-plasty.
  - Steinman pin through the third metacarpal.
  - Criticisms include continued radial drift with time and impaired growth at the distal ulna, wrist stiffness; salvage arthrodesis may be required. Long-term effects on function are unclear.
- **Buck–Gramcko – radialisation** of ulnar by placing the second metacarpal and radial carpus over the centre of the ulnar, if elbow movement is not good. This is a more recent alternative to centralisation; it avoids excision of carpal bones, and the axis favours active ulnar deviation whilst retaining wrist mobility. There is some debate regarding the choice between the two, with some saying that radialisation provides for better radiological appearance and clinical outcomes, but there is little evidence of any major functional difference.
- **Distraction lengthening** has been described to treat the deformed radius.
- **Pollicisation** before 3 years of age.

ULNAR DEFICIENCY

Ulnar deficiency is 4–10× less common than radial deficiency; it shows the 'reverse' skeletal abnormalities, though with much more variation. Seventy per cent are unilateral with the left side being much more frequently affected. It is often sporadic; other musculoskeletal abnormalities (short fibula) may be present, but **systemic syndromic associations are uncommon**. Functionally, **the wrist is good whilst the elbow tends to be worse** off. Thumb and carpal anomalies are also relatively common.

BAYNE'S CLASSIFICATION

- I – Hypoplastic ulna
- II – Partial aplasia – most common
- III – Total aplasia
- IV – Total aplasia with radiohumeral synostosis

TREATMENT

- Splinting and physiotherapy to improve passive movements.
- Generally, the functional status without resection of the anlage is very good, and thus resection is controversial. Fusing the proximal ulna to the distal radius (thus eliminating problems with bowing of the ulnar and dislocation of the radial head) to form a **one-bone forearm** may create a stable forearm. Tendon transfers are not usually needed.

CENTRAL DEFICIENCY

There is a range of deformity from total absence of middle ray to monodactyly. The bones are absent or malpositioned, but never rudimentary. Flatt AE (1977) described it as a **'functional triumph but a social disaster'** – despite its appearance, the wide central cleft allows for effective grasp and pinch and with normal sensation allows good function. 'Lobster claw hand' is a somewhat cruel term that should be avoided.

There may be some confusion with symbrachydactyly (Manske PR, *Plast Reconstr Surg*, 1993). In contrast to the symbrachydactyly-type of the cleft hand, which is usually ulnar, the radial side is more frequently affected in central deficiency. In addition, in severe forms, the only remaining digit is the little finger (whilst in severe symbrachydactyly, the only remaining digit is the thumb).

Barsky (after Lange) describes two types:

- **Typical ('V' cleft)** – bilateral **absence of the third finger** creating a deep palmar cleft between the central metacarpals, with syndactyly of the first and fourth web. There is skeletal hypertrophy adjacent to the cleft. The little finger is preserved. It is usually familial (**AD**); other abnormalities include cleft lip/palate.
- **Atypical ('U' cleft) – unilateral** deep cleft with complete/partial absence of central rays (**second, third and fourth**) with short radial and ulnar digits present with a shallow

cleft. There is hypoplasia adjacent to the cleft. The thumb is preserved. It is usually **sporadic** and may be associated with Poland's syndrome. This is often regarded as a form of symbrachydactyly and a failure of formation, whilst the typical cleft is failure of differentiation.

Another classification is that of Cole and Manske (1997) based on the quality of the thumb and the first web.

TREATMENT

Treatment centres on cleft closure with attention to avoid limiting the first web function – not all procedures that improve appearance will improve function. Syndactyly should be separated with care, as the blood supply is often tenuous.

Snow–Littler procedure ('reverse pollicisation' with palmar-based interdigital flap; an alternative is Miura–Komada with a dorsal interdigital flap) – basically shift the cleft to widen the first web space and bring non-thumb digits together.

- Palmar-based flap from the cleft that is inset into the first web space. The flap is often long, and distal viability may be tenuous.
- Correction of syndactyly between the thumb and the index.
- **Index metacarpal transposed ulnarly**, i.e. to the base of the third metacarpal (the middle finger).

TRANSVERSE DEFICIENCY

Transverse deficiencies can occur at any level, but usually it happens at the **proximal third of the forearm** ('short below elbow defect') or wrist. It may be difficult to distinguish transverse arrest at the arm from constriction band syndrome, which, unlike the former, tends to be unilateral and proximal parts tend to be hypoplastic. Some believe that vascular disruption may be part of the underlying mechanism.

- Proximal deficiency – usually treated with **prosthesis**; **Krukenberg's** procedure (sensate pincer by splitting the forearm bones) in selected patients.
  - Children with unilateral problems tend to discard/ignore prostheses, and the simple cosmetic arm is more likely to be accepted than a 'functional' myoelectric prosthesis.
- Distal (to MC) - distraction or bone grafting up to 1.5 cm from the toes. Free transfer is ideal for the thumb. The aim is to achieve a three-digit pinch.

PHOCOMELIA

This condition is rare. In contrast to amelia where no hand is present, a functional terminal hand is always present in phocomelia. It is often lumped into longitudinal deficiency category.

- Complete – absence of all arm and forearm bones; hand directly attached to the trunk

- Proximal – arm absent and forearm attached to the trunk
- Distal – forearm absent; hand attaches to the humerus.

Prosthetics (palmar plate or myoelectric) are the mainstay of management, though extremely short limbs may make this difficult; surgery is rarely indicated.

III. FAILURE OF DIFFERENTIATION OF PARTS

This includes syndactyly, camptodactyly, clinodactyly and arthrogryposis. Other conditions that fall into the category include synostoses (radio-ulnar) and carpal coalitions.

SYNDACTYLY

This condition occurs at an incidence of 1 in 2000 live births and is the second **commonest congenital limb abnormality** after polydactyly. It is due to failure of apoptosis (leading to failure of separation) in the seventh week, compared with acrosyndactyly, which is a result of the constriction band syndrome.

Eighty per cent are sporadic. There is a family history in 1/3 (highest incidence in a small cluster in Iowa), inheritance is AD with incomplete penetrance and variable expressivity described. It is not uncommonly associated with other anomalies, e.g. Apert's and Poland's.

- 50% bilateral.
- Twice as common in males.
- 10× more common in White patients compared with Africans.
- In order of decreasing frequency, the most affected web space is the **third web space**, then the fourth, second and first (3%). In the foot, the most affected space is the second.

PATHOLOGY

- There may be fascial interconnections (thickened Cleland's and Grayson's ligaments are coalesced and web-space/palmar fascia is thickened), shared flexor and extensor tendons or shared anomalous digital nerve and artery. Abnormal tendons are more common in Apert's syndrome.
- There are varying degrees of bone abnormalities.
- Individual joints are commonly preserved unless there is symphalangism (more common in syndromic cases) where joints remain incompletely differentiated and progress to ankylosis.

CLASSIFICATION

- **Complete** (digits united as far as DP) vs. incomplete.
- **Complex** (metacarpal or phalangeal **synostosis**) vs. simple (no synostosis). Conjoint nails are suggestive of joined bones, i.e. complex.

- **Complicated** syndactyly includes many forms including polydactyly, symbrachydactyly, acrosyndactyly; these are often associated with syndromes.
  - Acrosyndactyly – shortened digits that are united distally but with proximal fenestration – may be associated with congenital band syndrome (Streeter's dysplasia). It is usually isolated but may be associated with other anomalies, e.g. craniofacial abnormalities and spinal dysraphism.

SYNDROMIC

- Apert's spoon-like hand with conjoint fingernail for second to fourth
- Poland's – symbrachydactyly – short conjoint fingers

CONTRAINDICATIONS TO SURGERY

Minor degree of webbing, not cosmetically or functionally significant.

- Severe complex syndactyly; digits share common structures including digital nerves and arteries.
- Hypoplastic digits where one digit would function better than two.
- Adjacent webs should not be released simultaneously.
- The risk of hypertrophic scarring may be increased in feet and is a relative contraindication.

TIMING OF SURGERY

Flatt says that results are better with surgery after 18 months, but this is contradicted by Gesell who says that hand patterns are established by 24 months. Hand function is balanced against safety/fitness for surgery (>6 months); there is a wide range depending upon personal practice, but most operate 12–24 months, with a trend for earlier surgery at 9–12 months.

Indications for **earlier surgery (4–6 months)** in syndactyly:

- Border digits.
  - With multiple webs – border digits first, aiming to finish all by 3 years; only one side at a time
- Length discrepancy; there may be increasing deformity of longer digits.
- Complex syndactyly involving DP or producing flexion contracture.

Generally, one side of a digit is operated on at a time to reduce the risk of vascular insufficiency. Bilateral procedures can be performed in children less than 14 months of age but should be avoided in older children.

SURGICAL TECHNIQUE

There is always a shortage of skin (of 22% according to Kozin SH, *Plast Reconstr Surg*, 2015); one should resist the temptation to close flaps under tension to avoid grafting

except perhaps in cases of simple syndactyly that do not extend beyond the PIPJ. Revision cases in particular are not generally amenable to release without grafting.

- **Dorsal and palmar zigzag incisions** either to the midline of digits (*Cronin triangular flaps* 1956) or to the lateral borders (Zachariae). Mark dorsal zigzags (~60° angles) with bases over the PIPJ and the DIPJ of one finger, and then complementary volar flaps (a needle can be used to help plan volar flaps). Take care with the dorsal veins when raising flaps (Figures 6.19 and 6.20).
  - Colville – rectangular flaps with a pentagonal island flap for the web space.
  - Withey 'open-finger' techniques use seven to eight narrower flaps; these should not be defatted – tips are tacked into place with a single stitch and raw areas heal by secondary intention. Many advised against this due to the significant scars/contractures.
- Web space is usually created with a proximally based dorsal flap extending from the MCPJ to the PIPJ or just proximal to it, and inset into the palmar surface. Web flaps should be wide to allow spread and robust to avoid skin grafts around the web spaces. There are a variety of different flap designs.

Separation should proceed carefully bearing in mind that the arterial bifurcation may be more distal in these patients. The level of division of the NVB forms the limit of the web space. Defatting the flaps helps closure (Greuse M, *J Hand Surg Am*, 2001) and may allow grafts to be avoided in selected cases. Where grafts are needed especially near the web, FTSG is usually preferred over SSG and may be taken from the groin or instep, for example; the grafts should be tied in. Techniques that use all the skin to cover one finger, and graft the other, tend to have worse results.

- Buck–Gramcko technique for division of the syndactyly nail – use matching tongue flaps at the tip of the finger curled around the raw edge of the ipsilateral nail bed.

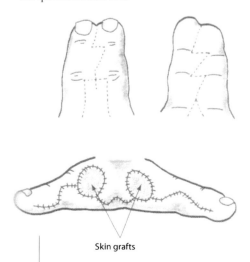

Skin grafts

Figure 6.19 Syndactyly repair usually requires skin grafts.

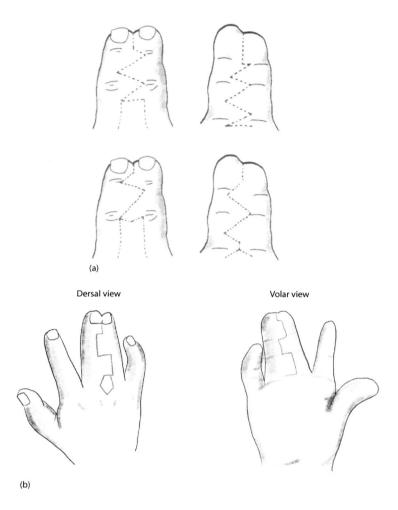

(a)

Dersal view   Volar view

(b)

Figure 6.20 Types of incisions used for syndactyly release. (a) triangular and (b) rectangular flap techniques.

- Deepening of web spaces (e.g. partial simple syndactyly or web creep) can be achieved by four-flap Z-plasty (120° Z-plasty provides 164% expansion compared with 75% with single Z-plasty) or jumping man flap.

POST-OPERATIVE COMPLICATIONS

Intra-operative and early

- Division of nerve or tendon
- Circulatory compromise (grafts too tight or digital artery injury)
- Haematoma, infection, graft loss

LATE

- Destabilisation of joints
- Deformity of the digit or web
- Web creep, particularly with growth spurt; splints tend to be of limited use

CAMPTODACTYLY

Camptodactyly was first described by Tamplin in 1846. It supposedly affects <1% of the population; it is painless and is usually of **no functional significance** in the majority (and thus may be under-reported). It is occasionally inherited as an AD trait; it may present in infants or in adolescence, particularly in **females**.

- I – **congenital,** isolated and unilateral. Most commonly little finger and apparent during infancy. F = M
- II – **adolescent form,** as above but appears as a progressive flexion deformity at 7–11 years of age with female predominance
- III – severe involvement of multiple digits and often associated with generalised conditions especially arthrogryposis

It is a congenital flexion deformity of the digit, usually involving the **little finger** (90%) and usually at the **PIPJ**. It is commonly **bilateral** but is rarely symmetrical. It is usually explained as an imbalance between flexion and

307

extensor forces at the joint; there is usually an abnormal insertion of lumbrical or FDS. Almost every structure around the PIPJ may be involved in the pathogenesis; surgery is most successful if associated with an abnormal lumbrical.

There may be secondary changes in the joint (X-ray may show a flattened dorsal ridge). The DIPJ is never involved, except if there is a secondary boutonnière deformity.

- If there is also brachydactyly ('short fingers') with a stiff PIPJ with anterior flexion/extension creases, it may be a case of symphalangism.

OPTIONS

- **Conservative treatment** in the form of **splintage and/or stretching** exercises is rarely successful except for cases with <15° contracture that is passively correctable. Half of adolescent patients may improve with this regime.
- In cases with a normal joint, passively correctable deformity >30°, surgery may help but probably will not achieve full correction, and results are largely unpredictable.
  - **Identify cause** – e.g. release of anomalous intrinsic insertion or lengthen FDS; but can be tethered by skin, fascia, tendon sheaths, intrinsics, collateral ligaments, volar plate, etc.
  - Correction of soft tissue contracture (see below) with stepwise release of tethering structures.
  - (Philippe) Saffar procedure – subperiosteal lift, division of collateral and accessory collateral ligaments and check rein ligaments.
  - Those with severe contracture (>90°) will need K-wires to maintain the PIPJ position.
- With a deranged joint, e.g. with long-standing contractures:
  - Dorsal angulation osteotomy.
  - Arthrodesis if severely contracted.

CLINODACTYLY

Kliner is Greek for 'to bend'.

Clinodactyly is the curvature of a digit in a radio-ulnar plane that in most cases is usually a **radial deviation at the PIPJ of the little finger** and usually bilateral. It is most commonly due to an abnormally shaped phalanx (usually MP) leading to abnormal longitudinal growth. The classic **'delta' phalanx** (Blundell Jones G, *J Bone J Surg*, 1964) – longitudinally bracketed epiphysis – is characterised by a trapezoidal or triangular phalangeal bone with a curved 'C'-shaped epiphysis, which makes angulation inevitable.

However, occasionally it is due to soft tissue problems, e.g. fibrous band on the ulnar side of the digit. In some cases, the phalanx may also be shortened (brachyphalangia). The abnormal phalanx may reduce mobility; pain is not a prominent feature.

It is more common in males. It is less common in Whites (~1%) compared with up to 19.5% in non-Whites. It can be sporadic but is often inherited with an AD pattern with variable penetrance. Marked clinodactyly may be associated with mental retardation including trisomy 21 (Down's); there are many other associations including Poland's, Treacher Collins and Klinefelter's syndromes, and its severity is often related to the severity of the other anomalies.

- Incidence in Down syndrome patients up to 80%
- Incidence in general population 1%–20%

OPTIONS

Surgery is essentially cosmetic; thus, leaving things alone is a choice except in cases of severe angulation.

- Bracket resection with horizontal growth plate preservation and fat graft to fill the defect, at 3–4 years.
- Closing wedge osteotomy (if phalanx normal length but trapezoid, best to wait until skeletal maturity).
- Opening wedge osteotomy plus bone graft (if the phalanx is short).
- Reversed wedge osteotomy (wedge from long cortex turned over and inserted into the shorter side).
- Vickers procedure – rongeur of delta-phalanx epiphysis and free fat graft, useful before 6 years of age.
- The use of distraction has been reported.

Clinodactyly may be mistaken for **Kirner's deformity** (dystrophy/ osteochondrosis of the fifth finger, acrodysplasia), which is a volar and radial incurvature at the DIPJ. The exact aetiology is unknown; there is a disruption of the growth plate due to an unknown mechanism.

- It is not as common as clinodactyly and is **often bilateral**. Family history is uncommon; it affects prepubertal females (7–14 years). It may be associated with Turner's syndrome.
- It starts as a painless swelling but can develop into an arthrogryposis, incurved joints with the appearance of a 'windblown' hand. The DP is shortened, swollen and deflected in a volar–radial direction and a dysmorphic nail.
- **Treatment.** There is usually no functional limitations that require treatment.
  - Splints (may need to be continued until school age) with variable results.
  - Surgery is reserved for severe deformities, e.g. soft tissue release and occasionally osteotomy with K-wire stabilisation.

SYMPHALANGISM

Symphalangism (Cushing's) is the **failure of segmentation** of the fingers (joint is represented by a cartilaginous bar), mainly at the **PIPJ** and rarely at the MCPJ, and usually the ulnar fingers are more frequently affected. The resultant fingers are stiff, lack flexion creases and are usually more slender.

Hereditary symphalangism is an AD trait. There may also be symbrachydactyly of the middle finger and it may be associated with hearing defects.

- True symphalangism – normal digital length.
- Brachysymphalangism – short digits.
- Syndromic, e.g. Apert's and Poland's syndromes; these tend to be non-hereditary types of symphalangism.

Reconstruction including arthroplasty tends to lead to poor results; osteotomy or arthrodesis (20°/30°/40°/50° for the digits) is usually the most practical option, but should be delayed until after skeletal maturity.

RADIO-ULNAR SYNOSTOSIS

This is fusion of the proximal radio-ulnar joint, leading to a **fixed pronation** deformity with compensatory hypermobility at the wrist. The radius is thickened and bowed with possible radial head agenesis or dislocation, whilst the ulnar is straight and narrow.

- Primary – radial head is absent.
- Secondary – radial head is dislocated.

It is bilateral in 60%. Synostosis can occur at a number of other sites in the hand, e.g. metacarpal synostosis. Due to the good functional status, it is often a late/under-diagnosis. Treatment options include

- Minor – good functional adaptation at the wrist/ shoulder; thus no treatment.
- Severe (fixed pronation >45°) – de-rotational osteotomy through the synostosis (risk to arteries and the PIN). In bilateral cases, one is placed in neutral, and the other in 20° pronation.

IV. DUPLICATION

POLYDACTYLY

This is the second most common congenital limb abnormality – affecting 1 in 300 Africans (more common) and 1 in 3000 White patients (and more likely to be syndromic). It may be inherited in an AD manner. It may be radial (preaxial), ulnar (post-axial) or central.

STELLING CLASSIFICATION

- I – Skin only, rudimentary mass
- II – Skeletal – part of a digit articulating with a phalanx or bifid metacarpal
- III – Complete duplication of ray, including metacarpal (rare)

CENTRAL DUPLICATION

Type I or II. Type II is invariably within what clinically appears to be a simple complete syndactyly.

ULNAR (POSTAXIAL) POLYDACTYLY

This is more common in Africans with a positive family history. It is normally unilateral and an isolated condition; it is unusual for it to be associated with other anomalies except in Whites.

Temtamy and McKusick classification (1978):

- Type A – well-formed digit usually contains bone and other elements. Patients generally need formal surgery like radial polydactyly, requiring muscle, tendon and ligament reconstruction, etc.
- Type B – with small digit, held on by skin bridge/tag, and usually treated by simple excision (tying off with suture often leads to a residual protuberance that may need subsequent removal). **More common.**

RADIAL (PREAXIAL) POLYDACTYLY (DUPLICATE THUMB)

Duplicate thumbs occur in 0.8 per 1000 live births; it is more common in Whites and in males (2.5×). Some cases may be associated with shh dysregulation. Radial polydactyly can be associated with other anomalies, i.e. part of syndromes (e.g. Carpenter's, Holt–Oram with Wassell type VII, ASD/ VSD/PDA, Fanconi anaemia) that can affect any organ system. The presence of a duplicate thumb should prompt a thorough work-up.

Wassell classification (primarily a radiological classification, describes bone features without considering soft tissues). Neither part is completely normal (Figure 6.21):

- I – Bifid DP (2%), most uncommon
- II – Duplicated DP

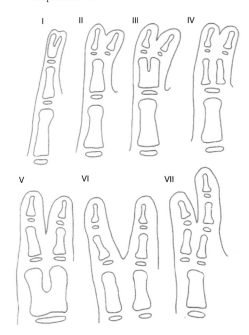

Figure 6.21 The types of thumb duplication (Wassell classification).

- III Bifid PP
- IV Duplicated PP (~50%), most common
- V Bifid MC
- VI Duplicated MC
- VII Partially duplicated M
- Other – hypoplastic duplicate thumb (pouce flottant) without skeletal elements, and **triphalangia** – strongest familial tendency (AD) and associations with Holt–Oram and Fanconi's.

Although both thumbs (on the one hand) tend to be hypoplastic, one of the 'duplicates' is often significantly shorter and thinner. There is hypoplasia of soft tissues and bone particularly in the central portion. The eccentric insertion of tendons tends to pull the thumbs together.

- Radial duplicate receives the hypothenar musculature, whilst the ulnar duplicate receives adductor pollicis and the first DIO. Absence or hypoplasia of these muscles is common.
- The anomalous insertion of FPL into the extensor expansion (Lister's tubercle) promotes abduction.

SURGERY

In some, one digit is dominant, whilst in others, they are similarly sized. Most often, surgery includes parts of both, and even when bones/joints are sufficient in one, the other can contribute soft tissue. Some would suggest that surgery is needed **before pinch grip develops** (10–12 months); this needs to be balanced by having structures large enough to facilitate surgery.

EXCISION (ABLATION)

Excision is appropriate where the duplicate is very rudimentary. Usually the radial (outer) digit is excised, with reattachment of the **radial collateral ligament** with a sleeve of periosteum and joint capsule. The UCL is both functionally more important and much more difficult to reconstruct and thus is usually kept on the main portion.

The nail and the growth plate(s) are preserved. Function is usually good, but the thumb is significantly smaller than the contralateral/normal digit.

COMBINATION (OF PARTS)

In most other cases, reconstruction is required to provide optimal function and cosmesis.

- **C1 (symmetric)** – **Bilhaut–Cloquet** procedure for types I and II (sometimes III; Figure 6.22).
  - Excision of adjacent marginal structures in the centre with merger of bone and soft tissue in a side-to-side fashion.
- **C2 (asymmetric)**, i.e. nearly all of one digit is retained and is augmented with selected tissues from the other digit, e.g. skin only and unused tissues from the 'spare part' are excised. It is most suited for Wassell type IV.
  - III and IV – remove smaller radial thumb, reconstruct RCL, osteotomies, rebalance tendons.
  - V and VI more complex with transfer of intrinsics and collateral ligaments.
- **C3 (on-top-plasty).**

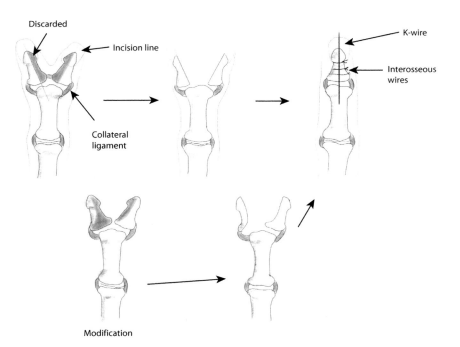

Modification

Figure 6.22 Bilhaut–Cloquet procedure and its common modification.

- V, VI and VII. Segmental digital transposition that brings the best distal segment of one duplicate onto the best proximal segment of the other.
- Technically difficult and limited application. Outcome studies have been limited.

REVISION

- Secondary surgery.
- Intrinsic transfer.
- Realignment of eccentric tendon insertions such as pollex abductus (where the FPL attaches to the EPL via an anomalous tendon that passes around the radial aspect of the thumb; it also occurs in thumb hypoplasia).

COMPLICATIONS

- Angulation – persistence or recurrence
- Stiffness
- Clinodactyly
- Instability

MIRROR HAND (ULNAR DIMELIA)

This is an extremely rare upper limb abnormality with duplication of the ulna and absence of the radius. There is polydactyly with midline symmetry, and there are usually seven fingers (5–4–3–2–3–4–5) sometimes eight with **no thumb**. It has been attributed to the limb bud having an additional progress zone. Elbow mobility may be limited.

Usually the post-axial side is more functional and regarded as dominant; accessory IV is pollicised, whilst accessories III and V are resected (Entin procedure). Six cases of multiple hand have been described in the literature.

V. OVERGROWTH

MACRODACTYLY

This is defined as congenital enlargement of a digit and is rare (2 in 100,000), making up approximately 1% of all upper limb congenital anomalies. It is a heterogeneous group that can cause confusion when interpreting the literature. The most common 'true' form is related to **lipofibromatous nerve** enlargement (harmatoma); 90% are unilateral, whilst 70% involve more than one digit, especially the index and the middle.

- Usually the metacarpals are of normal size, whilst the phalanges are enlarged.
- The tendons and blood vessels are of normal size (leading to ischaemia).

UPTON'S CLASSIFICATION

- I – macrodactyly with lipomatous nerve (especially median), most common and usually sporadic
- II – with neurofibromatosis (often bilateral) with gigantism with greater areas of upper and lower limbs

- III – with hyperostosis, i.e. multiple osseous osteochondral nodules/polyostotic fibrous dysplasia, very rare
- IV – with hemihypertrophy or Proteus syndrome (very rare, 1 in a million), generalised gigantism with hyperplasia of connective tissues, blood vessels and bone

The part usually has little movement. The deformity may be classed as

- **Static** – born with large digit and development of the digit keeps pace with the growth of the hand.
- **Progressive** – more common. There is rapid growth of what was a normal-sized digit at birth, increasing in size until epiphyseal closure. It is particularly debilitating.

ASSESSMENT

- Assess size discrepancy and effect on form and function.
- Investigations include X-ray of adjacent joints and angiography when vascular malformations are suspected.

TREATMENT

Amputation may be the best option; otherwise

- Debulking of soft tissues (best staged) and bones, i.e. reduction and longitudinal osteotomy.
- Nerve stripping, in some cases. It was once thought that nerve resection would reduce further overgrowth; Tsuge regarded it as being 'nerve-driven' overgrowth.
- Epiphyseal ablation/epiphysiodesis (when the digit is the same size as the same digit of the parent).

Surgical outcomes can be poor but are generally better than no treatment at all; secondary surgery is often required.

VI. UNDERGROWTH

HYPOPLASIA OF THE THUMB

This is usually an isolated anomaly, though there is often a hypoplastic/absent radius. The cause is unknown but may be related to a foetal neurogenic injury or reduced foetal oxygen tension or, in some cases, due to maternal thalidomide intake. There is an association with other anomalies that should be actively excluded, e.g. cardiac (Holt–Oram, VACTERL) and blood dyscrasias (TAR, Fanconi anaemia).

The condition commonly requires pollicisation of the index finger in the first year of life.

BUCK–GRAMCKO MODIFICATION OF THE BLAUTH CLASSIFICATION

- I – **Hypoplasia** – normal skeleton and musculature but all hypoplastic leading to reduced gross size but normal ROM.
- II – **Hypoplasia** – smaller thumb, bones narrow, reduced volume or absence of thenar muscles and **first**

web space adduction contracture due to adductor–abductor imbalance.

- III – **Hypoplasia** – even smaller thumb and the absence of thenar muscles lead to severe first web space contracture. There is **MCJP instability**, and bones/joints at the base are variably affected – there may be absence of the trapezium and the scaphoid.
- IV – **Pouce flottant** – a rudimentary appendage with bones/muscles except the trapezoid and the second metacarpal origin of the first DO. It is attached by a small skin bridge that may still have a neurovascular pedicle. Treat by amputation and pollicisation. Use of tissue in the floating thumb is rarely successful.
- V – **Total aplasia** with no skeletal or soft tissue elements. There are compensatory changes in the index finger (curvature, pulp widening, pronation and widened space between the index and the middle finger). Treat with pollicisation.

The tendon configuration can be quite variable, including the absence of intrinsic/extrinsic and anomalous connections, e.g. pollex abductus, musculus lubricalis pollicis (from the FPL to the index causing a tight web). Blauth divided **III into a and b** with stable and unstable CMC joints, respectively, which effectively differentiates those that can be reconstructed or require ablation/pollicisation. It can be difficult to differentiate between IIIa and IIIb in a child – the latter tends to lead to a thumb that is ignored with prehension developing between the index and long digits, and the index tending to pronate and rotate out.

THUMB RECONSTRUCTION

Principles

- Allow opposition.
  - The distal end of a pollicised digit must reach to the PIPJ crease of the MF when the thumb is adducted.
  - Good circumduction at the CMCJ.
- The thumb must be sensate with joints stable enough to allow pinch grip.

MANAGEMENT

- **Type I** does not require treatment.
- **Types II–IIIa**
  - **Opponensplasty** with ring finger FDS, may need to be augmented with Huber procedure (ADM transfer).
  - **Four-flap Z-plasty** to deepen the first web.
  - UCL stabilisation to stabilise the MCPJ.
  - May also need extensor indicis (EI) to EPL.
- **Types III(b)–V. Pollicisation (of index)** is usually utilised and is best performed between 6 and 18 months. There is a rearrangement of bones, muscles (interossei, IO) and tendons in various combinations/variations. The following are some suggestions:

- The MC head assumes the role of the trapezium; the **MC is shortened.**
- The 'thumb' is the index MC, which is dissected as an island flap pedicled on NVBs and long tendons and **fixed in pronation of 140–160°** and hyperextension at the MCPJ.
- First dorsal IO assumes the role of the APB; insertion transferred to the radial border of the index.
- First palmar IO assumes the role of the adductor pollicis – it is detached from the base of the PP and reinserted into the base of the MP.
- EDC to the index becomes the APL.
- EI becomes the EPL.

There have been reports of **microsurgical joint transfer** in types IIIb and IV, but results do not seem to be better than pollicisation. Second MTPJ transfer has been advocated by Shibata (*J Bone Joint Surg*, 1998), but proximal structures (bone, muscle, tendon, neurovascular) may be deficient. Options for reconstruction following trauma:

- Thumb replantation
- Finger replantation with pollicisation
- Distraction osteogenesis
- Web-space deepening
- Non-vascularised toe phalangeal transfer (keeping periosteum allows up to 90% growth) or other bone graft
- Vascularised toe–hand transfer/wrap-around (first or second toes)

VII. CONSTRICTION RING SYNDROME

Constriction ring syndrome is usually sporadic (~1 in 1200–15,000), and no known prenatal risk factors have been demonstrated. There may be oligohydramnios/premature rupture, and there is a strong association with **clubfoot and cleft lip/palate;** otherwise, there is a low incidence of associated anomalies.
There are two main theories:

- **Extrinsic – amniotic band** (partial rupture involving only amnion layer) may encircle extremity.
- **Intrinsic** (Streeter GL, *Contrib Embryol*, 1930) – internal defect in the embryo leading to apoptosis. Vascular disruption relating to an intrinsic defect of the circulation; this is often used to explain the association with cleft lip/palate.

PATTERSON CLASSIFICATION

There is a wide spectrum of anomalies. Proximal anatomy is usually normal.

- I – Simple constriction, i.e. grooving/indentation
- II – Constriction with distal deformity, i.e. lymphoedema
- III – Constriction with variable distal fusion, i.e. acrosyndactyly
- IV – Amputation from complete intrauterine disruption

Urgent release may be required to reduce venous obstruction and lymphoedema, e.g. multiple circumferential Z-plasty or W-plasty (though some suggest a partial 50%–65% release initially to reduce vascular embarrassment); otherwise, bands should be released before growth disturbances occur, i.e. before 2 years. In Upton's method, reverse skin and subcutaneous fat flaps are separately transposed and closed as two layers to reduce indentation.

ACROSYNDACTYLY

Acrosyndactyly is classified along with constriction ring syndrome and is seen in Apert's syndrome. It is attributed to disruption after the digits have already separated, to be united by scar tissue. There may be fistulae, clefts or sinuses distal to the band and should be explored with probes.

- Deepen web spaces especially the first and release small skin bridges. Staged smaller procedures are preferable to single procedures to reduce adversely affecting the vascularity.
- Amputation with delayed reconstruction may be needed.

VIII. GENERALISED ANOMALIES

Arthrogryposis, achondroplasia, arachnodactyly and diastrophic dwarfism are also included in this category.

ARTHROGRYPOSIS ('CURVED JOINT')

Approximately 1 in 3000 live births are affected by arthrogryposis multiplex congenita. This is the presence of **bilateral symmetric** joint contracture affecting at least two areas (i.e. **multiple**), joints that are **non-progressive** and are associated with (intrauterine) motor unit defect with muscle wasting (and replacement with inelastic fibrofatty tissue). The lack of movement means that there are no flexion creases; sensation is normal. There is a characteristic posture:

- Shoulder internal rotation and adduction
- Elbow extension, forearm pronation
- Wrist and finger flexion
- Thumb clasped into palm
- Lower limbs – hip dislocation, knee subluxation and club feet

It is not a specific disease entity; rather, it is a descriptive diagnosis of the clinical features and may result from 300 different conditions. Cases are usually sporadic. The cause is often unknown, though theories include multifactorial influences such as

- Obstruction of foetal movement – increased intrauterine pressure, oligohydramnios
- Viral infection, chronic cyanide intoxication, exposure to paralysing agents

It is associated with syndromes/anomalies such as

- Klippel–Feil syndrome
- Sprengel's deformity
- Hypoplastic mandible, cleft palate
- Dislocated radial head
- Renal and cardiac anomalies

MANAGEMENT

A multidisciplinary team is useful.

- Splintage and stretching, e.g. serial casting.
- Surgery should aim to bring the hands to the front of the body at the table level. It consists mostly of a combination of skeletal reorganisation and **muscle transfer**:
  - Shoulder – external de-rotational osteotomy of humerus
  - Elbow – triceps release, flexion by transfer (triceps to biceps, Steindler flexorplasty, free gracilis)
  - Wrist – carpectomy (total or proximal row), osteotomies of radius and ulnar, FCU to ECRB transfer
  - Fingers – osteotomy, FDS to extensor band transfer
  - Thumb (clasped)– thenar muscle release, four-flap plasty

DIFFERENTIAL DIAGNOSES OF A FLEXED THUMB (THUMB IN PALM)

Newborns have flexed thumbs until approximately 3 months of age (dominant flexor innervation has been proposed).

- Fixed flexion at the IPJ due to triggering related to Notta's nodule (a thickening of the FPL tendon). It is bilateral in 25%. It is not a true congenital abnormality as it actually develops in the first year or two of life. It is best to delay surgery as it may resolve spontaneously <2 years of age (30%) but should be differentiated from a clasped thumb.
- Clasped thumb involving the IPJ and the MCPJ may be due to weak or absent EPL tendon, and there may also be UCL instability. Other fingers may also be involved.
- Arthrogryposis.

SYMBRACHYDACTYLY

Symbrachydactyly (*sym* – together) is characterised by short, stiff-webbed fingers creating a U-shaped cleft (see also 'central deficiencies'). The cause is unknown but possibly related to a deficient blood supply, like **Poland's syndrome**, to which it has an association. It occurs in 1 in 32,000 cases and is not inherited.

There are four types (**Blauth**). Overall function tends to be reasonable as the condition is unilateral.

- Peromelic type – digits are nubbins.
- Short finger type – short fingers, telescoped due to the action of rudimentary long tendons.
- Cleft hand type (**ulnar side more affected**, absence of central finger).
- Monodactylous type.

SURGICAL OPTIONS

- **Phalangeal transfer** (non-vascularised) – a toe PP usually the third and fourth. There are potential problems with growth and thus transfer is usually performed before 2 years of age when there is a better chance of growth of the transferred parts. The toes are ultimately shorter, but there are a few problems with mobility.
- Distraction osteogenesis after 7 years old.
- Deepen web spaces.
- Toe–hand transfer.

MADELUNG'S DEFORMITY

This condition with AD inheritance is an abnormality leading to premature closure of the ulnar third of the distal radial epiphysis. (It is not the same as Madelung's disease, which is symmetrical non-encapsulated lipomatosis of the upper body.) It usually presents at ages 8–12 years (F>M); there is pain and decreased supination at the forearm, and limitation of wrist movement especially extension.

- Radius – short, radial inclination >20° with the horizontal
- Ulnar – dorsal subluxation, enlarged ulnar head
- Carpus – wedge shaped
- Widened interosseous space

Treatment options

- Excision of the ulnar head (prominent)
- Wedge osteotomies of the radius

D. ACQUIRED CONDITIONS OF THE HAND

I. DUPUYTREN'S DISEASE

GENERAL FEATURES AND ANATOMY

This was first described by Sir Astley Cooper and Henry Cline, then by Guillame Dupuytren in 1831. Dupuytren's disease (DD) is a benign fibroproliferative disorder characterised by abnormal thickening and contracture of the palmar fascia, affecting predominantly the longitudinal fibres and vertical fibres (of Skoog) resulting in palmar nodules and contractures of the fingers. It may be associated with other fibromatoses.

The disease is characterised by three phases (Luck's classification, 1959):

- Proliferative – no purposeful arrangement.
- Involutional – alignment of the myofibroblasts along lines of tension.
- Residual – the tissue becomes mostly acellular, devoid of myofibroblasts, and resembles a tendon.

GENETIC FACTORS

The disease affects mainly White men – classically those of Celtic descent in the middle age. The male/female ratio is ~14:1; Hueston suggested that this may be in part due to the fact that females tend to get the disease later and have a less severe form.

- It is less common in Afro-Caribbeans and Asians (though some parts of Japan and Taiwan have high prevalence; these [like diabetics] tend to have palmar disease without finger contractures, i.e. nodules without cord formation, and thus tend to require less surgery).
  - Those with RA have a reduced risk.

Cases can be sporadic or inherited in an AD manner with variable penetrance. Strong family history in some patients suggests a single gene defect, possibly affecting the expression of γ-interferon or high-affinity TGF-β receptors on fibroblasts.

- Other fibroproliferative conditions (Peyronie's, Lederhosen's) may be pleiotropic effects of the same gene.
- Possible link with trisomy 8.
- Increased relative risk 2.94 for those with HLA-DR3 (Neumuller J, *Clin Immunol Immunopathol*, 1994; but many others did not find HLA association).

DUPUYTREN'S DIATHESIS (HUESTON JT, *PLAST RECONSTR SURG*, 1963)

This is an aggressive form of Dupuytren's disease. It is often bilateral with more radial side involvement as well as diffuse dermal involvement.

- Younger age of onset (<40 years age) and rapid progression.
- Recurrence is more likely and tends to be early.
- Strong family history.
- Other areas of involvement:

  - Garrod's knuckle pads (PIPJ) occur in ~20% of patients, lying between skin and extensor tendon, attached to paratenon.
  - Plantar fibromatosis (Lederhosen) but no flexion contracture.
  - Penile curvature (Peyronie).
  - Frozen shoulder.
  - The first two rarely cause symptoms.

OTHER FACTORS

In other patients, environmental factors seem to play a role; it is important to realise that many have been put forward but few are confirmed.

- **Diabetes** – double the risk, but milder (and radial) disease and rarely need surgery. There is a 30% risk in those with diabetes <5 years, rising to 80% for

>20 years. It does not seem to be related to the need for insulin; possible link is micro-angiopathy.

- **Epilepsy/anti-epilepsy** drugs especially phenobarbitone – 2% of patients with DD are epileptic; incidence of DD in epileptics is two to three times higher than the general population.
- **Alcohol intake** – studies have shown correlation with the amount of alcohol consumed, though there is some controversy and is disputed (Gudmundsson KG, *Scan J Prim Health Care*, 2001).
- **Smoking** – affects glycosaminoglycan concentrations supposedly.
- **Occupations** involving the use of vibrating hand tools (possibly via an effect on the small vessels of the hand, e.g. micro-angiopathy or oxygen free radicals). The majority of evidence points against it.

PATHOPHYSIOLOGY

Controversy remains; the precise triggers for fibroblast proliferation and collagen deposition have not been clearly elucidated.

- **Intrinsic theory** (McFarlane) – perivascular fibroblasts within normal fascia are the source of disease. However, the central cord has no precursor.
- **Extrinsic theory** (Hueston) – disease starts with proliferation of fibrous tissue de novo (due to, say, trauma, diabetes mellitus or smoking) as nodules appear superficial to palmar fascia, and then spreads as cords.
- **Synthesis theory** (Gosset) – combines both theories with nodules arising de novo and cords from pre-existing fascia.
- **Murrell's hypothesis** – age, environmental and genetic factors cause microvessel narrowing leading to local tissue ischaemia and oxygen free radical formation, which stimulates fibroblasts. Subsequent increase in cell density and contracture exacerbates the ischaemia.

AETIOLOGY

Molecular factors: there has been a relatively large amount of literature on the subject, but as yet, there is no unifying theory.

- **Myofibroblasts** (Gabiani G, *Am J Pathol*, 1972).
  - Prostaglandin-F2α (PGF2α) and lysophosphatidic acid seem to promote myofibroblast contraction.
  - Expression of type VI collagen during the proliferative phase acts as a scaffold for DD fibroblasts.
  - Disturbed regulation of fibroblastic terminal differentiation (apoptosis).
- Abnormality of expression of matrix metalloproteins (MMP).

- Microangiopathy, **local ischaemia** and xanthine oxidase **free radical** production have been proposed.
- **Fibrogenic cytokines** (including IL-1), free radicals (via xanthine oxidase) and growth factors.
  - Increased levels of growth factors in the diseased palmar fascia including bFGF, PDGF and TFG-β.
  - Modulation of TGF-β receptor expression: DD fibroblasts express high-affinity type 2 receptors vs. low-affinity type 1.
  - Low levels of interferon in DD patients (also low in black patients with keloids).

The commonest affected digit is the **ring finger** (then the little, and then the middle); both hands are usually involved. Palmar nodules appear at the base of the digit first, then painless cords develop proximal to this, progressing to the MCPJ then PIPJ contracture; DIPJ joint hyperextension may occur, DIPJ contracture is rare.

Dupuytren's disease: An overview. (Saar JD, *Plast Reconstr Surg*, 2000)

The diseased tissue possesses the biological features of benign neoplastic fibromatosis. The major collagen type of normal palmar fascia is predominantly type I, although small levels of type III are present. In DD, there is an increase in the ratio of type III to type I collagen.

- Early stage – type III collagen; at high fibroblast density, type I collagen production is inhibited (Murrell GAC, *J Hand Surg*, 1991).
- Active stage – type III and type V
- Advanced stage – type I

ANATOMY OF THE PALMAR FASCIA (MCGROUTHER)

The palmar fascia is a complex three-dimensional structure.

- Transverse fibres (these are usually not involved in DD).
- Vertical fibres (of Skoog) attached to the MCs.
- Longitudinal (horizontal) fibres of palmar fascia merge with the deep fascia of the forearm, whilst distally they pass in three layers:
  - Layer 1 – inserts into the skin between distal palmar crease and finger crease.
  - Layer 2 – spiral band of Gosset, either side of the flexor tendon, deep to the NVB and insert to the lateral digital sheet (LDS).
  - Layer 3 – deepest layer flexor tendon sheath just beyond the PIPJ.

'Bands' are normal whilst 'cords' represent disease. It is unusual to have diseased cords on both sides of the finger.

- **Spiral band** passes from the pretendinous band at the base of the finger, beneath the NVB, and reattaches to the continuation of the **pretendinous band**, the **central band**, which itself attaches distally to the flexor sheath.

- **Spiral cord**, which causes PIPJ contracture, is formed from the 'PLSG (plastic surgeons look good)' – pretendinous band, spiral band, LDS, and Grayson's ligament (on the volar surface, Cleland's ligament is spared). This is important as the spiral cord can displace the **neurovascular structures** proximally, medially and superficially placing them at risk of injury during surgery (Figure 6.23).
- Change in the Grayson's ligament is said to be most dangerous, displacing the NVB towards the midline and also more superficially. The 'danger zone' lies between the MP and the middle of the palm.
- Spiral, lateral and central cords insert into the flexor sheath and the MP just distal to the PIPJ; thus all cause **PIPJ contracture.**
- **Pretendinous band** becomes pretendinous cord, which causes MCPJ contracture (without NVB displacement).
- **Natatory ligament** spans the web spaces and then bifurcates at each digit to form the lateral band (lateral to the NVB, intimately adherent to skin) and attach to the pretendinous band. Natatory cords cause web space/adduction contracture.
- **Lateral cord** runs from the natatory ligament to the LDS and is rarely seen.
- **Central cord has no fascial precursor** and is the most common cause of PIPJ contracture (but does not displace bundle).
- **Retrovascular band of Thomine** (formed by fascia just deep to the NVB, hence the name) lies just superficial to Cleland's ligament and attaches to the

periosteum of the PP, extending to insert into the periosteum of the DP causing **DIPJ contracture**.
- Cleland ligaments are said to be never involved.

Nodules are independent of the fascia; any adhesion to the aponeurosis is secondary. They show preference for pretendinous zones, e.g. the base of the phalanx distal to the first IP crease. There is a high density of myofibroblasts in these nodules.

In summary,

- Pretendinous cord causes MCPJ contracture.
- Central cord causes PIPJ contracture (and has no precursor).
- Lateral cord causes PIPJ (and DIPJ) contracture.
- Natatory cords adduction contracture.
- Spiral and lateral cords displace NVB.
- Cleland ligaments are not involved.

PATIENT ASSESSMENT

History

- Age, hand dominance, occupation or hobbies
  - Check for Dupuytren's diathesis – age of onset of disease, family history, rate of progression of disease and other affected areas.
- Functional deficit and social history particularly if the patient lives alone, as it has implications for post-operative discharge plans
- Drugs – aspirin/warfarin, oral hypoglycaemics, anti-epileptics
- Smoking history (affects graft take and skin flap viability)
- Previous hand surgery

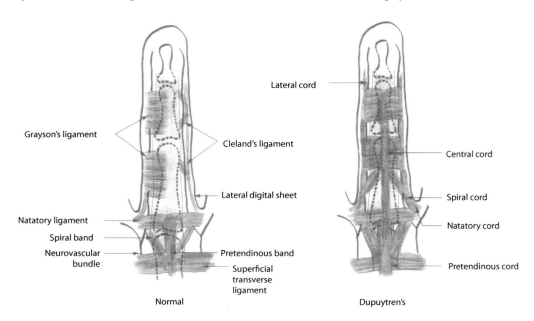

Figure 6.23 Comparison of normal structures and their analogues in a finger with DD. Grayson's ligament runs from the flexor sheath to the skin and is involved in DD, whilst Cleland's ligament runs from the bone to the skin, dorsal to the NVB, but is not involved in the disease. Note that the central cord has no precursor.

EXAMINATION

- Look
  - Garrod's pads (dorsum PIPJs)
  - Scars, swellings, sudomotor changes, skin lesions, wasting, attitude of the hand
- Feel – palmar nodules, thickening, degree of skin involvement, sensation distal to any site of proposed surgery
- Move
  - Active and passive ROM of the affected digits to quantify degree of contracture
  - Examination of each of the three nerves of the hand

INVESTIGATIONS

- There are no specific investigations. Plain X-rays may be used to determine the degree of joint changes in long-standing patients to predict results.

NON-OPERATIVE TREATMENT

- Splintage with a thermoplastic night splint pending any surgery.
  - Messina (*Plast Reconstr Surg*, 1993) used skeletal traction (TEC device) to get 2 mm lengthening per day over weeks, to soften cords and straighten fingers. Pipster (Hodgkinson) and Verona (Messina) devices were refinements. In 2000, Piza-Katzer described a non-invasive alternative extension procedure using a balloon coupled with a custom metal plate. None of these have really taken off in a big way. It may be useful to avoid amputation in severe cases.
- Steroid injections to nodules and pads may help pain.
- **Collagenase** (clostridium histolyticum) injections are promising. Xiaflex was approved by the FDA in February 2010 for use in DD with a palpable cord (FDA approval for treatment of Peyronie's disease in 2013). It may be best for MCPJ contractures, but the best indications and longevity remain unclear at this time. An average of 3 injections are needed, with or without 'finger extension procedures'.
  - 2014 announcement regarding risk of tendon rupture (3 cases of flexor tendor rupture in 1082 patients) and how to avoid it, as well as the potential for hypersensitivity/anaphylaxis (15% had pruritis after three injections).
- Regression has been noted in rare cases especially paralysed hands.

INDICATIONS FOR SURGERY

Surgery is still regarded as the gold standard treatment for DD.

- Contracture >30° at the MCPJ.
- Any contracture at the PIPJ, in practice >20°.

- Contractures of the first web space, i.e. thumb adduction.
- Painful palmar nodules or Garrod's pads.
- Hueston table-top test – place the palm on a table top; if it cannot be placed flat, then surgery is recommended.

The **rate of progression** is probably the best indication for surgery; also it is important to consider the severity of the functional limitation and its importance to the patient. Surgery should be avoided in those with arthritis, those with active infection/inflammation and those likely to be poorly compliant. MCPJ contractures are more correctable than PIPJ contractures.

TECHNIQUES

The fascia, skin and joint can be considered separately.

- It can be performed under general or regional anaesthesia.
- Make markings then inflate the tourniquet. Loupes should be used.
- Variety of incisions can be used – **Bruner** or multiple Z-plasty; transverse wounds may be left open if short of skin and to prevent haematoma – **open palm** (McCash) technique. Combination of palmar transverse incision and digital Z-plasty was first suggested by McIndoe and modified by Skoog.

MANAGEMENT OF THE FASCIA

- **Fasciotomy** (Sir Astley Cooper), which only releases tension in the fascia by **incising it**, e.g. for single band. Cline first proposed palmar fasciotomy as a surgical cure in 1787. It can be performed percutaneously (see 'needle aponeurotomy').
- Moermans described a **limited fasciectomy**, in which only short portions of fascia are **removed** – usually a limited fasciectomy of the pretendinous cord is sufficient to restore MCPJ function.
- **Regional (partial) fasciectomy is the most commonly** performed operation and entails removing all involved fascia in the palm and digit by a progressive, longitudinal dissection.
- **Extensive or radical fasciectomy** removes all involved fascia with the additional removal of **uninvolved fascia** to try to prevent disease progression or recurrence. This procedure is usually reserved for patients who have extensive disease or a diathesis. It has a higher rate of complications but still has a 50% long-term recurrence rate.
- **Dermofasciectomy with an FTSG** (Hueston, with the aim of removing dermis infiltrated by myofibroblasts) is often used to treat recurrent disease, skin involvement and diathesis patients. The **firebreak graft** aims to alter the tension line to reduce recurrence of disease, and inhibition of myofibroblast activity under the graft has been demonstrated in rat models. Advantages

need to be balanced against the risks of grafting as well as immobilisation.

- John Hueston (1926–1993) was an Australian surgeon and had worked with Archibald McIndoe at East Grinstead.

Needle aponeurotomy (NA), also known as needle fasciotomy, originated in France; NICE approval in the United Kingdom was gained in 2004. A needle bevel is used percutaneously to slowly saw through the cords (previously a blade was used) and can be performed under LA in outpatients. Some say that as recurrence is almost inevitable whatever treatment is used, safety is as important as efficacy.

Complication rates of <1% are quoted and include skin breaks, nerve injury, tendon injury and infection. The results of NA can approach those of open surgery (>50% recurrence at 5 years), and whilst the results are not as long lasting, the procedure can be safely repeated as required. In addition, recovery is quicker and patient satisfaction higher, although this has not been objectively compared. **In general, NA is suited to treatment of early-stage disease and is particularly recommended for the elderly**. It is not suitable for diffuse or severe disease, cases with tethered skin, MCPJ contracture or previous open surgery. Approximately 10%–15% of cases need open surgery rather than NA.

Comparison of treatment outcome after collagenase and needle fasciotomy for Dupuytren contracture. (Stromberg J, J Hand Surg, 2016)
This is a single-blinded RCT comparing collagenase treatment versus needle fasciotomy (NF) in 140 patients with disease at the MCPJ (palpable cord, deficit of at least 20°), with the primary endpoint being a straight joint (within 5°) being assessed by a blinded physiotherapist at 1 week and 1 year. The results at 1 week were 88% response in the collagenase group vs. 90% in the NF group; at 1 year, it was 90% in both. Procedural pain was 4.9/10 vs. 2.7/10, respectively. There was one recurrence in each group.

The follow-up period is rather short and did not include PIPJ contractures, which are more difficult to treat.

JOINT

One suggested protocol is that after excision of diseased fascia,

- If the PIPJ can extend to 30° or less from full extension, then it is deemed satisfactory (physiotherapy is likely to maintain/improve).
- If >30°, then manipulate.
- If still >30°, then capsule/ligament release can be considered.

PROCEDURES

- **Joint release** – incision of the flexor sheath, the accessory collateral ligaments and the check rein ligaments (proximal attachment of the volar plate). Release the

volar plate from the accessory collateral ligament. This tends to improve extension, i.e. reduce contracture but may cause reduced active flexion.

- **Joint replacement is very uncommon;** arthrodesis is a salvage procedure for severe recurrence (>70° at the PIPJ).
- **Amputation** is another choice for salvage.

Most benefit/extension is gained from the release of MCPJ contracture rather than IPJ contracture. The best predictors of post-operative correction/outcome are preoperative deformity and intra-operative correction.

POST-OPERATIVE MANAGEMENT

Rehabilitation should be started after the early inflammatory phase (3–5 days); after a dressing change/check, ROM exercises (to reduce oedema) are taught by therapists.

- A volar splint is applied at the end of the procedure.
- This is changed for a thermoplastic splint at ~3–5 days that is then kept for 2 weeks until sutures are removed.
  - Hand ROM exercises 1–2 hourly are initiated – all joints without excess wound tension, 12 repetitions five times a day.
- 2 weeks – non-absorbable sutures are removed and scars are massaged.
- Over the next 2 months, the aim is to strengthen during the day with exercises and to use a splint at night (up to 6 months).

COMPLICATIONS OF SURGERY

Complication rates are relatively high (McFarlane and McGrouther), up to 17%–19% overall.

- Intra-operative
  - NVB in 3% of patients. Division or over-stretching and arterial spasm may lead to ischaemia and temporary paraesthesia.
- Early post-operative
  - Haematoma (mostly in the palm), skin flap necrosis or graft loss and infection.
- Late post-operative
  - Inadequate release (inadequate fascia excision, failure to address joint contracture) or recurrent contracture (including poor compliance with physiotherapy). All patients should be advised that the disease will recur, with rates ranging from 26% to 80%, or more simply 50% at 5 years and 100% at more than 10 years. Dermofasciectomy should be considered for recurrent disease; arthrodesis, arthroplasty and amputation are salvage options.
  - Stiffness. DIPJ contracture is very difficult to improve due to tight lateral bands and ORL, and release of the PIPJ actually makes the latter worse. Usually treated conservatively.

- CRPS type 1 (4% of males, 8% of females), 5% of patients overall. The flare response is often regarded as a form of CRPS (see 'CRPS' above).
- Scar-related problems.

POOR PROGNOSTIC FACTORS

- Early age of onset
  - Gelberman (*Bone Join Surg*, 1980) found that recurrence is not related to age at onset, duration or severity of disease
- Presence of Garrod's knuckle pads
- Multiple rays involved
- Epilepsy or alcoholism
- Dupuytren's diathesis

Dupuytren's disease in children. (Urban M, *J Hand Surg Br*, 1996)

DD is very rare in children; this article presents two cases <13 years of age, and there were only seven other histologically confirmed cases of DD in this age group reported at the time. The authors suggest that DD in children should be treated aggressively, particularly early consideration of **dermofasciectomy**.

TRIGGER FINGER

This is a stenosing tenosynovitis of the flexor tendon, which can be primary (including congenital) or secondary (less common, usually due to RA, gout, diabetes). The ring and middle fingers are mostly frequently affected in adults (index rarely). It may co-exist with de Quervain's disease or with CTS.

In most cases, the primary event seems to be A1 pulley stenosis, which stimulates nodular change in the FDP that then becomes too big to slide through the pulley. Patients complain of either being stuck or being unable to flex the thumb actively. On examination, gentle pressure over the A1 pulley (distal palmar crease) reproduces the pain. The finger is not usually swollen; if it is – suspect another condition.

- Steroid injections (at the **A1 pulley** or flexor sheath at the PP) are usually beneficial in cases of short duration (60% chance of success, can be curative in 70% with three injections), but these have the tendency to recur frequently.
  - Adults who do not respond to injection or has <4 months of relief can be considered for surgery.
- Release of the A1 pulley offers operative cure, but caution is needed in RA patients as the A1 pulley attaches to the head of the metacarpal, and its release may exacerbate the tendency towards volar subluxation.

II. HAND TUMOURS AND MASSES

Malignant bone tumours are commonly metastases, especially bronchial carcinoma, which affects the DP most frequently. The most common malignant tumour of the upper limb is SCC.

GANGLION CYSTS

These are mucin-filled cysts continuous with the underlying joint capsule; they are the most common masses occurring in the hands. They are three times more common in **women** and 70% occur in those with age <40. There are some uncommon associations: metacarpal boss, de Quervain's disease (first extensor compartment ganglion) and Heberden's nodes (mucous cysts).

- Present due to a 'lump', pain or wrist weakness.
- There is a history of trauma in up to 10%, but there seems to be no correlation with occupation.
- They **transilluminate** unless deep and are thought to represent mucoid degeneration of fibrous connective tissue – histological examination demonstrates collagen without synovial or epithelial cells. The fluid contains glucosamine, albumin and hyaluronic acid.
- They are **not true cysts** as the lining is not composed of cells; rather the lining is made up of compressed and degenerate stromal tissues.

The pathogenesis is poorly understood (Gude W, *Curr Rev Musculoskelet Med*, 2008)

- Ball valve effect.
- Metaplasia produces microcysts and fibrous metaplasia forms mucoid cells.
- Embryonic rests (ganglions may arise away from synovial joints).
- Other theories include the following:
  - Ligament strain/capsular rent – there is little direct evidence to support this.
  - Capsule herniation – this has even less evidence as there is a lack of synovial lining; similarly, they are not inflammatory in nature.

It is an entirely benign condition; there have been no reported cases of malignancy. They have a tendency to subside with rest and enlarge with activity; most ganglia resolve spontaneously (50% in adults after 5 years, 75% in children).

COMMON TYPES

- **Dorsal wrist ganglia** (70%) lie directly over the **scapholunate ligament** (midline) or connected to it by a pedicle; it is most often found between the third and fourth MCs. Occult ganglions may only be identified by volar wrist flexion and may be associated with underlying scapholunate diastasis (e.g. RA). No treatment is required unless there is pain, functional disability or RSS: 60% of dorsal wrist ganglia will resolve. Surgery involves a transverse incision and exposure of the ganglion between the thumb and index finger extensors (ECRL, ECRB and EPL radially and EC and EI ulnarly). Note that the rare extensor tendon ganglions are located more distally over the back of the hand.

- **Volar wrist ganglia** (20% in adults, but most **common type in children**) arise mainly from the radiocarpal ligament, lying under the volar wrist crease between the FCR and the APL. It is important to take care to preserve the radial artery during surgery as it is often intimately attached to, or encircled by, the ganglion. Allen's test is needed before surgery; inadequate ulnar perfusion may contraindicate surgery.
- **Flexor sheath (seed) ganglia** (~10%) are small, firm, tender masses in the palm or base of the finger and arise from the **A1 pulley** or occasionally more distally. They may be related to direct trauma to the flexor sheath, and if excised, then a small portion of the flexor sheath is taken. Aspiration or steroid injection may be temporising measures.
- **Mucous cysts** are ganglia of the **DIPJ** found on the dorsum of the finger lying to one side of the central slip insertion of the extensor tendon. There may be **longitudinal nail grooving**. The overlying skin is often taut and thin and may necrose/rupture. They can be associated with OA (and osteophytes of the DIPJ, which need to be removed); occult cysts may exist on the other side. It is often found in older patients.

MANAGEMENT

Non-operative

- Aspiration and injection of steroid (small or occult dorsal ganglions)
- Extrinsic rupture ('bible' ganglions)

OPERATIVE

Operative treatment is indicated for pain, deformity or reduced function. There is a 30%–50% recurrence rate. 'Recurrence' is probably mostly related to inadequate excision; sometimes it may be related to occult intraosseous ganglions. Complications include scar tenderness or numbness and joint stiffness; 25% require up to 8 weeks to regain maximal function.

- Excision of the whole cyst with stalk and the joint surface at the point of attachment, closing the joint capsule, is not essential as it may lead to prolonged immobilisation and stiffness.
- Avoid injury to the superficial branch of the RN.
- No splintage is required.

DIFFERENTIAL DIAGNOSES: OTHER HAND/ WRIST MASSES

- **Carpometacarpal boss**. These are palpable bony lumps (exostosis) on the dorsum of the second/third MC bases that present as swellings, with pain and decreased extension at the wrist. The diagnosis can

be confirmed by X-ray. They are twice as common in women (especially 20–30 years) and twice as common on the right hand; 30% are associated with wrist ganglion, whilst many also have arthritis.

- After excision, a cast is needed for up to 6 weeks. Recurrence may occur; rongeuring the bone after excision may help.
- **Pigmented villonodular synovitis** (giant cell tumour [GCT] of the tendon sheath). This is a relatively common benign tumour that usually presents as a bossellated yellow swelling on the volar surface of the finger or around a joint, particularly the radial digits. It may be confused with a ganglion, but GCTs are fixed to deeper tissues, possibly eroding the bone.
  - Treat by excision, but typically there is a high rate of recurrence, either due to incomplete surgery or to satellite lesions.
- **Epidermoid inclusion cysts** may follow penetrating injuries that cause implantation of epidermoid cells. It presents as a firm, spherical mass on parts that are exposed to injuries, i.e. fingers and palm; the contents are a mixture of protein, cholesterol and fat. These should be excised completely to avoid recurrence.

BONE TUMOURS

Benign

Enchondromas are the commonest benign bone tumour (90% of bone tumours in the hand). They are well-demarcated swellings that are radiolucent, expansile lesions of the non-epiphyseal portions of tubular bones, usually the phalanges and metacarpals. Most are asymptomatic, but some present with a pathological fracture. Treat with curettage with or without cancellous bone grafts. There is a lifetime malignant risk of 10% in solitary tumours.

- Multiple enchondromas occur in Ollier's disease – a rare condition.
- Multiple enchondroma with vascular malformations is Maffucci's syndrome.
- Both can lead to chondrosarcoma (>25% before 40 years) and should be treated by wide excision.

Osteochondroma – are relatively more common in younger patients; they appear as bony protuberances with a narrow stalk arising from the **metaphyseal** cortex particularly the distal end of the PP. There is an association with EXT1 gene. Treatment should be wide excision.

- **Multiple osteochondromatosis.** There may be abnormalities of stature. There is a 1% risk of malignant transformation (more than solitary lesions).
- **Chondroma** – benign cartilaginous tumours that often arise from an abnormal focus of cartilage.

Aneurysmal bone cysts – these constitute 5% of all benign bone tumours and occur before the closure of the epiphyseal plates in the second decade, most commonly affecting the vertebrae and knee. The aetiology is unknown – it may be related to the vascularity of the bone; some lesions are associated with pre-existing bone conditions such as GCT (19%–39% of cases), fibrous dysplasia and chondro-/osteoblastomas. They appear as **painful radiolucent** expansile locally destructive lesions particularly the metacarpals in upper limb involvement (21% of total). X-rays are usually diagnostic; MRI/CT can add detail.

- Excision with bone grafting is most definitive but destructive.
- Curettage is associated with a high recurrence rate of up to 60%.
- As a compromise, to preserve joint surfaces, etc.
  - Intralesional excision, improving marginal control with measures such as liquid nitrogen, argon laser, PMMA (exothermic) and phenol (less common now)
  - Selective arterial embolisation or intralesional injection, e.g. Ethibloc, with or without prednisolone or calcitonin

OSTEOID OSTEOMA

These lesions (10% of benign bone tumours) usually occur in young adult males (two to three times more common than in females), are characterised by localised pain that is worst at night and are **relieved by NSAIDs**. The DP is most commonly involved. On X-ray, they show up as a radiolucent nidus with surrounding sclerosis and are 'hot spots' on a bone scan. Surgery involves curettage possibly with bone grafting – recurrences are usually associated with incomplete resection; some cases may be treated with percutaneous radiofrequency ablation (Ryan CB, Foster RCB, *Semin Intervent Radiol*, 2014).

Osteoblastomas are rare in the hand, but when they do occur, they are mostly restricted to the wrist, particularly the scaphoid, presenting as painful swellings. They are poorly mineralised swellings of immature neoplastic osteoid. Surgical wide local resection is usually successful; post-operative radiotherapy may be indicated in certain cases.

GCT of bone (osteoclastoma) was first described by Chassaignac in 1852 who thought they were neoplasms. These often occur around the knee rather than the hand (2%–5% of total) affecting mostly middle-aged females. The cause is unknown but probably reflects a reactive/regenerative hyperplasia associated with an inflammatory process (Jaffe); PCR shows them to be polyclonal proliferations. There have been sporadic reports of malignancy, but most are probably doubtful. Most lesions are histologically benign but **locally aggressive** with soft tissue involvement – some exhibit malignant-type behaviour and may metastasise to the lungs (5%, still histologically benign), even leading to death. GCTs of the distal radius may be more aggressive than in other areas.

They are solitary lesions with a dull ache and hindrance to movement. On X-ray they are lucent/lytic lesions often near to the epiphyseal regions, and their **lack of sclerosis**

differentiates them from other bone tumours. MRI is useful to assess soft tissue and medullary involvement prior to surgery, which is the preferred treatment modality (intralesional excision for stage I/II or en bloc with a wide margin for stage III), though radiotherapy may be used for non-resectable lesions. Pathological fractures should be allowed to heal before surgery.

- **Stage I** – benign latent GCT with no locally aggressive activity.
- **Stage II** – benign active GCT; imaging demonstrates alteration of the cortical structure.
- **Stage III** – locally aggressive; imaging demonstrates a lytic lesion, and there may be tumour penetration through the cortex into the soft tissues.
- **GCTs in bone are different from GCTs of the tendon sheath,** which are the second commonest swelling in the hand. The latter are areas of localised nodular synovitis and are composed of histiocytes from the flexor tendon sheath (usually the volar aspect of the DIPJ, bone GCTs are often found in the distal radius).

MALIGNANT

Chondrosarcoma – this is the **most common primary malignant bone tumour** in the hand, often arising in an older age group (60–80 years) with an association with osteochondroma and enchondromas. It is typically a painful mass around the MCPJ with a slow clinical course and only metastasises late. Amputation is the mainstay of treatment, but recurrence is not uncommon.

Ewing's sarcoma – this rarely affects the hand, but this subset may have a better prognosis than usual with good local control following surgery and chemotherapy with or without radiotherapy. It is typically a mass with a sclerotic reaction seen on X-ray affecting younger males (twice as common as in females).

Osteosarcoma – it is very rare in the hand (<0.1%) but is more frequent after irradiation, in those with Paget's disease, fibrous dysplasia, GCT of bone as well as osteochondromas/enchondromas. The immature osteoid is produced by the proliferating stroma (spindle cells). The typically rapidly growing painful mass has a **sunburst pattern** on X-ray. Excision with wide margins and adjuvant chemotherapy result in a 70% 5 year survival in the absence of metastasis (but this decreases to 10%–20% if there are metastases, which are uncommon).

Other soft tissue masses (see 'soft tissue sarcomas'):

- Glomus tumours.
- Peripheral nerve tumours (1%–5% of hand tumours).
  - Schwannomas.
  - Neurofibromas, neurofibromatosis, malignant peripheral nerve sheath tumour.
  - Intraneural non-neural tumours, e.g. lipoma, haemangioma or lipofibromatous harmatoma. The median nerve is the most commonly affected and

may be associated with macrodactyly. It is usually not possible to separate the tumour from the nerve.

- Skin tumours.
  - Squamous cell carcinomas (SCCs) are the most common malignancy of the hand; SCCs of the hand constitute 11% of all SCCs, typically affecting the dorsum in elderly individuals (with pre-existing actinic changes). Web-space lesions seem to have a higher risk of metastasis. Surgery is the main treatment method; recurrence ranges from 7% to 28% for well- to poorly differentiated lesions, respectively.
  - Basal cell carcinomas (2% of all BCCs). Palmar and subungual lesions may be a feature of Gorlin's syndrome.
  - Melanoma (10%–20% of all). Treat with wide excision or amputation to joint proximal to lesion.
- Sarcomas are uncommon in the hand, though 15% occur in the upper limb in younger patients. There is a high incidence of lymphatic spread and nodal metastasis. In general, they are treated by excision with a wide (2–3 cm) margin with or without adjuvant therapy. An important determinant of the prognosis is being treated in a **sarcoma centre;** thus it is important that referral is made for any soft tissue swelling, that is,
  - Deep to fascia, greater than 5 cm in size, painful/ hard with rapid growth.
- Types of sarcoma include the following:
  - **Epithelioid (most common)** – local recurrence and distant metastasis is common.
  - **Fibrosarcoma** – more frequent in the deep subcutaneous space. Haematogenous spread is common.
  - **Synovial** – typically a slow-growing palm mass, but the prognosis is relatively poor due to the high propensity for distant spread. Consequently, treatment is usually multifactorial with surgery, radiotherapy and chemotherapy.
  - **Clear cell** (uncommon) – typically a slow-growing deep mass that is attached to fascia and tendons. Prognosis is poor.
  - **Malignant fibrous histiocytoma** – may be superficial or deep, multiple or solitary. There is a tendency to extend along tissue planes; it may metastasise through lymphatics or bloodstream.
  - **Alveolar rhabdomyosarcoma** – this is a highly malignant lesion that usually affects the palm (thenar/hypothenar muscles) in children. Prognosis is poor.
  - **Kaposi's sarcoma** – these are dark blue macules (most frequently found on the lower limbs) that can be associated with AIDS/HIV.

III. OSTEOARTHRITIS

This condition affects females more frequently and is mostly secondary to general **ageing** and trauma, including the microtrauma of daily repetitive actions. There is primary joint destruction. In the hand, the most commonly affected joints are the **DIPJ, CMCJ**, PIPJ and scaphotrapeziotrapezoid joint (STTJ) in order of decreasing frequency.

- History – in contrast to RA, there is less **pain** in the morning and **more during the day**, and it may interfere with sleep – but it is still important to formally rule out RA and its variants. The main difficulty the patient has is with movements such as opening jars or wringing out clothes.
- Examination may show point tenderness and 'grind test' (CMCJ).
  - Heberden's nodes – osteophytes at the DIPJ, may be painful
  - Bouchard's nodes – osteophytes at the PIPJ
- Radiology – typical changes are narrowed joint space, subchondral sclerosis (eburnation), cysts, osteophytes, bony exostoses, etc. Appearance on X-rays does not correlate well with symptoms.
  - Robert's (A–P) view of the thumb with X-ray beam at 90°
  - Eaton–Littler stress view for the CMCJ

Alnot's classification of (hand) pain. (Alnot JY, *Ann Chir Main*, 1985)

- 0 – no pain
- I – pain during particular activities
- II – pain during daily activities
- III – episodes of spontaneous pain
- IV – constant pain

TREATMENT

General non-operative

Once the articular cartilage has been destroyed, healing is not possible. Non-operative treatment should be maximised before surgery is considered.

- Splinting and activity modification
- NSAIDs
- Intra-articular steroids (may lead to ligament attenuation)

SURGERY

- Basal osteotomy (wedge osteotomy, removing the radial cortex to change the vector of stress forces acting on the joint)
- Trapeziectomy with FCR sling (Burton–Pellegrini) – probably the gold standard for management of late-stage CMJ OA
- Joint replacement
- Arthrodesis

RADIOLOGICAL STAGING

Distal interphalangeal joint

- Mucous cysts (which may cause nail deformities) and **Heberden's nodes** are notable features. There may be gross joint destruction with little pain.
- A painful DIPJ can be treated with an **arthrodesis** (screw, Lister loop of K-wire) via a dorsal incision (H, Y or inverted Y).

PROXIMAL INTERPHALANGEAL JOINT

OA in this region is often post-traumatic and presents with pain, deformity and possibly impingement from the osteophytes (**Bouchard's nodes**).

- **Arthrodesis** is a good option particularly for the IF to provide a stable post for pinch. This relieves pain at the cost of the loss of mobility.
- **Arthroplasty** is preferred for the ring and little fingers to accommodate the power grip but requires reasonable bone stock. Options include Swanson's (silastic interpositional) or metal/carbon (pyocarbon – inert with good wear characteristics). Dorsal tendon splitting, volar, lateral or Charney approaches may be used.

THUMB CMCJ/BASAL JOINT

It is said that there is a high density of **oestrogen receptors** in the basal joint of the thumb (and in the hip), which have a role in degenerative changes (hence higher incidence in post-menopausal women).

Joint stability is dependent on the anterior oblique ligament (volar beak) from the trapezium to the volar ulnar metacarpal, which limits the dorsal movement of the metacarpal. Traditionally, it is thought that in OA, the ligament is attenuated/stretched, and the thumb will become adducted and hyperextended. The thumb will eventually collapse in a **zigzag**.

Symptoms include **pain** on the radial side of the wrist (differential diagnoses include scaphotrapeziotrapezoid [STT] OA, de Quervain's, Wartenburg's, CT), swelling and crepitus with a weak pinch. **Positive grind test** is strongly suggestive.

- Ask for Eaton (stress) views: thumbs against each other in resisted abduction, palms flat.

Eaton and Littler Classification of Thumb CMCJ Arthrosis. (Eaton RG, *J Bone Joint Surg*, 1973)

- I – <1/3 subluxation at the CMCJ
- II – 1/3 subluxation, osteophytes <2 mm
- III – >1/3 subluxation, >2 mm, minor joint narrowing
- IV – Advanced. Major subluxation, joint space narrowing, sclerosis and osteophytes >2 mm

REVISION: EATON AND GLICKEL CLASSIFICATION (1987):

- **Stage I.** Mild joint narrowing or subchondral sclerosis, mild joint effusion or ligament laxity. No subluxation or osteophyte formation. Treatment includes **NSAIDs and immobilisation**, which involves splinting the thumb in abduction.
- **Stage II.** Joint narrowing and small osteophytes. Besides CMCJ narrowing and subchondral sclerosis, there may be joint debris – osteophyte formation/loose bodies (<2 mm) at the ulnar side of the distal trapezial articular surface. Mild to moderate subluxation, with the base of the first MC dislocated radially and dorsally. Treatment: ligament reconstruction tendon interposition (LRTI).
- **Stage III.** Significant CMCJ destruction. Further joint space narrowing with cystic changes and bone sclerosis. Larger joint debris >2 mm, including prominent osteophytes at the ulnar border of the distal trapezium. The first MC is moderately displaced radially and dorsally. There could be a hyperextension deformity of the CMCJ. The scaphotrapezial joint (STJ) appears normal. Treat by **LRTI.**
- **Stage IV.** Involvement of both the CMCJ and the STJ. The destruction of the CMC joint is similar to that in stage III, whilst the STJ has evidence of destruction with sclerosis and cysts. The CMC joint is usually immobile, and often patients have little pain. Treat by **LRTI.**

TREATMENT

Indications for surgery: failure of conservative management, pain, disabling joint instability and first web contracture – **never for deformity alone.** The CMCJ is the most commonly reconstructed area in the OA of the upper limb.

- Rest/immobilisation.
- Oral anti-inflammatories/steroid injections – may provide temporary relief, but **permanent relief when the joint surfaces are destroyed can only be obtained by separating the damaged surfaces:**
  - **Trapeziectomy** with interposition and ligament reconstruction is the commonest. It is a simple procedure and is effective in relieving pain. Disadvantages include thumb shortening, weak pinch and reduced thumb adduction. It is probably the gold standard for late disease; by comparison, the best management of early disease is less certain.
    - **LRTI** (Burton and Pellegrini). Trapezium is excised and a distal FCR slip is tunnelled through the base of the thumb metacarpal and sutured back onto itself and anchored into the trapezial space. The Weilby technique uses the APL. The exact indications for LRTI are not well defined.

- **Implant arthroplasty** – spacers of various materials (silicone abandoned due to high complications), prosthetics (e.g. Swanson silicone trapezium implant or titanium) with possible complications of instability and prosthesis dislocation.
- **Arthrodesis** is used in isolated cases – for painful instability particularly following Bennetts fracture. There will be stiffness.
- **Metacarpal osteotomy** – particularly for stages I and II.

Scaphotrapeziotrapezoid (STT) OA (pain and swelling at the scaphoid pole in anatomical snuffbox and on wrist motion – **radial grind test**) should be carefully excluded as an involved joint generally excludes CMC arthroplasty. The main complication of treatment is non-union; a good outcome can be expected if union is achieved.

- Trapeziectomy for pantrapezial disease
- For isolated STT OA – fusion of STT with 6 weeks in plaster to decrease wrist movement, to reduce the significant non-union rate
- Excision arthroplasty – excise distal scaphoid, 3 weeks in plaster
- Interposition arthroplasty

METACARPOPHALANGEAL JOINT

MCPJ degeneration causes subluxation of the MC base, and the first web is narrowed by MC adduction deformity. There may be hyperextension deformity and instability. The aim of the treatment is to provide good pinch and stability:

- If hyperextension is >30°, then MCPJ arthrodesis (15° flexion and 10° pronation), volar plate capsulodesis and APL advancement.
- If hyperextension is >30°, then K-wire.

PISOTRIQUETRAL OA

There is typically pain over the volar ulnar wrist, and symptoms may be elicited by the hand resting on hard surfaces, e.g. **writing**. One-third of patients also have ulnar neuropathy.

- Provocation – compression with side-to-side movement that will elicit severe pain over the joint.
- Treat with steroid injection, splint wrist in slight flexion – if there is no relief after two injections, then consider pisiform excision with or without minimal triquetral excision.

CARPUS AND WRIST

The radial side is more frequently involved; involvement of the middle row is rare.

- 90% involve scaphoid.
- 50% SLAC pattern.
- 20% STT pattern.
- 10% combination.

SLAC WRIST

This refers to a specific pattern of OA and subluxation resulting from untreated chronic scaphoid non-union or chronic scapholunate dissociation (SLD). There is a predictable pattern of changes in the areas of abnormal loading (Watson stages). The radiolunate joint is spared.

- Stage I – distal radioscaphoid arthritis – attenuation of carpal ligament
- Stage II – proximal radioscaphoid arthritis – scaphoid mal-alignment
- Stage III – capitolunate arthritis

Watson's scaphoid shift test for SLAC – dorsally directed pressure is applied over the distal scaphoid tubercle with the examiner's thumb; if the scapholunate ligament is torn, then there is pain when the scaphoid proximal pole subluxes out of the scaphoid fossa of the radius as the hand is passively moved from ulnar to radial deviation.

- SNAC (scaphoid non-union advanced collapse) wrist can be difficult to differentiate from SLAC.
- The commonest treatment is arthrodesis (see below).

TREATMENT

- **Denervation.**
- **Joint excision** (scaphoid, proximal row carpectomy).
- **Arthrodesis.**
    - Total wrist fusion – relieves pain (not always totally) whilst sacrificing function.
    - Limited carpal fusion (LCF) – four-corner fusion – if the articular surface of the proximal lunate is intact, i.e. radiolunate changes exclude the use of LCF. This is often combined with scaphoid excision.
    - Scaphoid excision and intercarpal arthrodesis.
    - Radioscaphoid, radioscapholunate.
- **Arthroplasty.** Numerous types of implants have been used, but implant wear and loosening are common complications.

Free and island vascularized joint transfer for proximal interphalangeal reconstruction. (Foucher G, *J Hand Surg Am*, 1994)
Options for stiff and arthritic PIPJ are as follows:

- Arthrodesis
- Skoog perichondrial arthroplasty
- Silicone joint replacement (reversed Swanson's)
- Non-vascularised joint transfers (in young children)
- Islanded vascularised joint transfers:
    - Heterodigital joint including collateral ligaments, volar plate, extensor tendon and vascular pedicle, e.g. the PIPJ or DIPJ from a non-functioning finger.
    - Homodigital, e.g. islanded DIPJ transfer (the DIPJ contributes 15° to the flexion arc, whereas the PIPJ contributes 85°); thus, DIPJ transfer can be an option following complex trauma to the PIPJ.

This is then followed by DIPJ arthrodesis and reinsertion of FDP.

- Free vascularised joint transfer – joints harvested from a non-replantable finger, or toe donor, along with skin island and extensor tendon with a common example being joint transfer from the second toe

IV. RHEUMATOID ARTHRITIS

RA is a systemic autoimmune phenomenon mediated by B and T lymphocytes affecting mainly synovial tissues within joints but can affect many other tissues/organs. Rheumatoid factor (RF) is a circulating macroglobulin (IgM) present in 70% of RA patients (15% of normal population); there is increased ESR, CRP and reduced haemoglobin. It affects 1% of the population. It tends to affect females (4:1 males) in their 20s–40s.

The American College of Rheumatologists state that there must be at least four of the following seven signs for at least 6 weeks.

- **Morning stiffness** lasting for 1 hour
- Arthritis of more than three joint areas
- Arthritis of hand joints – MCPJ, PIPJ
- Symmetrical arthritis
- Subcutaneous nodules (on extensor surface)
- Positive RF
- X-ray evidence of erosions, cysts or osteopaenia, reduced joint space, carpal ankylosis

STAGES (LISTER)

- **Proliferative** – synovial swelling, pain, restricted movement, nerve compression
- **Destructive** – tendon rupture, capsular disruption, joint subluxation, bone erosion
- **Reparative** – fibrosis, tendon adhesions, fibrous ankylosis, fixed deformity

PATTERN

- Monocyclic – one episode, spontaneous remission, 10%
- Polycyclic – remissions and relapses, 45%
- Progressive – inexorable course, 45%

There is a mixture of soft tissue and articular changes. T cells (CD4) are important in joint destruction; collagenases and prostaglandins damage cartilage.

SOFT TISSUES

Tendons

Tenosynovitis (>50% in RA); synovitis is a synovial inflammation with formation of pannus and release of erosive enzymes. It may occur before joint involvement.

- It may manifest as tender boggy swelling dorsum of the wrist and around flexor tendons, leading to tendon ruptures and disruption of the stabilising structures

around joints. When a joint persistently adopts angulation, the joints either side tend to go in opposite directions due to the change in tendon mechanics, i.e. Z deformities such as Swan neck or boutonnière.

- **Tenosynovitis** of flexor tendons and triggering. The A1 pulley should be preserved:
  - Release worsens volar subluxation of proximal phalanges.
  - Flexor tendons are held by the pulley to the volar plate and to the head of the MC; release increases the lever arm of the tendon increasing the MCPJ flexion deformity.
- **Tendon ruptures** may be due to **synovitis**, e.g. EDC 4/5, EDM – sometimes known as a **Vaughan–Jackson lesion,** or due to **attrition**, e.g. ulnar head (EDM, EDC), scaphoid tubercle (FPL, Mannerfelt lesion) and Lister's tubercle (EPL). Ischaemic degeneration due to devascularisation may have an additional role. The rupture of juncturae allows ulnar subluxation into metacarpal gutters. EDM rupture can be tested for with the 'horn sign', asking the patient to extend the index and the little finger with the ring and middle flexed – this requires intact EI and EDM tendons.
  - The **Vaughan–Jackson** is the commonest tendon rupture in RA; the FPL (Mannerfelt) is the commonest flexor tendon rupture.

SKIN

- **Rheumatoid nodules** (foci of fibrinoid necrosis) are the most common extra-articular manifestation (25%) and a poor prognostic factor. They are most commonly found on the subcutaneous border of the ulna.
- **Palmar erythema.**
- **Vasculitic ulcers.**
- **Nerves:**
  - Nerve compression due to tenosynovitis/joint synovitis, e.g. CTS, also cubital and radial tunnel
  - Polyneuropathy
- **Muscle** – atrophy of intrinsics, inflammation, myopathy (or nerve compression).
- **Cardiovascular.**
  - Vessels – obliterative arteritis, vasculitis and Raynaud's
  - Cardiac – valvular, pericarditis/myocarditis
- **Respiratory** – nodules, pleuritis.
- **Eyes** – uveitis, iritis.
- **Haematological** – anaemia, Felty's (splenomegaly, lymphadenopathy).

JOINTS IN RA

The most common joints/upper limb deformities are

- Elbow – posterior subluxation of elbow
- Wrist and hand:
  - Palmar subluxation of the wrist, radial deviation of the wrist
  - Ulnar translocation of the carpus

- Fingers:
  - **Ulnar drift** of the fingers (MCPJ), **palmar subluxation** of the MCPJ
  - **Swan neck and boutonnières** of fingers and thumbs
  - Lateral dislocation of the IPJ
  - Z deformity of the thumb

OA VERSUS RA

The MCPJ and PIJP are most commonly involved in RA, whilst it is the DIPJ and thumb basal joint in OA.

Note also the neck joints, with implications for patients requiring general anaesthesia/intubation. There is a 25%–50% incidence of atlanto-axial instability – screen with X-rays with flexion and extension views.

- Atlanto-axial subluxation
- Superior migration of the odontoid peg into the foramen magnum
- Anterior subluxation of vertebral bodies

MANAGEMENT

Non-surgical treatment is the mainstay of RA management and usually consists of NSAIDs, steroid injections and splints. **In general, the increasing use of disease-modifying antirheumatoid drugs (DMARDs) has reduced the need for surgery in RA.**

- Drugs:
  - NSAIDs are first line – aspirin, indomethacin, naproxen.
  - Corticosteroids – systemic and injections.
  - **DMARDs:**
    - Immunomodulators – azathioprine, metho trexate, hydroquinones, cyclosporin
    - Antimonoclonal antibody compounds – etanercept, infliximab
- Splinting to counteract deforming forces
- Non-weight-bearing exercise programme

The primary aims of treatment are pain relief and function restoration, and to improve the appearance of the hand. Surgery in RA is only indicated where there is pain and loss of function – **deformity alone is not an indication**. The abnormal soft tissue tends to compromise surgery and arthroplasty in particular.

- **Preventive** – to prevent further deformity, e.g. early synovectomy if medical therapy fails after a 6 week trial – this aims to reduce risk of tendon rupture and flexor tendon triggering; also decompression of median nerve.
- **Reconstructive** (to restore function, i.e. stability and mobility) – tendon transfers.
- **Salvage** – e.g. **pain relief**, replacement/fusion. The process should be staged, addressing **proximal joints before distal ones**. It is important that cases are

carefully selected to proceed with those known to have high rates of satisfaction; for example:

- Thumb MCJP fusion (can often be achieved by pinning for 4–6 weeks)
- External synovectomy and ulnar head excision
- Stabilise wrist
- Flexor synovectomy
- PIPJ fusion
- MCPJ arthroplasty

ELBOW IN RA

- Articular disease, i.e. posterior subluxation – synovectomy and radial head excision for pain relief (90%); elbow arthroplasty is controversial due to the high complication rate and lack of studies.
- Extra-articular disease, i.e. nodules that can be injected with steroids (risk of ulceration), whilst synovitis and bony spurs may lead to nerve compression.

WRIST IN RA

The distal radio-ulnar joint (DRUJ) is the most commonly affected area in RA of the wrist – typically synovitis along with erosive changes.

The **DRUJ** is the area between the sigmoid notch and the head of the ulnar that is responsible for the majority of forearm rotation. The TFCC (triangular fibrocartilage complex) is the most important stabiliser of this area with an **articular disc** of triangular fibrocartilage that originates from the medial border of the distal radius inserting into the base of the ulnar styloid (5 mm thick on the ulnar side and 2 mm at the radial side; the central 3/4 is avascular and thus tears can present a healing problem) and also dorsal and volar radio-ulnar ligament, ulno-carpal ligament and ECU sheath. The TFCC also transmits about 20% of the load across the wrist.

The proximal row of carpal bones forms the **mobile intercalated segment.**

- Scaphoid becomes longitudinal/extended with ulnar deviation, whilst it is transverse/flexed with radial deviation.
- All tendons moving the wrist (except the FCU) insert beyond the carpus; therefore, ligaments that connect the metacarpals to carpus and carpal bones to each other are very important.

ULNA CAPUT (HEAD) SYNDROME – CAPUT ULNAE

This is seen in up to one-third of RA patients undergoing surgery. Synovitis around the ulnar head causes erosion of the TFCC and the ligamentous supports to the wrist. This causes **pain, instability** and limited wrist dorsiflexion aggravated by pronation of the forearm; **the wrist is the keystone of the hand.**

- **Prominent ulnar head due to dorsal dislocation,** disruption of the radio-ulnar ligament and DRUJ instability – which can be detected by the 'piano key test' – depress the ulnar head and release to see it spring back.

- **Supination of the carpus** on the forearm due to damage to the TFCC, which also causes ulnar translocation of carpus (may see as the prominent ulnar head), limiting wrist dorsiflexion and supination on the forearm. This also increases risk of CTS.
- **Volar subluxation** of ECU reducing its extensor function, making it more of a wrist flexor causing radial deviation of the wrist and promoting attritional rupture of ulnar extensors over the prominent ulna head.

RADIUS

- **Radial carpal rotation** (increase in Shapiro's MCP angle between the radius and the index MC, normally ~112°) due to erosion of the sling ligament (radioscaphocapitate). This causes the scaphoid to adopt a volar-flexed position with secondary loss of carpal height.
- **Radial scalloping** at the sigmoid notch (as well as around the ulnar head – both are highly indicative of DRUJ instability with increased risk of extensor tendon rupture).
- **Larsen index scoring single X-ray changes compared with the Amos index that looks at the progression**. The Wrightington system is another classification system for the rheumatoid wrist with good interobserver reliability.

OPTIONS FOR ULNAR WRIST PROBLEMS IN RA

Tenosynovectomy, tendon transfers (ECRL to ECU to reduce radial carpal rotation) and joint synovectomy.

ULNAR HEAD SURGERY

- **Sauvé–Kapandji procedure** fuses the distal ulna to the radial head after removal of a 10–15 mm segment of ulna proximal to this (the gap can be filled with PQ, effectively creating a **pseudoarthrosis**). It aims to allow forearm rotation for better mobility whilst preventing abnormal movements at the DRUJ as well as unloading the ulnar, allowing more force to be transmitted across the radius, which is not damaged. This procedure is suited to **younger patients** with an arthritic painful DRUJ limiting movement. Specific complications include instability of the ulnar stump and fusion of the ends reducing mobility (Figure 6.24).
- **Darrach procedure** for relief of pain in DRUJ arthritis in the **elderly** with low functional demands (younger patients, e.g. after Colles' mal-union, will do better with distal radial osteotomy). The distal

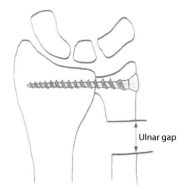

Figure 6.24 Schematic representation of a Sauvé–Kapandji procedure.

1–2 cm of the ulna is excised (minimised to restore full motion whilst avoiding instability) via a dorsal incision. If the distal ulna is unstable, then it can be stabilised either by an ECU tendon strip passed through a drill hole and sutured to itself or ECU/PQ arthroplasty. Complications are more common in younger patients with instability or subluxation; radio-ulnar convergence (impingement) that is exacerbated by power grip/PQ contraction and is related to the amount of bone excised.

WRIST ARTHRODESIS

Fusion may be offered to **low-demand patients** with advanced disease, providing predictable pain relief.

- **Limited wrist fusion** is an option for early collapse with destruction limited to radiocarpal joints. This involves synovectomy and removal of articular cartilage from affected joints, with cancellous bone graft and K-wires for 6 weeks.
  - Proximal row fusion – radius, scaphoid and lunate
  - Mid-carpal fusion – all joints surrounding the capitate
- **Total wrist fusion** may be necessary for young patients with high, long-term stresses on joints, with already significant wrist deformity/instability, poor wrist extensor function and poor bone stock.
  - The ulna head is excised, and the cartilage is removed from the distal radius and proximal carpal row. A Steinman pin is introduced through the third MC and passed via the carpus into the radial medulla with the wrist in neutral.
  - Cancellous bone graft and arthrodesis using a plate allow for 50° dorsal angulation to be created, which may be more functional than the neutral wrist position.
  - Complications include pseudoarthrosis, pin migration, nerve injury and fracture of healed fusion at the ends of the pin.

WRIST ARTHROPLASTY

This may be suited for high-demand patients; complications include implant failure, loosening and infection.

- Bi-axial total wrist devices (a plastic polyethylene spacer fixed to metal carpal component rocks on the flatter radial component, and can be cemented or non-cemented).
- Silicone (Swanson's) total wrist implants – for very low-demand patients with poor bone stock, who are willing to trade reduction in mobility for pain relief.

HAND IN RA

Whilst the wrist is radially deviated, there is ulnar deviation at the MCPJs.

- Anterior subluxation of the wrist renders the flexor tendons less effective and promotes the **intrinsic-plus position**; hence, the fingers adopt a **swan neck** deformity.
- First DIO **wasting**, which may be masked by an adduction deformity of the thumb.

EXTENSOR TENOSYNOVITIS AND TENDON RUPTURE

Tendon rupture in RA can be due to direct synovial infiltration, attrition or ischaemia, and will lead to extension lag. Differential diagnoses include

- **Dislocation** of the extensor tendon into the ulnar metacarpal valley/gutters
- Volar dislocation/subluxation of the MCPJ
- **Paralysis** of extensor musculature, e.g. PIN compression/radial tunnel syndrome due to synovitis at radiohumeral joint
- Flexor synovitis and triggering

TREATMENT

- **Synovitis** – dorsal tenosynovectomy ± wrist joint synovectomy ± osteophyte excision. Complications include skin necrosis exposing tendons, haematoma and bowstringing if a strip of extensor retinaculum is not preserved.
- In cases of **rupture, tendon transfer** is needed.
  - Isolated EPL rupture due to hamate/radius attrition and tenosynovitis – EI to EPL transfer (tighten so that with wrist extended, the thumb can still oppose to the little finger)
    - Or EDM transfer, APL slip transfer or IPJ arthrodesis
  - Rupture of finger extensors (little, ring then middle, i.e. Vaughan–Jackson) due to ulnar head
    - Single tendon – 'buddy' suture to an adjacent intact extensor tendon

- Two tendons – suture to EDC, EI to EDM/EDC
- Multiple – ring finger FDS transfer (Boyes') to motor several tendons

- **Normal 'rules'** regarding tendon transfers do not always apply in RA patients because of the following:
  - Hostile territory.
  - Motor tendons may be weak.
  - Full range of passive movement may not be available.

FLEXOR TENOSYNOVITIS AND TENDON RUPTURE

The symptoms and signs of flexor tendon problems are similar to the extensor tendon as described above with the additional possibility of triggering. Common sites of attrition rupture are

- Ridge of the trapezium – FCR
- Hook of the hamate – FCU
- Scaphoid bone osteophyte – FPL (Mannerfelt lesion)

MANAGEMENT

- Conservative treatment as above
- Synovitis – flexor tenosynovectomy plus CTR, ± osteophyte excision
- Rupture:

  - FPL (Mannerfelt) is the most common rupture in RA due to scaphoid attrition and tenosynovitis – PL tendon graft or FDS ring/middle transfer (Bunnell).
  - FDP – DIPJ arthrodesis is often the best option, alternately adjacent FDP transfer.
  - FDS and FDP rupture (usually caused by direct effects of pannus) – adjacent FDS transfer to ruptured FDP.

METACARPOPHALANGEAL JOINT

The MCPJ is the key joint for finger function, yet it is also the joint **most commonly involved in RA**.
Radiologically, the MCPJs can be viewed with Brewerton views: the MCPJ flexed to 60° with the extensor surfaces of the fingers flat on the X-ray plate.

INTRINSIC MUSCLES

These are responsible for MCPJ flexion and IP extension, and have a crucial role in the RA hand. Intrinsic muscle tightness can contribute to **swan neck deformity.**

- **Interosseous muscles** (all supplied by the ulnar nerve with an occasional variant where the first DIO is supplied by the median nerve).
  - **Palmar IO adduct** towards the axis of the middle finger (PAD). They arise from the MF side of their

own MC and insert into the same side of the extensor expansion and PP.

- **Dorsal IO abduct away** from the axis of the MF (DAB). They arise by two heads, one from each MC bordering the interosseous space and insert into extensor expansion and PP on the side away from the MF. The MF has a DIO on each side.
- **Lumbricals** arise from the radial parts of the FDP tendons and pass radial to the MCPJ and insert into the dorsum of the extensor expansion at the sagittal bands, distal to the insertion of the interossei. **They have no bony insertion.**
  - The lumbricals to the IF and MF are innervated by the median nerve, whilst those to the RF and LF are innervated by the ulnar nerve. The latter are bicipital, i.e. arise by two heads from adjacent FDP tendons, whilst median-innervated lumbricals are unicipital.

SEQUENCE OF EVENTS DESTABILISING THE MCPJ IN RA

Ulnar deviation is caused by normal use/anatomical predispositions:

- Thumb pressure during pinch grip
- Ulnar inclination of MC heads
- ADM action as a strong ulnar deviator

On the other hand, **ulnar drift describes a pathological force** once the normal configuration/stability is lost:

- **Radial wrist deviation** leading to ulnar drift of the MCPJ (Z deformity).
- **Ulnar shift of extensors** (extensors sublux into the intermetacarpal sulcus and thus tend to become ulnar deviators).
  - **Ulnar** rotation with ulnar shift of the phalangeal base at the MCPJ in the fingers due to synovial erosion of the radial sagittal bands of the extensor tendons causing extensors to dislocate in an ulnar direction (the radial collateral ligaments **are thinner than the ulnar**, lax collateral ligaments due to synovitis allow ulnar deviation).
- **Ulnar vector forces of flexors**.
- **Intrinsic tightness** – test by attempting to flex the PIPJ with the MCPJ hyperextended, which is not possible with tight intrinsic muscles.
  - This reduces power grip.
  - This increases ulnar drift, palmar subluxation of the MCPJ and swan neck deformity.

Volar subluxation of the base of the PP.
  - Weakening of the dorsal capsule and volar subluxation of extensor tendons.
  - Weakened attachment of the membranous part of the volar plate to the metacarpal head due to synovial erosion and loosening of the collateral and accessory collateral ligaments. This allows the pull of the flexor tendon on the A1 pulley to be

transmitted to the base of the PP (instead of to the head of the metacarpal).
- Palmar subluxation leads to telescoping.
- Joint destabilisation following damage to cartilage and bone from synovitis.

HARRISON'S GRADING OF MCPJ IN RA

- 1 – dislocation of the extensor tendon without medial shift
- 2 – ulnar drift and medial shift
- 3 – reducible subluxation of the MCPJ
- 4 – irreducible subluxation of the MCPJ

NALEBUFF CLASSIFICATION

- I – synovial proliferation
- II – recurrent synovitis without deformity
- III – moderate articular degeneration, ulnar and palmar digital drift that is passively correctable
- IV – severe joint destruction with fixed deformities

MANAGEMENT

- After an adequate trial of conservative treatment including splints and steroids, **synovectomy** can be offered for persistent MCPJ synovitis in the presence of
  - Minimal radiological changes
  - Little or no joint deformity
- It is often combined with soft tissue reconstruction, e.g. **relocation of extensor tendons** and **intrinsic release** particularly if ulnar drift >30°; however, there is a high incidence of recurrence.
- Those with pain and loss of function may warrant joint surgery.

INTRINSIC SURGERY

Treatment options for intrinsic tightness include

- **Intrinsic release** – division of the insertion of intrinsics into the ulnar sagittal band ± bony attachment.
- **Crossed intrinsic transfer** – restores finger alignment with long-term correction of ulnar drift and is usually combined with other soft tissue or joint procedures. The intrinsic insertions on the ulnar side of the ring, middle and index fingers are released and the tendons are mobilised up to musculotendinous junction. The insertion is then relocated and sutured to the RCL of the MCPJ.

ARTHROPLASTY

The common indications for surgery are primarily pain and loss of function. The aims of joint surgery are

- Painless stable joint
- Functional range of movement ~ 70°
- Better cosmesis

Types of arthroplasty (see Tupper JW, *J Hand Surg*, 1989)

- **Perichondrial arthroplasty** – useful for young patients, restores cartilage.
- **Resection arthroplasty**, e.g. basal joint of the thumb.
- Silicone joint replacement – metacarpophalangeals and interphalangeals.
- **Volar plate interpositional arthroplasty** – aims to restore joint stability by tightening the ligamentous support. It is useful for those with poor bone stock and thus unsuited for joint replacement. See below.
- **Vascularised joint transfer** – in children, the transfer of an epiphysis allows continued growth.

Long-term follow-up of Swanson's silastic arthroplasty of the metacarpophalangeal joints in rheumatoid arthritis. (Wilson YG, *J Hand Surg*, 1993)

Swanson's prosthesis (1972) is essentially a dynamic joint spacer that maintains alignment. The joint is stabilised with fibrous encapsulation and relies upon a telescoping effect. Long-term follow-up shows the majority of patients have sustained improvement in pain and ROM, though there is a **gradual deterioration** in the latter with time.

- Complications include infection (1.3%), bone resorption (14%) and giant cell reactive synovitis (no patients in this study). The deformity may recur, or the implant may fracture/dislocate, thus requiring revision (3.2%).

The metacarpophalangeal volar plate arthroplasty. (Tupper JW, *J Hand Surg* 1989)

- **Resection arthroplasty** – transverse incision, ulnar release, capsulotomy with division of the collateral ligaments (preserving RCL for later repair), followed by synovectomy and excision of the metacarpal head.
- **Vainio method** – cut the extensor tendon proximal to the MCPJ and attach the distal end to the volar plate to provide interpositional tissue whilst reinserting the cut proximal end to the dorsal surface of the extensor at the proximal edge of the PP.
  - The author's criticism of the Vainio method is that the interpositional substance is not robust enough and that it also impairs extensor function as it does not correct the volar pull of the flexor on the base of the PP via the A1 pulley.
- **Tupper method** – incise the volar plate at the proximal end at the junction between fibrocartilaginous and membranous areas, and then separate the attachment of the A1 pulley from the volar plate. The proximal end of the volar plate is reflected into the joint and attached to the dorsal edge of the cut metacarpal. The proposed advantages are that it provides thick interpositional substance and also elevates the base of the PP and re-establishes anchorage of the volar plate to the metacarpal.

FINGERS IN RA

The fingers may acquire a **swan neck deformity** or **boutonnière deformity**

BOUTONNIERE VS. SWAN NECK (TABLE 6.8)

Boutonniere is usually due to a central slip problem at the PIPJ.

Swan neck deformity is PIPJ hyperextension and DIPJ flexion secondary to imbalance of the IPJ forces. As volar subluxation of wrist renders the flexor tendons ineffective, an **intrinsic plus deformity** is adopted – the intrinsics hyperextend the PIPJ via the lateral bands. It tends to be more debilitating than boutonniere deformities. Swan neck may originate at any of the affected joints:

- DIPJ – extensor tendon problem (chronic Mallet finger)
- PIPJ – **PIPJ synovitis** leading to laxity of the volar plate and the FDS rupture
- MCPJ – subluxation of the MCPJ, which **tightens intrinsics**

Intrinsic tightness (effects are like contraction of intrinsic muscles) may cause characteristic flexion at the MCPJ with hyperextension of the PIPJ with secondary flexion of the DIPJ.

- Intrinsic tightness will restrict PIPJ flexion when the MCPJ extends, whilst extrinsic muscle tightness will limit PIPJ flexion when MCP joints are flexed (when intrinsics at shortest).

Table 6.8 Comparison of swan neck and boutonnière deformities

	Thumb	Fingers
Swan neck:	Flexion deformity at CMCJ	Volar plate attenuation
PIPJ hyperextension, DIPJ flexion		Intrinsic tightness or mallet FDS rupture
Boutonnieres:	Rupture of EPB	Rupture of central slip of EDC
PIPJ hyperflexion,		
DIPJ hyper extension		

- In **mallet finger**, with secondary hyperextension of the PIPJ and attenuation of TRLs allowing dorsal subluxation of lateral bands. The intrinsic muscles tighten as the lateral bands sublux dorsal to the axis of PIPJ rotation.

NALEBUFF CLASSIFICATION OF SWAN NECK DEFORMITY

The type of treatment depends on the stage of the condition:

- I – **PIPJ flexible** in all positions. Treat with swan neck **extension block splint** to correct PIPJ hyperextension with the DIPJ free so that lateral bands can move back dorsally and distally. If the primary cause is volar plate laxity, then this usually results in a flexible deformity that does not usually need surgery.
  - **Sublimis/superficialis sling** (Urbaniak) – FDS slip transected in palm and looped over the A2 pulley to be sutured to itself; it aims to keep the PIPJ flexed/reduce hyperextension; 6 weeks of post-operative extension block is required (Figure 6.25).
  - **FDS hemitenodesis**. One slip of the FDS tendon is divided 2 cm proximal to the PIPJ and attached to the tendon sheath at the base of the MP to limit PIPJ hyperextension.
  - **Dermadesis** – excision of loose skin over the flexor surface of the PIPJ; the long-term results tend to be poor.
  - **Littler (retinacular ligament reconstruction)**.
- II – deformity is position-dependent, i.e. **limited PIPJ flexion when the MCPJ extended** (intrinsic tightness). Treat with **intrinsic and lateral band release** ± arthroplasty if the joint has subluxed.
- III – **Limited PIPJ flexion in all positions but** joint is preserved. Treat by correcting MCPJ subluxation by arthroplasty, mobilisation and release of lateral bands or hemitenodesis.
- IV – **Stiff PIPJ** with poor radiographic appearance, i.e. bone changes that occur late. Treat by **arthrodesis** (index or middle, or if flexor tendons have ruptured) or **arthroplasty** (ring or little).

BOUTONNIERE DEFORMITY

Flexion at the PIPJ with hyperextension of the DIPJ and MCPJ is usually due to PIPJ synovitis causing **central slip** attenuation/erosion to the central slip. The lateral bands fall volarly, becoming fixed with the ORL and thus tend to cause flexion; there is less resistance against FDS action, which flexes the PIPJ, extends the DIPJ (secondary to Z mechanism), whilst the MCPJ also develops compensatory hyperextension.

NALEBUFF AND MILLENDEN CLASSIFICATION

- **Stage 1 – Mild** – 10–15° extensor lag at the PIPJ, which is passively correctable. Treat with Capner splint, lateral band reconstruction (relocate dorsally) or Fowler's **terminal extensor tenotomy** over MP allowing lateral bands to slide proximally to improve DIPJ flexion (ORL extensor action at the joint prevents mallet formation).
- **Stage 2 – Moderate** – 30–40° lag, passively correctable and joint space preserved. These patients often have MCPJ hyperextension. Treatment results are somewhat unpredictable: reposition the lateral band with TRL release, shorten the central slip – holding the PIPJ in extension with a K-wire for 3 weeks.
- **Stage 3 – Severe** – fixed PIPJ deformity, tight TRL (maintains lateral bands in volar position, PIPJ flexion) and ORL (DIPJ extension and block to flexion). Treat by arthrodesis (if cartilage damaged) or arthroplasty (soft tissue attenuation makes results unpredictable) as above, but only after splinting/ serial casting to restore full passive extension to the PIPJ. These patients may have little functional deficit and surgery may not help.

Arthrodesis – is an option mainly for DIPJ disease (or intra-articular fractures). The PIPJ is arthrodesed at angles of 20°, 30°, 40° and 50° for the index, middle, ring and little fingers, respectively. In general, the PIPJ of the index does better with arthrodesis than arthroplasty – a stable index can be used in pinch, whilst the mobile middle finger can be used in grasp.

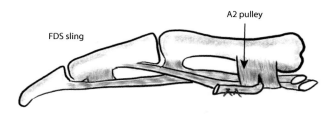

Figure 6.25 Flexor superficialis sling.

THUMB IN RA

The thumb may have swan neck or boutonnière deformities.

NALEBUFF CLASSIFICATION OF RHEUMATOID THUMB DEFORMITY

The most common types are I and III.

- I – **Boutonnière,** IPJ hyperextended, rupture of EPB at the level of the MCPJ (i.e. MCPJ disease).
- II – **Boutonnière plus metacarpal adduction** (CMC subluxation). This is rare.
- III – **Swan neck deformity** (extended MCPJ, flexed IPJ) volar subluxation of the thumb at the level of the CMC joint; it is often due to CMCJ synovitis.
- IV – **Gamekeeper's thumb.** UCL rupture with radial deviation of the thumb at the MCPJ, with adduction contracture.
- V – **Isolated swan neck** (MCPJ hyperextension with IPJ flexion) and no CMCJ subluxation. Treat with MCPJ fusion and IPJ palmar plate advancement or MP arthroplasty with IPJ fusion.
- VI – **Arthritis mutilans.**

BOUTONNIÈRE DEFORMITY

The basic deformity is MCPJ flexion with IPJ hyperextension; most are type I (MCPJ disease), whilst type II with CMCJ disease/subluxation is rare. Disease at the MCPJ and attrition of EPB causes loss of MCPJ extension and flexion deformity.

- Intrinsics (AP and APB) exacerbate flexion at the MCPJ and extension at the IP joint.

TREATMENT

- Stage I – supple and passively correctable.
  - Synovectomy at the MCPJ.
  - Reconstruct the extensor apparatus to reposition it dorsal to the joint – dorsalise lateral bands and re-route EPL to the base of the PP, silicone arthroplasty.
- Stage II – fixed MCPJ and supple IPJ. Treat with MCPJ fusion if other joints are not degenerated; otherwise, MCPJ arthroplasty is preferred.
- Stage III – fixed MCPJ and IPJ. Treat with IPJ fusion and MCPJ arthroplasty.

SWAN NECK DEFORMITY

This is more common in OA than RA; a 'true' swan neck does not occur at the thumb as it has one less joint. There is disease at the CMCJ leading to subluxation and metacarpal adduction contracture. The patient is unable to extend at the CMCJ, and extension forces are transmitted to the MCPJ instead leading to hyperextension of the MCPJ and flexion of the IPJ.

- Stage I – CMCJ subluxation with no MCJP hyperextension. Treat with CMCJ arthroplasty.

- Stage II – CMCJ subluxation with MCPJ extension. If the articular surfaces are satisfactory and other joints are not damaged, then treat with CMCJ synovectomy, ligament reconstruction (FCR/ECRL) and soft tissue stabilisation with palmar capsulodesis/tenodesis plate, or fusion if the joint has degenerated and is unstable.
- Stage III – web-space contracture. Treat as above along with web release – release adductor pollicis and first DIO. The MC base may need to be resected.

GAMEKEEPER'S THUMB

MCPJ disease leads to chronic UCL rupture and thus radial deviation of the thumb at the MCPJ and secondary adduction of the metacarpal.

Treatment options include the following:

- If the articular surfaces are intact (rare), then reconstruct the UCL with APL or a free FCR tendon graft.
- MCPJ arthrodesis ± IPJ arthrodesis if the joint surfaces are poor.
- Correction of adductors, release adductor pollicis and first dorsal interossei, ± Z-plasty web.

DIFFERENTIAL DIAGNOSES OF ARTHRITIDES

JUVENILE RA

This is the commonest connective tissue disorder in children. It is characterised by a proliferative synovitis that affects the knees and wrist most frequently. Diagnostic criteria include the following:

- Onset under 16 years of age.
- First episode lasting more than 6 weeks.
- Arthritis in more than one joint with two or more signs (joint tenderness, stiffness, pain on motion and inflammation) and other rheumatoid disease has been excluded.
- Juvenile RA patients may have non-RA features – ulnar deviation of wrist and metacarpals, radial deviation of the MCPJ, abnormal ring and little finger metacarpals (secondary to accelerated maturation of epiphyses), short ulnar and narrow small tubular bones of the hand.

Subtypes include

- **Polyarticular** (40%). This form is similar to adult RA with minimal systemic involvement and tends to continue into adulthood. Those with RF tend to have a worse prognosis.
- **Monoarticular** (40%). Affects less than or equal to four joints within the first 6 months. It affects the lower limb more frequently and eye problems are common – many are RF-negative and antinuclear antibody (ANA) positive. The younger age group (<6) tend to be female, whilst the second older age group are males.

- **Systemic onset** (Still's disease, 20%). These have intermittent pyrexia, rash, hepatosplenomegaly, lymphadenopathy, anaemia, myalgia/arthralgia and eye involvement; 25% progress to severe arthritis.

Treatment is mainly supportive with the aim of preventing deformities – upper limb deformities may result due to abnormal epiphyseal growth and ankylosis especially the wrist. Surgery may damage growth plates and is avoided unless necessary.

- Splintage, physiotherapy
- Synovectomy for pain

ANKYLOSING SPONDYLITIS

This condition is characterised by these main features:

- Back pain of insidious onset in males (10× more frequent than females) under 40 years of age.
- Morning stiffness, and the stiffness improves with movement/exercise.
- Present for more than 3 months.

It affects the sacroiliac joints and back in particular; 20% have peripheral arthritis similar to RA but only 10% are RF positive; 90% of patients are HLA B27 positive.

SYSTEMIC LUPUS ERYTHEMATOSIS

Systemic lupus erythematosis (SLE) is the commonest of the connective tissue diseases (but RA is 20× more common). It is especially prevalent in pigmented races. On average, it affects 1 in 250, mostly women (10× more than men) 20–40 years of age.

- 90% have joint involvement, although SLE arthritis affects mainly the soft tissues rather than joint surfaces. This is a **non-erosive arthritis** with ligamentous laxity, particularly the hands and wrists, and may lead to subluxation. In extreme cases, fusion should be considered.
- Antinuclear antibody and anti-dsDNA positive.
- Other features include the following:
  - Butterfly rash on face
  - Raynaud's phenomenon
  - Liver palms, purpuric rash in fingers
  - Vasculitis affecting heart, lungs and kidneys
  - May also have neurological and GI manifestations

PSORIATIC ARTHRITIS

A key feature of psoriatic arthropathy (5%–30% of psoriasis sufferers) is **fibrosis** along with **osteolytic destruction** leading to phalangeal erosions and periosteal new bone formation – progressive bone loss may lead to 'pencil in a cup' (tapering of the proximal bone whilst the distal bone proliferates) and **arthritis mutilans** in 5%. It tends to begin 10 years after the skin disease manifests itself; in a minority (10%–15%), the joint disease precedes the skin disease. It differs from RA in that

- It is seronegative (HLA-B27) positive and asymmetric.
- Nail pits in 80% (>20 for diagnosis in the absence of typical skin changes).

- Absence of skin nodules/rash.
- Synovitis is rare whilst stiffness is frequent; dactylitis due to inflammation of soft tissues.
- **Arthritis mutilans** may follow RA or psoriatic arthritis and can affect any joint. It is characterised by considerable amounts of bone loss – treatment is generally fusion with lengthening by bone graft, which will tend to stop bone loss; arthroplasty is contraindicated in all but the MCPJ as bone loss will continue, but preserving MCPJ mobility is important.

Disease in the DIPJ is more likely to be psoriatic arthritis than RA – in RA, DIPJ deformity is usually secondary to PIPJ deformity. A subtype is often called distal interphalangeal predominant (DIP) (5%) and is characterised by disease localised to DIPJs of fingers and toes along with marked nail changes.

NALEBUFF CLASSIFICATION

- I – spontaneous ankylosis predominates, especially at DIPJ and PIPJ.
- II – osteolytic, bone loss predominates – arthritis mutilans. Early fusion with lengthening, avoid arthroplasty.
- III – RA-like features.

Management is primarily medical: NSAIDs, steroid injections (for those with pauci-articular involvement), with second line being immunosuppression that also deals with the skin disease. More recently, etanercept and infliximab (TNFα inhibitors) have been used for severe cases.

Surgery may be required and includes corrective osteotomies, arthrodesis (IPJ) and arthroplasty (MCPJ, PIPJ for ring and little fingers). Overall expectations are lower compared with RA with less motion, along with a higher infection rate; the goal is large object grasp.

OTHERS

- **Systemic sclerosis/scleroderma** is a rare multi-organ disease, affecting women three to six times more often. There is a polyarthritis in some patients (40% of whom are RF positive). Erosive arthritis is rare, but joint deformity may occur secondary to fibrous contracture. There are associations with the CREST syndrome, i.e. calcinosis circumscripta, digital ischaemia, etc.
- **Ulcerative colitis** – transient seronegative arthritis in 10% that seems to be related to ulcerative colitis disease activity.
- **Behçet's syndrome** – oral and genital ulcers and iritis associated with arthritis of the elbow and wrist. This seems to be a form of cell-mediated autoimmunity.
- **Reiter's syndrome** – polyarthritis, urethritis and conjunctivitis in patients who are HLA-B27.
- **Reactive arthritis** – secondary to *Salmonella, Brucella, Neisseria gonorrhoeae*.

7

Lower limb

I. RELEVANT ANATOMY

SENSATION

- Lateral calf – sural nerve
- Medial calf – saphenous nerve
- Dorsum of foot – superficial peroneal nerve
- First web space – deep peroneal nerves
- Sole of foot – medial and lateral plantar nerves from posterior tibial

DERMATOME TESTING

- L2 – lateral thigh
- L3 – knee
- L4 – medial calf
- L5 – lateral calf/first web
- S1 – lateral foot
- S2 – posterior middle thigh

II. CLASSIFICATION OF LOWER LIMB TRAUMA

There are many systems; however, crucially none of them reliably predict which injuries do better with reconstruction and which do better with amputation.

Gustilo and Anderson Fracture Classification
Prevention of infection in the treatment of 1025 open fractures of long bones. (Gustilo RB, *J Bone Joint Surg Am*, 1976)

The first classification had subtypes I–III for long bone fractures, which was subsequently modified and applied mostly to open tibial fractures. The classification below was published in 1990 (Gustilo RB, *J Bone Joint Surg Am*, 1990); the subtypes were added in 1984.

- **I – clean wound <1 cm**
- **II – wound 1–5 cm** but without significant tissue disruption
- **III – wound >5 cm** with significant tissue disruption
  - IIIA local tissues provide adequate soft tissue coverage.
  - IIIB extensive soft tissue loss, contamination, periosteal stripping.
  - IIIC arterial injury requiring repair.

The classification **does not actually consider the bony injury**; it is widely used and relatively simple; however, inter-observer reliability is not high and is best applied *after* wound excision.

- By definition, IIIB and IIIC need soft tissue reconstruction.
- Francel (1992) *Plast Reconstr Surg*, found that at a mean of 3.5 years, IIIB patients who had limb salvage took longer to full weight bearing and had a lower return to work rate than those who had BKA (28% vs. 68%). However, at 10 years, those with salvaged limbs had a higher return to work rate (60% in IIIB/C; Laughlin RT, *J Orthop Trauma*, 1993) – social factors and pending litigation were some variables. Both patients and surgeons should be aware just how long is needed to rehabilitate.
  - The degree of complexity of limb salvage obviously has an effect.

Byrd classification. (Byrd HS, *Plast Reconstr Surg*, 1989)

- I – low energy (spiral oblique fracture with relatively clean wound, laceration <2 cm)
- II – moderate energy (comminuted/displaced fracture with wound >2 cm, with moderate muscle and skin contusion)
- III – high energy (severe comminution/displacement or bony defect with extensive soft tissue injury, deviatisation muscle)
- IV – extreme energy (degloving or vascular injury requiring repair)

Mangled extremity severity score (MESS; simplified) Objective criteria accurately predict amputation following lower extremity trauma. (Johanssen K, *J Trauma*, 1990)

- **Skeletal and soft tissue injury** (1, 2, 3, 4)
  - Low/medium/high/very high energy with gross contamination
- **Limb ischaemia** (1, 2, 3 – double if greater than 6 hours)
  - Pulseless but perfused
  - Pulseless, paraesthetic with prolonged capillary refill
  - Devascularised – cool, paraesthetic, insensate
- **Shock (0, 1, 2)**
  - No hypotension SBP >90 mmHg
  - Transient hypotension
  - Sustained hypotension
- **Age (0, 1, 2)**
  - <30 years
  - 30–50 years
  - >50 years

The MESS is specific but **not that sensitive**; it may have a role in the decision of whether or not to amputate a severely traumatised leg. A score of 6 or less suggests a salvageable limb; with 7 or more, salvage is unlikely to be successful. However, some parts are subjective, e.g. contamination in consideration of energy.

There are many more complicated systems including the AO score, which has a better predictive value but is rather complex, and may be most suited for audit/data collection rather than everyday clinical use.

Classification of soft-tissue degloving in limb trauma. (Arnez ZM, *Br J Plast Surg*, 1999)

- Type 1 – non-circumferential degloving
- Type 2 – abrasion but no degloving
- Type 3 – circumferential degloving
- Type 4 – circumferential degloving plus avulsion between deep tissue planes: intermuscular and muscle–periosteum planes

Type 4 injuries require serial conservative debridements and delayed reconstruction as early radical debridement usually results in a functionless limb.

BAPS/BOA working party report on open tibial fractures. (BAPS/BOA Working Party, *Br J Plast Surg*, 1997)
This report emphasised early cooperation between senior plastic and orthopaedic surgeons.

- Half of open tibial fractures are Gustilo grades IIIA or B.
  - 70% of Gustilo grade IIIB injuries require flap cover.
- 4% are Gustilo grade IIIC – these often proceed to amputation so rarely involve plastic surgery input.

Fractures can be classified as **low or high energy** (e.g. RTA, fall from a height and missile injuries); the latter have poorer prognosis.

- Clinical signs of a high-energy injury:
  - Large/multiple wounds.
  - Crush or burst lacerations.
  - Closed degloving – tissues feel loose and boggy.
  - Signs of nerve or vascular injury.
- Radiological signs of a high-energy injury:
  - Multiple bony fragments especially more than one fractured bone in the same limb
  - Widely spaced fragments or segmental injury

The wound should be examined at once by the surgeon of the responsible team – digital photographs taken, and the **wound dressed and left until theatre**. Open tibial fractures should be closed within a maximum of 5 days:

- **Wound excision and irrigation** (6 litres normal saline pulsed lavage; antiseptics are not necessary).
  - Debride to healthy tissues, with a view to check at a 'second look' within 48 hours.
    - ICG, fluorescein and Woods lamp can be used as adjuncts to assess tissue perfusion.
    - Muscle colour and contraction are unreliable.
- **Fracture stabilisation**.
  - Remove loose bone fragments – it is easier to manage bone defects than to deal with the sequelae of inadequate bone debridement.
  - External fixation, ensuring that potential skin flaps are not compromised.
  - **Definitive stabilisation that is immediately covered**
    - Diaphyseal open tibial fractures – intramedullary (IM) nail.
    - Metaphyseal open tibial fractures – plate or external fixation, pin sites should avoid compromise of fasciocutaneous flaps or free flap pedicle/recipients.
    - For bone gaps that cannot be fixed and covered (see below).
- **Soft tissue reconstruction** ideally as soon as possible – wounds closed within 72 hours have the highest success rate and the lowest complication rate. However, immediate closure is not always required, and delayed closure may enable serial debridements and compartment monitoring.

Standards for the management of open lower limb fractures. (BOA/BAPRAS, *Royal Society of Medicine Press*, 2009)

A review 'upgraded' the guidelines into a set of standards. They emphasised that timely surgery by specialists was preferred over emergency surgery by the less experienced. A combined plan is formulated and documented; centres without combined care should arrange early transfer. The best method of skeletal stabilisation was still up for debate.

Selected recommendations include

- IVAB within 3 hours – co-amoxiclav or cefuroxime or clindamycin (if allergic to penicillin).
- Vascular impairment needs restoration of circulation (shunts as needed) within 6 hours, preferably within 3–4 hours.
- Decompress compartment syndrome (CS) immediately – access four compartments via two incisions.
- Urgent surgery is required in the multiply injured with open fractures, or grossly contaminated.
- Minimise wound contact. The wound is handled only to remove gross contamination and allow **photos** to be taken; it is covered with wet gauze and film.
- **Wound debridement** (soft tissue and bone) should be performed by a combined team during scheduled hours within 24 hours of injury (unless grossly contaminated). Thoroughly irrigate with saline. Give co-amoxiclav and gentamicin perioperatively for 72 hours or until definitive wound closure.
  - If definitive closure is not possible, use negative pressure wound therapy (NPWT) or antibiotic beads. NPWT is not used for definitive wound management.
  - Aim for closure by 72 hours, no later than 7 days.

GENERAL CONSIDERATIONS

'Debridement' was described first by Pierre-Joseph Desault (*French surgeon*, 1744–1795) in the treatment of traumatic wounds. Advances in the management of lower limb trauma include

- Debridement, with antibiotics/asepsis
- Bone fixation

- Vascular repair
- Soft tissue coverage, with flaps as necessary

GENERAL MANAGEMENT OF LOWER LIMB TRAUMA

Adhere to ATLS principles for immediate management, i.e. ABC. The first priority is the airway with C-spine control – continue with the primary survey, treating life-threatening injuries, and then perform the secondary survey. Once the patient is stable, take a history and examine the limb.

- AMPLE history including 'Event' – the time and mechanism of injury, high energy vs. low energy, etc.

INVESTIGATIONS

- X-rays
- Angiography if the limb is pulseless following fracture reduction

Determining salvageability of the limb:

- Is revascularisation needed? Consider on-table angiogram.
- Is there a nerve injury? The results of nerve repair and grafting in the lower limb are poor except in children. Nerve injury per se does not preclude salvage if it is distal enough, but patients with complex injuries with nerve damage will rehabilitate faster with an amputation.
  - Peroneal nerve – foot drop, sensation distal foot (superficial) branch or first web (deep) branch
  - Tibial nerve – sensation heel/plantar midfoot
  - Sural nerve – sensation lateral midfoot
- Is the soft tissue defect treatable with local flaps or free flaps? (Table 7.1)
- Is there any bone loss and is it reconstructable?

In assessing the **patient** suitability for salvage – is there any concomitant life-threatening injury and what are the needs and wishes of the patient? Below knee amputation (BKA) greatly reduces the work of walking compared to above knee amputation (AKA; 25% increase vs. 65% increase over no amputation), and the quality of life is significantly better. Patients can often return to work earlier if amputated.

Table 7.1 Comparison of fasciocutaneous flaps and muscle flaps for soft tissue reconstruction

	Fasciocutaneous flaps	Muscle flaps
Advantages	Quick	Better in terms of providing well-vascularised tissue (greatest capillary density for tissue) that is flexible and compliant (less likely to leave a dead space). More effective against infection (Mathes SJ, *Plast Reconstr Surg*, 1982).
Disadvantages	Higher complication rate (partial loss, infection) Poor donor site cosmesis Restricted by pedicle location May be compromised by external fixation	May be in zone of trauma.

TIMING OF SOFT TISSUE COVER

- **Emergency** – within 24 hours
- **Early (under 3 days)** – associated with less infection and less flap failure (Godina M, *Plast Reconstr Surg*, 1986). See Table 7.2.
- **Delayed** – <3/12.
- **Late** >3/12 (Arnez ZM, *Clin Plast Surg*, 1991).

There is a '5 day rule' that many adhere to, but the evidence for this exact cut-off is lacking; according to the BAPRAS/BOA standards (2009), microsurgery is best performed within a week before the vessels become friable or fibrosed.

FIRST LOOK

The wound is extended as required for access preferably longitudinally, taking care not to damage tissue that may be needed for flaps particularly the medial and lateral perforators.

RECONSTRUCTIVE PLAN

- Reduce and stabilise the fracture (this often alleviates any vasospasm).
- Restore perfusion by arterial reconstruction if necessary.
  - Consider bypass shunt if ischaemic time is/will be prolonged, then fix bones to avoid disruption during fracture next manipulation/fixation. Some prefer to connect the vein before the artery whilst others prefer the reverse.
- Fasciotomy for crush, reperfusion injuries.
  - CS is not uncommon in tibial fractures, even open ones. The anterior compartment is most commonly involved (McQueen MM, *J Bone Joint Surg Br*, 2000); this may be due to the mass of muscles in a tight compartment as well as its proximity to the tibia.
- Debridement of all non-viable tissue and pulsed lavage under tourniquet – muscle that is dark, is non-contractile and does not bleed is dead (though the converse is less reliable, i.e. a muscle that is contractile may be dead/dying).
- Soft tissue cover.
  - Nerves should be repaired where possible, but the distances involved limit the results. Although sensation is important, tibial nerve injury resulting in loss of sensation to the sole of the foot is **not** an absolute contraindication to salvage.

- **Intramedullary nailing**
  - Reamed nails with proximal and distal locking provide very stable fixation and allow early mobilisation. However, they may be difficult to use in comminuted fractures.
  - **Unreamed nails** avoid disruption of the endosteal blood supply.
- **Internal fixation** – exacerbates periosteal stripping and increases infection risk
- **External fixation**
  - This is often the method of choice, using Ilizarov frames that allow easy access for repeated debridement. Pins must be sited carefully to avoid compromising local flap options and track infections may occur.

MANAGEMENT OF BONE GAPS

If there is no bone loss, then reduce and stabilise using either external fixator or unreamed IM nail.

- **Non-vascularised bone grafts** are suitable for small defects (<4 cm) in well-vascularised graft beds, though they will still take about 9 months to heal. It is common to wait 6–12 weeks post-trauma before introducing non-vascularised bone graft into the defect; gentamicin impregnated MMA spacers may be used temporarily.
- **Distraction osteogenesis** is useful where the traumatic bone gap is >4 cm.
- **Vascularised bone graft** – although it is a potentially complex reconstruction in the early post-trauma phase, use of either DCIA or free fibula can effectively reconstruct large segmental defects >8 cm. The transferred fibula has been shown to hypertrophy with use. **Good soft tissue cover is needed**.

ILIZAROV TECHNIQUES

- **The fracture gap (4–8 cm)** is compressed causing limb shortening, followed by **distraction osteogenesis**, which often compensates for inadequate soft tissue for primary closure.
  - Shortening more may kink vessels.
- **For larger defects (8–12 cm)**, the limb can be held to length followed by **bone transport**, with a corticotomy

Table 7.2 Summary of results of Godina M

	Group I	Group II	Group III
Time since injury	<3 days	3/7 to 3/12	>3/12
Flap failure rate %diabetic	0.75	12	9.5
Infection %	1.5	17.5	6
Bone healing time, months	6–8	12.3	29

Source: *Reconstr Surg*, 1986.

to develop the **mobile segment** – preserving medullary and periosteal blood supply. Adequate soft tissues are needed, i.e. may need a flap. This method avoids the vessel kinking, and the soft tissue contracture that may otherwise occur in a shortened limb. Bone transport was more complicated requiring 2.2 additional operations compared with only 1 for compression–distraction (Saleh M, *J Bone Joint Surg*, 1995). Problems with this technique include docking non-union due to the leading edge being relatively avascular or obstructed by soft tissues; most cases of non-union required a bone graft.

- **A latent period** of ~5 days is needed following corticotomy before commencing distraction at one-quarter turn four times a day to lengthen 1 mm/day.
- The rate of distraction is monitored by serial X-rays to avoid premature fusion or the appearance of lucency indicating that distraction is too fast. When the required length is achieved, the frame is left for ~2 months to allow for **consolidation** of the distracted segment.
- **For defects >12 cm**, the bone can be held out to length with external fixator and reconstructed secondarily with vascularised bone flap (free fibula), which hypertrophies but is never as strong as the tibia (double barrelling may help). Patients get to weight bear after about 15 months.
  - Alternatively, double Ilizarov distraction (bifocal lengthening) from each bone end can be considered. This halves the time required to span defect and can be used for defects >12 cm.

COMPLICATIONS

- Length discrepancies
- Incomplete docking/non-union requiring secondary bone grafting
- Pin track infections
  - Minimise tension at the interface between pin and skin, particularly with bone transport.
  - Recalcitrant infection may necessitate removal of the wire.

PHYSIOLOGY OF DISTRACTION HISTOGENESIS

- **Tension–stress effect** – tissues under tension respond by forming more tissues.
- Distracted bone regenerates by **intramembranous ossification** orchestrated by the periosteum–osteoblastic differentiation of periosteal mesenchymal cells and hence is not analogous to endochondral ossification, which would normally occur at a fracture site.
  - Patients with fibrous dysplasia cannot do this; therefore, this technique cannot be used as the new bone will also be dysplastic (but osteogenesis imperfecta can be treated in this way).

CHRONIC OSTEOMYELITIS

There is a 4.5% incidence in Gustilo III fractures, but the risk can be minimised by thorough debridement.

Adult chronic osteomyelitis – An overview. (Cierny G, *Orthopedics*, 1984)

CLASSIFICATION

- Superficial
- Localised
- Diffuse
- Medullary

INVESTIGATIONS

- Plain X-rays – these still provide the best screening for acute and chronic osteomyelitis (Lazzarini J, *Bone Joint Surg Am*, 2004).
  - Other imaging modalities may be better for diagnosis and guiding management decisions. **MRI is useful** if the diagnosis is doubtful on plain radiographs, with **bone scans** (leucocyte for acute, technectium for chronic) if metalwork precludes the use of MRI. CT may be useful to establish surgical plans.
- Wound swab/culture.
  - Swabs should be taken **after the wound has been cleansed** with sterile saline to remove debris and extraneous microorganisms. The aim is to detect what is left growing on the burn after cleaning, which is most likely to cause infection.
- Arteriography.

TREATMENT

Operative treatment may not be feasible for all patients.

- Radical wound debridement (remove necrotic soft tissue and sequestrum).
- Bone graft the bone defect (free or vascularised) and immobilise.
- Free muscle flaps bring in a good blood supply and obliterate dead space.
- Antibiotics – local delivery systems/systemic for 2–6 weeks; consult with a microbiologist.

IV. SOFT TISSUE COVERAGE

SOFT TISSUE CLOSURE

LOCAL FLAPS

Fasciocutaneous flaps harvested on the perforators have fewer complications than free flaps, though they may be problematic in the elderly and in diabetics.

All three major vessels in the lower leg give off perforators: medially, the PTA gives two to five fairly predictable perforators, whilst anterolaterally, there are four to five perforators from the ATA and four to five from the peroneal artery (less predictable/consistent). Using a single sturdy perforator facilitates rotation for propeller flaps; twisting is more likely with two or more vessels. Some have described **perforator plus** flaps, which keep a skin attachment – supposedly to enhance venous return.

MUSCLE

Muscle flaps are reliable and provide bulk, and are useful for dealing with deep infection (supposedly). One of the commonest choices is **gastrocnemius** (plus skin graft) for knee and proximal third of tibia defects but may cause some functional loss. **Soleus** has a supply from the proximal perforators of posterior tibial and peroneal arteries.

Local flaps tend to require a large amount of tissue to be elevated in order to cover relatively small defects.

FREE FLAPS

Flaps such as LD or ALT can cover large and distal defects. They can also bring in new blood supply; end-to-side anastomoses allow distal run off, whilst other options include a 'T' anastomosis or 'flow-through' flaps, e.g. RFFF or ALT, to reconstruct **short vascular gaps**. Preoperative angiograms are generally not necessary if the distal pulses are normal. Advanced age per se, or diabetes, are not contraindications.

- **Recipient vessels.** It is often useful to choose flaps with longer pedicles, which allows anastomoses outside of the zone of injury; vein grafts may be needed. Actual vessel damage may not be visible.
  - **Popliteal artery** and its continuation via posterior midline muscle splitting approach (Godina M, *Plast Reconstr Surg*, 1991).
  - **Posterior tibial artery** (PTA) is usually well protected and thus available. On the other hand, although the anterior tibial artery is often damaged, some prefer it for reasons of easy accessibility.
  - **Geniculate vessels** in popliteal fossa or vein grafts to **superficial femoral artery**.
  - **Cross-leg flaps** are rarely used as immobilisation is required for 4 weeks (with risk of DVT, contracture) before division, and still need a vascular wound bed for healing. Thus, they should be regarded only as a salvage option in young patients.
    - Cross-leg free flaps have been described by Chen (*Trauma*, 1997) one in eight flaps failed. It is a salvage procedure in the young; no significant long-term stiffness was reported.
- **Timing of free tissue transfer.**
  - Emergency free flap – at the time of first debridement, within 24 hours
  - Early – 24–72 hours post-injury
  - Delayed – more than 72 hours

The advantages of early or emergency cover of open fractures are as follows:

- Less infection. Infection rates increase after 5 days and major complications increase after 15 days.
- Earlier mobilisation.
- Fewer operations with shorter hospitalisation time and lower treatment costs.

Healing by secondary intention (Papineau) has been described for situations where no local flap option exists and the patient is unsuitable for free flap surgery. The cortex can be drilled and kept moist to encourage granulation tissue formation, which is then covered by skin graft. It may take 3–4 months to heal. It is mostly of historical interest; a better option now is probably to use NPWT and/or dermal matrices. **Degloved skin** can be harvested as an split skin graft (SSG) only on the day of injury and stored for later use, but dead skin cannot be salvaged.

- Vein, artery, nerve, split skin and bone grafts may all be harvested as spare parts. Large sections of skin based on septocutaneous perforators leading to the anterior and posterior tibial arteries were harvested and anastomosed to recipient vessels in the salvaged limb in two cases (Southern SJ, *Injury*, 1997).

AMPUTATION

BKA (6 cm below the tibial tuberosity) is vastly superior to AKA in terms of rehabilitation (25% vs. 65% increase in energy requirements over normal). Midfoot amputations (Symes) have little functional advantage over BKA. The ideal length is at least 6 cm of tibia below the tubercle, but in practice, as much as soft tissue possible is preserved for cover. Free FC flap salvage for a BKA stump may be needed, but the best tissue with the best sensation is probably a pedicled fillet of sole flap or a free sole flap with tibial nerve repair.

- Muscle flaps tend to shrink as the muscle tissue atrophies and may lead to late bone exposure.

Attempted salvage of 'unsalvageable' legs may be detrimental in the long term. The patient has to be aware of high failure rates, increased mortality, prolonged disability/rehabilitation and other potential long-term problems.

- Pelissier (*Plast Reconstr Surg*, 2003) demonstrated that patients with salvaged limbs had longer hospital stays, more surgeries, longer time to bony union and more long-term stiffness and pain.
- Tomaino (*Am J Orthop*, 2001) showed that amputees and those with salvaged limbs after IIIB/C fractures had similar QOL in the long term.

Consider early amputation, particularly if the patient is not fit for reconstructive surgery; it avoids psychological trauma of late amputation. General predictors for poor salvage results include

- Prolonged ischaemia.

- Nerve injury (insensate foot). Higgins (*Orthop Clin North Am*, 2010) found that the absence of plantar sensation at presentation is not a good predictor of eventual plantar sensation, functional outcome or an indication for amputation per se.
- Crush/degloving/multiple-level injury.

Defects can be considered according to their location:

Upper third
- **Proximally based FC flap** that was first described by Ponten
- **Gastrocnemius muscle** (medial and/or lateral)
    - Type I flap based on sural artery from the popliteal artery. The **medial head is larger, has a longer reach** and is suited for the upper third of tibia and knee defects. Using the lateral head may cause compression of the common peroneal nerve.
    - After splitting the muscle, the plane between the medial head and the soleus is developed with blunt dissection, taking care to identify and protect the sural nerve and the muscle pedicle. Divide the distal tendon and reflect; the arc of rotation can be increased by releasing the origin whilst the aponeurotic undersurface can be scored for a little more length.
- **Free flap**

Middle third
- **Proximally/distally based FCs flaps** based on perforators of peroneal or posterior tibial arteries
- **Soleus muscle**
    - Type II muscle flap with dual supply, medial (posterior tibial) and lateral (peroneal artery) and can be used either wholly or a single half. Separate the muscle tendon from the Achilles and then reflect upwards, dividing the attachments as needed to allow rotation into the defect. Scoring the aponeurosis may increase the reach.
- **Free flap**

Lower third
Early flaps were raised in a subcutaneous plane and based on the subdermal plexus. Subsequent perforator-based flaps, e.g. Ponten, were more reliable and could be longer.
- **Adipofascial turnover flap**, which leaves a better donor defect than fasciocutaneous flaps and is particularly suited for young female patients.
- **Sural artery island flap** sacrifices the nerve and is relatively small and unreliable being based on a small artery and vein supplying the sural nerve. The pivot point (peroneal perforator) is 5 cm above the midpoint of a line joining the lateral malleolus to the Achilles tendon.
- **Distally based fasciocutaneous flap** based on perforators of peroneal or posterior tibial arteries that can be islanded for greater arc of rotation to reach the ankle. Sometimes called 'reverse flow'.

- The main perforators of the PTA perforators are 6, 9 and 12 cm above the medial malleolus and are situated in the intermuscular septum between soleus and flexor hallucis longus (FHL) (NVB is deep to soleus) with venous drainage via venae comitantes accompanying the perforating arteries. The skin paddle can be rotated through 180°; rotation is facilitated by having a single good perforator.
- **Free flaps** (good success rate and flexibility with a donor site remote from the trauma zone but is a more complex procedure). Choices include
    - Sole of foot – free lateral arm flap (sensate using lateral cutaneous nerve of the arm)
    - LD, gracilis, ALT with or without vastus lateralis

Tissue expansion has more complications in the lower limb but can still be useful to close more superficial defects in non-acute wounds.

A five-year review of islanded distally based fasciocutaneous flaps on the lower limbs. (Erdmann MWH, *Br J Plast Surg*, 1997)
Fasciocutaneous flaps replace like with like in the lower limb. In this study, flaps based on perforators of the PTA were used preferentially in males and older females.

- Although suitable for IIIB fractures, 20% of flaps failed. Heavy smoker suffered more tip loss.
- Three quarters of flaps were used to close lower-third defects, but are also capable of covering Achilles/heel defects.
- Flaps raised on lateral perforators from the **peroneal artery are less reliable** because of the larger number of perforators: more must be divided to create the required arc of rotation.

ANKLE/HEEL

- **Distally based islanded fasciocutaneous flaps** as above
- **Medial plantar island flap** based on a cutaneous branch of the medial plantar artery.
- **Dorsalis pedis flap**, a fasciocutaneous flap based on dorsalis pedis artery used as pedicled or free flap.
- **Exposed Achilles tendon** – use a thin flap or graft after granulation; NPWT may be useful.

PLANTAR/SOLE RESURFACING

Sole skin is rather special with a complex network of fibrous septa that is adapted to its purpose and is essentially irreplaceable and so should be preserved, whenever possible. Reconstructing weight-bearing surfaces is often proposed as a priority, but it has been established that patients will generally change gait/stance (heel walking vs. head of toe walking) to avoid walking on reconstructed areas, **unless forced to** when there is very little/no sole left. Thus, the choice of reconstruction is very much individualised, depending on the defect, local tissues and the ambulatory status of the patient.

- **SSG** – hyperkeratosis and fissuring especially at the borders can be a problem.
- **Fillet toe flap** via dorsal incision.
- **The medial plantar artery flap** is an FC flap. It is versatile with a wide arc of rotation able to reach the heel and medial ankle, providing a **sensate flap** (cutaneous branch of medial plantar nerve) as large as 6 × 10 cm. Patients have to be prepared for a long time off their feet and work, whilst persistent pain is not uncommon.
- **Free flaps**
  - Sonmez (*Plast Reconstr Surg*, 2003). FC flaps provided better sensation and vibration outcomes compared to skin-grafted muscle flaps (gracilis, LD, serratus).
  - Skin-grafted muscle flaps were better at withstanding shear compared to myocutaneous flaps.
- **Sensate free flaps**
  - Free flaps can have their nerves coapted to the sural or medial calcaneal nerves to fabricate potentially sensate flaps.
  - Kuran (*Plast Reconstr Surg*, 2000). Sensory flaps provided early return of pressure sensation but long-term functional results (after a year) similar to non-sensory flaps.
  - Santanelli (*Plast Reconstr Surg*, 2002). Both innervated and non-innervated RFFF provided adequate protective sensation.

Selective use of preoperative angiography in free flap reconstruction of the lower extremity. (Dublin BA, *Ann Plast Surg*, 1997)

In this study, 38 patients had angiography before free flaps for lower limb trauma.

- In 23 patients with normal distal pulses, there was one abnormal angiogram.
- In 15 patients with abnormal distal pulses, all had abnormal angiograms.

The authors therefore suggest that there is no need to perform angiography if **distal pulses** are intact.

Computed angiography in the planning of free tissue transfer in the post-traumatic setting. (Duymaz A, *Plast Reconstr Surg*, 2009)

This study examined 76 patients with lower extremity trauma who had computed tomography angiography (CTA) before flap reconstruction. The CTA demonstrated normal vascular anatomy in 52.6%, anatomical variants in 9.2% and atherosclerotic occlusive disease in 7.9%. The limb salvage rate was 94.7%, and all four of the amputated limbs had at least single artery occlusion on pre-operative CTA.

CTA can provide useful information without the 1%–3% risk of vessel injury (pseudoaneurysm, dissection, haematoma) associated with groin puncture for conventional angiography. There is debate over when to use either CTA or angiography in lower limb trauma – they do not seem to be indicated when there are two **palpable** pedal pulses (PT and DP).

Others (e.g. Gonzalez MH, *Plast Reconstr Surg*, 2002;109:592) use arteriograms almost routinely. They found that >1/3 of lower limb trauma patients have abnormal vessels, and these have 33% risk of free flap failure compared with 12% in those with normal arteriograms.

The fate of lower extremities with failed free flaps. (Benacquista T, *Plast Reconstr Surg*, 1996)

In their review, the free flap failure rate in trauma patients (mainly Gustilo IIIB and C) was about 10% compared with ~7% in non-trauma patients. The commonest cause of failure was venous thrombosis.

Although vessel spasm, scarring and granulation tissue may make delayed reconstruction more difficult and increase the need for vein grafts, the timing of surgery did not affect the rate of failure *in this study* – results were no worse in those flaps performed on day 1 compared with later time points, which contrasts with Godina (flaps before 72 hours had <1% failure, whilst those performed later had a 12% failure rate).

- Overall, ~80% of patients with a failed flap had their limb salvaged by other methods whilst the other 20% had amputation.
- Culliford (*Ann Plast Surg*, 2007) reported an 8.5% failure rate with an 18% amputation rate in their patients.
  - Second free flaps had a failure rate approaching half.
  - In particular, there was a high failure rate for acute free bone flaps; thus, it is recommended that the soft tissues are closed first, leaving bone reconstruction for later.

Long-term behaviour of the free vascularized fibula following reconstruction of large bony defects. (Falder S, *Br J Plast Surg*, 2003)

This is a retrospective review of free fibula flaps used to reconstruct a mean bone gap of 12 cm in limb long bones following either trauma or tumour; they note a trend towards more use of Ilizarov bone fixation. There were three failures. Bone union was achieved in 74%, taking a median time of 4.75 months. Flap **hypertrophy** of 76.5% was noted in the lower limb similar to Erdmann (*Br J Plast Surg*, 2002).

Stress fractures (21%) required plating and bone grafting in two-thirds; double-barrelled flaps were less likely to suffer stress fracture (compare with Muramatsu K, *Br J Plast Surg*, 2004 – double-barrelled fibular flaps do not prevent stress fractures).

V. COMPARTMENT SYNDROME

This is a limb-threatening and potentially life-threatening condition: when perfusion pressure falls below tissue pressure/compartment pressure, this will lead to tissue necrosis, renal failure and death if untreated. It can occur in any compartment, but the common ones involved are the lower limb, abdomen, buttocks and upper limb. It can happen in 'open' tibial fractures as some compartments may still be closed.

- Volkman (1881) – paralytic contracture of the forearm with tight bandages. Volkman's ischaemic contracture is the final state of ischaemic necrosis and fibrosis.
- Thomas (1909) – extrinsic compression not necessarily required.
- Mubarak (1976) – CS results from raised interstitial pressure in a closed compartment.

Tissue perfusion = capillary perfusion pressure (CPP) – interstitial perfusion pressure (IPP)
- CPP and IPP are approximately 25 and 4 mmHg, respectively; as IPP rises above 30 mmHg, the capillaries will collapse.
- Anaerobic metabolism causes lactic acid accumulation and failure of sodium pump to maintain gradients that further increases oedema and compression.

CLASSIFICATION

- Acute – recognised symptoms and signs
- Subacute – without easily recognisable symptoms and signs but may progress to acute
- Recurrent – found mostly in athletes
- Chronic – unrelieved acute, ischaemia progressing to fibrosis and Volkman's contracture

AETIOLOGY

CS can develop late (>3 days) after injury depending on the mechanism. The ischaemic injury is proportional to the pressure elevation and the duration. Pressure >40 mmHg for >2 hours causes irreversible necrosis.

- **Fractures** – In the lower limb, the FDP and FHL are often affected first; 6% of Gustilo grade IIIB fractures may be complicated by CS. In a lower limb fracture, there may also be components of crush injury, vascular injury/haemorrhage, soft tissue swelling and reperfusion.
  - **Vascular injury** including extravasation injuries, bleeding from fractures. There is a case report of an anticoagulated patient sustaining an intracompartmental haemorrhage due to acupuncture needles (Smith DL, *West J Med*, 1986). CS has also been reported after inversion ankle injuries causing peroneal haematomas, after knee arthroscopy and even after vein puncture in the anticoagulated.
- **Swelling** of soft tissue, e.g. excessive exercise (increases muscle volume) or tetany/fits, **electrical injury** or **reperfusion** (with generation of free radicals), virus-induced myositis, leukaemic infiltration, nephrotic syndrome (low osmolality).
- **Prolonged extrinsic compression** including anti-shock trousers and POPs, prolonged lying in one position, e.g. drug overdoses (head on forearm 48 mmHg, leg under the other 72 mmHg, forearm under trunk 178 mmHg).
- **Combination**, e.g. **burns** with thick constricting eschar and soft tissue inflammation/swelling.

SYMPTOMS AND SIGNS

The five 'P's of ischaemia are **not reliable.** The clinical impression/suspicion is important; the presence/absence of pulses is not a good discriminating sign.

- **Pain**, especially on **passive stretching, out of proportion to the injury**. Reduction of pain may herald necrosis rather than recovery. An increasing need/demand for analgesia is a classic sign.
- Tense swelling in the compartment.
- Paraesthesia/hyperaesthesia (remember to compare both sides).
- Pallor and capillary refill >2 s, pulselessness (late) and poikilothermia.
- Weakness of compartment muscles (late), contracture (very late).

INVESTIGATIONS

- **Compartment pressure measurement** (ideally of all compartments)
  - Tissue P >30 mmHg in a normotensive patient (some cite 45 mmHg).
    - Tissue P >20 mmHg in a hypotensive patient
    - If high risk of progressing to dangerous intracompartmental pressure i.e. looking at the trend.
  - **Delta-p** (diastolic BP minus intracompartmental pressure) as a measure of perfusion pressure; 30 mmHg is the cut-off and anything below this requires decompression (McQueen MM, *J Bone Joint Surg Br*, 1996).
- **Doppler/arteriography/MRI** – may be more useful for non-acute forms
- **Serum potassium**, CK, clotting profile
- **Urine myoglobin**

Clinical suspicion must be followed by operative exploration of all the compartments in the area concerned.

MANAGEMENT

- Release any extrinsic compression and place limb at heart level (over-elevation may be counterproductive – it reduces mean arterial pressure [MAP] but has no effect on compartment pressure).
- Decompression with fasciotomy then splint in a position of function with elevation.
  - Burn wounds may require escharotomy and fasciotomy. The emphasis is on successfully achieving **decompression**.
- It is important to anticipate rhabdomyolyis/myoglobinuria; treat it aggressively.
  - IV hydration to promote urine output 1–2 mL/kg/hour to reduce myoglobin accumulation.
  - Mannitol.
- Definitive wound closure when swelling has gone down; either direct closure or skin grafting. Complete recovery is expected if decompression occurs within hours, although this depends on the actual injury/mechanism.
- The role of HBO to protect against reperfusion injury is controversial; it is not widely available.

Fasciotomy should be performed under controlled conditions, i.e. in an operating theatre with full asepsis when circumstances allow.

LOWER LIMB

BAO/BAPRAS 2009 standards advocate a **two-incision** decompression for the leg (Table 7.3 and Figure 7.1).

Incisions should be placed anterior to the line of perforators both medially and laterally to preserve fasciocutaneous flap options.

- **Lateral incision** – decompress **anterior and lateral compartments** via an incision 2 cm anterior to the fibula (or halfway between the fibula and tibia) and aim for the intermuscular septum going between peroneus longus, EHL/tibialis anterior. Take care to avoid the superficial peroneal nerve as it becomes superficial 10 cm above the ankle.
- **Medial incision** – decompress superior and deep posterior compartment via an incision 1–2 cm behind the medial tibial border. Release the fascia over the soleus and then aim for the FHL in the deep compartment.

Table 7.3 Compartments of the lower leg and their contents

Compartment	Anterior	Lateral	Posterior superficial	Posterior deep
Muscles	EHL, EDL, TA, PT	PL and PB	Gastrocnemius plantaris, soleus	FHL, FDL, TP
Main function	Dorsiflexion	Eversion	Plantar flexion	
Nerve	Deep peroneal nerve	Superficial peroneal	Tibial nerve	
Artery	Anterior tibial artery	Peroneal artery	PTA	

Note: Extensor hallucis longus (EHL), extensor digitorum longus (EDL), flexor hallucis longus (FHL), flexor digitorum longus (FDL), tibialis anterior (TA), tibialis posterior (TP), peroneus longus (PL), peroneus brevis (PB) and peroneus tertius (PT).

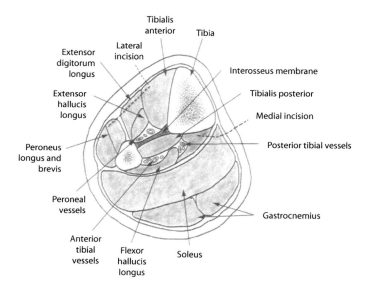

Figure 7.1 A cross-sectional diagram of the lower leg demonstrating the incisions used for decompression in CS.

Take care to avoid the perforators from the PTA as well as the neurovascular bundle itself. Watch also for the long saphenous vein and nerve.

ONE INCISION TECHNIQUE

One long incision over lateral compartment directly over or slightly posterior to the fibula extending just distal to the head of the fibula to 3–4 cm proximal to the lateral malleolus; it is important to identify (and spare) the common peroneal nerve proximally.

- Undermine skin anteriorly whilst avoiding the superficial peroneal nerve; longitudinal fasciotomy of anterior and lateral compartments is performed.
- Undermine skin posteriorly, perform fasciotomy of superficial posterior compartment then define the interval between the soleus and the FHL; subperiosteally dissect the muscles from the fibula and retract muscle and peroneal vessels posteriorly to reach the deep posterior compartment.

OTHER COMPARTMENTS

- Foot – two dorsal incisions along the lines of the second and fourth intermetatarsal spaces, and release all compartments – interosseus, central lateral and medial.
- Thigh – medial and lateral incisions to release the medial and anterior/posterior compartments, respectively.
- Upper arm.
  - Medial incision for medial compartment and lateral incision for posterior compartment.
  - Take care to avoid the ulnar and radial nerves.
- Forearm.
  - Dorsal – from the lateral epicondyle to the line of middle metacarpal.
  - Volar – starting with the carpal tunnel release (if necessary), proximally curve to the ulnar border, curving back radially at the elbow to **avoid the ulnar nerve**.
- Hands.
  - Dorsum – two incisions along the second and fourth intermetacarpal spaces (interossei and adductor pollicis).
  - Volar – release thenar, hypothenar eminences and carpal tunnel.

Comparison of fasciotomy wound closures using traditional dressing changes and the vacuum-assisted closure device. (Zannis J, *Ann Plast Surg*, 2009)
This is a retrospective review of 804 fasciotomy wounds; 438 were treated exclusively with VAC, 270 saline dressings only and 96 with both. They found a shorter time for primary closure in the VAC group.

Rogers (*J Plast Reconstr Aesthet Surg*, 2013) found that delayed primary closure is superior to grafting in terms of aesthetics, and actually involved a shorter hospital stay.

A comparison of fasciotomy wound closure methods following extremity compartment syndrome at a regional trauma centre. (Price G, *Eur J Plast Surg*, 2016)
This is a retrospective review comparing delayed primary closure (on the third day, n = 66), skin grafting (7) and dynamic closure (which seem to involve a hotchpotch of suture/sloop techniques, n = 109). Primary closure had the shortest time to wound closure and overall hospital stay, with a complication rate of 15%. Skin grafting had no complications but took the longest time. Dynamic closure took 6 days to close wounds on average but had a 55% complication rate. However, there was not a clear description of these techniques.

There have been many published methods for fasciotomy closure.

- Shoelace technique – Cohn (*Orthopedics*, 1986)
- Vessel loop technique – Harris (*Injury*, 1993)
- Steristrips – Harrah (*Am J Surg*, 2000)
- STAR (suture tension adjustment reel) – McKenney (*Am J Surg*, 1996)
- Sure-closure device – Narayanan (*Injury*, 1996)
- VADER (vacuum-assisted dermal recruitment) – Van der Velde (*Ann Plast Surg*, 2005)

Long-term sequelae of fasciotomy wounds. (Fitzgerald AM, *Br J Plast Surg*, 2000)
The study demonstrates that 10% and 7% of patients have persistent pain and muscle herniation, respectively.

- Altered sensation at wound edges (77%)
- Dry skin (30%) and pruritis (40%)
- Discoloured scars (30%), tethered scars (25%) and tethered tendons (7%)
- Recurrent ulceration (13%)
- Swollen limb (25%)

VI. CHRONIC LEG WOUNDS

This is generally defined as **lack of wound closure after 3 months** and is often due to diabetes, venous hypertension, ischaemia or pressure. There are derangements of the cytokine response including decreased EGF, PDGF and increased Il-1, IL-3 and TNFα. **There are decreased tissue inhibitor of metalloproteinsases (TIMPs) and increased matrix metalloproteinases (MMPs).** Wound debridement removes MMPs, helping to convert it to an acute wound.

Free flap coverage of chronic traumatic wounds of the lower leg. (Gonzalez MH, *Plast Reconstr Surg*, 2002)
The authors describe their results using free flaps to cover open lower leg wounds following trauma with a mean

duration of 40 months (over half had established osteomy-elitis). Flaps (LD and RA) were used after an average of 2.3 debridements.

- Most underwent pre-operative angiography (36% abnormal).
- 19% (8) flap loss – 3/8 of these due to infection, 5/8 had normal angiograms and 6/8 had chronic osteomyelitis.

They conclude that diffuse chronic osteomyelitis and an abnormal angiogram increase the risk of flap failure. They recommend the use of vein grafts to ensure that anastomoses are performed outside the zone of trauma or vicinity of the chronic wound.

VENOUS LEG ULCERS

These account for 80% of leg ulcers and are related to valvular incompetence and venous hypertension that lead to fibrin deposition in the soft tissues and increase in the oxygen diffusion barrier. There is often oedema, lipodermatosis and haemosiderin deposits.

The mainstay of treatment is **compression therapy** (30–40 mmHg at the ankle and 18 mmHg just below the knee, arterial disease having been excluded) and allows 93% of patients to heal by 5.3 months, but the recurrence rate is high, partly due to issues with compliance. Compression bandaging is usually painful but gets better as healing occurs, taking up to 10–12 days.

Surgery includes vein stripping and subfascial ligation of incompetent perforating veins; skin grafting is more successful if venous surgery is also performed.

DIABETIC FOOT

There are multiple reasons that diabetic patients have problems with their feet.

- Sensory neuropathy and loss of protective sensation, derangement of joints; they may have pressure sores over metatarsal heads.
  - Reduced endoneurial blood flow
  - Effect of glycosylated products
- Increased risk of infection due to
  - Autonomic neuropathy (AV shunting) leading to dry, cracked skin
  - Peripheral vascular disease causing tissue hypoxia
  - Decreased cellular and humoral immunity

Prevention is possible to a certain extent with effective glycaemic control and proactive chiropody/diabetic foot-care regimes.

MANAGEMENT OF DIABETIC FOOT WOUNDS

- Wound debridement including bone where necessary.
- Systemic antibiotics as needed.

- Hyperbaric oxygen therapy (HBOT) (Faglia E, *Diabetes Care*, 1996). HBOT is covered by Medicare (since April 2003) for treatment of diabetic wounds that meet three criteria:
  - The patient has diabetes and has a lower limb wound due to diabetes.
  - Wound is Wagner grade III or higher.
  - A course of standard wound therapy has failed.
- Revascularisation if the ulcer is predominantly ischaemic.

Lack of effectiveness of hyperbaric oxygen therapy for the treatment of diabetic foot ulcer and the prevention of amputation. (Margolis DJ, *Diabetes Care*, 2013)
A retrospective observational cohort study found that 6259 patients who had HBOT for their diabetic foot ulcers did not have increased healing rates or reduced amputation rates. The authors suggest that the evidence for skin substitutes, rhPDGF and total contact casting was more convincing.

A 2015 Cochrane study (Kranke P, *Cochrane Database Syst Rev*, 2015) looked at 12 RCTs with 577 patients with chronic foot ulcers (mostly diabetic). They found that HBOT improved the chances of healing in the short term (up to 6 weeks) but not in the longer term. The major amputation rate may be reduced. They commented on design flaws in the studies; their conclusion was that they could not confirm nor refute HBOT benefits.

Innovations in diabetic foot reconstruction using super-microsurgery. (Hyun SS, *Diabetes/Metab Res Rev*, 2016)
JP Hong (senior author) described their surgical approach for successful diabetic foot reconstruction. Debridement, infection and vascular intervention are needed to stabilise and prepare the wound before free flap reconstruction. They have a low threshold for angioplasty/bypass surgery to improve the vascular status just prior to reconstruction. They use small flaps based on small perforators >0.8 mm, e.g. SCIP, posterior interosseous, etc., usually described as supermicrosurgery, that can be anastomosed to **collateral vessels**.

AMPUTATION/ARTHRODESIS

- Amputation of non-viable toes
  - At the level of tarsometatarsal (TMT) joints (Lisfranc)
  - At the level of talonavicular joint (Chopart)
  - Just above the ankle joint (Symes)
- Metatarsal phalangeal (MTP) joint arthrodesis for dorsal ulceration as a result of motor imbalance.

SOFT TISSUE CLOSURE

- Trial of dressings to allow healing by secondary intention.
- Granulation tissue may accept an SSG.

- Consider local flap options first, e.g. medial plantar flap or distally based FC flaps to heel defects, but with a significant risk of distal flap necrosis (flap delay may help).
  - Kelahmetoglu. (*Plast Reconstr Surg*, 2015). It is postulated that elevated VEGF levels in the edge of a chronic wound lead to the enlargement of perforators. **Wound edge-based perforator (WEBP) flaps** could be harvested; 3 out of 25 flaps had venous congestion.
- Free flaps to larger defects.
  - FC, e.g. lateral arm flap for dorsum of the foot.
  - Muscle flap plus SSG for heel/ankle (this combination is less bulky than myocutaneous flaps, whilst the use of SSG provides a surface that is just as stable).

VII. LYMPHOEDEMA

Lymphoedema is the accumulation of protein-rich interstitial fluid in subcutaneous tissues; the deep muscle compartments are uninvolved. The skin becomes thick and brawny, and fissuring and ulceration result. Women are more frequently affected than men. Genital lymphoedema in men may lead to impotence and infertility from swelling, fibrosis and raised testicular temperature.

- Lower limb > upper limb

PATHOGENESIS

- Accumulation of proteins into the interstitium raises the tissue oncotic pressure and disruption of Starling's equilibrium.
- The increased interstitial protein and fluid causes relative tissue hypoxia with cell death and a chronic inflammatory response.
- Intralymphatic pressure increases, valves become incompetent and there is **dermal backflow**, increasing the amount of fluid and proteins in the tissues further.
- The accumulated fluid also acts as a medium for bacterial growth.
- Fibrosis eventually obliterates lymph channels.

CLINICAL FEATURES

- Initially pitting, then non-pitting, oedema due to fibrosis of soft tissues.
- Skin ulceration.
- Pain (see below).
- **Lymphangiosarcoma** may develop >10 years following the onset of lymphoedema and carries a poor prognosis. Stewart–Treves syndrome is lymphangiosarcoma developing in a lymphoedematous arm following mastectomy.

PAINFUL LYMPHOEDEMA

Pain is not a major feature in most cases of lymphoedema but can occur.

- Inflammation/infection – antibiotics are needed in higher doses and for longer courses.
- Compression/fibrosis of tissues.
- Stress on joints/bones.
- Others causes, e.g. neuropathic (radiation, recurrence), myofascial (trigger points) and vascular.

PRIMARY LYMPHOEDEMA

Primary lymphoedema where no precipitating cause can be found and is less common (10% in the United States) than secondary lymphoedema. It is effectively a diagnosis of exclusion. Primary lymphoedema can be either sporadic or inherited. The swelling in primary lymphoedema generally shows slower progression; it tends to begin distally and progress proximally (often it is the distal lymphatics that are most malformed/underdeveloped), whilst secondary lymphoedema often begins near the trunk and progresses distally.

- **Congenita (10%)** involves the lower limb/below knee most frequently, and 1/3 of cases are bilateral. The condition is usually apparent before 2 years of age, most often at birth, but this category includes cases up to 14 years old. It tends to be **non-progressive** but may be complicated by recurrent infections. There are associations with Turner's syndrome and Noonan's syndrome (web neck and cystic hygroma)
  - Some define **Milroy's** as the **inherited form of congenital lymphoedema** (Milroy WF, *NY State J Med*, 1892) It shows AD inheritance with incomplete penetrance (up to 10% have no symptoms). There is a defect in a tyrosine kinase receptor VEFGR3 (FLT4 gene on locus 5q35.3, required for lymphatic development). It is one of the **rarest** causes of lymphoedema (2%) and the actual aetiology is unknown – **lymphatic aplasia** is implicated, though Mellor (*Microcirculation*, 2010) says that dysfunction (of absorption) contributes, as well as saphenous reflux. Patients have ski-jump toenails, toe papillomatosis and wide calibre leg veins (Brice G, *J Med Genet*, 2005).
    - The term has been applied inappropriately to congenital or primary lymphoedema in general. Milroy described the condition in 1892, in a missionary and his mother, but the name came from Osler.
  - Hypotrichosis lymphoedema telangectasia syndrome (HLTS) with mutations in SOX18 gene. Hair is lost in infancy; vascular lesions affect palms/soles in particular.
- **Praecox (80%)** – sometimes called Meige's lymphoedema (1898) and is much more common in females

(10:1). The swelling usually begins at puberty but can occur from ages 14 to 35. It is particularly severe below the waist affecting the dorsum of the foot first; it is often unilateral (70%), even though the underlying lymphatic anomalies (hypoplastic distal lymphatics) are bilateral. It may worsen with activity, sometimes presenting with symptoms of acute inflammation.

- **Lymphoedema distichiasis** (*di* and *stichos*, Greek for 2 and row): There is a mutation in chromosome 16q24.3 FOXC2 gene in patients with a double row of eyelashes; the extra set is usually soft and pale, placed in the meibomian gland openings. Irritation tends to be the presenting complaint before the pubertal onset of lower limb oedema. Vessels tend to be hyperplastic with reflux and may be associated with clefts, heart defects, ptosis and vertebral anomalies.
- **Tarda (10%)** is a less common variant with later onset of bilateral swelling, typically after 35 years of age. Vessels are usually hyperplastic – tortuous and abnormal.

SECONDARY

The commonest cause of secondary lymphoedema worldwide is filariasis due to infection by *Wuchereria bancrofti*. This condition is rare in developed countries where lymphoedema is most commonly related to malignant disease particularly its treatment with surgery and/or irradiation. Upper limb lymphoedema most often follows the treatment of breast cancer; 77% of cases present within 3 years of surgery (latent period), but it can arise at any time. Lymphoedema may also follow gynaecological/pelvic malignancy and melanoma (post node dissection).

- Neoplastic – malignant nodes, extrinsic compression
- Infective/inflammation – tuberculosis, Wuchereria bancrofti; prolonged inflammation from wounds/ulcers, DVT, trauma
- Iatrogenic
  - **Radiotherapy** (delayed for a year or so) causes scarring, fibrosis and reduces lymphangiogensis.
  - **Lymph node surgery** (including harvesting nodes for vascularised lymph node transfer) with lifelong increased risk surgery. Lymph vessels do have some regenerative capacity and not all patients undergoing surgery and/or radiotherapy develop lymphoedema; it may be related to some underlying susceptibility, which is as yet undefined, though possibly genetic. Even nonlymphatic surgery may increase risk through damage of lymphatics, scar, infection, etc. In general, the more extensive the surgery, the greater the damage.
- MRM + lymph node surgery ~20% risk.
- ALND ~15%, with RT 30%–45%.
- SLNB ~5%–8%, with RT ~15%.

Morbidity of sentinel lymph node biopsy (SLN) alone versus SLN and completion axillary lymph node dissection after breast cancer surgery. (Langer I, *Ann Surg*, 2007)

A prospective Swiss study with 659 patients demonstrated a lymphoedema risk of 19.1% after completion of nodal dissection compared to 3.5% following SLNB. Irradiation causes fibrosis and inhibits lymphangiogenesis, and approximately doubles the risk of developing lymphoedema after nodal surgery.

DIFFERENTIAL DIAGNOSES

Lymphoedema needs to be differentiated from

- **Lipoedema** (lipodystrophy) – suitable for liposuction. See below.
- **Klippel**–Trenaunay syndrome – varicose veins, limb elongation, vascular malformations, limb oedema (some have lymphatic abnormalities).
- **Venous hypertension** – exclude deep venous thrombosis (DVT) (Doppler/venogram).
- **Oedema due to hepatic**, renal or cardiac causes.

LIPOEDEMA

Lipoedema (Allen EV, *Proc Staff Meet Mayo Clin*, 1940) is sometimes called **painful fat syndrome** and is commonly mistaken for lymphoedema, but it is not a lymphatic disease (Van Geest AJ, *Phlebologie*, 2003). There is a lower risk of skin infections and lymphoscintigraphy will show a flame-like pattern.

It can be heritable. Patients are mostly females with problems of swelling starting at puberty; it is symmetrical and usually spares the feet with a characteristic fold at the ankle – **Stemmers sign** (picking up the fold of skin over the dorsum of the second toe) is negative, i.e. the examiner can pick up the fold, whereas it is positive in lymphoedema forming a bulky lump.

Fat accumulates around the pelvis, hips down to the thighs ('jodphurs'), up to but not including the ankles. The fat is not responsive to dieting, but patients often gain significant weight due to their condition; low esteem may be evident. Pain and tenderness are characteristic features – often in medial thigh; easy bruising may also be seen, but the skin itself is normal in character. Treatment can be problematic:

- Gentle massage and compression like lymphoedema therapy can help but may be limited by discomfort (and in theory there is little to decongest). It is important to avoid the occurrence of **lipolymphoedema** (secondary lymphoedema due to the enlarging fat occluding fine lymphatics), which is the major serious sequelae in addition to weight gain and joint tissue strain.
- Medications including diuretics are not useful.
- Liposuction.

STAGING OF LYMPHOEDEMA

Accurate staging is vital to monitor and to assess the efficacy of treatment. The International Society of Lymphology (ISL) staging is the most commonly used system, but it is somewhat flawed in that it is based only on physical findings. Some suggest incorporating measures of QOL to improve its usefulness. The classification offered by Campisi (*World J Surg*, 2004) shows congruence with ICG dermal backflow patterns (see below), which provides an indication of lymphatic function.

ISL staging 2003/2009 consensus document. Stage 0 (latent lymphoedema) is a recent addition.

ISL stage	Features
0/la	No oedema but lymphatic impairment present.
I	Mild oedema that is reversible with appropriate limb position. May pit.
II	Moderate oedema that is not reversible with limb elevation. Pits except in late stage II as more fibrosis occurs.
III	Lymphostatic elephantiasis with trophic skin changes such as acanthosis, deposition of fat and fibrosis, warty overgrowth.

Campisi staging 2010.

Campisi stage	Features
1A	No oedema but lymphatic impairment is present; no difference in volume/consistency between limbs.
1B	Mild oedema that is reversible with appropriate limb position.
2	Persistent oedema that is partially reversible with appropriate limb position.
3	Persistent oedema that continually becomes more severe; recurrent acute lymphangitis.
4	Fibrotic lymphoedema with lymphostatic warts; **column-shaped limbs**.
5	Elephantiasis with severe limb deformation, scleroindurative pachydermatitis, widespread lymphostatic warts.

INVESTIGATIONS

In most cases, the diagnosis can be made clinically, though in some, comorbidities may co-found the clinical pictures. Generally, one may need to exclude other causes of swelling, e.g. heart/renal/hepatic failure, DVTs, etc.

- The most commonly used method of objectively assessing the swelling is some form of **conal measurement**, e.g. measuring the circumference at intervals, which is more

practical than **water displacement methods** but is supposedly similar in accuracy.

- **Bioimpedance spectroscopy** uses electrical current to measure the degree of tissue fluid retention and is useful in detecting early-stage lymphoedema including stage 0 disease.
- **CT/MRI** shows a honeycomb appearance of subcutaneous tissues but are generally nonspecific/nondiagnostic. They may be useful for general purposes, e.g. image pelvis for tumours. Similarly, Doppler USG may be used to exclude DVT.
- **Lymphography/lymphangiography** involves direct cannulation of a lymphatic vessel in the foot/hand (under magnification). An oil-based contrast material is then injected through this vessel, and serial plain radiographs of the limb are taken; this allows the lymphatics to be precisely delineated. Due to the potential for damage to the lymphatic vessels, it can theoretically worsen lymphoedema and has largely been replaced by:
- **Radionuclide lymphoscintigraphy** (also called isotope lymphography). Technetium-labelled colloid is injected into the web spaces, and proximal drainage of the colloid is then recorded using a gamma camera. Delayed or absent radiotracer transport suggests lymphatic abnormalities. It is 'minimally' invasive and enables both qualitative and quantitative analyses to be made.
  - **SPECT/CT** may be useful.
  - **Magnetic resonance lymphangiograms** may in time replace lymphoscintigraphy as it avoids direct injection of contrast and use of ionising radiation, but is able to provide a sharp image of lymphatic vessels.
- **Indocyanine green** (ICG) scan can give dynamic information; it can be used to stage the disease based on dermal backflow patterns.
- **Genetic testing** in some with primary lymphoedema (VEGFR3, FOXC2, SOX18).

MANAGEMENT OF LYMPHOEDEMA

Remove the precipitating cause, if any. No form of treatment is curative, though early treatment may reduce deterioration; neglected cases tend to get progressively worse with more skin changes, more episodes of infection and fluid weeping/leakage. Patients are best treated in a specialised clinic; inexperienced staff may delay treatment or, worse, advocate inappropriate remedies.

GENERAL ADVICE

The vast majority of this is no more than anecdotal, but seems simple enough to implement without being too onerous.

- **General care** – patients are advised to avoid even minor degrees of trauma, e.g. venepuncture, insect bites, acupuncture, etc.

- **Air travel** – reduced cabin pressure will lead to more swelling; compression garments, hydration and mobilisation are recommended.
- **Avoid blood pressure taking by sphygmomanometer on the affected arm** – automated machines may be more traumatic.
- **Needlesticks** – some evidence supports the idea that they should be avoided. Patients can wear medical alert bracelets to warn others.
- **Exercise** – gentle stretching, resistive and aerobic exercises advised, avoiding overexertion to fatigue.
- **Avoid extremes of temperature**.
- **Diet** – reduce BMI, some suggest flavanoids, selenium and bromelain.

MEDICAL

- **Skin care** – prevention of ulceration and infections, especially fungal. Be careful of even minor trauma, e.g. nail cutting, shaving hairs.
- **Elevation.** It does not improve drainage per se but will decrease venous pressure, which, in turn, decreases filtration pressure, hopefully to levels that drainage can 'cope' with.
- **Compression garments.**
- **Drugs.**
  - **Antibiotics.** Treat lymphangitis and cellulitis aggressively.
  - Dimethylcarbazine to kill Wuchereria bancrofti.
  - **Benzopyrone** (a class of drug originally used in patients with vascular disease, e.g. coumarin) can induce phagocytosis by binding to interstitial proteins, but clinical results have been mixed. Overuse with coumarin can cause hepatotoxicity; Paroven (an oxerutin) is supposedly less hepatotoxic. Daflon (a bioflavinoid) is similar, and a 500 mg twice daily dose has been shown to be more effective than placebo; but, in general, poor quality data prevent its recommendation (Badger C, *Cochrane Database Syst*, 2004).
- **Physical**
  - **Low level laser therapy** (LLLT) generates low intensity light (650–1000 nm) that is believed to promote lymph vessel regeneration and increase lymph pumping. It is FDA-approved, but long-term results are lacking. Near infrared (NIR) light therapy aims to increase nitric oxide to improve tissue repair and lymph regeneration but has not received FDA approval. Electrical stimulation is not recommended based on current evidence.
  - Heat treatment has been used in traditional Chinese medicine and has been applied in some Western treatment regimes. It is said to soften up the tissues and may induce macrophage activation. Exacerbations have been reported.

COMPLETE DECONGESTIVE THERAPY

This is the standard of care and if properly applied, reductions in volume of 50%–60% are expected. It is the specific **combination** of components (manual lymphatic drainage [MLD], compression bandaging, pressure garments, exercise and skin care) applied in two phases, though local regimes may vary. Systematic reviews support the use of CDT and MLD; failure of CDT is usually due to misdiagnosis, noncompliance or inadequate therapy.

- **Phase one** – Inpatient (or intensive outpatient) 'decongestive phase' takes weeks:
  - MLD aims to **lightly** massage lymph away from the swelling towards healthy channels. This needs to be preceded by emptying the proximal areas on the trunk.
  - Compression bandaging and exercise. Exercises are performed whilst in bandages, which oppose the filtration pressure and provide a counterforce to muscle contraction. Nail/skin care.
- **Phase two** – outpatient. The effects of phase 1 are temporary without **lifelong** stockings/compression garments, and a regular exercise regime is needed to maintain effects; ~50% maintain volume reduction at 3 years; obviously compliance can be a problem.

Caution is required to avoid excessive pressures that may occur with pneumatic compression (over 45 mmHg), which can rupture fragile lymphatic vessels or displace fluid to the trunk and genitalia (thus contraindicated in active infection, heart failure and DVTs).

SURGERY

Surgery is not a common option (<10%); it should always follow CDT or equivalent. For one reason or another such as concerns over scarring or lack of effect, surgery has often been regarded as a 'last resort', meaning that there is often a delay before patients are referred for surgery by which time they may only be suited to 'salvage' type procedures. Whilst initial attempts at 'physiological' reconstruction or restore function were met with disappointing late results, improved understanding of the pathophysiology accompanied by improved microsurgical techniques have seen the development of newer techniques that seem to offer improved outcomes.

EXCISIONAL SURGERY

- **Charles** (1912) – excision of all soft tissue down to fascia and covered with SSG. The aesthetic results are poor, with unstable grafts and keratotic overgrowths, and so this is usually reserved for swelling with severe skin changes.
  - Wrongly attributed by McIndoe to Sir Richard HH Charles who treated many patients with scrotal oedema but apparently never treated lower limb oedema.

- **Thompson buried dermal flap** – subcutaneous tissue is excised, and a dermal flap is buried into the uninvolved muscle compartments. Theoretically this creates a lymphatic communication allowing drainage of the skin via the deep compartment, but this has not been substantiated and only a few good results have been reported. It is rarely performed.
- **Homans** (1936; modification of Sistrunk procedure 1918) – subcutaneous excision of lymphoedematous tissue down to muscle fascia, preserving overlying skin flaps 1 cm thick, which are trimmed for direct closure. It is usually staged, i.e. medial side then lateral side whilst taking care to preserve vital structures such as the common peroneal and sural nerves. It is capable of producing good results and is consequently the **most commonly performed surgery** for lymphoedema. It can be repeated if necessary.
  - A variation on this is described as **radical reduction with preservation of perforators**; the flaps are elevated with 'microsurgical' preservation of perforators from posterior tibial and peroneal arteries (pre-Dopplered); the aim is to allow thinner flaps (~5 mm).
- **Liposuction** for lymphoedema was pioneered by Brorson, (*Scand J Plast Reconstr Surg Hand Surg*, 1997), and it probably counts as an excisional method. It is based on the observation that there is adipose hypertrophy in lymphoedema. Patients have to be prepared to wear pressure garments thereafter. Practice has evolved from the initial dry suction to tumescent-type liposuction; jet-assisted liposuction (Waterjet) may be gentler.
  - Treated patients have better QOL and suffer fewer episodes of cellulitis. Preliminary results with laser Doppler scanning seem to support the theory that liposuction can reduce the lymphatic load without damaging the lymph function. Though Brorson's results have been difficult to reproduce, NICE suggests that liposuction may be considered in those patients with severe disease (massive incapacitating disease, nonresponsive to conservative therapy).
  - More recently, Schaverian, *J Plast Reconstr Aesthet Surg* (2012) used Brorsons technique and demonstrated 101% reduction compared to normal limb at 1 year; this effect was maintained at 5 years.

The proven benefits of excisional surgery are often ignored, in part due to misconceptions of morbidity and complications that were mostly related to overly aggressive use of the techniques, leading to almost total abandonment of procedures in the mid-twentieth century. Recently, Karri (2011) demonstrated that good results are possible with modern application of the Charles procedure that may also be combined with NPWT. Similarly, Lee (2008) modified the Homans procedure and combined this with postoperative pressure garments to achieve good results.

PHYSIOLOGICAL SURGERY

Physiological techniques aim to increase the return of lymphatic fluid into the circulation, by reconnecting the lymphatic pathways above and beyond the obstruction, either directly (lymphatic to lymphatic) or indirectly via another segment such as veins/venules.

- **Lymphatic bridges**
  - Pedicled omental or stripped ileal segments on a vascular pedicle have been used in the hope that lymphatics connections will form between the flap and the recipient bed, but clinical results were poor.
  - Withey (*Br J Plast Surg*, 2001) described a case of severe head and neck lymphoedema ameliorated by the inset of a tubed deltopectoral flap to act as a lymphatic bridge.
- **Microsurgical lymphovenous** and lympholymphatic shunts, the 'derivative' techniques and 'reconstructive' techniques of Campisi, respectively.
- **Lympholymphatic**/lymphatic grafting (Baumeister) aims to overcome a local blockade, e.g. after surgery or trauma. In the lower limb, a long segment of lymphatic vessel is dissected out from the upper inner thigh and tunnelled over to affected contralateral leg for a lymphatic–lymphatic anastomosis. The dissection is technically challenging.
- **Lymph-vein anastomosis or bypass (LVB)**
  - Campisi (2010) described **lymphovenous anastomoses** connecting larger venules to one or more lymphatics (1800 cases in 30 years with 10 follow-up); he reported 67% average volume reduction and 87% reduction in cellulitis. Boccardo (*Lymphology*, 2009) reported on his results with LVB performed at the time of breast surgery with the aim of preventing lymphoedema but found that there was no difference in limb volume compared to controls up to 18 months.
- **Lymphaticovenous anastomoses** (LVAs) are popular, partly due to relatively atraumatic surgery that can be performed under LA. In Koshima's opinion, one of the inherent problems in LVB was that the higher venous pressure led to thrombosis at the anastomotic site. LVAs offered better vessel size match and lower venous pressures in the submillimetre vessels ('supermicrosurgery').
  - Empirically, it seems to be most effective in early stage (0/1) disease where some healthy lymphatics still remain, before the fibrotic stage when damage is irreversible. Proper staging, e.g. with ICG, is important.
  - Koshima (*J Reconstr Microsurg*, 2003) reports persistent reductions at an average follow-up period of 3.3 years. Some surgeons such as Damstra (*Breast Cancer Res Treat*, 2009) found no improvement in those with post mastectomy lymphoedema, with minimal improvement in reported QOL.

– Undoubtedly some patients improve, but the **longevity is in doubt**; as such, some suggest it as a treatment to reduce limb size prior to excisional surgery or as an adjunct to VLNT. Invariably studies involve relatively small numbers with short follow-up.

- **Vascularised lymph node transfer**. Proponents of node surgery say that LVAs eventually become occluded – possibly due to the effect of interstitial pressure on low-pressure thin vessels.

  - It seems that the transplanted nodes develop new drainage pathways – proposed theories for this drainage include nodes acting as suction/internal pumps, whilst others suggest they are a source of VEFG-C that promotes lymphangiogenesis.
  - Becker (*Clin Plast Surg*, 2012) describes the transfer of lymph nodes from the groin to the axilla in patients with postmastectomy lymphoedema; 62.5% of patients were said to be 'cured' and were able to discontinue physiotherapy.
  - Lin (2009) anastomosed superficial circumflex iliac nodes at the wrist to treat upper limb lymphoedema and reported a 55% reduction of volume at 56 months, with fewer episodes of cellulitis.
  - Cheng (*Plast Reconstr Surg*, 2014) used ICG to show lymph flow in a vascularised lymph node flap into the pedicle vein in both rats and humans.
  - Some transfer lymph nodes as part of a breast reconstruction procedure – there may be several other

benefits of such a procedure including release of scar tissue in the axilla and the provision of vascularised tissue that may act as a lymphatic bridge.

- Overall, good long-term functional data are lacking. Some authors have had difficulty reproducing published results; there may be a significant learning curve and some series found 38% risk of complications.

Minimal invasive lymphaticovenular anastomosis under local anesthesia for leg lymphedema. (Koshima I, *Ann Plast Surg*, 2004)

In this study, an average of 2.1 LVAs per patient were performed in 52 patients under LA. At a mean follow-up of 14.5 months, there was an average 41.8% reduction in leg circumference; there were beneficial effects even in stages III and IV disease.

Lymphatic venous anastomosis (LVA) for treatment of secondary arm lymphedema. (Damstra RJ, *Breast Cancer Res Treat* 2009)

This is a prospective study of 11 LVAs in 10 patients with **lymphoedema related to breast cancer, which is estimated to occur between 7% and 35%.** The patients had been unresponsive to conservative treatment. After surgery, they showed a 4.8% reduction of lymphoedema at 3 months and 2% after a year. There was a minimal improvement in the reported quality of life; non-operative treatment including elastic stockings was preferred by the patients particularly in the early stages of disease.

8

Skin and soft tissue

A. OVERVIEW AND SKIN, SUBCUTANEOUS AND APPENDIGEAL TUMOURS

I. OVERVIEW

A neoplasm is an abnormal mass of tissue with a growth rate exceeding that of the normal tissue. The excessive growth is **uncoordinated** and persists after cessation of the stimulus that evoked the change. According to the multistage carcinogenesis model, the following steps are involved.

- **Initiation** – a change in the genome of a cell follows exposure to a mutagen such as X-rays, ultraviolet (UV) radiation, chemical carcinogens or viruses.
  - The cellular change does not cause significant change in the cell/tissue morphology but does confer a long-term risk of developing cancer.
- **Promotion** – the change is made permanent by cellular division. The promotion stage requires a non-mutagenic stimulus, such as chronic inflammation, which enhances cellular proliferation resulting in the formation of a localised tumour that displays self-limited non-malignant growth and may regress if the stimulant is withdrawn.
- **Progression** – further cell division to form an invasive tumour.

A **malignant neoplasm** is one that invades surrounding tissues and has a propensity to metastasise. Tumours may arise due to

- Inappropriate activation of normal cellular proto-oncogenes that encode growth factors, growth factor receptors or transcription factors, to become oncogenes.
- Inactivation of tumour suppressor genes, e.g. p53 tumour suppressor gene is mutated in the majority of human cancers.

UV LIGHT

UV radiation is an important mutagenic factor – it causes mutations in cellular DNA and a failure of DNA repair (see 'Non-melanoma skin cancer').

MELANIN

Upon stimulation, melanocyte tyrosinase converts tyrosine to 3,4-dihydroxyphenylalanine (DOPA) and then to dopaquinone, forming black brown eumelanin or red-yellow pheomelanin (less UV absorptive capacity) with different proportions between different ethnic/skin types.

- Albinos have faulty tyrosinase enzyme (see below).
- In those with phenylketonuria (PKU), there is a lack of enzyme (phenylalanine hydroxylase) that converts phenylalanine to tyrosine, leading to a build-up of phenylalanine and metabolites that are toxic to CNS. Patients tend to have light skin, blond hair and blue eyes.
- In vitiligo, there is a lack of melanocytes due to an active 'depigmentation' process, e.g. with depleted melanocyte reservoir in hair follicles. This makes the

condition difficult to treat and the mainstay tends to be medical, e.g. PUVA and psoralens. Some have described surgical procedures, e.g. dermabrasion and very thin SSG or pulverised graft; so-called melanocyte transfer (some say that the dermabrasion may be enough by itself to stimulate dormant follicular melanocytes). Before surgery, it is best to have stable disease for 2 years (otherwise, a halo effect may result); some cases are relentless and never become stable.

There are no tanning pills; the only proven effective substance Melanotan (not FDA approved) is similar to MSH and works only when injected. Fake tan creams are usually based on DHA (dihydroxyacetone) that reacts with keratin protein and is temporary due to continual sloughing; better manufacturing techniques allow better quality (less orange, more brown) and more predictable colouring. The major problem is risk of allergy.

- β-Carotenes offer no protection as their absorption spectrum is outside the UVB range.
- Certain 'tanning pills', e.g. canthaxanthin, deposit colour in tissues (similar to carotene are fed to salmon to make them a more appetising colour), especially in the subcutaneous fat layer. These are FDA-approved as food additives, but not as tanning agents; but are widely sold online and in tanning salons. There is significant risk of complications at the dosages used for tanning, as visual disturbance/loss from retinal deposits and a plastic anaemia (at very high doses). The colour and coverage are unpredictable; it will stain all excreta. They are sometimes used to reduce sunlight sensitivity in patients with erythropoietic protoporphyria.
- Psoralens make skin darker with UV exposure, but are hazardous and are usually utilised only for major conditions, such as severe psoriasis. They increase skin sensitivity to UV, damaging DNA and forcing melanocytes to increase melanogenesis.

II. BENIGN SKIN AND SUBCUTANEOUS LESIONS

EPIDERMAL NAEVI

Naevi (Latin for blemish or spot) are best defined as **cutaneous hamartomas,** usually incorporating a proliferation of sebaceous glands (sebaceous naevus, SN), melanocytes (melanocytic naevus) or vascular tissue (vascular naevus).

Epidermal naevus syndromes are associations of epidermal naevi with developmental anomalies in other organ systems, especially of the CNS, eye and skeleton. Examples include the following:

- Proteus syndrome – overgrowth syndrome affecting multiple sites and tumours may develop.
- Sebaceous naevus syndrome.
- Becker's naevus syndrome – occurrence of Becker's naevus with unilateral pectoral hypoplasia and skeletal anomalies.

SEBACEOUS NAEVUS OF JADASSOHN (JADASSOHN'S DISEASE II)

This is a hamartomatous lesion present at birth in 0.3% of neonates – histologically, there is an accumulation of mature sebaceous glands with overlying epidermal hyperplasia. The condition usually presents at birth as flat pink plaques in the scalp/head, i.e. alopecia and neck, though there is significant variability in appearance with some forms being particularly florid; the lesion tends to become more nodular/verrucous with age.

The lesions tend to enlarge at the time of adolescence, and there is a risk of malignant transformation in 10%–20% in middle age (wide range quoted in literature) – classically to BCC, but also SCC, sebaceous and apocrine carcinomas. Namiki (*Case Rep Dermatol*, 2016) described a case where 4 different tumours arose in a single SN. However, a French series (Jaqueti G, *Am J Dermatopathol*, 2000) states that the risk of malignant transformation is probably nearer 1% and previous lesions identified as BCCs were actually trichoblastomas.

- **Sebaceous naevus syndrome** – in this rare disorder, there is a large sebaceous naevus often in the lines of Blaschko associated with other organ anomalies including neurological features such as seizures, developmental delay, palsies (cranial nerves, hemiparesis) and structural anomalies of the brain.
  - Josef Jadassohn (1863–1936) was a German dermatologist who also introduced patch testing for contact dermatitis.

TREATMENT

Excision is a common option with the aim of preventing malignant transformation or for cosmesis. Larger lesions may need serial excision, tissue expansion or dermal substitutes with thin SSG.

Should naevus sebaceous be excised prophylactically? A clinical audit. (Barkham MC, *J Plast Reconstr Aesthet Surg*, 2007)
This study/review concluded that prophylactic excision of all lesions is not warranted (due to a very low rate of transformation, 0.8% or less) and is only recommended when neoplasms are clinically suspected or for cosmetic reasons.

Serial excision is a useful technique for excision of benign lesions when applied correctly. If a lesion is going to require more than three excisions, then consider tissue expansion – the risk–benefit balance will depend on individual cases.

A user's guide for serial excision. (Quaba O, *Br J Plast Surg*, 2008)

- Excise early – skin elasticity is greatest and joints respond better, particularly if an enforced position is needed.

- Keep scars within the lesion and align parallel to relaxed skin tension lines if possible. In the limb, this should be along the longitudinal axis.
- In unscarred lesions, consider excising the outer part of the lesion first before closing with undermining and a purse-string suture.
- Undermine but avoid excision of subcutaneous tissue that may lead to contour defects.
- Close under **moderate tension** to maximise the excision as well as to recruit more skin. Sutures can be kept in longer to minimise stretching in between procedures; consider using non-absorbable buried/subcuticular sutures that do not need removal but will be excised during the next stage.

MELANOCYTIC NAEVI

Melanocytes are derived from neural crest cells. Melanin is synthesised in these cells (spindle-shaped with dendritic processes); from tyrosine, it accumulates and is then distributed to keratinocytes via the processes. The number of melanocytes between different races is not significantly different; rather it is the activity or **melanin production per cell** that differs – this is stimulated by sunlight and melanocyte-stimulating hormone (MSH) from the pituitary. Naevus cells (melanocytes leaving the epidermis to go into the dermis) are rounder and have no dendritic processes and gather in 'rests'.

Common **epidermal** lesions are as follows:

- **Freckles** – these have normal numbers of melanocytes but with increased melanin content in each. These tend to regress with reduced exposure to sunlight.
- **Lentigo** – there is an **increased number** of melanocytes in these lesions and they do not regress with sunlight avoidance.
- **Macules (CALM)** – normal melanocyte numbers with increased production (macromelanosomes).
- **Becker's naevus/melanosis** – irregular light-brown pigmentation, classically on the shoulder/torso of pubertal males that gradually enlarges, thickens and becomes hairy. It is generally regarded as an acquired condition of unknown cause (a quarter are associated with sun exposure).
  - Fehr (*Dermatologica*, 1991) reported nine cases of melanoma in patients with Becker's naevus, but only one actually occurred in the naevus itself. Becker's naevus is regarded as a benign disease, though it should be monitored; treatment is primarily cosmetic – laser hair removal is more successful than laser depigmentation, which has variable results.
  - Samuel Becker (1894–1964) was an American dermatologist.

Note the difference:

- **Melanocytic** – means more cells.
  - **Lentigines** – this may explain why these lesions do not go away even with sun avoidance. These

can be reliably treated with QS switched laser (PIH is a common complication) or IPL. Also respond to cryotherapy/peels/'Triple therapy'.
  - Naevus of Ota (see below) Mongolian Spot
- **Melanotic** – means more melanin with the same number of cells; most clinical lesions fall into this category.
  - Epidermal – freckles, CALM, Becker's and conventional sun tanning
  - Dermal – haemachromatosis, drug related
  - Mixed/either – PIH, melasma
    - PIH is due to inflammatory stimulation of epidermal melanocytes as well as disruption of the basal layer leading to dermal melanin that is subsequently trapped.
- **Chromatosis** is non-melanin pigmentation.

Melanocytes transfer melanin to neighbouring cells via cytoplasmic processes; these recipients may end up containing more pigment than the producers. Thus, skin colour is not directly related to melanocyte numbers.

The **level of the pigmentation** can be estimated by its colour:

- Upper epidermal – black
- Epidermal – brown
- **Papillary dermal – blue grey,** classically slate grey
- Reticular dermal – steel blue, 'grey ' – 'blue' naevus
- Mixed – brown grey

The reasons are not fully understood, but it helps to explain some phenomena such as why Mongolian spots appear bluer when the patient is younger before there is significant overlying melanin in the epidermis. According to Anderson RR (1987), if you take the epidermis from a patient with Naevus of Ota (NOO), it will appear grey/brown in reflected light and brown/yellow in transmitted light. If you take the underlying dermis (without epidermis), it will look blue in the reflected light. **The melanin in the dermis absorbs the incident visible light such that diffuse reflectance in the longer (red) wavelengths is reduced giving the pigment a blue appearance.** Some ascribe it to the Tyndall effect where blue light (shorter wavelength) is reflected more through scattering by particles. Melanin in the epidermis does the opposite reducing diffuse reflectance at shorter wavelengths, giving it a yellow to dark brown colour. Reflected light from the dermis reaches the observer after passing through the epidermis; hence, the degree of blueness of dermal melanin depends on the amount of epidermal melanin.

ACQUIRED NAEVI

- **Junctional naevus** – this is a melanocytic proliferation at the dermo-epidermal junction and the lesion is flat (macular) and deeply pigmented. They are found at any site, but benign acral or mucosal lesions are usually junctional naevi. Junctional naevi appear during childhood or adolescence with the tendency to progress to compound or intradermal naevi with age.

- **Compound naevi** – these are maculopapular pigmented lesions that appear in adolescence due to junctional proliferation of melanocytes forming nests and columns of dermal melanocytes.
- **Intradermal naevi** – cessation of junctional proliferation and clusters of dermal melanocytes. These are papular faintly pigmented lesions found in adults.

CONGENITAL NAEVUS (CONGENITAL HAIRY MELANOCYTIC NAEVUS)

Congenital melanocytic naevi (CMN) are histologically similar to a compound naevus and are large, pigmented, hairy and verrucous. There is an arbitrary definition of what constitutes 'giant', but this is usually taken to be 2% body surface area or 20 cm in the largest diameter (in adult or 'predicted' size). There are widely varying rates of malignant transformation in the literature, but recent systematic reviews suggest the figure to be probably close to 4%–5% or less, and usually within the first 5 years of life. Lesions overlying sacrum may be associated with meningocoele or spina bifida. It can be difficult what to advise patients/parents, but in most cases lesions are excised if feasible. The **risk of malignant change is reduced, not eliminated** – some melanomas arise from the dermis or deeper tissues, and there is a risk of extracutaneous melanomas (CNS, GI and retroperitoneal).

Although lesions tend to be well demarcated, the border may be more irregular than acquired naevi, and skin markings/appendages, including hair and piloerector apparatus (causing goose bumps), are exaggerated; pigmented cells may extend into fat/muscle layers; 80% of patients with giant CMN have satellite naevi. From a practical point of view, if a treatment cannot allow the patient to pass a 'stare test' – stop a passer-by from staring, then the usefulness is limited even if there has been objective improvement.

- **Skin grafts** have been popular in the past and may provide children and adolescents with a scar that is 'easier' to explain away as a 'burn scar', but long-term follow-up has usually shown regret and dissatisfaction; the grafted skin is dry, insensate and fragile compared to naevus skin. Contour defects on the limb are more obvious with more proximal lesions/defects. Skin substitutes, e.g. Integra, Nevelia, can be used, but there are no large studies on their long-term results.
- **Tissue expanders** have the potential for the best cosmesis particularly in those with few/no satellite naevi. Expanders can be reinserted if any naevus remains, but generally a period of rest of at least 3 months is recommended to allow flaps to adhere; there is a 20%–40% risk of complications if two or more surgeries are required (see 'Tissue expansion').
  - Expanders can be used to expand FTSG or flap donor sites to allow closure.
- **Serial excision** is a reasonably good choice if the excision can be completed in three stages or less

(6 months rest between); it is relatively simple with few complications (see above).
- **Less common:**
  - Dermabrasion – the hair follicles are often deep, and there is often 'seep-back' of pigment and regrowth of hairs. Some suggest that the best patients are the very young with very superficial naevi, particularly on the face. Success with phenol peels was reported by Hopkins, but a few have replicated their results.
  - Laser especially QS ruby and long pulse alexandrite has been used, but the response is unpredictable; in some cases, the pigment darkens. CO_2 laser 'dermabrasions' have been reported, though (sublethal) laser effects on melanocytes are unclear. Another concern is that laser therapy may partially treat dysplastic areas and delay diagnosis.

Congenital melanocytic nevi – When to worry and how to treat. (Price HN, *Clin Dermatol*, 2010)

- Risk of melanoma in small- and medium-size CMN is low and is nearly zero before puberty.
- Risk of melanoma in giant CMN is ~5%, with half in the first few years of life.
- **Melanoma and neurocutaneous melanosis (NCM) are most likely when size or predicted size >40 cm, numerous satellites (>20) and truncal/midline lesions.**
  - NCM is found in ~1/3 of GCMN, with 1/3 of these being symptomatic, e.g. raised ICP, hydrocephalus, development delay or space-occupying lesion; most die within 2–3 years of the development of symptomatic disease.
  - The management of asymptomatic NCM remains controversial, and the role of MRI screening is also debatable, except perhaps before major surgery.
  - Some suggest a baseline MRI at the age of 4–6 months before normal brain myelination obscures small lesions.

Large congenital melanocytic nevi: Therapeutic management and melanoma risk: A systematic review. (Vourc'h-Jourdain M, *J Am Acad Dermatol*, 2012)

Literature review shows only two prospective studies with enough data to accurately evaluate melanoma incidence of 2.3 per 1000 person-years (Egan C et al., *J Am Acad Dermatol*, 1998; Kinsler VA, *Br J Dermatol*, 2009). The cosmetic benefit was greatest in those with smaller lesions and those in the head and neck. They conclude that **the risk of MM is related to size (>40 cm), trunk and satellites** (but only one case of MM in a satellite). Half of MM were fatal. Mean diagnosis age was **12.6**, i.e. childhood.

- Kinsler (*Br J Dermatol*, 2009) showed 12% MM rate in bathing trunk LCMN >60 cm.
- A Singaporean study with 39 GCMNs (>5%) surface area demonstrated no malignancies (mean 19 years; Chan YC, *J Am Acad Dermatol*, 2006).

SPECIAL TYPES OF NAEVI

Spitz naevus – this is a benign melanocytic tumour with **cellular atypia** occurring predominantly in childhood (3–13 years old) but has been reported as congenital and also occurring at >70 years of age (i.e. wide age range). It is uncommon and accounts for less than 1% of melanocytic naevi in children. Typically, these are solitary reddish-brown nodules, occasionally deeply pigmented, found on the face and legs most commonly. There is rapid initial growth before remaining static. Bleeding after minor trauma is not uncommon. It resembles a compound naevus with spindle-shaped or epithelioid cells at the dermo-epidermal junction – there are multinucleated giant cells, abundant melanin, acanthosis and atypia, and it may be **difficult to differentiate from melanoma on histopathological examination**. These were previously called juvenile melanomas, but this is a misnomer and the lesions are generally regarded as benign and are managed more conservatively.

- Sophie Spitz (1910–1956) was the pathologist that described the condition (as juvenile melanoma) in 1948.
- **Spindle cell naevus** – these are typically dense black lesions occurring most commonly on the thigh particularly of females. There are spindle cell aggregates and atypical melanocytes at the dermo-epidermal junction. Their malignant potential is unclear. It is sometimes regarded as a variant of Spitz naevus.

Halo naevus – there is a pale zone around a pigmented naevus due to inflammatory infiltration (especially T lymphocytes and CD8 lymphocytes) and lack of melanocytes (thus, some suggest a similarity to vitiligo). They are most commonly found on the trunk, and often multiple. Halo naevi are benign.

Dysplastic naevus (2%–5% of the population, usually occur in sun-exposed areas) – this is an irregular proliferation of **atypical melanocytes** around the basal layer. Clinically, they are nodules >5 mm in diameter with variegated pigmentation and irregular border, sometimes described as a **'fried egg'** appearance. If there are multiple lesions, then it may be part of a **dysplastic naevus syndrome**, which has familial inheritance with a 5%–10% risk of **malignant change** to the SSM type of melanoma.

DERMAL MELANOCYTOSIS

Mongolian spot – macular pigmentation (a blue–grey patch up to 10 cm in diameter) present at birth on the sacral area of >90% of Mongoloid and ~1% of White neonates. Histologically, there are ribbon-like melanocytes around the neurovascular bundles of the dermis with a lack of melanophages. The pigmentation increases after birth but regresses by the age of 4–7 years, and no treatment is required. Some 'persistent' Mongolian spots may be larger and persist for longer.

Blue naevus – nodular benign blue–black pigmentation due to a collection of dermal melanocytes gathered around dermal appendages, which is said to represent arrested migration of melanocytes bound for the dermo-epidermal junction. The presence of melanophages distinguishes it from Mongolian spots. They are found on the extremities, buttocks and face, with 80% occurring in females and 60% present during infancy. They can be excised, but malignant transformation into melanoma is very rare.

Naevi of Ota – are commonest in the Japanese and Chinese females. They are blue–brown patches of pigmentation due to (upper) dermal melanocytosis of the skin around the eye (ophthalmic and maxillary divisions of the trigeminal nerve), sometimes involving the sclera (**glaucoma** is a rare association). Histologically, the lesions demonstrate similar features to Mongolian spots. They are not usually present at birth; they darken during childhood and persist in adult life. The development of malignant melanoma (MM) is very rare. Q-switched laser (with nano second pulse widths) is the treatment of choice; there may be temporary hyperpigmentation. New pico second 755 and 1064 nm lasers have shown good results for NoO as well as tattoos (Ohshiro T, *Laser Ther*, 2016).

- Naevus of Ito is a similar lesion distribution on the shoulder/upper arm.

BENIGN EPITHELIAL TUMOURS

Seborrhoeic keratosis (SK, basal cell papilloma, seborrhoeic or senile wart)
These are very common lesions from the fifth decade onwards with equal sex distribution. They have a warty appearance, but no viruses have been isolated from them – the cause is unknown, but it may run in some families (AD inheritance has been described) and is sometimes associated with pregnancy or oestrogen therapy.

They seem to represent an accumulation of immature keratinocytes between basal and keratinising layers – despite the name, they are not really caused by sebaceous glands nor limited to seborrhoeic distribution; also, they are **not** strongly associated with UV light exposure. Malignant transformation has been reported but is extremely rare.

- They are verrucous plaques with fissures and/or horn pearls, and a 'stuck-on' appearance due to the edge being slightly elevated and not attached to skin.
- They may be heavily pigmented (but this is very variable) – the proliferating keratinocytes produce melanocyte-stimulating cytokines.
- Multiple lesions are typical on the face, hands and upper trunk; lesions can be itchy, may bleed and become inflamed.

TREATMENT

- Shave, excision or curettage (alone or in conjunction with electrodesiccation)
- Cryotherapy, ablative laser

- Chemical peels, e.g. trichloroacetic acid (TCA) or 70% glycolic acid
- Combinations, e.g. cryotherapy or glycolic acid before curettage

Variants include the following:

- **Stucco keratosis** – non- or lightly pigmented flat keratosis more often found on the distal parts of the limbs.
- Dermatosis papulosa nigra – multiple facial lesions, usually pigmented tags, that are histologically similar to SK, found in darker-skinned races. They have an earlier age of onset. The cause is unknown (but there is a family history in half) and they are harmless.
  - This is not the same as the **Leser–Trélat sign**, which is a sudden explosion of multiple inflammatory itchy SKs that may be associated with visceral malignancies (gastrointestinal, breast, etc.) and may coexist with acanthosis nigricans. It is very rare. A sudden crop may also occur with inflammatory dermatoses such as sunburn or eczema.

KERATOACANTHOMA (MOLLUSCUM SEBACEUM)

This is a rapidly evolving tumour that is composed of kera-tinising squamous cells originating in pilosebaceous fol-licles and classically resolves if left untreated (over a few months). There has been a recent change in viewing it as pseudo-malignant to pseudo-benign – i.e. a cancer that resembles a benign lesion, and some have suggested a name of SCC-KA type. Similarly, some view it as a malignancy that rarely progresses; however, 2% show no regression and can become invasive.

- Weedon (*ANZ J Surg*, 2010) disputes that they are variants of SCC and suggests that they are distinct lesions that can be separated morphologically, specifically by their pattern of keratinisation Watanabe (*Medicine*, 2015) found lower levels of proliferation marker Ki67 in KA compared to SCC.
- A small number of cases of metastases from KA have been reported in the immunocompromised; in other patients, this phenomenon may arise due to SCC arising within the KA, which may occur in up to 10% of KAs occurring in those over 80 years old.

Typical lesions are smooth and globular with a central keratin plug or horn, and are most common on the face and dorsum of hand. Histopathologically, there are rapidly dividing squamous cells derived from skin appendages with atypical mitoses and loss of polarity; keratin-filled crypts are another feature. Variants are less likely to regress.

- Giant (>2–3 cm).
- Multiple lesions are rare (2%).
- Grzybowski's eruptive keratoacanthomas, hundreds to thousands of very itchy lesions on mucosa as well as skin, which generally **do not involute**.

- Ferguson-Smith familial keratoacanthoma that can be rather large ulcerated lesions that are ultimately self-healing. Lesions start appearing in early adulthood; more common in men.
- Keratoacanthoma marginatum centrifugum is an uncommon variant with central healing whilst the periphery continues to grow. It can reach large sizes and be difficult to treat.

In Whites, it is three times less common than SCC and is three times more common in males. The aetiology is mostly unknown, although there may be some similari-ties to SCC and Bowen's disease, e.g. role for sun exposure from epidemiological studies, and other carcinogens such as coal, tar and carcinogenic hydrocarbons (which tend to cause multiple lesions).

- Some cases involve sites of previous trauma including skin graft donor sites, excisional scars and previous cryotherapy sites.
- Human papilloma virus (HPV) has been isolated in some cases, and virus DNA sequences have been detected by PCR (Forslund O, *J Cutan Pathol*, 2003) but no types/subtypes predominated. The role of HPV is controversial.
- Up to 1/3 have chromosomal defects, but their significance is unclear.
- Immunocompromise and deficient cell-mediated immunity may be factors.

Keratoacanthoma may be a marker for **Muir–Torre syn-drome**: multiple internal malignancies and sebaceous ade-nomas, but the association of keratoacanthomas themselves with other malignancies is more controversial. Muir–Torre is a rare AD condition associated with a defect in the DNA mismatch repair (MMR) gene. Screening for internal malig-nancies particularly proximal colonic carcinomas with colo-noscopy is recommended. In ~1/3, the skin tumour precedes or is synchronous with the internal malignancy.

TREATMENT

The current standard of care for suspected keratoacantho-mas is active treatment; they should not be left to regress spontaneously, and it is a myth that spontaneous resolution does not leave unsightly scars.

- Generally, it is good practice to excise the lesions to provide a good histological specimen – shaving often produces only non-diagnostic keratin fragments. **Without information regarding invasion, it cannot be distinguished from frank SCC.**
- 5-FU and radiotherapy may shorten the time to resolution, but radiation in young people may leave poor results in the longterm.
- Alternatives include cryotherapy for small lesions, curettage and cautery for thicker lesions, leaving scabs that come off several weeks later to leave a slightly depressed scar.

- There have been some (essentially anecdotal) reports for intralesional methotrexate, bleomycin, interferons, topical imiquimod and oral retinoids.

DIGITAL FIBROKERATOMA

This is an uncommon benign tumour of fibrous tissue that presents as a papillary or keratotic outgrowth in the region of a finger joint found in adults (more commonly males). The cause is unknown, and though trauma has been implicated, there is little evidence to support this view. Histologically, there is hyperkeratosis and acanthosis (thickening of the epidermis, specifically the stratum spinosum). Its fleshy colour and finger-like appearance on occasion means that it should be distinguished from supernumerary digits. It is treated by excision.

III. HAIR FOLLICLE TUMOURS

TRICHOEPITHELIOMA

This is a relatively rare benign epithelial tumour differentiating towards **hair follicle cells.** Macroscopically they are pinkish nodules found most commonly around the nose, i.e. cheeks, eyelids and nasolabial folds. Typically they appear at puberty and can occur in non-familial solitary forms and familial (AD) multiple forms; a third variant is the desmoplastic trichoepithelioma. The tumour suppressor gene associated with the familial form has been located at 9p21, whilst the sporadic form has been associated with deletions at 9q22.3.

Solitary forms are typically larger and they are often diagnosed as BCC, whilst pigmented lesions are mistaken for melanoma. There have been reported cases of malignant change into BCCs in those with the multiple-familial form.

They are treated by excision. Histologically, there are rounded masses of fusiform cells and lacunae filled with keratin; tumour islands may connect with hair follicles. Immunohistochemistry may be needed to distinguish it from BCCs.

TRICHOLEMMOMA

A tricholemmoma is a hair-follicle tumour often misdiagnosed clinically as BCC; it is relatively common, though the true incidence is difficult to determine. The cells of origin come from the **outer root sheath**, and histologically there are plaques of squamous cells containing glycogen.

The lesions occur on the face as smooth asymptomatic papules in the middle-aged/elderly with equal sex distribution. The cause is unknown, although multiple lesions may be associated with the rare **Cowden disease** (multiple hamartoma syndrome with increased incidence of breast and thyroid carcinoma, AD type inheritance and more common in women). Confirmed lesions can be treated with shave biopsy or laser ablation.

Pilomatrixoma. (Benign Calcifying Epithelioma of Malherbe, 1880)

Pilomatrixoma is a benign appendigeal tumour that most probably arises from **hair matrix cells**. Part of it is composed of dead calcified cells (this **calcification** may be demonstrated by ultrasound or X-ray) and presents as a dermal/subcutaneous tumour with stony hard consistency and often with an angulated shape – the 'tent sign'– due to stretching of overlying skin. It is most common in the head, neck and upper extremity.

Histologically, it is a well-circumscribed tumour in the lower dermis and subcutaneous layer, composed mainly of basophilic cells along the periphery of tumour nests and ghost cells, lacking basophilic granules and nucleus. Calcium deposits are found in 75%.

It is uncommon but probably more common than previously thought, particularly in adults (bimodal incidence, first peak at 5–15 years and a second peak at 50–65 years) and slightly more common in females. The cause is unknown. An association with myotonic dystrophy has been reported, whilst one study shows positive immunostaining of bcl-2, a proto-oncogene that suppresses apoptosis in tumours. Another study demonstrated CTNNB1 mutations in 75%, but the significance of this is unknown.

Lesions grow slowly but may grow to a large size in some cases, and in very rare cases, malignant change has been reported. Excision is the commonest treatment; recurrences are rare and if they do occur may indicate a malignant variant.

TRICHILEMMAL CYST (PILAR CYST)

These keratin-filled cysts arise from the **outer root sheath** of the deeper hair follicle. They occur in areas of high follicle concentration, and thus most are situated on the scalp. They are more common in women than men; they are often multiple (70%) and in such cases may be familial (AD, though the responsible genes have not been found).

They are often erroneously referred to as 'sebaceous cysts', but there is **no punctum**. Furthermore, the cyst wall has follicular cells and thus can be histologically distinguished from epidermoid (sebaceous) cyst by presence of a granular layer in the lining epithelium of the latter. Rupture may cause cell proliferation to form the so-called proliferating trichilemmal cysts or **pilar tumours**, which may become large and ulcerated but are histologically benign. Neoplastic change is very rare.

Treat trichilemmal cysts by excision in a similar fashion to epidermoid cysts – either by complete excision with an ellipse or a more conservative approach, first decompressing the cyst with a punch biopsy, evacuating the contents and then pulling out the wall – larger cysts with thicker walls are more amenable to this type of treatment that leaves a shorter scar.

TRICHOFOLLICULOMA

This is an uncommon harmatoma arising from hair follicles with a dilated primary follicle, which may be connected to the epidermis – the cause is unknown but may be due to abortive hair-follicle differentiation. They are flesh-coloured or white papules found mainly on the face particularly around the nose, classically with a **central pore** or dot from which **white vellus hairs** may emerge.

IV. SEBACEOUS AND SWEAT GLAND TUMOURS

TUMOURS OF SEBACEOUS GLANDS

Benign sebaceous tumours are uncommon and difficult to classify. The following are generally not considered as true tumours:

- Sebaceous hyperplasia, which is sebaceous gland proliferation
- Sebaceous naevus, which is a congenital harmatoma
- Fordyce spot, which is the occurrence of ectopic sebaceous structures in lesions other than hair follicles

SEBACEOUS ADENOMA

This is a benign tumour affecting the face (including eyelid) or scalp, most frequently composed of incompletely differentiated sebaceous cells. It is rare and affects mainly the elderly with equal sex incidence. Grossly, these are small, shiny, yellowish multi-lobular tumours of the upper dermis, and histologically, there are small basophilic sebaceous matrix germinative cells in the periphery and more numerous, larger sebocytes with a foamy, bubbly appearance. Excision or other ablative modalities is the commonest treatment; incomplete excision generally leads to recurrence.

- Some patients who have multiple sebaceous adenomas (or epitheliomas or carcinomas) may have **Muir–Torre syndrome** (see above).

SEBACEOUS CARCINOMA

Sebaceous carcinomas are malignant tumours differentiating towards sebaceous epithelium and are rare (slightly more common in women). They comprise only 0.2% of skin cancers, though they are more common in Asians. In the Chinese population, it is the second most common periocular cancer after BCC with HPV being implicated. They tend to be aggressive with tendency for recurrence and metastasis. The aetiology is mostly unknown, but some follow radiodermatitis.

They present usually as yellowish nodules anywhere where sebaceous glands are distributed, e.g. scalp and face, whilst 75% are periocular (half said to arise from Meibomian glands of the tarsal plate). Tumours tend to deeply set in the dermis; the epidermis usually uninvolved, but Pagetoid spread is possible (clinically invisible involvement of adjacent epidermis beyond obvious tumour). They are often mistaken for benign lesions clinically; histologically, they differ from adenoma by the presence of dermal aggregates of poorly differentiated tumour cells with central necrosis.

Evaluation for **Muir–Torre syndrome** is suggested. The skin lesions are excised with 5 mm of normal tissue; exenteration may be needed if the orbit is involved. Up to one-third will recur and thus some propose Mohs micrographic surgery (MMS). Radiotherapy is usually viewed as non-curative and is reserved for palliation.

EPIDERMOID CYST ('SEBACEOUS CYST' BUT ARE NOT OF SEBACEOUS ORIGIN)

The term encompasses inclusion cysts due to implantation of epidermis into the dermis as well as infundibular cysts that originate from proliferation of epidermal cells from the infundibulum of hair follicle.

- Milia ('milk spots') are like mini epidermoid cysts with keratin trapped under the epidermis.
- Dermoid cysts occur in lines of cleavage and are distinct.

Epidermoid cysts are most common in young and middle-aged adults, whilst earlier presentation is seen in **Gardner syndrome** (multiple lesions, preceding the polyps in over half). The actual aetiological mechanism is unclear, though proposals include embryonic sequestration or acquired occlusion of hair follicle unit or implantation (post-injury or surgery). Some speculate on a role for HPV especially for lesions of palms and soles.

Clinically, they present as spherical cysts in the dermis, tethered to the epidermis at the punctum. Histologically, the cyst is lined by stratified squamous epithelium and filled with birefringent **keratin**, often laminar and breakdown products. They enlarge slowly but may become infected/inflamed secondarily (often colonised with *Staphylococcus epidermidis* and Propionibacteria) and suppurate. Malignant change is a very rare occurrence (to BCC, SCC, Bowen's disease), and recent studies show malignancies in 0.01% rather than 1%–4% from earlier smaller studies.

They are excised with an elliptical incision designed around the punctum. Some authors suggest mini incisions or a punch biopsy to drain the contents before removing the lining – this technique is associated with a recurrence rate of 4%–9%, and scarred lesions are more difficult to remove in this way. Cysts in certain areas, especially genital and umbilical, may extend deeply; intracranial intraosseous lesions have been described especially around the fontanelle regions.

SWEAT GLAND TUMOURS

Types of sweat glands (Figure 8.1)

- **Apocrine glands** release lipid secretions in membrane-bound vesicles by **decapitation**, where apical portions of cytoplasm pinch off (e.g. secretion in breast). Apocrine sweat glands are found in the **axilla**, pubic and perineal areas, labia major and around the nipples. The coiled gland lies in the deep dermis and the ducts terminate in the upper part (or isthmus)

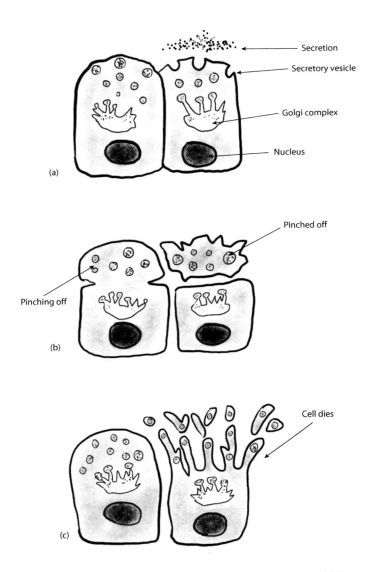

Figure 8.1 Modes of secretion. (a) Merocrine, e.g. salivary gland. (b) Apocrine, e.g. mammary gland. (c) Holocrine, e.g. sebaceous gland. Mitosis in underlying cells replaces lost cells.

of **hair follicles**. The lumen is much bigger than in eccrine glands; the secretions are **more viscous** and less copious. They are functional from puberty onwards with the hormonal changes, but their exact function is unclear; they secrete sialomucin, which is initially odourless but may become transformed by bacteria.

- Apocrine glands are affected in **hidradenitis suppurativa**.
- Lactation.
- **Eccrine glands** release secretions by **exocytosis** into ducts; this is also called merocrine secretion. Eccrine sweat glands are smaller than apocrine glands, and the ducts open **directly onto the skin surface** (unlike apocrine). They are found in highest density in the palms, soles and axilla. The initially isotonic secretions are modified by active NaCl and HCO_3 reabsorption in the ducts (which patients with cystic fibrosis are unable to do) to become hypotonic. Their primary function is thermoregulation with sympathetic cholinergic innervation; emotional stressors tend to induce sweating in the palms/soles.

- **Holocrine glands** discharge whole cells, which then disintegrate to release secretions, e.g. **sebaceous glands** of skin and meibomian glands. Sebaceous glands produce sebum and are closely associated with hair follicles and thus are absent in hairless skin (palms, soles and glans penis/clitoris); under androgenic stimulation, sebum is released onto the skin surface.

- Hybrid-type apoeccrine glands in the axilla may have a role in hyperhidrosis, being present in large numbers in those affected. They also respond to cholinergic stimuli, open directly onto the skin but have 10× the sweat production of eccrine glands.

BENIGN ECCRINE SWEAT GLAND TUMOURS

The commonest examples are syringoma, acrospiroma and cylindroma.

SYRINGOMA (PAPILLARY ECCRINE ADENOMA)

Syrinx is Greek for 'pipe' or 'tube', reflecting the characteristic appearance of convoluted ducts in the upper dermis. A syringoma is a benign tumour of eccrine sweat gland origin and is uncommon. They affect females more often with onset during adolescence.

They appear as small, yellowish dermal papules on the chest, face and neck, usually ~3 mm. They may appear cystic and injury may cause release of a small amount of clear fluid. Each lesion is generally small, but they may erupt in crops typically on the chest to lower abdomen; this form is more common in Asians/darker skins. Eruptive forms may not be true neoplasms, but rather dermatitis-type responses to inflammation/fibrosis, e.g. scalp lesions.

- Multiple tumours may be associated with Down syndrome.
- They must be differentiated from BCCs and trichoepitheliomas.

Although benign, they are a cosmetic concern, particularly on the lower eyelids.

- Excision is best for small isolated lesions (which may be left to heal secondarily).
- Electrocautery (with needle).
- Alternatives include electrodesiccation or laser ablation, cryotherapy, dermabrasion or TCA peel.

ECCRINE ACROSPIROMA (HIDRADENOMA)

This is a benign tumour derived from eccrine sweat duct epithelium from the distal parts of the gland. Their appearance is of hyperkeratotic plaques on the sole or palm (i.e. acral, hence the name) that may ulcerate. Patients are middle-aged with equal sex distribution.

They can be pigmented and thus resemble a melanoma. Actual malignant change (to a malignant eccrine acrospiroma) is rare but has been reported with propensity for local recurrence and distant metastasis. Excision is the commonest treatment.

POROMA

This is a benign tumour of skin adnexae (the malignant counterpart is porocarcinoma). They are often referred to as 'eccrine poroma', but recent reports show that they can be either eccrine or apocrine, with the latter possibly being more common.

They present usually as solitary skin-coloured (rarely pigmented), well-circumscribed lesions and affect males and females of any ethnicity equally. Lesions are mostly slow-growing and asymptomatic, though pain may be a feature in some.

Poromas are related to acrospiromas, with similar cytological features, but are more superficial being confined to the epidermis and upper dermis, whilst acrospiromas are found in the deep dermis or upper hypodermis. They are satisfactorily treated by simple excision/ablation.

DERMAL CYLINDROMA (TURBAN TUMOUR, SPIEGLER'S TUMOUR)

These uncommon tumours are derived from the coiled part of sweat glands (part secretory, part duct) and are most commonly found in the scalp and the forehead. They appear in early adult life, though solitary forms typically affect an older age group. They were previously thought to be apocrine in nature, thus distinguishing it from 'eccrine' spiroadenomas, but there is probably a fair overlap between the two. It is a **dermal tumour** with no attachment to epidermis; histologically, there are columns of cells interspersed with hyaline material.

Typically, they present as a slow-growing rubbery lesion with pinkish, fleshy appearance on the scalp – multiple lesions may eventually coalesce together like a 'turban', hence the name. Multiple lesions may be inherited (AD), whilst solitary lesions are not. Treatment is typically by surgical excision, although ablative lasers have been used with some success. Malignant change is very rare but has been reported; the tumour is then locally aggressive with significant risk of metastasis.

- **Brooke–Spiegler syndrome** shows AD inheritance with variable expression, with a predisposition to develop multiple appendigeal tumours, e.g. trichoepitheliomas, spiradenomas and cylindromas, etc. The gene CYLD has been localised to the 16q chromosome and encodes a deubiquinating enzyme whose exact biological function is yet to be elucidated.

SWEAT GLAND CARCINOMA

Malignant epithelial tumours of the sweat glands (i.e. adenocarcinoma within the dermis) form a rare heterogeneous group and categorisation can often be difficult. Most benign sweat gland tumours have a malignant counterpart, and the diagnosis depends on identification of a residual benign portion. There are eccrine or apocrine varieties, though the former is more common and frequently metastasises.

- Porocarcinoma.
- Syringomatous carcinoma.
- Ductal carcinoma.

- Mucinous carcinoma.
- Syringocystadenocarcinoma papilliferum is very rare.

In general, sweat gland carcinoma affects patients in their middle age onwards (no sex difference). The most common presentation is of a painful, firm/hard, reddish nodule within the dermis with an irregular border. They can occur anywhere, but mainly affect the scalp and the face. Growth is typically slow but may metastasise; excision should be wide, whilst the nodes should be assessed and monitored.

EXTRAMAMMARY PAGET'S DISEASE

Extramammary Paget's disease (EMPD) is a rare **intraepithelial adenocarcinoma** with a predilection for apocrine gland bearing skin. It is morphologically identical to Paget's disease of the nipple described by Sir James Paget in 1874; the first extramammary variant was in the penoscrotal area (Radcliffe Crocker, 1889) followed by vulval EMPD (Dubreuilh, 1901). Other reported sites of involvement include the perineum, axillae, groin, umbilicus and even the eyelid. Unlike mammary Paget's disease, most cases of EMPD represent primary epithelial disease, and in some, the intraepithelial disease then becomes invasive. Some cases are associated with carcinoma of the bladder, colon, kidney (renal cell) and prostate; although there is physical continuity between the skin and these internal sites, the anatomical route of spread is not easily explained. It is important to distinguish true associations from coincidental occurrences; studies should use immunohistochemistry to confirm the cell of origin for both EMPD and internal malignancy. Screening protocols in asymptomatic patients have not been definitively established but usually involve rectal exam, sigmoidoscopy and cystoscopy. Schmitt (*Mayo Clin Proc*, 2018) found 17 noncontiguous tumours in 15 out of 161 patients with EMPD – mostly affecting prostate, urinary tract and breast. They recommend urine cytology, colonoscopy, PAP smears, mammograms and PSA.

The commonest presenting symptom is pruritis; the lesion is typically erythematous, eczematous and scaly. It is often mistaken for inflammatory or infective conditions such as lichen sclerosus, Bowens, psoriasis, eczema, tinea cruris, etc. A **high index of suspicion** is needed in persistent lesions and definitive diagnosis requires biopsy. Cell markers such as carcinoembryonic antigen, CAM 5.2, epithelial membrane antigen and cytokeratin 7 can enhance diagnostic accuracy. Differential metalloproteinase distribution and mucin gene expression have also been noted in those with or without underlying carcinoma.

Clearance by surgical excision with adequate margins with skin grafting remains the treatment of choice. However, the disease tends to extend beyond the visible clinical extent diffusely/possibly multifocally, making lateral margin control a problem. Reflectance confocal microscopy (RCM) has been used to look at EMPD margins in vivo with 75% sensitivity and 100% specificity (Yelamos O, *JAMA Dermatol*, 2017).

- Even MMS still has a recurrence rate of 27% in vulval EMPD (Fanning J, *Am J Obstet Gynecol*, 1999).

- Wide local excision (WLE) is a common alternative, though a 3 cm resection (Pitman, 1982) had positive margins in 47%. WLE with frozen sections of the margins is commonly used with a recurrence rate of ~30% over 2.5 years (Chiu T, *World J Surg*, 2007).
- Non-surgical modalities such as radiotherapy, chemotherapy, CO_2 laser ablation and photodynamic therapy have been used as primary and adjuvant treatment, with reasonable results. Primary radiotherapy has a lower efficacy (50% recurrence) but may be suitable for selected patients.
- Imiquimod has been used with some success especially in women but represents off-label use; PDT with aminolevulinic acid.
- CO_2 laser and cavitational ultrasonic surgical aspiration have been used in small numbers.
- The disease mortality is 50% if an internal carcinoma is found compared to 18% in patients without. Those with a concurrent adnexal carcinoma in the skin also have increased risk of distant metastasis and death.

ADENOID CYSTIC CARCINOMA OF THE SCALP

This malignant tumour usually arises in the salivary glands and less commonly in the lacrimal glands and mucous glands of the upper respiratory tract. It rarely arises in the skin, with most cases affecting the eccrine sweat glands of the scalp – though this remains disputed with some shown to arise from apocrine glands.

Clinically, this is a slow-growing, skin-coloured tumour in the middle aged, which invades fascial planes, nerves and bone. It has a characteristic lattice-type appearance microscopically. It tends to run an indolent course of ~10 years before diagnosis. It is treated by excision with histological control of margins (requires wide excision) but tends not to spread distantly. It is not radiosensitive.

B. MALIGNANT MELANOMA

I. EPIDEMIOLOGY AND OVERVIEW

MM is a malignant tumour of epidermal melanocytes that accounts for 5% of all skin cancers but >75% of deaths from skin cancer. It was first described by John Hunter in 1799 as a 'cancerous fungous excrescence' behind the jaw in a 35-year-old man.

INCIDENCE

- 1 per 100,000 per year in Hong Kong
- 6 per 100,000 per year in the United Kingdom
- 33 per 100,000 per year in Australia

It is the commonest cancer in young adults (but rare before puberty), and the incidence is increasing rapidly, especially in men. This means that even though survival is increasing, there is an increase in absolute mortality figures. The lifetime risk in the United States is 1.4%; it is estimated that people born in 2000 will have a 1:75 risk of developing MM sometime during their lifetime.

- It is more common in Celtic races ('classically') and uncommon in black populations; the risk is related to the Fitzpatrick skin type (highest in types I and II).
- Female/male ratio is 2:1.
- There is a family history in 10% and the familial type tends to present younger.
- Some cases are associated with gene mutations:
  - BRAF gene mutation found in about half of the cases; vemurafenib is a specific monoclonal antibody targeting this. BRAF, RB1 and PTEN mutations are associated with metastatic disease.
  - Some familial forms have mutations of P16 (tumour suppressor protein), which inhibits CDK4.

OTHER RISK FACTORS

- **Sunlight** – it is more related to non-occupational **ultraviolet light** (UVB) exposure, i.e. **short, intense episodes** of sun exposure particularly resulting in sunburn (at a young age), rather than total or occupational exposure.
  - **Sunbed use** and adult exposure in the unacclimatised, e.g. going on 'sunny' holidays (some studies have shown a connection with higher socioeconomic group).
  - The incidence of melanoma is higher in those **who tend to burn** rather than tan. Note, however, that up to 75% of MM occurs on relatively unexposed areas and has been difficult to produce experimentally with UV light.
  - Case–control studies have not shown a reduction with sunscreen use, though in Australia, the incidence of MM among young Australian adults declined from 1983 to 1996. A relatively small (1621 adults) study with long follow-up (10 years) after a 4.5 year randomization to daily SPF 16 or their usual practice, found that the former group had 11 new melanomas compared to 22 in the latter, i.e. halved the risk (Green AC, *J Clin Oncol*, 2011).
- British Association of Dermatologists (BAD) guidelines (Marsden JR, *Br J Derm*, 2010) recommend limiting recreational exposure (level I evidence), and people who are at risk the most are those with freckles, those with red/blond hair, those who burn, those with increased numbers of naevi and those with a family history of melanoma. It is also recognised that insufficiency of vitamin D in the United Kingdom is becoming more common, and thus, those not in the risk categories above should still be careful about sun exposure but not greatly limit it (vitamin D supplementation may be needed).
- Immunosuppression.

PREDISPOSING CONDITIONS

- **Significance of a pre-existing naevus**. The vast majority of melanocytic naevi are benign – each adult has 30 naevi on average. Only ~10% of melanomas arise in a pre-existing naevus, i.e. **most tumours arise de novo**. The lifetime risk of malignant change in an individual naevus is difficult to quantify, with the highest risk in congenital and dysplastic naevi. Prophylactic excision of naevi or small congenital naevi (~5 cm) in the absence of suspicious features is **not** recommended (BAD 2010, level III, grade B).
- **Dysplastic naevus syndrome**. Multiple dysplastic moles can occur anywhere but are often found in covered areas particularly the back. These patients should have life-long screening (~50× relative risk or 11% 10-year risk); there is a **spectrum of risk** from those with few atypical moles and no family history to those with hundreds of moles and a positive family history. Monthly self-examination with regular total skin (dermatoscopic) examinations by a physician beginning around puberty is advisable; baseline photography is useful. Prophylactic excision is not useful as most tumours arise de novo, i.e. it is a marker of risk.
  - About 20%–40% of hereditary MM has a germline mutation in **CDKN2A**, a tumour suppressor gene on chromosome 9. By comparison, it is found in 0.2%–2% of sporadic MMs.
  - Dysplastic naevi (see 'Naevi'). In non-syndromic patients, they are often single and usually insignificant though are often removed.
- **Giant congenital melanocytic naevus**. Current BAD guidelines recommend lifetime monitoring by an 'expert' (BAD 2010, level III, grade B; see 'Congenital naevus').
- **Lentigo maligna (LM)**.
- **Xeroderma pigmentosum with faulty DNA repair** (1000× incidence; see below).
- **Albino** patients are very sensitive to UV effects, but very few cases of melanoma have been described.
  - **Albinism** (*albus*, Latin for 'white') is an AR inherited lack of melanin due to tyrosinase defects (but a normal number of melanocytes) that greatly increases the risk of SCC in particular. There is no sex or race predisposition. The most common forms are oculocutaneous albinism (Types 1–4 with differing levels of pigment) and ocular albinism (five forms). Eye disorders are common in albinism, particularly nystagmus and strabismus. It may be part of a syndrome, e.g. Chediak–Higashi.

CLINICAL FEATURES

There are commonly described characteristic features that should alert suspicion: ABCD rule (Stolz W, *Eur J Dermatol*, 1994). Up to 10%–20% of melanoma arise from pre-existing lesions.

- **Asymmetry**. One-half is not the same as the other half.
- **Border irregularity** – this feature is most commonly found in superficial spreading melanoma (SSM) and LM melanoma (LMM), whilst nodular melanomas are often symmetrical with a well-defined border.
- **Colour irregularity**, i.e. variegated (two different colours or more) pigmentation and irregular surface.
  - Typically a melanoma has a haphazard array of brown–black, though nodular lesions are often blue–black.
  - Red lesions indicate a host inflammatory response.
  - Depigmentation indicates either an amelanotic area or a focus of regression; an asymmetric halo around an asymmetrical lesion is strongly indicative of a melanoma.
- **Diameter** >6 mm.
- E could be included to stand for **'evolving'** – particularly significant is a recent history of changing size or pigmentation ('major signs' with a good positive predictive value). Absolute size or the presence of bleeding or itching is less predictive ('minor signs'). Ulceration is suggestive of malignancy.
  - Note that 'E' is not part of the original criteria, neither is 'F', which stands for something that looks 'funny'.

MAJOR VS. MINOR CRITERIA

The original seven-point checklist (7PCL; Mackie RM, *Clin Exp Dermat*, 1991) gave equal weighting to the criteria. It was revised in 1989 to a Weight 7PCL (a score of 3 or more suggests referral):

Major criteria (2 points)	Minor criteria (1 point)
Change in size	Inflammation
Irregular pigmentation	Itch/altered sensation
Irregular border	Diameter >7 mm
	Oozing/crusting

GROWTH PHASES

The growth of an MM is described as having two phases.

- **Radial growth phase** – this is the proliferation of neoplastic melanocytes within the epidermis above the epidermal–dermal junction, with only focal invasion of the papillary dermis. This is typical of SSM, LMM and acral lentiginous MM.
  - The tumour is said to lack metastatic potential during this phase.
- **Vertical growth phase** – this is the invasion of malignant melanocytes into papillary and reticular dermis and is typical of nodular MM and late LMM. Invasive melanocytes are spindle-shaped and infiltrate along neurovascular structures.

II. MELANOMA SUBTYPES

SSM (PAGETOID MELANOMA)

This is the **most common** type of melanoma (50%–70% of all) in White patients and may arise from **pre-existing naevi**. There is a stronger association with UV light. It is usually found on the backs and legs in women, whilst in men it is more common on the trunk. The radial growth phase may be as short as 6 months or as long as 6 years. The lesions are often flat with irregular border, pigmentation and surface; there may be areas of regression. Invasion is usually heralded by ulceration. Dense lymphocytic and fibroblast aggregations indicate regression. It can be difficult to distinguish histologically from Paget's disease when located at the nipple.

NODULAR MELANOMA

These comprise 20% of all melanomas and are characterised by concurrent radial and vertical growth – the relatively early vertical growth phase means that these lesions tend to have a shorter history, and **better demarcated (due to a relative lack of horizontal growth)**. The ABCD signs are often missing; these lesions often occur de novo with less association with UV exposure.

It is twice as common in men, whilst 5% are amelanotic; amelanotic lesions will still stain positively for tyrosinase.

LMM (5%–10% OF ALL MELANOMA)

These are most commonly found on sun-exposed skin (**strongest UV** association), especially the face, of **older patients** (more in women). Lesions have a prolonged radial phase and may take up to 30 years before the vertical growth phase begins, which coincides with the development of LMM and the formation of a nodule.

LMM is said to be the invasive counterpart of LM (**which is in situ melanoma, also known as Hutchinson's melanotic** freckle). Atypical cells do not penetrate beyond the epidermis; 3%–5% of LM will become invasive (lifetime risk), appearing as darkened nodules/foci within areas of pre-existing LM. Standard excision of LM with 5 mm margins will be insufficient in 50%, and MMS is recommended (McKenna JK, *Dermatol Surg*, 2006). The use of cryotherapy or imiquimod has been described but probably should not be the first line. Close follow-up is recommended after surgery.

- Johnathan Hutchinson (1828–1913) was a Yorkshire-born surgeon who trained at St Bartholomew's and was mentored by James Paget.
- Lentigo simplex/solar lentigo is very common and a different entity.

ACRAL LENTIGINOUS MELANOMA

Acral lentiginous melanoma (ALM) comprises 2%–8% of melanoma in White patients but up to 60% in dark-skinned patients. In the former group, it usually affects the elderly (>60 years) with lesions most commonly found on palms, on soles, on mucocutaneous junctions and in subungual locations (black streaks in nails – melanonychia). Radial growth is followed by vertical growth after ~2 years. It is histologically similar to LMM but is more locally aggressive and more likely to metastasise.

- **Subungual melanoma** (1%–3%) affects the great toe in ~50% of cases with the thumb the next most common. It is typically a pigmented lesion of the nail bed, often with splitting of the nail and nail dystrophy – it can be difficult to distinguish from the pigmented naevus of the nail matrix. Hutchinson's sign – broad streaks of variegated pigmentation within the nail plate are associated with subungual melanoma. It is treated by amputation of the affected digit. There is a higher incidence of amelanotic lesions in subungual melanoma (~30% vs. 5%–7%).
- Quinn (*J Hand Surg Am*, 1996) found that the mean duration of symptoms before diagnosis was ~12 months, often having been treated for a 'fungal' infection. The authors recommend distal amputation, either through the neck of the proximal phalanx of the thumb or through the PIPJ of the fingers. Prior to this, many proposed amputation at the CMCJ.
- Finley (*Surgery*, 1994) confirmed that more distal amputations preserved hand function without compromising survival or local control.
- Isolated limb perfusion (ILP) reduces local recurrence but does not affect survival (Lingam LK, *Br J Surg*, 1995).

Functional surgery in subungual melanoma. (Moehrle M, *Dermatol Surg*, 2003)

The authors described their results with 64 patients with stage I and II melanoma. They recommend 'functional surgery' with partial resection of the DP only and three-dimensional histology to ensure clearance, and their figures suggest that it does not negatively affect the prognosis whilst improving function and cosmesis. Patients with amputation at or proximal to the DIPJ did not fare better. However, there is selection bias as the decision for conservative excision was based on the pathological results of the initial excision.

Subungual melanoma: Management considerations. (Cohen T, *Am J Surg*, 2008)

This series describes the Memorial Sloan Kettering experience with 49 patients with subungual melanoma treated after they began to use SLN mapping (30 patients).

- Female patients were more common (63%) in contrast to the Quinn study.
- Toe lesions were thicker with an average Breslow depth of 2.1 mm.
- SLNB positive rate was 17%, and all underwent complete node dissection.
- For the majority of invasive lesions, they performed amputation at the MTP for the toe and the PIPJ/MP for digit lesions as their standard operation. In their experience, WLE was associated with local recurrence and eventual formal amputation.

DESMOPLASTIC MELANOMA

This rare subtype (1%) occurs most commonly in the head and neck and may be non-pigmented. Histologically, there is desmoplastic spindling stroma with melanocytic dysplasia; special stains may be needed for the diagnosis. There is a tendency for local recurrence due to perineural infiltration and lymphatic spread.

MELANOMA WITH UNKNOWN PRIMARY

In these cases, it is assumed that the primary lesion has regressed. This accounts for ~3%–5% of melanomas, usually presenting as lymph node disease, though non-node metastatic sites including skin, brain, lung, bone, spinal cord and adrenals have been described. Abdominal presentation of MM is most commonly with obstruction or intussusception, due to a metastatic deposit that is usually amelanotic. Radiotherapy may offer effective palliation of brain metastases, whilst surgery may be indicated for a solitary brain metastasis.

TUMOUR MARKERS

Tumour markers are substances produced (in higher quantities) by tumour or other cells in response to tumours. At present, there is no true 'tumour marker' that is of value in the early detection of melanoma, but other tests may be helpful in other ways.

- **Diagnostic**
  - Immunohistochemical – HMA-45, Melan-A, tyrosinase, Sox10, microphthalmia transcription factors, S-100. There is actually diminishing sensitivity with advanced disease, particularly the first three. These biomarkers cannot distinguish malignant melanocytic lesions from non-malignant melanocytic lesions.
    - Polymerase chain reaction assay of tyrosinase activity is often used to assess occult (micrometastasis) tumour burden, e.g. in sentinel nodes. Specificity of tyrosinase is very good (97–100) for distinguishing MM from nonmelanocytic tumours.
    - S-100 has been used on tissue samples to aid the histopathological diagnosis of melanoma. Serum S-100 may be helpful in detecting progression (increased volume of disease; Chung MH, *Ann Surg Oncol*, 2002). Although it is sensitive, it is **not specific** to MM; it also stains Schwann cells, chondrocytes, etc.
- **Prognostic**
  - Immunohistochemical – ki-67, BRAF (V600E), MCAM, CD10.

III. EXCISION

The initial excision biopsy should be excised with **2 mm normal skin** and a cuff of fat, with the axis orientated **along**

the axis of limbs if possible. Shave or incisional biopsies (including punch) are not recommended; the latter may be acceptable in larger lentiginous lesions or ALM, but should only be performed by those within the melanoma multidisciplinary team.

- Over-excising may hinder sentinel node biopsies (though this is disputed by an MD Anderson study).
- Incisional biopsies are prone to sampling error and may theoretically cause deeper implantation of tumour cells.

Excision margins in high risk malignant melanoma. (Thomas JM, *N Engl J Med* 2004)

This study presented outcome data from the UK Melanoma Study Group trial (*n* = 900, >2 mm thick) assessing 1 cm vs. 3 cm margins, and found that 1 cm margin was associated with a significantly increased risk of local recurrence, but overall survival was similar in the two groups. This is commonly referred to as the BAPS/MSG study.

Surgical excision markings for primary cutaneous melanoma. (Sladden MJ, *Cochrane Database Syst Rev*, 2009)

Included trials are as follows:

- **BAPS/MSG (Thomas JM**, *N Engl J Med*, 2004)
- French study (Khayat D, *Cancer*, 2003)
- Intergroup study (Balch CM, *Ann Surg Oncol*, 2001)
- Swedish study (Cohn-Cedermark G, *Cancer*, 2000)
- WHO study (Cascinelli N, *Sem Surg Oncol*, 1998)

This systematic review summarises the evidence regarding the width of excision margins for primary cutaneous melanoma. None of the five published trials, or the meta-analysis, showed a statistically significant difference in the **overall survival** between narrow or wide excision.

- The summary estimate for **overall survival** favoured wide excision by a small degree (hazard ratio 1.04; 95% confidence interval 0.95–1.15; *P* = 0.40), but the result was **not significantly** different.
- The summary estimate for **recurrence-free survival** favoured wide excision margins (hazard ratio 1.13; 95% confidence interval 0.99–1.28; *P* = 0.06), but again the result did **not reach statistical significance** (*P* – 0.05 level).

The conclusion was that current randomised evidence is insufficient to address optimal excision margins for primary cutaneous melanoma. However, a small (but potentially important) difference in survival between wide and narrow excision margins cannot be confidently ruled out.

In the main, a 2 cm wider excision margin is often the upper limit for most lesions with 3 cm used in certain circumstances (particularly in UK practice). There is no evidence to suggest that >3 cm needs to be excised.

Current national guidelines are given in Tables 8.1 and 8.2. Recently, there has been a shift to wider margins with in situ disease from 5 to 5–10 mm.

Wide versus narrow excision margins for high-risk, primary cutaneous melanomas (Hayes AJ, *Lancet Oncol*, 2016). This was a follow-on from the 2004 Thomas MSG study; 900 patients with melanoma greater than 2 mm thick were assigned to either a 1 or 3 cm margin. At median follow-up of 8.8 years, there were 194 deaths (out of 453) in the 1 cm group compared to 165 (out of 447) in the 3 cm group. The difference was not significant; the conclusion was taken to be that 1 cm was inadequate. Surgical complications were greater in the 3 cm group (15% vs 8%).

Relevant studies are summarized in Table 8.2.

IMAGING

Taking account of both sensitivity and specificity of an investigation is important; a high false-positive rate increases patient anxiety, prompts more investigations and reduces overall cost effectiveness.

- **CXR** (equivalent to 3 days of natural radiation) has a low yield (approximately 0.1%) in **asymptomatic** patients with a relatively high false-positive rate (FPR) 4.4%.
  - It does have a role as a preoperative screen in symptomatic patients as well as in the asymptomatic advanced T-stage.
- **Ultrasound** – is very much operator-dependent with an FPR of 6%. It can be used to assess the skin, nodes, and abdomen/pelvis.
  - High-frequency probes (20 mHz) can differentiate MM from other pigmented lesions, such as BCC and by providing additional depth of information may potentially allow a single-stage excision (i.e. use ultrasound thickness to guide wider excision

Table 8.1 Summary of recommendations for wider excision margins for melanoma.

Breslow thickness	UK (BAD, 2010)	Australia (Sladden MJ, *Med J Aust*, 2018)	US (AAD, 2011)
In situ	2–5 mm	5–10 mm	0.5–1 cm
≤1 mm	1 cm	1 cm	1 cm
1.01–2.00 mm	1–2 cm	1–2 cm	1–2 cm
2.01–4.00 mm	2–3 cm	1–2 cm	2 cm
>4 mm	3 cm	2 cm	2 cm

Note: There is no evidence that wider excision is an urgent surgery – a matter of weeks rather than days; it affects local recurrence rather than survival The SIGN 2017/ NICE 2018 guidelines state that 0.5 cm is recommended for in situ (stage 0) melanoma; imiquimod or RT could be considered in certain cases. For stage I and II MM, clinical margins of at least 1 and 2 cm, respectively, are offered.

Table 8.2 Summary of the important tumour trials relevant to excision margins

Trial	Design	Number of patients	Follow-up (years)	Local contol	Overall survival
Veronesi WHO 1988	1 vs. 3 cm WLE for MM <2 mm	612	5 years	ND	ND
Cohn-Cedermark (Swedish Melanoma Study Group) 2000	2 vs. 5 cm WLE for primary MM 0.8–2.0 mm trunk or extremities	989	11 years	ND	ND
Balch Intergroup Melanoma Surgical Trial 2001	2 vs. 4 cm WLE for primary MM 1–4 mm trunk/upper limb	468	10 years	ND	ND
Khayat French Co-operative Study 2003	2 vs. 5 cm WLE for primary MM <2.1 mm	337	16 years	ND	ND
Thomas MSG Study 2004	1 vs 3 cm WLE for MM >2 mm	900	5 years	Increased local recurrence in 1 cm group	ND
Hayes 2016 Cancer Research UK study	1 vs 3 cm for MM >2 mm	900	8.8 years		More MM deaths in 1 cm group but NS

Abbreviation: MM, malignant melanoma; ND, no difference; WLE, wide local excision.

at the first surgery), though this is still being evaluated.

- USG with FNA may allow detection of sentinel nodes and is the best alternative if SLNB is not available. It has a significant false-negative rate (FNR), with limits of deposits of 2 mm.
- **CT chest/abdomen and pelvis** – this involves radiation equivalent to 400/500 CXRs with a calculated mortality risk from radiation-induced cancer of 1 in 2000. It is not good for small deposits; the yield is relatively low in the asymptomatic and has an FPR of 12%–22%.
- **MRI** – provides better contrast resolution but a problem with movement artefact in chest/lung/heart due to the scan time whilst others complain about it being loud and claustrophobic. It is usually associated with high cost and longer waiting times particularly in public hospitals.
- **PET–CT** – it is sensitive but has an FPR of ~20%, making overall accuracy 85%, though this can be improved by careful exclusion of infection, inflammation and recent surgery. It cannot be used to assess the brain as it has high background activity. The spatial resolution is 4 mm. The combination with CT (lower resolution and without contrast) is synergistic and improves localisation.
  - PET-18FDG scan is less commonly used due to its disadvantages compared to PET-CT. The radiation dose is comparable to bone scans and CTs.
- **The relative costs for CXR–USG–CT–MRI are 1–3–7–11, respectively.** Several studies have demonstrated

that >80% recurrences are found by clinical means with half by examination, i.e. clinical examination is the most useful 'investigation'.

WORK-UP

Stage III and IV disease has poor prognosis (see below). Defensive medicine should be avoided, but imaging in the **symptomatic** may reveal disease that can be palliated or dealt with on an individual basis, e.g. **whole body CT/MRI/PET** may characterise equivocal lesions such as in the liver in those with resectable stage IV, as well as to evaluate occult disease in other sites, e.g. to avoid futile surgery if other disease foci present. American Association of Dermatology (2011) suggests that **no imaging should be done in the asymptomatic with localised melanoma;** investigations are guided by history and examination.

NICE GUIDELINES

Patients with stages I–IIIA do not need routine investigations (this includes blood tests).

- Offer CT staging (head, chest, abdomen and pelvis with contrast) to those with stage IIC who have not had SLNB, and to those with stage III or suspected stage IV.
- Consider whole body MRI for children and the young (up to 24 years of age) with stage III or suspected stage IV.

FDG–PET SCANNING FOR STAGING OF MELANOMA

18F-Fluorodeoxyglucose–positron emission tomography (FDG–PET) is being used increasingly in MM. The volume threshold for sensitivity seems to be 80 mm³ of tumour (Wagner JD, *J Surg Oncol*, 2001); it detects all nodal metastases ≥10 mm in diameter, 83% 6–10 mm in diameter and 23% of those less than 5 mm in diameter (Crippa F, *J Nucl Med*, 2000). It has relatively low sensitivity for detecting micrometastases; the threshold of 80 mm³ volume or 3 mm in one dimension.

- Havenga (*Eur J Surg Oncol*, 2003) – FDG-PET was compared with SLNB in staging 55 patients with primary cutaneous melanoma **>1.0 mm thickness and no palpable regional lymph nodes**. FDG– PET scan was performed before SLNB and detected metastases in 2 of the 13 positive SLNBs, and the explanation was that SLN biopsy reveals regional metastases that are **too small** to be detected by FDG-PET. In addition, in some patients, FDG accumulation was recorded in node basins where the SLNB was negative (five) and increased activity at a site of possible distant metastasis (eight) with metastatic disease confirmed in only one patient. FDG-PET has significant false postives and false negatives.

It is neither as sensitive nor as specific as SLNB for nodal metastases, but as it provides a wider area of imaging than CT and MRI, it can detect distant metastasis that may alter patient management. The AJCC recognises the use of FDG-PET as a staging tool in selected patients with recurrent or metastatic disease (stage III/IV), but the bulk of **literature does not support its role for stage I/II.**

The role of fluorine-18 deoxyglucose positron emission tomography in the management of patients with metastatic melanoma: Impact on surgical decision making. (Gulec SA, *Nucl Med*, 2003)

Forty-nine patients with known or suspected metastatic MM underwent extent-of-disease evaluation using CT of the chest, abdomen and pelvis, and MRI of the brain. After formulation of an initial treatment plan, patients underwent FDG-PET imaging, and more metastatic sites were identified in 27 of 49 patients (55%). In six of these, PET detected disease outside the fields of CT and MRI; 44 of the 51 lesions that were resected were confirmed to be melanoma. All lesions >1 cm were positive on PET, whilst 2 of 15 lesions smaller than 1 cm were detected. The results of PET led to treatment changes in 24 patients (49%).

The authors suggest that FDG-PET provides a more accurate assessment than conventional imaging in patients with **metastatic carcinoma.**

F-18 fluorodeoxy-D-glucose positron emission tomography scans in the initial evaluation of patients with a primary melanoma thicker than 4 mm. (Maubec E, *Melanoma Res*, 2007)

This is a prospective study in 25 patients newly diagnosed with T4 melanomas who had FDG-PET as well as SLNB in those without palpable nodes. After correlation of results, they found

that the scan detected 1 of 6 primary melanomas, 0 of 6 nodal micrometastases, 4 of 4 nodal macrometastases (palpable) and no distant metastases. FDG-PET also led to an unnecessary node dissection, i.e. false-positive and three other sites of false-positive distant metastasis. **They conclude that PET is not useful for the initial work-up of patients with melanoma, even for thick lesions**.

Head and neck malignant melanoma: Margin status and immediate reconstruction. (Sullivan SR, *Ann Plast Surg*, 2009)

Immediate reconstruction is safe except for patients with locally recurrent, ulcerated or thick (T4) tumours as the risk of a positive margin after WLE is increased in these cases. The tendency to be more conservative with resections in the head and neck leads to higher rates of incomplete excision and subsequent recurrence (9% and 13%, respectively) compared with the extremities (1% and 6%). Immediate frozen sections are generally regarded as not being that reliable; thus, in these cases, temporary coverage was needed until paraffin sections confirmed clearance of tumour. Some have suggested (delayed) skin grafting to facilitate monitoring, but tissue transfer has not been found to hinder follow-up for recurrences.

IV. PROGNOSIS AND PROGNOSTIC INDICATORS

CLINICAL VARIABLES

Better prognosis in

- Thinner tumours.
- Without ulceration.
- Node negative.
  - The number of, rather than the size (pre 2002) of, lymph nodes.
  - Satellite lesions are considered together with intransit lesions as part of nodal disease (N2) being regarded as intralymphatic metastases and a poorer prognosis; both can be subcutaneous and nonpigmented.
- Women.
- ~50 years old (but the elderly tend to have thicker lesions and more ALM).
- From pre-existing naevus (20% of cases).
- The significance of upper back, posterior arm, posterior neck, and posterior scalp (BANS) lesions is disputed.

PATHOLOGICAL VARIABLES

- **Tumour thickness** (Breslow – Breslow A, *Ann Surg*, 1970) – measured from the stratum granulosum to the deepest part of the tumour. This is a continuous variable.
  - pT1, <1 mm; pT2, 1.01–2 mm; pT3, 2.01–4 mm; pT4, >4 mm
- **Level of invasion** (Clark – Clark WH, *Cancer Res*, 1969). Limited use in the current system; was used for T1 lesions in AJCC 2001, but in 2009, it was only considered when the mitotic rate could not be determined.
  - I – confined to the epidermis
  - II – invasion of papillary dermis

- III – filling of papillary dermis
- IV – invasion of reticular dermis
- V – invasion of subcutaneous fat
- **Ulceration** upstages the tumour, as it represents aggressive behaviour, i.e. poor differentiation in a locally advanced tumour.
- **Neurovascular invasion**.
- **Microscopic satellites** are defined as discontinuous nests of tumour cells more than 0.05 mm in size and separated from the main invasive tumour by at least 0.3 mm normal dermis.
- **Mitotic activity**.

It is worth taking a closer look at the past few AJCC staging manuals to see how things have changed.

Final version of the AJCC staging system for cutaneous melanoma. (Balch JM, *J Clin Oncol*, 2001)

Drawing on a database of 30,450 patients with full data on 17,600 available for production of survival data, this paper produced updated staging information for the 2002 staging system. The **main differences** between this and the previous edition can be outlined. New parameters in bold.

- **Histological level of invasion**.
  - Was – used as alternative to thickness.
  - Now – not used except for T1 lesions.
- **Ulceration**.
  - Was – not used.
  - Now – a secondary determinant of T and N staging; it implies locally advanced disease and upstages tumour.
- **Nodes**.
  - Was – size.
  - Now – number. Best fit data grouped patients as N1 (one node), N2 (2–3 nodes) and N3 (4 or more).
- **Metastatic volume in nodes**.
  - Was – not used.
  - Now – included as the secondary determinant of N staging. **Micrometastases** are detected by SLNBs, whilst macrometastases are palpable nodes confirmed pathologically or nodes with gross extracapsular spread.
- **Lactate dehydrogenase** (LDH).
  - Was – not used.
  - Now – used in M category.
- **Satellite lesions**.
  - Was – considered separately from in-transit.
  - Now – merged with in-transit lesions in N category and considered stage III disease.
    - **In-transit metastases** are non-nodal cutaneous or subcutaneous deposits between the primary site and draining nodal basin, i.e. in transit to the node. Rapid development of in-transit metastases often coincides with development of distant disease.
    - **Satellite lesions** by definition are those that occur within several centimetres of the

site of the primary lesion (i.e. satellite of the primary) but are probably biologically the same entity as in-transit disease, and thus grouped together. Some say 5 cm (Messeguer F, *Actas Dermosifiliogr*, 2013), MD Anderson (1983) used 3 cm and AJCC (1997) 2 cm.

- **Pathological staging**. There is a large variability between clinical and pathological staging; the latter is recommended before patients are entered into melanoma trials.
  - Was – not used.
  - Now – SLNB results incorporated into the definition of pathological staging.

Pathological staging is based upon further information about the regional nodes following SLNB and completion of lymph node dissection (LND) and thus subdivides stage III disease by N stage. **Positive SLNB upstages the patient to stage III,** irrespective of tumour thickness, but survival in a patient with a non-ulcerated melanoma and micrometastases in the sentinel node only (stage IIIa) is likely to exceed survival in a patient with stage IIc disease, i.e. a thick, ulcerated primary (69% and 45% survival at 5 years, respectively).

AJCC STAGING MANUAL 7TH EDITION

Final version of the 2009 Melanoma staging and classification. (Balch JM, *J Clin Oncol*, 2009)

The staging system was updated again and was effective from 1 January 2010. The main differences between this and previous edition are as follows. New parameters in bold.

- **Histological level of invasion**.
  - Was – used only for defining T1 lesions.
  - Now – is used only in the unusual circumstances of the mitotic rate being indeterminate, e.g. in very thin lesions.
- **Mitotic rate per mm^2**.
  - Was – not used.
  - Now – used for T1 lesions; a rate of greater than or equal to 1/mm^2 defines **T1b**. From the data, its predictive value is almost as strong as thickness and better than ulceration.
    - T1a 10 year **mortality** is 5%; T1b is 12%.
- **Immunochemistry for nodal metastasis**.
  - Was – not used.
  - Now – used; at least one marker, e.g. HMB-45, Melan-A, MART-1 with cellular features of malignant morphology.
- **Threshold of defined N+**.
  - Was – implied to be 0.2 mm and required formal H&E staining.
  - Now – deposits – 0.1 mm with histological or immunohistochemical criteria, i.e. there is no lower limit.
- **Elevated serum LDH**.
  - Was – a secondary determinant of M staging.

- Now – same; a repeat confirmatory test is recommended if elevated.
- **Clinical vs. pathological staging**.
  - Was – SLNB results incorporated into the latter.
  - Now – SLNB/staging encouraged as standard care and is required before entry into clinical trials.

Other comments included the following:

- The staging committee recommends that the **microsatellite** be retained in N2c.
- Metastatic disease from an unknown primary arising in nodes, skin or subcutaneous tissues is stage III rather than stage IV.
- **Stage III disease is very heterogeneous** and depending on the number of nodes, presence of ulceration and nodal tumour burden (micro- vs. macrometastases), 5 year survival may range from 81.5% (single micrometastasis in node, non-ulcerated

tumour) to 29% (four or more macroscopically involved nodes with an ulcerated primary tumour).

- The removal of a lower limit for the definition of nodal and the acceptance of immunohistochemistry for the diagnosis means that **even one metastatic cell** is enough and many more patients will be diagnosed as stage III. This is likely to be the point that is most debated – some feel that micrometastases smaller than 0.1 mm carry a prognosis almost as good as no micrometastasis at all.

AJCC TNM 8TH EDITION

It comes formally into effect 1 January 2018; the main changes are as follows (Tables 8.3, 8.4 and 8.5):

- **T1 staging has changed (to nearest 0.1 mm).**
  - T1a if non-ulcerated, <0.8 mm.
  - **T1b if 0.8–1.0 mm or <0.8 mm with ulceration.**

Table 8.3 TNM (tumour node metastasis) staging for melanoma – primary tumour staging. AJCC 8th edition 2017

T category	Thickness	Ulceration status (unknown/unspecified, a or b)
Tx: cannot be assessed		
T0: no evidence of primary tumour		
Tis: in situ		
T1	≤1.0 mm	a: <0.8 mm no ulceration
		b: 0.8–1.0 mm no ulceration OR ≤1.0 mm with ulceration
T2	1.1–2.0 mm	a: no ulceration
		b: with ulceration
T3	2.1–4.0 mm	a: no ulceration
		b: with ulceration
T4	>4.0 mm	a: no ulceration
		b: with ulceration

N stage	Features	Clinical detectability/micrometasis status MSI comprise any satellite, locally recurrent or in transit lesions
Nx	Regional nodes cannot be assessed, e.g. previously removed for another reason	
N0	No regional metastases detected	
N1	0–1 node	a: clinically occult, no MSI
		b: clinically detected, no MSI
		c: 0 nodes, MSI present
N2	1–3 nodes	a: 2–3 nodes clinically occult, no MSI
		b: 2–3 nodes clinically detected, no MSI
		c: 1 node clinical or occult, MSI present
N3	>1 nodes	a: >3 nodes, all clinically occult, no MSI
		b: >3 nodes, ≥1 clinically detected or matted, no MSI
		c: ≥1 nodes clinical or occult, MSI present

M stage	Features	LDH subclassification
M0	No detectable evidence of distant metastases	
M1a	Metastases to skin, subcutaneous or distant lymph nodes	0: normal LDH
		1: elevated LDH
M1b	Metastases to lung	
M1c	Metastases to all other visceral sites	
M1d	Metastases to brain	

Table 8.4 Clinicopathological staging for melanoma

Anatomic stage/prognostic groups							
Clinical staging				**Pathologic staging**			
Stage 0	Tis	N0	M0	0	Tis	N0	M0
Stage IA	T1a	N0	M0	IA	T1a	N0	M0
Stage IB	T1b			IB	T1b		
	T2a				T2a		
Stage IIA	T2b	N0	M0	IIA	T2b	N0	M0
	T3a				T2a		
Stage IIB	T3b			IIB	T3b		
	T4a				T4a		
Stage IIC	T4b			IIC	T4b		
Stage III	Any T	≥N1	M0	IIIA	T1-2a	N1a	M0
					T1-2a	N2a	
				IIIB	T0	N1b-c	M0
					T1-2a	N1b-c	
					T1-2a	N2b	
					T2b-3a	N1a-2b	
				IIIC	T0	N2b-c	M0
					T0	N3b-c	
					T1a-3a	N2c-3c	
					T3b-4a	Any N	
					T4b	N1a-2c	
				IIID	T4b	N3a-c	M0
Stage IV	Any T	Any N	M1	IV	Any T	Any N	M1

Table 8.5 Melanoma stage III subgroups

	T Category								
N category	**T0**	**T1a**	**T1b**	**T2a**	**T2b**	**T3a**	**T3b**	**T4a**	**T4b**
N1a	N/A	IIIA	IIIA	IIIA	IIIB	IIIB	IIIC	IIIC	IIIC
N1b	IIIB	IIIB	IIIB	IIIB	IIIB	IIIB	IIIC	IIIC	IIIC
N1c	IIIB	IIIB	IIIB	IIIB	IIIB	IIIB	IIIC	IIIC	IIIC
N2a	N/A	IIIA	IIIA	IIIA	IIIB	IIIB	IIIC	IIIC	IIIC
N2b	IIIC	IIIB	IIIB	IIIB	IIIB	IIIB	IIIC	IIIC	IIIC
N2c	IIIC	IIIC	IIIC	IIIC	IIIC	IIIC	IIIC	IIIC	IIIC
N3a	N/A	IIIC	IIIC	IIIC	IIIC	IIIC	IIIC	IIIC	Stage IIID
N3b	IIIC	IIIC	IIIC	IIIC	IIIC	IIIC	IIIC	IIIC	Stage IIID
N3c	IIIC	IIIC	IIIC	IIIC	IIIC	IIIC	IIIC	IIIC	Stage IIID

- Use of the mitotic rate has been dropped, e.g. a 0.9 mm non-ulcerated MM with 1 mitosis/mm^2 and negative SLNB is T1bN0M0, stage IB in 2017 but T1bN0M0, stage IA in 2018.
- Tumour thickness is measured to nearest 0.1 mm, not 0.01 mm, taking into account the inherent lack of precision.
- T0 if there is no evidence of primary tumour, Tis for in situ MM and TX when thickness cannot be determined, e.g. shave biopsy.
- **N category is more complicated.**
  - Micrometastasis is now a 'clinically occult disease'.
  - Macrometastasis is a 'clinically detected disease'.
  - There are subcategories for N3 depending on the number of nodes involved. There are four stage III groups instead of three – pathologic stage IIID is T4b, N3 a or b or c, and M0.
- **M category.**
  - LDH status is more elaborate.
  - **M1d** is new for patients with distant metastasis to the CNS. M1d if LDH is not recorded, M1d(0) if not elevated and M1d(1) if elevated.

SLNB is not recommended for MM in situ, stage IA/B disease 0.75 mm thick or less; the probability is too low at ~3%. Routine imaging or laboratory tests are also discouraged in these patients.

- 0.76–1 mm, no ulceration, mitosis less than 1/mm^2 – probability is 7%, can **discuss and consider SLNB**
- **Discuss and offer**

- 0.76–1 mm, ulceration or mitosis 1/mm^2 or more
- >1 mm thick
- Probability up to 35%

V. MANAGEMENT OF LYMPH NODES IN MELANOMA

CLINICALLY PALPABLE LYMPH NODES

The 5 year survival after **therapeutic lymph node dissections** (TLNDs) ranges from 13% to 45%; some studies show that up to 3/4 of these patients will already have occult distant metastasis depending on the primary disease. There is no evidence of improved survival, but there is a risk of increased morbidity especially oedema (others dispute this). The current guidelines are surgery by an experienced surgeon with a prior CT except if it means undue delay. See 'Groin dissection'.

- Clinical nodes below the inguinal ligament can be adequately treated with subinguinal node dissection of the femoral triangle.
- Gross involvement of subinguinal (>1 or matted nodes), metastases in Cloquet's node or imaging suggestive of pelvic nodal disease is a justification for an extended dissection to the iliac and obturator nodes.
- Axillary dissection aims to clear levels I–III.

CLINICALLY IMPALPABLE LYMPH NODES

Clinically impalpable nodes are more difficult to manage in an evidence-based manner. The argument for **elective lymph node dissection** (ELND) assumes that it identifies nodal metastases and that surgery prevents subsequent recurrences in the same (dissected) basin and prevents subsequent spread to distant sites.

- ELND is not indicated for **thin lesions** (<1 mm) because the yield will be very low.
- Conversely, ELND will be of little use in **thick lesions** (>4 mm) because of the **high chance of occult distant** metastasis (66%), and will have no effect on prognosis, although it may offer better local control; the risks of distant disease outweigh any benefit of ELND.
- In **intermediate thickness lesions**, the risk of metastasis is 50%. ELND may theoretically be useful but has not been shown to provide any significant survival benefit.
  - Early non-randomised retrospective studies found that patients who had positive nodes in ELND specimens do slightly better than those who have TLND for clinical nodes. However, subsequent randomised prospective trials did not confirm this.

Immediate or delayed dissection of regional nodes in patients with melanoma of the trunk: A randomised trial. (Cascinelli N, *Lancet*, 1998)
This multicentre trial had 240 patients with truncal melanoma >1.5 mm randomised to either ELND or observation and TLND. The 5 year survival in positive ELND patients was 48.2% compared to 26% in patients undergoing TLND when nodes became clinically obvious. Their interpretation was that node dissection may increase survival in patients with nodal metastasis only.

- Other series indicate that ELND begins to offer a survival advantage over TLND only if <10% of the node basin harbours occult disease.
- The argument against ELND was mainly based on the Veronesi (WHO) study in 1977; however, this had a gender bias (women > men) and lesion bias (mostly lower limb – better prognosis in women).
- The **Intergroup Melanoma Surgical Trial** (1983–1989; Balch CM, *Ann Surg Oncol*, 2000) prospectively randomised 740 patients with intermediate thickness MM to ELND or observation groups. Ten-year survival rates favoured those with ELND with approximately 30% survival benefit for non-ulcerated melanomas, tumours 1–2 mm and tumours of the limbs. With thicker (>4 mm) ulcerated lesions, the risk of distant metastatic disease offsets the potential benefits of ELND.

Most agree that the pick-up rate is ~20% (Morton DL, *Ann Surg*, 2003), i.e. 80% will have undergone unnecessary surgery. Neither ELND nor delayed TLND has become universally accepted, and it was partly as a result of this controversy that Morton (*Arch Surg*, 1992) devised a selective node biopsy based on intra-operative lymphatic mapping, i.e. SLNB.

SENTINEL LYMPH NODE BIOPSY (SLNB) AND STAGING OF MM

The sentinel node is the first LN to which lymph drainage from the area of the lesion is received. Afferent lymphatics drain in a **compartmentalised fashion** into the node. Truncal melanoma exhibits unpredictable drainage patterns in up to 32%; in head and neck lesions, 10% may drain contralaterally.

- **Incubator hypothesis of spread** – in most patients, SLN harbours MM cells allowing distal passage after a critical mass and a latent period (Morton DL, *Br J Dermatol*, 2004), i.e. precursor for systemic spread. A critical mass of cells must be achieved in order to allow passage of cells along the lymphatic chain (via a postulated generation of immunosuppressive factors).
- **Marker hypothesis of spread** – in some other patients, MM cells in the sentinel nodes are a marker for metastatic disease that will pass through/bypass the node. This may be the case in very thick lesions, making SLNB not useful.

The microanatomic location of metastatic melanoma in sentinel lymph node predicts nonsentinel lymph node involvement. (Dewar DJ, *J Clin Oncol*, 2004)
Positive SLNs were examined for intra-nodal location of metastases, which was correlated with non-sentinel node involvement at completion LND. They suggest that in those

with only subscapular deposits (26% of cases in this series) in the sentinel node, completion node dissection may be safely avoided.

Further studies showed that this micro-anatomic classification according to Dewar would prove not to be useful in predicting survival and non-SLN involvement (Saadi A, *J Cancer Therap*, 2013). Van Akkooi's Rotterdam criteria (2008) would prove to be much more useful.

According to McMasters (*J Clin Oncol*, 2001), the main benefits of SLNB in melanoma are as follows:

- **Accurate staging** (for prognostic assessment). **SNLB** is the best modality for assessment of nodal status; USG with FNAC is adequate if SLNB is not available. PET/CT is not a proven substitute but is being used more often. There is a learning curve, and SLNB should be undertaken in centres with experience of the procedure.
  - The hazard ratio for survival for those with a positive SLN was 6.53 compared with 1.23 for tumour thickness and 1.62 for tumour ulceration. The 3 year survival rates for patients with negative and positive SLNB are 96.8% and 69.9%, respectively.
  - **Positive SLNB upstages the patient to stage III**; they are up to six times more likely to die during the follow-up period than patients with negative nodes (Topping A, *Br J Plast Surg*, 2004; see below).
- Morton (*N Engl J Med*, 2006) concluded that SLNB may identify patients with nodal metastases whose survival may be prolonged potentially by immediate therapeutic nodal surgery.
- Identification of those who may benefit from adjuvant therapy, e.g. IFN-2-α.
- Delineation of populations for trials.

Complications (Kretschmer L, *Melanoma Res*, 2008).

The overall incidence of at least one complication **after SLNB was 13.8%** (all were mild – wound problems, e.g. seroma [6.9%] and infection [3.6%], haematoma [2.5%]) vs. **65.5% after completion LND** – including swelling (37.1%) and functional deficit (16.8%).

SLNB RECOMMENDATIONS

The **risk of metastasis to nodes is directly proportional to the thickness** of the primary tumour. Tumours less than 1 mm have a low incidence of sentinel metastasis, whilst intermediate thickness lesions may have sentinel-only metastasis (non-sentinel nodes not involved), whereas thicker lesions may have additional nodes and distant sites involved.

There is **no evidence to suggest that SLNB itself affects prognosis**. Over 10 years, 1 in 10 will die if the SLNB is negative compared to 3 in 10 if the SLNB is positive. The current UK guidelines suggest that it can be considered for stage IB to IIC melanoma with **patients being informed** that it has no proven therapeutic value and the risk of procedure (quoted as 4%–10% risk of complications) and of false negatives (quoted as 3 in every 100 negative SLNBs will

develop a nodal recurrence). Nonetheless, the psychological comfort of a negative result is significant.

- SLNB is recommended for T2–3 tumours (1–4 mm). See also 'AJCC 8th edition guidelines'.
- There may be indications for
  - Thin/T1 with adverse features
  - Thick tumours T4 with no nodal involvement

PROCEDURE

- **Preoperative formal lymphoscintigraphy is** performed after a radioisotope Tc-99m is injected intradermally to the scar or lesion in two to four divided doses, 2–4 hours before surgery. This should identify the nodal groups likely to drain lymph from the melanoma and may also demonstrate identify intransit lesions
- **Perioperative** (at the time of preparing the patient in OT) injection of **blue dye** (e.g. lymphazurin, patent blue). **After 20 minutes**, the 'hot' blue node is found and resected. Timing is important to avoid spill-over into second echelon nodes. Warn the anaesthetist as the dye can interfere with oximetry.
  - There is much debate concerning **frozen sections**; they are not recommended in many studies because they only have a sensitivity of 50%–60%; instead, formal 'paraffin' sections and immunohistochemistry (S-100, Melan A) are preferable as they increase detection. Standard pathology techniques have a 70% detection rate; serial sectioning with H&E increases this to 94%.
  - RT-PCR facilitates detection of micrometastases that are missed by serial sectioning (with 12–20 sections, this represents about 1% of the total node volume).

PATTERNS OF RECURRENCE AFTER SLNB

- **SLNB-negative** patients have fewer nodal recurrences and better disease-free survival than SLNB positive (stage III disease; Morton DL, *N Engl J Med*, 2014). Tables 8.6 and 8.7.
  - SLNB-negative patients had better disease-free survival at 3 years (75% vs. 58%) and fewer recurrences (14% vs. 40%) compared with SLNB-positive patients (Clary BM, *Ann Surg*, 2001). **Re-evaluation** of selected negative SLNB samples by PCR in patients developing recurrent disease showed that most (7/11) **actually had metastatic disease** that was undetected at the time.
  - Those with negative SLNB had a higher rate of nodal recurrence (17% vs. 9%) but lower incidence of in-transit and distant disease (35% vs. 41%). The overall survival at 5 years was 92% in SLN-negative compared with 67% in SLN-positive (Vuylsteke RJ, *J Clin Oncol*, 2003).

Table 8.6 Summary of recurrence rates after negative SLNB

Negative SLNB	Biopsied nodal basin	In-transit	Distant
Gershenwald, 1998	4.1%	5.8%	7.4%
Essner, 1999	4.8%	2.6%	4.0%
Clary, 2001	4.4%	2.8%	5.6%
Chao, 2002	0.4%	1%	2.7%
Wagner, 2003	2%	5%	5.9%
Doting, 2002		4%	
Estourgie, 2003	6%	7%	12%
Vuylsteke, 2003	2.4%	6.5%	4.8%
Topping, 2004	2%	0.7%	2.8%

Table 8.7 Summary of recurrence rates after positive SLNB

	Positive SLNB rate %	Recurrence		
		Biopsied nodal basin	In-transit	Distant
Essner, 1999	15.7%	12%	10%	16.7%
Cascinelli, 2000	18%	6%	4%	7%
Clary, 2001	17%	5.4%	12.5%	17.9%
Chao, 2002	19.7%	0.4%	2%	10.3%
Doting, 2002	24%		8%	
Estourgie, 2003	24%	8%	23%	42%
Vuylsteke, 2003	19%	0%	32%	22.5%
Wagner, 2003	20.8%	4.7%	9.4%	16.5%
Leiter, 2016	11.2%	7.3%	8.3%	5.5%

- Predictors of recurrence included lesion thickness, ulceration, positive SLNB and the number of positive nodes at SLNB (Chao C, *Am J Surg*, 2002). After positive SLNB, patients had a lower rate of recurrence in the nodal basin (after completion), but a higher rate of in-transit and distant recurrences, compared with patients with negative SLNB.
- **False-negative** SLNB – The rate of FNR is low, ~1%–5% (lower if PCR is used), though this depends in part on the follow-up period. Vuylsteke (*J Clin Oncol*, 2003) found a 9% FNR when followed up for 5 years. Doting (*Eur J Surg Oncol*, 2002) postulated potential causes of FN including biological failure (cells yet to reach node), technical failure (wrong node harvested) or pathological failure (cells not identified; Doting MH 2002, *Eur J Surg Oncol*; see below). Others ascribe this to obstruction of lymphatics by metastatic melanoma (Lam TK, *Melanoma Res*, 2009) and suggest that ultrasound of the nodal basin may reduce this occurrence.
- Analysis of overall survival in 287 pairs of patients matched for clinical/pathological stage showed **improved survival in the SLNB/completion LND group** compared with delayed LND (73% and 51% survival at 5 years, respectively; Morton DL, *Ann Surg*, 2003). However, this study has been described as being flawed in its calculations and definition of disease-free interval.

- In the study of Morton (*N Engl J Med*, 2006), 1269 patients with intermediate (1.2–3.5 mm) thickness MM was randomised to observation, with lymphadenectomy for nodal relapse, or SLNB with immediate completion lymphadenectomy if positive. There was no difference in the 5 year survival rates, contradicting Morton (2003), but there were subgroups:
  - In the SLNB group, the 5 year survival was 72.3% in those with positive SLNB compared with 90.2% in those with negative SLNB.
  - Those with positive SLNB had better survival than those with nodal relapse during observation (72.3% vs. 52.4%, respectively). They conclude that SLNB may identify patients with nodal metastases whose survival may be potentially improved by immediate nodal surgery.

The question of **survival benefit with SLNB** has been controversial and is unlikely to be resolved soon.

- The MSLT-1 final report (Morton DL, *N Engl J Med*, 2014) concluded that patients (with MM 1.2–3.5 mm) who had positive SLNB and completion LND had better 10 year survival than those assigned to observation and therapeutic LND when nodes appeared. This generated a great deal of discussion.
- DeCOG-SLT study (Leiter U, *Lancet Oncol*, 2016; see below) in contrast found that those who had completion

LND did not show any difference in the 3 year survival, distant metastasis free survival or recurrence free survival compared to the observation group. However, it is underpowered.

- The results of the MSLT-II trial (2022) with the same design as DeCOG-SLT are expected to provide more answers.

Five years experience of sentinel node biopsy for melanoma: The St George's Melanoma Unit experience. (Topping A, *Br J Plast Surg*, 2004)

This was the largest UK series at the time of publication with prospective data on 347 patients undergoing SLNB (1996–2001). The indications were Breslow thickness >1 mm or <1 mm if > Clark III. Positive SLNB was followed by completion LND within 3 weeks in all patients; the false-negative rate was 2%.

- The rate of positive SLNB was 17.6% and 87% had no further disease in the same node basin; 11 patients subsequently died of disseminated disease; two of these had further disease in the nodal basin at completion lymphadenectomy.
- Patients with a positive SLNB were six times more likely to die from their disease than patients with a negative SLNB during the follow-up period; it is an independent prognostic indicator for survival but was not as significant as tumour thickness.

Complete lymph node dissection versus no dissection in patients with SLNB-positive melanoma (DeC)G-SLT): A multicentre randomized trial. (Leiter U, *Lancet Oncol*, 2016)

Some feel that an SLNB may be 'curative' in some patients – completion LND would not be needed in these patients. In this phase III trial, 483 patients with **micrometastasis** (<1 mm) on SLNB were randomised to CLND or observation. No survival benefit was seen; 77% metastasis-free survival in the observation group at 3 years vs. 74.9% in the CLND group.

This study had a mean follow-up of 35 months, which may not be long enough; it can take 10 years or more. Some feel that CLND offers a survival advantage and that it is easier than a therapeutic lymphadenectomy.

VI. AXILLARY DISSECTION

Some suggest that radical LND should only be performed by those who do a minimum of 15 cases a year of axillary and groin dissections for skin cancer.

- The risk of locoregional recurrence is 16%–32% despite radical surgery.
- The number of positive nodes is predictive – 5 year survival 53% vs. 25% for one positive node vs. more than four (White RR, *Ann Surg*, 2002).
- 29% of LND patients developed in-transit metastases (Kretschmer L, *Melanoma Res*, 2002); this was more likely with thicker primaries and lower limb primaries. The 5 year survival was 0%.

ANATOMY

The axilla contains the axillary artery, axillary vein, lymph nodes and brachial plexus.

- Floor – axillary fascia
- Anterior wall – PM, pectoralis minor, subclavius and clavipectoral fascia
- Posterior wall – subscapularis, teres major, tendon of LD
- Medial wall – serratus anterior
- Lateral wall – the intertubercular sulcus of the humerus
- Apex – outlet/inlet bounded by outer edge of first rib medially, clavicle anteriorly and scapula posteriorly

AXILLARY ARTERY

There are three parts to the artery relative to the **pectoralis minor** muscle, with the second part behind the muscle, which arises from the third, fourth and fifth ribs to insert into the coracoid process and assists serratus anterior in protraction of the scapula but is of no great functional significance.

- Superior thoracic artery arises from the first part, which is superior to the muscle.
- From the second part, there are the thoraco-acromial and lateral thoracic arteries; this part of the artery is clasped by the cords of the brachial plexus.
- Third part – subscapular artery (largest branch), which runs down the posterior axillary wall and divides into the circumflex scapular and the thoracodorsal arteries, and the medial and lateral circumflex humeral arteries.

The axillary vein lies on the medial side of the axillary artery in the apex of the axilla and is not invested by the fascia projected off the paravertebral fascia – the axillary sheath, and hence is free to expand. It receives the cephalic vein in its first part (above the pectoralis minor).

LYMPH NODES

There are between 35 and 50 in number that are arbitrarily divided into surgical groups I, II and III, lying lateral, beneath and medial to the **pectoralis minor**, respectively.

ANATOMICAL GROUPS

- Anterior (pectoral) – medial wall of axilla, along the lateral thoracic artery at the lower border of pectoralis minor, drain the majority of the breast (level I)
- Posterior (subscapular) – medial wall of axilla in its posterior part, along the subscapular artery, drain the posterior trunk and tail of the breast (level I)
- Lateral – along the medial side of the axillary vein, drain the upper limb (level II)
- Central – within the fat of the axilla, receive lymph from all the above groups (level II)
- Apical – at the apex of the axilla, receive lymph from all the above groups (level III)

BRACHIAL PLEXUS; NERVES IN THE AXILLA

- **Long thoracic nerve C5, 6, 7** supplies serratus anterior.
- **Thoracodorsal nerve C6, 7, 8** enters latissimus dorsi on its deep surface.
- **Intercostobrachial nerve**. This is the lateral cutaneous branch of the second (occasionally third) intercostal nerve that supplies an area on the medial aspect of the upper arm.
- **Lateral pectoral nerve C6, 7, 8**. Arising from the lateral cord, it crosses the axillary vein to enter the deep surface of the pectoralis minor, and then through to the PM to end up being positioned more medial than the medial pectoral nerve.

TECHNIQUE

- A skin flap is raised with an inverted U-shaped incision with the arm in abduction, and the fat is swept off the PM, continuing on its deep surface whilst taking care to preserve the lateral pectoral nerve.
- The arm is then flexed to relax the PM and allow access to the apex of the axilla and the pectoralis minor (dividing its insertion).
- The fat is dissected off the axillary vein, following it from medial to lateral, tying off tributaries. The specimen is swept downwards and off the medial wall of the axilla, preserving the long thoracic nerve anteriorly and the thoracodorsal nerve and subscapular artery posteriorly.

VII. GROIN DISSECTION

ANATOMY

Femoral triangle

The boundaries of the femoral triangle include the inguinal ligament superiorly, the medial border of sartorius laterally and the medial border of adductor longus medially, i.e. **a small triangle**. The gutter-shaped floor is formed by adductor longus, pectineus, psoas and iliacus (from medial to lateral). The femoral sheath containing the femoral vessels (artery in lateral compartment, vein in intermediate) lies in this gutter, but the nerve is lateral to and outside the sheath. In the medial compartment of the femoral sheath is the **femoral canal**, which allows dilatation of the medially placed vein as well as transmitting lymphatics from the deep inguinal nodes to the iliac nodes. **Cloquet's node** lies in the femoral canal and drains the lymph of the clitoris/glans penis.

Femoral artery, vein and nerve

The **femoral artery** has four branches in the thigh, arising just below the level of the inguinal ligament:

- Superficial circumflex iliac
- Superficial epigastric
- Superficial external pudendal
- Deep external pudendal

The **femoral vein** receives four tributaries corresponding to the arterial branches as above plus the long saphenous vein (LSV).

The **femoral nerve** gives off

- Muscular branches to the extensor compartment of the thigh
- Sensory branches – intermediate and medial cutaneous nerves of the thigh
- Saphenous nerve

Other nerves that are nearby include

- The lateral cutaneous nerve of the thigh, which passes deep to the inguinal ligament at the origin of sartorius at the lateral upper corner of the femoral triangle.
- The femoral branch of the genitofemoral nerve (L1), which pierces the femoral sheath to supply the skin overlying the femoral triangle.

Lymphatics and lymph nodes

Lymphatics accompany the LSV. The superficial inguinal nodes include the following:

- Vertical group along the termination of the LSV drains the leg.
- Lateral group below the lateral inguinal ligament drains the buttocks, flank, etc.
- Medial group below the medial part of the inguinal ligament drains the anterior abdominal wall below the umbilicus and the perineum.

Deep inguinal nodes lie medial to the femoral vein and communicate with superficial nodes at the cribriform fascia at the saphenous opening.

TECHNIQUE

The patient is positioned with the hip extended, slightly abducted and externally rotated. There are various types of skin incision described, each with their pros and cons. In general, **vertically orientated** incisions allow wider access particularly if a deeper/higher dissection is needed, but skin flap necrosis may be a problem; whilst horizontal incisions parallel to the inguinal ligament have better vascularity, access is more limited.

- For vertical incisions, begin 5 cm above the inguinal ligament, two-thirds along its length from the pubic tubercle and curve down to the inferior apex of the femoral triangle.
- Flaps are raised to include the fascia. Fat is cleared to the margins of the femoral triangle working from above inferolaterally; some recommended tying off of the lower portions of the dissection (LSV) rather than using diathermy to reduce lymph leak.
- **'Sartorius switch'** procedure is recommended by many surgeons to cover the femoral vessels and two large drains are commonly used. Avoid closing with excessive tension, which will lead to a dead space forming underneath.

Whilst other superficial vessels are usually sacrificed during a groin dissection, the superficial circumflex iliac and deep external pudendal arteries are usually preserved as they lie deeper along the floor of the femoral triangle, and this may help reduce skin necrosis.

COMPLICATIONS OF LYMPHADENECTOMY

- Intra-operative – accidental damage to vessels and nerves
- Early post-operative – skin necrosis, dehiscence, infection, seroma, DVT/PE
- Late post-operative – numbness and dysaesthesia, lymphoedema, hernia

DEEP GROIN DISSECTION

The deep lymphatic system is less developed and relatively independent of the superficial system; there are few deep-to-superficial connections, mostly connecting at nodes. Retrograde flow does not occur unless there is proximal obstruction.

SUPERFICIAL VS. RADICAL INGUINAL NODE DISSECTION

- Inguinal node clearance includes the femoral triangle up to the inguinal ligament, also called superficial inguinal node dissection.
- Iliac node clearance includes the iliac and obturator nodes up to bifurcation of the common iliac artery (or further up to aortic bifurcation if nodes are clinically enlarged), and is also called deep or extended dissections.

Patients with positive deep inguinal (iliac) nodes have a poor prognosis (reduced 5 year survival from 47% to 19%; Hughes TM, *Br J Surg*, 2000) with a high likelihood of distant disease, and iliac node dissection may significantly increase morbidity particularly of lymphoedema. In particular, the data are conflicting on the survival benefit following radical clearance of deep nodes (see Kretschmer L, *Acta Oncol*, 2001).

- If there is gross inguinal disease, there is 36%–40% risk of the iliac nodes being involved; with microscopic inguinal disease, the risk is 14%–19%.
  - Other prognostic factors were extracapsular spread and the number of positive superficial nodes.
- Some prefer to predict the likelihood of pelvic nodes using either Cloquet node histology (79% risk of pelvic node if positive) or the number of inguinal nodes involved (12% for one to three nodes compared with 44% for more than three positive superficial nodes).

The benefit of deep LND (DLND) continues to be debated; one set of guidelines recommend a pelvic/iliac dissection in those with

- More than one clinically palpable inguinal node
- CT/MRI or ultrasound evidence of deep node involvement

- >1 microscopically involved node at SLNB
- A conglomerate of inguinal or femoral triangle lymph nodes
- **Microscopic or macroscopic involvement of Cloquet's node (level III, grade B)**

Superficial inguinal and radical ilioinguinal lymph node dissection in patients with palpable melanoma. metastases to the groin. (Kretschmer L, *Acta Oncol*, 2001)

Thirty-five per cent of 69 patients undergoing extended clearance had positive iliac nodes, which correlated with a significant increase in mortality compared with iliac node negative patients (5 year survival 6% vs. 37%). As there was **no difference in the overall survival between extended and superficial dissection groups**, on this basis, the authors recommend that unless there is evidence for pelvic nodal disease, a superficial node clearance is preferred.

Prognosis and surgical management of patients with palpable inguinal lymph node metastases from melanoma. (Hughes TM, *Br J Surg*, 2000)

Retrospective analysis of 132 patients with positive pelvic nodes. There was no significant increase in morbidity following extended dissections in comparison with superficial lymphadenectomy, whilst providing additional prognostic information and optimal regional control.

Pelvic lymph node dissection is beneficial in subsets of patients with node-positive melanoma. (Badgwell B, *Ann Surg Oncol*, 2007)

This study from the M.D. Anderson reviewed the records of 235 patients who underwent SLND, and 97 who underwent combined SLND and DLND. They found that age ≥50 years, the number of positive superficial nodes and positive imaging were predictors of deep nodes. The 5 year survival was 51% for those with negative deep nodes vs. 42% for positive deep nodes (much better than Hughes TM, *Br J Surg*, 2000). The overall survival of those with three or fewer deep nodes (treated) was comparable to those with no deep nodes, and the authors suggest that deep pelvic disease should be classed as stage III and not stage IV (distant) disease. Those with risks factors for deep node involvement may benefit selectively from a combined node dissection.

VIII. DISTANT METASTASIS

IMAGING AND INVESTIGATIONS OF STAGE III/IV MELANOMA

Current BAD guidelines are as follows:

- **Stage III** – CT of the head, chest, abdomen and pelvis will adequately exclude metastases in most cases and is most useful in stage III disease **before planning a regional LND or regional chemotherapy**.
- **Stage IV** – CT of the head and whole body when stage IV disease is suspected; PET/CT potentially increases

yield, but results are unlikely to be clinically relevant (level III, grade D) – **except** where metastectomy is planned and a PET/CT may exclude other disease that may make such surgery inappropriate.

- There is no indication for bone scans in the absence of bone symptoms.

TREATMENTS

For stage III disease, the aim should be to increase the survival or quality of life in these patients with a high risk of metastasis (80%). The Cochrane review in 2004 concluded that there were no adjunctive treatments of proven benefit for melanoma; however, there have been recent developments.

STAGE III (NODAL DISEASE)

- Positive SLNB – completion LND slightly better than waiting for TLND.
- Clinical nodes – TLND offers no survival benefit but controls disease better. Adjunctive treatment often offered.
- **In transit disease** or local recurrence after excision – generally palliative.
  - Excision (narrow margins acceptable) or CO_2 laser therapy.
    - Kandamany (*Lasers Med Sci*, 2009) suggests laser as a first-line therapy and described a subgroup that did not show systemic progression for unknown reasons.
  - ILP with good response rates reported. Also isolated limb infusion (see below).
  - Radiotherapy with 52% response rate reported by Fenig (*Am J Clin Oncol*, 1999).
  - Chemotherapy for widespread truncal or head and neck in-transit disease, which is not amenable to surgery (Hayes AJ, *Br J Surg*, 2004).
  - Amputation can be considered for palliation of fungating disease or exsanguinating haemorrhage.

In general, **regional/local techniques are preferable**, having better control and reduced operative morbidity, whilst systemic therapy has considerable toxicity and marginal response (Gimbel MI, *Cancer Control*, 2008).

ISOLATED LIMB PERFUSION

This involves the regional administration of high-dose chemotherapeutics and can be used for palliation of locally advanced disease, particularly as an alternative to amputation. The main agent used is **melphalan**, but alternatives include cisplatin, IF-γ and recombinant TNF-α. It has a significant risk of side effects: erythema, myopathy, peripheral neuropathy, 1% death, amputation and severe leukopaenia.

- Under GA, a pump oxygenator perfuses the drugs under conditions of **mild hyperthermia** (38–43°C); the limb is flushed out with a unit blood at the end. There seems to be **no significant survival benefit**,

but it offers better local control for symptomatic extremity melanoma.

- An alternative is **isolated limb infusion (ILI)**, whereby a solution is manually infused, without an oxygenator, via cannulation of contralateral vessels under radiological guidance to site the tip in the affected limb; it seems to offer comparable results, but can be done under LA and sedation with fewer side effects.
  - Better responses seen in patients aged >70 years (Lindner P, *Ann Surg Oncol*, 2002); the median response duration is 16 months and the median patient survival is 34 months.

Management of in-transit melanoma of the extremity with isolated limb perfusion. (Fraker DL, *Curr Treat Options Oncol*, 2004)

A limited number of in-transit metastases (1–3 nodules) can be managed by simple surgical excision with minimal negative margins (no role for wide excision) plus staging of distant disease. Indications for ILP include

- Rapidly recurrent in-transit disease
- Disease out of local surgical control

The authors report partial response rates between 80% and 90%, though complete response rates are lower, between 55% and 65%; ~1/4 have sustained complete responses, typically 9 to 12 months.

RADIOTHERAPY (RT)

Survival gains from adjuvant RT may be limited because patients with involved nodes usually die from distant metastasis. A review of the literature by Ballo (*Surg Clin North Am*, 2003) suggests that there is a possible role for RT in certain situations:

- **Primary** treatment in LMM with response rates of 95%, or as an adjunctive treatment for aggressive (e.g. desmoplastic) or recurrent tumours.
- Or **after LND** especially if there is widespread extracapsular spread (not recommended by the SIGN). Chang (*Int J Radiat Oncol Bio Phys*, 2006) described a prospective trial comparing adjuvant RT to the node basin vs. observation; RT reduced the recurrence rate with significant (grade 2–4) toxicities but there is no survival benefit.
- It can also be used for palliation particularly in the head and neck, where extensive resection or isolated perfusion is not possible. The optimal dosages have not been established.
- **Metastatic disease** (see below):
  - A retrospective review of 100 patients with brain metastases demonstrated that an overall median survival time was 4.8 months (Meier S, *Onkologie*, 2004). Aside from tumour thickness, radiotherapy (partial and whole brain), chemotherapy and especially surgery and stereotactic radiosurgery significantly prolong survival.

STAGE IV (DISTANT METASTATIC DISEASE)

Those with elevated LDH are unlikely to benefit from systemic treatments. The median survival is 8.5 months; the most common cause of death is from lung metastases (respiratory failure) followed by brain metastases.

- **Surgical resection** offers no survival benefit but may palliate pain/ulceration and can be considered in oligometastatic disease.
- **Chemotherapy** response is generally poor (partial and temporary) and at best is palliative (see 'Isolated limb perfusion').
  - New options include ipilimumab and vemurafenib (see below).
- **Radiotherapy** can offer useful palliation for cord compression and symptomatic bone, viscera and brain metastases. The primary melanoma is radioresistant, but probably not as resistant as once thought.

SYSTEMIC TREATMENTS

There have been recent developments offering a few new options.

- **Chemotherapy** can be given as a single agent or in combination; however, there is little evidence for any survival benefit in patients with disseminated disease.
- **Dacarbazine** was once the most commonly used drug for advanced disease. Tumours could shrink 15%–20% for 6 months before resuming growth; to date, it has not been shown to significantly prolong survival. Combination regimes (e.g. Dartmouth or CVD) have not been shown to be significantly more effective than dacarbazine alone but have more side effects (Chapman PB, *J Clin Oncol*, 1999).
  - **Paclitaxel.**
  - **Temozolomide** is a well-tolerated oral alkylating agent with activity in the CNS (Agarwala SS, *J Clin Oncol*, 2004). Overall, the early promise has not been borne out by more recent trials.
- **Immunotherapy** uses the patient's own immune system, directly or indirectly, to act against the tumour. Many have shown initial promise but have subsequently fallen from favour, e.g. Canvaxin (produced from whole tumour cells) and antibody to GM2.
  - Interferon α and interleukin-2 (IL-2, aldesleukin) are the most studied. The small benefit needs to be weighed against the significant side effects and cost.
  - **Interferons (IFN α-2b)**. IFN α-2b was given FDA approval in 1995 as immunotherapy for IIB/III melanoma.
    - Meta-analysis of phase III trials has concluded that IFN α reduces recurrence by 26% and improves survival by 15% (NS, $P = 0.06$; Wheatley K, *Cancer Treat Rev*, 2003).
    - Results of the ECOG 1690 trial showed relapse-free survival advantage **but no**

survival advantage in stage IIB/III (Riker AI, *Expert Opin Bio Ther*, 2007).
- In the study of Bottomley (*J Clin Oncol*, 2009), 1256 patients with stage III melanoma post-lymphadenectomy were randomised to either observation or pegylated (PEG) IFN α-2b. After a median follow-up period of 3.8 years, for the primary end point of recurrence-free survival (RFS), risk was reduced by 18% in the treatment arm (a significant improvement), but there was a **negative effect on health-related quality of life** (HRQOL).
- In Janku (*J Clin Oncol*, 2010), the price (side effects and reduced QOL) is too high for the delay in disease recurrence (in a small subset, many for less than a year).
- BAD (2010) does not recommend IFN as a standard of care for stage III melanoma (level Ia, grade A).
- **Interleukin 2** (IL-2) is FDA-approved (1998) for metastatic melanoma; it has a low but consistent response rate of 13%–17%. Optimal dosage regimes have not been determined, and there is no way to predict which patients will or will not respond.
- **Ipilimumab** (Yervoy, MDX-010/MDX-101, monoclonal antibody targeting cytotoxic T lymphocyte antigen 4, CTLA-4; blocking this aims to potentiate antitumour T-cell response). A large phase III trial with patients with inoperable metastatic disease (Hodi FS, *N Engl J Med*, 2010) showed improved survival of 24% after 2 years vs. 14% with other treatments. It was the first time a treatment has been shown to improve overall survival in advanced melanoma. When administered with dacarbazine to patients with previously untreated metastatic melanoma, it improves overall survival compared to dacarbazine plus placebo (11.2 months vs. 9.1 months; Robert C, *N Engl J Med*, 2011), though a small subgroup had a much more dramatic response due to, as yet, unknown reasons. FDA approval was gained in 2011 for treatment of metastatic melanoma. Despite initial excitement, its use has been decreasing since the advent of PD1 inhibitors.
- **Vemurafenib** (i.e. PLX4032) is a form of targeted therapy working as a BRAF inhibitor. It can shrink tumours in advanced melanoma patients with the **BRAF V600E gene mutation** (~60%) 48% vs. 5% with dacarbazine and improved **6 month survival** (84% vs. 64%, respectively) in a phase III trial. However, the effect on long-term/overall survival is unclear as tumours can switch to other pathways and become **resistant** to the drug (Chapman PB, *N Engl J Med*, 2011). It increases the risk of keratoacanthomas/SCCs. Others include dabrafenib and trametinib (MEK inhibitor).
- **TK (tyrosine kinase) gene mutation inhibitors** such as imatinib mesylate (Gleevec, used previously

in CML) showed efficacy in tumours with KIT mutations (Hodi FS, *J Clin Oncol*, 2013). However, the duration of disease control is rather short and, overall, its utility as a single agent seems limited.

- **Programmed death 1 (PD1) protein inhibitors.** Nivolumab and pembrolizumab are monoclonal antibodies targeting PD1, which when bound to its ligand often found on tumour cells downregulates the immune response.
  - Received FDA approval in 2014 for metastatic melanoma.
  - In 2016, FDA expanded its approval as **first-line treatment** for metastatic or unresectable melanoma, regardless of mutational status.
  - Pembrolizumab versus ipilimumab in advanced melanoma (Schachter J, *N Engl J Med*, 2015).
- **Anti-PD1 and anti-CTLA therapies** are being tested in combination.
- **Targeted cancer therapies** are drugs that block the growth, progression and spread of cancer; they are deliberately chosen/designed to interact with specific targets. In contrast, standard chemotherapy acts on all rapidly dividing cells, normal and cancerous. Targeted therapy is often cytostatic whilst chemotherapy is usually cytotoxic.

OUTPATIENT FOLLOW-UP

Recurrence of thin melanoma: How effective is follow-up? (Moloney D, *Br J Plast Surg*, 1996)
A total of 602 patients were followed for a minimum of 5 years following excision of thin primary lesions (<0.76 mm). There was recurrence in 14 within 5 years with mean time to recurrence of ~4.5 years. Only 5/14 were treatable (1% of all patients) including a need for TLND.

- In four of the five treatable cases, treatment resulted in survival beyond 5 years and all of them presented within 2 years of primary excision.
- The other nine patients with recurrence returned with disseminated disease.

After 5 years, there were a further 10 recurrences (4 treatable and 6 non-treatable), but none survived >10 years. Hence, the total number of recurrences was 24/602 (4%). Their conclusion was that as the **treatable recurrences were all detected within 2 years of primary excision,** the need for continued follow-up beyond this point can be debated.

Others would disagree and offer long-term surveillance. There is currently no consensus for follow-up, and little in the way of evidence to support one practice over another. NICE recommendations are as follows:

- Stage 0 – discharge, with advice.
- Stage IA – two to four times in the first year and then discharge. Do not offer routine screening investigations.

- Stage IB–IIB, or Stage IIC with negative SLNB – every 3 months for 3 years, then 6 monthly for 2 years. Discharge after 5 years.
- Stage IIC with no SLNB or Stage III – as above. Consider surveillance imaging as part of the trial or if local funds allow (6 monthly for 3 years)
- Stage IV – offer personalised follow-up.

The best way to detect metastatic disease is to take a thorough history. A full examination of the skin and regional lymph nodes is needed at follow-up appointments.

Robert, *N Engl J Med*, 2011 (5.2%) developed a second primary whilst 5 developed three (particularly those with multiple dysplastic naevi). In 30%, this occurred within 1 month and was considered to be synchronous. First primaries were between 0.2 and 6.0 mm thick, but all subsequent primaries were in situ or <1 mm (which the authors suggested may be due to earlier diagnosis or some altered host immune response). The patient's prognosis is related to the thickness of the thickest lesion, and thus developing more than one melanoma does not necessarily change the prognosis.

C. NON-MELANOMA SKIN CANCER

I. RISK FACTORS AND PREMALIGNANT CONDITIONS

The causes tend to be multifactorial, with an interaction between host-related and environmental factors.

IMMUNOLOGICAL FACTORS

Cell-mediated immunity is a major host defence mechanism against subdermal invasion of cutaneous malignancies.

- Ageing reduces the effectiveness of immunity and DNA repair.
- Immunosuppression, e.g. after organ transplants, increases risks of malignancies, possibly by depressing immune surveillance against newly transformed cells.

ULTRAVIOLET LIGHT (UVL)

UVL causes formation of pyrimidine dimers that are usually dealt with by nucleotide excision repair (NER) – excision of the damaged sequence by endonucleases, then repaired by DNA polymerase and sealed by a ligase. Radiation absorption by the ozone layer means that 95% of UVA, 5% of UVB and ~0% of UVC reach the surface. SCC is primarily associated with cumulative exposure, BCC has an association with intermittent (over)exposure, whilst MM is related to intense exposures leading to burning, particularly when young.

- **UVA radiation** (320–400 nm) generates oxygen free radicals that damage cell membranes and nuclear DNA, contributing to erythema, photoageing and **carcinogenesis** – initially regarded as relatively harmless but now regarded as a potentiator of the effects of UVB (co-carcinogen). Its longer wavelength means greater penetration.

- Sunbeds, PUVA
- Stimulates MMPs that degrade collagen, cathespin G and other elastolytic enzymes
- **UVB radiation** (290–320 nm) is said to be responsible for **sunburn,** tanning, local and systemic immunosuppression, photoageing, **skin cancer** and precancer. UVB tends to cause direct photochemical damage (to DNA and DNA repair mechanism), whilst UVA acts through other molecules.
- **UVC** is completely blocked by the ozone layer and thus is not normally a cancer risk, although it is a potent carcinogen.

UV effects can lead to increases in production of immunosuppressive cytokines, depletion and alteration of antigen-presenting lymphocytes and systemic induction of T-suppressor cells by altered lymphocytes, inflammatory macrophages and cytokines.

Other environmental factors may act as **co-carcinogens**, increasing the sensitivity to UV radiation.

- Ionising radiation – accumulated dosage also important.
- Chemicals, e.g. polycyclic aromatic hydrocarbons, psoralens (and UVA, PUVA therapy for psoriasis), arsenic. These may also be direct carcinogens.

PUBLIC EDUCATION

The long lag time of the disease means that any prevention scheme needs to be sustained and will take many years before effects are evident. UV exposure depends on the following:

- Geographic factors – elevation, latitude and cloud cover (halves it); water/sand/snow can reflect UV and increase exposure.
- Time of the day – UV intensity 3 hours before or after the peak is halved.

It is common to divide sun exposure into

- Occupational, e.g. farming, construction.
- Non-occupational/recreational, e.g. sunbathing, sports, fishing. Skiers should be aware that UVB increases 10% for every 1000 feet of elevation.

SUNSCREENS

- A cotton T-shirt provides the equivalent of less than SPF 10.
- Chemical sunscreens absorb UV radiation. SPF > 15 is needed before a reduction is seen in actinic keratoses (AK) and malignancies. SPF 30 is usually the most recommended.
  - SPF applies to UVB protection, up to a maximum of SPF 50+.
- Physical or reflective sunscreens reflect radiation and are usually opaque, e.g. zinc oxide; they provide the best protection.
  - Most sunscreens have both.

Sunscreen should be applied generously and frequently; it needs to be reapplied after swimming or sweating. However, outcome data on cancer reduction through sunscreen show only limited success; programmes designed to increase awareness have little measurable effect on behaviour including that of medical students. 'Broad spectrum' sunscreens also offer UVA protection – the UVA-PF system is used in some Asian countries. Issues with FDA approval limits the choice in the United States. Patients should also be given advice regarding avoiding vitamin D depletion.

Patients should also be given advice regarding avoiding vitamin D depletion.

CONDITIONS ASSOCIATED WITH SKIN CANCER

Xeroderma pigmentosum (XP)

Kaposi first described the condition in 1874, though he did not coin the term until 1882. XP is a group of rare familial disorders (2 in a million, AR) in which there are deficiencies in the **DNA repair processes** especially NER, and DNA damage becomes cumulative and irreversible. This leads to **photosensitivity** and a predisposition to cutaneous malignancy – BCC and SCC (median age 8 years compared with 58 in the normal population) and a 2000× risk of melanoma; 80% have eye problems whilst 20% have neurological problems.

There are eight subtypes based on the specific repair defect (A is the 'classical' form, but C and D are most common, whilst V is a 'variant'). It is usually detected at age 1–2 after having apparently healthy skin at birth.

- First stage – at 6 months, erythema, actinic changes and freckles/lentigines on exposed areas initially, followed by other areas – the **skin is dry and pigmented, hence the name**. There is sensitivity to sunburn, e.g. first sun exposure of the baby.
- Second stage – poikiloderma – skin atrophy, telangiectasia and dyspigmentation.
- Third stage – malignancies as early as 4–5 years and then relentless thereafter. Most die in their 30s from SCC and melanoma (Kraemer KH, *Arch Dermatol*, 1987); 90% survive to 13 years, 70% to 40 years; overall life expectancy is reduced by 28 years.

MANAGEMENT

- Patients need to adhere to strict sun avoidance – sunscreens, clothing and eye care – and caution even with fluorescent and quartz halogen lights.
- Frequent skin, eye and neurological examinations.
- **Treat lesions early** – AK may be treated with 5-FU or cryotherapy; isotretinoin may be considered in those with multiple tumours, but side effects include irreversible calcification of tendons and ligaments.

Some studies have been conducted with DNA repair enzymes delivered via liposomes, but these are a little way from clinical use; gene therapy is still pretty much experimental/theoretical.

Gorlin's Syndrome (Gorlin–Goltz Syndrome, Naevoid Basal Cell Carcinoma Syndrome, Basal Cell Naevus Syndrome)

This affects 1 in 100,000 and demonstrates AD inheritance (40% are new mutations). There are multiple BCCs, odontogenic keratocysts and pits of the palm and soles (three or more), calcification of the falx cerebri and a first-degree family history of the syndrome – these are major criteria (Kimonis VE, *Am J Med Genet*, 1997). The diagnosis is made with two major criteria or one major with one minor. Other features include sebaceous cysts, medulloblastoma, lymphomesenteric cysts, hypertelorism, widened nose, frontal bossing and abnormalities of ribs (e.g. bifid) and vertebrae (scoliosis). There may be partial agenesis of the corpus callosum with learning difficulties.

There is an abnormality of the PTCH gene on chromosome 9q.

- Patients usually present in their 20s for removal of jaw cysts; BCCs do not appear until 30–40s. These are treated in the usual manner, but radiotherapy should be avoided as patients are very sensitive to radiation (imaging with ionising radiation should also be minimised). Isotretinoin may be used as chemoprevention to reduce the risk of future tumours. The so-called basal cell naevi are true BCCs.
- Robert J. Gorlin (1923–2006) described it in 1960 along with R. Goltz.

POROKERATOSIS

Porokeratosis is an uncommon AD inherited condition characterised by abnormal skin keratinisation that leads to malignant degeneration – risks ~7.5%–11%. Typical lesions are annular plaques with horny borders and flattened centres. There are various forms with disseminated superficial actinic porokeratosis (DSAP) being the most common. Experience with 5-FU, imiquimod, oral retinoids and PDT has been described, but none are entirely satisfactory.

EPIDERMODYSPLASIA VERRUCIFORMIS

Colloquially known as 'Tree Man' disease, it is an inherited (AR) disease with a high risk of skin cancer. They are characterised by chronic HPV infection, with widespread eruptions over their bodies, especially the extremities.

PREMALIGNANT SKIN CONDITIONS

Actinic (solar) keratosis (AK)

AKs are the commonest premalignant skin lesion, seen in almost half of the White patients over 40 living in Australia. These are patches of keratosis (thickened, rough, dry, scaly skin) in sun-damaged skin that also features telangiectasia and sometimes keratin/cutaneous horns. It is most commonly found on the face and dorsum of hands. Histopathologically, the cardinal feature is epithelial **dysplasia**.

These are the earliest identifiable lesions that can eventually develop into invasive SCC. Clinical conversion into SCC occurs after 10 years (~10% progress in a 5 year study; Marks R, *Lancet*, 1988). These tumours tend to be slow-growing and are unlikely to metastasise. **Sunlight is the strongest aetiological factor** – UVB-specific p53 mutations have been found; they are increased in the immunosuppressed/transplant patients and the association with HPV is unclear.

BCCs are often found in areas of previously diagnosed AKs, but the cells of origin are different.

TREATMENT

Generally, treatment is conservative; treatment if required includes cryotherapy or non-surgical topical therapies. There is FDA approval for 5-FU, imiquimod, topical diclofenac and PDT D-ALA; these are preferred to excision/curettage, but surgery is needed when SCC is suspected or lesions fail to respond. There is actually a lack of evidence to show that treating AKs reduces the number of invasive SCCs. Parentheses in the following list show 2017 BAD guidelines with strength recommendation and level of evidence scores.

- **Skin care** (sun avoidance and sunblocks, with or without emollients). Some evidence that up to **25% will regress** within 1 year (A, 1++). Applying block twice daily may help prevent further lesions after treatment.
- **5-fluorouracil (5-FU, 5%)** twice daily for 6 weeks is effective for up to a year (A, 1++). It inhibits thymidylate synthetase and causes death in proliferating cells. It may cause irritation reducing its popularity; though some suggest diluting it or using concomitant topical steroids.
  - Topical **salicylic acid** ointment (A, III) is sometimes used before 5-FU to remove superficial keratin (2%). Facial peels or other resurfacing techniques may be helpful but are not adequate by themselves (C, III).
- **Imiquimod** may be used for 4 months (2 or 3 times a day) or more (A, 1++), but the longevity of its effects are unclear with some studies suggesting that two thirds recur after 12 months (compared to one third with 5-FU) and there may be irritation similar to 5-FU. It upregulates the cytokine response, and there may be a memory effect with regards to upregulation of T cells, thus reducing the risk of recurrence. It costs almost 20× the price of 5-FU with similar side effect and is thus used mostly on a named patient basis.
- **Topical diclofenac gels** (3%) twice daily for 3 months have moderate efficacy and low morbidity (A,1+). The exact mechanism is unknown; the duration of benefit is unclear.
- **Tretinoin cream** (B,1+). Some evidence of benefit but probably needs to be used for about a year. **Systemic retinoids** (C, 2+) can be used for high-risk,

e.g. immunosuppressed or organ-transplant, patients. There is a rebound effect if discontinued.

- **Cryotherapy** (A, 1++) for thicker lesions that would be less responsive to topical creams, but often leaves hypopigmented scars.
- **Photodynamic therapy (PDT)** (A, 1+) has good results with superficial and confluent AKs, with a similar efficacy to 5-FU, though optimal protocols have not been definitively established. It is expensive, but good healing makes it preferable for sites known for poor healing, e.g. lower leg.
- **Ingenol mebutate cream** (A, 1+) contains a plant-derived ester. It works well in about half of early AKs with one-half relapsing after a year. A 2015 FDA update described complications such as allergies and zoster.

BOWEN'S DISEASE

This is **intra-epidermal carcinoma** (basement membrane is intact) and thus strictly not a premalignant lesion. Lesions are usually red well-demarcated hyperkeratotic plaques in elderly patients. The limbs are particularly affected, but it can occur anywhere on skin or mucosal surfaces including non-sun-exposed regions. The potential for transformation into an invasive SCC (which tends to be fairly aggressive) is ~3%–5%; **appearance of ulceration is often an indication of invasion**. There is squamous proliferation, acanthosis and atypia (nuclear and cellular pleomorphism, hyperchromatism and frequent mitoses). It may be difficult to distinguish from full thickness AKs.

- Erythroplasia of Queyrat is Bowen's disease of the glans penis, with 20% risk of SCC. It can also affect the inner prepuce (more common in uncircumcised), vulva or oral mucosa.
- Up to half of patients also have NMSC

The main aetiological factor seems to be sun damage; others include exposure to arsenicals (including medical solutions such as Fowler solution previously used to treat psoriasis), immunosuppression and viral infection (HPV). Contrary to some reports, there does not seem to be an association with internal malignancy (Lycka BAS, *Int J Dermatol*, 1989), i.e. Bowen's disease is not paraneoplastic and extensive investigation is not required.

Suspicious lesions should be biopsied and a full skin examination performed. Confirmed lesions should be excised (A, II-iii) with margins of 5 mm or more, Mohs surgery and also for selected lesions, curettage (A, II-ii) and ablative lasers. Alternatives include 5-FU applied one to two times a day for 6–16 weeks with a margin around the lesion (B, II-i), PDT (A, I), imiquimod (B, I) and cryotherapy (B, II-i) with caution in the pretibial area of the elderly. Radiotherapy is not a common therapy currently, but it is reported to be radiosensitive (B, ii–iii).

- JT Bowen described the disease in 1912.

CUTANEOUS METASTATIC MALIGNANT TUMOURS

This is relatively uncommon but may arise from, in order of frequency: breast, stomach, lung, uterus, large bowel, kidney, prostate, ovary, liver and bone. The trunk and scalp are the most commonly affected areas of the skin, whilst para-umbilical metastases may occur secondary to intra-abdominal malignancy (Sister Joseph's nodule).

- Histologically, these tumours are usually poorly differentiated and may resemble a primary lesion; a foreign body-type inflammatory reaction may be present.
- Tumour deposits can be treated by excision or laser to prevent fungation.

II. BASAL CELL CARCINOMA

This is a malignant tumour composed of cells derived from the pluripotential cells of the epidermis or outer root sheath of the hair follicle. It is the commonest malignant skin tumour in White patients; the estimated lifetime risk in this group is 23%–39%. It is less common in non-Whites, but the tendency for pigmented variants (up to ¾ in Chinese) is increased. The face is at much greater risk than other sun-exposed areas (this may be partly related to the density of pilosebaceous follicles).

RISK FACTORS

Sun exposure: UVB causes changes in DNA (p53 tumour suppressor 9q22). The strongest association is seen with repeated sunburn in childhood (either recreational or occupational, up to 20 years of age) with a lag time of 20–50 years; the field effect is demonstrated by the almost 50% risk of developing a further BCC in the subsequent 5 years. Those with type 1 skin (never tan, always burn) are most vulnerable. Educating children and parents on sun exposure is particularly important. PUVA treatment for psoriasis is a modest risk factor. Others include

- Ionising irradiation.
- **Immunosuppression**, e.g. transplants (up to 10× risk) – the highest risk is for Kaposi's sarcoma (KS) (>200×); other transplant-related tumours include PTLD (post-transplantation lymphoproliferative disorders).
- Malignant change in **sebaceous naevi** and other adnexal hamartomas.
- Exposure to carcinogens such as hydrocarbons/ **arsenic** (occupational, medicinal or environmental) – contaminated water supplies are often implicated.
- Occasionally there is familial inheritance or is syndromic, e.g. genetic conditions such as XP or syndromes such as Gorlin's. Patients with Gardner's syndrome (SOD) have soft tissue tumours such as BCCs, osteomas and dermoids. Albinism and Bazek's (multiple BCC with follicular atrophoderma and local anhidrosis).

Classically, the tumour cells with varying degrees of atypia are arranged in **palisades** with a well-organised surrounding stroma. Mucin accumulation and central necrosis are characteristic of cystic lesions. BCCs are usually slow growing and very rarely metastasise. Long-standing tumours may invade deep into subcutaneous tissues, and in combination with central ulceration gives rise to the appearance of a **rodent ulcer**.

Subtypes (there are 26 different types identified in the literature and a third may have a mixed pattern) Table 8.8: The common subtypes include the following.

- **Nodular** – most commonly a pinkish, pearly nodule (50%–60%), with telangiectasia, and may be ulcerated or encrusted. Some may also be
  - **Cystic**
  - **Pigmented** (~5%), more common in Asian patients and may resemble melanoma
- **Superficial** – (10%–15%) often multiple and found on upper trunk/shoulders as red scaly patches.
- **Infiltrative** (7%).
- **Morpheaform/sclerosing** – uncommon (2%–3%). The scar-like appearance seems to come from fibroblast proliferation.
  - Highest risk of positive margins

Basisquamous BCCs show elevated levels of collagenase enzymes that may account for more aggressive behaviours; however, there is no consensus that it forms a separate subtype.

TREATMENT

- **Excisional biopsy – 3–5 mm margins** depending on the location and on how well demarcated the border is. Some recommend antibiotic cover if the tumour is ulcerated. The deep margin includes some subcutaneous fat.
  - For well-defined lesions **up to 2 cm** in size, a 3 mm margin will clear the tumour in 85%, **whilst 4–5 mm will increase this to 95%** (BAD guidelines; Telfer NR, *Br J Dermatol*, 1999, updated 2008). Morphoeic lesions, in particular, may require 13–15 mm to achieve >95% clearance (Breuninger H, *J Dermatol Surg Oncol*, 1991), though in practice, most use 5 mm for larger BCCs.

- A meta-analysis concluded that a **3 mm surgical margin** can be safely used for non-morpheaform BCC, with a 95% cure rate in a lesion <2 cm. The recurrence rate for positive margins is 27% (Gulleth Y, *Plast Reconstr Surg*, 2010).
- **Mohs micrographic surgery** gives a 99% cure rate. This may be most useful in recurrent cases, nonnodular, size >2 cm in high-risk sites such as ear, eyes, lips, nose and nasolabial folds.
- **Radiotherapy** in the older age group with a cure rate of 92%, but late results can be poor due to contraction.
- **For selected lesions:**
  - **Curettage and electrodesiccation** – overall cure rate 75% but for selected small tumours (<2 mm), it approaches 95%. No margin information but commonly used by non-surgeons.
  - **Cryotherapy** or CO_2 ablation for low risk lesions.
  - 5-FU (primarily for AKs), imiquimod (6 weeks treatment) or PDT for superficial BCCs and AKs.
- **Anti-SMO agents**, e.g. cyclopamine, vismodegib (FDA approved 2012) may be of use in advanced or metastatic disease.

Imaging is rarely needed; incidence of metastasis is very low (<1%). Recurrence is more likely with

- Larger lesions
- Histologically aggressive, e.g. morpheaform, infiltrative
- Sites, e.g. perinasal/auricular/orbital

FOLLOW-UP

There is a 35% risk of developing another non-melanoma skin cancer in 3 years, 50% in 5 years. Recurrence may take up to 5 years. In one large review (Rowe DE, *J Dermat Surg Oncol*, 1989):

- 1 year – less than 1/3 recurrences present.
- 2 years – 50%.
- 3 years – 66%.
- i.e. 1/3 recurrences occur after 3 years.

Current European guidelines (second edition, 2012) recommended follow-up for at least 3–5 years to detect recurrences/new lesions particularly in those with high-risk lesions, but there are a wide range of 'protocols' depending on resources. Patient attendance tends to be low, particularly after the first visit – thus, they must be properly counselled

Table 8.8 Prognostic factors in BCC

	Poor prognosis	Intermediate prognosis	Good prognosis
Clinical form	Morpheaform or ill-defined	Superficial recurrent	Superficial primary Pinkus
	Nodular:	Nodular:	Nodular:
	>1 cm in high risk area	<1 cm in high risk area	<1 cm in intermediate risk area
		>1 cm intermediate risk area	<2 cm in low risk area
		>2 cm low risk area	
Histology	Aggressive		
	Recurrent		

Source: After Dandurand M., *Eur J Dermatol.*, 2006;16:394.

on this occasion regarding sun protection, the risk of recurrent/new lesions and the need for self-monitoring.

INCOMPLETELY EXCISED BCCS

Depending on the series, this occurs in about 4.5% (Kumar P, *Br J Plast Surg*, 2002) to 11.2% of cases (Yu SY, *Plast Reconstr Surg*, 2007). The lowest published result is 0.7% (Emmett AJJ, *Aust NZ J Surg*, 1981) with two experienced surgeons operating on 1411 private patients.

- **More common for periorbital and nasal lesions**; the lateral margin(s) is involved most frequently (~1/2) compared to the deep margin (~1/3). Other risk factors include location on the head, non-nodular subtypes (morphoeic, superficial, infiltrative), lesions larger than 2 cm, multiple lesions and recurrent/incompletely excised lesions.
- **About 30%–41% of incompletely excised tumours recur** and re-excision of incompletely excised tumours shows residual tumour in only 54% of cases (Griffiths RW, *Br J Plast Surg*, 1999). When offered a choice, older patients are more likely to opt for observation over re-operation. Current European guidelines recommended re-excision particularly in high-risk lesions.

Incompletely excised basal cell carcinomas: Our guidelines. (Longhi P, *Onco Targets Ther*, 2008)
Out of 116 with margin involvement, 36 were re-excised whilst the others were followed up.

- 72% of re-excision margins had residual tumour.
- 16 of the observation cases had recurrences, with several after 5 years.
  - They recommend immediate re-excision in cases of margin involvement.
- They found that those with **clear but close margins (<1 mm) were safe** for follow-up with only 1 in 40 recurring after 6 years of follow-up.
- NCCN (USA) – 4 mm for lesions less than 2 cm; >4 mm for bigger lesions. MMS recommended for high-risk lesions.
- European Dermatology Forum – 3–4 mm for lesions less than 2 cm; 5–10 mm or MMS for higher-risk lesions.
- Cancer Council Australia – 2–3 mm for simple lesions (small, nodular, not in central face) and 3–5 mm for complex (location, histology or ill defined).

Nahhas (*J Clin Aesthet Dermatol*, 2017) found little consensus amongst the different guidelines.

III. SQUAMOUS CELL CARCINOMA (SCC)

SCC is a malignant epidermal tumour whose cells show maturation towards keratin formation. **It has the strongest association with UV irradiation** particularly total and occupational exposure; it is uncommon in dark-skinned races. SCCs appear from late middle age onwards; males are affected twice as often as females.

Other causes include the following:

- Premalignant conditions (see above).
- **Burn scar (Marjolin)** or other chronic scar/wounds (~1%–2% risk in burn scars with latency of about 30 years) including osteomyelitis sinuses, granulomatous infections, HS and venous ulcers. These tend to behave more aggressively, and 30% have lymph node metastasis at the time of presentation, <10% 5 year survival.
- **Immunosuppression** (>200× risk in renal transplant patients).
- Industrial carcinogens and oils.
- Viruses, e.g. HPV; their exact role is unclear.
- SCCs of the lip are associated with (pipe) smoking.

Histopathologically, there are variable degrees of cellular atypia and differentiation; well-differentiated tumours exhibit parakeratosis and keratin pearls. The clinical appearance also varies significantly depending on the level of differentiation. The wide range of lesions in 'primary' SCCs makes controlled study difficult.

- Scaly red patches resembling Bowen's.
- Classic keratotic papule, with or without a keratin horn or ulceration/crust.
- Verrucous form looks like a wart – slow growing and less likely to metastasise.
- Keracanthoma may be regarded as a well-differentiated SCC.

CLASSIFICATION

There are several different methods:

- Broder's grade based on the level/ratio of (un)differentiation
- Tumour thickness/depth – 2 mm or less (low risk of recurrence and metastasis), 4–10 mm (high risk), more than 10 mm (very high risk)
- Histological subtype, e.g. verrucous
- Growth pattern

TNM staging (that is also applicable to BCCs).

TREATMENT

- **Excision** with clear margins is the standard care. Margins according to Broadland (*J Am Acad Dermatol*, 1992) are **4 mm for low-risk tumours and 6 mm for high-risk tumours (see below)**; this provides an overall 95% cure. SIGN (2014) recommendations are the same.
  - The reported rates of incomplete excision range from 0% to 10% with experience of the surgeon and difficulty of the anatomical sites being two commonly cited factors.

- Mohs surgery is used less than it is for BCCs; a recurrence rate of 2% has been reported. Conventional frozen sections are not recommended particularly in high-risk lesion due to false positives and negatives.
- **Radiotherapy** is generally not a primary treatment modality, but there is a response rate of up to 90% in T1 lesions (and some choose it as an adjuvant for incomplete excision); the long-term cosmetic outcome can be poor. It may be more useful for sites such as the lip, nasal vestibule and ear, where reconstruction would be challenging.
  - Radiotherapy may be palliative in large inoperable or recurrent SCC.
- **Chemotherapy** has little role in SCC.
  - Systemic low-dose acitretin may be considered for secondary prevention, in immunosuppressed patients with multiple lesions.
- **Curettage or cryotherapy** may be indicated for small early lesions.
- **Topical treatments** such as 5FU, PDT and imiquimod are only suited for AK/Bowens rather than frank SCC.

NODAL DISEASE

Lymph node metastases may be present; always examine the regional nodes. TLND may be needed for clinical node disease.

The risk of occult nodes is 2%–3% – SLNB is not routine practice but can be considered as part of a trial. ELND has been proposed for skin SCC thicker than 8 mm, but the evidence is rather weak (strength of recommendation is C).

Overall, the risk of metastasis is low (<5%), but if involved, the 5 year survival is reduced from >90% for small tumours to 25%–40%. The risk of metastases seems to be related to the location of the primary:

- Trunk and metastases 2%–5%
- Face and dorsum of hand 10%–20%
- Scars 38%

Multiprofessional guidelines for the management of the patient with primary cutaneous squamous cell carcinoma. (Motley R, *Br J Plast Surg*, 2003)
This is a review of the overall management of SCC including surgical and adjuvant treatment modalities that was also published in the *British Journal of Dermatology*. The metastatic potential of SCC is determined by the following:

- **Location of tumour** – highest in sun-exposed areas including lip and ear.
- **Diameter of tumour** – tumours >2 cm are twice as likely to recur locally and three times more likely to metastasise than smaller tumours (Day CL, *J Am Acad Dermatol*, 1993).
- **Depth of invasion** – tumours >4 mm thick most likely to metastasise (>45% incidence; Day CL, *J Am Acad Dermatol*, 1993).

- **Histological differentiation** – poor differentiation and perineural involvement correlate with local and distant recurrence.
- **Host immunosuppression**.

These are often described as **'high-risk SCC'**. SIGN 2014 also includes extension into subcutaneous fat and desmoplastic subtype. There are some biomarkers, e.g. E-cadherin (Bosch FX, *Int J Cancer*, 2005), EGF (Ch'ng S, *Hum Pathol*, 2008) and CD147 (Sweeny L, *J Cutan Pathol*, 2012), but as yet do not form part of routine practice.

FOLLOW-UP

Early detection and treatment of recurrent disease improve patient survival. **Three-year risk of a second lesion is 18%**. SIGN (2014) recommends 3–6 monthly review up to 2 years for patients with high-risk lesions; a final third year review can be considered. Those with low-risk lesions can be taught self-surveillance or be followed up by GPs.

MANAGEMENT OF PRIMARY CUTANEOUS SQUAMOUS CELL CARCINOMA

SIGN (Scottish) guidelines, June 2014
They comment that there are no guidelines for optimal clearance margins, the main debate being the subsequent management of close margins (itself being a rather arbitrary term, from 0.5 to 3 mm). A study (Bovill ES, *J Plast Reconstr Surg*, 2012) looking at re-excision of positive margins found tumour recurrence in 29% of those with tumour in the re-excisions compared to 5% without. There is insufficient evidence for guidelines, but they suggest that <1 mm clearance should be considered for further excision (or RT) in high-risk lesions that should have a clinical margin of 6–10 mm. Low-risk lesions may not require further treatment.

D. SOFT TISSUE SARCOMAS

I. GENERAL

Soft tissue sarcomas (STSs) are relatively rare, comprising 1% of all cancers (in adults, up to 15% in children). They are ranked as the 21st most common cancers in the United Kingdom with 2.5 cases per population of 100,000 per year. Non-specialists may see only one or two in their career, and it is well established that STSs are more effectively treated in specialist centres, particularly true for large (>10 cm), high-grade and trunk/retroperitoneal tumours (Gutierrez JC, *Ann Surg*, 2007).

Sarcoma means a tumour of connective tissue (or mesenchymal tissue), from the Greek words *sarkos* (for flesh) and *sarcoma* (for fleshy substance). There are various histopathological subtypes that have their own characteristics, and it is difficult to make sweeping statements that apply to all. Overall, it is a heterogeneous group (WHO-STT 1994 classified 15 subtypes), and only the commonest types will be discussed.

- It is important to note that STSs (80% of sarcomas) demand a very different approach from primary bone sarcomas.
- They tend to behave in a similar fashion despite the different cells of origin; the **histological grade** is one of the most important prognostic indicators, hence its use in most staging schemes.
  - Larger tumours have a greater risk of **de-differentiation.**
  - Nodal and distant metastasis have a similar prognosis. N1 also being stage IV (A in AJCC GTNM).

AETIOLOGY

In most cases, there is no clearly defined aetiology; however, in some cases, STSs are related to genetic conditions:

- **Neurofibromatosis** – NF1 (schwannoma, benign and malignant, 5% risk) and NF2 (meningiomas and schwannomas) and neurofibrosarcomas.
- **Retinoblastoma** – the original eye cancer can often be cured, but survivors are at high risk of developing another cancer decades after, particularly osteosarcoma or other sarcomas. This is probably due to the RB-1 gene mutation as well as the RT given (though tumours may occur outside the radiation field, e.g. leiomyosarcoma [LMS]).
- **Li–Fraumeni syndrome** – this is a rare AD condition that increases cancer susceptibility due to germline mutations of the p53 tumour suppressor gene. There is an increased risk to a wide variety of cancers including sarcomas (STS and bone) or breast, brain, leukaemias, often at a young age (below 45) and at multiple times.
- **Familial adenomatous polyposis** (FAP) is one of the polyposis syndromes (FAP, Gardeners, AAPC); typical features include (abdominal) desmoids and osteomas.
  - **Gardner's syndrome** (Eldon Gardner, 1909–1989, was a geneticist who described the condition in 1951) – mutation of APC gene on chromosome 5q21 (AD inheritance) is associated with epidermoid cysts, desmoid tumours (15%), osteomas and colonic polyps, which are numerous and have malignant potential (100% risk unless the colon is removed). It is phenotypically distinct from the more common FAP but shares the same gene that is mutated, but in a different way.
  - Risk is related to the number of polyps (e.g. more or less than 1000) as well as the specific mutation. Screen (FOB, or barium or scope) – every 1–2 years from age of 18–20 years usually treat with prophylactic surgery of various types.

- **Gorlin's syndrome** (gene PTC [chromosome 9q22.3]) with increase in mediastinal sarcomas – fibrosarcoma and rhabdomyosarcoma (RMS) particularly.

Genetic alterations (mostly due to unknown causes) are relatively common in sarcomas including

- Alterations in cell regulatory genes, e.g. Rb-1 and p53 detected in substantial proportion of sarcomas
- Translocation in Ewing's sarcoma
- Presence of TLS-CHOP fusion protein, which is now a definitive diagnostic tool for myxoid liposarcoma

ACQUIRED CONDITIONS

- **Radiation exposure** particularly in treatment of carcinomas of breast and cervix, as well as lymphoma, typically appearing 7–10 years afterwards. Such tumours (most commonly MFH and osteosarcomas) tend to have a poor prognosis.
- **Lymphoedema** (lymphangiosarcoma) – **Stewart–Treves syndrome** – aggressive lymphangiosarcoma (often multifocal) in those with post-mastectomy lymphoedema. Such sarcomas are not regarded as radiation-induced as they are usually found outside the irradiated zone. The incidence ranges from 0.07% to 0.45% of 5 year survivors. The most common cause of death (8–16 months after diagnosis) is metastasis to lungs and chest wall; metastasis and local recurrence are common even after radical excision.
- In some, **chemical agents** are important, such as phenoxyacetic acids (herbicides), vinyl chloride and liver angiosarcoma (thoratrast, thorium dioxide), arsenic, chlorophenols (wood preservatives) and thorotrast (radioactive contrast agent).
- **Virus**, e.g. HPV8 in KS.

AGE AND SEX

Sarcomas are slightly more common in males than females, and in general, the incidence increases with age. Some subtypes are more common in certain age groups:

- Malignant fibrous histiocytoma (MFH) – elderly
- Liposarcoma – middle age
- LMS – young
- RMS – children

ANATOMICAL SITE

The most common sites involved are the extremities particularly for liposarcoma, MFH, fibrosarcoma and tendosynovial sarcoma.

- 60% are found in the limbs; the remainder are trunk/retroperitoneal/intra-abdominal.
  - Limbs – generally **painless mass** – suspicious signs include **>5 cm** for more than 4 weeks. Overall 5 year survival is 75%.

- Retroperitoneal – liposarcoma, LMS. Tend to present with vague symptoms and a palpable mass; late presentation reflected in relatively poor median survival of 6 years.
  - Trunk – desmoid tumour, liposarcoma.
- 20% are found in the head and neck, with a higher proportion in adults compared with children.

The most important prognostic variables are **grade, size and location of tumour**. To a certain extent, these determine the mode of presentation, e.g. superficial tumours as a mass, deep tumours due to compression/distortion that will cause pain.

II. ASSESSMENT, BIOPSY AND STAGING

Definitive diagnosis usually requires biopsy, which should **follow imaging** to avoid distortion of the architecture. Histological grade is one of the best predictors of clinical behaviour, except in RMS.

CLINICAL ASSESSMENT

- Size of tumour and skin involvement (and likely defect)
- Pulses and sensation (for vascular and nerve reconstruction)
- Involved muscle groups (for tendon/vascularised muscle transfer)
- Age and fitness for surgery
- Lifestyle (for limb preservation)

RADIOLOGICAL ASSESSMENT

- Ultrasound may exclude benign soft tissue swellings such as lipomata or Baker's cysts.
- **MRI (with gadolinium) provides most useful information** particularly the size of tumour and its relationship to surrounding structures, e.g. nerves and vessels. Fatty tumours can be identified by suppression on T2 images.
  - There is no way to detect microscopic spread preoperatively; MRI is the most useful method to define the limits of detectable residual disease but can be falsely negative in up to one quarter. In the end, about half will turn out to have no residual tumour on re-excision.
- CT is required for assessment of bone involvement, whilst it is also useful for staging (chest and abdomen/pelvis).
- PET can also be used for staging.

REFERRAL TO AN STS SERVICE

The Department of Health UK advises urgent referral (within 2 weeks) if a patient presents with a palpable lump that has the following characteristics:

- Mass >5 cm
- Deep to fascia, fixed or immobile

- Enlarging
- Painful
- Recurrent

Ten per cent will have regional metastasis at the time of presentation particularly for high-grade lesions. **Delays in referral** may lead to a poorer prognosis; medical professionals are the source of greatest delay (Brouns F, *Eur J Surg Oncol*, 2003; Hussein R, *Ann R Coll Surg Engl*, 2005). Furthermore, **inadequate excision by non-specialists** results in a difficult situation with regards to further surgery.

- Clinical evaluation of STS is often inaccurate due to a variety of factors including vague history (often with misleading history of trauma) and inaccurate palpation.
- Imaging can often be non-specific – the majority of soft tissue masses/tumours are post-traumatic, inflammatory or benign.

In general, the advice is that suspected sarcomas **should not be biopsied** prior to referral to a specialist sarcoma centre. **Large masses below the level of the fascia** should be considered malignant until proven otherwise, and referred onwards.

Biopsy in itself is simple, but the following points should be borne in mind:

- Biopsies should be **large enough** to obtain adequate tissue without interfering with definitive surgery. The decision is often between open (incisional/excisional) or closed (FNA/trephine/core) biopsy. The biopsy tract, particularly for Tru-cut, should be planned so that it is incorporated in the resection; thus, it is ideally performed by the operating surgeon.
  - **Trephine/core biopsy** preserves the architecture and has an overall accuracy of 80%, providing ample tissue for diagnosis, which is particularly useful for low-grade and uncommon tumours. Directed core biopsies, e.g. by high PET activity, may be useful in heterogeneous lesions.
    - **Open biopsy** is often used after failed core biopsy.
  - **Closed techniques** are popular due to their ease and the apparent low risk of complications such as haematoma and infection and reduced need for anaesthesia/hospitalisation. However, interpretation is more difficult and thus should not be used in centres that see these tumours only occasionally.
    - **FNA** is less accurate diagnostically but should still be able to differentiate malignant from benign in 90%, and provide information on the grade in 75%. Positive reports are more useful than negative.
  - Excisional biopsy can be considered for lesions under 3 cm in size.

Ideally, biopsy should be the final step in the evaluation of the patient with all local imaging done – this will provide the maximum information for the person doing the biopsy of the mass and for the pathologist examining the specimen, and will reduce artefacts affecting imaging. In some situations, biopsy may be CT-guided to target the most suspicious or most representative areas.

PRINCIPLES OF BIOPSY

- Choose a site in the tumour that (along with tract) can be excised en bloc with the tumour.
  - The most frequent site is usually at the vertex of the tumour away from vital structures. Avoid breaching the deep border or otherwise transgressing compartments, potentially upstaging tumours.
  - The best area to sample is around the pseudocapsule–tumour interface where the tumour is most viable, i.e. the periphery.
- Longitudinal incisions in the limbs are preferable.
- Good haemostasis is vital to avoid **contaminating haematomas.**
- Drains, if necessary, should be closed and in line with the incision.
- Light compression and elevation.

POTENTIAL HAZARDS

- Bad planning.
- Complications, e.g. haematoma, infection, contamination.
- Studies have shown that there are **more problems if biopsy is performed outside of specialist centres**. Open biopsies are more likely to cause problems that significantly alter management.

AJCC STAGING 2002 – TUMOUR, NODE, METASTASIS, GRADE (TNMG)

- Based on tumour grade, size and location.
- Lymph node metastasis is uncommon but is associated with a poor prognosis.
- **Grade** is one of the most important prognostic factors – a pathologist with expertise is vital, but this may be difficult because of the low incidence – pathologists may only see one case per year.

Primary

- TX – cannot be assessed.
- T0 – no evidence of primary tumour.
- T1 – tumour 5 cm or less in greatest dimension (a superficial, b deep).
- T2 – tumour more than 5 cm in greatest dimension (a superficial, b deep).

Regional nodes

- NX – cannot be assessed.
- N0 – none.
- N1 – regional nodes.

Distant metastases

- MX, M0, M1

Histological grade G (G1/2 would be low grade)

- GX – cannot be assessed.
- G1 – well differentiated.
- G2 – moderately differentiated.
- G3 – poorly differentiated.
- G4 – undifferentiated.
- This basically describes how (ab)normal the cells look; instead many institutions use a three-tiered system such as the FNCLCC or French system looking at
  - Differentiation
  - Mitotic count
  - Tumour necrosis

MEMORIAL SLOAN-KETTERING STAGING 1992 (TABLE 8.9)

Stage is related to the number of favourable features:

- 0 – 3 favourable
- I – 2 favourable
- II – 1 unfavourable, or 1 favourable and 2 unfavourable
- III – 3 unfavourable
- IV – metastasis

ENNEKING STAGE 1980 TMG

It is similar to the TNM staging except that **nodal status is ignored**; it is the most commonly used system. Most tumours present at stage IIB/III.

- T1 – intracompartmental. Size itself is not important.
- T2 – extracompartmental, i.e. breaching periosteum.
- G1 – low grade.
- G2 – high grade.
- M0 – no metastasis.
- M1 – metastasis (regional or distant).

TREATMENT

Planning of treatment should happen within a multidisciplinary team environment.

Surgery is the mainstay of treatment – consider anatomical margins of excision and requirements for flap reconstruction, e.g. skin, nerve and functional muscle. See 'Adjuvant therapy'. Frozen sections can be used for histological control of the margins.

Table 8.9 Favourable versus unfavourable features for sarcomas

	Favourable	Unfavourable
Size	<5 cm	>5 cm
Depth	Superficial	Deep
Grade	Low	High

- **Small/low-grade lesions** can often be treated with wide excision only; larger/higher-grade lesions may benefit from adjuvant treatments.
- **Compartectomy** means to excise a whole musculofascial compartment (corresponds to 'radical'). Muscles are excised from origin to insertion where possible. Main arteries are dissected free unless encased by tumour as they are rarely invaded by tumour in comparison to veins, which are usually sacrificed unless it is a major vein. Tumour is dissected off nerves taking along the perineurium.
- **Different types of resection** – the aim is R0 (no tumour at margin); R1 and R2 denote microscopic and macroscopic tumour at margins, respectively.
  - Intralesional – partial removal of tumour.
  - Marginal – through reactive zone and may leave residual microscopic disease.
    - **Reactive zone** is the zone around the tumour that is discoloured due to haemorrhage, scar, degenerating tissue and oedema.
  - Wide – entire tumour with cuff of the normal tissue (usually 3–5 cm).
  - Radical – entire compartment containing tumour.
- **Amputation** is reserved for otherwise unresectable tumours (sometimes for recurrent tumours). Studies have shown no survival advantage over limb-sparing surgeries (Willard WC, *Surgery*, 1992). See 'Isolated limb perfusion'.

A barrier in this context is any tissue (fascia, periosteum, epineurium, etc.) that provides resistance to penetration by tumour and is either thin, being equivalent rather arbitrarily to 2 cm of the tissue margin, or thick, equivalent to 3 cm of the margin.

Whilst the aim of surgery is always obtaining negative margins, there is no consensus on what actually constitutes *adequate margins*. According to Popov (*Plast Reconstr Surg*, 2004), the general aim of surgery is to preserve function whilst excising widely. If **wide excision** is impossible, then perform a **planned marginal excision** (clear but <2.5 cm) supplemented by adjuvant RT. Local recurrence is not directly correlated with survival. Reoperation for positive margins was performed where possible. With this protocol, at 5 years, there was 79% overall local control rate and 68% overall metastasis-free survival.

- There was no difference in recurrence rates between wide excision and marginal excision plus radiotherapy.
- Some have suggested SLNB in RMS and synovial sarcoma.

RESECTION MARGINS

If positive margins are re-resected, residual tumour is found in ~55% (Zagars GK, *Cancer*, 2003; see below), and margin status is an important predictor. Local recurrence does not always have to be strongly related to a positive resection margin

(particularly if planned and if low grade; Gerrand CH, *J Bone Joint Surg Br*, 2001; see below) due to adjuvant therapies (Eilber FC, Ann Surg, 2003; see below).

Otherwise, local recurrence is often taken to be a marker of an aggressive tumour that is more likely to metastasise, but the exact relationship is yet to be fully defined.

Classification of positive margins following resection of soft tissue sarcoma of the limb predicts the risk of local recurrence. (Gerrand CH, *J Bone Joint Surg Br*, 2001)
The authors suggest that **positive surgical margins** may occur after limb-sparing excision of STS for the following reasons:

- **Group 1** – **Planned marginal excision with likely positive margins with**, for example, **low-grade** liposarcomas that often present as large tumours. This will help to preserve vital structures with the rationale that the lesion seldom recurs locally and rarely metastasises.
- **Group 2** – Planned positive margins in tumours **other than low-grade** liposarcoma after decision to accept positive margins to preserve vital structures **agreed at MDT planning meeting**.
- **Group 3** – **Unplanned** positive margin at re-excision of an incompletely excised and **previously unrecognised** sarcoma (first attempt at excision usually by a non-sarcoma surgeon).
- **Group 4** – **Unplanned positive margin** due to primary surgery performed by the sarcoma team but surgical margins (unexpectedly) found to be histologically positive – further excision always considered in such cases.

Their retrospective review of 566 STS patients at Mount Sinai Hospital showed 87 patients with positive margins after limb-sparing surgery for extremity STS. All had had neoadjuvant RT and a post-operative RT boost. The local recurrence rate (at mean follow-up of 5.4 years) was 3.6%–4.2% vs. 31.6%–37.5% in groups 1 and 2 (planned) and groups 3 and 4 (unplanned), i.e. there was a low rate of recurrence following excisional surgery with planned positive margins.

High grade extremity soft tissue sarcoma: Factors predictive of local recurrence and its effect on morbidity and mortality. (Eilber FC, *Ann Surg*, 2003)
This was a retrospective review of 753 patients treated for intermediate- to high-grade extremity sarcoma at UCLA.

Microscopically positive margins (2%) were treated by additional local re-excision, additional RT, amputation or no further treatment. Of the 92 patients who developed locally recurrent disease, only 5 had positive resection margins – i.e. **positive resection margin was not a significant risk factor for the development of local recurrence**. Instead significant risk factors for development of local recurrence in order of hazard ratio were as follows:

- Malignant peripheral nerve sheath tumour (MPNST).
- High histological grade.
- Age >50 years.
- Failure to receive neoadjuvant treatment was the only risk factor in patients treated for already locally recurrent disease.

Significant risk factors for decreased survival in order of hazard ratio:

- Local recurrence.
- High histological grade.
- LMS.
- Size.
- Age >50 years.
- Lower extremity location.
- Male gender was a risk factor in patients treated for already locally recurrent disease.

Surgical margins and re-resection in the management of patients with soft tissue sarcoma using conservative surgery and radiation therapy. (Zagars GK, *Cancer*, 2003)

This paper reviewed the MD Anderson Cancer Centre experience of 666 patients in whom macroscopic tumour clearance had been achieved prior to tertiary referral. Some required re-excision. Negative margins achieved by re-resection still qualified as negative, and patients in whom negative margins were not achieved by re-resection had shorter disease-free and overall survival.

- Predictors of local recurrence were as follows:
  - Age >64 years
  - Positive or uncertain resection margins (primary or re-excision)
  - Recurrent tumour at presentation to the specialist unit
  - Tumour size >10 cm
- Predictor of lymph node recurrence
  - Histopathological tumour type – epithelioid sarcoma, RMS and clear cell sarcoma
- Predictors of distant metastases.
  - Tumour size >5 cm, tumour gade and margin status

ADJUVANT THERAPY

- **Post-operative RT** for marginal excisions and high-grade, deep, tumours >5 cm; consider brachytherapy if radiosensitive tissues are nearby. The general effect is to reduce local recurrence with little improvement in overall survival.
  - There is no consensus on deciding between preoperative RT (to reduce tumour size for limb-sparing surgery) or post-operative RT, and the choice depends largely on the preference of individual centres. Preoperatively, tumour cells are

better oxygenated and thus more responsive, but neoadjuvant therapy may delay surgery, complicate histological evaluation and increase wound complications.
  - Liposarcomas (and Ewing's) are very sensitive to radiation.
- **Post-operative chemotherapy** for high-grade tumours and chemosensitive tumours; possible role in palliation. There are many different regimes, including combinations that may be preferred in rapidly progressive disease, but at the cost of increased toxicity. The most commonly used agents include the following:
  - Doxorubicin – cardiotoxicity may be reduced by continuous infusion or liposomal formulations.
  - The use of Olaratumab with doxorubicin in adult STS is being appraised by NICE; evidence suggests that it can increase survival by 11.8 months. It is a recommended option if they have not had any previous chemotherapy, if they cannot have curative surgery or if their disease does not respond to radiotherapy.
  - Ifosfamide – prodrug activated by liver metabolism, urothelial toxicity.
  - Paclitaxel – good response rate in angiosarcoma.
  - Gemcitabine, methotrexate, cisplatin, mitomycin C.
  - Anthracycline – dermatofibrosarcoma.
  - Trabectedin is also being appraised by NICE for use in patients who have failed treatment with anthracyclines and ifosamide.
- ILP with melphalan, TNF-α and interferons has been effective (albeit transiently) and may be useful to reduce tumour size for limb-sparing surgery.

PROGNOSIS

Tumours in proximal or deep sites, especially large lesions and with positive nodes are associated with poor survival.

The average rate of metastasis is 5% for low grade and 40% for intermediate/high grade STS the vast majority (80%) are pulmonary, whilst other sites are rare – lymph nodes (10%), bone (8%) and liver (1%). Metastatic risk is increased in high-grade tumours, after limb sparing surgery or when margins are 'close'. However, local recurrence after incomplete excision does not necessarily correlate with earlier development of distant disease.

- Local recurrences can be treated with further surgery, if there are no metastases (Zagars GK, *Cancer*, 2003).
- Consider the risk of nodal metastases (10%) – SLNB reported for RMS, epithelioid and synovial sarcoma.
- Metastatic disease is usually incurable, but some benefit is still possible from chemotherapy or local control methods; higher-grade lesions respond better to chemotherapy.
  - Metastectomy can be considered for limited lung metastasis with up to 30%, 5 year survival.

FOLLOW-UP

- Clinical assessment – 3 monthly for 2 years then 6 monthly for 3 more years, and then annually if appropriate until year 10.
- Radiological follow-up
  - Local tumour site (MRI)
    - Superficial tumours – only if clinical suspicion of recurrent disease.
    - Deep tumours – baseline scan, post-operative imaging at 6–12 months with further imaging annually for up to 5 years.
  - Distant site imaging
    - For high-grade tumours, a plain chest X-ray at each clinical review with CT chest if any change from previous film, or annual CT chest.
    - Low-grade tumours rarely metastasise and an annual chest X-ray is sufficient.

III. TUMOURS OF FIBROUS TISSUE

- Benign – fibrous histiocytoma, dermatofibroma
- Intermediate – atypical fibroxanthoma, DFSP
- Malignant – storiform pleomorphic tumour, myxoid tumour

Nodular fasciitis is a benign subcutaneous tumour due to reactive proliferation of fibroblasts. Lesions consist of spindle-shaped fibroblasts in a myxoid stroma that can infiltrate fat or muscle bundles. It presents as a rapidly growing (<2 weeks), often tender mass (1–3 cm diameter) beneath the skin, most commonly in the forearm. It can occur at any age but is commonest in middle age. Treatment of choice is excision; resolution may still follow incomplete excision.

HISTIOCYTOMA

Histiocytes are monocytes derived from the bone marrow that populate areas of acute or chronic inflammation of the skin. Histiocytomas are closely related to foreign body giant cells and epithelioid cells. Histologically, they are proliferations of histiocytes, fibroblasts and vascular endothelial cells with iron inclusion bodies and foam cells.

Histiocytomas show a predilection for females and often occur on the lower extremities, presenting as a firm brownish nodule with smooth or warty surface up to 3 cm diameter. Around 20% may be preceded by trauma or insect bite. A **dermatofibroma** is a histiocytoma with maturation of cells towards fibroblasts.

Treatment of choice is excision; resolution may follow incomplete excision but 5%–10% may recur.

MALIGNANT FIBROUS HISTIOCYTOMA

MFH may represent malignant change in a benign histiocytoma or may arise de novo; >80% have cytogenetic abnormalities such as 7q32, which may predict a worse outcome. It is one of the commonest STSs, comprising about 20% of all diagnoses and mostly affecting patients in late adult life with a slight male predominance.

MFH is most common in the abdomen and extremities especially the thigh (only 1%–3% in the head and neck). It has been reported to arise in burn scars; although many report preceding trauma, but trauma does not seem to cause MFH – it may draw attention to the lesion. Typically there is a **subcutaneous nodule** that is composed of histiocytes and fibroblast-derived cells in different proportions with storiform-pleomorphic, myxoid, giant cell and inflammatory subtypes. More recent evidence has shown no true histiocytic differentiation and that **MFH may be a final common pathway in tumours that undergo undifferentiation** (in 2002, the WHO declassified it as a diagnostic entity, renaming it undifferentiated pleomorphic sarcoma NOS), but the MFH name continues to be widely used.

MRI is the best investigation before biopsy.

Treatment of choice is **wide excision** (compartmental or 3 cm margins) with post-operative RT for close/positive margins; chemotherapy (doxorubicin) may be offered for distant metastasis (or at high risk of), in the context of a trial. However, local recurrence (20%–40%) and metastases (20% especially if high grade and >5 cm) are common. Overall mortality is 40%, but it is age related (70% for over 70s, 30% for under 40s).

ATYPICAL FIBROXANTHOMA

This is a locally aggressive cutaneous tumour of the head and neck that may represent a superficial variant of pleomorphic MFH. It occurs most commonly on the ears and cheeks of elderly people, with a predilection for sun-damaged skin and areas of previous RT. A typical lesion is a red, fleshy mass with granuloma-type appearance consisting of fibroblasts, histiocytes and multi-nucleate giant cells and may become ulcerated. Histologically, it is a diagnosis of exclusion after immunohistochemistry, looking very similar to melanomas, spindle cell SCC and LMSs. It has invasive potential; lesions may recur locally after excision, though metastasis is rare. Lesions should be excised with margins >1 cm.

DESMOID TUMOUR (AGGRESSIVE FIBROMATOSIS)

The name comes from *desmos* (Greek for band- or tendon-like); the tumour was first described in 1832 by McFarlane and named in 1834 by Müller. The estimated incidence is 1–2 per 500,000. These are firm, irregular tumours arising typically from the **muscular aponeurosis of the abdominal wall**, especially below the umbilicus. The mean size at presentation is 7 cm. It can be regarded as an aggressive fibromatosis with fibroblast proliferation, variable collagen deposition and mucoid degeneration. It is prone to aggressive local invasion and local recurrence if inadequately excised but is unlikely to metastasise (however, death can still result from the aggressive local invasion). Desmoid tumours have a predilection for parous women in their

30s–50s and have an association with Gardner syndrome. The aetiology is unknown but possible aetiological factors include the following:

- **Trauma** – reports of desmoid tumours arising in scars, e.g. Caesarean section and desmoid reported in the capsule surrounding a breast implant.
  - Some say that surgical trauma may stimulate tumour growth particularly in FAP.
- **Hormonal factors** – extra-abdominal desmoids may express oestrogen receptors and increased growth is observed during pregnancy, with a peak incidence in post-pubertal and pre-menopausal women. Tumours may regress during menopause, after tamoxifen or combined oral contraceptive (COC) treatment.
- **Genetic factors** – Gardner syndrome or FAP with APC gene mutation –desmoid tumours are 1000× more common (incidence of 10%–15%). Familial multicentric fibromatosis – desmoid tumours usually occur singly in non-FAP patients but can occur multifocally without evidence of Gardner syndrome in some patients.

TREATMENT

Tumours tend to be large with diffuse margins. Local control is equivalent to cure, although local recurrence after wide resection is not uncommon even with supposedly 'negative margins'. Several series show ultimate local control rates (surgery with salvage surgery and/or RT) approaching 90%, but factors affecting this are not consistent amongst studies.

- **Surgery** – where possible, surgery is the treatment of choice and WLE is recommended; positive histological margins increase the risk of local recurrence, but it is not inevitable. Musculoaponeurotic lesions are more likely to be multifocal. Recurrence after surgery alone is relatively high (25%–40%).
- **Intralesional injections**, e.g. acetic acid, radio-frequency ablation reported.
- **Radiotherapy** is useful in those who cannot have surgery (it will slow down growth but prolonged follow-up is mandatory), or as an adjunct, except for intra-abdominal tumours. Radiographic evidence of an effect may take many months to be evident.
- **Medical – NSAIDs (especially sulindac)** and anti-oestrogens (e.g. **tamoxifen** at breast cancer doses – there is no evidence to support higher dosages). These two types of drugs are often used in combination – they will improve symptoms in approximately half but chances of major shrinkage are low. There is **greater tendency to treat desmoids conservatively** due to the tendency for local recurrence after surgery.
  - Some have even proposed wait-and-see-type policies for stable lesions (Fiore M, *Ann Surg Oncol*, 2009) with a 50% rate of non-progression at 5 years, and most cases with progression were picked up in the first 2 years.

- **Chemotherapy** – generally low-toxicity regimes, e.g. of methotrexate and vinblastine; most reserve high-dose regimes for tumours unresponsive to other therapies.
- **Beta-catenin gene (CTNNBI) mutations** are prevalent in sporadic cases and have been implicated in pathogenesis and may correlate with local recurrence (Lazar AJF, *Am J Path*, 2008).

DERMATOFIBROSARCOMA PROTRUBERANS

Dermatofibrosarcoma protruberans (DFSP) is an uncommon tumour of dermal fibroblasts – constitutes 6% of all soft tissue STS. There may be a history of preceding trauma, but the actual aetiology is unknown. There is no overall sex preference, though it is reported to be hormone-sensitive with accelerated growth during pregnancy. More than 90% have a reciprocal **chromosomal translocation t(17:22),** a rearrangement that leads to constitutive activation of the PDGF receptor (fusion with COL1A1 collagen gene), thus providing a rationale for therapy in those with advanced unresectable disease, i.e. **imatinib**, a selective inhibitor of PDGFR tyrosine kinases. Imatinib (Gleevec) is FDA approved.

Histologically, it is a locally malignant tumour of dermal fibroblasts with a distinct storiform (cartwheel) pattern extending from the dermo-epidermal junction into subcutaneous tissues. Lesions are generally low grade and well differentiated. It spreads in an infiltrating manner laterally, but metastasis is rare (5%, usually to lungs).

- There are reports of potential progression into tumours with **fibrosarcomatous differentiation** (fibrosarcoma [FS] or malignant fibrous histiocytoma [MFH], i.e. transformed DFSP) with greater risk of recurrence and metastasis, but the actual risk is uncertain (Gorgu M, *Eur J Plast Surg*, 2011).
- Some say that recurrence is related mainly to adequacy of excision, and lesions with fibrosarcomatous change are not different, if excision is adequate.

Typically, DFSP appears in early adult life, and though rarely diagnosed during childhood, congenital DFSP has been reported (Weinstein JM, *Arch Dermatol*, 2003). Typical lesions are red dermal nodules with a firm/rubbery touch and are intimately fixed to the overlying skin. It can look like a scar/keloid, but has a giveaway deeper component.

Most commonly they appear on the front of the trunk or on the extremities as a painless (<15% have pain) mass that tends to grow slowly but may enter a more rapid growth phase, which usually prompts the patient to seek attention. The risk of metastasis is generally regarded as being low 1%–4%. DFSP is fairly resistant to chemotherapy and RT; thus, the mainstay is surgery.

- **Local recurrence is common** if inadequately excised.
  - Historically, **margins as high as 5 cm** were used; recent guidelines suggest 2–4 cm (NCCN, National Comprehensive Cancer Network 2007 and 2014)

along with complete circumferential peripheral and deep margin assessment (CCPDMA, of which **Mohs surgery** is an example) – taking the **deep and lateral faces for complete frozen section** examination to avoid the false-negative error inherent in 'bread loafing'.

- Positive margins should be followed by another 2–3 cm of excision.
- **Margins of 2.5 cm clears all lesions**, whilst 1.5 cm is sufficient for lesions less than 2 cm wide (Parker TL, *J Am Acad Dermatol*, 1995).
  - In other studies, 3 cm margins have been associated with 11% recurrence.
- **Anti-CD34** immunohistochemistry may be useful but not 100%.
  - **Factor XIIIa** is usually negative. Other markers include nestin, cathepsin K and apolipoprotein D; they may be useful in equivocal cases.
  - **FISH/PCR** for the COL1A1 translocation has been described.

Efficacy of Mohs micrographic surgery for the treatment of dermatofibrosarcoma protuberans: Systematic review. (Foroozan M et al., *Arch Dermatol*, 2012)
The review found no RCTs comparing WLE with MMS. There is no consensus – there is weak evidence for MMS or other margin control as **first-line therapy** especially in areas prone to recurrence. Five-year follow-up is recommended. With MMS, an average of 2 stages/layers is needed at 0.5–1 cm each time, median maximum tumour margin of 1–2 cm, i.e. **potentially tissue sparing**.

- Paradisi (*Cancer Treat Rev*, 2008) compared two cohorts of patients treated with WLE of 2 cm+ (*n* = 38, Italy) vs. MMS (*n* = 41, Germany). There were five recurrences in the WLE patients but none in the MMS group (follow-up 4.8–5.4 years).

FIBROSARCOMA

This is a relatively uncommon malignant tumour consisting of cells resembling fibroblasts that mostly affects patients in their 30s–60s (slightly more common in males). It may be more common in irradiated skin (10 year delay), burns scars (30 year delay) and patients with XP.

Histologically, lesions show atypical fibroblasts with generous blood supply; there may be large amounts of mucin (low-grade fibromyxoid sarcoma). Less well-differentiated tumours may be best described as anaplastic sarcomas. Better techniques have shown that many lesions previously labelled as fibrosarcoma were actually MFH, synovial sarcoma, etc.; this means that **earlier literature should be interpreted cautiously**.

Fibrosarcomas usually present as painless slow-growing masses of the tissues of the thigh or the trunk; if close to the skin, it is usually a red–purple nodule with a smooth surface. There may be **some fluctuance due to intralesional haemorrhage**, whilst anaplastic lesions tend to ulcerate. Lesions tend to be locally aggressive with lung and bone metastasis; 5 year survival is ~50%.

The treatment of choice is **wide excision**, though local recurrence can still occur even after apparent complete excision with negative margins. RT has also been used primarily for close or positive margins. Poor prognostic factors include high grade, >5 cm, positive margins (with invasion to vessels, nerves, bone or skin). The variant that occurs in infants (<5 years old) has a much better prognosis.

EPITHELIOID CELL SARCOMA

This is a malignant connective tissue tumour composed of epithelioid cells; tumours are often multifocal. It is found most commonly in adolescents and young adults, mainly in the subcutaneous and deep tissues of the extremities, especially the palm/flexor surface of fingers. Deeper nodules may be associated with fascia, periosteum, tendon and nerve sheaths. They ulcerate sometimes and then are commonly mistaken for ulcerated SCCs. Prognosis is poor with local recurrence common and metastases frequent.

IV. TUMOURS OF VESSELS

GLOMUS TUMOUR

Glomus is Latin for 'ball'. A **glomus body** is a highly convoluted arteriovenous shunt (i.e. no intervening capillary bed) with rich sympathetic innervation. It is involved with thermoregulatory activity. The central coiled endothelial canal is surrounded by smooth muscle and rounded specialised pericytes called glomus cells; there are numerous unmyelinated nerve fibres. A **glomus tumour** is an encapsulated dermal tumour (strictly a hamartoma) of sheets of proliferating glomus cells surrounding small vascular channels. They arise from the arterial portion of the glomus body. These were originally described as 'painful subcutaneous tubercles' by William Wood in 1812.

Glomus tumours arise from late childhood onwards, most commonly in the 30–40s, with a female preponderance (two to three times) for subungual lesions, whilst extradigital lesions tend to have equal sex distribution. They are relatively rare (1% of all hand tumours), whilst the malignant counterpart, glomangiosarcoma, is exceptionally rare.

- They are usually solitary (75%) small lesions ~10 mm in size and occur spontaneously (some report a history of prior trauma) as pink-purple **painful nodules** on the extremities (75%), especially **subungual** (most common, 'haemangioma like lesion' with nail deformity), deep palm.
  - **The classic triad** is of pinpoint tenderness, severe paroxysmal pain and extreme cold sensitivity (place finger in ice water for a minute, 100% specific) in decreasing order of frequency; the diagnosis is primarily clinical.
  - **Love's test** is the provocation of pain isolated to the area of a pin head/paper clip on nail over tumour, with relief when released. It is supposed

to be 100% sensitive (Bhaskaranand K, *J Hand Surg Br*, 2002).

- **Hildreth's test** (92% sensitive, 91% specific) – exsanguinate arm by elevation then apply a tourniquet inflated to 250 mmHg (pain and tenderness should be reduced) – the test is 'confirmed' if release of the tourniquet causes sudden increase in pain (Giele H, *J Hand Surg Br*, 2002).
- There is an AD familial inheritance in some cases with multiple tumours – these are often painless and may be associated with limb malformations.
- Rarely, larger tumours may be situated elsewhere, e.g. stomach, sinuses where glomus bodies do not normally exist and may not be painful.

Imaging has variable success: X-ray may show erosion of bone with a thin reactive **sclerotic margin** (van Geertruyden J, *J Hand Surg Br*, 1996). **Ultrasound is inconsistent, CT is useful whilst high-resolution MRI is regarded as the gold standard** with a high signal on T2 images and enhancement with gadolinium.

TREATMENT

Excision (with capsule to reduce local recurrence) provides relief in all cases. Use Love's test to localise the tumour and then excise under direct vision. Subungual lesions will need nail removal with meticulous nail-bed repair afterwards, but a lateral paronychial approach may be better for deeper or more lateral lesions. Incisions through the hyponychium may cause nail deformity.

KAPOSI'S SARCOMA

KS is a malignant, multifocal tumour of proliferating capillary endothelial cells and perivascular connective tissue cells, with lymphocytic inflammatory response. The original description was of a very aggressive tumour that killed patients within 2–3 years, but then came to describe a less common, more indolent tumour found in older people of Mediterranean origin that often involutes spontaneously but may be associated with leukaemia/lymphoma.

The tumour is now more commonly due to AIDS/HIV (non-classic or 'epidemic') – it develops in up to 50% of these patients, presenting as multifocal blue–purple macular plaques on skin and sometimes mucosa, which grow and coalesce. They usually appear on the extremities, which become lymphoedematous; tumours may develop in internal organs without skin manifestation. Lymphadenopathy may be a feature.

- Type 1 – chronic, originally restricted to eastern European Ashkenazi Jews and Mediterranean races, i.e. **'classic KS'**. Patients usually die of other causes.
- Type 2 – lymphadenopathic.
- Type 3 – **transplant immunosuppression associated**, affects <1% of transplant patients. Similar to HIV type.

- Type 4 – related to HIV infection (**epidemic KS**). At its peak, it was the presenting symptom for undiagnosed AIDS in 14%, affecting up to 40% overall. Antiretroviral therapy has reduced the overall prevalence to 15%. It is more aggressive than classic KS with a significant mortality rate due to disseminated disease or opportunistic infection.

TREATMENT

The disease runs a variable course; lesions may involute or ulcerate and fungate. Excision is a common treatment but other options include:

- Localised lesions – local injection with cytotoxic agents or cryotherapy. Laser/cryotherapy may palliate mucosal lesions.
- Extensive localised disease – radiotherapy.
- Systemic or aggressive disease – liposomal anthracycline or liposomal doxorubicin. In AIDS, neutropaenia is a limiting factor for this type of treatment. Interferons and β-HCG have been used with some success.

ANGIOSARCOMA

Angiosarcoma is one of the least common STSs (<1%) with very poor prognosis generally. It is more frequent in men (three times). The tumour is derived from endothelium (vascular – haemangiosarcoma or lymphatic – lymphangiosarcoma). Histologically, endothelial cell markers such as factor VIII will be positive and there will be Weibel–Palade bodies (endothelial storage granules) on electron microscopy (if well differentiated). There are four clinicopathological types:

- Cutaneous angiosarcoma – uncommon type that affects scalp/face in elderly patients especially post-RT. Lesions are often well differentiated.
- Angiosarcoma of the breast – that may follow RT for breast cancer. These tumours are often high grade.
- Angiosarcoma of the deep soft tissue.
- Angiosarcoma of the parenchymal organs, e.g. liver lesions that may be related to vinyl chloride exposure (not associated with angiosarcomas of other regions).

Other risk factors include extremity lymphoedema >10 years (e.g. Stewart Treves syndrome). High-grade lesions tend to present with pain and bleeding from multiple ulcerated lesions, whilst low-grade lesions tend to be asymptomatic painless red nodules. Adjacent satellite lesions are common, which suggests **multifocality,** which partly explains the high recurrence rate.

The usual treatment is excisional surgery (>3 cm) and RT. Some recommend regional LND. The role of adjuvant chemotherapy is unclear, though there have been recent reports of reasonable results with paclitaxel. Overall, there is a recurrence rate of over 50%.

V. TUMOURS OF NERVES

NEUROFIBROMA (MOLLUSCUM FIBROSUM: A REALLY OLD TERM)

NFs are benign tumours derived from peripheral nerves and supporting stromal cells including neurilemmal cells, i.e. a mixed cell population – Schwann cells and fibroblasts. Tumours usually appear at an early age, e.g. before age 10, and are usually soft and fleshy; they can be sessile or pedunculated.

- Visceral – appendix, gastrointestinal tract, larynx.
- Peripheral – from the peripheral nerve, usually solitary and not associated with neurofibromatosis (and its other features).
- Plexiform, usually in association with the fifth cranial nerve – this is a diffuse type of NF arising from a superficial/cutaneous nerve and characterised by myxoid degeneration. These can be very disfiguring and their vascularity can make surgery difficult.

Riccardi's classification describes two typical forms (NF1 and NF2) and six atypical forms. NF7 is late onset (after the third decade) NF, which may have a higher risk of malignant transformation. **Neurofibromatosis is the occurrence of multiple NFs.**

Neurofibromatosis type 1 (NF1) – 1 in 3000, AD inheritance with half due to a new mutation affecting the NF1 gene at **chromosome 17q11.2;** the gene encodes a protein known as neurofibromin. Diagnosis is made from two or more of the following criteria:

- Six or more café au lait spots – >5 mm pre-puberty, >15 mm post-puberty
- Two or more NF or one plexiform NF
- Axillary or inguinal freckling
- Two or more Lisch nodules (pigmented iris harmatoma)
- An osseous lesion, e.g. sphenoid dysplasia or long bone cortical thinning
- Optic glioma
- First-degree relative with NF1
- Friedrich Von Recklinghausen (1833–1910) was a German pathologist who studied under Virchow.

Other associated features include

- Neural – meningioma, phaeochromocytoma, mental disability
- Cardiovascular – obstructive cardiomyopathy, renal artery stenosis, orbital haemangioma, pulmonary fibrosis
- Bony – scoliosis, fibrous dysplasia

Generally patients present with skin lesions for excision, with large facial mass/asymmetry (plexiform NF) or rarely, **sarcomatous change** (<1%). Most individuals with NF1 lead healthy and productive lives. NFs can be excised with primary nerve repair if possible.

Neurofibromatosis type 2 (NF2) or 'central NF' due to involvement of intracranial tumours is less common (1 in 50,000) and is also AD (95% penetrance), but is due to a gene defect on chromosome **22q12** (encoded protein is called merlin). It is more commonly associated with **acoustic neuroma** (actually more accurately a vestibular schwannoma).

- Bilateral VIII nerve masses confirmed on MRI/CT
- First-degree relative with NF2 and either unilateral VIII mass or two of the following:
  - NF, meningioma, glioma, schwannoma
  - Juvenile posterior subscapular lenticular opacity

The condition usually presents in adolescence with hearing loss or tinnitus. NFs and café au lait spots may also be present but in fewer numbers than NF1. Some lesions can lead to functional abnormalities such as paraesthesia, whilst some may be associated with gigantism. There is a risk of sarcomatous change (3%–10%, especially if >10 years), which is usually manifested by an increase in size and pain; this is commoner in non-cutaneous lesions (15%) than cutaneous (1%). The prognosis of malignant nerve sheath tumours/neurofibrosarcomas is poor (20% 5 year survival) even after radical surgery.

NEURILEMMOMA (SCHWANNOMA)

These benign nerve sheath tumours are most common in the middle aged (equal sex distribution), presenting as an asymptomatic eccentric slow-growing nodule extrinsic to a nerve; it can be excised/separable except for the one that involved fascicle. The aetiology is unknown, but many show genetic aberrations, e.g. ring chromosome 5 (this chromosome includes the NF2 gene on band **22q12**).

They are the **commonest nerve tumour** and are usually solitary (multiple in neurilemmatosis, which is a variant of neurofibromatosis NF2); the head and neck, and flexor surfaces of limbs are the commonest sites. Occasionally, there may be paraesthesia, numbness (sensory nerves are more commonly affected) or weakness. They resemble NFs but there are no neurites within the tumour; there are Antoni A and B areas.

- Imaging with MRI or ultrasound is usually diagnostic. Indications for excision include enlargement causing concern or disfigurement, symptomatic, e.g. pressure effects, or neurological. They can usually be removed without sacrifice of the main nerve. NFs occur in the substance of a nerve, whilst neurilemmomas occur on the surface, and thus the latter can usually be 'shelled out' whilst the former need excision.
- Recurrence is rare and malignant transformation is practically zero.

Some have described NF3 (schwannomatosis) that is clinically and genetically distinct from NF1 and NF2. There are multiple nerve sheath tumours without involvement of the vestibular nerves; there may be dyasethesia/paraesthesia.

MPNST (MALIGNANT SCHWANNOMA)

Malignant peripheral nerve sheath tumours form 2%–3% of malignant tumours and affect adults between 20 and 50 years of age. They may arise de novo or in pre-existing NFs. There are three groups:

- Neurofibromatosis related (neurofibrosarcoma)
- Post irradiation
- Solitary

Most are associated with the major nerves of the extremities or trunk. They are typically clinically aggressive with high metastatic potential, with up to 90% mortality. Solitary lesions tend to have a better prognosis. They are treated with wide excision, as sensitivity to radiotherapy or chemotherapy is poor.

CUTANEOUS MENINGIOMA

These are typically soft dermal or subcutaneous masses (2–10 cm) found in the scalp and paraspinous regions in children and young adults. The histological features are similar to the intracranial type of meningioma (i.e. psammoma bodies).

MERKEL CELL CARCINOMA (MCC)

The Merkel disc is the expanded cutaneous nerve ending responsible for **mechanoreception**. Merkel cell tumours (or trabecular cell carcinoma, small cell carcinoma of the skin) are aggressive malignant **neuroendocrine** tumours arising from dermal Merkel cells; tumours are masses of small dark cells with positive immunostaining for neuroendocrine differentiation.

They are typically found in elderly females (four times more common than in males), presenting as a reddish-blue nodule most often on the head and extremities. It is usually an aggressive tumour with early lymphatic spread, though spontaneous regression has been reported occasionally.

- Some recommend 2 cm margins with SLNB for lesions >2 cm.
  - Senchenkov (*J Surg Oncol*, 2007) found that LND did not offer any survival benefit but helped predict the risk of regional recurrence. They also found that MMS did not reduce recurrent rates compared to WLE.
- MCCs are more responsive to RT than melanoma. Al-Ghazal (*Br J Plast Surg*, 1996) suggested the combination of RT after WLE to reduce the high recurrence rate seen after surgical excision alone. RT did not improve survival.
- Friedrich Sigmund Merkel (1845–1919) was a German anatomist. He described the large clear oval cells intimately associated with nerve endings in vertebrate skin in 1875 and named them 'Tastzellen' (touch cells).

VI. TUMOURS OF MUSCLE

LEIOMYOSARCOMA

LMS is a malignant tumour of smooth muscle composed of spindle-shaped cells containing myofibrils with cytological atypia. Typical patients are >60 years of age. The most frequently affected site is the **uterine wall**, but it may also be found in the retroperitoneum where it typically presents as a metastatic deposit. The tumour invades muscle and spreads along fascial planes and blood vessels. Distant spread occurs by both haematogenous (20% at presentation) and lymphatic routes (less common). The average length of survival is 2 years. Treatment of choice is WLE with adjuvant therapy where indicated.

- **Leiomyoma** is the benign counterpart. It arises from the erector pili muscle (leiomyoma cutis) most commonly on the extremities. It may also arise from the tunica media of blood vessels (angiomyoma) or the panniculus carnosus of the genitalia or nipple (dartotic myoma). Lesions present as painful/tender pinkish dermal nodules, and adjacent nodules may coalesce to form plaques. Excision is curative. Familial lesions are often multiple.
- **Cutaneous LMS** is a distinct biological entity from LMS, presenting as a smooth reddish dermal nodule. They tend to run a more indolent course than subcutaneous or deep lesions. These account for 1%–2% of all STSs and may be associated with premalignant leiomyomas, physical trauma and radiation. They arise from dermal smooth muscle, erector pili and the smooth muscle surrounding eccrine glands. There is a relatively high risk of local recurrence, but metastases have never been reported.

RHABDOMYOSARCOMA

Rhabdo is Greek for 'rod'.

STSs account for approximately 7% of all childhood cancers, and RMS alone accounts for over half of these. **It is the most common STS in children** (still only 2%–3% of total childhood tumours and uncommon in adults) with 40% arising in those under 5 years of age. The incidence in Asians is lower than in White patients. Small studies have demonstrated an association with parental use of marijuana or cocaine (Grufferman S, *Cancer Causes Control*, 1993), but the aetiology is otherwise unknown. Most cases are sporadic, but after a thorough assessment, some (10%–20%) are associated with identifiable **genetic risk factors**:

- **Li–Fraumeni** cancer susceptibility syndrome (germline p53 mutations), 20–30× risk of sarcomas, breast cancer, leukaemia.
- Beckwith–Wiedemann syndrome – also risk of Wilms tumour.
- NF1 (4%–5%).
- Costello syndrome (germline HRAS mutations) is very rare; it is characterised by postnatal growth

retardation, typical coarse facies, loose skin and developmental delay.
- Noonan syndrome.
- Gorlin syndrome.

Tumours generally present as painless enlarging masses with or without localised symptoms and signs such as overlying erythema. They tend to be rather locally aggressive. The commonest sites are orbit, nasopharynx, temporal bone and sinonasal. Parameningeal tumours may cause indirect symptoms such as facial nerve or other palsies, ear/nasal discharge, etc. Tumours arising from the orbit, non-parameningeal head and neck and the genital tracts are often considered to be **'favourable'**.

- **One-third in the head and neck** region particularly orbital.
- Genitourinary tumours (1/4), bladder, vagina, testes. More common in males (three times).
- Extremity tumours (1/5) with inguinal node involvement in up to 50%. These tend to be the most aggressive types growing to a large size within weeks.

PATHOLOGY

The tumours arise from **skeletal muscle** precursors; some tumours may exhibit skeletal muscle and nerve differentiation (Triton tumours). There are five main pathological subtypes with different behaviours, e.g. alveolar has a much poorer prognosis with high risk of metastasis; botryoid (shaped like a bunch of grapes) has the best prognosis.

- Embryonal (60%) – primitive spindled rhabdomyoblasts
- Spindle cell embryonal
- Botryoid embryonal – genitourinary tumours and other mucosal cavities (5%)
- Alveolar (cancer cells form hollow spaces or 'alveoli'; 20%) – increasing in proportion with age, i.e. adolescents, and are common in larger muscles of extremities.
- Anaplastic, previously known as pleomorphic – the rarest at 1% (higher proportion of adult RMS at 20%).

INVESTIGATIONS

- CXR, CT, MRI especially head and neck
- Biopsy – with cytogenetics/FISH, RT-PCR if available

STAGING SYSTEMS

There are several systems in use.

SURGICOPATHOLOGICAL CLINICAL GROUP

Intergroup RMS clinical grouping system

- Group I – localised disease, completely resected (10%–15%)
  - A. Confined to site of origin
  - B. Beyond site of origin, negative nodes

- Group II – gross total resection (20%)
  - A. Microscopic residual disease in tumour bed or
  - B. Microscopic disease in regional nodes or
  - C. Both
- Group III – incomplete resection, gross residual disease (>50%)
  - A. Biopsy
  - B. Resection/debulking of more than half
- Group IV – distant metastatic disease (15%–20%)

TNM

Pathological staging using pre-treatment TNM:

- T stage is determined by site, size and degree of confinement to anatomic site. T1 and T2 are differentiated by confinement to site of origin or otherwise.
  - T1 confined to site of origin, T2 extension to local tissue
  - A – <5 cm; B – 5 cm or more
- Nodal and distant metastasis, 1 to denote presence.

Clinical staging with Arabic numerals based on TNM:

- Stage 1 – localised disease **in favourable regions**, e.g. orbit, head and neck (not parameningeal), genitourinary (not bladder or prostate)
- Stage 2 – other locations, N0/X, tumour less than 5 cm
- Stage 3 – nodal involvement or tumour larger than 5 cm
- Stage 4 – metastasis

TREATMENT

Local surgical therapy in the form of complete resection with 2 cm clear margins provides the best chance of cure, but in the head and neck, narrower margins may have to be accepted, whilst in the extremities, compartectomy is preferred to amputation; in such situations, **radiotherapy as well as chemotherapy** play a major role in the control of patients with microscopic or gross residual disease, whilst avoiding mutilating surgery. SLNB may be used for staging.

MULTIMODALITY

Multimodality management can lead to a 5 year survival in up to 70% and is the preferred treatment; durable remissions are possible even in metastasis. The risk of late relapse increases in those with gross residual disease in unfavourable sites, or with metastatic disease at diagnosis. The very young (under 1 year of age) who cannot withstand the full course of therapy have poorer results.

- **Induction (neoadjuvant) chemotherapy.** There has been a shift towards giving combination chemotherapy first, followed by surgery and RT. In particular, orbital, vaginal and bladder RMSs show good response, and this facilitates more limited surgery.
- Radiotherapy may be complicated by growth disturbance and induction of secondary tumours.

- Adjuvant chemotherapy – mainstay is VAC (vincristine, actinomycin D, cyclophosphamide). Stem cell reconstitution seems to have no survival benefit.
- Cases of local recurrence may still be curable with salvage surgery particularly if primary therapies were complete. Chemotherapy for metastatic disease usually only has temporary effects (slows progression) and 5 year survival is ~30%.

VII. MISCELLANEOUS SARCOMAS

LIPOSARCOMA

Liposarcomas are relatively common (20% of all STS) and are found in patients in their **middle age** onwards, affecting males more frequently (in comparison, benign lipomas tend to be more common in females). Liposarcoma arising in pre-existing lipomas has been described, but most believe that the majority are distinct lesions with separate origins. The aetiology is unknown, but a variety of cytogenetic abnormalities have been described.

It is a malignant tumour of mesenchymal cells resembling fat cells. It appears as a diffuse nodular swelling of subcutaneous fat, most commonly the lower limb or buttock. Lesions can spread haematogenously, but well-differentiated lesions are unlikely to metastasise. **The histological grade** has predictive value and is usually the single most important criterion. Histologically, there are uniglobular and multiglobular fat cells and undifferentiated sarcoma cells. There have been reports of de-differentiation to high-grade MFH.

Treatment of choice is excision with a wide margin (3–5 cm; despite an apparent capsule, most lesions are infiltrative); tumours are relatively **radioresistant**, but radiotherapy may have a role as an adjunct for well-differentiated or myxoid subtypes. Local recurrence and survival is related to the pathological subtype.

SYNOVIAL SARCOMA

This is relatively rare (6%–10% of all STS) but most common in adolescents and young adults (males two times more frequent) where it is second to RMS. It arises from soft tissues in the vicinity of large joints of the extremities. However, it has **no relation to synovium** per se and is called synovial because of its histological appearance. A reciprocal translocation t(X;18)(p11.2;q11.2) has been identified.

All synovial sarcoma are classified as high grade by the AJCC. Lymph node metastases are rare (5%–15%), and SLNB can be used to assess nodal status; but distant metastases (usually lungs) are fairly common (50%). Prognosis is generally poor.

- Excision with adequate negative surgical margins and post-operative RT is the commonest treatment (Andrassy RJ, *Am J Surg*, 2002). RT reduces recurrence rates from 60%–90% to 28%–49%. Chemotherapy (ifosfamide) has limited use but may be beneficial for distant metastasis.
- Late relapse is not uncommon; therefore, long-term follow-up is advocated.

CLEAR CELL SARCOMA

This mainly occurs in young adults and typically presents as a subcutaneous mass around the knee. Histologically, lesions are S-100 and HMB45 positive, and some regard it as a variant of MM. The prognosis is poor, with local and distant (including lymphatic) recurrence being common.

E. VASCULAR LESIONS

Mulliken and Glowacki (1982) demonstrated that there are only two major types of vascular birthmarks. The histological features are the most important differentiating factors. An expanded classification was proposed by the International Society for the Study of Vascular Anomalies (ISSVA), with an update in 2014. Clear differentiation is important as the clinical behaviours are very different. Often, there is an inadequate appreciation of the distinction (and its implications) **particularly amongst radiologists**, leading to terms being used interchangeably, i.e. incorrectly and causing confusion.

- **Haemangiomas** – increased turnover of endothelial cells; lesions have plump endothelia, increased mast cells (produce heparin) and multilaminated basement membranes.
- **Vascular malformations (VMs)** – these arise due to inborn errors of vascular morphogenesis and are thus permanent. They are classified according to their flow characteristics and their composition – capillary, lymphatic, venous, arterial, combined.
  - VMs have flat endothelia, normal mast cell numbers and a thin basement membrane.

I. INFANTILE HAEMANGIOMAS (IHS)

Haemangiomas are the most common tumours of infancy (1%–3% of live births) and the most common birthmark (20× more common than port wine stains, PWSs) and are seen in up to 10% of White children. The exact cause is unknown, but hypoxia seems to be an important factor (Gurtner); prematurity and/or **low birth weight** are one of the most significant risk factors (30% of infants <1 kg in weight). Most occur in the **head and neck** (60%); visceral lesions can occur without cutaneous lesions. The most common parotid tumour of childhood is a haemangioma; there is a risk of ear canal obstruction with conductive hearing loss.

IHs are more common in **females**, whilst VMs tend to have equal sex incidence (except PWS). Although they can be subdivided by their depth, their clinical behaviour is similar.

- **Superficial**, also known as capillary haemangioma/naevus, strawberry haemangioma/naevus due to its colour.
- **Deep**, also known as cavernous haemangioma; these have a bluish colour and may be confused with venous VMs.

IHs are **benign neoplasms** of vascular tissue with a well-defined life cycle of **rapid proliferation and slower involution**.

- Ninety per cent appear within the first month of life, though up to one-third may be seen at birth. **Precursor lesions** that appear prior to the actual proliferation of the haemangioma include telangiectasia, macular erythema or bluish discolouration that may be confused with PWSs.
- **Proliferation.**
  - These lesions **grow rapidly** in the first year of life, and then intravascular thrombosis and fibrosis results in regression with a colour change from bright to dull red, then with central greying, leaving a pale pink wrinkled scar. **Anetodermia** is an indented scar with a loss of elastic dermis.
  - Proliferating lesions are fleshy and **do not empty** as easily as venous malformations **due to the parenchyma**.
  - Doppler ultrasound may demonstrate high vessel density and 'shunting' with decreased arterial resistance and increased venous flow. MRI is the gold standard investigation but, in children, will require a GA.
- **Involution** also corresponds with mast cell infiltration, and as a general rule, 50% involute aged 5 years, 60% aged 6 and 90% aged 9. The final appearance is unpredictable; early onset of involution may lead to a better final cosmetic outcome, but this is largely anecdotal. The rate of resolution is generally unaffected by ulceration, size or depth of lesion.
  - Most will end up with (near-) normal skin and no serious sequelae; one-third will have a residual patch of loose grey fibrofatty tissue. There is increased fibrous tissue and anti-angiogenic factors during this phase.
  - **Congenital haemangiomas** (CHs) are rare; they are either rapidly involuting (RICH, within a year or so) or non-involuting (NICH), which may mimic a VM. They are largely similar to infantile haemangiomas but fully formed at birth; there some discernible histological differences, and markers are not elevated, e.g. GLUT-1. Some have also described partially involuting congenital haemangiomas (PICHs) that leave a plaque of variable thickness.

This cycle is accompanied by a changing cytokine/cellular profile:

- Increase in markers such as **GLUT1** or Lewis Y antigen.
- Levels of **matrix metalloproteinases (TIMP-1) and bFGF** seem to be correlated with proliferating lesions.
- **Mast cell population** dramatically increases in involuting lesions.
- **VEGF expression** decreases with resolution, but **bFGF** levels remain high.

Most haemangiomas are single localised lesions (80%), but larger lesions may occupy a dermatomal-type distribution and are called **segmental haemangiomas**. These larger haemangiomas may be associated with other anomalies (**PHACE syndrome** – posterior fossa abnormalities, e.g. Dandy–Walker malformation, haemangiomas of head and neck, arterial cerebrovascular anomalies, cardiac defects and eye anomalies – some add an 'S' for sternal clefts; 8% of PHACE/S patients have strokes in infancy and should have MRI brain scans). Associated syndromes are less common.

- Multiple haemangiomas are more common in multiple births and may be associated with internal haemangiomas of the CNS and viscera, e.g. the liver. It is rarely associated with other malformations, but examples include the following:
  - Maffucci enchondromatosis with multiple cutaneous haemangiomas with risk of chondrosarcomas.
  - In **diffuse neonatal haemangiomatosis**, there are multiple, small uniform cutaneous lesions that may be associated with internal lesions. These may be asymptomatic, but there may also be high-output cardiac failure, obstructive jaundice or haemorrhage/coagulopathy. Lesions (both cutaneous and visceral lesions) tend to involute by age 2 years.
    - Those with more than four skin haemangiomas should have a CT (liver) to rule out visceral involvement.
  - Cervicofacial, thoracic and lumbosacral haemangiomas, especially if large, may be associated with underlying structural abnormalities.

COMPLICATIONS

- **Ulceration** – more common in rapidly growing lesions and in the lip and diaper areas. Recurrent problematic bleeding is rare (5%) as these are low flow lesions.
  - **Ulceration tends to be painful.**
- Obstruction.
  - **Eye** (upper lid three times more often) – amblyopia, obstruction of visual axis or direct compression.
  - **Airway** – stridor, obstruction; note that neonates are obligate nose breathers for a few months.
- Large/diffuse complex lesions may be associated with **skeletal distortion** or high-output **cardiac** failure (see above).
- Late complications include scarring, residual colour/mass, redundant skin, telangiectasia and hypopigmentation

NON-OPERATIVE TREATMENTS

- **Observation only** with dressings for minor bleeding, etc. Reassurance after explanation of the condition is sufficient in most cases; showing photographs of other cases may be useful. The child is reviewed in regular follow-up visits.

- **Propanolol.** This has become first-line medical treatment following the fortuitous discovery of haemangiomas shrinking in patients given propranolol to treat the cardiac (HOCM) side effects of corticosteroid given to treat the original haemangioma. See below.
  - Typically 2 mg/kg/day; although caution is always advisable, the need for hospitalisation is controversial. Effects can be rapid, but treatment may need to be prolonged e.g.18 months.
  - Side effects include bradycardia/hypotension, bronchospasm, fatigue, sleep disturbance and hypoglycaemia. **Hypoglycaemia** seems to be the most commonly reported complication (Bonifazi E, *Ped Dermatol*, 2010).
- **Corticosteroids.**
  - **Oral steroids** are very effective in **rapidly proliferating lesions**. Regimens vary, but typically, 2–4 mg/kg/day is used for several weeks, with tailing off to reduce rebound on withdrawal. Some patients may require an additional course. Side effects are usually transient but include increased appetite, change in sleep patterns, increased risk of infection and adrenal suppression; it should be used under close supervision, e.g. by a paediatrician.
    - Steroids seem to offer a more consistent result than propranolol, but the two have not been formally compared.
  - **Intralesional steroid** injections (Mulliken) have been used for periorbital haemangiomas but with significant local complications (including blindness), and systemic absorption can still be significant.
- Some have reported good results with **lasers**, e.g. Achauer (*Plast Reconstr Surg*, 1997).
  - **Pulsed-dye lasers** (PDL, yellow light, 585 nm with cooling) will only produce a slight surface lightening by acting on small vessels in the superficial component of the lesion, but may help in ulceration.
  - Burstein (*Ann Plast Surg*, 2000) – 46% had >90% reduction in size, whereas 54% had a 50%–90% reduction. The surface was treated with PDL in 68 cases; 76% had surgery. Complications included small burns in two and facial weakness in another two.
  - **Intralesional lasers** have also been used but generally do not work as well as expected and are often complicated by ulceration. The overall effect of ablative lasers is similar to surgery, although some report more atrophy and hypopigmentation in laser-treated lesions. IPL has also been used but seems to have more complications.
  - Achauer (*Plast Reconstr Surg*, 1999) – periorbital haemangiomas were treated with bare-tip KTP or Nd:YAG laser. Two-thirds had a >50% reduction in bulk at 3 months without affecting the overlying skin, though there was ulceration in four patients.

- A NICE review in 2004 concluded that intralesional photocoagulation is of uncertain efficacy; facial nerve damage is an important potential complication
- **Interferon** (anti-angiogenic, anti-proliferative agents and enhanced apoptosis) **can be used for lesions not responsive to corticosteroids** including non-proliferating lesions. Due to the side effects, it is generally reserved for use in life-threatening lesions only, e.g. systemic haemangiomatosis and liver lesions, Kasabach–Merritt syndrome. There is a 10%–25% incidence of potentially severe side effects including fever, neutropenia, spastic diplegia (5%, potentially permanent but may be reversible with early discontinuation) and motor delay.
- **Radiation** has been used in the past; it may be effective but is no longer appropriate due to the risks and complications including angiosarcoma, skin atrophy and hyperpigmentation.
- **Sclerosants** work better in vascular malformations.

INDICATIONS FOR SURGERY

Uncomplicated haemangiomas should, in general, be left alone until complete involution and late scar revision are performed if required. However, selected lesions may be excised, e.g. very small lesions, with psychological morbidity (including anxious parents), that can be easily excised and directly closed. A **short trial of propranolol** (Li YC, *Clin Exp Ophthalmol*, 2010) or oral high-dose steroids may be still worthwhile before surgery. Other indications include the following:

- Obstruction, e.g. oral cavity, visual axis, airways.
  - Subglottic lesions are sometimes associated with multiple cutaneous lesions.
- Impingement on visual axis (mechanical ptosis) causing secondary amblyopia, whilst deformation of the growing cornea may cause astigmatism.
- Severe bleeding or ulceration unresponsive to conservative treatments.

Propranolol for severe hemangiomas of infancy. (Leaute-Labreze C, *N Engl J Med*, 2008)

In this letter, the authors report on their experience with the use of oral propranolol in 11 children with haemangiomas. They report discernible changes within 24 hours of starting treatment.

Since then, multiple reports have appeared in the literature – many have described successful use of the drug, though the optimal dosage is not yet known, whilst others are concerned about the potential side effects. In a review by Storch (*Br J Dermatol*, 2010), the early effects seem to be related to vasoconstriction due to reduced nitric oxide release, intermediate effects due to inhibition of angiogenic signals (VEGF, bFGF and matrix metalloproteinases [MMPs]) and long-term effects may be due to induction of apoptosis.

Propranolol for infantile hemangiomas: Early experience at a tertiary vascular anomalies center. (Buckmiller LM, *Laryngoscope*, 2010)

This paper reports on 32 children treated with oral propranolol (2 mg/kg/day in three divided doses). Ninety-seven per cent showed improvement (50% excellent responders). Therapy continued until 1 year of age, or until observable benefit ceased – tailing off was required when stopping. Side effects were reported in 10 patients including somnolence, gastro-oesophageal reflux and a rash. Patients had baseline investigations including ECG; history of asthma, cardiovascular illness or hypoglycaemia was specifically elicited from parents.

Lawley (*J Eur Acad Dermatol Venereol*, 2010) suggests that older children can be treated as outpatients (with baseline ECG and blood glucose) but recommends inpatient treatment for those <3 months of age. Yamada (*J Eur Acad Dermatol Venereol*, 2010) suggests starting at 0.5 mg/kg/day in three divided doses for a week and then 1 mg/kg/day for another week before going to 2 mg/kg/day. The rapid action makes it suited for more urgent situations such as airway or orbital haemangiomas (Li YC, *Clin Exp Ophthalmol*, 2010).

KASABACH–MERRITT SYNDROME (KMS)

KMS is a sequestration of platelets leading to thrombocytopaenia, localised consumption coagulopathy and DIC with a mortality rate of 30%–40%. It is associated with haemangioendothelioma or tufted angioma and **not** the common types of IH.

The term KMS is also often misapplied to bleeding disorders seen in some slow flow VMs; those with extensive venous anomalies can exhibit chronic haemorrhagic diathesis due to consumptive coagulopathy within the malformation.

- Localised intravascular coagulopathy can be demonstrated by analysis of blood taken from the lesion; platelets are minimally depressed, prothrombin time/ activated partial thromboplastin time (PT/APTT) is prolonged, fibrinogen is low and D-dimer is elevated with evidence of fibrinolysis.
- **In true KMS, platelets are very low (10 or less), PT and APTT are within normal limits and fibrinogen levels are decreased, if there is a superimposed consumptive coagulopathy**.
  - Treatment options include excision, interferons or systemic corticosteroids.
  - Transfusion may be required; administering heparin may exacerbate the problem by increasing tumour growth.

PYOGENIC GRANULOMA

Pyogenic granulomas are vascular nodules composed of proliferating capillaries in a loose stroma, although histologically, they are 'haemangiomas' – they are reactive rather than neoplastic. They often follow trauma with rapid growth and the tendency to bleed easily. The exact cause is usually

unknown, but targeted tumour therapy is an increasingly frequent drug-induced form of the disease (others being COC and retinoids). The proliferating vessels extend deep into the dermis; thus, recurrence is likely after simple cautery, e.g. with silver nitrate sticks, laser, curettage or cryotherapy and excision is preferred. Imiquimod may be useful in children; Neri (*Pediatr Dermatol*, 2017) reported on the use of total propranolol – 59% responded after 66 days.

II. VASCULAR MALFORMATIONS

MULLIKEN AND GLOWACKI CLASSIFICATION, 1982

- Low flow – capillary (PWS), venous and lymphatic
- High flow – arterial and arteriovenous

VMs occur in 1.4% of live births. There may be a family history in up to a quarter of patients.

PORT WINE STAIN (PWS)

PWSs are capillary VMs related to developmental weakness of vessel walls leading to progressive ectatic dilatation of mature superficial dermal vessels. The vessels are very heterogenous. Most lesions occur in the head and neck; 50% of facial PWSs are restricted to one trigeminal sensory region. The frequent distribution along with the branches of the fifth cranial nerve suggest a neurogenic pathogenesis.

PWSs occur with an incidence of about 0.3% of neonates with equal sex and racial predilection. They are almost always present at birth with growth in proportion to the child. They start off as a flat patch with a red–purple colour but may progress to become nodular (cobblestoning) and hypertrophic over time (supposedly related to altered/ reduced density of sympathetic innervation – relative deficiency causes slow growth, whilst an absolute deficiency causes an aggressive, rapidly growing lesion).

Differential diagnoses:

- **Flat haemangioma**.
- **Naevus flammeus neonatorum.** This is a fading macular stain that affects up to 50% of neonates, in the supratrochlear or supraorbital nerve territories; one-half resolve spontaneously, whilst the remainder persist but never progress.
- **Salmon patch.** These are pink patches found most frequently on the nape of the neck; they occur in up to 50% of infants but usually disappear within a year. Transient flushing may be seen during crying and exertion. The lesion is composed of ectatic superficial dermal capillaries and is thought to reflect persistence of foetal-type dermal circulation.

Some PWS are associated with syndromes:

- **Sturge–Weber syndrome** is classically a triad of facial PWS (particularly V1), ipsilateral parieto-occipital leptomeningeal angiomatosis (causing neurological symptoms) and ocular choroidal malformations/congenital glaucoma (Sturge, 1879). There may be epilepsy in the first year of life (80%) and mental retardation (60%). Imaging may demonstrate railroad track calcifications.

- All those with a V1 PWS should have ocular and neurologic evaluation; there is an 80% risk of eye or CNS involvement (as compared to 9% average for all facial PWS) and a 45% risk of glaucoma, if V1 and V2 are involved. Conversely, lesions involving V3 without V1/2 never have ocular/CNS involvement.
- With CNS involvement, medication is not started until a seizure occurs. Focal motor seizures are the most common manifestations; in some cases, these are intractable and lead to motor and mental decline. Routine brain imaging of asymptomatic patients is probably not indicated.

- **Klippel–Trenaunay syndrome (KTS)** – two out of the following three: soft tissue and bony **hypertrophy** of an extremity (95% lower limb), varicosities and a capillary malformation (**CLVM**). The overgrowth is not present at birth but may eventually lead to significant limb length discrepancy. There are no associated CNS or visceral anomalies.
  - Abnormal lateral leg varicose veins (with abnormal valves of variable length; pathognomonic marginal vein of Servelle) may be present in up to two-thirds and may be painful/tender with thrombophlebitis. Conventionally, ligation was contraindicated (hindering debulking surgery), as it was thought that they represent the only venous drainage for the limb. However, experience has demonstrated that resection is safe and that deep veins are present in most cases, but are simply not filled by normal techniques.
  - Generally, the treatment is conservative, e.g. compression garments with X-rays to follow limb length, whilst hypertrophy may need limb shortening surgery or epiphysiodesis. Eventual resection/amputation may be needed.
- **Parkes Weber's syndrome** is the association of a mixed malformation, e.g. **CM-AVM, AVF**, with bony and soft tissue overgrowth. It may look similar to KTS, but the malformations are usually patchy and separated (vs. KTS, where they are often multiple but contiguous). There is usually more haemodynamic compromise and overall greater morbidity and mortality. Healing (after surgery) may be poor. Some have a mutation on the RASA1 gene on chromosome 5; inheritance is AD.
- **Blue rubber naevus syndrome** (usually arise sporadically) – **painful** blue blebs that are actually multiple venous malformations (VeMs) in the skin and other tissues, particularly the gut. Gastrointestinal haemorrhage is a common cause of death. Blebs can be treated with excision, sclerosant or laser. Steroids are ineffective.
- **Mafucci syndrome** is the occurrence of VeMs with enchondromatosis particularly on fingers and toes;

bones are deformed, shortened with exostoses. Visceral malformations are also present. Malignant change, e.g. chrondosarcoma, angiosarcoma, may occur in up to 25%.

- **Proteus syndrome** with capillary, lymphatic, venous and capillary–venous malformations in association with overgrowth (macrocephaly, macrodactyly), lipomas and naevi.
- **Wyburn–Mason syndrome** – retinal and CNS AVM, facial PWS.
- **Riley–Smith syndrome** – cutaneous VeM, macrocephaly.
- **Cobb syndrome** – VeMs of spinal cord, truncal PWS.
- **Bannayan–Zonana syndrome** – subcutaneous/visceral VeMs, lipomas.
- **Gorham's syndrome** – venous and lymphatic malformations involving skin and skeleton – osteolytic bone disease.

TREATMENT OF PWS

Early laser therapy used continuous-wave lasers, e.g. ruby and argon, which caused significant collateral damage. As such skin grafting and cosmetic camouflage were common alternatives prior to PDL.

PDLs (585 nm) were a major breakthrough and remain the treatment of choice for PWS. Modern machines with selective epidermal cooling permit the use of higher light dosages for better clearing. Although multiple treatments are required (average 6.4), there are few side effects; however, only 10% of lesions will be completely ablated, 60%–70% will have improved but 20% will have no benefit. The response to the first treatment is often predictive of overall response.

- No anaesthesia is needed for treatment of smaller lesions in adults. There seems to be evidence that aggressive treatment of infants and young children at **earlier ages improves PWS clearance**; early treatment is said to exploit the 'optical' advantages to allow deeper penetration into tissues. However, a GA is required. Children often complain of **increasing pain** with each treatment, i.e. as it lightens, which is a little counterintuitive – one theory is that recovering vessels acquire a more normal vessel innervation.
  - Less cumulative UVL exposure means less epidermal melanin to compete for the absorption of laser light.
  - Less collagen in the skin results in less scatter.
- Purpura is the end point and thus to be expected. It may last for 1 or 2 weeks, and there may be some hypopigmentation (less evident with cooling).
  - The response does seem to vary according to anatomical area – the face responds better than elsewhere, whilst the central face responds less well compared with the lateral face.
  - Alegre-Sanchez (*Ped Dermatol*, 2017) described tips to avoid GA when treating PWSs in children with PDL such as using EMLA, larger spot sizes and higher frequencies to reduce the total treatment time. Having a parent present can also be useful.

- Some reports suggested that up to 50% may 'recur' or redarken (Huikeshoven M, *N Engl J Med*, 2007) after 4 years, but this is probably due to deeper vessels (not affected by the initial PWS) becoming larger/more obvious rather than the previously treated vessels 'reforming', i.e. not a true 'recurrence'. Criticisms made against the Huikeshoven study include the fact that the patients were treated with older machines without cooling and that the average age of the patients was 13.
  - Long-term follow-up suggests that at 10 years after treatment, the PWS will have an appearance that is halfway between pre and post treatment. This may be useful when counselling patients prior to treatment. Use of PDL with PDT or topical angiogenesis inhibitors has been described but is considered investigational.

RESISTANT PORTWINE STAINS

The PDL parameters can be adjusted, e.g. larger spot size, or change to 595 nm.

- **Intense pulsed light** (IPL; Drosner M, *Med Laser Appl*, 2008) – this German study showed that superior clearing by IPL was found in 57.5% vs. 13.8% for PDL; patients elected to continue with IPL in 59% vs. 19% preferring PDL.
- KTP 532 nm (penetrates deeper, does not cause purpura but may have more scarring).
- Cynosure Multiplex – combination PDL and Nd:YAG.
  - Thermal penetration of Nd:YAG is 6–10 mm (Yamagami T, *Neurosurg Rev*, 1984).
- Gemini – combination Nd:YAG and KTP.

Ablative CO_2 lasers have been used for the nodules/hypertrophy found in some PWSs.

VENOUS MALFORMATIONS (VEMS)

These are soft blue sub/cutaneous swellings composed of superficial or deep venous lakes that **empty with compression (i.e. no parenchyma** distinguishing them from haemangiomas) and elevation, and demonstrate no pulsation. They are often multiple; 85% occur in the head and neck. The lips are commonly involved, usually laterally, as well as the tongue. Most cases are sporadic, but some are associated with syndromes (see below). They are non-proliferative and thus generally non-progressive but may enlarge with episodes of trauma or infection, or straining/Valsalva manoeuvre. Lesions seem to be somewhat sensitive to the hormonal environment.

Large facial lesions may show deep involvement of soft tissues such as the masseter and parotid, but bony involvement is rare. It is generally a cosmetic deformity in the main, though functional sequelae are possible, e.g. orbital venous malformation can cause enophthalmos or exorbitism (depending upon filling) or may communicate with the infratemporal fossa via the inferior orbital fissure. Some patients, particularly those with large/multiple lesions, may have a coagulopathy due to decreased fibrinogen.

VASCULAR MALFORMATION VERSUS HAEMANGIOMAS

- VMs grow in proportion to rest of the child. There is no involution.
- Their colours tend to be consistent, while haemangiomas change colour.
- There may be thrombosis (causing pain and swelling).
- **VMs are compressible** (venous/lymphatic) and are easily emptied with slow refill/engorge with dependent position, whilst haemangiomas are more firm and doughy due to the parenchyma.
- Skeletal deformities and tissue overgrowth are more common in malformations, especially lymphatic.

Imaging

- USG/Doppler can demonstrate the speed of flow and can usually adequately diagnose venous lesions, but are less useful when assessing the extent.
- CT appearance of VeMs is typically more heterogeneous than haemangiomas, which are well circumscribed and homogeneous. **Phleboliths** are often described as the pathognomonic sign of VeMs but may only appear later in life (on T2 MRI, they are dark holes, whilst the lesion is hyperintense).
- MRI is used more often, as it avoids irradiation and is multiplanar; **signal voids indicate high flow**; no flow signal indicates a capillary malformation. VeMs have no parenchyma.
  - T1-weighted image – isointense with muscle.
  - T2-weighted image – hyperintense; phleboliths appear as dark holes. Fluid–fluid levels may be present.
- **Arteriography is rarely indicated** (often only if surgery is considered), and it often underestimates the amount of normal tissue.
  - MRA can be useful and avoids the use of contrast.

TREATMENT

- **Conservative.** Compression garments can help with pain and oedema Analgesia.
- **Intralesional.**
  - Pappas (*Ear Nose Throat J*, 1998). Sclerotherapy with **95% ethanol** is effective in reducing the size of the lesion with immediate coagulation, followed by an intense inflammatory response that causes late fibrosis. Sclerotherapy is contraindicated if malformations communicate with the ophthalmic veins to avoid cavernous sinus thrombosis. At least 4 months should elapse before judging the results.
    - Alternatives include sodium tetradecyl sulphate, hypertonic saline, polidocanol, Ethibloc, etc.
  - High recurrence rates are quoted, but the procedure can be repeated fairly safely; complications are uncommon and include skin necrosis or nerve injury.
- Discrete lesions can be considered for **surgical excision** – with or without a prior course of

sclerotherapy up to 4 weeks before surgery. For more complex lesions, the extent of involvement should be carefully defined with preoperative MRI.

- Laser, e.g. Nd:YAG, is not curative, but may be an option for debulking, e.g. intraoral lesions. The results with intralesional lasers have been variable.

ARTERIOVENOUS MALFORMATIONS (AVM)

Schobinger classification

International Workshop for the Study of Vascular Anomalies 1990.

- Stage 1 – AV shunting – quiescence
- Stage 2 – thrill, pulsation, bruit – expansion
- Stage 3 – ulceration, bleeding, pain – destruction
- Stage 4 – high-output cardiac failure – decompensation

AVMs are due to errors of angiogenesis during weeks 4–6. Although present at birth, at least at a microscopic level, they may not be immediately obvious. The **shunting is low pressure**, occurring at a capillary level. AVMs may be localised or diffuse, with the middle of the upper lip a common site; intracranial lesions are more common than limbs, trunk or viscera. The epicentre is called the nidus.

They may be first noticed following puberty, with skin discolouration or a pulsatile mass. Puberty or pregnancy may provoke progression from stages 1 to 2 or 3. AVMs are generally high flow, warm, pulsatile with thrills/bruits. They may ulcerate causing bleeding in one-third (either spontaneously or after trauma such as after dental extraction – a loose tooth in a bleeding socket should be treated with caution) and pain.

- Microfistula – usually multiple and do not cause ischaemia; usually on lower limb
- Macrofistula – more likely to have ischaemia; parasitic steal phenomenon

Treatment

Treatment is directed predominantly at stage 3/4 lesions.

- **Embolisation alone** causes recruitment of other feeding vessels and so is inadequate as a standalone treatment. It can be used (repeatedly) as a way to delay surgery (up to 8 years).
  - **Ligation of feeding vessels** complicates the management in the long term as the low-resistance nidus/lesion remains and stimulates development of collaterals from normal vessels, making the lesion more extensive and complex. Distal embolisation may reduce/slow recurrence from collateral flow.
- Commonly, preoperative angiography and super selective embolisation is followed by **surgery** within 24–48 hours. Some recommend excision early in life (Kohout MP, *Plast Reconstr Surg*, 1998).
  - AVMs need to be excised completely (determined from frozen sections or the pattern of bleeding) with vascular control, including use of hypotensive anaesthesia, quilting sutures or coagulative aids

such as argon plasma. High-grade lesions may involve skin; skin excision was then mandatory to reduce recurrence. Reconstruction with a free flap is often needed.

- Similarly, resection of scalp AVMs **must include the periosteum** to avoid recurrence (Bradley JP, *Plast Reconstr Surg*, 1999). They noted that neighbouring tissues are often hypovascular, making them of dubious reliability for expansion.

LYMPHATIC MALFORMATIONS

The head and neck region is most commonly affected, particularly the posterior triangle.

CLASSIFICATION

- **Microcystic** (previously known as lymphangioma) – tend to be diffuse firm lesions that violate tissue planes. Commonly facial or cervicofacial.
- **Macrocystic** (previously known as cystic hygroma, tend to be soft) are localised and respect tissue planes, and thus tend to shell out easily.
  - 75% occur in the neck with predilection for the left side, mainly in the posterior triangle (Ardenghy M, *Ann Plast Surg*, 1996).
- **Mixed.**

Lymphatic malformations (LMs) are foci of abnormal development of lymphatics that grow in proportion with growth of the child. Usually, they are **sequestrations** of abnormal vessels, i.e. do not usually directly communicate with normal lymphatic vessels but may have connections to larger anomalous cisterns at the interface with dermis/subcutaneous tissues.

- LMs will be present at birth, though sometimes they may only manifest themselves during late childhood or adolescence.
- **LMs do not involute** – they fill and empty, and any sudden enlargement may be due to intralesional bleeding or in response to infection, e.g. upper respiratory tract infection or secondary to minor trauma. One in five will have an episode of infection.
- Some may have a significant venous component, i.e. lymphovenous malformation, though intralesional bleeding may cause confusion. Phleboliths seen in some patients may be secondary to intralesional bleeding.
- Massive cervicofacial lesions account for ~3% of LMs and are more likely to cause local mass effects such as airway obstruction and difficulty feeding.
- Tissue overgrowth – LMs are the commonest cause of **macroglossia/macrocheilia** in children. Dental caries may occur secondarily to difficulty in access for cleaning and speech problems.
  - Secondary bony hypertrophy, especially mandible, may lead to abnormal bite. Osteolysis may also be a feature (Lopez-Gutierrez JC, *Lymphat Res Biol*, 2012).

- Thoracic LMs involving the mediastinum may cause pleural and pericardial effusions, whilst lesions in the groin can cause lymphoedema and limb hypertrophy.

INVESTIGATIONS

- **Transillumination test**.
- Fluid levels on MRI scan are diagnostic – 'rim enhancement' (gadolinium) and hyperintense (T2). MRI or CT may help to define the relationship of the lymphatic malformation with surrounding tissues.
- USG demonstrates multiloculated cysts.

MANAGEMENT

- Antibiotics and NSAIDs if inflamed; prolonged courses (6–8 weeks) may be needed due to the slow clearance of bacteria.
- Support garments if needed.
- **Sclerotherap**y with doxycycline, 95% ethanol (significant complications) or sodium tetradecyl sulphate 3%. Often used before surgery. Alternatives include OK-432 (denatured group A *Streptococcus pyogenes*, limited availability).
- **Surgical excision** should be carefully planned after imaging has defined the full extent as recurrence is almost inevitable following incomplete excision as the lymphatics 'regenerate' (Lille ST, *J Paediatr Surg*, 1996). Complete macroscopic excision may still have a 20% recurrence rate. Vesicles 'bubbling' through around the incision site is not uncommon.
- Laser (Nd:YAG) has been used for cutaneous lesions.

ACQUIRED VASCULAR MALFORMATIONS

- **Campbell de Morgan spots** are tiny AV fistulas at the dermal capillary level found mostly in sun-exposed skin in older patients.
- **Spider naevi** are angiomas appearing at puberty and disappearing spontaneously; They also affect two-thirds of pregnant women and disappear in the puerperium.
  - Those with vessels that can be cannulated with a fine needle (32G) should be treated with sclerotherapy – hypertonic saline before 1% sodium tetradecyl (3% increases scarring). This may cause brown discolouration that lasts for months, and extravasation may cause necrosis.
  - Laser or electrocautery can be used for smaller vessels.

F. MISCELLANEOUS

I. HYPERHIDROSIS

Hyperhidrosis is excessive sweating, mostly from the eccrine sweat glands affecting axillae, palms and soles of feet. Patients complain about social embarrassment and staining of clothing.

- Primary hyperhidrosis affects up to 1% of the population, predominantly young adults.
- Secondary hyperhidrosis may be due to the following:
  - Endocrine disorders, e.g. hyperthyroidism, menopause
  - Neurological disorders, e.g. syringomyelia
  - Drugs, e.g. antidepressants
  - Neoplastic disease, e.g. Hodgkin's lymphoma, carcinoid, phaeochromocytoma

TYPES OF SWEAT GLANDS (SEE 'SWEAT GLAND TUMOURS')

- **Eccrine sweat glands** are found on almost the entire body surface and secrete a salty, watery solution under control of cholinergic sympathetic nerves.
- **Apocrine sweat glands** are found in places such as the axillae, periareolar area, perianal area are eyebrows. They secrete a mixture of fat, cholesterol and salt onto hair shafts under adrenergic sympathetic nerve control.
  - They are present in equal numbers as eccrine glands in the axilla.

ANTIPERSPIRANTS ARE OFTEN USED AS FIRST-LINE TREATMENTS

- **Aluminium hexachlorhydrate in alcohol** is the first choice in most cases. Concentrations of up to 20% may be used (e.g. Drysol). The maximum effect comes from regular application to dry skin. The exact mechanism of action is unknown but may involve damage of the terminal duct lining by aluminium ions. There may be irritation that is related to aqueous contamination leading to the active ingredient slowly decomposing to hydrochloric acid.
- **Iontophoresis** probably works by blocking sweat ducts with ions or coagulated surface proteins. The hands (or feet) are soaked in tap water (if water is too soft, then minerals in the form of baking soda can be added) with or without anticholinergics such as glycopyrronium (more effective). A weak electric current is passed through for 30 min (reversed once halfway). The beneficial effects begin immediately and last for 3–4 days, and thus need to be repeated two to three weekly; when the full effect is achieved (~15 treatments), it lasts longer (about 1 month). It can be performed at home and works in up to 85% cases. It is often a first-line treatment and can be combined with other modalities.
  - Kavanagh (*Br J Dermatol*, 2004) – botulinum toxin has been added to iontophoresis solution to provide 3 months' effect after one treatment, but this does not seem to be cost effective.
- **Systemic agents** such as anxiolytic drugs, e.g. benzodiazepines, to reduce anxiety-provoked symptoms and glycopyrronium bromide (anticholinergic side effects).

Botulinum toxin (BTX) has been a major development in hyperhidrosis treatment. The effect on sweat glands may last longer (14 months) than on muscle, possibly reflecting the differences between autonomic and motor nerves. The use of BTX for hyperhidrosis came from observations of the side effects of treatment of hemifacial spasm. Several reports published in 1997 demonstrated beneficial effects lasting 9–14 weeks with a slight decrease in hand grip force in one study (Naumann). The initial dosages used were high, whilst further studies showed that a single treatment of around 50 U (of botulinum toxin A) can reduce sweating after 2–4 days and completely stop it by 3–7 weeks, lasting up to 16 weeks. Eighty per cent of patients respond compared to 20% in placebo controls.

- FDA approval for onabotulinumtoxinA for severe primary axillary hyperhidrosis in 2004.
- There were no effects on unpleasant odours (i.e. adrenergic apocrine glands)
- It is 80%–90% effective for palmar sweating; touch-up injections are required after 6 months or so. The finger pulps are usually not treated to avoid deleterious effects on grip (and such injections would be very painful).
- There is a low risk of developing immunity (<4% from data in the treatment of cervical dystonia where large doses were used).

The area to be treated should be mapped out, e.g. with **Minor's starch iodine** method. Patients should NOT shave underarms for a few days, abstain from use of over-the-counter antiperspirants for 24 hours prior to the test and avoid precipitating activities such as exertion ~30 minutes prior to the test.

- Dry the area and paint it with iodine solution (Betadine works); when dry, lightly sprinkle with starch powder (flour), and the hyperhidrotic area will develop a deep blue–black colour over a few minutes.
- Each injection site has a ring of effect due to diffusion of up to approximately 1 cm radius (depends on dilution/volume). Ink can be used to mark sites, but do not inject through ink to avoid tattooing.
- Inject evenly at a 2 mm depth with a 45° angle, with the bevel up to ensure intradermal placement which is preferable to subcutaneous injection. Avoid patching gaps before 3 months.

The main problems are as follows:

- Injection pain that is not reduced by EMLA, i.e. usually requires injected LA either as local infiltration or nerve block. Nerve blocks are usually not needed for axillary injections (ice or vibration analgesia suffices) but are recommended for the palm. Dermojet (needleless injection system of 2% lignocaine) have been used to reduce pain but are usually not effective enough–there will still be pain dependent on the volume and

pressure used. It also interrupts the workflow. Others have tried to use jet injection of BTX but there is at least a 10% wastage.
- Muscle weakness is uncommon.

Hyperhidrosis: A review of current management. (Atkins JL, *Plast Reconstr Surg*, 2002)

Surgery

- Excision of skin and/or subcutaneous tissue (direct closure, Z-plasty or S-shaped closure) is effective, but significant scarring, risks of wound infection/dehiscence, haematoma, delayed healing common. Not a frequent option.

Alternatives include the following:

- **Curettage/shaving** of glands via incisions (see 'Bromidrosis').
- **Axillary liposuction,** particularly superficial (subdermal) liposuction. UAL may be more effective (Commons GW, *Aesthetic Plast Surg*, 2009).
  - Hong (*Plast Reconstr Surg*, 2004) used very superficial UAL with cold irrigation externally to reduce thermal injury; the end point was bloody aspirates and erythema of the skin. It could be done under sedation. With an average follow-up of 18.8 months, 91.7% had satisfactory reduction of odour. Complications included mild skin sloughing (3.2%), haematoma (1.3%) and temporary sensory alteration of the hand (0.3%).
- **Subdermal Nd:YAG laser.**
- **Thoracoscopic sympathectomy** is more suited to palmar than axillary hyperhidrosis; response rates are good, but Horner's syndrome, thoracic duct injury and phrenic nerve injury are reported, and the skin tends to be vasodilated, dry and fissured. Furthermore, **compensatory sweating** on trunk, limbs or face may occur in up to 50% of patients, especially if sympathectomy is bilateral (treat dominant hand only).
  - Eleven per cent regret the procedure in some series.

The efficacy of a microwave device for treating axillary hyperhidrosis and osmidrosis in Asians. (Lee SJ, *J Cosmet Laser Ther*, 2013)
MiraDry is a microwave-based device. There was a reduction of sweating in 83% at 7 months, and 94% had reduced osmidrosis. Histology from one case showed fibrotic destruction of eccrine and apocrine glands. There was one case of temporary alteration of lateral forearm sensation.

MiraDry was FDA **cleared** (equivalent to another device) in 2015 for elimination of axillary hair, sweating and odour, in addition to its initial indication for hyperhidrosis. A systematic review by Hsu (*J Cosmet Laser Ther*, 2017) found five clinical trials including Lee SJ; the sample sizes were small and follow-up periods short (1 year maximum).

However, they seemed to suggest some efficacy; balanced against this were relatively common side effects of swelling and altered sensation.

II. BROMIDROSIS

Bromidrosis is an offensive odour due to the bacterial degradation of apocrine sweat gland secretions. Alternative terms include 'bromhidrosis' or 'osmidrosis'. Some say that osmidrosis is the problem of odour and bromidrosis is the combination of osmidrosis and hyperhidrosis.

Sweat itself is relatively odourless, but modifications may make it pungent:

- Propionic acid from amino acid breakdown by propionibacteria ('vinegary')
- Isovaleric acid from *Staphylococcus epidermis* ('cheesy')

Surgical management of axillary bromidrosis – A modified Skoog procedure by an axillary bipedicled flap approach. (Wang HJ, *Plast Reconstr Surg*, 1996)
Parallel incisions are made in the axilla to allow a bipedicled strip of skin to be turned inside out for careful thinning with scissors, which divides sweat gland ducts and generates fibrosis. The authors report good resolution of symptoms in their series of 110 patients, with reduction in sweating in 92% of operated axillae at 30 months. Complications include haematomas in four patients and mild dehiscence in six.

- Technique is similar to that originally described by Skoog 1963 – raised four flaps (staggered).
- Qian (*J Plast Reconstr Aesthet Surg*, 2010) used a single 3 cm incision in the axilla to elevate the skin flaps that were thinned/defatted. In this series, up to 97% had reduction of odour after surgery; all reported reduction in sweating. A side effect was reduced hair growth in 95% that seemed particularly welcomed by the female patients. Complications include haematoma, seroma and wound infection in 1% each roughly but **superficial epidermal necrosis of 37%** (the surgeons seemed to thin out the skin significantly).

III. HIDRADENITIS SUPPURATIVA

This is an inflammatory disease of apocrine sweat glands causing recurrent deep abscess-like swelling in axillae and groins.

- Early lesions are tender subcutaneous nodules that are deep and round without pointing. They may resolve or progress to discharge to the skin, forming a sinus.

It affects mostly young females (three times) with peak incidence in the second and third decades. It is still poorly understood.

- It may be familial in some patients (AD inheritance).

- Disease seems to be associated with obesity (exacerbating rather than causative, weight loss may help), acne and hirsutism (i.e. androgen related).
- Strongly linked with smoking.

The condition can be classified as active or inactive, with primary lesions in a number of 'designated sites', e.g. axilla, groin, Hurley clinical stages (I–III):

- Stage I – solitary or multiple isolated nodules
- Stage II – recurrent lesions with sinuses and scars
- Stage III – diffuse branching sinuses

Traditionally, surgery consists of **excision** (limited vs. wide – including 2 cm margin around hair-bearing skin), with reconstruction as indicated by the defect. Soldin (*Br J Plast Surg*, 2000) reviewed their experience with 94 axillae.

- Healing by secondary intention
- Primary closure of small defects
- Reconstruction of larger defects, e.g. split skin graft +/– NPWT, pedicled flaps especially from scapular region.

Radical excision was associated with much fewer recurrences, but wound breakdown was observed in all modalities of closure; most importantly, **scar contracture** observed in one-third of axillae reconstructed with SSGs.

Hidradenitis suppurativa: Pathogenesis and management. (Slade DE, *Br J Plast Surg*, 2003)
Non-surgical management

- Oral clindamycin 300 mg twice daily (including perioperative infection prophylaxis).
- Cyproterone acetate (antiandrogen) improves symptoms in females.
- Acitretin 25 mg twice daily (retinoids reduce sebaceous gland activity).
- Laser treatment with CO_2 laser with healing by secondary intention.

HiSCR (Hidradenitis suppurativa clinical response). (Kimball AB, *JEADV*, 2016)
This is a short report on improved outcome indicators evolved during a phase 2 clinical study on the use of adalimumab (Humira®) for HS.

This is a new indication for this medication. Starting at 160 mg on the first day, the dosage is titrated down to 40 mg a week. Antibiotics and antiseptic wash can be used in combination.

PYODERMA GANGRENOSUM

Pyoderma gangrenosum is an uncommon condition characterised by cutaneous ulceration with a purple undermined border; in some, there are multiple skin abscesses with necrosis that continues to enlarge. It can occur in any part of the skin but most often in the pretibial area. Histologically, there are intense dermal inflammatory infiltrates composed of neutrophils with little evidence of a primary vasculitis.

Gram-negative streptococci are frequently cultured from wounds, but their role is unclear.

Classic pyoderma gangrenosum may be associated with symptoms of pain, fever, malaise, myalgia and arthralgia. The aetiology is unclear but seems to be related to **altered immunological reactivity**. Approximately 50% of cases are associated with a specific systemic disorder: inflammatory bowel disease, rheumatoid arthritis, non-Hodgkin's lymphoma, Wegener's granulomatosis (especially head and neck lesions) and myeloproliferative disorders. The other 50% have no identifiable risk factors.

- The diagnosis is based on clinical and histopathological findings (characteristically a neutrophilic infiltration). There is no specific test; biopsy is used mainly to rule out other causes.

Pyoderma gangrenosum has also been reported in the following:

- Fasciocutaneous flaps and complicating breast reduction (Gudi VS, *Br J Plastic Surg*, 2000)
- DIEP flap breast reconstruction (Caterson SA, *J Reconstr Microsurg*, 2010)

MANAGEMENT

- Surgery may exacerbate the disease and is usually avoided.
- The commonest reported treatments include steroids, azathioprine and cyclosporine.

9

Genitourinary and trunk

A. PRINCIPLES OF SURGICAL MANAGEMENT OF HYPOSPADIAS

I. RELEVANT ANATOMY AND EMBRYOLOGY

EMBRYOLOGICAL DEVELOPMENT OF THE PENIS AND URETHRA (SADLER TW. LANGMAN'S MEDICAL EMBRYOLOGY, 11TH EDN.)

During the third week of development, primitive streak mesenchymal cells migrate around the cloacal membrane to form the cloacal folds, which fuse cranial to the membrane to form the genital tubercle.

- The foetus is **sexually indeterminate** until the sixth week of gestation when the cloacal membrane divides into urogenital and anal membranes, whilst the cloacal folds also divide into urethral folds anteriorly and anal folds posteriorly with genital swellings lateral to them (these form the scrotal swellings in the male and labia majora in the female).
- During the 6th to 11th weeks, the genital tubercle elongates to form the phallus under the influence of androgens. As the phallus develops, it pulls the urethral folds forwards to form the lateral walls of the urethral groove, which extends only up to the distal part of the phallus – here the epithelial lining is of **endodermal origin and is known as the urethral plate** (glanular urethra).
- During the 12th week, the urethral folds come together and close over to form the penile urethra (the glanular part of the urethra has not canalised at this stage).
- During the 13th week, the glanular urethra becomes canalised by the inward migration of ectodermal

cells to form the external urethral meatus, and the genital swellings enlarge to form each half of the scrotum.

BLOOD SUPPLY

There are three pairs of arteries that are all branches of the internal pudendal artery (internal iliac artery).

- Artery to the bulb – supplies the posterior part of the corpus spongiosum.
- Dorsal artery of the penis – supplies the corpus spongiosum, skin, fascia and glans (hence an anastomosis exists between the artery to the bulb and the dorsal artery). The arteries run either side of the deep dorsal vein in the groove between the corpora cavernosa.
- Deep artery – supplies corpus cavernosum and its sole function is erectile.

Although some venous drainage from the penis follows the venae comitantes draining into internal pudendal veins, most of it flows along the **deep dorsal vein deep to Buck's fascia**, draining into the prostatic venous plexus.

- The superficial dorsal vein drains skin only and joins with the superficial external pudendal and great saphenous veins.
- Lymphatic channels accompanying the superficial dorsal vein drain into the superficial inguinal nodes, whilst the glans and corpora drain into the deep inguinal nodes/internal iliac nodes.

Internal preputial skin is vascularised from the Dartos fascia whilst external preputial skin is vascularised from the subdermal plexus (larger vessels), and a plane that is readily dissectable exists between these two layers. Hence, the internal preputial skin may be islanded as a flap and tubularised to form neo-urethra, whilst the external skin may be raised as a cutaneous flap to resurface a ventral defect. Obviously, preputial flap techniques cannot be used if the child has been circumcised.

ANATOMY OF THE MALE URETHRA

The urethra is lined by transitional epithelium except for the part just proximal to the external urethral meatus, the navicular fossa, which is lined by stratified squamous epithelium and has blind-ending lacunae. The empty urethra is horizontal in cross section, whilst the external meatus forms a vertical slit, and hence the urine stream spirals. The urethral glands of Littré open into the urethra on its anterior and lateral aspect, 'against' the stream.

There are three points of constriction along the urethra: the internal meatus (bladder neck), the proximal end of navicular fossa and the external meatus. The three dilatations are prostatic urethra, bulb and navicular fossa.

II. ASSESSMENT OF HYPOSPADIAS

Hypospadias results from incomplete closure of the urethral folds during the 12th week of development and may represent abnormal fusion between endodermal and ectodermal processes. It occurs in **1 in every 300** live male births and seems to be **increasing**; it is characterised by

- Ventral meatal dystopia, i.e. ventral position of the meatus
- Dorsal hooded foreskin
- Ventral curvature on erection (**chordee**)
  - This is a fibrous remnant of the corpus spongiosum causing ventral penile curvature that may occur without hypospadias. Dissection of the urethral plate alone will not correct the curvature. In >90% of cases, chordee is due simply to ventral skin shortage; the aetiology is uncertain.
    - Artificial erection test. See below.
- Deficiency of ventral skin
- Clefting of the glans, and in the most severe cases scrotal bipartition

Seventeen percent of cases have associated urogenital abnormalities including undescended testes and inguinal hernia; these patients may have intersex conditions and should be referred for karyotyping and exclusion of congenital adrenal hyperplasia. Patients with proximal hypospadias should be screened for abnormalities of the urinary tract (renal ultrasound, isotope renogram). Routine investigation is not indicated in the absence of other anomalies.

CLASSIFICATION

Classification is based on the position of the abnormally proximal opening of the urethral meatus, from distal to proximal.

- Distal or proximal
  - 85% are distal (glandular, coronal, subcoronal, distal penile shaft).
- 15% are proximal (midshaft, proximal penile shaft, penoscrotal, scrotal and perineal).

It can be subdivided into several ways:

- Glanular/coronal/subcoronal
- Distal shaft/mid-shaft/proximal shaft
- Penoscrotal/scrotal or perineal

AIMS OF CORRECTION OF HYPOSPADIAS

- Allow micturition whilst standing with a non-turbulent stream
- Achieve a natural appearance with slit-like meatus located at the distal extent of the glans
- Allow normal sexual function

AETIOLOGY

Studies have shown that maternal age >35 years and maternal obesity increased the risk of having a baby with hypospadias.

- Environmental (oestrogenic chemicals – DDT, soya beans); ingestion of progestin for pregnancy complications such as luteal phase defects, but not oral contraceptives (Norgaard M, *Urology*, 2009). It is five times more common in IVF children.
- Androgen hyposensitivity (especially if associated with micropenis, severe hypospadias, hypogonadism, undescended testes and inguinal hernia).
- Genetic – with an affected male, his sons will have an 8% risk whilst his brothers have a 14% risk (Bauer SB, *Urol Clin N Am*, 1981); **identical twins do not necessarily both have hypospadias**; hence, the aetiology is multifactorial.
- Intersex states – the severest forms of hypospadias are strongly associated with 'disorders of sexual development' (DSD).
- There is a link with cleft palate and hypertelorism, i.e. Schilbach–Rott syndrome, which is very rare (Joss SK, *Am J Med Genet*, 2002).

HISTORY

- Family history of hypospadias
- Maternal drugs, occupation of the father, etc.
  - Kallen, *Teratology*, 2002. This Swedish study showed a negative association between hypospadias and maternal smoking but a positive association with primiparity.
  - Pierik, *Environ Health Perspect*, 2004. Risk factors include being small for age, paternal smoking.
- Any urinary tract infections (which may be manifested as failure to thrive) or known abnormalities of the upper genitourinary tract
- Any curvature during witnessed erections

EXAMINATION

- Penis – size, degree of meatal dystopia, i.e. position of meatus, depth of urethral groove, chordee, dorsal hooding
- Preputial involvement (circumcision or preputial reconstruction)
- Assessment of associated anomalies
  - Position of testes – descended/undescended, size – cryptorchidism in up to 10%
  - Inguinal hernia/open processus vaginalis 9%–15%

INVESTIGATIONS

Investigations should include general examination and exclusion of an intersex state in severe anomalies with ambiguous genitalia (genetic and endocrine work-up). Otherwise, no investigations are necessary in the common forms of hypospadias.

- Urinary stream.
- Urea and electrolytes (U&Es), renal ultrasound or isotope renogram if concerned about **upper genitourinary tract** (not affected except in very severe forms of hypospadias).

III. SURGICAL PRINCIPLES

TIMING OF SURGERY

This is quite variable and opinion is divided. Traditionally (up to the 1970s), surgery was deferred until 3 years of age or soon after (before children went to school, and so could urinate standing up at school), but it is often suggested that earlier repair **(6–18 months)** will reduce psychological impact of the condition and young children will have little memory of their hospital stay. However, Weber (*J Pediatr Urol*, 2009) found no difference in terms of psychological adjustment whether surgery was performed before or after 18 months. There is no true data/evidence base regarding timing – protocols are mostly based on expert opinion.

- Single stage – the Action committee for American Academy of Paediatrics (1996) recommended surgery between 6 and 12 months.
  - In selected cases with normal sized phalluses, a distal repair (and selected proximal repair) can be considered at 3 months.
  - Those with proximal hypospadias or small glans can start hormonal treatment and are reassessed at 6 months.
- Two stage – stage 1 at 12 months and stage 2 at 18 months.

Waiting much longer makes little difference to the **size** as the penis grows less than 1 cm during the first 3–4 years. Administering pre-operative testosterone, DHT or β-chorionic gonadotropin may be useful for those with a small penis (particularly small glans) or for repeat surgery.

TECHNIQUES

There have been several hundred different techniques described in the literature:

- 1932 Mathieu (flip–flap one stage)
- 1949 Browne (modified Duplay)
- 1952 Cecil–Culp (modified Duplay)
- 1962 Cloutier (two-stage preputial FTSG)
- 1963 Devine and Horton (modified Mathieu)
- 1965 Mustarde (modified Mathieu)
- 1977 Van der Meulen (modified Duplay)
- 1980 Duckett (transverse preputial island flap)
- 1981 Duckett (meatoplasty and glanuloplasty – MAGPI)
- 1984 Harris (split preputial flap technique)
- 1987 Elder and Duckett (onlay island flap)
- **1994 Snodgrass (tubularised incised plate, most common worldwide)**
- **1995 Bracka (modified Cloutier)**
- 1997 Turner–Warwick (bulbar elongation and anastomotic meatoplasty – BEAM)

SURGICAL TECHNIQUES

Use of loupes is common. Techniques to repair hypospadias can be divided into one-stage or two-stage repairs. The early techniques were two-staged, but technical developments allowed a single-stage procedure to be performed safely and applied to the vast majority of cases of hypospadias. There is renewed interest in two-staged repair, as it can improve results in most severe forms of hypospadias.

One-stage repairs can be classified as follows:

- **Urethral advancement** techniques (see below)
- **Inlay** techniques in which tissue, usually a buccal mucosal graft, is inset into a longitudinal split in the dorsal urethral that is then **tubularised** in a Thiersch–Duplay fashion, i.e. one-stage dorsal inlay TIP
- **Onlay (incomplete tube)** techniques in which tissue is transposed onto the ventral urethral defect to close the tube, usually a vascularised flap, e.g. Mathieu/Flip flap or onlay island flap (OIF) from inner preputial skin
- **Tubularisation** after a central relaxing incision e.g. Snodgrass, or where a tubed flap of tissue is transposed into the defect to reconstruct the whole circumference of the tube, e.g. Ducketts tubularised preputial island flap

The terms 'inlay' and 'onlay' can be a bit confusing sometimes. An alternative way to classify the techniques are vascularised flap vs. graft, augmentation vs. substitution urethroplasty:

- Vascularised flap
  - Augmentation, e.g. Mathieu
  - Substitution, e.g. Ducketts
- Free grafts
  - Augmentation, e.g. Dorsal onlay TIP
  - Substitution – most commonly used in two-stage surgery

One-stage surgery involves fewer operations for the patient, costs less overall and is said to cause less psychological trauma. However, there are some advantages to a two-stage repair (particularly Bracka):

- Greater versatility for dealing with a wider spectrum of hypospadias and thus less need to master a greater number of techniques.
- Surgery is technically easy and offers reliable results, with a low fistula rate of ~3%.
- It avoids a circumferential anastomosis, a potential site of stricture, and achieves a more natural-looking and distal slit-like meatus.
- Some argue that psychosexual adjustment is more related to final appearance than the number of operations.

ADVANCEMENT TECHNIQUES

These techniques best treat **very distal** hypospadias that would probably have been ignored previously; it can also be applied to the residual meatal deformity (retrusion) following some older techniques, e.g. Thiersch–Duplay, Byars.

- **MAGPI (Duckett)** is suitable for glanular hypospadias only; subcoronal hypospadias is better treated by other techniques. A longitudinal incision is made distal to the abnormal meatus and closed transversely to provide some advancement, then glans tissue is closed over the advanced meatus in two layers. Careful patient selection is important to avoid complications; there is a tendency to cause a 'fish mouth' deformity when applied inappropriately.
- **Bulbar elongation and anastomotic meatoplasty (BEAM)** – the meatus is advanced by dissecting free a length of penile urethra.

TYPICAL CHOICE OF REPAIR (FIGURES 9.1 AND 9.2)

- Distal meatal dystopia
  - MAGPI (Duckett)
  - BEAM (Turner–Warwick)
- Mid-shaft to coronal meatal dystopia

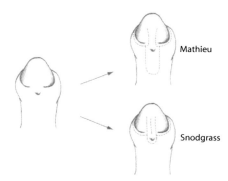

Figure 9.1 Common techniques for more distal types of hypospadias.

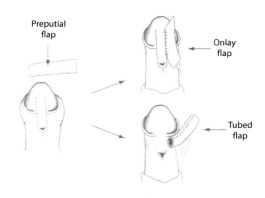

Figure 9.2 Other techniques for hypospadias using preputial flaps.

- Tubularised incised plate (TIP/Snodgrass, most common technique – in a supposedly worldwide survey, it was used in 71% of distal hypospadias; Springer A, *Eur Urol*, 2011)
- Ventral skin flip–flap (Mathieu, particularly popular in France) better than TIP when a healthy urethral plate is not available
- Transverse preputial island flap (TPI, Duckett)
- Two-stage repair (Bracka)
- Penoscrotal meatal dystopia
  - Two-stage repair (Bracka, preferred technique as reported by Springer)
  - TPI
  - Two-stage repair (Cecil–Culp)

ANAESTHESIA

General anaesthesia may be supplemented with

- **Dorsal penile block** – fails to fully anaesthetise ventral skin/glans.
- **Penile ring block**.
- **Caudal block** – also anaesthetises mucosa and there is less bladder neck spasm; it allows a lighter general anaesthetic to be administered with lower opiate requirements but causes a semi-erection.

RELEASE OF CHORDEE

Orthoplasty is chordee correction.

- **Artificial erection test** (Horton) – saline injected via 25G butterfly cannula inserted into corpus cavernosum with tourniquet applied.
- Deglove penis in between Bucks and Dartos (releases **skin chordee** due to ventral skin shortage). Some more release may come from
  - Fairy cuts in Bucks
  - Dissection of spongiosum
- Excision of **genuine chordee** (fibrous tissue on ventral penis); the urethral plate does not cause curvature in most cases. This precludes use of a Snodgrass-type

surgery; conversion to a two-stage with grafting of the defect is common.

- Otherwise, tubularised inlay islanded preputial flap (complete tube)
- Flip flap at a pinch
- Residual chordee is usually due to **disproportion of the corpora** (usually spongiosum too short due to defect of midline differentiation) and requires straightening by dorsal orthoplasty (modified Nesbit).

PRESERVING THE URETHRAL PLATE

The mainstay of surgery is to preserve the well-vascularised urethral plate and to utilise it for urethral reconstruction. From an embryological perspective, the urethral plate is always abnormal in hypospadias.

- If the plate is wide, it can be tubularised as per Thiersch–Duplay.
- If the plate is too narrow for tubularising, then a midline relaxing incision can be used as per the Snodgrass technique.
  - There is a significant complication rate when using this technique for proximal defects.
- If the plate is too narrow or too unhealthy:
  - For proximal defect – onlay technique.
  - For distal defects – many choices, e.g. Mathieu, urethral advancement, etc.
  - If the continuity of the plate cannot be preserved, then an islanded tubularised flap is used. A two-stage technique may be useful.
  - If preputial/penile skin is not available (e.g. balanitis xerotica obliterans, BXO), then buccal mucosa can be used if onlay or two-stage.

POST-OPERATIVE MANAGEMENT

There is a wide range of practice for dressings and drainage, and there is not a strong evidence to make any specific recommendations.

- **Diversion of urinary stream away from the suture line** for 2–6 days.
  - Silicone catheter – fix carefully.
  - Urine can be drained with a transurethral dripping stent or suprapubic catheter, but some do not drain after distal repairs.
- Circular dressings with slight compression, keeping penis pressed against the abdomen.
- Ketoconazole 400 mg tds – start 2 days before surgery for control of erections (Evans KC, *Int J Impot Res*, 2004).
  - DeCastro (*J Urol*, 2008) found little difference from placebo.
- Cyproterone acetate can be given 10 days prior to surgery in young adults to reduce postoperative erections.
  - A sharp icy blast of freeze spray can be kept on the bedside locker for emergency use.

- Treat bladder neck spasm with oxybutynin 1 mg 8 hourly.
- 0.75% plain marcaine continuous dorsal penile block, 1 mL 4 hourly.
- Antibiotics.

Is prophylactic antimicrobial treatment necessary after hypospadias repair? (Meir DB, *J Urol*, 2004)

This is a prospectively randomised clinical trial evaluating the role of oral cephalexin in hypospadias repair by TIP urethroplasty, with a urethral catheter in situ for a mean of 8 days post-operatively. The incidence of bacteriuria was halved in the cephalexin group, and there was lower frequency of urinary tract infection, fistulae and meatal stenosis. There was also a difference in pathogens – *Pseudomonas aeruginosa* was the commonest in the prophylaxis group, whilst in the control group, it was *Klebsiella pneumoniae*. The author recommends broad-spectrum prophylaxis.

STENT OR NO STENT

Generally as long as there is a watertight repair without overlapping suture lines, drainage is not necessary in **distal repairs**.

- The original **Mathieu** operation was performed **without stents**, but the batch of studies following this showed an almost four times increase in complications with stent-less repairs. Subsequent experience showed that there was **little/no difference** in complication rates.
  - Some studies have shown success with the use of stents without suprapubic catheters (which are regarded as a bit over the top).
  - Similarly, traditionally after a TIP repair, a catheter is left in for 7–14 days, but some studies have shown that early removal of the catheter does not affect the final results or increase the risk of complications.

COMPLICATIONS

The main aim of follow-up is primarily to monitor for stenosis (also fistula and aesthetics) – the **onset of spraying** is usually indicative of a stenotic process. Patients are seen regularly for ~3 years and then intermittently until after puberty.

- Early – haematoma, infection (uncommon with antibiotic prophylaxis), dehiscence (all of which may lead to fistulae)
  - Dehiscent wounds are probably better repaired after a delay.
- Late
  - Fistula (salvage surgery 10%; primary surgery 3%). See below.
  - Stenosis (early 2%; overall 7%; late strictures mainly due to BXO developing in preputial FTSGs).
  - Poor aesthetics.

FISTULAE

The suture lines in a hypospadias repair may be under adverse conditions, being continually bathed in urine under pressure, and the skin may be under tension due to oedema, erections and post-operative haematomas. In addition, multiple operations may have left tissues friable or scarred. There is probably also an element of infection. All this means that there is a significant risk of fistula formation; 90% are detectable within 1 week of operation.

- Early fistulae due to post-operative obstruction, extravasation, haematoma, infection.
- Late fistulae are usually said to be due to turbulent flow. They rarely close by themselves.

Generally, for **primary surgery**, the defect in the urethra should be closed carefully (e.g. Lembert inverting sutures) and avoid overlapping suture lines. Some suggest that the skin is closed in a double-breasted manner with one side de-epithelialised for 5 mm and sutured to the undersurface of the other side. Some propose using an interpositional dartos/fascial flap.

When repairing the fistula, it is important to ensure that there is no distal obstruction prior to reoperation; it is generally advisable to wait for the tissues to soften and for inflammation to settle.

Preputioplasty (foreskin reconstruction) is usually possible with most distal hypospadias, and some midshaft repairs, unless flap urethroplasty leaves insufficient skin.

IV. SPECIFIC TECHNIQUES

ONE-STAGE REPAIRS

Flip–flap one stage [original article in French]. (Mathieu D, *J Chir*, 1932)

This is a turnover of a ventral penile skin flap, distally based at the meatus and with parallel incisions, into the glanular groove to form the neo-urethra. However, as it uses abnormal urethral plate in the repair (which tends to be scar-like tissue), it is prone to problems with wound healing. It is suited for **distal hypospadias**. The technique has withstood the test of time, though its main drawback is the meatus that tends not to be very natural/aesthetic.

Transverse preputial island flap technique for repair of severe hypospadias. (Duckett JW, *Urol Clin N Am*, 1980)

This technique is described as being suitable for anterior urethral defects of 2–6 cm. The authors used **suprapubic catheters** for diversion.

- Subcoronal incision, release of chordee and erection test.
- Transverse preputial rectangle is marked out on inner preputial skin, as long as the anterior urethral defect and 12–15 mm in width. This island flap is tubularised around a catheter (suture line facing inwards against

tissue) and raised with Dartos fascia; it is anastomosed to the native urethra (spatulated) and then channelled through glans.

Onlay island flap in the repair of mid and distal penile hypospadias without chordee. (Elder JS, *J Urol*, 1987)

The senior author of this paper is Duckett. The urethral plate is preserved by U'-shaped incision around the meatus and along glandular groove lines. The penile skin is mobilised, fibrous chordee removed – if curvature persists, then dorsal tunica albuginea plication is performed.

- The thin/hypoplastic proximal urethra is excised.
- A TPI flap is raised, but instead of tubularising, it is inset into the 'U'-shaped incision as an **onlay** island flap.
- Closure of the lateral glans flaps and ventral penile skin using preputial skin flaps.

Tubularized incised plate urethroplasty for distal hypospadias. (Snodgrass W, *J Urol*, 1994)

This technique is suitable for distal hypospadias, or in conjunction with other modern techniques when urethral closure might otherwise be too tight. It is currently one of the most popular techniques for distal (and midshaft) hypospadias.

- Subcoronal degloving incision and chordee correction by tunica albuginea plication (Nesbit).
- Parallel longitudinal incisions at the edges of the urethral plate are made to create glans wings, and a midline incision is made in the urethral plate. The epithelial strips are closed ventrally leaving the dorsal defect to re-epithelialise.
- Waterproofing layer is closed followed by closure of glans wings.

MAGPI (meatoplasty and glanuloplasty): A procedure for subcoronal hypospadias. (Duckett JW, *Urol Clin N Am*, 1981)

This is used to produce a more terminally located meatus in cases of subcoronal hypospadias, especially where the glans is broad and flat. An incision is made in the cutaneomucosal junction of the prepuce. A deep vertical incision in the glans groove is made and then closed transversely with advancement of the meatus. The ventral lip of the meatus is lifted up with a stay suture and glans flaps closed beneath the elevated meatus.

Bulbar elongation and anastomotic meatoplasty (BEAM) for subterminal and hypospadiac urethroplasty. (Turner-Warwick R, *J Urol*, 1997)

This technique relies upon mobilisation of the bulbar urethra to gain sufficient length to allow advancement of the distal urethra to the glans tip. Ventral penile curvature may result from over-ambitious stretching; 2–2.5 cm in children and 4–5 cm in urethral length in adults may be gained.

- The meatus is wrapped by glans flaps or is tunnelled through, to a new terminal position. A slit-like meatus may be achieved by a Parkhouse procedure (double-spatulate the urethra at 6 and 12 o'clock positions and partially resuture, face to face).

Analysis of meatal location in 500 men. (Fichtner J, J Urol, 1995)

Analysis of meatal location in 500 men showed that 13% had hypospadias (glanular/coronal ratio = 3:1), and two-thirds of these were unaware of a penile anomaly; all but one (homosexual) had fathered children and all were able to micturate whilst standing. Only one case of subcoronal hypospadias was associated with penile curvature. Given these observations, the need for meatal advancement for distal hypospadias, potentially complicated by meatal stenosis and fistula formation, is questioned.

TWO-STAGE REPAIR

Duplay described the technique of **tubularisation** of the urethral plate (in French) in 1874, the general principle being that it can be tubularised as far as the tip of the glans. (The Snodgrass technique aimed to overcome difficulties in tubularising a narrow plate by incising it longitudinally.) In two-stage repair, preputial skin flaps are brought ventrally with second-stage tubularisation.

- Stage one – Subcoronal incision, release of chordee and glans split. The dorsal prepuce is split in the midline and brought ventrally around either side of the penis with skin closure in the midline.
- Stage two – Two vertical incisions from the native meatus to the neomeatus at glans tip and free edges sutured together to tubularise a neo-urethra. Direct ventral skin closure over this tube is possible due to previously imported preputial skin; closure in a double-breasted fashion.

MODIFIED CLOUTIER TECHNIQUE

Hypospadias repair: The two-stage alternative. (Bracka A, Br J Urol, 1995)

Stage 1 at 3 years of age (now usually about 1 year of age): tourniquet, 8F urinary catheter, erection test.

- Subcoronal incision and release of chordee; verify with repeat erection test.
- The glans is split and inner preputial FTSG placed with Jelonet tie-over dressing (buccal mucosal graft is preferred in the presence of BXO, harvested 1:1 vs. bladder mucosa that tends to shrink). FTSG restores the thin skin layer firmly adherent onto the glans tissue that flap techniques cannot achieve. The catheter is left in for 2 days with trimethoprim antibiotic prophylaxis. The patient is kept in hospital

until dressing change at 5 days under GA or sedation + EMLA cream.

Stage 2 – 6 months later:

- The grafted skin is tubularised around an 8F catheter, starting with a 'U'-shaped incision beneath the native meatus and allowing a width of 14–15 mm of skin for tubularising with minimal undermining.
- Close in two layers and cover with a waterproofing pedicled flap of Dartos fascia/subcutaneous tissue from the prepuce.

In very proximal repairs, insufficient tissue may be available for the waterproofing layer; in this situation, an anteriorly based fascial flap from the scrotum can be used. In most cases, the penis is circumcised rather than attempting to reconstruct the foreskin, which can often become tight and uncomfortable. The catheter is left for 6 days and augmentin antibiotic prophylaxis is given.

There is a significant **learning curve** the fistula rate is halved after the first 40 repairs (5% for all primary repairs but >20% for salvage procedures). It leaves a natural-looking meati, no suture marks and no stenosis.

Satisfaction with penile appearance after hypospadias surgery. (Mureau MA, J Urol, 1996)

There was no correlation between patient and surgeon satisfaction. Patients were less satisfied in general; patients with a glanular meatus were more satisfied than those with a retracted meatus. Satisfaction did not correlate with penile length.

Long-term follow-up of buccal, mucosa onlay grafts for hypospadias repair. (Fichtner J, J Urol, 1995)

This is a retrospective review of 132 patients with buccal mucosal onlay graft for hypospadias repair with an average of 6.2 years of follow-up. The overall complication rate was 24%, almost all occurring in the first year; thereafter the results were stable and long term.

Most surgeons agree that buccal mucosa has its advantages and, contrary to Hensle (J Urol, 2002), is a good choice in BXO patients. It is relatively thick, mechanically stiff and elastic; the lamina propria allows rapid graft take.

B. PERINEAL RECONSTRUCTION

I. EPISPADIAS AND EXSTROPHY OF THE BLADDER

EPISPADIAS

Epispadias is embryologically different from hypospadias. It is a developmental **abnormality of the abdominal wall that reflects abnormal development of the cloacal membrane** due to failure of rupture and mesenchymal ingrowth. Epispadias proximal to the bladder neck leads to incontinence. Other features include diastasis of recti, low-set umbilicus and widening of the pubic symphysis.

- In males – short penis, dorsal chordee, epispadic meatal dystopia, divergent corpora
- In females – short vagina, wide separation of the labia, bifid clitoris

EXSTROPHY OF THE BLADDER

It is a multisystem disorder with anomalies that fall along a spectrum – **bladder exstrophy epispadia complex**. Features of bladder exstrophy include abdominal wall defect, separation of the symphysis pubis and absent anterior bladder wall and eversion of the bladder. There is an increased risk of carcinoma if left untreated due to cystitis glandularis.

- Exstrophy plus epispadias (commonest combination) occurs in 1 in 30,000.

STAGED FUNCTIONAL RECONSTRUCTION

It may be diagnosed prenatally by ultrasound at 15–32 weeks. Treatment is often staged, but the optimal timing is unknown.

- Bladder and abdominal wall closed as a neonate – 1 week. Surgery within the first 72 hours may avoid osteotomy by virtue of maternal relaxin that facilitates manipulation and stabilisation.
  - Otherwise, osteotomies (bilateral anterior innominate and vertical iliac) are needed to allow closure of the symphyseal defect, whilst abdominal wall closure may need rectus muscle flap.
- Epispadias repair at 1–2 years of age. Surgery for epispadias is virtually the same as for hypospadias but conducted on the dorsal surface, and most common options are flip-flap types of procedure (Devine–Horton) or preputial island flap (Duckett). The phallus is usually small and hormonal treatment is often used.
- Bladder neck reconstruction at 3–4 years of age, e.g. Young–Dees–Leadbetter technique.

II. PEYRONIE'S DISEASE AND BXO

PEYRONIE'S DISEASE (PD)

The majority of patients with this condition have upward curvature with **thickening on the dorsal surface** of the tunica albuginea, with fibrosis extending into the septa between corpora; it is a similar phenomenon to Dupuytren's disease. It is rare before 40 years of age and may be related to repetitive trauma, especially to the semi-erect penis. Some suggest a causative role for TGF-β over-expression.

MEDICAL TREATMENT

- Xiaflex (collagenase) FDA approved in 2013
- Off label – pentoxifylline, verapamil (injections or topical), interferon α-2b
- Steroid injections/iontophoresis

- Ultrasound/shockwave
- Traction/vacuum devices
- Many others used, mostly lacking quality data:
  - Potassium aminobenzoate (Potaba, related to vitamin B complex) often used as first line but requires high dosage and may cause GI upset. Lacks data.
  - Vitamin E (lacks data), colchicine (significant side effects, RCT by Safarinejad MR, *Int J Impot Res*, 2004, showed no difference), tamoxifen (conflicting results, Teloken C, *J Urol*, 1999, no difference from placebo).

SURGICAL TREATMENT

Spontaneous resolution may occur in 50% – thus, it is uncommon to operate within 1 year of presentation. Surgery is indicated if the patient is unable to have intercourse; a penile prosthesis is a choice if the patient is bordering upon impotence.

- Nesbit procedure to plicate the ventral tunica; however, this shortens the penis and may cause erectile dysfunction (ED).
- Excision (or incision) of plaque and grafting of tunica defects with dermis (the use of dura, fascia lata, Alloderm, etc. has been reported); however, these materials can resorb or produce ballooning of the corpora and compromise erection.

An analysis of the natural history of Peyronie's disease. (Mulhall JP, *J Urol*, 2006)
PD when left untreated for at least 12 months: 12% improved in terms of angle, unchanged 40% and worsened in 48%. Pain tends to resolve after 12–18 months without treatment – and thus is not a good clinical endpoint.

BALANITIS XEROTICA OBLITERANS

BXO is a male genital form of lichen sclerosis of unknown aetiology, though some viral and HLA associations have been reported. It typically occurs in obese patients; a warm, moist uriniferous environment increases the risk. BXO accounts for many hypospadias cripples; chronic BXO may lead to SSC. There is a white stenosing band at the end of the foreskin, whilst a haemorrhagic response to minor trauma leads to phimosis and distal urethral stenosis – which may lead to higher pressures proximally.

- Early – dyskeratosis and inflammatory changes progressing to
- Late – fibrosis and skin atrophy, prepuce becomes adherent to glans

Treatment

- **Trial of steroid creams for early disease in children**. Slows progression but does not offer a definitive treatment.
- For disease restricted to the prepuce or glans, **circumcision** (allows glans to dry out) and/or meatoplasty.

Urethral dilatation or meatotomy is simple but will restricture. Often used as a temporising measure, but those with meatal/urethral disease will inevitably need definite excision and reconstruction.

- Narahari (*Cochrane Database Syst Rev*, 2008): no difference between dilatation or urethrotomy. Insufficient data to compare with urethroplasty.
- **Substitution urethroplasty**. Surgical excision of advanced disease and thick SSG; alternately may use buccal/lingual mucosal grafts, bladder mucosal grafts (fail to keratinise and tend to retain an ugly fleshy appearance). Recurrence can occur:
  - Genital FTSG – 18 months to 2 years
  - Postauricular FTG – >5 years
  - Buccal mucosa – none yet recorded

PENILE ENHANCEMENT

- Liposuction (of pubic fat pad), fat injection into shaft
- Partial/complete division of suspensory ligament (drops angle of erection)
- V–Y skin advancement from the pubic area
- Dermofat onlay grafts around tunica to increase girth
  - Tissue-engineered scaffolds, e.g. Maxpol-T (mostly PLGA), with or without cografted autologous fibroblasts, implanted under Buck's fascia through a circumcision incision (Jin Z, *J Androl*, 2011;32:491).

III. VAGINAL RECONSTRUCTION

PATHOLOGY

- Congenital absence (Meyer–Rokitansky–Kuster–Hauser syndrome) or segmental (imperforate hymen, long segment atresia)
- Congenital malformation – female hypospadias (1 in half a million) when urethral opening is in the anterior part of the wall
- Surgical ablation – e.g. tumour, mid-section excision for prolapse
- Radionecrosis – hostile tissues

SURGICAL OPTIONS

- **Local tissue**, e.g. vagina, vulva, skin. Vulval tissue expansion provides appropriate tissue with minimal donor defect and high success rate. However, treatment requires two stages and hospitalisation for 6–7 weeks during expansion.
- **SSG** (e.g. McIndoe technique for vaginal agenesis; however, skin graft take may be poor and requires a donor site).
- **Pedicled flaps** – bilateral groin flaps, TRAM (pedicled through the pelvis on IEA) or pedicled ALT or gracilis.
  - Bowel (jejunum, sigmoid colon) but tends to get stenosis at mucocutaneous anastomosis.

With post-radiotherapy defects, well-vascularised tissue on its own blood supply needs to be imported.

VAGINAL RECONSTRUCTION FOR HYPOPLASIA

Vaginoplasty in childhood usually has poor results; procedures are best deferred until after puberty.

- Pressure dilation – often first line
- Vaginoplasty

PRESSURE DILATION TECHNIQUES

Vaginal oestrogen creams or pessaries are useful; it results in a 'plumping' up and cushioning of the vaginal tissues, making it more comfortable to use dilators. Systemic HRT does not always produce an improvement in vaginal symptoms (dryness and atrophy), and local vaginal oestrogen may also be needed.

- **Intermittent pressure** (Frank method, 1938). Self-dilation is carried out with rounded rod-shaped appliances, and gentle pressure is applied (enough to cause mild discomfort), once or twice per day for 30 minutes. It can take from less than a month to over a year to complete; a motivated patient is needed.
  - Ingram (*Am J Obstet Gynecol*, 1981) developed a set of Lucite appliances and a specialised stool (the 'bicycle seat') that allows dilation to be carried out whilst the patient is clothed and in a sitting position. Modern dilators are also designed to be used in a seated position, but on an ordinary chair, thus removing the need for the cumbersome stool. The length can be increased in very small increments, which helps make the process less uncomfortable.
- **Continuous pressure (Vecchietti procedure).** The Vecchietti operation (1965) is well accepted in Europe. Pressure is applied in the vaginal area by a dilation 'olive', a plastic bead through which traction sutures or threads are threaded, and run up through the abdominal cavity to a traction device placed on the outside of the abdomen (this can be done with laparoscopic assistance). It is a true dilation-type neovagina. However, in contrast to the intermittent pressure technique using dilators by hand, which requires considerable patient, effort and time, the Vecchietti method applies constant round-the-clock traction to create a functional vagina (10–12 cm length) in 7–9 days. Intercourse is said to be possible after 3–5 weeks. The Vecchietti procedure is useful when manual dilation is excessively uncomfortable, or when progress is poor. Its relative advantages over manual dilation are greater when the vagina is initially represented by only a very shallow dimple. It does require flexible/elastic skin and thus is not suitable for those with scarring from previous operations.

VAGINOPLASTY

The **McIndoe** method is the most common surgical technique used and is variably attributed to McIndoe, Reed and Abbe. The neovaginal cavity is lined with split skin graft that is held in place with a stent for 7 days. The main problem is the strong tendency for the graft to contract, necessitating the conscientious use of dilators (or inter-course) daily. The graft donor site is also a concern for some patients. Variants include lining with FTSGs (Sadove) or with amnion (Sharma D, *J Gynecol Surg*, 2008), which is gradually replaced by vaginal epithelium.

- Davydov technique uses peritoneum freed from the pelvic side wall to line a newly excavated vagina; it can be performed laparascopically.
- Intestinal transposition and variants – A vagina is formed from a transplanted length of pedicled sigmoid colon (colovaginoplasty). This is possibly the most invasive of the techniques used and is not recommended as first-line treatment. It has a lower contracture rate compared with the McIndoe procedure, but there may be a problem with prolonged unpleasant mucous discharge (may respond to irrigation with short-chain fatty acids/steroids). In rare cases, adenocarcinoma in the segment of bowel has been reported.
- Fasciocutaneous flaps, e.g. Singapore (internal pudendal artery), vulvoperineal fasciocutaneous flaps (Malaga flaps), ALT, etc. at the expense of external donor scars. Avoid circumferential incision line at the introitus.

Classification of vaginal defects (Cordeiro PG, *Plast Reconstr Surg*, 2002) and common options:

- Type IA – anterior and lateral vaginal walls: Singapore flaps (Wee, 1989)
- Types IB – posterior wall: RA flap
- Type IIA – circumferential upper two-thirds: RA or sigmoid
- Type IIB – circumferential: bilateral gracilis

Comparison of two methods of vagina construction in transsexuals. (Van Noort DE, *Plast Reconstr Surg*, 1993) MTF surgery is three times commoner than FTM. An epithelium-lined cavity must be created between prostate/urethra/seminal vesicles and the rectum. Inversion of penile or penile and scrotal skin flaps is the most commonly used technique; scrotal skin is incorporated into neovagina or used to fashion labia. Other techniques include SSG, pedicled flaps or intestinal segments. Regular dilation post-operatively is achieved by stent and then intercourse. Complications include hair growth and skin prolapse.

C. DEFECTS OF THE CHEST WALL, ABDOMINAL WALL AND TRUNK

I. CHEST WALL AND STERNUM

Chest wall defects, fistulae and empyemas are the common problems.

- Clearance of cancer including breast or other chest wall malignancies – palliative surgery may be acceptable for advanced lesions.
- Radiation-induced ulceration. Of note, irradiated tissues tend to be stiffer and show fewer tendencies

for paradoxical chest movements post-resection. It may be difficult to distinguish between radiation ulcers and tumour on biopsy – the whole area should be resected, which would also remove tissues of poor vascularity. Vascular tissue in the form of pedicled or free muscle flaps is preferred.
- Congenital defects, e.g. pectus and Poland's syndrome.
- Trauma or post-operative, e.g. sternotomy wound dehiscence.

BRONCHOPLEURAL FISTULA

- **Millers** (*Ann Thorac Surg*, 1984) – Close cavity using as many flaps as necessary, using the same thoracotomy incision.
- **Arnoid and Pairolero** – use a separate incision, aim mainly to cover the fistula, rather than filling the space, which is left to close secondarily (*Plast Reconstr Surg*, 1989). The current consensus is that **filling is not necessary (and extremely difficult) as long as the cavity is clean.**

EMPYEMA

Empyema treatment is more successful if instituted early – surgery is easier, lung more likely to re-expand, etc. Others prefer to wait for the cavity to 'mature'. The basic strategies are

- **Space filling**, e.g. Miller (see above).
- **Space sterilising**
  - **Eloesser procedure** – use Eloesser flap (U-shaped flap folded into the cavity to allow drainage and packing, i.e. marsupialisation); irrigation with anti-biotic solution until the cavity granulates and is clean (can take a year). Originally left open but now can fill with antibiotic solution and close; 60% success rate.
    - Originally used for TB empyema in patients unfit for flaps.
  - **Clagett procedure** – multistage – inferolateral window of the chest wall with rib resection to allow drainage/irrigation; any fistulae are covered with flaps and when the cavity is clean, it is closed.
- **Space collapsing – thoracoplasty** is rare in modern practice; it is often a last resort if flaps are not suitable/available; staged removal of ribs (two to seven usually, keeping intercostal muscles intact) allows the chest wall to collapse down to obliterate/reduce the dead space. Additional delay will allow the volume of the cavity to reduce further through granulation, contraction of soft tissues and mediastinal shift.

FLAPS FOR CHEST WALL RECONSTRUCTION

Mostly local flaps are used.

- **PM** – advancement based on the thoracoacromial axis or turn-over flaps based on parasternal IMA perforators (type V). Both sides may be used.
  - Effective reach is rather limited.
  - IMA vessels may be compromised by CABG.

- **Pedicled TRAM/VRAM** for sternal wounds, in particular. The superiorly based rectus can still be harvested after use of the IMA (for CABG), being supplied by the eighth intercostal, but the inferior portion below the umbilicus is less reliable.
  - The flap can reliably reach the ipsilateral nipple/sternal notch, but the amount of muscle available is rather meagre.
- **Pedicled LD** (type V) – originally described by Tansini in 1906 for closure of a chest wall defect. Central back defects can be closed using bilateral advancement flaps.
  - It has a good arc of reach, which can be lengthened by about 5 cm if the tendon is cut; however, the distal portion is rather insubstantial.
  - It can be combined with other flaps based on the subscapular artery, e.g. SA.
- **Serratus anterior** (SA) for intrathoracic transposition (type III). It may cause shoulder discomfort and winging of the scapula in some.
  - The LD and SA may have been injured by prior surgery, i.e. axillary incision/thoracotomy.
- **Trapezius** is based on the transverse cervical artery (type II, minor pedicles from occipital artery and posterior intercostals) and can be harvested down to ~5 cm below the scapula. It can be used to cover defects of the upper back/nape.
  - Longer flaps can be used but are less reliable.
  - Shoulder weakness may occur if most of the muscle is harvested.
- **Breast sharing** (see below).
- **Omentum** (based on right gastro-epiploic artery) can be harvested trans-diaphragmatically or trans-abdominally (with or without laparoscopes). Incisional herniae are common sequelae. They are often a salvage choice.
- **Free flaps** may be considered in selected cases; bulky flaps such as LD, TRAM. Recipient vessels include thoracodorsal, IMA, intercostals and innominate veins.

SKELETAL RECONSTRUCTION

Paradoxical chest movement (with reduced efficiency of ventilation) may follow multiple rib removal, though the actual threshold for reconstruction is rather arbitrary. Dingman says **four ribs** will result in a significant flail segment; Pairolero says resection of four to six ribs can be tolerated, whereas some use **absolute size**, e.g. >5 cm (McCormack). In general, the young and fit are more tolerant of defect than the elderly; similarly, those with underlying lung disease will be less tolerant of a chest wall defect, whilst those with prior irradiation will be more tolerant due to tissue stiffness. Tolerance to chest wall surgery is largely determined by preoperative pulmonary function.

Options for skeletal support include the following:

- **Alloplastics.** These become semi-rigid and are generally satisfactory even if they need to be removed later (preferably wait for at least 6–8 weeks to allow a capsule to form). Meshes can be prone to complications particularly in irradiated wounds.
  - **Marlex mesh (polypropylene)** forms a fibrous capsule that is semi-rigid. Prolene mesh is double weave and stiff in both directions; it has a tendency to wrinkle (and fracture).
  - **Gore-Tex** is usually thick and does not conform well; it is characterised by a lack of tissue ingrowth/incorporation. It is more waterproof and thus potentially useful to separate cavities. It is more expensive and more prone to seroma formation.
    - **Dualmesh®** is textured on one side, smooth on the other.
  - **Methyl methacrylate** (MMA) sandwich with a cement layer ~ 0.5 cm thick – the tissues have to be protected from the exothermic chemical reaction as it is being fabricated. It can be reinforced with Marlex. The infection and extrusion rates are moderately high, but there is usually adequate strength from the capsule after half a year.
  - **Titanium**.
- **Autologous.**
  - **Bone** (little indication for rib grafts now, bone healing is unlikely given that there is usually very little cancellous bone to bone contact – the usual fibrous type of union does not offer effective support) or fascia grafts (often stretches, and is not resistant to infection).
  - **Muscle or fascial flaps**.

Design of the 'cyclops flap' for chest wall reconstruction. (Hughes KC, *Plast Reconstr Surg*, 1997)
This is essentially an axial pattern flap based upon the lateral thoracic artery, and breast tissue is advanced across the midline to leave the nipple in a more central position. The aesthetic result is poor but it is worth keeping in mind, being useful in situations where

- Scarring in the axilla may preclude a pedicled LD or microvascular anastomosis.
- Chest wall defect, e.g. full thickness excision of the chest wall precludes use of the internal mammary arteries or may be lost due to previous cardiac surgery.
- The patient may be unfit for a major procedure.

STERNAL WOUND DEHISCENCE

Sternotomy wound infections occur in 5% of cardiac procedures particularly after IMA harvest – 0.3% of unilateral harvests and 2.4% with bilateral harvests. The historical treatment was to lay open the wound and allow granulation; this had a high mortality rate – in addition to the sepsis, the paradoxical movement was extremely energy consuming. Shumaker (*Arch Surg*, 1963) used debridement and closed irrigation to reduce mortality to 20%; further advancement came in the form of debridement and **dead space closure** with vascular tissue, e.g. omentum (Lee AB, *Surgery*, 1976) or muscle flaps.

PAIROLERO CLASSIFICATION

- **Type 1** – within the first 3 days. There is a serosanguinous discharge with negative cultures. This is often minor and due to superficial wound infection, which can be treated with exploration, debridement and closure. Wires may need to be removed.
- **Type 2** – presents within the first 3 weeks, presenting with a purulent mediastinitis with positive cultures; there may be chondritis, with or without osteomyelitis.
- **Type 3** – presents late, usually months to years afterwards, typically with a draining sinus that connects to a focus of chronic osteomyelitis. There is often a dehiscence of the sternum itself. These should be treated with flap coverage after debridement.

STARZYNSKI CLASSIFICATION (STERNAL DEFECTS)

- Loss of upper sternal body and adjacent ribs – minimal physiological effect
- Loss of entire sternal body and adjacent ribs – moderate physiological effect
- Loss of manubrium and entire upper sternal body and ribs – severe effect

Exposed cartilage should be removed even if 'healthy'-looking as it is likely to be infected due to its poor vascularity. NPWT has become a good adjunct in the management of chest wounds, particularly of the sternal area; it temporises the wound, offers a closed wound management system obviating the need for frequent dressing changes and improves the wound condition both in terms of size and vascularity. Initial concerns that it reduces cardiac output (30% according to sonometric studies) were allayed by fMRI that showed much lower (10%) impairment. On the other hand, the splintage effect of NPWT aids ventilation and lung function.

RECONSTRUCTIVE OPTIONS (SEE ABOVE)

The wound tends to stiffen and dead spaces are almost impossible to close down just by approximation – they usually **need to be filled** with vascular soft tissue in the form of flaps that often also provide skin for the central defect. The PM and RA are first-choice flaps. The PM flap tends to fail in the lower part whilst the rectus tends to fail distally, i.e. superiorly, the salvage option being the other flap. **Delay may improve distal reliability**.

- **PM** – The muscle can cover the upper two-thirds of the sternal defect fairly reliably when pedicled on the thoracoacromial trunk.
  - The muscle is elevated off the ribs and pivoted on the thoracoacromial trunk (TAT); the humeral insertion can be divided, if necessary, via an additional incision in the deltopectoral groove. It can easily close the midline but is less suited filing a big dead space (Schulman NG, *Plast Reconstr Surg*, 2004).

- Turnover flap based on the IMA perforators is supposedly better for filling the dead space, but some length is 'wasted' in turning over. IMA harvest would make a turnover less reliable, but could effectively serve as a delay for the PM based on the TAT pedicle.
- Perkins (*Br J Plast Surg*, 1996) described bilateral PM advancement whilst keeping the IMA perforators intact to maintain chest wall/breast perfusion.
- **RA** – can cover the lower two-thirds of the sternal defect reliably. The most distal portion is least reliable, and thus the flap should be trimmed ruthlessly.

Second-line flaps include the LD (can cover the lower one-half of the sternum) and omentum, which can be very thin in typical patients, and Wening suggests preoperative laparoscopy (*Br J Clin Pract*, 1990). Other recently described flaps include

- Infra-areolar pectoralis major myocutaneous island flap (Simunovic F, *Plast Reconstr Aesthet*, 2012)
- Supraclavicular flap (Moustoukas M, *Plast Reconstr Surg*, 2012)
- Superior epigastric artery perforator flap (Saleh DB, *J Plast Reconstr Aesthet Surg*, 2014)
- Second IMA perforator flap (Koulaxouzidis G, *J Plast Reconstr Aesthet Surg*, 2015)

Free flaps anastomosed to neck or axillary vessels can be used in salvage situations, e.g. when lateral thoracotomy precludes use of pedicled LD.

- Used free muscle flaps to fill in persistent cavities; 8.7% had persistent empyema (Perkins DJ, *Br J Plast Surg*, 1995).
- Multiple flaps are needed to close the chest cavity completely; an average of 2.1 flaps were used in patients (Micheals BM, *Plast Reconstr Surg*, 1997) along with thoracoplasty in some cases.

II. CHEST WALL DEFORMITIES

POLAND'S SYNDROME

The chest defect was first described in a post-mortem examination by Alfred Poland at Guy's Hospital in 1841 of a convict called George Elt, without seemingly noticing the hand anomalies. The name was coined by Clarkson PW in 1962 who described a case with similar chest features and hand anomalies. It occurs in 1 in 25,000 live births affecting males three times more, and is on the right side in 75% of cases. There are many theories regarding its aetiology:

- Intrauterine vascular insult (subclavian artery disruption) or hypoxia during the stage of limb bud development (weeks 6 and 7).
- Genetic – familial tendency has been reported, although most cases are sporadic.

ESSENTIAL FEATURES (FLATT, 1994)

- Unilateral hand hypoplasia
- Syndactyly
- Brachydactyly of index, middle and ring fingers
- Absence of the sternocostal part of the PM (100%)

There may be many other features:

- **Chest wall defects**
  - **Deficiency of PM** (total aplasia or isolated loss of sternocostal head); variable deficiencies of **pectoralis minor, SA, LD** (thus may not be a reconstructive option), deltoid, supra- and infra-spinatus.
    - Isolated PM aplasia is more frequent and is not Poland's syndrome (Flatt, AE 1994); 13.5% of these have the full syndrome.
  - **Breast hypoplasia** or aplasia with a small NAC or absent nipples. The nipple is often higher.
  - **Others:**
    - Abnormalities of the anterior portion of the second to fourth ribs.
    - Deficiency of subcutaneous tissue.
    - Contraction of the anterior axillary fold.
    - Thoracic scoliosis, pectus excavatum, Sprengel's deformity.
- **Limb abnormalities**
  - Shortening of digits and syndactyly (simple, complete) – **brachysyndactyly** – the MPs are most affected.
  - **Hypoplasia** of the hand and forearm.
  - Foot anomalies.
- **Cardiovascular abnormalities**
  - Dextrocardia.
  - Hypoplastic or absent vessels (subclavian, thoraco-acromial, thoracodorsal).
  - **Consider angiography before reconstructing** breast with LD.
- **Other associated abnormalities**
  - Renal hypoplasia.
  - Congenital spherocytosis.
  - Increased incidence of leukaemia and NHL (should be ruled out).

Patients usually present for chest wall management at adolescence or early in adult life. The functional problems are usually minor. For optimal aesthetics, more severe skeletal deformities should be corrected before the breast.

- Women usually complain of breast maldevelopment.
  - The anterior axillary fold can be recreated with LD muscle transposition, inserting the tendon into the bicipital groove (Hester TR, *Plast Reconstr Surg*, 1982).
  - The LD muscle should be inset into the IMF inferiorly whilst avoiding an infraclavicular depression superiorly.
  - In the absence of a normal ipsilateral LD, a free contralateral LD can be considered, though ipsilateral recipient vessels may be hypoplastic also.

- Male patients tend to complain of a deficient axillary fold. Classically, the LD is used with or without customised silicone implants (alternatively a de-epithelialised flap).
  - The LD will atrophy somewhat unpredictably even if the innervation is kept intact.

PECTUS EXCAVATUM (FUNNEL CHEST)

Pectus excavatum tends to present in early childhood with a progressive worsening of the deformity – retrodisplacement of the **lower** one-third to one-half of the sternum, affecting males three times more often. This is **the most common** chest wall abnormality (90%–95%), occurring in ~8 in 1000 live births (some say 10× more common than pigeon chest). Most patients are asymptomatic, but some may have cardiopulmonary compromise. Psychological morbidity can be significant.

Early repair is advocated, with better results between the ages of 2 and 5 years; some believe that physiological impairment may be reversible before puberty. Others believe that damage to cartilaginous growth centres may lead to failure of growth (acquired asphyxiating chondrodystropy; Haller JA, *Ann Thorac Surg*, 1996). Many operations have been described; the actual indications are unclear as function is usually unaffected.

- **Sternal turnover**, e.g. Wada (*Ann Thorac Surg*, 1970): the devascularised sternum is at risk of **avascular necrosis** and infection.
  - Variations, e.g. leave one IMA intact (Ishikawa S, 1988).
- **Cartilage resection/remodelling**
  - **Ravitch technique** – sternal osteotomy, removal of deformed cartilages (leaving the perichondrium intact for regrowth, which takes 6 months or more) and **retrosternal strut for support**. It is a well-documented procedure with good long-term results. Originally described in 1949, there have been many modifications, particularly more conservative cartilage resection:
    - **Leonard modification** (2003) – removal of four to five cartilages whilst the perichondrium is left in place; a **wedge osteotomy** of the sternum is performed and a sheathed wire (instead of a bar) placed behind the sternum.
- **Cartilage remodelling without resection**
  - **Nuss procedure** (1998) – a 'minimally invasive technique' using 1 inch incisions on the lateral chest wall. A curved stainless-steel bar (moulded to the chest beforehand) is placed thoracoscopically behind the sternum and then 'flipped' 180°C to push the anterior chest out; fixation/stabilisation is usually needed. The bar is removed after 2–4 years, and long-term follow-up has shown ~5%–8% recurrence.
    - It is less likely to work well in adults or those with a marked deformity. There is a significant learning curve, and some studies have shown a longer hospital stay/greater analgesic requirements compared to the Ravitch (see Nasr A, *J Ped Surg*, 2010).

- Camouflage with silicone implant for less severe deformity/asymptomatic – 3D reconstructive CT can be used to design custom-made implants, often with Dacron backing. A submuscular plane is preferred.
  - Fat injection – though typical patients often lack the fat.

There is some evidence that surgery **reduces** lung function/capacity (Wynn J, *Thorax Cardiovasc*, 1990), which may be related to failure of growth of the thoracic wall after extensive surgery. Kaguraoka (*J Thorac Cardiovasc Surg*, 1992) found a 10% decrease in VC and F_{Exp} flow at 2 months, but these had recovered by a year. Some more recent studies with more dynamic or exercise studies seem to suggest less deleterious surgical effects. The cosmetic results and psychological benefits are not in doubt. Less extensive surgery such as the Nuss may improve cardiac function with less respiratory restriction.

Comparison of the Nuss and the Ravitch procedure for pectus excavatum repair: A meta-analysis. (Nasr A, *J Ped Surg*, 2010)

In this study, data were extracted from nine studies (there were no randomised trials). There was no difference in patient satisfaction; there were also no differences in overall complications, time to ambulation and length of hospital stay.

The rate of reoperation and haemo/pneumothorax was higher in the Nuss procedure. There was a trend towards a higher analgesic requirement in the Nuss procedure.

PECTUS CARINATUM (PIGEON CHEST)

Pectus carinatum is more common in males, with a family history in one-third; there is an **association with scoliosis** and heart disease (MVP) in 15%, as well as developmental conditions such as Noonan syndrome. The problem presents later in life than funnel chest, with one study reporting that half are found after about 10 years of age – it is mostly a cosmetic problem with only a minority with pulmonary problems. The mechanism seems to be related to overgrowth of the costal cartilages with displacement and buckling of the sternum.

- Chondrogladiolar protrusion – anterior displacement of the sternum, with protrusion of the ribs – most common, 90%.
- Lateral depression of ribs on the other side, which tends to be more common in those with Poland's syndrome (mixed carinatum and excavatum).
- Chondromanubrial (pouter pigeon chest) – upper prominence with inferior depression (a distal anterior displacement gives it a characteristic Z on lateral X-ray). This is the least common (3%) form and is often noted at birth. Patients should have echocardiogram to look for occult cardiac lesions (Fokin AA, *Chest Surg Clin N Am*, 2000).

TREATMENT

Orthotic bracing may work in younger patients.

SURGERY

- Ravitch-type procedures, e.g. Lester's method (1953) – partial costal cartilage resection/overlapping and wedge osteotomy of the sternum to achieve sternal depression. It is rather radical and is associated with significant blood loss.
  - Shamberger and Welch (*J Pediatr Surg*, 1988) with double or single wedge osteotomies.
- Ambramson (*J Pediatr Surg*, 2009) used a subcutaneous bar to apply pressure on the anterior chest wall, i.e. similar to Nuss. Works better in children.
- Breast augmentation in female patients may disguise the deformity, but there is a tendency for the nipple divergence to get worse.

III. ABDOMINAL WALL AND PERINEUM

The aim of reconstruction is the restoration of functional integrity of the abdominal wall; it is important to determine which components are missing. In addition, whilst immediate closure is usually desirable, it is also important to consider the implications of relocating abdominal viscera that may be swollen into an enclosed space – thus, consider pre-operative pulmonary function tests and assess the effect on respiration of closing the abdominal wall (e.g. for large incisional hernias).

Reconstructive options can be 'definitive' closure or as a temporising stage, i.e. debridement and SSG with or without the intervening stage of allowing granulation/NPWT. The latter option may be more suitable to allow local tissue inflammation (due to bowel fistulae, trauma, surgery or infection) to subside before attempting definitive reconstruction. Fabian (*Ann Surg*, 1994) suggested staging – (I) insertion of prosthetic mesh material that is allowed to granulate over 2–3 weeks; (II) remove mesh and approximate if possible; otherwise (III) SSG 2–3 days later to allow discharge home; and (IV) 6–12 months later for definitive reconstruction (mesh or components separation).

- NPWT will assist in increasing granulation tissue, reducing the defect size whilst stabilising the wound. However, whilst NPWT may simplify surgery, it is rarely able to provide definitive closure by itself.
- NPWT can be combined synergistically with tension devices, e.g. VADER, Topclosure or Proxiderm. They are a good option when the problem is mainly due to swollen viscera with little/no actual abdominal wall loss. See 'Closing difficult wounds'.
- SSG can be applied directly to viscera, but the results will be less stable, are prone to adhesions/herniation and will need to be replaced eventually.

INDICATIONS FOR ABDOMINAL WALL RECONSTRUCTION

Acquired:

- Tumours
- Traumatic including burns or iatrogenic, e.g. wound dehiscence, incisional hernia

- Necrotising fasciitis
- Post-radiation ulcers, etc.

Congenital

- **Diaphragmatic hernias** – ECMO has been an important development. Alloplastic mesh, e.g. PTFE, is commonly used for repair, but these do not have the capacity of growth and may lead to secondary deformities. Wung JT suggests that a short delay for surgery improved survival from 82% to 94% by waiting 100 hours instead of operating at 6 hours (*J Pediatr Surg*, 1995). Muscle flaps are probably better as the definitive repair.
- **Umbilical hernias** – many small hernias (<1 cm) close spontaneously after 1–2 years.
- **Omphalocoeles** – this is a persistent defect connecting (embryologically) the yolk sac to the midgut. It is usually >4 cm in diameter and often contains liver and midgut structures. After resuscitation, mesh can be used as a temporary measure before definitive reconstruction; a 'silo' can be made from silastic sheets if the contents are too large with gradual displacement back into the abdominal cavity over 3–4 days. Tissue expansion between the internal oblique (IO) and transversus abdominis or anterior to the rectus has been described.
- **Gastroschisis** – defect of abdominal wall to the right of the normal location of the umbilical cord due to mesoderm failure embryologically. Intestines are usually swollen and matted as the loops have been floating in the amnion for a period. Treatment is similar to omphalocoele.

- **Beckwith–Wiedemann** syndrome has a variety of midline abdominal defects; mutation on chromosome 11.

COMPONENTS SEPARATION TECHNIQUE (FIGURE 9.3)

- **Elevate skin flaps** from medial to lateral up to the anterior axillary line.
- **Incise the EO aponeurosis 1 cm lateral to linea semilunaris** and elevate in the relatively avascular plane between the obliques to the mid axillary line taking care to avoid damaging the IO fascia (dissecting to the posterior axillary line may give additional mobility).
  - **Check that you are in the right plane by stimulating the muscle and looking at their direction.**
- If necessary, release the **posterior rectus sheath** from the muscle, incise along the medial edge of the posterior sheath and release the rectus muscle from the sheath – this contributes to 2 cm of the advancement above and around the umbilicus.
- **Suture anterior rectus sheath and muscle in mid-line** with 0 nylon, and then advance skin flaps, with suction drains in the planes of dissection. Intraperitoneal mesh is often needed, whilst others suggest that any lateral fascial incisions should be covered by another mesh (with at least 5 cm overlap).
- **It is much easier to advance at the waist than the upper and lower thirds.**

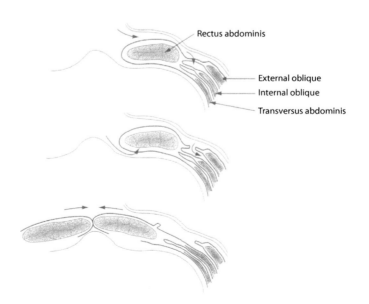

Figure 9.3 The components separation technique (CST) involves dissecting the plane between the oblique muscles, and then incising the rectus sheath to allow advancement of the rectus as a unit with the two inner muscle layers. This was described by Ramirez (*Plast Reconstr Surg*, 1990). Bilateral dissection allows advancement of 10, 20 and 6 cm at the epigastric, umbilical and suprapubic areas, respectively (i.e. very little movement inferiorly). Similar techniques had been described by Young (*Br J Surg*, 1961), but CST is a bit more nuanced.

FOR THE PERINEUM AND GROIN

In simple terms, muscle flaps will bring the best blood supply, but fasciocutaneous flaps are thin and potentially sensate. There are a number of pedicled flaps that are usually available.

- RA muscle, TRAM (high skin paddle including peri-umbilical perforators) or VRAM flaps. This is useful for reconstructing large perineal defects and can be transferred through the pelvis or subcutaneously; dis-insertion from the pubis allows greater mobility.
- The rectus femoris (RF) myocutaneous flap can be applied to most situations of perineal reconstruction but leaves a relatively poor donor site scar.
- ALT.
- Tensor fascia lata (TFL).
- Gracilis muscle or myocutaneous flap.
- Posterior thigh fasciocutaneous flap.

Free flaps – there are a wide choice including LD and TRAM – can be anastomosed to inferior gluteal vessels or vessels around the groin.

- Full thickness abdominal wall reconstruction using an innervated LD flap (Ninkovic M, *Plast Reconstr Surg*, 1998) or autologous fascial grafts (Disa JJ, *Plast Reconstr Surg*, 1998).

An algorithm for abdominal wall reconstruction. (Rohrich RJ, *Plast Reconstr Surg*, 2000)

ASSESS SIZE OF DEFECT

- Small defects can often be closed directly by undermining and local advancement, small random pattern fasciocutaneous flaps or skin grafts.
  - Larger defects may be reduced by NPWT then managed as above.
- Defects >15 cm may require axial flaps, tissue expansion or distant pedicled or free flaps. Distant flap from the **thigh** region, e.g.
  - TFL, RF, sartorius, gracilis.
  - Often limited by the size and arc of rotation, only suitable for lower defects. Large anterior thigh flaps based on either anterolateral or anteromedial perforators have been used to cover large defects of the anterior abdomen up to the level of the xiphisternum (Lin SJ, *Plast Reconstr Surg*, 2010).

FASCIAL RECONSTRUCTION

- **Prosthetic materials**, e.g. nylon/polypropylene mesh (**Marlex/Prolene**), can be used on clean wounds; granulation tissue comes through the mesh that will be graftable, offering a temporising option. There are many varieties, but eventual herniation should be expected in all. Marlex is said to be stronger (like autogenous fascia) than Gortex but with a higher risk of adhesions.

- **Gore-Tex** elicits little foreign body reaction, supposedly producing fewer adhesions and being easier to remove. Strength is about the same according to Law (*Acta Chir Scand*, 1990), though it requires a larger overlap. Similar strength at 8 weeks confirmed by Jenkins (*Surgery*, 1983).
- Composite meshes are becoming popular – combining incorporation on one side with reduced adhesions on the other, e.g. Dacron/Mersilene coated with vicryl or different porosity Gore® **Dualmesh** (ePTFE/Gore-Tex with a smooth surface and a 'corduroy' surface).
- Meshes are generally not recommended in infected wounds, even absorbables such as Dexon or Vicryl (90 day lifespan in clean wounds, much shorter in infected wounds).
- Stoppa (*World J Surg*, 1989) suggests retroparietal preperitoneal positioning of a patch of ample size.
- Free or vascularised **fascia lata** (TFL flap or thigh flaps). If mesh is contraindicated by the presence of potentially contaminated tissue, autologous fascia lata grafts can be used instead, though supply is limited; take care to leave the tendon of the iliotibial tract to maintain lateral knee stability. The fascia, even when 'vascularised', tends to be remodelled over a year or more.
- Collagen substitutes or acellular dermal matrices (ADMs), e.g. Permacol™ – acellular porcine collagen, Alloderm (decellularised human dermis).
  - Synthetics are stronger but less resistant to infection, and are likely to have more tissue adhesion/fistulae.
  - There has been a decreasing trend in the use of allogeneic materials. Porcine collagen is most frequently used; processing by crosslinking is not that helpful.
  - Long-term outcome depends largely on fascial continuity; if the ADM is 'bridging' a fascial defect, then it will fail in about half of the cases; but if it does not need to bridge, i.e. fascial continuity can be established and the mesh is a reinforcing layer, then the failure rate is ~10%.

DIAGRAM OF ONLAY/INLAY

Wound closure in large defects

Midline defects

Components separation or lateral releasing incisions to advance fasciocutaneous flaps medially. Alternatively, Thomas (*Plast Reconstr Surg*, 1993) describes fascial partition/release, with parasagittal incisions in the EO and TA fascia, and closure reinforced with mesh.

The donor defect after a **bipedicled TRAM** harvest is a special case. Some suggest that it is important to leave as much anterior sheath attached to the linea alba as possible. Hartrampf (*Plast Reconstr Surg*, 1985) says the linea semilunaris is also important; the full width of muscle and sheath should not be removed below the lowest tendinous intersection to leave a fixation point and avoid muscle retraction; mesh was used in one-fourth of his cases. Some surgeons routinely use mesh in this repair.

Lateral defects

Upper third
- Superiorly based RA from the other side
- External oblique (EO)
- Extended LD flap
- Extended TFL, subtotal thigh

Middle third
- RA (including extended deep inferior epigastric flap)
- EO
- TFL, RF, subtotal thigh

Lower third
- Inferiorly based RA (including extended deep inferior epigastric flap)
- Internal oblique (IO)
- TFL, RF, vastus lateralis (VL), gracilis, groin flap, subtotal thigh

FREE TISSUE TRANSFER

The freedom of movement with free flaps means that they may be applied to upper, middle and lower third defects.

- Free LD myocutaneous flap, which can be anastomosed to the superior epigastric pedicle and re-innervated by coaptation of the thoracodorsal nerve to intercostal nerves supplying rectus abdominis, which in theory provides muscle contraction to the abdominal wall and can avoid using mesh.
- Alternatively, TFL innervated muscle transfer as described by Ninkovic.
- Subtotal thigh flap/ALT with pivot point about 2 cm below the inguinal ligament.
- Other recipient vessels include
  - Deep inferior epigastric vessels
  - Deep circumflex iliac vessels
  - Internal mammary vessels

GROIN RECONSTRUCTION

Soft tissue coverage of the groin may be needed following complications of surgery in this area:

- Infected prosthetic vascular grafts
- Complications following groin node dissection

GRAFT INFECTION

Despite precautions, such as strict aseptic technique and prophylactic antibiotics for the placement of prosthetic vascular grafts, infections may still occur particularly in the groin.

The reasons for this are possibly multifactorial: superficial location of graft, bacterial colonisation, proximity to the perineum and severed lymphatics leading to collections.

In the past, the gold standard treatment has been graft removal followed by extra-anatomic bypass; however, the risk of death or subsequent amputation is high, and total eradication of the infection cannot be guaranteed. The need for graft removal has been challenged and current recommendations are less dogmatic. Consequently, others have tried less radical treatments, particularly in situ replacement with veins, arterial homografts or prosthetic grafts; rifampicin and silver compounds bonded with the graft placed in an anatomic position have similar mortality and limb loss rates according to some studies. Other measures include the following:

- **Wound preparation** – the infection needs to be controlled through adequate debridement with removal of all necrotic tissue. Some have used NPWT, but patients need to be carefully selected.
- **Antibiotics** – the use of antibiotics is almost universal, but choices and protocols are variable – it is common to give 4 weeks intravenously followed by 6 weeks orally. Before positive identification of organisms, empirical treatment usually consists of vancomycin and a third-generation cephalosporin.
- **Local muscle flaps** have proved invaluable in treating infected wounds; the muscle bulk fills the 'dead' space after debridement and provides well-vascularised tissue that is resistant to infection, reduces bacterial count and improves wound healing. It also increases antibiotic delivery, local tissue oxygenation and phagocytic activity. The local outcome is excellent in most studies with reduced hospital stay. See 'Individual flaps'.
  - Sartorius
  - Gracilis
  - RF
  - RA
  - TFL
  - Vastus lateralis (VL)

OTHER FLAP-RELATED ISSUES

- **Fasciocutaneous (FC) flaps** – it has been demonstrated in certain cases that muscle is not always necessary for the treatment of infected wounds. FC ALT perforator flaps have successfully treated osteomyelitis wounds and graft infections. It is emerging that as long as the flaps used are well vascularised, and the basic concepts of adequate debridement and dead space obliteration are adhered to, then the actual type of flap is less important.
- **Free flaps** – there may be uncommon situations when suitable local tissues become unavailable, and in such cases, there are a wide range of free flaps available. These flaps have been shown to have reasonably good success rates even in patients with peripheral vascular disease, though careful planning is needed and vein grafts are often necessary.

IV. POSTERIOR TRUNK

Apart from tumours and infections, defects of the posterior trunk may result from

- Spina bifida/dysraphism with myelomeningocoele the commonest – associated with hydrocephalus (VP shunt) and neurogenic bladder in over 90%. Protect with damp non-adhesive dressings and then close in a tension-free manner with vascularised tissue, e.g. LD for upper defects (there are fewer options for lower trunk).
- Spinal surgery wound dehiscence.

Flap choices depend on the location of the defect:

- Upper third – trapezius myocutaneous flap based on transverse cervical artery
- Middle third – LD based on thoracodorsal pedicle
- Lower third:
  - LD turnover flap
  - Lumbar artery perforator flaps
  - Gluteus maximus or S-GAP flap
  - Bipedicled fasciocutaneous flaps, keystone flaps

Other options include

- Tissue expansion
- NPWT and SSG

Management of massive thoracolumbar wounds and vertebral osteomyelitis following scoliosis surgery. (Mitra A, *Plast Reconstr Surg*, 2004)

This is a review of a series of 33 patients with large thoracolumbar wounds following scoliosis surgery with exposed metalwork, osteomyelitis and large dead spaces.

PRINCIPLES OF MANAGEMENT

- Expedient return to theatre
- Wound irrigation
- Thorough excisional debridement of non-viable bone and soft tissue
- Specimens for culture
- **Vascularised tissue cover**
  - Superior wounds:
    - Myocutaneous extended LD flap – the fasciocutaneous extension of the flap, beyond the inferior muscle edge, is de-epithelialised and turned into the defect to help obliterate dead space. The donor site is grafted.
  - Inferior wounds:
    - Whole gluteus maximus muscle islanded on the superior gluteal vessels and rotated into the defect after insertions on the iliac bone, sacrum and gluteal fascia are divided, and also released laterally from the iliotibial tract and the femur.
      - This flap was only used in non-ambulatory patients.
      - Some wounds also required inferiorly based FC flaps to supplement closure.
      - The metalwork was able to be retained in all patients.
- Closed suction drainage

10

Aesthetic

I. LASERS: PRINCIPLES AND SAFETY

- 1916 – Einstein's theory of stimulated emission of radiation.
- 1957 – Townes, Schawlow and Gould laid down the principles for **light amplification by stimulated emission of radiation** (LASER). As always, at the time there was a side story with patents, lawsuits etc. between the protagonists.
- 1960 – Maiman built the first laser using a synthetic ruby crystal placed inside a coiled flashlamp inside a Fabry–Pérot etalon (two parallel flat semi-transparent mirrors in a tube – light that enters is reflected multiple times, and the resulting interference modulates the beams).

Soon after this, developments came quickly; the helium neon, neodymium:yttrium aluminium garnet (Nd:YAG), CO_2 and argon lasers were all developed in the early 1960s.

COMPONENTS OF A LASER

- Energy source
  - Electricity (argon laser)
  - Flashlamp (pulsed-dye laser)
  - Another laser (CO_2 laser)
- Laser medium – solid or gas
- Laser cavity (resonator)

The laser medium is energised to excite electrons into a higher energy state (singlet state in an unstable orbit around the nucleus). As electrons move back into a stable orbit, a photon of light of a particular wavelength is emitted. Photons hitting excited atoms generate more photons, i.e. **stimulated emission**. Photons move randomly in the resonator, but through the action of a pair of mirrors, they become a parallel or **collimated** laser beam all with the same wavelength. Thus, laser light travels in the same direction (without spreading out), same phase and wavelength – these characteristics are in decreasing order of importance to the clinical effect.

Continuous wave lasers may have their output interrupted intermittently by a mechanical shutter to form a pulsed wave (pulsed-dye laser) with higher energy and peak temperature.

- Q-switching (QS) – electromagnetic switch produces ultra-short pulse duration in the nanosecond range; newer lasers have picosecond pulse duration.
- Pulsing and ultra-pulsing deliver higher energy.

When the laser beam contacts the target, the light can be

- **Reflected** (by the same colour).
- **Transmitted** – passes through unchanged.
- **Refracted** – passes through with a directional change.
- **Scattered** – by dermis (collagen).
- **Absorbed** – clinical effects occur when laser light is absorbed by 'chromophores'. Different **chromophores** maximally absorb light at different wavelengths; they are of the opposite/complementary colour. Absorbed laser light is predominantly converted to heat (photo-thermal), i.e. a laser is a very precise, controllable source of heat; sometimes there are photomechanical or photochemical reactions.
  - Matching peak absorption of the target chromophore to the laser wavelength increases efficacy; however, some other chromophores will also absorb the laser light to a lesser extent, leading to collateral damage.

The shorter the wavelength, the more scatter and reflectance, or the corollary is that **longer wavelengths allow better penetration**. The absorption coefficient of tissues also determines penetration. The depth of penetration is proportional to the following:

- Degree of scatter
- Absorption by chromophores
- Energy delivered
- Wavelength of the laser beam

Gaussian distribution of heat within the laser spot means that 10% overlap is usually not harmful. **Multiple passes do not produce additive effects** – the first pass causes coagulation and changes the optical properties of the tissue; thus, a second pass achieves only 50% coagulation compared with the first.

Selective photothermolysis: Precise microsurgery by selective absorption of pulse radiation. (Anderson RR, *Science*, 1983)

The principle of **selective photothermolysis** (Anderson and Parrish) aims to target the following:

- Wavelength of laser light specific to chromophores of that tissue with sufficient energy to destroy the target
- Pulse width to maximise destruction of chromophores without collateral damage:
  - A pulse width less than the **thermal relaxation time** of the tissue (Tr = time to cool to 50% of initial temperature achieved) limits thermal diffusion and thus minimises unwanted collateral damage.
    - If the rate of heating is slower than the rate of cooling, then the thermal energy is spread to the surrounding tissue. The effects (including side effects) are spread out instead of being localised.
  - Diameter of a vessel determines its thermal relaxation time.
  - Fluence above threshold for destruction of that chromophore.

For example, the argon laser (457–514 nm) aims to target haemoglobin (and cause coagulation), but the chromophore absorption peaks and Tr are as follows:

- Melanin (500–600 nm) – 1 μs
- Haemoglobin (577–585 nm)

Thus, if an argon laser is used to treat VMs, it will cause depigmentation because melanin also absorbs this wavelength. The darker a patient's skin colour, the more likely that there will be pigmentation changes after laser treatment.

LASER SAFETY

- Laser plume can contain viable bacteria and viruses including human papillomavirus (HPV), HIV and hepatitis B (HBV), although the actual infection risk is difficult to quantify. Good smoke evacuation systems and protection in the form of masks and gloves are needed.
- Tissue splatter with Q-switching.
- Goggles are needed for eye protection (patient and doctor) and are not interchangeable between lasers.
- Fire and electrical shock hazards.

INDIVIDUAL LASERS

CO_2 LASER

The CO_2 laser was one of the first medical lasers.

- Gas mixture includes helium and nitrogen – helium provides targeting beam as for laser pointers. The 10,600 nm wavelength is in the infrared spectrum and is absorbed by water in the tissues and leads to vaporisation of the superficial layers of skin.
- It is often used as a surgical scalpel in neurosurgery and ENT surgery or for superficial ablation/rejuvenation. Leukoplakia, warts with no pigmentation, and other superficial cutaneous or mucosal lesions can also be ablated with CO_2 laser.

ARGON LASER

- 457–514 nm **blue–green** light, continuous wave and mechanical shutter.
- Usual target chromophores are haemoglobin and melanin. It is effective in treating PWS but
  - Shallow penetration depth ~1 mm and increased energy required, increases risk of scarring

PULSED-DYE LASER (PDL)

- Fluorescent dye absorbed in water or alcohol; flashlamp stimulates emission of light that is tuned to 400–1000 nm depending upon the dye used, but is usually 577–585 nm (**yellow**) for most clinical applications.
  - The pulse duration is very short.
  - Penetration 1.2 mm at 585 nm.
- It is good for VMs with a high concentration of oxyhaemoglobin; there will be transient purple discolouration when used in the treatment of PWS.

ND:YAG LASER

- Laser media consists of yttrium aluminium garnet (YAG) crystals in which neodymium is an impurity (YAG crystals can also be grown in erbium – Erb:YAG 2940 nm). It emits light at 1064 nm; it is poorly absorbed by haemoglobin, melanin and water, allowing **greater penetration**. Machines are usually Q-switched with nanosecond pulses; newer picosecond lasers offer good results in tattoo removal.

- 1064 nm (infrared) wavelength is useful for pigmented lesions and hair removal, particularly in darker-skinned patients.
- 532 nm (green yellow, frequency doubled) has been used for haemangiomas and VMs, also used in ophthalmology for retinal photocoagulation.

RUBY LASER

- Flashlamp stimulation produces 694 nm **(red) light.**
- May be used for tattoos or hair removal (only safe for those with very pale skin).

ALEXANDRITE LASER

- Emits light at 755 nm **(red).**
- It can be used for hair removal but is not safe for darker skins.

II. LASERS IN PLASTIC SURGERY

If the properties of a laser can be matched to a particular clinical problem, then they will be effective with relatively few side effects.

LASER TREATMENT OF VASCULAR LESIONS

- The most commonly treated vascular lesions are PWS (see also Chapter 8, Section E), a practice that seems well established.
- Use of lasers for haemangiomas is more controversial. There may be a role in superficial or ulcerating lesions but probably not in those with significant deeper components.
  - Rizzo (*Dermatol Surg*, 2009). Haemangiomas in patients with median of age 3 months were treated with 595 nm long-pulse PDL with dynamic cooling device (DCD) at 2 to 8 week intervals. They reported near-complete/complete clearance of colour in 81% and reduced thickness in 64%. There were pigmentation problems in 18%.
- **Warts** can be treated with PDL (being relatively vascular, and may be preferred to CO_2); shaving the top off beforehand may help penetration – note that HPV particles may be found 1 cm away from the visible wart.
- Hypertrophic scars can also be treated with PDL (Alster TS, *Plast Reconstr Surg*, 1998).

Choice of laser depends on the vessel size of the target:

- Small vessels 30–40 µm, e.g. PWS, can be treated with argon (488 nm), PDL.
- Medium-sized 100–400 µm, e.g. haemangioma, with a KTP laser.
- Large vessels >400 µm, e.g. VeM, with a Nd:YAG laser (>100 ms).

Note that lesions such as PWS may have variable appearances in terms of colour, texture and distribution, probably representing different vessel configurations; these will respond differently to specific lasers, e.g. light pink-red lesions respond much better to PDL than darker lesions.

Surface cooling has been useful to reduce superficial damage whilst allowing higher energies to be delivered. Candela's VBeam is a PDL (595 nm for deeper penetration) with a DCD that delivers a pulse of cryogen spray just before the laser pulse. Other methods of tissue cooling include gels, contact and air-cooling; the timing may be pre-, parallel or post-cooling.

- Excessive cooling can cause epidermal damage and hyperpigmentation (Handley JM, *J Am Acad Dermatol*, 2006).

Randomised controlled study of early pulsed-dye laser treatment of uncomplicated childhood haemangiomas. (Batta K, *Lancet*, 2002)

One hundred twenty-one infants (<14 weeks) were randomised to PDL treatment or observation only. Large, deep or complicated (obstructing vital structures) lesions were excluded. Follow-up at 1 year showed no difference between observational and laser-treated groups in terms of clearance of haemangioma, but skin atrophy and hypopigmentation rates were **higher in the treatment group**. The authors concluded that PDL is **not better** than 'wait-and-see' in simple lesions.

PDL penetrates to ~1.2 mm and so is only effective for superficial early haemangiomas; 93% were apparently <1 mm in height in this study.

Kolde (*Lancet*, 2003) criticised the study for including infants that were too young. In his opinion, early haemangiomas have solid cell nests that are not yet perfused and thus less susceptible to PDL. Results from other studies suggest that matured lesions (at least 11 weeks old) and slightly nodular lesions responded better than initial macular lesions. On the other hand, some suggest that early treatment when lesions are still flat would be better, emphasising the need for more controlled studies.

Treatment of pulsed-dye laser-resistant port wine stain birthmarks. (Jasim ZF, *J Am Acad Derm*, 2007)

This paper reviewed the options for PWS that do not respond to 577/585 nm PDL – most studies suggest that **less than 20% can be lightened almost completely**, 70% will lighten by half or more whilst 20%–30% respond poorly, particularly the central face and the limbs. The reasons for variable response are unclear but may be related to the vessel configurations and depth. Strategies to improve PDL treatment include use of 595 nm with cooling, longer pulse duration/larger spot sizes for deeper lesions and pulse stacking. Other options discussed include intense pulsed light (IPL) with cooling, alexandrite (755 nm), diode (810 nm) and Nd:YAG (1064 nm).

LASER TREATMENT OF PIGMENTED LESIONS

Melanin has absorption peaks lying within 500–600 nm; towards the red end, there is less haemoglobin absorption. For laser treatment to be successful, the pigment must be within the range of the laser. QS-Nd:YAG has deeper penetration but has relatively poor absorption by melanin; thus, **higher energies are required**. On the other hand, QS-532 has good absorption by melanin but only superficial penetration and is also absorbed by haemoglobin; thus, there is purpura and possibly pinpoint bleeding.

- **Dermatoses**, e.g. naevus of Ota (NoO), naevus of Ito and blue naevus can be treated with QS ruby laser or QS-Nd:YAG.
  - A similar condition is acquired bilateral naevus of Ota-like macules (ABNOM), aka Hori's macules, seen as a bluish hyperpigmentation of bilateral malar regions. It is more resistant than NoO to QS lasers and often needs repeating before repigmentation occurs with the rationale of treating deeper chromophores.
- **Naevi** – two-thirds of benign naevi respond to laser, but dysplastic naevi should not be treated by laser. Some have used lasers to treat congenital naevi, but the malignant potential still exists, and complete clearance is very unlikely.
- **Lentigines.** Ablative or QS lasers (Nd:YAG, KTP 532). Inflammation, purpura and post-inflammatory hyperpigmentation (PIH) are seen in 10%–25% of cases. Melanin has a very broad absorption spectrum, and if longer wavelengths are used (600–1200 nm), there is reduced absorption by haemoglobin, and consequently less purpura.
- Also see 'Tattoos and hair removal'.

Some lesions are known to **respond well to laser**, e.g. café au lait macule (CALM); the response in others can be first observed in a test patch.

- Best results – freckles, **NoO, lentigines**
- Variable results – CALM (recurrences are common, whilst some lesions may darken), Beckers
- Controversial, somewhat – acquired naevi, melanocytic naevi (see above)

Successful treatment of a giant congenital naevus with the high-energy pulsed carbon dioxide laser. (Kay AR, Br J Plast Surg, 1998)

Pulsed CO_2 laser, i.e. ablation, was used to treat a giant congenital naevus in a 44 day old infant who had been unsuccessfully treated by curettage. Near-full healing was achieved by 2 weeks.

Arons (*Br J Plast Reconstr*, 1998) responded to the article above to highlight the point that it was premature to say that the lesion had been 'successfully' treated after only 4 month follow-up.

Combined use of normal and Q-switched ruby laser in the management of congenital melanocytic naevi. (Kono T, Br J Plast Surg, 2001)

Normal mode ruby light (NMRL) was used first to remove the epidermis and facilitate greater penetration of the QS ruby laser (QSRL) that effectively destroys naevus nests.

A similar strategy was used in giant congenital melanocytic naevi by Michel (*Eur J Dermatol*, 2003). Kishi (*Br J Dermatol*, 2009) used early QSRL alone, and it took an average of 9.6 treatments to reduce the colour of lesions in their nine patients to within 0%–20% of the baseline.

MELASMA ('MASK OF PREGNANCY')

Melasma may be caused in part by hormones such as thyroid hormones, MSH from stress as well as UVL. The dyspigmentation is due to the presence of more cells that are more active; a Wood's lamp enhances epidermal pigment, but not dermal (which tends to be blue/black).

- **Bleaching creams** (see below) do take a while to have an obvious effect, but are first-line treatment, because other treatments are not terribly effective and have significant risk of complications. Chemical peels may also be considered.
- In persistent cases, treatment is challenging; **cautious light treatment** may be tried (after pretreatment with sunblock and topical bleaching for at least 6 weeks). There is a risk of PIH or of converting epidermal melasma to dermal melasma, which is even more difficult to treat.
  - Lasers generally have poor results and high risk of complications particularly PIH (due to stimulation of hyperactive melanocytes), even when using long-pulse Nd:YAG.
  - IPL may lead to improvements of ~30%–40%, but there is a 10%–15% risk of PIH.
  - Early promise from fractional lasers, e.g. Fraxel Re:store (which had FDA approval), was tempered by high recurrence rates and inconsistent results.

TRIPLE THERAPY

- **Hydroquinone** (HQ, 2%–4%) blocks the tyrosinase enzyme (dopamine to melanin) of the melanogenesis pathway. Increased concentrations have increased effects but with more complications – skin irritation and phototoxicity. Treatment breaks are required to maintain effectiveness.
- **Tretinoin** (0.05%–0.1%) (trans-isomer) increases keratinocyte turnover, thus limiting transfer of melanosomes to keratinocytes. Full effects take 6 months.
  - Steroid antagonist; therefore, may reduce steroid side effects.
  - Irritation may improve HQ and alpha-hydroxy acid (AHA) penetration.

- Complications include photosensitivity – it should only be applied at night. It should be avoided during pregnancy due to teratogenic effects.
- **Azelaic acid** 20%. The effectiveness is similar to 2% HQ, but with fewer side effects; the precise mechanism of action is unknown. It is anti-microcomedogenic and possibly antimicrobial; it can be used to treat acne and lentigines. The combination of tretinoin and AHA is well tolerated.

The classic mix is the **Kligman formula** – HQ 5%, tretinoin 0.1% and dexamethasone 0.1% (steroids reduce irritation). A proprietary pre-mix is Tri-luma® (0.01% fluocinolone, 4% hydroquinone and 0.05% retinoic acid), which is FDA approved (2002) for treatment but not maintenance; in controlled trials, 63% of patients had at least one adverse event, most commonly erythema and desquamation.

Predicting the outcome of laser treatment for pigmented lesions. (Grover R, *Br J Plast Surg*, 1998)
This study used 2 mm punch biopsy and immunohistochemistry in 32 patients to predict outcome following laser treatment. They found that unfavourable indicators were depth of melanocytes >0.3 mm and significant amelanocytosis (>20%) – amelanotic melanocytes are refractory to treatment but, following treatment, may form melanin and be a cause of hyperpigmentation.

Treatment of minocycline-induced cutaneous pigmentation with the picosecond alexandrite (755 nm) laser. (Rodrigues M, *Dermatol Surg*, 2015)
Minocycline-induced pigmentation is a rare side effect that can take years to resolve. The mainstay treatment has been QS alexandrite laser, usually requiring several treatments. The authors found that 1-2 treatments with the 755 nm picosecond laser was sufficient.

TATTOOS

Ink/pigment is implanted into the skin during tattooing. After approximately 1 month, the tattoo fades slightly due to clearing of epidermal ink, and ink then becomes sequestered into cells — keratinocytes, macrophages and fibroblasts – and in a fibrous granulation tissue. At first, the distribution is diffuse; then the ink aggregates together, moving deeper into the dermis where it cannot move back into the epidermis once the basement membrane reforms. Thus, most ink in stable tattoos is **intracellular and immobilised**.

- Professional tattoos can involve a wide variety of inks, but in general, they are fairly inert, and reactions are rare (those that do react usually involve red/yellow – they may disappear spontaneously). The reaction to laser can be unpredictable, and a test patch is advisable.
- Amateur tattoos are generally easy to remove with lasers – the blue-black ink typically used is placed in small amounts, relatively superficially, but it can be quite inconsistent.

- Traumatic tattoos can contain a variety of debris, e.g. gravel or metal. Caution is required in treating firework injuries.

TATTOO REMOVAL

A variety of mechanisms can be used to remove the superficial layers of skin for patients who do not mind the scarring.

- Salabrasion is one of the oldest methods.
- Surgery – e.g. dermabrasion or tangential excision and skin grafting.
- Thermal infrared coagulator – results are similar to other nonspecific methods, i.e. scarring and incomplete response.
- Ablative lasers such as CO_2 target water in the tissues; one treatment to vaporise 30%–50% of the overlying skin (often combined with urea paste over 10–14 days to leach out the remaining pigment), leaving a patch like a superficial burn scar.

LASER TREATMENT OF TATTOOS

Different lasers with different wavelengths are needed for different pigments; thus, multicoloured professional tattoos will need repeated treatments with different machines. The majority of lasers used for tattoo removal are Q-switched lasers (QSLs; see below). New picosecond laser machines e.g. Picosure® are promising.

Q-SWITCHED LASERS

QSL can deliver pulses in the nanosecond range with high peak energies that cause photomechanical fragmentation of the pigment (rapid expansion and rupture of melanosomes) that can then be phagocytosed, facilitating clearance.

- The immediate effect is whitening of the skin without blistering or bleeding. One problem is **splatter** due to the force of the shock wave, and the debris may contain cells, viable viruses or other microorganisms with infectivity.
- Several treatments (6–8 weeks apart) may be needed. **Nitrogen bubble** formation from the rapid expansion and causing whitening is said to prevent further laser light penetration; thus, only one pass is possible at a time.
- The wavelength of the laser light needs to be matched to the pigment, but the exact composition of the ink is often unknown, contributing to the variable and inconsistent responses seen.

Red and black are easiest to remove, green and purple more difficult and yellow/orange tattoos tend to respond most poorly. Particularly bright-coloured tattoos may only be partially removed (laser light is reflected). In general, with the exception of simple blue-black tattoos, most cases require a long treatment period, and the clearance will most likely be incomplete. However, even if the pigment can be removed somewhat selectively, there will be some **residual textural and pigmentary differences** from normal skin. Hypopigmentation (10%) and scarring are potential complications.

- **Blue/green** – QSRL (red light, 694 nm, high risk of complications) or QS-alexandrite (purple red, 755 nm). QSRL is effective, but the higher frequency of complications, such as hypopigmentation and textural changes, reduces its usefulness in clinical practice.
- **Red** – QS frequency doubled Nd:YAG (green light, 532 nm).
- **Black** – Nd:YAG (infrared, 1064 nm); all lasers are effective for black pigment. The longer wavelength of the Nd:YAG laser and its poor absorption by melanin allow deeper penetration; avoiding superficial structures makes it useful, especially in darker skin, but at the expense of more splatter and bleeding, although healing is usually satisfactory. It works very well for black pigment, but effectiveness with other colours is limited as compared to other lasers.
- **Yellow** – all poor. The required wavelengths are in the UV range that tends to be absorbed by melanocytes (damaging them as well as hindering penetration)

Tattoos may undergo **colour shifts** following laser treatment (Peach AH, *Br J Plast Surg*, 1999), e.g. conversion of ferric oxide (Fe_2O_3 found in eyeliner tattoos) to ferrous oxide (FeO) in red pigments may darken tattoos; test patch first. Titanium oxide (TiO_2) is white but may turn black (TiO).

Successful and rapid treatment of blue and green tattoo pigment with a novel picosecond laser. (Brauer JA, *Arch Dermatol*, 2012)

The authors used a picosecond 755 nm alexandrite laser to clear 12 recalcitrant tattoos with blue and green after one to two treatments, with more than two-thirds approaching 100% clearance.

Laser treatment of tattoos. (Bernstein EF, *Clin Dermatol*, 2006)

The pitfalls:

- Using the wrong device – only QSL should be used.
- Using too high an energy, resulting in complications – often trying to remove residual pigment that is probably deeper in the skin. A better strategy would be to switch to another laser or accept partial removal.
- Failing to consider endogenous melanin – darker-skinned patients are prone to dyspigmentation after laser treatment.
- Allergic reactions to pigment – **most often red** – these areas are usually nodular and scaly to begin with; check with the patient for skin reactions when the tattoo was first applied. Reactions may be due to the laser causing 're-exposure' or altering the antigenicity of the tattoo pigment
- Tattoo darkening, e.g. permanent eyeliners.

- There have also been reports of burns with MRI scans (Ross JR, *Sports Health*, 2011).

COMPLICATIONS

- Scarring is uncommon with QSL, but textural changes may persist.
- Incomplete response especially if there are bright and light colours; **yellow** is notoriously difficult to clear.
- Chemical reactions may occur, e.g. changing colour or nature – mercury may be released from some red inks, whilst chromium and cobalt can cause hypersensitivity. Allergies are rare.

LASER HAIR REMOVAL

- **Hypertrichosis** is hair growth in a non-androgenic distribution that is excessive for the age, sex and race of the patient. It may be congenital or acquired, commonly due to drugs such as minoxidil, cyclosporine and phenytoin.
- **Hisutism** is growth of hair in a male pattern in female patients. It is usually due to androgen sensitivity; there is a genetic predisposition in some.

There are many laser systems available, and most current options focus on **long-pulsed lasers** that seem to reduce interactions with the epidermal melanin.

- Ruby (694 nm) – 50% reduction at best, less commonly used.
- Alexandrite (755 nm) – only safe for lighter-skinned patients.
- Diode (810 nm), Nd:YAG (1064 nm) and IPL are more commonly used at present.

The target cells are the pluripotential cells responsible for hair growth in the bulge/bulb region, which are 4 mm or so below the skin surface; they are destroyed indirectly by heat conducted from the melanin in the follicle. Anagen follicles are most sensitive to laser energy, whilst telogen (resting) hairs are least susceptible; thus, repeated treatments are needed to catch hairs in the most vulnerable state. Usually, two to three treatments are needed to catch most hairs.

Although there can be good results in well-selected patients, e.g. dark hair in lighter skinned patients, individual responses cannot be predicted/guaranteed. Painless treatment (without any anaesthesia, including topical) is not likely to be effective. Sublethal energies may push hairs in telogen and/or cause miniaturisation. The FDA discourages claims of painless or permanent removal. The term 'permanent reduction' is preferred to clearly that that there may be a permanent reduction in the total number of hairs, permanent removal of all hairs cannot be guaranteed.

The clinical end-point is to see immediate vaporisation of the hair shaft, and then after a few minutes' delay, perifollicular oedema and erythema; immediate epidermal damage is not expected.

- Ejection of hairs occurs for 2 weeks after treatment.
- After an initial set of six to eight treatments spaced 2–4 months apart, further maintenance therapy may be required about once a year.
- 'Touch-ups' of stray hairs with electrolysis or other methods as they may be too fine for laser treatment.
- The commonest complication is hyperpigmentation that may last for months.
- Laser hair removal at home has become popular. Most FDA cleared (which is slightly different to 'approved') 'laser' devices, e.g. Sik'n (RRP 220 USD for the Flash&Go compact), usually use IPL (sometimes called HPL – home pulsed light). The Tria Laser 4X is the first and only diode laser designed for home use and remains popular (RRP 450 USD).

NON-LASER HAIR REMOVAL

- **Shaving** – simple but needs to be performed regularly; risk of cuts, etc. It does not seem to increase the number of hairs.
- **Epilation** – the whole shaft is removed, e.g. waxing, plucking/threading. Hairs that return tend to be finer, possibly due to damage to the follicle.
- **Electrolysis** – fine needle electrodes ablate follicular germ cells. It is time consuming but is the only method that is FDA approved for permanent hair *removal*.
- **Depilation** – topical treatments; often have thioglycates that break hairs by disrupting disulphide bridges in keratin.
- **Eflornithine hydrochloride** (Vaniqa®, FDA approved in 2000 for facial hair in women) was developed initially as an antitumour therapy and then used in forms of sleeping sickness (trypanosomiasis) with hair loss being a noted side effect. It is rather expensive, discontinuation will lead to regrowth; it can cause local skin irritation.
- **Dianette** works by androgen suppression. It is licensed for use in hirsutism in the United Kingdom.

LASER SCAR TREATMENT

Just as not all lasers are the same, not all scars are the same.

- Ablative lasers may be suited for acne scarring.
- PDL lasers may treat hypertrophic scars with some success.

FRACTIONAL LASERS

Fractional lasers are a relatively new development in lasers. A tiny array of laser energy delivery produces microthermal treatment zones (MTZs) that extend into the dermis and consist of a microscopic ablation zone (MAZ) surrounded by a zone of remodelling. Leaving intact tissue in between the minute cores of coagulative necrosis results in faster, better healing, i.e. less downtime. The dermal remodelling around the MAZ is the basis of the treatment of wrinkles, scars and photodamage, i.e. **non-ablative skin rejuvenation**.

- Manuskiatti (*J Am Acad Dermatol*, 2010) – patients with type IV skin and **atrophic acne scars** were treated with fractional CO_2 laser. After 6 months, 85% of patients rated at least 25%–50% improvement, whilst objective measures of scar volume and surface smoothness also improved. There was temporary hyperpigmentation in 92%.
- Hedelund (*Lasers Med Sci*, 2010) – this study used a fractional erbium YAG laser – although it is strictly ablative, but due to the low level of epidermal disruption, it is classified as non-ablative fractional resurfacing. Ten patients with **acne scarring** were treated; improvements in scars were noted on blinded clinical evaluations. Half of the patients noted moderate improvement in their scars.
- Fractional laser improves **post-burn hypertrophic scars** (Dhepe N, *Lasers in Surgery and Medicine*, 2011).
- Ozog (*Arch Dermatol*, 2011) – fractional CO_2 **at time of surgery** reduces scarring in 10 patients who had half scar treated.

Pulsed-dye laser treatment of hypertrophic burn scars. (Alster TS, *Plast Reconstr Surg*, 1998)

Forty hypertrophic scars (half due to burns and half following CO_2 laser resurfacing) were treated with 585 nm PDL and had symptomatic improvement after only one treatment. After 2.5 treatments, there was decreased redness, and scars were softer and more pliable.

- Kono (*Ann Plast Surg*, 2005) noted similar improvement in hypertrophic scars in Japanese patients treated with 585 nm PDL with cryogen cooling, with 40.7% and 65.3% improvement in scar height and redness, respectively.
- Parrett (*Burns*, 2010) discussed the use of PDL in post-burn hypertrophic scarring (see Chapter 2, Section D).

OTHER NON-ABLATIVE REJUVENATION MODALITIES

INTENSE PULSED LIGHT

Intense pulsed light (IPL) is not laser light, but rather, it is light in a broad range – 500–1300 nm with multiple potential effects:

- 550–580 nm targets water and haemoglobin
- 550–570 nm – superficial pigment
- 590–755 nm – deeper pigment

Filters can be used to target components more selectively depending on the effect required. IPL was derived from the use of infrared light for the treatment of tattoos and vascular lesions. IPL can be useful for a variety of problems, particularly the following:

- **Vascularity** – telangiectasia, rosacea, flushing, **hypertrophic scars** and **PWS** (particularly those unresponsive to PDL).
- **Pigmentation** – lentigo, melasma, freckles (and **hair removal**).
- **Photorejuvenation** – improve skin texture, e.g. reduction of pore size.

Pretreatments are not required. No analgesia is usually needed; cooling by 'gel' is sufficient. There is usually **erythema** for several days – possibly with some purpura, oedema or scabbing. Repeated treatments are needed with sun avoidance/block in between. Contraindications include tanned skin or Fitzpatrick skin type VI (V is a relative contraindication).

SKIN TIGHTENING

The market for noninvasive/non-ablative skin tightening, i.e. without the trauma and downtime of surgery or dermabrasion/laser resurfacing, is very large. These mostly act by causing collagen contraction (for an immediate tightening effect) followed by collagen remodelling (denaturation and new production) providing a delayed additional tightening effect. Some have demonstrated histological changes with these modalities, but it does not correlate directly with clinical effects.

- **Radiofrequency.** The aim is to remodel the dermis through RF energy and so bring about skin tightening; it is often used for the lower face and neck. The energy is applied by a probe onto skin with simultaneous cryogen cooling to reduce pain (which is often the limiting factor). As expected, it is not as effective as ablative resurfacing, and multiple treatments are needed, but the downtime is minimal (24 hours of mild erythema).
  - **Thermage®** – bulk healing 2–4 mm vs. ~1 mm with lasers
- **High-frequency focused ultrasound (HIFU)**
  - **Ulthera®** – deep effects up to 4.5 mm (FDA approval 2010)
- **Infrared heating**

III. FACIAL RESURFACING

CAUSES OF FACIAL AGEING

It is conventional to divide up ageing into intrinsic and extrinsic components, but there is overlap, and the relative contributions can be difficult to define.

- **Chronological or intrinsic ageing** – histologically there is thinning of the dermis, reduced papillae, reduced collagen/elastic fibres/ground substance, reduced blood vessels, fibroblasts and mast cells.

Gravitational forces cause soft tissue descent and deep furrows, whilst the contractile forces of the underlying muscles cause wrinkles.

- **Extrinsic** (i.e. related to environment, particularly sunlight, thus often called **actinic damage**) – characterised by fine rhytids, skin laxity and dyschromia; keratoses; elastin accumulates in abnormal arrangements, whilst collagen content is both reduced and more disorganised.
  - Actinic skin is thicker than normal.
  - Greek *rhytis* for 'wrinkle'.

As the two are somewhat interrelated, an alternate view of ageing is as follows:

- **Weathered skin**, i.e. ageing skin, in terms of its superficial features.
- **Loss of structure**, i.e. sagging face. The laxity of the soft tissue envelope can be caused by volume resorption, tissue laxity and thinning of the skeleton, i.e. facial bones. In addition, weakness of muscles around the eye contributes to protrusions around the eyelid.

Thus, the 'ageing face' for an individual patient is a **combination of effects** with different contributions. The issues that need to be or can be corrected fall into the following categories:

- Soft tissue descent – re-drape with lifts
- Volume loss – treat with augmentation
- Dermal elastosis – treat with resurfacing

Some conditions predispose to ageing, e.g. progeria, Ehlers–Danlos, cutis laxa and pseudoxanthoma elasticum.

AGEING CHANGES

Choosing between surgery (see below) and non-surgical methods of facial rejuvenation comes after discussion; the patient has to accept realistic goals including the following:

- Non-operative methods are generally not as effective as, nor have the longevity of, surgery.
- Resurfacing will be especially useful for actinic damage and aims to initiate dermal collagen reorganisation and new collagen synthesis, but has a significant downtime that increases with deeper resurfacing.

LASER RESURFACING

FITZPATRICK SKIN TYPES

The Fitzpatrick classification categorises patients according to their skin response to UVL; the skin type also impacts on their response to laser treatment and scarring after surgery (Table 10.1).

GENERAL POINTS

(Resurfacing) lasers can be non-ablative or ablative – the common examples being Er:YAG or CO_2, respectively. The CO_2 laser is an alternative to dermabrasion or chemical peels

Table 10.1 Fitzpatrick skin types

Skin type	Skin colour	UV sensitivity	Sunburn history
I	White	Very	Always burns, never tans
II	White	Very	Usually burns, sometimes tans
III	White	Sensitive	Burns sometimes, tans gradually
IV	Light brown	Moderately	Burns minimally, tans well
V	Brown	Minimally	Never burns, tans easily to dark brown
VI	Black	Insensitive	Never burns, deeply tans

(such as the 35% trichloroacetic acid or 50% Baker–Gordon phenol), but with more control and predictability. It is often regarded as the 'gold standard'; however, there is no evidence that it is markedly superior.

CARBON DIOXIDE LASER

The light energy targets water as the 'chromophore'. It vaporises the entire epidermis with the first pass, and the whitish eschar needs to be removed with a damp swab; otherwise, it will act as a heat sink, increasing thermal damage. Significant dermal collagen shrinkage begins with subsequent passes. Laser resurfacing is painful. Topical anaesthetics are usually insufficient; thus, nerve block or local infiltration with intravenous sedation may be needed for larger areas.

- Collagen shrinkage (by 10%–30%) at 55–60°C; relative shrinkage decreases with successive passes.
- Some collagen remodelling and laying down of new shorter collagen over several months post-treatment. The damaged disorganised collagen of the papillary dermis is replaced by normal compact collagen.
- Erythema can lasts for several months. The most common adverse reaction is hypopigmentation, particularly in the fair skinned.
- Fractional lasers (see above) – Tierney (*J Drugs Dermatol*, 2009) described safe and effective use of fractional CO_2 laser for neck resurfacing in 10 patients.

Histological changes in the skin following CO_2 laser resurfacing. (Collawn SS, *Plast Reconstr Surg*, 1998)
Post-operative progress:

- Seven to ten days – re-epithelialisation from adnexal structures
- Three months post-treatment:
  - Epidermal atypia corrected, polarity restored.
  - Melanocyte numbers back to normal with even distribution of melanin.
  - Neocollagen formation, elimination of elastoses and decreased glycosaminoglycan (GAG) ground substance.
- Six months post-treatment:
  - Resolution of inflammatory changes.
  - Fibroblasts are hypertrophic.

ERBIUM:YAG LASERS

The pulsed erbium:YAG laser was introduced in 1996 with infrared wavelength 2940 nm. It is closer to the peak absorption for water than a CO_2 laser and thus is absorbed 12–18× more efficiently and with less thermal diffusion. There is less collateral tissue damage. The penetration depth of 2–5 μm is much less than the 20–30 μm for the CO_2 laser, meaning a faster recovery/shorter downtime and fewer side effects (erythema lasts for 2–4 weeks only).

- However, as it is less coagulative, there will be more bleeding (which is the clinical endpoint).
- Less collagen shrinkage and less stimulation of remodelling mean less pronounced and shorter-lasting effects.

It is used less frequently; Er:YAG is usually reserved for milder photodamage, rhytids and dyspigmentation (Alster TS, *Plast Reconstr Surg*, 1998).

CONTRAINDICATIONS TO LASER THERAPY

Patients should be encouraged strongly to give up smoking.

- Absolute
  - Isotretinoin (used in the treatment of acne) within the last 2 years
  - Infection (bacterial, HSV)
- Relative
  - Collagen, vascular or immune disorder
  - Keloid tendency
  - Ongoing UV light exposure

SKIN PRECONDITIONING

Preconditioning regimens with topical vitamin A (retinoic acid), hydroquinone or glycolic acid are often **used before laser resurfacing or chemical peels** to increase the effectiveness of these therapies. These agents increase the metabolism of the skin, accelerate cellular division, boost collagen synthesis and reduce the thickness of the stratum corneum.

RETINOIC ACID

Topical tretinoin (all-trans retinoic acid) increases papillary dermal collagen, glycosaminoglycan (GAG) synthesis and angiogenesis and exfoliates the stratum corneum.

It thus makes the **skin more sensitive** to peels, for example. Pretreatment with topical retinoids may help to reduce post-treatment hyperpigmentation but may contribute to erythema. Overall, it is not proven as a worthwhile pretreatment and is also contraindicated during early pregnancy due to its teratogenicity.

Different formulations/products are available.

- **Tretinoin 0.05%** (Retinova) topical cream for photo-damaged skin and mottled pigmentation – excellent treatment for solar-induced lentigines on the dorsum of the hands.
- **Tretinoin 0.025%** (Retin-A) topical cream for acne treatment.

Note that **isotretinoin** is 13-cis-retinoic acid and known as Roaccutane/Accutane in the United States. It is an isomer of tretinoin used for acne treatment and is not used as a pretreatment. Delayed **healing and atypical scarring**, thus typically, patients are asked to stop the medication at least 6 months (many insist on a much longer interval) before laser therapy as it inhibits re-epithelialisation from adnexal structures. Some suggest that recovery of dermal appendages from effects of drug may be gauged by the return of skin oiliness or acne. However, more recent literature reviews (Wootton CI, *Br J Dermatol*, 2014) show a lack of evidence to support this practice. Any risk is likely to be small, and (semi) urgent surgery should not be delayed – for the prudent, stopping isotretinoin before the surgery and waiting for satisfactory wound healing before resuming should be adequate.

COMPLICATIONS OF LASER RESURFACING

Resurfacing with two passes of the CO_2 laser at 500 mJ results in healing at 7–10 days. Most patients get good to excellent results; complications are relatively uncommon.

- **Pigment changes** – hypo- (3%) or hyperpigmentation (7%).
  - **Hyperpigmentation is more common** especially in darker-skinned individuals (Fitzpatrick types IV–VI) but is generally temporary, whilst **hypo-pigmentation** is less common but more **liable to be permanent**.
  - Pretreatment bleaching with hydroquinone (toxic to melanocytes/inhibits tyrosinase) may reduce hyperpigmentation, although it is not licensed for this use in the United Kingdom.
  - Cut UV exposure post-operatively – sunscreens, avoiding strong sunlight for 3 months.
- **Prolonged erythema** >10 weeks (6%) may occur. It is important to warn patients of this; it will also get redder when they blush. Topical steroids (1% hydrocortisone twice daily for 6 weeks) may help.
- **Superficial infection.**
  - **Acne/milia** due to greater production of sebum – the latter in particular is self-limiting. Treatments include retinoic acid, glycolic acid and hydroquinone at night (comedolysis).

- Post-treatment antibiotics (broad spectrum, e.g. cephalexin); fluconazole is less commonly used.
- **Flare-up of herpes simplex** may occur with or without a history of herpes. Some give acyclovir to **all patients** pre- and post-operatively until re-epithelialised (or 1 week), whilst others limit the use to those with a history of herpes infection.
- **Hypertrophic scarring** (1%), which in some cases may lead to ectropion.

CHEMICAL PEELS AND DERMABRASION

A chemical peel is a controlled chemical burn that removes the surface layers and stimulates collagen remodelling in the residual dermis, thus treating dyschromia, rhytids and uneven skin. They are classified according to the chemical composition as well as the depth of peel. Resurfacing of various sorts (chemical, laser, dermabrasion) work well due to the excellent healing potential of the facial skin with its plentiful skin appendages, vascularity, etc. They should be used with caution in non-facial areas.

- **Superficial** – **alpha-hydroxy acids** (AHAs), Jessner's solution, salicylic acid
- **Medium** – trichloroacetic acid (TCA)
- **Deep** – phenol

The depth of the peel required is related to the level of actinic damage (**Glogau classification** of photoageing). Those with skin types IV–VI are at greatest risk of PIH, and this modifies the type of treatment administered. Peels are cheaper than laser resurfacing with less dermal thinning but more erythema and early swelling.

CHEMICAL PEEL

SUPERFICIAL PEELS

The 'normal' reaction is similar to **exfoliation** (removal of dead outer skin layers) via **keratolysis** (dissolution of intercellular attachments), and includes immediate erythema and gradual whitening hours later, although some may have crusting. The skin is red, with peeling like mild sunburn 2–5 days later. Multiple treatments are often needed for maximum benefit. Light peels will not address deep wrinkling, offering more a 'fresh look'. Shallow rhytids that disappear on light stretching respond to a 'skin tightening' (more superficial) peel, whereas those that do not disappear require a 'skin levelling' (deeper) peel.

- **Glycolic acid** (40%–70%) is an AHA from sugar cane, similar to lactic (milk), tartaric (grapes), malic (apples) and citric acids. Hence, the alternative collective term is 'fruit acids' (but most can be synthesised in the laboratory). Kojic acid peels are more irritant and are thus second-line treatment. The effects are less dramatic than dermabrasion/chemical peel/facelifts but with less risk. The depth of effect is related to concentration and time of contact (neutralising with bicarbonate/rinsing with water). There is no significant downtime (i.e. typical 'lunch time peel', although some get crusting several days later). There may be temporary irritation and thinning of skin that needs sun protection.

- **Retin-A (tretinoin)** increases keratinocyte turnover and thins the stratum corneum but thickens the dermis with increased collagen synthesis and elasticity. It binds to DNA receptors that bind to activator protein-1 (AP-1) transcription factor, leading to inhibition of metalloproteinase action.

MEDIUM PEELS

Trichloroacetic acid (TCA) was one of the earliest agents used; it remains very versatile, whilst the lack of systemic toxicity makes it particularly safe. TCA causes a **coagulative necrosis/protein denaturation**, and the surface layers slough off subsequently. The 'classic' medium peel is 35% TCA; **different concentrations result in different depths of peel**. This variation can be used according to skin thickness, e.g. 35% for face, 20% for neck and the following for different effects:

- 10%–25%: light – epidermis
- 30%–40%: medium – into papillary dermis; classic TCA peel
- 50%–60%: deep – more scarring risk than phenol, laser or dermabrasion

The usual technique is to wait for the desired effect, and then wipe and rinse thoroughly with water. It is usually possible to judge depth approximately by the appearance – erythema (superficial), pink/**white frost** (intermediate and the usual endpoint appearing after 30 min), denser white (deeper) and grey white ([too] deep). However, it is usually better to repeat treatments than overdo the concentration of TCA at one sitting.

- Patients should expect some darkening of the skin and peeling (as for sunburn) afterwards.
- On average, a medium peel results in half the dermal penetration and half the collagen remodelling seen after a deep peel.

TCA-based blue peel: A standardised procedure with depth control. (Obagi ZE, *Dermatol Surg*, 1999)

The rationale for this technique was the observation that the variable results associated with chemical peels were due to lack of control over the depth of peel. The TCA blue peel (30% TCA diluted by an equal volume of blue peel base) facilitates treatment of the papillary and immediate reticular dermis (junction of reticular and papillary dermis). An even blue colour confirms the evenness of application, whilst it also allows the endpoint of the peel to be easily recognizable.

DEEP PEEL

The term 'deep peel' is generally synonymous with a **'phenol peel'**, which uses phenol or carbolic acid (C_6H_5OH) with or without croton oil as an irritant to increase inflammation and soap (glycerine) as a surfactant to decrease surface tension and emulsifier. The Baker–Gordon formula was first described in the 1960s and is still the most common one in use. Phenol peels are painful, and conscious sedation is often needed; they produce protein coagulation with a very predictable depth of peel (upper reticular dermis) that is long lasting (years). It is pretty much an all-or-nothing-type response, and it is difficult to vary the depth of peel. The phenol peel is approximately twice the depth of a TCA peel.

- Indications include treatment of actinic changes, fine wrinkles and superficial acne scars. It has also been used for actinic and seborrhoeic keratosis, lentigo/lentigines, melasma and even for superficial BCCs.
- Phenol peels are restricted to use in types I–III skin. There is a marked inflammatory response; epidermal regeneration is complete by 1 week.
- It should not be used in non-facial areas (with poorer healing) and must be used with caution around eyes, as it can cause serious corneal damage. Phenol is absorbed and detoxified to HQ and pyrocatechin in the liver, or excreted by the kidneys. High levels are toxic to the liver, kidneys and cardiac tissues (arrhythmias). Thus, it is contraindicated in patients with a history of cardiac disease or renal disease.

COMPLICATIONS OF MEDIUM/ DEEP PEELS

The general effect of a peel is to thin out the epidermis; therefore, the skin will look **erythematous** due to increased transparency and telangiectasia, and blotchy pigmentation may be more pronounced due to increased contrast. Medium peels, e.g. TCA and dermabrasion, do not significantly change elastin (but phenol does).

- **Erythema** may persist for 3–6 months, but most patients can go back to work after 2 weeks. The erythema occurs especially around the upper cheeks and lower eyelids; steroids may help but may in turn cause telangiectasia.
- There may be **itchiness** that may require treatment to reduce scratching and scarring.
- **Dyspigmentation**
  - Hypopigmentation proportional to increasing depth of peel – almost invariable after phenol peel, may be permanent
  - Hyperpigmentation – inflammatory melanocyte response that usually resolves
- **Viral and bacterial infections** are rare but potentially serious and can generally be prevented by meticulous care.
- **Milia** for 2–3 weeks after re-epithelialisation due to occluded sebaceous glands. It can be treated with gentle abrasion, incision or retinoic acid.
- Scarring.

SPECIFIC TO AGENTS

- **Arrhythmia – phenol** is absorbed and is toxic to the heart and CNS (TCA is not), with no antidote. Dilution may actually increase absorption by reducing coagulation. The risk may be reduced by gradual application.
- **Scarring** – particular caution is needed when using phenol and trichloroacetic acid at more than 50% concentration; the neck has fewer skin appendages and is at greater risk of poor healing.

DERMABRASION

This is the gradual removal of layers of skin using a diamond burr on a drill, or even sandpaper, i.e. a mechanical peel. The indications are similar to chemical peels and ablative lasers, working well for fine rhytids and providing minor skin tightening, but it is also useful for focal problems such as uneven superficial scars. It is a useful adjunctive treatment of rhinophyma.

The depth of resurfacing is controlled by the coarseness of the abrasive, pressure on the skin and the speed and length of treatment – the usual clinical endpoint is **pinpoint bleeding** from the superficial papillary dermis. Some use gentian violet to paint the area and guide treatment for spot dermabrasion (Gold MH, *Am J Clin Dermatol*, 2003). **Results tend to be quite operator dependent.** The side effects and complications are similar to laser resurfacing – over-dermabrasion will lead to hypertrophic scarring; thus, it is important not to extend through the reticular dermis.

IV. TISSUE FILLERS AND BOTULINUM TOXIN

TISSUE FILLERS

Volume loss is a significant component of ageing; thus, volume restoration through the use of tissue fillers can improve facial appearance, e.g. filling hollow cheeks or deep folds without the need for surgery. Fillers can also be used to treat static wrinkles; in Asians, wrinkle lines are not a major problem, and fillers are primarily used for nose, chin and lip augmentation.

The 'ideal filler' does not exist. There are many products to choose from; important factors to consider include safety and ease of use with predictable results that are potentially reversible if needed.

CLASSIFICATION OF TISSUE FILLERS

Tissue fillers can be classified according to their source (animals, humans, etc.), nature (synthetic or biological), composition (collagen, hyaluronic acid) or longevity (temporary, semi-permanent, permanent).

- **Autologous fillers**
  - These were not commonly used due to the expense and time required, as well as the wide choice of alternatives.
    - **Isolagen** – made of cultured autologous fibroblasts prepared from a 3 mm punch biopsy. It takes about half a year for the effects to become apparent and lasts for about a year and a half.
      - Company reorganised into Fibrocell, and product became Azfibrocel-T (laViv) – cultured fibroblasts from a patient's postauricular tissue; requires 3 months. FDA approval for nasolabial fold in 2011.
    - **Autologen** – collagen prepared from a biopsy of the patient's own skin, taking about 2 months. The manufacturer Collagenesis went out of business in 2006.
  - **Autologous fat** enhances subcutaneous volume and is thus strictly **not a dermal filler**.
- **Collagen fillers were once widely used.** Zyderm I was the only FDA-approved dermal filler for over a decade from 1981. Almost all collagen fillers had been voluntarily removed from the US market by 2010 due to decreasing demand.
- Zyderm I was made from **bovine dermal collagen;** it had a very short effect. Zyplast was a better product with collagen cross-linkage by glutaraldehyde, making it less immunogenic/more resistant to biodegradation.
  - **Skin testing** with two sets of subcutaneous injection in the forearms; two tests, 2 weeks apart, 4 weeks prior to beginning treatment. One to three percent developed sensitivity on definitive injection even with negative testing.
  - **CosmoDerm and CosmoPlast** – human bioengineered.
  - **Evolence** – porcine collagen.

Hyaluronic acid (*hyalos* from Greek for 'vitreous'; it was first isolated in Greece)

- Hylaform (Genzyme), one of the first products in the United States (FDA approval 2004), is made from rooster combs.
- Restylane (QMed, Sweden) was made from bacterial (equine streptococci) fermentation; often referred to as a **NASHA** (non-animal source hyaluronic acid). It had been widely used in Europe before it gained FDA approval.
- Juvederm (Allergan) gained FDA approval in 2006 to treat moderate to severe facial wrinkles and folds.
- The list is continually increasing. Hyaluronic acid (HA)–based products have become the most commonly used tissue filler, reflecting their longer duration of action (6–12 months), ease of use and good safety record with minimal risk of infections or allergy, and most complications are easily treated, e.g. with hyaluronidase.

HA is plentiful in the skin, being part of the ground substance; it has a very well conserved structure. It is composed of large random coils of a linear sugar polymer of two saccharide subunits (D-glucuronic acid and D-N-acetylglucosamine). In the body, HA has an average half-life of 2 days, with one-third of the body's HA being turned over every day. Modifications to injected HA, such as particle size, cross-linkage, etc., are used to increase their longevity.

Injections of HA are (more) **painful**; some mild redness and swelling is not uncommon, often limiting social activities on the day of treatment. Hypersensitivity reactions are much less common with modern formulations.

- The most serious complication relates to **vascular accidents** related to either direct intravascular injection and/or compression, which can lead to skin necrosis or blindness or cerebral events.
  - Management options include aspiration, use of hyaluronidase, nitroglycerine patches, HBO, etc.

SEMI-PERMANENT FILLERS

Longer-lasting fillers are obviously more cost effective, but the actual duration of action in a given case really depends on the individual.

- **Radiesse** is made up of calcium hydroxyapatite microspheres in a gel carrier. Collagen fibrosis (supposedly neocollagenesis) occurs around the microspheres as the gel is absorbed. It is particularly useful for augmenting the cheek and filling in the 'tear-trough' area. It is approved for use in the treatment of deep folds and HIV lipoatrophy; other uses are off-label, e.g. malar, chin.
- **Sculptura** (New Fill in Europe) is made of poly-L-lactic acid particles in a cellulose matrix; it is cleared by hydrolysis and macrophage action. Volume enhancement comes from increased collagen synthesis as the material is replaced – thus, it may take weeks (and a second treatment) before obvious results appear. It usually lasts about 2 years. It was approved for correction of **facial lipoatrophy in HIV** patients but more recently (July 2009) has also been approved for aesthetic indications. It can be injected deeper (deep dermal, subcutaneous or periosteal). There are some cases of **granuloma** formation.
  - It needs to be reconstituted well in advance; practitioners advise at least overnight, preferably 48 hours if not more.

OTHERS (RARELY USED)

- **Cymetra** (micronised Alloderm: decellularised processed dermis, i.e. cadaveric collagen matrix, making it less immunogenic) in the form of dry particles with antibiotic supplementation, which has to be hydrated with 1% lignocaine. Like Alloderm, it has been classed as human tissue; thus, specific FDA approval is not required. It has found limited appeal in cosmetic use; some have reported success in vocal cord (and penile) augmentation.
  - **Fascian** (Fascia Biosystems) is made from micronised cadaveric fascia; it is freeze-dried, irradiated and antibiotic-supplemented. Availability doubtful.

- **Permacol** (Medtronic, micronised porcine dermal collagen, used primarily to treat urinary incontinence but is often used off-label). Cross-linking is said to increase mechanical strength but may delay incorporation, increasing infection risk, i.e. behave more like a synthetic.
- **Selphyl (PRP) 'Vampire facelift'.** PRP is platelet-rich plasm; it was very popular for a while, but results from controlled studies have been disappointing. It does not work well as a filler**.**

PERMANENT FILLERS

- Polymethylmethacrylate (PMMA) **ArteFill®** (was ArteColl) is composed of PMMA beads (20%) in **bovine** collagen; it is regarded as a permanent filler for deeper lines; FDA approval (2006) is limited to nasolabial folds. The initial corrections last up to 6 months until the collagen component is absorbed, followed by tissue growth around the beads that may last >5 years. Skin testing is recommended (1%–3% risk). The most serious side effect seems to be granuloma formation (<0.1% risk).
  - Others are uncommon but include silicone, polyacrylamide hydrogel (PAAG), etc.
    - PDMS **silicone oil** is FDA approved for HIV retinopathy, creating a source of medical-grade silicone that is often used off label. Silicone oil has been used extensively for augmentation but is associated with significant complications.
    - **PAAG** hydrogels are banned in some countries, due to inflammatory/infective complications especially when used for breast augmentation. There are also (theoretical) concerns about the toxicity of the monomer.

COMPLICATIONS OF TISSUE FILLER INJECTION

Although seemingly simple, the optimal results are very much dependent on the surgeon's technique and experience. There is a low incidence of complications, and these are either temporary or easy to treat, e.g. hyaluronidase injection. By comparison, the complications with semi/permanent fillers may be persistent and more difficult to treat with no natural 'antidotes'. Fillers should be used cautiously in certain areas, e.g. around the eye or nose, due to reports of vascular occlusion or skin necrosis.

- Early – infection, hypersensitivity (true hypersensitivity is rare), lumpiness, vascular accidents, light blue discolouration due to **Tyndall effect** due to light scattering by the suspension.
- Late – delayed hypersensitivity infection, foreign body reaction/granulomas and migration. Nodules may or may not represent a foreign body reaction (with other symptoms of inflammation, e.g. redness) or may be due to uneven or incorrect distribution/injection.

FAT GRAFTS

The injection of the patient's own fat is theoretically an ideal method of tissue filling; it is totally biocompatible with potential for full integration. It remains soft and changes in proportion to the patient's weight gain/loss. However, early results were poor, and it was largely abandoned (particularly with the advent of other fillers), until better results were demonstrated with changes in the technique. It is important to realise that fat cells are very fragile and each step (harvest, purification, injection, etc.) can potentially increase damage; thus, graft survival is very technique dependent and somewhat unpredictable. The amount retained is generally quoted to be ~50% (stabilising after 4–5 months). There are many variables; something close to a standard is the **Coleman technique.**

TECHNICAL POINTS

- **Harvest** – donor areas are infiltrated with a 'wetting solution' at ~1:1; though some have reported that LA reduces cell viability. The exact composition does not seem to be vitally important. Low suction harvest by hand with a syringe and blunt needle is recommended.
- **Processing – centrifugation** (typically 3000 RPM for 3 minutes) has the definite effect of removing more water, thus 'concentrating' the fat, but whether this is actually useful is unclear – it can make injection more difficult for example. Others leave the fat to stand and separate by gravity (sedimentation and decant); others let the liquids pass through gauze/mesh, Telfa/cotton gauze rolling (Fisher C, *Plast Reconstr Surg*, 2013); whilst some use commercial kits, e.g. lipodialysis kits, Puregraft®, Revolve®, etc. It is probably desirable to keep the fat cool and minimise exposure to the air before it is injected.
  - Whilst in general, one aims to minimise trauma to fat cells during the whole process, Rubin (*Plast Reconstr Surg*, 2002) suggests an alternative – **'survival of the fittest'** – stressing the cells with sterile water washing and centrifugation at 6000 RPM selects out the most resilient cells for injection. This is naturally quite controversial.
  - Note that it is the relative centrifugal force (in g) that is more important than the RPM; It depends on the radius of the rotor as well as the speed – 3000 RPM translates to 1200 g vs. 1800 g for a 12 or 18 cm radius, respectively. Kim (*Aesthet Surg J*, 2009) found that cell survival was much lower when centrifuging for longer (>5 minutes at 1200 g) or at higher speed (>3000 g at 1 minute).
- **Placement** – a 1 mL fat sphere will probably undergo necrosis of 60%. The theory is that injecting **small aliquots** (through blunt needles) increases revascularisation through greater contact surface area, but this requires time and patience. Some use specialised dispensers, e.g. MAFT gun.

- Some suggest a degree of overcorrection to compensate for absorption, but it should not be excessive, particularly for the face. Gross injection (beyond capacity of pocket) will tend to compromise blood supply.
- Pre-expanding the soft tissue envelope, e.g. with Brava® 4 weeks before injection and 1 week after, is said to increase graft survival (Khouri RK, *Plast Reconstr Surg*, 2010).
- **Post-operative** – expect swelling with significant tissue oedema that lasts for 3–4 days. Some suggest that fat survives better in static areas, leading to the suggestion that survival will be improved by using botulinum toxin in combination with fat injection.

Like most grafts, it is more successful in younger than older patients. In general, studies that have examined the various variables on cell viability numbers have not followed this through on **clinical outcomes**, i.e. graft/volume retention, and thus should be interpreted with caution.

- The choice of donor site does not seem to matter, but this is often debated.
- Storage – harvested fat should be used immediately. Some studies show reduced stem cell numbers after more than 24 hours of 4°C; some studies suggest that cryopreservation (−80°C fridge) may be viable.
- Complications include damage to structures, intravascular embolisation, contamination causing infection, etc. and lumpiness at donor and injection sites. Migration of injected fat is unusual unless excessive amounts have been injected into very mobile areas. Thaunat (*Plast Reconstr Surg*, 2004) described a case of cerebral fat embolism after facial fat injection.
- Cell-augmented/assisted lipoinjection (CAL) and platelet-rich plasma (PRP) are relatively new strategies that are being reported increasingly frequently, in order to improve fat survival/results of fat grafting. PRP is probably not so useful.

Adipose-derived stem cells (ADSCs, also adipose stromal cells, ASCs). Adipose tissue is a richer source of mesenchymal stem cells (MSCs) than bone marrow and is being studied in a number of wound-healing scenarios including repair of radiation damage. It seems that these stem cells are mostly located around the perivascular areas that are mostly left behind after liposuction; thus, in theory, there is a relative paucity of stem cells in suctioned fat, hence the rationale for supplementing injected fat with an aliquot of stem cells or a stromal vascular fraction (SVF).

- Bartisich (*Wounds*, 2012) – fat grafting in combination with skin grafting allowed healing of chronic sickle cell ulcer.
- Riggotti (*Plast Reconstr Surg*, 2007) is one of the pioneers in the use of fat grafting to ameliorate the effects of irradiation in breast cancer treatment.
- Salgarello (*Plast Reconstr Surg*, 2012) – breast implants were placed after two to three sessions of fat grafting in an irradiated patients ('lipobed' technique).

BOTULINUM TOXIN

Botulinum toxin is the exotoxin of the spore-forming anaerobe *Clostridium botulinum*, which has a similar structure to tetanus toxin; it has a heavy chain (HC, binding) and light chain (LC, active moiety) connected by disulphide bridges. Seven serotypes have been isolated (A–G), of which 'A' is the most potent and commonly used sub-type. It is a potentially lethal toxin with a lethal dose of about 3000 U for a 70 kg male (extrapolated from LD50 in 20 g Swiss Webster rats intraperitoneally).

MECHANISM OF ACTION

- The toxin binds to presynaptic cholinergic receptors (via HC) and then becomes internalised, entering lysosomes.
- The toxin is cleaved to release the LC into the cytoplasm and catalyses proteolytic cleavage of membrane proteins responsible for exocytosis of acetylcholine.
  - For botulinum A, SNAP-25 is the cleaved protein, which then prevents fusion of acetylcholine-containing vesicles with the terminal membrane.
- The result is presynaptic inhibition of acetylcholine release.

CLINICAL EFFECTS

The blockage of cholinergic transmission leads to the following:

- Denervation of striated muscle – useful for certain neurological disorders as well as in aesthetics where dynamic wrinkles caused by the contraction of underlying facial muscles can be improved.
  - It can be used to balance out the face in unilateral facial palsy.
- Anhidrosis – useful for hyperhidrosis and Frey's syndrome.

TIMING

- Onset of dose-dependent activity after 1–3 days (toxin needs to be internalised, cleaved, etc.), peak 7–14 days and lasting for several months, until the sprouting of motor axons and formation of new motor-end plates.
- Reassess patients after 2 weeks and touch up if necessary.
- Formation of neutralising antibodies may gradually reduce efficacy.

BOTOX®

Botulinum toxin (BTX), in general, is often referred to as 'Botox'. However, Botox® is a brand name (Allergan, 100 U per vial) of a particular formulation of the A toxin. Note that most products, particularly Botox®, have undergone several

reformulations in particular, a reduction in neurotoxin complex proteins from 25 to 5 ng per 100 units in 1998, which have changed the effect and side-effect profile (in this case, immunogenicity).

- Reconstitute with normal saline (NS with preservatives or not does not seem to make any clinical difference) – keep refrigerated and use within around 4 hours of reconstitution according to the manufacturer, though many report efficacy when stored in the fridge for several weeks.
  - Avoid in pregnancy/lactation and patients with myasthenia gravis, with areas of active infection, with known allergy to human albumin solution or taking aminoglycoside antibiotics (may potentiate clinical effect).

An alert was issued by the FDA in 2009 regarding reports of death, mostly in paediatric patients with cerebral palsy being treated for spasticity. Additional names were given to reinforce the differences between products, particularly potencies, and boxed warnings were included.

- Botox® (Allergan) onabotulinumtoxin A.
  - Approved for strabismus (1989, the **original indication** per Scott A), blepharospasm (1989), cervical dystonia (2000), axillary hyperhidrosis (2004), urinary incontinence (2011), chronic migraine (2010).
  - Approved aesthetic indications – glabellar lines (2002, side effect noticed by Carruthers J and published 1992), crow's feet (2013), axillary hyperhidrosis. **All other aesthetic uses are off label** (see below).
- Dysport® (Ipsen) abobotulinumtoxin. Four times less potent (thus a bottle contains 500U); there is more diffusion (see below). It may act quicker than Botox.
  - Approved for cervical dystonia and glabellar lines.
- Xeomin® (Merz) incobotulinumtoxin A. It is free of complexing proteins and does not require refrigeration, with shelf life of 2–3 years. Units are of equivalent potency to Botox and seem to act quicker.
- Myobloc®/Neurobloc® rimabotulinumtoxin B.
  - Approved for cervical dystonia by FDA in 2000.
  - Less potent than toxin A, faster onset of action but shorter duration.

Areas commonly treated in cosmetic practice:

- Glabellar lines – procerus and corrugator supercilii
- Forehead creases – frontalis
- Periorbital rhytids (crow's feet) – orbicularis oculi
- Less commonly used to treat perioral rhytids and platysma bands

MASSETER HYPERTROPHY

Hypertrophy of the muscle may arise due to emotional 'clenching', which is usually bilateral, although most cases are 'idiopathic'. The hypertrophy seems to be more of a concern for Asians possibly due to their shorter wider faces in general. Atrophy following botulinum toxin injection has been shown to last for up to 25 months in a study with volunteers in 2001, possibly related to reduction in habitual chewing or bruxism. The peak effect is a 30% reduction at 3–6 months when assessed by CT.

- Injections (total 30 U [females]/50 U [males] units per side) are usually given **deep** in the most prominent parts. Note that optimal doses have not been carefully scrutinised by objective criteria, e.g. a 2007 study showed no differences giving 25 U or 35 U in women or men.
  - Paralysing the superficial portions only will often lead to the deeper portions bulging through.
- Avoid injecting too high (stay below a line from tragus to oral commissure) to reduce unwanted zygomatic prominence and to avoid important structures. The common side effects are temporary headache, swelling, pain and muscle weakness.

SIDE EFFECTS OF BTX

- Pain, swelling, bruising and redness at injection sites. Reduce bruising through the following:
  - Use fine-gauge needle (30) that is changed frequently (every three to four injections).
  - Look carefully for visible vessels, no matter how fine, and avoid them.
  - Avoid unnecessary medications including herbal remedies that may affect clotting (see 'Complications'), e.g. stop aspirin 14 days prior if possible.
- Unwanted muscle weakening.
  - Intrinsic muscles of the hand (when treating palmar hyperhidrosis).
  - Extraocular musculature (causing ptosis in 3%, diplopia) and dry eyes when treating periorbital rhytids. Adrenergic eye drops, e.g. **apraclonidine** 0.5% (α2-adrenergic), can be used for unintended ptosis.
  - **'Diffusion'** is the passive movement of toxin from the injection site (over several days), whilst **'spread'** is a function of volume of injection, needle size and injection technique.
- Anaphylaxis has not yet been reported following cosmetic injection in humans (two cases of severe reaction after injection for spasticity).
- Blocking antibodies (5%–15%) may cause reduced/lack of efficacy after repeated, particularly high, dosages. It seems to be less common than in previous reports, which may be related to alterations in formulations as well as changes in practice due to the problem. This is often solved by switching to another formulation.
  - The maximum recommended dose in a 70 kg adult is 400 U of Botox®; commonly used cosmetic doses are around 25 U Botox® or 125 U Dysport® per patient.

FACELIFTS

CLINICAL CHANGES WITH AGE

- Skin changes – thinner, more fragile and less elastic.
- Soft tissue and skeletal volume loss – the maxillary may undergo significant resorption and loss of projection (Mendelson B, *Aesthetic Plast Surg*, 2012).
  - There is also muscle laxity, attenuation of ligaments and descent of the fat pads that produce **apparent** volume loss.
- Apparent volume loss – fat transfer may fill the midface hollows but increases the weight and further descent.

HISTOLOGICAL SKIN CHANGES WITH AGEING

- Changes in the collagen composition of the dermis – loss of type III collagen.
- Loss of elastin – elastin production ceases after ~70 years.
- Reduction in glycosaminoglycans (GAGs).
- Flattening of the dermo-epidermal junction.
- Depletion of Langerhans cells and melanocytes (will lead to immunological changes).

Skin creases on the face may arise due to the following:

- Animation – found perpendicular to the direction of muscle pull
- Loss of skin elasticity – fine and shallow
- Solar elastosis, epidermal atrophy, soft tissue descent – coarse and deep

In simple terms, facelifts address the gravitational effects on the face and are not a treatment for fine wrinkling; deep wrinkles may be improved but not eliminated. There is redistribution but not removal of fat (e.g. removal of the buccal fat pad, which makes the patient look older). It 'sets the clock back but does not stop it ticking'.

The **midface is the focus of facelifts** in particular; it is a complex zone that is 'shared' by several regions with different tissue characteristics (periorbital, perioral and malar) and the borders may form grooves (palpebral malar, nasojugal and midcheek grooves). The facial muscles are different from other muscles in that they exist more in the soft tissues of which they are a part. Their function in the control of the 'spaces' of the orbital and oral cavities means that a balance exists between mobility and stability.

ANATOMY

The blood supply comes almost completely from the external carotid artery (ECA); there is a small contribution from the ophthalmic artery.

- Anterior – musculocutaneous perforators from the facial artery (and its labial branches), and supratrochlear and supraorbital arteries.

- Forehead and scalp – superficial temporal, posterior auricular and occipital.
- Lateral – fasciocutaneous perforators from the transverse facial, zygomatico-orbital, anterior auricular and submental arteries. These are divided in a typical facelift operation; thus, the face becomes dependent on the first group.

Sensation to the mid and lower face is supplied mostly by the maxillary and mandibular divisions of the trigeminal nerve.

- **The great auricular nerve (C2, 3) is the most commonly injured nerve** during facelifts and may result in earlobe numbness.
- The auriculotemporal nerve (secretomotor to parotid) may also be at risk.
- Facial nerve (see below).

FACIAL NERVE

This innervates the muscles of facial expression on their deep surfaces, except for buccinator, LAO and mentalis.

- Seventy percent of subjects have communicating branches between buccal and zygomatic branches. The former is the most common facial nerve branch injured during a facelift but rarely causes a noticeable deficit.
- The marginal mandibular nerve may lie above the inferior border of the mandible (20%) at its posterior extent behind where the facial vessels cross the border.
- The temporal branch runs beneath a line drawn from the tragus to a point 1.5 cm above the lateral margin of the eyebrow and, along with the superficial temporal vessels, lies beneath the TPF/superficial temporal fascia. It is vulnerable at the zygomatic arch.
- The muscles of the face are arranged in four layers.
    - DAO, zygomatic minor, orbicularis oris.
    - Depressor labii inferioris, risorius, platysma.
    - Zygomaticus major, LLS alaeque nasi.
    - **Mentalis, LAO, buccinator – the facial nerve is superficial to these** (and deep to the three other layers).

LAYERS IN THE FACE

The facial soft tissue consists of five **layers** similar to the scalp, but there are some modifications particularly in the musculo-aponeurotic and areolar/space layers (3 and 4, respectively) related to the function of the musculature. The muscles have a superficial flatter layer consisting of muscles such as frontalis, orbicularis and platysma, whilst deeper muscles have a wider skeletal attachment. These layers are condensed over the zygomatic arch.

- **Layer 1. Skin**.
- **Layer 2. Subcutaneous fat.**
- **Layer 3. SMAS** (Mitz and Peyronie 1976) – the superficial musculo-aponeurotic system layer (i.e. superficial fascia) in the face is continuous with the

TPF in the temple, the platysma in the neck and the galea in the scalp. The SMAS is an extension of the superficial fascia; it is a mobile fibrous support system lying between facial skin and bone that is the key element for suspension in most facelifts. Some suggest that SMAS should be regarded as a facial muscle ('facial' part of the platysma); it invests the superficial muscles, namely, orbicularis oculi, platysma, zygomaticus major and minor, and risorius. It is a clearly identifiable structure lateral to the zygomaticus major.

- **Sensory nerves run above.**
- **Motor nerves run deep** – the facial nerve supplies the muscles of facial expression via their deep surfaces, except for mentalis, LAO and buccinator.
- The SMAS can be safely elevated from the preauricular region to the anterior border of the masseter.
- **Layer 4. Retaining ligaments and spaces** (see below).
- **Layer 5. Deep fascia** (parotid fascia, deep temporal, cervical fascia) **and periosteum/pericranium.**

There are a number of additional components:

- A **retinacular system** of connecting fibres links skin and skeleton; they start off as single trunks deeply and then divide and subdivide to form a fine network of fibres in the dermis.
    - There are spaces or gaps of attachment in layer 4, which is the **gliding plane**; there are septae in the boundaries where vessels and nerves move.
- **Retaining ligaments** are zones of adhesion between the skin and the deeper tissues.
    - Osteocutaneous – **zygomatic ligament** (aka McGregor's patch) from zygoma to malar fat and dermis, **mandibular ligament.**
    - Musculocutaneous – **parotid ligament, masseteric ligament.**
    - The last three lie parallel to each other, becoming increasingly anterior.
- **Fat pads**
    - Malar – superficial to SMAS layer and prone to descent that contributes to the deepening of NLF.
    - Buccal – composed of a larger central mass (like an egg yolk in size and colour) with temporal, pterygoid and buccal extensions. It contributes to the cheek contour.

Raising the facial tissue in layer 4 is comparable to raising scalp flaps in the sub-galeal layer. It can be regarded as **safe** as nothing travels through per se, but it also is the most complex and dangerous with the retaining ligaments/boundaries, and the facial nerve is most vulnerable when it moves from deep to layer 4 in the lateral lower face to the underside of layer 3:

- The temporal branch reaches undersurface of layer 3 immediately after exiting the parotid under the zygomatic arch to the supraorbital rim.

- The marginal mandibular branch lies in the lower border/boundary of the premasseter space close to the mandibular ligament.

ASSESSMENT OF THE AGEING FACE

Preoperative photographs are essential. Relevant history includes a patient's complaints and expectations; medical history should include smoking, diabetes, hypertension, drugs affecting coagulation and wound healing including herbal remedies.

- General
  - Skin quality, thickness, elasticity and laxity
  - Asymmetry, distribution of excess tissue, distribution of wrinkles
  - Facial movement and sensation
- Forehead
  - Level of hairline and quality of hair
  - Ptosis and wrinkles
  - Glabellar lines and contraction of corrugator supercilii and procerus muscles
- Midface
  - Nasolabial folds, marionette lines
  - Ptosis of the malar fat pad and jowls
- Jaw
  - Submental fat deposits, 'witch's chin'
  - Platysma bands, divarication

Patients in whom lifts are to be avoided are the following:

- Increased bleeding risk with patients suffering from hypertension and those on aspirin, steroids, warfarin, etc.
- Smokers
- Poor skin quality/keratoses
- Thick, glabrous skin with deep creases
- Collagen/connective tissue diseases

Ultimately, those with unrealistic expectations, particularly those who have had significant previous facial surgery, should be counselled against having surgery.

FACELIFTS

There are many variants in terms of level of dissection, undermining, incision length and adjunctive measures.

- Incisions
- Vectors
- Level of lift

INCISIONS

- Temple
  - In front of hairline – for repeat lifts and those with short sideburns
  - Behind hairline – often used as continuation of open coronal brow lift
- Preauricular

- Pretragal usually safer and faster. For men, the sideburn area will be distorted; the alternative would be to place the incision more anteriorly, which would be more visible.
  - Retrotragal – scar is hidden but may evert/alter contour of tragus, with risk of necrosis.
- Postauricular
  - High for moderate skin redundancy.
  - Low for moderate to excessive skin redundancy.
  - Occipital hairline for excessive skin redundancy.

VECTORS

- SMAS fixed
  - Vertical to improve jawline and perioral creases
  - Diagonally to improve neck and submental crease
- Skin fixed
  - Posterior
  - Vertical

LEVELS OF LIFT

Infiltrate with adrenaline for haemostasis; hypotensive anaesthesia may be associated with more bleeding postoperatively. Muscle relaxants/paralysis should be avoided. Suction drains are often used.

Generally, those with moderate middle-third face laxity with jowls will need some form of SMAS lift, whilst those with marked laxity and deep NLF creases will need a deep-plane or composite lift. However, there are those who regard the risk to the facial nerve and oedema as not being worth it. Minimal-access cranial suspension (**MACS**, Verapaele 1999) is a useful technique that suspends the platysma to the temporalis fascia vertically. Minimal-scar techniques are more suited for younger patients with less tissue laxity.

SUBCUTANEOUS FACELIFTS

These techniques involve subcutaneous undermining from the incision line laterally, to within 1 cm of the lateral orbital rim, to the NLF, within 1 cm of the oral commissure.

- Subcutaneous only – relies on skin tension only for the lift; early recurrence is to be expected.
- Subcutaneous facelift with SMAS plication/imbrication (incise SMAS – advance for suturing with overlap, without significant elevation; see below). This is a commonly performed procedure.
  - SMAS elevation allows better fixation than imbrication, potentially offering longer-lasting results.
  - The key points for skin fixation are 1 cm above the ear and at the apex of the postauricular incision.

SMAS LIFT (SKOOG 1974)

In the original description, SMAS and skin are elevated as a single unit and advanced posteriorly – elevating the SMAS from the underlying structures including release of retaining ligaments distinguishes it from techniques that only plicate the SMAS (see above). The original procedure was designed to address NLFs by releasing the SMAS medial to them.

There are many variants on the SMAS lift: a **skin and SMAS lift** (of some sort) is the standard operation for many, particularly for **younger patients,** who do not yet have significant laxity in more superficial tissues. In older patients, the results on the midface may be unpredictable; there may be exacerbation of hollowing of the lower eyelid and a lateral sweep appearance.

- **Low SMAS technique** – below the zygomatic arch. This addresses the lower face only with no effect on the midface or eyes.
- **High SMAS technique** (popularised by Barton) – above the zygomatic arch, therefore addresses the midface and the periorbital area.
- **Composite facelift** (Hamra), which carries platysma, subcutaneous fat and orbicularis oculi to the lower lid as a **single unit**, suspending the malar and periorbital areas. The skin and subcutaneous tissues are not elevated separately, maintaining more skin vascularity.
- **Foundation facelift** (Pitman), formerly known also as a deep-plane lift, is characterised by elevation of composite musculocutaneous flaps of face and upper neck soft tissue that are rotated to a more lateral and superior position. It is particularly effective in treating the NLF.
- **Lamellar high SMAS lift** – the skin and SMAS are elevated as two separate layers and advanced to different degrees, along different vectors and suspended under different tension. The high incision allows a more vertical lift vector for the SMAS to be attached to the deep temporal fascia whilst the skin is pulled more obliquely.
- **Finger-assisted malar elevation (FAME,** Sherrel Aston) – the index finger is used to separate the lateral orbicularis oculi around the lateral canthus from the temporal fascia. The malar fat pad is repositioned.

SUBPERIOSTEAL LIFT (TESSIER)

This aims to rejuvenate the **upper and mid face** by lifting all of the facial soft tissue in relation to the bone whilst avoiding extensive skin undermining; it only addresses the upper two-thirds of the face. It is more suited to the younger patient who accepts or desires a possible change in eye appearance to an 'almond' eye shape.

- Gingivobuccal sulcus and/or subciliary incisions are also required for elevation of periosteum over the maxilla including periorbital areas and the anterior arch of the zygoma.
- The midface periosteum is elevated as a single unit without SMAS or skin dissection as a separate unit.

- Endoscopic subperiosteal lifts have been described (Byrd HS, *Plast Reconstr Surg*, 1996).

There is a ~5% risk of complications.

- Nerve injuries – particularly temporal and infraorbital nerves (Heinrichs HL, *Plast Reconstr Surg*, 1998), which are usually transient and largely avoidable with careful dissection
- Prolonged facial oedema
- Haematoma

MINI-LIFTS

It was realised that larger operations did not necessarily produce better results; many variants of a more conservative technique exist. The modern facelift has become more a facial sculpturing, combining tension-free skin re-draping with suturing and judicious liposculpture with volume addition. Generally these techniques are unable to change the neck contour significantly.

Short-scar facelift with lateral SMASectomy. (Baker DC, *Aesthet Surg J*, 2001)
A strip of SMAS overlying the anterior parotid and parallel to the NLF is excised. A sling of inferiorly based SMAS is created and sutured to the mastoid fascia to give a pull vector perpendicular to NLF. Avoidance of the postauricular incision is aimed at reducing flap ischaemia. Critics say that the vector may give an unnatural 'pulled' appearance; there may also be flattening in the lateral cheek.

Types of patients, according to authors:

- Type I – **ideal candidate**: a female in her early to late 40s with ageing primarily in the face; early jowls with or without submental and submandibular fat.
- Type II – good candidate.
- Type III – fair candidate.
- Type IV – **poor candidate**: 60s to 70s with significant jowls and active lax platysmal banding. There is severe cervical skin laxity and deep skin creases below the cricoid. These patients are not suitable for any type of minimal incision procedure and require extensive dissection and re-draping of the platysma, necessitating a larger incision.

The MACS-lift short-scar rhytidectomy. (Tonnard P, *Aesthet Surg J*, 2007)
In the **minimal-access cranial suspension** (MACS) short-scar facelift, the skin–subcutaneous tissue is dissected from the SMAS–platysma layer, which is suspended vertically (using microimbrications of fat and SMAS with pursestring sutures) to the deep temporal fascia through a temporal hairline incision to prevent sideburn elevation. The skin is directed along different vectors.

Overall, the incision line is similar to standard pattern except for the absence of the postauricular scalp component. There is a risk of damage to facial nerve branches as the purse-string is placed blindly.

UNFAVOURABLE RESULTS, I.E. 'FACELIFT STIGMATA'

- Unnatural pulled-up appearance – this is due to excessive skin tension and/or poor choice of vector giving a **lateral sweep**.
  - Joker's lines pulling the oral commissures onto the cheek
  - **Lateral sweep** (Hamra) – excessive lateral pulling on the lower face without treatment of the midface, which sags over the lower tighter tissues; can avoid with more vertical vectors
- Visible scars (too anterior or too wide) – either due to poor placement or excess tension.
- Ear.
  - Tragal deformity with blunting of the pretragal depression or anterior displacement, due to excessive tension.
  - Pixie ear deformity – the lobule is pulled inferiorly by tension.
- Hair.
  - Hairline distortion/displacement – the temporal hairline should be 3–4 cm away from the lateral orbit.
  - Transient alopecia is not uncommon. Incisions in the hairline should be made parallel to the hairline; dissection should be deep to the level of the follicles. Avoid excessive tension in the suture line.

COMPLICATIONS OF FACELIFTS

The risk of complications is small, but caution is required given the consequences. With repeated lifts, the risk of hairline distortion is increased, but the risk of haematomas is reduced, and less necrosis is expected as the skin flap has been 'delayed'.

- Intraoperative – facial nerve injury, bleeding
- Early
  - **Skin necrosis** (1% and 4%, for sub-SMAS dissection and subcutaneous dissection, respectively) particularly in the retroauricular area, with a 12× higher risk in **smokers** – they should stop smoking several weeks before surgery. Superficial slough heals quite well even for larger areas, but full-thickness slough will scar and contract (which may be beneficial). Thus, generally treated conservatively with late scar excision.
  - **Haematoma** – this **is probably the commonest complication** (see below).
  - **Nerve injuries** (see below).
  - **Infection** – low incidence with routine use of prophylaxis.
  - **Salivary fistula** – the duct is at risk with extensive undermining of the SMAS layer. Fistulae (or subcutaneous salivary collections or pseudocysts) can be managed by the following:
    - Aspirate and test fluid for amylase to confirm diagnosis and to exclude haematoma – early aspiration may prevent fistulation (McKinney P, *Plast Reconstr Surg*, 1996).
    - Insert a suction drain.
    - Antibiotics.
    - Compressive dressing.
    - Fistulous tract may need to be excised (Wolf K, *Plast Reconstr Surg*, 1996).
- Late
  - Alopecia 1%–3%
  - Hypertrophic scarring
  - Hyperpigmentation

Preoperative risk factors and complication rates in facelift: Analysis of 11,300 patients. (Gupta V, *Aesthet Surg J*, 2015)

This prospective study took data from the CosmetAssure database. The commonest complications (overall 1%–2%) were haematoma and infection; the most significant risk factors were being male, having BMI >25 and performing an additional procedure. Smoking or diabetes was not associated with more complications in this study.

Effect of steroids on swelling after facelift. (Rapaport DP, *Plast Reconstr Surg*, 1995; Owsley JQ, *Plast Reconstr Surg*, 1996)

Both studies were prospectively randomised double-blind studies assessing the impact of steroids on facial swelling after SMAS facelift in a total of 80 patients. Neither demonstrated any advantage related to steroid medication in terms of a reduction in immediate or early post-operative swelling.

NERVE INJURIES

If nerve branches are not cut during surgery, they will usually recover. Most injuries involve sensory nerves. Numbness around the incision is almost universal and will fade (4–6 months) in most but not all cases.

- **Great auricular nerve** (C2,3) – usually injured where it crosses the sternomastoid at the midpoint, 6.5 cm below EAM (McKinney's point). Injury to this nerve is largely avoidable but is the most common symptomatic nerve injury (3%–5%).

  There is an average of 2% risk of injuries to facial nerve branches – deeper-plane lifts have a higher rate of facial nerve injury (4%) versus 1% in subcutaneous lifts.
- The **temporal branch** (often called frontal) of the facial nerve runs superficially along Pitanguy's line from 0.5 cm below the tragus to 1.5 cm (or more) above the lateral eyebrow, with the anterior branch of the superficial temporal artery (STA). It runs just under the TPF/superficial temporal fascia; thus, one must dissect either under the superficial layer of the deep temporal fascia (above superficial temporal fat pad), when above the zygomatic arch in the temporal area, or in the subcutaneous plane.
- The **buccal branch** is commonly involved but, due to overlap, is well compensated; the effect is subtle

(a slight difficulty elevating the upper lip) and is often unrecognised.

- The **marginal mandibular branch** of the facial nerve: cadaveric studies suggest that posterior to the facial artery, it lies above the inferior border of the mandible 80% of the time, and in others, always within 1 cm. However, dynamic studies suggest that it may be 3–4 cm below the inferior mandibular border in the living. Injuries are less common but are usually more obvious due to the lack of overlap.

HAEMATOMAS

Most haematomas occur in the first 12 hours after surgery (often in the recovery room), presenting as painful swelling, and should be evacuated by releasing some sutures. Small haematomas are more common (10%) but may not be apparent until the oedema has subsided. They can be aspirated after ~10 days, when they begin to liquefy or will subside on their own over a few months, but with the risk of prolonged firmness and haemosiderin discolouration. Major haematomas require formal drainage in theatre. The risk of developing haematomas seems to be increased by the following:

- **High preoperative systolic blood pressure** – most common.
- Male sex – 8% vs. 4% overall, possibly related to greater blood supply to the beard and sebaceous glands, and hypertension.
- Anterior platysmaplasty.
- Non-steroidal medication within 2 weeks of surgery, smoking. Also be cautious of herbal remedies.
- Vomiting.

Late haematoma (>5 days post-operative) is usually due to bleeding from the superficial temporal vessels and is often associated with physical exertion.

The prevention of haematoma following rhytidectomy. (Grover R, *Br J Plast Surg*, 2001)

In this review of an initial group of 1078, the incidence of major haematoma was 4.4%, and no significant difference was observed with or without the use of the following:

- Tumescent solution (~200 mL each side)
- Adrenaline with or without bupivacaine/lidocaine
- Triamcinolone, hyaluronidase in 500 mL Ringer's lactate
- Fibrin glue sealant
- Suction drains (four concertina suction drains used typically)

The subsequent group of 232 patients received tumescent solution as above but without adrenaline. There was a **significant decrease in haematoma formation** amongst patients who did **not** receive adrenaline. There were 11 major and 6 minor haematomas in the adrenaline group vs. 0 and 1, respectively, in the non-adrenaline group.

Deep vein thrombosis and pulmonary embolus after facelift. (Reinisch JF, *Plast Reconstr Surg*, 2001)

Abdominoplasty is probably the most high-risk aesthetic procedure for thromboembolic complications (TECs) (Grazer FM, *Plast Reconstr Surg*, 1977). TECs – deep vein thrombosis (DVT)/pulmonary embolism (PE) – were responsible for 5% of operative deaths in the hospital (incidence of 1.2% and 0.8%, respectively).

DVT/PE reported by 31 surgeons in this survey gave incidences of 0.35% and 0.14%, respectively; this is much lower than for abdominoplasty. A plastic surgeon could expect a TEC once in every 200 facelift cases.

- General anaesthesia significantly increases risks compared with local anaesthesia.
- Operative time is longer in patients developing DVT/PE (5.11 hours compared with 4.75 hours).

The surgeons were also surveyed for their thromboembolic prophylaxis protocols:

- 60.7% of surgeons had no protocols.
- 19.6% used pressure stockings.
- 19.7% used intermittent compression devices.
  - **Only these devices** have been shown to significantly decrease the risk of TEC. They are supposed to prevent venous stasis, induce fibrinolytic activity in veins and stimulate release of antiplatelet aggregation factor from endothelial cells.

The Caprini risk assessment model (Caprini JA, *Dis Mon*, 2005) has been validated to predict DVT/PE risk in plastic surgery patients within 60 days. Those with Caprini scores of >7 have a risk of 11.3% and should have prophylactic enoxaparin. In higher risk (>7) patients, there is no evidence that the risk is limited to the immediate post-operative period (Pannucci CJ, *J Am Col Surg*, 2011). The Million Women study (Sweetland S, *Brit Med J*, 2009) demonstrated that there is an **elevated risk for 90 days** or more after surgery in middle-aged women.

BROW LIFT

BROW ANATOMY

The frontalis muscle forms a continuous layer with the galea. It inserts into the supraorbital dermis and interdigitates with the orbicularis oculi, whilst the posterior part of the galea passes deep to the muscle and inserts into the periosteum at the supraorbital rim. Other brow muscles include the following:

- The **corrugator supercilii** with its oblique head (supraorbital rim to medial eyebrow dermis and thus acts as a brow depressor forming the oblique glabellar lines) and transverse head (from medial supraorbital rim to middle-third eyebrow dermis, thus moving the brow medially and forming vertical glabellar lines).

- The **depressor supercilii** runs from the medial supraorbital rim to the medial brow dermis, thus depressing the brow and forming oblique lines.
- The **procerus** runs from the medial supraorbital rim to the dermis of the medial brow, thus depressing the brow forming the nasal root lines that are oblique and horizontal.
- **Orbicularis oculi**, orbital part – the medial part causes medial brow depression whilst the lateral portion causes lateral brow depression and crow's feet.

These are all depressors of the medial brow; they are all affected to a certain degree during brow lift surgery, thus leading to **medial brow elevation**.

Brow sensation is provided by the supra-trochlear and supraorbital nerves (superficial branch to the forehead and deep branch to scalp posterior to the hairline – this is transected with sub-galeal and coronal incisions, leading to paraesthesia).

BROW AESTHETICS

The normal eyebrow position (Figure 10.1) is as follows:

- Male – at the level of the supraorbital rim, 6 cm from hairline.
- Female – just above the level of the supraorbital rim, 5 cm from hairline.

The normal eyebrow shape is as follows:

- The medial limit forms a ~vertical line joining the inner canthus with the lateral alar groove.
- The lateral limit forms an oblique line joining the outer canthus with the lateral alar groove.
- The lateral brow end lies slightly above the medial end. The medial brow is more club shaped, whilst the lateral brow tapers out to a sharper end.
- The highest part of the eyebrow lies directly above the outer limbus of the iris (junction of medial two-thirds and lateral one-third of the brow).

BROW LIFT SURGERY

Brow lift surgery is indicated for brow ptosis (commonly due to degenerative changes) and transverse furrows. It may also be needed before upper lid blepharoplasty (see below).

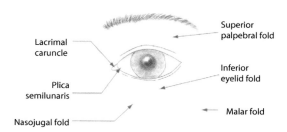

Lacrimal caruncle

Plica semilunaris

Nasojugal fold

Superior palpebral fold

Inferior eyelid fold

Malar fold

Figure 10.1 Features around the eye.

Patients with facial palsy may benefit from skin excision above the eyebrow (direct brow lift).

PREOPERATIVE EVALUATION

- Assess brow (may have been modified by plucking).
- Assess hairline position (high or low) and quality (thick or sparse, which may make scar concealment difficult).
- Assess wrinkles.
  - Dynamic wrinkles – on animation, are best treated with BTX, but surgery may improve them by weakening the responsible muscles.
  - Static wrinkles – present at rest. May be partly due to sustained muscle activity and may thus be partially improved by surgery to the muscles but probably benefit from some form of skin re-draping.
    - Superficial wrinkles are amenable to treatment with fillers or resurfacing.
- Assess eyelids – about 3 cm of the upper lid is required for proper upper eyelid function. If excessive eyelid skin has been excised, then not only will the aesthetic results be poor as thicker brow skin is dragged down to the lid; the brow cannot be lifted without flaps or grafts.

If the brow is truly low, it can be 'lifted' by pulling the tissues back up, and the effect of such an operation can be roughly assessed by using the palms to pull upwards either side of the forehead. There are two main ways of performing the surgery – open or endoscopic – although there are many minor variations, and they may be combined with other surgeries (facelifts and blepharoplasty).

INCISIONS

- Direct/supraciliary – with excision of a strip of skin above the brow; it is useful particularly in males with thick brows.
  - **Direct brow lift** is a useful and simple technique in certain circumstances, e.g. where the patient refuses more extensive surgery involved in a full lift or in conditions such as established facial palsy in the elderly (Ueda K, *Ann Plast Surg*, 1994), where there is localised lateral brow hooding.
- Transblepharoplasty – can be used to tack the brow to the periosteum as well as excise the corrugator and procerus. Internal brow elevation (Burroughs JR, *Arch Facial Plast Surg*, 2006).
- Midbrow – will advance the hairline as well as lift the brow; useful for males, and those with deep wrinkles.

These incisions may be useful in balding patients, but the **coronal incision** or endoscopic approaches are the more common techniques in use.

- Coronal approach - the incision should be made **at least 3 cm behind the anterior hairline**. This will lengthen the forehead and therefore is most suited for those with short foreheads.

- Bevel the incision parallel to the hair follicles and elevate the flap in a sub-galeal (or subperiosteal) plane.
- Connell suggests using an extreme bevel (like trichophytic closure) to allow camouflage of the scar.
- Pretrichial/hairline incisions shorten the forehead and are indicated in those with a long forehead.

PLANE OF DISSECTION

Temporal fusion line between galea, temporalis and periosteum at the temporal crest

- **Subcutaneous** – allows preservation of sensation of posterior scalp but at the expense of reducing flap vascularity; it is also a tedious dissection. Not commonly used.
- **Sub-galeal** – quick dissection with direct access to muscles; galea can be fixed to the periosteum.
- **Subperiosteal** (Ramirez) – requires release of arcus marginalis for a better and supposedly a more sustained lift; however, some say this is more related to the fixation rather than the dissection. Less blood loss and less distortion of the hairline.
- **Biplanar/dual plane** (Ramirez) – subcutaneous dissection of the flap from muscle in the upper part of the flap combined with endoscopic/open subperiosteal dissection (and muscle excision) at the orbital rim. This is said to allow the hairline to stay in its original position whilst improving forehead rhytids.

OPEN SURGERY

The **orbit (retaining) ligaments (Knize)** are zones of **attachment that must be released** to allow a long-lasting lift. They are classed as 'true' dermal to periosteal retaining ligaments, approximately 6–8 mm in length and centred over the ZF suture, tethering the lateral orbital rim to the superficial temporal fascia and dermis. More medially, there is a **periosteal zone of adhesion** that is a wing-shaped band about 2 cm wide running above the supraorbital rims, and because it represents an adherence between the deep galea and periosteum, it is described as a 'false' retaining ligament.

- After flap elevation and ligament release, the flap is raised and turned over; it is important to protect the eyes from pressure.
- Identify supraorbital and supra-trochlear nerves deep and superficial to the corrugator, respectively, and then resect the muscle to reduce vertical creases.
  - **Direct excision,** e.g. corrugator, frontalis (2 cm of frontalis should be left above the brow to maintain animation); some suggest fat grafting to correct the depression from excision.
  - Scoring.
  - BTX.

- Pull back the forehead flap and excise any skin excess before closure; **1.5 mm of flap retrodisplacement translates to ~1 mm of brow lift**. Although part of the lift is due to skin resection, the **majority of the lift comes from fixation** of the flap.
  - There will be potentially more wound problems with more skin excision. Resecting less skin medially will help to avoid the surprised look that is difficult to correct.
  - The **elastic band principle** (Flowers) states that the further away the suspension point is from the part to be lifted, i.e. the brow in this case, the less effective the lift becomes.
    - Sutures – cortical tunnels, temporalis fascia
    - Devices – **Endotine** (absorbable fan-shaped anchor device, dissolves after 6 months), Mitek anchor, screws
- Whilst the result may be a **lifted** brow, often, the brow may lie at a similar level but is **relaxed** with fewer (forehead/glabella) wrinkles.

COMPLICATIONS

- Haematoma.
- Skin necrosis.
- Alopecia.
- Frontalis paralysis due to injury to the temporal branch is rare and usually recovers within 12 months.
- Injury to sensory nerves (supraorbital/supra-trochlear) will lead to forehead numbness; numbness posterior to the skin incision is to be expected.
- Chronic pain/supraorbital nerve dysaesthesia particularly if the patient has a history of migraines.
- Poor cosmesis, e.g. asymmetry, displacement of lateral brow.

ENDOSCOPIC BROW LIFT

A wide coronal-type incision can be avoided with an endoscopically assisted lift. The number of incisions varies, but usually, there are two parasagittal and two temporal sites (Ramirez O, *Plast Reconstr Surg*, 1995, see below). The central dissection is raised in the subperiosteal plane, whilst dissection in the lateral zones is just deep to the TPF; thus, there is a **transition zone** where the periosteal layer has to be divided to join the two planes together. It is important to take care at the orbital rim to identify and preserve the nerves whilst carefully debulking the corrugator and procerus.

Chiu (*Plast Reconstr Surg*, 2003) noted a progressive decline in the number of endoscopic procedures compared with open brow lift from a survey of plastic surgeons. They speculate that the decline may possibly be due to the following:

- More selective use of the technique, recognising that endoscopic brow lift is ineffective in many patients
- Increased use of BTX

Endoscopic brow lift: A personal review of 538 patients and comparison of fixation techniques. (Jones BM, *Plast Reconstr Surg*, 2004)

This was a review of 538 endoscopic brow lifts using a technique based upon that of Oscar Ramirez (*Plast Reconstr Surg*, 1995). Eighty percent of patients had a simultaneous facelift:

- Lift vector is marked preoperatively; two parasagittal and two temporal incisions are made.
- Hydrodissection of the plane beneath the TPF with tumescent solution, followed by surgical dissection with endoscopic elevators to within 2 cm of the supraorbital rim.
- Sub-galeal fascial flap is raised from the temporal incisions.
- The fascia at the temporal crease is divided and dissection extended subperiosteally along the zygomatic process of the frontal bone.
- At the supraorbital rim, the supraorbital and supra-trochlear nerves are identified and the corrugator supercilii and procerus muscles debulked.
- The brow is then elevated and secured. Initially, fibrin glue was used before they changed to sutures passed through drill-hole bone tunnels with longer-lasting results.

COMPLICATIONS

- Alopecia and hairline distortion
- Asymmetry
- Prolonged forehead paraesthesia and frontal branch paralysis
- Implant infection

VI. BLEPHAROPLASTY

Excessive overhang of the upper eyelid results in a tired appearance; actual visual impairment is rare. It is important to differentiate true **dermatochalasis** from other problems such as brow or eyelid ptosis, which would not benefit from a simple blepharoplasty.

- **Blepharochalasis** is a rare AD condition affecting young adults where there is atrophy and stretching of upper lid tissues following recurrent episodes of atopic eyelid oedema. Antihistamines and steroids do not help.
- **Steatoblepharon** – excess fat protruding through a lax septum.
- **Blepharoptosis** – drooping of upper lid, i.e. 'ptosis'.
- **Pseudoblepharoptosis** – the eyelid is in a normal position but has the appearance of ptosis due to brow ptosis.

EYELID ANATOMY

- **Tarsal plates.** The tarsus is composed of fibrous connective tissue with meibomian glands, i.e. **not cartilage**; approximately 2 mm thick.

- Upper tarsus 7–11 mm tall (in White patients) – Müller's muscle and some fibres of the levator are attached. The upper tarsus is narrower in Asian patients.
- Lower tarsus 4–5 mm tall – the capsulopalpebral fascia is attached.
- The **orbital septum** is composed of fibrous tissue and can be viewed as an extension of the orbital periosteum and lies posterior to the orbicularis oculi muscle (OOM). It acts as a fascial barrier.
  - Upper septum – superior orbital rim to levator aponeurosis
  - Lower septum – inferior orbital rim to capsulopalpebral fascia
- **Canthal tendons** are extensions of the preseptal and pretarsal OOM. They act as check ligaments for the lateral and medial recti muscles.
  - The lateral canthal tendon (LCT) attaches to Whitnall's tubercle, which is 1.5 cm posterior to the lateral orbital rim.
  - The medial canthal tendon (MCT) is more complex – it is tripartite (anterior horizontal, posterior horizontal and vertical) and is important for the lacrimal pump.

FAT

- **Preseptal fat.**
  - Upper lid – ROOF (retro-orbicularis fat)
  - Lower lid – SOOF (suborbicularis fat)
- **Orbital fat** is physiologically different from other body fat – the cells are smaller; the fat is more saturated and has less lipoprotein lipase activity, is less metabolically active and is only minimally affected by diet/obesity. The medial fat is usually more vascular, but paler with smaller lobules and more fibrous tissue.
  - Upper lid (two pads) medial and central that are separated by the trochlea of the superior oblique (SOB).
  - Lower lid (three pads) medial, central and lateral. The medial and central fat pads are separated by the inferior oblique (IOB). The IOB lies relatively anterior and is thus vulnerable during fat resection, which may cause (temporary) diplopia.

MUSCLES

- **Upper lid retractors**
  - The **levator palpebrae superioris** (LPS, oculomotor) is the main retractor with 10–15 mm excursion; it arises from the lesser wing of the sphenoid, runs to Whitnall's ligament (where it changes direction) and courses inferiorly as an aponeurotic sheet to the tarsal plate with some fibres to the dermis.
  - **Müller's muscle** (sympathetic) provides 1–2 mm retraction, which is lost in Horner's syndrome; it

originates from the lower surface of the LPS and inserts to the superior tarsal margin.

- **Lower lid retractor**
  - **Capsulopalpebral fascia** – arises as two sheets around the IOB to fuse anteriorly as Lockwood's ligament, which runs to the lower lid septum some 5 mm below the tarsal plate. There is 1–2 mm of downward pull from the action of the inferior rectus muscle, **thus retracting the lower lid in synchrony with inferior globe rotation when looking downwards.**

LACRIMAL APPARATUS

The lacrimal gland has palpebral and orbital portions, separated by the levator aponeurosis. Tears help to lubricate the lid movements over the globe and contribute to the nourishment of the corneal epithelium, whilst some components are antibacterial. There are three layers:

- Lipid layer from the meibomian glands and sebaceous glands of Zeiss and Moll
- Mucoid layer from goblet cells
- Aqueous layer from the lacrimal gland

Reflex secretion comes mainly from the lacrimal gland under parasympathetic control, whilst passive/baseline tear production comes mainly from the accessory lacrimal glands, mucin goblet cells and meibomian glands.

The tears flow from lateral to medial, to the puncta of inferior and superior canaliculi that join the lacrimal sac, which empties via the nasolacrimal duct to the inferior meatus.

HISTORY

- Age, smoking, general health, e.g. diabetes, hypertension, coagulopathy
- Eye disease, e.g. dry eyes (sicca syndrome), epiphora, glaucoma
- Drug history especially anticoagulants
- Previous scars – quality?

EXAMINATION

- Specifically exclude **compensated brow ptosis** (CBP) – most patients have this to some degree when constant frontalis activity masks the ptosis. The need for a brow lift should always be considered. Mild to moderate CBP may not be that obvious in young or Asian patients with thicker forehead tissue.
  - **Look** at the brow position relative to the supraorbital ridge; there may be frontalis creases due to contraction.
  - **Ask the patient to look ahead and close his/her eyes.** Descent of the brow and relaxation of corrugator frown suggest CBP.

- **With the eyes still shut, immobilise the frontalis** and ask the patient to open his/her eyes again. A drop in the brow indicates that there was brow compensation. Performing a blepharoplasty in such a patient will cause the frontalis to relax, leading to a drop in the brow, which is unattractive and unwanted.
- **Brow ptosis can be corrected at the same operation**, or prior to the blepharoplasty to avoid excessive skin resection. Staging is preferred if there are concerns over dry eye.
- **Eye examination.**
  - Upper lid
    - Ptosis and lagophthalmos, skin laxity especially lateral hooding
    - Position of supratarsal fold (with downward gaze) 8–10 mm from lash line (in white patients)
    - Degree of fat herniation (press gently on the globe)
  - Baseline examination including vision
  - Bell's phenomenon
- **Facial nerve function**.

COUNSELLING

It is important to ascertain the patient's expectations both aesthetically and functionally. They should be advised of the following:

- Scars and bruising; time off work
- Possibility of reoperation
- Gritty/sticky eyes or scleral show

STANDARD BLEPHAROPLASTY TECHNIQUE

- Patients should be **marked in an upright position** with the upper lid under closing tension. The lower line is marked 9–10 mm above the lash line; the upper line varies – the skin is pinched with a pair of Adson forceps to determine the amount of skin to be removed at various points along the lid. There should still be 10–12 mm remaining between the upper incision line and the eyebrow. Extend the lower line laterally so that closure occurs within a wrinkle line.
- **Conservative skin/muscle excision.** The skin is removed, followed by an underlying strip of orbicularis (up to 3 mm) to reduce the bulk of the lid whilst preserving the pretarsal portion.
  - There must be 30 mm remaining between the lashes and the lower margin of the eyebrow; if too much is removed and then brow ptosis is corrected, (permanent) lagophthalmos will result.
  - Lagophthalmos that lasts for a week is not unusual. If it lasts longer (and excessive skin was not resected), suspect problems such as inadvertent tethering of the septum.
- **Incise the orbital septum high up to avoid LPS injury**. Gentle pressure on the globe may lead to

fat herniation from medial and lateral upper lid compartments through the incisions, which can then be removed with bipolar cautery.

- Prolapsing 'fat' far laterally is likely to be the lacrimal gland; consider glanduloplasty/gland suspension.
- Meticulous haemostasis with bipolar diathermy is very important to avoid retrobulbar haematoma.

COMPLICATIONS

- Infection.
- Inadequate correction.
- Muscle injury.
  - Ptosis due to LPS injury.
  - The most commonly damaged extraocular muscle is the **IOB**, resulting in diplopia looking up and out.
- Retrobulbar haematoma and blindness are thankfully rare.

ASIAN BLEPHAROPLASTY

Asians have an absent supratarsal crease due to the lack of dermal insertion by the levator aponeurosis (Figure 10.2).

- Shorter tarsal plates
- Increased fullness due to increased amounts of ROOF and SOOF
- Epicanthal folds – tarsalis (more prominent in the upper lid, 'normal' variant of Asian eyelid); palpebralis (upper and lower equally); inversus (predominant in the lower lid, feature of blepharophimosis ptosis epicanthus inversus [BPEI] syndrome). There are several common epicanthoplasty methods (Figure 10.3)

In Asians without a fold ('single eyelid'), the 'double eyelid' is created 4–7 mm from the lash line, i.e. lower than in the eyes of white patients. There are many different techniques described in the literature; most are variations of either the 'closed' or 'open' techniques.

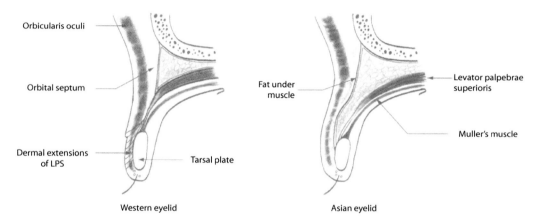

Figure 10.2 Anatomical differences between eyelids of Asians and whites accounting for the lack of an upper eyelid fold, often referred to as a 'double eyelid'. The tarsal plate in whites' eyelids is 8–11 mm, whereas it is 6.5–8 mm in Asians.

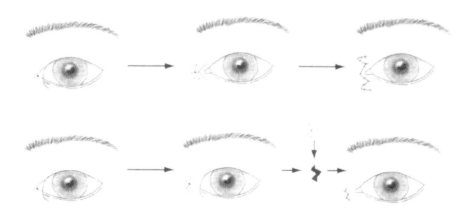

Figure 10.3 Two different methods of dealing with the epicanthal fold. None are entirely satisfactory due to the potential prominent scar; some suggest that the best way of treating epicanthal folds is to augment the nasal dorsum.

CLOSED TECHNIQUE OR SUTURE METHOD

The suture technique was first described in 1896 (Mikamo), and despite numerous modifications, the principles have remained the same. The closed technique uses two to three sutures to provide static fixation resulting in a **static fold**, i.e. visible when the eye is closed as well as open. Two to three small stab incisions are made with a no. 11 blade along the chosen line, and double-ended sutures are passed from the conjunctival side that has been marked at the same distance (some prefer to re-enter the same hole, others are less precise at 2–3 mm away, whilst others 'cheese-wire' the conjunctiva).

- This option is said to be more suited to younger patients, particularly those with thin lids, with no need for fat removal.
- The main disadvantage is that it tends to be temporary – some studies show 7% loss at 1 year. As there is no rearrangement of internal structures, some describe the technique as being non-physiological.
- It is less predictable, and asymmetry is more likely.

FULL OPEN TECHNIQUE OR INCISIONAL METHOD

The full open technique is 'definitive' in theory as it changes the internal anatomy and provides a dynamic fold, i.e. only seen with the eyes open. The incision is similar to a standard blepharoplasty and thus is more suited to older patients with fatter, puffier eyelids that have some tissue excess. It is still important to be selective and conservative with any excisions. In most of these techniques, the key sutures are those that bring together the dermis, tarsal plate and levator aponeurosis for secure fixation. The first suture at the mid-pupil point is tied, and the patient is asked to open his/her eyes in a forward gaze; the crease will be slightly higher than the final result due to intraoperative oedema.

LOWER LID BLEPHAROPLASTY

There is more debate and controversy regarding lower lid blepharoplasty.

LOWER LID EXAMINATION

- **Skin**. Examine for **lower lid tone** (it should **snap back** quickly – within one blink – after being pulled away from the globe; >1 second indicates significant laxity). **Scleral show** may be due to tarsal laxity, exophthalmos or middle lamellae contracture.
  - **Repair of lower lid laxity** is an important component of lower lid blepharoplasty; some propose that it is an integral problem in many patients that should be fixed prior to determining if skin excess exists.
    - Minimal lid laxity (1–2 mm distraction) can be treated with orbicularis repositioning.
    - For 3–6 mm of distraction, a **canthopexy** (retinacular suspension) is needed as well and/or muscle suspension (the fibrous lateral part of the orbicularis oculi is tacked up to a point lateral to the LCT). It is less invasive than a canthoplasty; it does not involve disinsertion of the lCT (i.e. no cantholysis) but provides only mild lid tightening and canthal elevation.
    - For more severe laxity (>6 mm), a **canthoplasty** with cantholysis is required, often called a lateral tarsal strip procedure.
    - Tarsal shortening (Kuhnt–Szymanowski procedure) – split-level excision of muscle (shield) and posterior lamellae lateral to lateral limbus and skin muscle via blepharoplasty incision. This is a good option if there is true tarsal excess.
- **There are a variety of lower lid lines/grooves/swellings to note**, and the inconsistent use of the terminology can be confusing. They often coexist.
  - **Palpebral/eyelid bags** (common eyebags) are the most common and are usually caused by fat protrusion (Castanares). The fat/swelling lies directly under the eyelid and becomes apparent as the ageing eyelid loses tone (attenuation of orbital septum). This is often bounded inferiorly by the arcus marginalis tethering ('dark circles').
    - These should be distinguished from malar bags as the latter are rarely corrected by blepharoplasty and probably represent chronic regional oedema related to chronic sun damage. Malar bags sit lower and more lateral on the cheek.
  - **Tear trough** refers to the groove/depression at the boundary of the eyelid and cheek, which is most prominent medially and continues down as the nasojugal groove; it runs between the eyelid and malar bags. The name comes from the observation that tears now run obliquely across the face instead of straight down. More severe forms may be called a tear trough depression, whilst a more widespread form, i.e. spreading laterally, is sometimes called 'suborbital volume deficiency'.
  - **Festoons (malar bags)** describe the redundant folds that hang from canthus to canthus encroaching on the cheek; they are soft tissue (usually skin and muscle but may include orbital septum and fat). The term is usually taken to refer to the sagging of the orbital and malar segments of the muscle of the lower lid. A festoon (Latin *festo*,

'festival garland') is a garland that hangs loosely from two points of attachment. They are said to feel typically 'squishy' and easy to move.

- Festoons squinch test – forcible closure of eyes will improve appearance of 'true' muscle festoons, i.e. ptotic orbicularis oculi (muscle contraction that also pushes any protruding fat back), though the skin redundancy remains.
- **Eyelid bags tend to become more prominent when looking upwards whilst festoons are minimally affected.**
- **Globe position.** Check for a **negative vector orbit** (most anterior part of the infraorbital rim lies behind the plane of the front of the globe), i.e. prominent eye, which increases the risk of ectropion. These patients may benefit from canthoplasty or malar augmentation.
  - Beware of excessive scleral show. Proptosis can be a feature of thyroid disease.
  - Enophthalmos may be post-traumatic, e.g. orbital fractures.
  - Perform **lacrimal function tests** in the elderly and those with dry eye symptoms.
  - Schirmer's test 1 – basic and reflex secretion; paper on lateral sclera; >10 mm in 5 minutes is normal.
  - Schirmer's test 2 – basic secretion (~40% of above) after topical local anaesthesia.
  - Others are more advanced – tear film break-up, Rose Bengal stain, tear lysozyme electrophoresis.

Reducing problems in lower lid blepharoplasty

- Avoid over-dissecting (to reduce contracture) and over-resecting – skin excision is generally not needed, but when it is being considered, patients should be marked upright and not supine to avoid lateral scleral show; only skin redundancy seen after the lateral canthus is placed in its proper position can be regarded as truly 'redundant'.
- Modest fat bulges are best removed via a trans-conjunctival approach or very small skin incisions. Overzealous removal causes a hollow appearance; it is better to tighten the septum by judicious plication (avoiding excessive tension, which can shorten the lid).

In general, there are three groups of patients:

- Young (20–30) with 'bags' due to premature fat herniation, with little skin laxity – these are typically treated with a trans-conjunctival fat resection.
- Middle aged (40–60) with excess of skin/muscle and fat herniation but good lid turgor and snapback – these can be treated with subciliary incision.
- Older (>60) with skin/muscle excess and lid laxity (lid can be pulled 8 mm or more from globe, normally 3–5 mm) and delayed snapback – these patients need a lateral canthoplasty (lid shortening) or canthopexy in addition to a 'traditional' blepharoplasty.

BLEPHAROPLASTY SURGICAL TECHNIQUE

Traditionally, lower lid blepharoplasty was an operation to remove skin and fat in the lower eyelid to deal with the wrinkling and bulging from orbital fat herniation (Figure 10.4).

- Elevate **a skin–muscle flap** with the skin incision just below the lashes (i.e. subciliary scars, which heal best out of the lower lid incisions).
  - A variant is to raise a **skin-only** flap over the preseptal orbicularis. This can be used in cases of skin excess, but the dissection is rather tedious and may cause scarring of the skin/muscle and lymphatic issues.
  - Excision of skin/muscle is determined by re-draping the flap without tension over the lash line. This may be estimated preoperatively by asking the patient to look up with the mouth open. Minimal/no skin resection is the norm; if in doubt, do not resect. However, lid retraction is multifactorial in aetiology and thus may still occur **even if no skin has been excised.**
    - Despite this, some lagophthalmos may still occur due to oedema; reduce post-operative oedema with cool packs and head elevation.
  - A strip of muscle may be positioned lateral and superior to provide some support. With more pronounced **lower lid laxity,** formal canthopexy or Kuhnt–Szymanowski may be needed (see above).
- Excise fat conservatively to avoid a 'hollowed-out' appearance.
  - The orbital septum and fat can be re-draped forwards and downwards over the infraorbital margin to diminish any tear trough.

The traditional skin–muscle lower lid blepharoplasty was a standard technique until recently but did have problems with ectropion, hollowing of the orbit and denervation atrophy of the muscle. It is still the standard approach if significant skin and muscle needs to be removed/re-draped; it also provides good access for fat transposition and midface procedures.

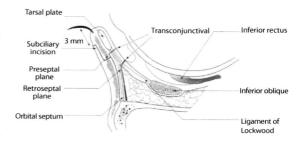

Figure 10.4 Lower eyelid anatomy and approaches for lower blepharoplasty. The trans-conjunctival approach can be preseptal or retroseptal and avoids an external skin scar.

The **trans-conjunctival approach** gained popularity as it avoided post-operative lower lid retraction from the scar; it is most suited to the younger patient with little skin laxity.

- The incision is made on the conjunctival surface at or just below the tarsal plate, stopping at least 4 mm lateral to the punctum.
- Division of the lower lid retractors allows access to the plane behind the septum, i.e. a **retroseptal approach**, which allows better visualisation of the fat.
  - Exposure is limited compared to a transcutaneous approach.
  - Fat could still be removed via an incision above the fornix if skin excision is not needed.
  - CO_2 laser resurfacing could offer some skin tightening whilst avoiding scars. A limited 'skin pinch' excision is possible for those with more skin excess; the thinking was that by avoiding undermining, there would be less scarring and contraction.

COMPLICATIONS

- **Asymmetry.**
- **Ectropion, excessive scleral show and lagophthalmos** – usually due to overcorrection; store removed skin in case it is needed later.
  - Lagophthalmos is usually temporary; treat with massage and taping; persistent cases may need skin grafts.
- **Blindness due to retrobulbar haematoma** (~1 in 40,000) – presents as pain, proptosis, ecchymosis, reduced eye movement, dilated pupil, scotomas and raised intraocular pressure. Emergency treatment includes head elevation, rebreathing bag (to raise CO_2), release of sutures, lateral canthotomy/cantholysis and administration of mannitol, acetazolamide, steroids and beta blockers. Emergency exploration; consult ophthalmologist.
  - Other causes of blindness are central retinal artery occlusion and optic nerve ischaemia.
- **Corneal injury** – check with fluorescein stain; treat with topical antibiotics and eye patch.
- **Muscle injury** – LPS (leading to ptosis), IOB and SOB (leading to diplopia); most cases are due to oedema and resolve.

TREATMENT OF TEAR TROUGH

This is a difficult area to treat. The problem is most certainly multifactorial with soft tissue deficiency/descent being the most significant; other factors include bony depression/deficiency. Some have identified it as a gap in the muscle cover below the inferomedial border of the OOM or a tight attachment of the muscle to the bone by retaining ligaments, and it may also occur in combination with fat herniation.

- Tissue fillers and autologous fat have been used to treat the folds and depressions under the eye; the effect is often temporary.

- Many surgical techniques for the tear trough have been described, including the following:
  - Repositioning of bulging lower orbital fat into the area of hollowness, e.g. Goldberg's repositioning of subseptal fat into a subperiosteal pocket formed after trans-conjunctival arcus marginalis release. The **septal reset** is similar to this (Hamra, Loeb).
  - Implants, particularly for bony deformities.
  - Mid-facelift.

VII. RHINOPLASTY

ANATOMY

See also Chapter 3, Section C:III (Figure 10.5).

- **Skin** over the upper two-thirds (dorsum and side walls, upper two zones) is thin with little subcutaneous tissue, whilst skin over the lower third (lower zone, tip and alar) is thick, sebaceous and more fixed.
- **Muscles**
  - LLS alaeque nasi – keeps the external nasal valve open

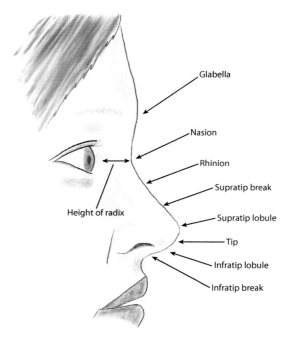

Figure 10.5 Lateral view of the nose. The nasion corresponds to the position of the nasofrontal suture, whilst the sellion is the deepest part of the nasofrontal angle and can be thought of as the soft tissue equivalent of the nasion. The radix is an area, being the root of the nose, centred on the nasion and extending down to the lateral canthus level and upwards for an equivalent distance. The height of the radix is measured from the plane of the anterior cornea.

- Depressor septi nasi – hyperactivity shortens the upper lip and reduces tip projection with smiling

NASAL VAULT

- **Bony vault** – paired nasal bones and frontal process of maxilla.
- **Upper cartilaginous vault** – paired upper lateral cartilages (ULCs) that lie under the bones by 6–8 mm. This overlapping zone is called the **keystone area**. It is the widest part of the dorsum and is important for the **dorsal aesthetic line**. They join the septum in the midline.
  - The female nose often has an hourglass shape, being narrowest in the middle third.
- **Lower cartilaginous vault** – paired lower lateral cartilages (LLC) with medial (middle) and lateral crura. The lateral crus (scroll area) overlaps the ULC in three-fourths of cases, with the reverse pattern in 11%.
  - Weak and soft triangles (Converse)
- **Frankfurt line** – horizontal line from the top of EAM to the lowest part of the orbital rim that also marks the middle of the nose (bone cartilage junction); it is the 'halfway' line.
- **Leonardo quadrilateral** – horizontal lines from the top of the ear to the upper eyelid, bottom of the ear to the base of the nose, with parallel slopes.

ASSESSMENT

A careful assessment of the problem and the patient, and his/her expectation(s), is essential. The nose should be consistent with the ethnic identity of the patient and in harmony with the face. Attempts to bring objectivity to 'harmony' include the use of 'Ideal proportions' such as the Thirds, as well as 'Ideal' lengths and angles (see below). Generally, rhinoplasty is not performed in children; the nose grows significantly until at least 16 years of age.

HISTORY

- Previous trauma or surgery. Older rhinoplasties often over-reduced the dorsum to match a nonprojecting tip.
- Symptoms of nasal disease such as nosebleeds, allergic rhinitis and olfactory disturbances.
- Drug history – aspirin, warfarin, steroids and recreational drugs.
- Medical problems, e.g. diabetes, hypertension, smokers.
- **Beware the male SIMON patient.**

EXAMINATION

Photographs are vital.

- **Skin quality and thickness** – specifically telangiectasia (which can get worse). The thicker the skin, the stronger and more angular the framework required to be visible through the skin envelope.

- **Assess proportions and symmetry** of the nose and relationship to thirds of the face. Note that micrognathia will make the nose look bigger and, in this case, is best treated by chin augmentation or genioplasty. The nose needs to match the ethnicity of the patient.
  - Width of the alar base approximates to the intercanthal distance (wider alar may be due to flaring or a truly wide base).
- **Evaluate the nasal lines.**
  - **Nasal deviation** – look at the dorsal line from the middle of the glabellar to the middle of the philtrum (to mentum).
  - Consider the **dorsum** and the presence of any hump, supra-tip deformity, etc.
    - Female dorsum is slightly concave; male dorsum is slightly convex/straight.
- **Evaluate the tip:**
  - **Alar rim symmetry.** On a basilar view, the alar rim and tip should approximate an equilateral triangle with the ratio of one-third lobule to two-thirds columella.
  - **Tip defining points** – one on each side, forming the lateral corners of a vertical rhombus/diamond (two equilateral triangles) with the supra-tip break and columellar break forming the upper and lower angles.
  - **Tip projection** – tip to alar cheek junction. In the 'aesthetic tip', 50%–60% of this line is anterior to the upper lip.
  - **Tip rotation** – columellar/**nasolabial angle**: males, 90–95°; females, 95–105°.
- Examine the **septum** for deviation and check for collapse of the internal valve (see below) and turbinate hypertrophy.

AIRWAY OBSTRUCTION AND RHINOPLASTY

Inferior turbinate (IT) hypertrophy is the commonest anatomic cause of nasal obstruction (Figure 10.6).

The relative importance of septal and nasal valvular surgery in correcting airway obstruction in primary and secondary rhinoplasty. (Constantian MB, *Plast Reconstr Surg*, 1996)

Four factors may cause **airway obstruction:**

- **Septal deviation** – septoplasty for more anterior deviations; submucous resection (SMR) is more suited for more posterior problems.
- **Inferior turbinate hypertrophy** – IT infracture/diathermy/resection: chronic exposure to air flow may cause mucosal changes leading eventually to atrophic rhinitis or ozena.
- **Internal valve problem** – The nose accounts for 50% of upper airway resistance, and a major contributor is the internal nasal valve, which lies at the angle (usually ~15°) made by the caudal edge of the ULC with the septum. Note that according to Poiseuille's law, air

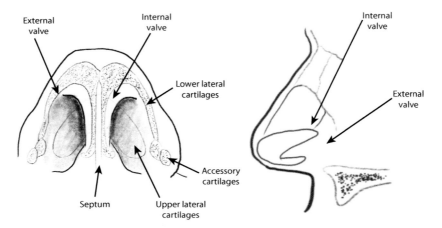

Figure 10.6 Nasal valves. The internal valve lies at the angle between the lower border of the upper lateral cartilage and the septum.

flow increases to the fourth power of the radius, and the converse is also true. Lateral traction on the cheeks (**Cottle's manoeuvre**) or spring devices worn by athletes open up the internal nasal valve and reduce airway resistance.

- Narrowing the nose by dorsal resection, osteotomy and infracture may render the internal valve too narrow (<10°); treat by insertion of **dorsal spreader grafts** between the ULC and the septum. The matchstick-shaped grafts maintain the valve whilst also buttressing/straightening up a slightly deviated septum and smoothing the profile. Alar batten grafts may be used for lateral wall supra-alar pinching.
- **External valve problem**. The external valve is formed by the alar rim (lateral crus of the alar cartilage, soft tissue of the alae), membranous septum and the nasal sill. The nasalis dilates the valve during inspiration. Malposition or over-resection of the alar cartilages may compromise the external valve mechanism; treat by insertion of **onlay tip lateral crural grafts** to stiffen the LLC or support the alar rim **with alar batten grafts** (septal or conchal cartilage inserted in a tight pocket in the area of collapse).

ASSESSMENT

- Test each nostril separately by occluding from below rather than by pushing on the ala from the other side; a cold metal speculum can be used to check for misting.
  - Bilateral obstruction that has variable severity suggests a mucosal problem (most commonly allergic or viral rhinitis), whilst a constant obstruction suggests a fixed, i.e. skeletal, problem such as septal deviation.
  - Nasal cycle – the IT undergoes a 3- to 4-hourly cycle of congestion and decongestion in 80% of the population. This is a normal phenomenon;

persistent congestion due to turbinate hypertrophy may warrant turbinectomy.
  - Cottle's manoeuvre.
- Assess alar rim including collapse.
- Examine the septum.

APPROACHES

The **closed approach**, i.e. endonasal, has the advantages of no external scar, and dissection is limited to the area needed with a precise pocket for graft insertion and fixation; this reduces post-operative oedema. It is adequate for most surgeries except for tip modification. However, the learning curve is significant, and the view (for surgeon and student) is limited (Figure 10.7). The incision placement depends on the problem that needs correction:

- **Inter-cartilaginous** – between the ULC and the LLC (alar); evert to deliver the alar cartilage. This is the standard route to the dorsum.
- **Trans-cartilaginous/intra-cartilaginous** – through the alar cartilage, as determined by the amount of cephalic trim required (the part above the incision is usually discarded), reducing volume. Five to seven millimetres of lateral crus is required for stability. This allows access to the alar cartilage and better exposure for tip surgery.
- **Marginal/infra-cartilaginous** – caudal to alar cartilage (will also need inter-cartilaginous incision to **deliver** the lateral alar crus into wound). Provides good access for domal suturing/scoring. It is commonly used for open rhinoplasties in combination with a columellar incision. A true 'rim' incision is rarely used.

The **open approach is useful for tip work** and is often the preferred routine approach for patients with cleft nose deformity or needing a **secondary** rhinoplasty. Note that the contribution to the tip from the columellar artery from the superior labial artery will be lost, leaving it supplied mostly by the external nasal artery (anterior ethmoidal) and lateral nasal artery (angular artery).

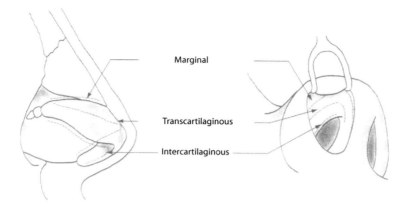

Figure 10.7 Types of incision for rhinoplasty.

CLOSED VERSUS OPEN RHINOPLASTY

Greater exposure is afforded by the open approach:

- This makes **diagnosis** of deforming factors easier.
- Repositioning of cartilaginous framework and application of grafts can be secured under **direct vision** including dorsal spreader grafts and onlay grafts to the dorsum and the tip.
- Allows excellent haemostasis.
- **Facilitates teaching**.

However, the main disadvantages of the open approach are the longer operative time, prolonged tip oedema and the **transcolumellar scar**. Patterns include the following: Gruber – step, Toriumi – central peak transverse or V or W, whilst some propose inverted V with lateral transverse components to reduce the vertical component.

Generally, **the closed approach is sufficient for most surgeries** (especially if no tip work is needed) but involves significant retraction required with the limited exposure, as well as the significant learning curve. Under certain circumstances, the closed approach may be contraindicated:

- Cantilever graft is needed.
- Excess skin needs to be excised.
- Extreme cephalic malposition of lateral crura, which makes alar dissection difficult with a closed approach.
- Severe deviation/deformity.
- Cocaine nose.

Alterations in nasal sensibility following open rhinoplasty. (Bafaqeeh SA, *Br J Plast Surg*, 1998)
The nerve supply to the nasal skin is derived from the following:

- Infra-trochlear nerve (V1, branch of nasociliary) – over nasal bones
- External nasal nerve (V1, terminal branch of the anterior ethmoidal) – over ULCs, tip and upper columella
  - The nerve emerges between the nasal bones and the ULCs and is at risk when elevating lateral nasal skin.
- Infraorbital nerve (V2) – over LLC and columella

Following open rhinoplasty, altered sensation at the nasal tip and upper columella was recorded at 3 weeks and had recovered by a year.

SEPTAL INCISIONS

- **Complete transfixion** – this is usually made as a continuation of the inter- or trans-cartilaginous incisions. It separates the membranous septum (and medial crura) from the caudal septum to free the tip, exposing the nasal spine and depressor septi muscles. The septum is also free for mucoperichondrial flaps to be raised. However, as the attachment of the medial crural footplates to the caudal septum is disrupted, there is a loss of tip support and potential loss of tip projection (which may be a desirable outcome in some cases).
- **Hemitransfixion** (Cottle M, *Arch Otolaryngol*, 1960) – this is a unilateral incision at the junction of the caudal septum and columella. Typically, this is used for procedures in which the caudal septum is deviated and needs resection for tip rotation or columellar adjustment.
- **High septal transfixion** (Kamer FM, *Laryngoscope*, 1984) – this transcartilaginous incision does not violate the junction of the caudal septum and medial crura/membranous septum and so does not alter tip support.

NASAL TIP

Tip projection depends on the supporting structures; some have likened the tip to a **tripod** (Anderson) with each lateral crus forming a leg, and the third leg from the conjoined medial crura. The medial crura are shorter and have additional support by attachments to the septum.

- Upward rotation of the tip occurs if the lateral limbs are shortened or if the central limb is lengthened. With short noses, the aim is to de-rotate the tip.

- Volume can be reduced by resection of the top portion of the lateral crus of the alar cartilages, though some say this also reduces support.

The support structures to the tip are often divided into **major** (alar cartilages and their attachments, particularly the medial crural footplates to the caudal septum) and **minor** (domal suspensory ligament, anterior septal angle, nasal spine and caudal septum, sesamoid cartilage complex).

Increasing tip projection – columellar strut grafts and suture techniques are used before cartilage tip grafts that may be palpable in thinner-skinned patients.

- **Columellar strut grafts**.
  - **Floating** – able to increase tip projection by 1–2 mm; place it 2–3 mm anterior to the nasal spine and secured in the pocket between the medial crura.
  - **Fixed grafts are used if >3 mm extra projection is needed.** Rib cartilage is often used and placed on top of the nasal spine.
- **Suture techniques** can increase projection by 1–2 mm and can help refine/define tip. Shield or umbrella grafts can camouflage the tips, especially after suturing.
  - **Medial crural septal sutures** – between the medial crura and the septum, cause rotation of the nasal tip, which increases tip projection and corrects drooping nose, e.g. ageing.
  - **Medial crural sutures** – stabilises the columellar strut and refines the nasal tip. These are different from the above; they are horizontal mattress sutures placed between the medial crura that bring the LLCs together and stabilise the columellar strut, reducing medial crural flare.
  - **Inter-domal sutures** – i.e. dome binding, increases infra-tip columellar projection and refines the tip.
  - **Trans-domal sutures** between the medial and lateral parts of the same alar cartilage, which allow the correction of domal asymmetry and increase tip projection.
- **Tip graft.**
  - **Infra-lobular** (hexagonal or rhomboid/diamond) (Sheen)
  - **Onlay graft** – provides tip projection and refinement, can be doubled up (or more) (Peak)
  - **Combinations** (Gunter)

Reducing tip projection – a maximum of 2 mm can be reduced without noticeable columellar bowing or alar flaring.

- **Closed approach** – transfixion incision to separate the alar cartilage from the septum and reduce support.
- **Open approach** – resection of attachment of the medial crura to the septum to remove support from inter-cartilaginous ligaments.
  - Volume reduction of the alar cartilage leaving at least 6–8 mm to prevent external valve collapse.

- To reduce projection further, then transect the lateral crura and overlap them; repeating this with the medial crura can reduce projection further – interrupted strip technique/crural overlay.

NASAL DORSUM

- **Dorsal hump reduction** – the hump is 57% cartilage and 43% bony. Separate the ULCs from the septum and shave down the septum with a blade (this avoids reducing the ULC, which may lead to collapse of the internal nasal valve and an irregular dorsum). If the ULC protrudes, it can then also be shaved flush. The bony hump is reduced with a down-biting rasp or osteotome. If there is an **open roof deformity** (the gap between the septum and the bone), then it can be closed with infracture/osteotomies (see below).
- **Dorsal augmentation.** Whilst Western rhinoplasty is usually concerned with reduction, Chinese patients have a flatter bulbous nose with less tip projection. Thus, the most requested operations are the augmentation of the dorsum and increased tip projection.
  - **Cartilage grafts** – septal, costal cartilage or ear (elastic) cartilage. Some have described the use of wrapping diced cartilage (conchal or septal) in deep temporal fascia or Surgicel. Cartilage has a memory effect but also the tendency to warp if damaged (Gibson).
  - **Bone** – iliac, calvarium, rib (10th and 11th have straight segments), but has the tendency for more resorption compared to cartilage (which has low metabolic activity).
  - **Alloplastic**, e.g. silicone, is popular in Chinese patients and, despite the theoretical problems with infection risk, seems to be well tolerated – this may be due in part to the thicker skin. A donor site is avoided. Medpor allows some vascular ingrowth, but the advantages of this property are unclear. The use of Alloderm has also been described. When choosing a material, it is also important to consider how difficult it would be to remove, if complications arise:
    - Infection can occur years after implant surgery. If an implant is extruding, the sterility has been compromised, and it should be removed. Occasionally, it can be salvaged with broad-spectrum antibiotics and irrigation, but most need removal eventually. Further surgery should ideally be delayed for 6–9 months.
    - Migration can occur.
    - If an implant is extruding, the sterility has been compromised, and it should be removed.
- Injections of paraffin or liquid silicone are rarely performed now. Modern alternatives include hyaluronic acid (may not be stiff enough), Radiesse or Sculptra.

Osteotomies

The bony vault is likened to a pyramid with the paired nasal bones and maxilla, and the shape can be altered with osteotomies (but may lead to ULC collapse). Relative contraindications include the following:

- Elderly patients with thin bones
- Patients who need to wear heavy spectacles
- Ethnic nose that is particularly flat and broad

Lateral osteotomies can narrow the side walls of the dorsum as well as close an open roof deformity and straighten a deviated nasal pyramid. Periosteal dissection should be limited to maximise support to the nasal bones, and osteotomy should not be carried above the inter-canthal line where the bone becomes thicker. Take care to avoid damaging the angular artery (Figure 10.8).

- **Low–high osteotomy** (most common) can be used to mobilise moderately widened nasal bones or a small open roof with a hinged greenstick-type fracture of the side wall. **It does not allow major movements.** The osteotomy starts low (lateral) to the piriform aperture and extends upwards to the inter-canthal line ending high (medial) on the dorsum. This tends to narrow the

airway slightly and thus should be avoided in those with narrow internal nasal valves.

- **Low–low osteotomy** can be used for wide nasal bones or a large open roof. It begins low and continues low to the dorsal region at the inter-canthal line.
- **Double-level** – for excessive lateral wall convexity or lateral nasal wall deformities. A lateral osteotomy is performed along the nasal wall along the nasomaxillary suture and combined with a low–low osteotomy.

'Low start' means start inferiorly at the side of the nose at the cheek–nose junction; 'high end' means end just below the medial canthus on the side wall of the nose above the junction with the cheek, whilst 'low end' means ending nearer to the junction of the cheek and the nose. 'Low–low' osteotomy generally needs a transverse osteotomy (and liable to collapse), whilst 'low–high' does not. 'High–high' osteotomies tend to produce a step deformity.

Medial osteotomies separate nasal bones from the bony nasal septum and may be used in cases of traumatically narrowed vaults or for patients with widened nasal bones to create a line for a controlled fracture. They should be performed before lateral osteotomies, advancing with a two-tap technique.

NASAL ALAE

Collapse of the alar rim may cause external nasal (valve) obstruction. The main support to the rim comes from the lateral crural attachments to accessory cartilages (lateral crural complex) and to the piriform aperture, ULC and suspensory ligament of the tip. The posterior 50% of the alar rim is made of fibrofatty tissue and **devoid of cartilage**.

- **Non-anatomic alar contour grafts** can be used in selected cases with minimal vestibular lining loss and at least 3 mm of the alar cartilage still remaining. A pocket is created above the rim for a 2–6 mm graft, verifying that the rim contour is corrected without the graft being visible.
- **Lateral crural strut grafts** are placed on the deep surface of the lateral crura and may be used for cases of malpositioned or misshapen lateral crura, as well as alar rim collapse or retraction. These are usually harvested from the septal cartilage (3 × 4 × 20 mm) and positioned during an open rhinoplasty in a pocket under the lateral crus and sutured in.

ALAR BASE

The problem should be analysed in terms of its components. Note that altering the alae may alter the smile and may make the tip look relatively bigger. Nostril thinning can be performed via rim/marginal incisions but is fraught with difficulties and complications such as dimpling and scarring.

The width of the alar base is approximately equal to the inter-canthal distance; a wide alar base may be due to a truly wide alar base or to **excessive alar flare** (>2 mm difference between the base and the maximum width). Alar base excision can be considered in the latter group – a wedge of tissue

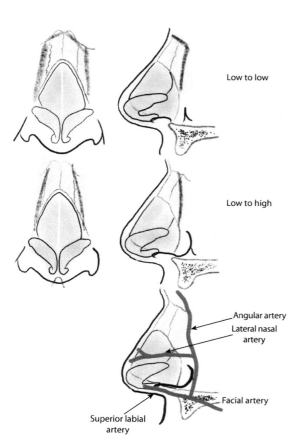

Low to low

Low to high

Angular artery

Lateral nasal artery

Facial artery

Superior labial artery

Figure 10.8 Lateral osteotomies of the nose. It is important to avoid the terminal branches of the facial artery.

is excised (wider skin side and not carried into vestibule, but can pass under the nasal sill) preserving 1–2 mm of the alar base above the groove. This is often called a Weir excision, although he described many variations.

For a wide alar base:

- A wedge excision of the alar base that extends to the vestibule.
- Excision of the nasal sill either as parallelogram or diamond.
- Some have described an 'alar cinch' stitch with a non-resorbable suture on a straight needle, which is passed through a hypodermic needle passed from stab incisions at the alar bases/creases under the soft tissue of the base of the nose.

'TYPICAL' OPEN RHINOPLASTY

EXPOSURE

- GA or LA including nasal block/sedation; topical xylometazoline/cocaine pack/spray. Shave vibrissae.
- Evert nostril with a double hook and make a curved **infra-cartilaginous** incision in the nasal mucosa connecting the two sides with a stepped columellar incision at its narrowest part.
- Lift the columellar skin and nasal tip soft tissues off the cartilage framework and then separate the LLCs from each other and the septum.
- Dissect the mucosa off the septum and create extramucosal tunnels beneath the ULCs; use scissors to separate the ULCs from the septal cartilage.

IDENTIFY AND REDUCE THE BONY HUMP

- Trim the upper edges of upper lateral and septal cartilages (soft hump) and then use an osteotome to cleanly excise the bony hump (save the bone as it may be needed for radix graft).

CLOSE THE 'OPEN ROOF'

- Make a stab incision in the inner canthus, and then use a periosteal elevator to dissect a subperiosteal tunnel down the side of the nasomaxillary angle for maxillary osteotomy.
- Introduce a 2 mm osteotomy and create a series of perforations along the proposed osteotomy line; then infracture the nasal bones with digital pressure and correct any irregularities by rasping.

RETURN TO THE TIP (I.E. SHOULD BE LAST OR NEARLY THE LAST STEP)

- Excise a portion of the cephalic edge of the LLCs to refine the tip and approximate with 6/0 ethilon.
  - Bulbous tip – excise a wedge or dart.

- Bifid tip – widely separated medial crura should be plicated in the midline.
- Hanging tip due to columella lacking adequate skeletal support (e.g. after over-resection of the caudal edge of the septum) – needs a T-shaped cartilage graft, e.g. from the septum.

CLOSURE

- Close mucosa with 5/0 vicryl rapide and skin with 6/0 ethilon.

POST-OPERATIVE CARE

Patient should expect to have a painful swollen nose with black eyes; nasal obstruction may last weeks to months. Head elevation and ice packs may help.

- Nasal packs (24–48 hours) – not usually necessary and certainly do not need to be placed all the way in.
- Plaster of Paris or other external splints (1–2 weeks). Remove sutures at 1 week.
- Avoid nose blowing for 2 weeks.
- Avoid wearing glasses or playing contact sports for 4–6 weeks.

COMPLICATIONS

The commonest complaint is the **lack of tip definition** (which takes time to become evident).

- Infection, haematoma/epistaxis
- Under-correction (residual deformity) or overcorrection (new deformity)
  - **Saddle deformity**. Excessive removal of the dorsal bone and cartilage.
  - **Pinched-tip deformity** from the fracture of the lateral crura.
  - **Supra-tip deformity** may be due to several reasons.
    - Inadequate septal dorsal hump reduction
    - Inadequate correction of a bulbous tip
    - Over-reduction of the cartilaginous skeleton
- Persistent nasal tip oedema (up to 2 years) and numbness that may include the upper teeth
- Scars (inner canthus, columella), palpable step at the lateral maxillary osteotomy site
- Airway obstruction – internal valve problem
- Alloplast infection/extrusion

RHINOPHYMA

Greek: *rhis* is 'nose'; *phyma* is 'growth'.

This is a severe form of acne rosacea and affects up to 10% of the population, more commonly males of Celtic races. There is a familial component in around half of patients. The nasal tip is affected more than the rest of the nose, although other areas may also be affected: mentophyma, otophyma and zygophyma.

Apart from the appearance (often unfairly stigmatised as being caused by alcoholism), lesions can have a foul odour and are prone to superficial infection. Malignant degeneration to BCC has been described but is rare.

Non-surgical treatment for mild cases:

- Antibiotics – metronidazole, tetracycline.
- Retinoids – tretinoin and isotretinoin – however, as it impairs re-epithelialisation, concurrent surgery should be avoided.

SURGICAL TREATMENT

For more severe cases, ablative CO_2 lasers can debulk the hypertrophied sebaceous glands, leaving sufficient remnants to heal (usually within 3 weeks). Skin grafts are rarely needed; contracture of the healed skin also helps to reduce the size of the nose. Lasers are more precise than, say, dermabrasion/tangential shaving, and the procedure is relatively bloodless. An **old photograph** is useful to help gauge the endpoint.

VIII. LIPOSUCTION

Charles Dujarier (1870–1931) is unfortunately credited with the first attempt at aesthetic fat removal from the calves of a model, Suzanne Geoffre, ostensibly to show off the new fashion of skirts stopping at the knee. Unfortunately, he removed too much skin during his procedure, and being unable to close the wound even after muscle resection, bound the legs, which led to gangrene. The patient successfully sued and received 200,000 Francs' compensation. He died soon after his appeal failed. Plastic surgery in France was practically outlawed in the immediate aftermath.

In modern liposuction, fat is sucked into the openings in the cannula tip and then avulsed as the suction cannula moves back and forth. The fibrous stroma surrounding neurovascular bundles remains relatively intact, preserving blood supply and sensation to the overlying skin.

The use of **blunt tip cannulae** (Illouz, also invented the 'wet' technique) was an important development over the early sharp curettes. Early cannulae were of large diameter to allow aggressive fat removal, but as the procedure evolved from 'mass removal' to **contouring**, smaller cannulae (2–5 mm) are used, allowing greater control.

FAT ANATOMY

- The fat above Scarpa's fascia is compact with many fibrous septae.
- The fat below Scarpa's fascia is globular with fewer fibrous septae; its distribution is responsible for the typical sex-related body shapes.

It is usually said that the number of fat cells in adults is fixed and moderate **weight gain is accompanied by fat cell hypertrophy** – cell hyperplasia usually only occurs in massive weight gain.

FAT DISTRIBUTION

- **Superficial fat.** The fat in this layer tends to be a lighter yellow in colour.
- **Deep fat.** In men, there is often fat under the muscle fascia that cannot be easily liposuctioned. There is also intra-abdominal fat.

Twin studies have shown that there is a significant genetic/gender influence on fat distribution, e.g. around the 'hips' – in males, it tends to be manifest as 'love handles' at the true hip area (android), whilst in females, the problem is largely lower down the lateral thigh (gynoid). There also seems to be redistribution with age; there is a greater proportion of intra-abdominal and intra-/inter-muscular fat tissue. Asking the patient to tense his/her abdominal muscles may help to distinguish between them.

INDICATION

The commonest indication is cosmesis – the removal of localised deposits of fat that are not responsive to dieting/exercise. Other indications are as follows:

- Applied for reduction of fatty tissue in other situations, e.g. flap thinning, debulking lipomas, treating gynaecomastia (and selected cases of female breast reduction, or as part of Lejour technique)
- Treatment for fat necrosis and extravasation injuries
- Harvest fat for injection
- Axillary hyperhidrosis (superficial liposuction, usually ultrasound assisted)

Liposuction is not for weight loss, but the reduced body size may act as a stimulus for further weight loss. Others have warned that liposuction may actually increase the proportion of visceral fat and negatively impact on the health of the patient, although this has been disputed.

Absence of an effect of liposuction on insulin action and risk factors for coronary heart disease. (Klein S, *N Engl J Med*, 2004)
Fifteen obese females had liposuction, with a 44% reduction of adipose volume in non-diabetics vs. 28% in diabetics. Liposuction did not alter lipid levels or insulin sensitivity.

Prospective clinical study reveals significant reduction in triglyceride level and white cell count. (Swanson E, *Plast Reconstr Surg*, 2011)
It was found that triglyceride levels decreased in 62% of those with elevated preoperative levels, whilst those with normal preoperative levels tend to remain the same. The mean reduction in TGs was 26%, whilst cholesterol levels were unaffected. There were decreases in mean white blood count.

Fat redistribution following suction lipectomy. (Hernandez TL, *Obesity*, 2011)
There is some evidence to suggest that in patients who have thigh liposuction and do not change their lifestyle, there may be more fat distribution to the abdomen.

ASSESSMENT

- Establish the patient's expectations and concerns.
- History including weight changes.
- Medical history including anything suggesting a bleeding disorder, use of medication affecting bleeding including herbal remedies.
  - Medications metabolised by liver cytochrome p450 such as erythromycin and cimetidine may increase the risk of lignocaine toxicity, though the effect in those with healthy livers is rather limited (Orlando R, *Br J Clin Pharmacol*, 2003).

EXAMINATION

The body mass index (BMI) should be documented.

- Skin – striae, scars and cellulite. Pinch testing and tissue elasticity.
  - As a rough guide, one should be able to 'pinch an inch' or more of fat for liposuction to be worthwhile.
- The typical appearance of cellulite arises due to the fibrous septae in the superficial fat layer that anchors the skin whilst the fat hypertrophies and the skin loses elasticity with age. Liposuction is not a treatment for cellulite (although some try); some use smaller cannulae with more incisions and cross tunnelling, or special probes, e.g. VASERsmooth®.
- **Tissue tone.** Patients with significant skin laxity may not benefit from liposuction alone. Good skin tone allows for better results.
- Fat distribution.

UNSUITABLE PATIENTS

- It is not suitable for those with significant loose excess skin with poor rebound, stretch marks and overhang, as liposuction is likely to exacerbate these problems, i.e. massive-weight-loss (MWL) patients.
- Patient satisfaction is predictably low in certain situations:
  - Legs and ankles where results are relatively poor and post-operative discomfort may be prolonged.
  - Medial thigh responds poorly and usually is better treated with lifting.
  - Male patients with more intra-abdominal fat and are thus more likely to be dissatisfied (15% vs. 2.8%).
  - **Zones of adherence** (Rohrich) where skin is adherent to the underlying fascia and liposuction may cause irregularities (Figure 10.9):
    – Lateral gluteal depression.
    – Gluteal grease.
    – Distal posterior thigh.
    – Medial mid thigh.
    – Inferior lateral iliotibial tract.
    – There are some sex differences: men have a zone of adherence along the iliac crest that defines the lower margin of the trunk, whilst this is absent in women, and fat continues as a mass to the lateral gluteal depression.

PROCEDURE

Full DVT/PE prophylaxis according to local protocols is given. The risk of TED increases in patients who are

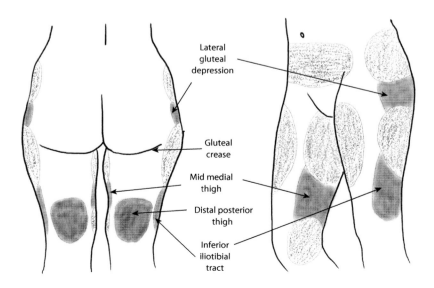

Figure 10.9 Zones of adherence. Liposuction in these areas in the crosshatched areas (lateral gluteal depression, gluteal crease, mid medial thigh, distal posterior thigh and inferior iliotibial tract) should be avoided to prevent contour deformities. The stippled areas are areas commonly treated with liposuction.

immobile for more than 2 hours, >60 years of age, on hormone therapy or overweight.

- Preoperative topographical markings are used to outline areas of proposed fat removal.
- Fluid is infiltrated according to the surgeon's preference (see below).
- Incisions are made in inconspicuous areas agreed with the patient: the areas are '**pretunnelled**' without suction – too many passes under suction can cause focal over-resection.
- Endpoints include bloody aspirate, loss of resistance or achieving final contour.

Whilst many may be treated as day cases and can go home with simple oral analgesia, it is suggested that those with large volumes aspirated should be monitored overnight/24 hours with blood tests. The use of urinary catheters is not universal but would facilitate monitoring and administration of IV fluids.

- Spinal or epidural anaesthesia is not recommended in the office setting due to the risks of vasodilatation, hypotension and fluid overload.

TUMESCENT TECHNIQUE

Prior to the use of 'wetting' solutions, liposuction was a procedure with significant blood loss. The tumescent technique was introduced by Klein in 1985 as a measure to reduce operative pain and bleeding whilst assisting the passage of the cannula as a lubricant of sorts. Most use something that lies between 'superwet' and tumescence, the latter requiring more time for infiltration and a potential for fluid overload.

The 'classic' **tumescent formula** combines 1 L of normal saline with 50 mL of 1% lidocaine, 1 mL of 1:1000 adrenaline and 2.5 mL of 8.4% sodium bicarbonate. The solution is injected until the tissues are swollen, firm and under pressure ('fountain sign'). Blanching is seen after 10 minutes, but the vasoconstriction is more effective after waiting for another 10 minutes. There are many different formulae in use.

- Blood loss is reduced to 1%–3% of aspirate volume compared with >40% without infiltration.
- Adrenaline is effective in dilutions of up to 1 in a million (though it takes longer to work).
- Large doses of local anaesthetic are infiltrated, but it is absorbed slowly, and some is re-aspirated. Ostad (*Dermatol Surg*, 1996) showed that using 55 mg/kg of lidocaine produces peak serum levels of only 1.9 mcg/mL, but this is attained quite slowly. As a corollary, this means that toxicity (albeit uncommon) may be delayed, for up to 8 hours. **The generally accepted maximum safe dose is 35 mg/mL** for tumescent infiltration (Klein JA, *Dermatol Clin*, 1990).
  - Some dispute the usefulness of lignocaine; its use does not seem to affect analgesic requirements, either intra- or post-operatively (Hatef DA,

Aesthet Surg J, 2009). Certainly there is a case for it to be omitted in cases being performed under GA.
- Bupivacaine provides long-lasting anaesthesia and is sometimes combined with or replaces lidocaine (Failey CL, *Plast Reconstr Surg*, 2009), but in general, the cardiotoxicity means that it should be used with caution.

Overall, ~70% of the total volume of tumescent fluid remains in the tissues and intravascular space at the end of the procedure; thus, it is important to avoid infiltrating large volumes in the elderly or those with congestive heart failure.

Tumescent technique: The effect of high tissue pressure and dilute epinephrine on absorption of lidocaine. (Rubin JP, *Plast Reconstr Surg*, 1999)
During routine liposuction, the 'safe' dose of lidocaine is often exceeded four- to fivefold (35 mg/kg, peaking at about 12 hours, i.e. long after surgery). In this study, 7 mg/kg lidocaine was injected with or without 1:1 million adrenaline into healthy volunteers, and serum levels were measured.

- There was a **slower rise in serum levels in adrenaline solutions**, but the peak concentration was the same with or without adrenaline.

Although lidocaine has vasodilatory properties, the vasoconstrictive effect of adrenaline is greater. Dilution of both lidocaine and adrenaline in the tumescent solution causes net vasoconstriction as 1 in 1 million adrenaline has a biological effect, whereas 0.1% lidocaine has little or none (in terms of vasodilation). The reduction in local blood flow to the area inhibits absorption, thus showing that high total doses of lidocaine are safe.

Strategies for reducing fatal complications in liposuction. (Cardenas-Camarena L, *Plast Reconstr Surg Glob Open*, 2017)
This literature review found that the most common cause of death was from thromboembolic disease, and the greatest risk for a fatal event was on days 3 to 7 postoperatively. Perforation of viscera was another serious complication, injury in the ileum most frequently, followed by the jejunum and spleen. The authors formulated a safety checklist, paying particular attention to fluid status, dosages of lidocaine and adrenaline.

TYPES OF LIPOSUCTION

- **Conventional liposuction** includes a blunt tip cannula attached to a vacuum pump (~1 ATM); alternatively, suction can be generated by a syringe (see 'Coleman technique').
- **Ultrasound-assisted liposuction (UAL).**
- **Power-assisted liposuction** uses a special probe that vibrates at about 4000 cycles per minute; it is not ultrasonic and uses smaller cannula and incisions. It may be slightly quicker and safer than UAL (due to less heat generation and shorter

operation and anaesthetic time), but substantive studies are lacking. It is, however, very noisy. It tends to produce coarse results and is not suited for fine-tuning.

ULTRASOUND-ASSISTED LIPOSUCTION

UAL was pioneered by Zocchi (*Aesthet Plast Surg*, 1992). Ultrasonic waves are converted into mechanical vibration (20,000 cycles per second) at the tip of the titanium cannula causing cavitation 1–2 mm from the tip, which induces fragmentation of fat, whilst the collagen network, vessels and nerves (Howard BK, *Plast Reconstr Surg*, 1999) are left relatively intact. The proposed advantages are reduced energy expenditure by the surgeon, more skin contraction and being able to disrupt fibrous tissue, e.g. in gynaecomastia.

However, the overall volume removed is not significantly greater, and there is a **risk of burns** (0.07%) at the deep surface of the overlying skin ('tip hits'); it is therefore important to keep the cannula moving with slower strokes, and the need for heat-insulating sleeves means that larger incisions are needed. The **extra liquefying step** before suctioning means that it can take a little longer than conventional liposuction.

A common error is to overtreat with UAL (endpoint is loss of tissue resistance rather than the final contour/pinch thickness with traditional liposuction), which will cause contour deformity otherwise.

- UAL produces some (perhaps desirable) skin contraction.
- Causes more seroma.

VIBRATION AMPLIFICATION OF SOUND ENERGY AT RESONANCE – VASER

The acronym **VASER** (Vibration Amplification of Sound Energy at Resonance) is a trade name for a (third-generation) UAL system. The ultrasound energy is pulsed and delivered from specially designed **probes with grooves** along the sides that are said to allow ultrasound energy to be delivered in a safer manner. Blondeel (*Br J Plast Surg*, 2003) was one of the first to come to this conclusion by comparing UAL vs. conventional liposuction prior to removing skin and fat as an abdominoplasty procedure. It is often used for sculpting of body contours, particularly the 'six-pack' (Vaser Hi Def™).

- Initially, it was thought that fat was 'melted', but it seems to work by a combination of microthermal and micromechanical mechanisms. The latter causes cavitation and micro-bubble formation from alternating pressure wave that leads to fat fragmentation into suspension of largely **intact cells**. Thus, VASER fat can be used for fat injection (although energies and pressures need to be adjusted).

Tissue temperatures during ultrasound-assisted lipoplasty. (Ablaza VJ, *Plast Reconstr Surg*, 1998)
Subcutaneous temperature probes were used to measure tissue temperatures during UAL.

- Infiltration of tumescent fluid at room temperature dropped tissue temperature to ~24°C, but this rapidly recovered to ~32°C; thus, tumescent fluid may reduce elevation of tissue temperature during UAL, though it had no effect on core temperature, which remained in a narrow range (35.7–36.3°C).
- During the procedure, tissue temperatures remained stable except when treating the thighs, when temperature rose to 41°C, but this did not result in a burn.

LARGE-VOLUME LIPOSUCTION

The definition of large-volume liposuction is rather arbitrary, but ASAPS strongly recommends a **maximum limit of 5 L** per session. There is an average 4-unit haemoglobin drop with 8 L liposuction; there may be an increased risk of TED. It may be better/safer to stage liposuction procedures.

- The old Illouz 'rule' of 1.5–2 L at one sitting and to avoid combining with other surgical procedures is not as relevant with modern practices. Greater volumes can be safely performed as long as patients are carefully selected, and have meticulous surgical, anaesthetic and post-operative care.
- Intravenous fluids have been recommended for cases where 4–5 L has been aspirated. It is important to avoid volume overload; many regimens have been suggested:
  - Rohrich recommends fluid one-fourth of the volume over 5 L aspirated.
  - Trott (*Plast Reconstr Surg*, 1998) suggests (for superwet) that maintenance fluids alone is adequate if aspirated volume <4 L, and if >4 L is aspirated, then give maintenance fluids, plus one-fourth of the aspirated volume over 4 L.
    - The authors state that 70% of the infiltrated volume is absorbed into the intravascular space. Fluid overload is a danger; **urine output is a useful indicator** of volaemic status.
  - Pitman (*Clin Plast Surg*, 1996) – if infiltrated volume is more than twice the aspirate, then no resuscitation needed.
  - Others have suggested that the liposuction 'wound' is like an 'internal burn' and that it is the area suctioned rather than the volume aspirated that is more significant, and if >15% body surface area, then the risk of haemodynamic problems increases.
- Reduce total lignocaine dosage.
- Monitor especially urinary output.
- Watch for perioperative hypothermia.

POST-OPERATIVE CARE IN LIPOSUCTION

Patients should expect bruising, numbness and swelling – the latter may take months to settle, meaning that the full benefit may not be evident for up to 6 months. Post-operatively, **support garments** to extremities are worn for at least 2 weeks – **most suggest 6 weeks**, whilst some say that 3 months is required for the best results.

- A 'strong–weak' compression regimen is often called 'bimodal' compression and is most easily achieved by having two garments – wearing both sets when drainage is still active and then only one afterwards for 3–8 weeks.
- Patients can resume gentle activities when leakage stops; normal activities and exercise can be resumed after 3 weeks. On average, patients should expect to have 1 week off from work for a large-scale liposuction under GA.

COMPLICATIONS OF LIPOSUCTION

Complications are more likely with **large-volume liposuction** (see above) and when performing other surgery concomitantly, e.g. abdominoplasty (×15), other surgery (×7).

- Infection, bleeding.
- Contour irregularity requiring further liposuction or fat injection.
- Lax skin especially in MWL patients.
- Haematoma, seroma – may be more common after UAL.
- Injury to nerves, major blood vessels and overlying skin. The risk of inadvertent entry into the body cavity, e.g. bowel perforation, is extremely small. Paraesthesia usually settles after a couple of months.
- Death – 1 in 50,000 (compared with 1 in 3000 when combining liposuction with abdominoplasty). Isolated reports of death have implicated PE and fat embolism.
  - DVT/PE 0.03% in white patients
  - LA toxicity

Some studies show that all patients with a sizeable liposuction procedure (>900 mL) have fat particles in their blood (i.e. **'fat embolism'**), but overt 'fat embolism syndrome' (tachypnoea, tachycardia, cerebral dysfunction, petechiae with severe hypoxaemia leading to death) is extremely rare. Furthermore, despite the name, fat embolism per se may not actually be the causative agent in what is often described as 'fat embolism syndrome'; presence/amount of fat does not correlate with symptoms. Fluid overload, aspiration pneumonia, etc. should be excluded. Treatment is largely supportive; steroids may help.

NON-SURGICAL LIPOLYSIS

There is a big demand for treatments that are less invasive, less technically demanding, particularly those that can be administered by non-surgeons.

Laser lipolysis (Smartlipo™) uses laser energy of three wavelengths (Triplex™) to disrupt fat, with a potentially beneficial skin tightening effect. The temperature needs to be monitored carefully to minimise the risk of burns. The results are very operator dependent; irregularity is a common complaint. Unfortunately, it was often sold to inexperienced doctors, and there were many cases of patient injuries. Purported advantages of less bleeding and faster healing remain anecdotal and unsubstantiated, nor is there any evidence of any difference over SAL.

Body contouring with external ultrasound. (Kinney BM, _Plast Reconstr Surg_, 1999)
External ultrasound is used in the presence of tumescent fluid before liposuction with the aim of causing fat cavitation. Constant motion of the ultrasound paddles and application of hydrogel are required to prevent burn injury to the skin (which has been reported).

The use of external ultrasound was introduced by Silberg in 1998. The paper above was a safety report and concluded that further data were awaited. There was a rash of papers soon after, but overall, external UAL is not widely used, and evidence of its usefulness is conflicting.

FOCUSED ULTRASOUND

High-intensity focused ultrasound (HIFU) may reduce the waistline by an average of 4 cm after three passes (single treatment) compared to 1.3 cm in a sham group (Jewll M, _Plast Reconstr Surg_, 2011). Branded products include Ultrashape™ and Liposonix™; the former is a multi-treatment procedure with less discomfort.

OTHERS

- **External laser lipolysis** – iLipo™: use of low-level laser energy (650 nm) supposedly to activate lipase.
- **Cryolipolysis** – Coolsculpting.
- **Kybella®** (Allergan) is deoxycholic acid, a secondary/synthesised bile salt. Like mesotherapy (phosphotidylcholine and deoxycholate), it is injected into the fat, which is 'dissolved'; the Kybella itself is metabolised and then excreted in the stool. It has gained FDA approval in 2015 for the treatment of double chins.

IX. ABDOMINOPLASTY

Some anatomical details are useful:

- **Umbilicus.** The umbilicus is exactly in the midline in only 17% (Rohrich RJ, _Plast Reconstr Surg_, 2003), lying halfway between the xiphoid and pubis at the level of the superior iliac crest. The shape is extremely variable (outie vs. innie, etc.), though many regard the ideal umbilicus to have superior hooding and inferior retraction and be relatively shallow and narrow in the vertical axis (resulting in an almost 'T' shape sometimes).

- Sensation comes from T10 (the whole abdomen is T7–12) with nerves running in the plane between the internal oblique and transversalis abdominis muscles.
- Normal waist (the narrowest part of the trunk) is usually 1 inch above the umbilicus
- The umbilicus takes a more transverse orientation in women after childbirth.
- During an abdominoplasty, the umbilicus relies on perfusion from the ligamentum teres and median umbilical ligament (Stokes RB, *Plast Reconstr Surg,* 1998).
- **Hip** – in many, there is a gentle double curve with a minor fullness at the iliac crest with a larger mound at the trochanter. Many want this double curve to become a smooth single curve. For patients with tight skin, excess fat would be better removed by liposuction, whilst abdominoplasty is more suited for cases with skin excess and laxity.

ABDOMINAL WALL BLOOD SUPPLY

The supraumbilical blood supply comes from T7–10 vessels running deep to the surface of the rectus muscle and is thus safe with flap undermining to the costal margin. The infraumbilical supply comes from T11–L1, and vessels travel superficial to Scarpa's fascia and are thus vulnerable to damage during abdominoplasty.

Huger's zones (1979) of blood supply to the anterior abdominal skin can be used as a guide in planning a safe operation:

- Zone I – the central zone supplied by the vertical deep epigastric arcade.
- Zone II – the lower abdomen is supplied by superior epigastric, external pudendal and circumflex iliac arteries.
  - DCIA supplies skin over the iliac crest.
  - SCIA supplies skin over ASIS.
- Zone III – the lateral zone/flanks supplied by the six lateral intercostal arteries and four lumbar arteries.

During an abdominoplasty, zone I and II supplies are divided with the **flap dependent on zone III** (i.e. lateral). Liposuction in this zone III may theoretically interfere with perfusion to the upper skin flap and thus should be used judiciously. Matarasso wrote about the 'safe zones' for liposuction in abdominoplasty; **unrestricted** (SA4) in the infraumbilical zone, **cautious** (SA3) in the epigastrium, **limited** (SA2) in the lateral areas of the flap and **safe** (SA1) in the flank and inferior to the abdominoplasty incision (Figure 10.10).

MATARASSO CLASSIFICATION

The majority of abdominoplasty procedures carried out are type IV (see Table 10.2). There is a trend that moves

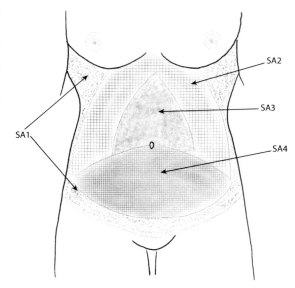

Figure 10.10 Safe/danger zones of liposuction during an abdominoplasty (Matarasso). SA1 is a safe area for liposuction, SA2 limited liposuction, SA3 liposuction with caution and SA4 unrestricted liposuction (i.e. the area usually discarded).

away from the 'traditional' method of wide flap elevation – instead, elevation is restricted to a central column just wide enough to allow rectus plication (thus reducing the elevation in the subcostal region).

ASSESSMENT

The aims of an abdominoplasty are to improve contour whilst minimising scarring and maintaining a natural umbilicus.

- The patient's complaints and expectations should be elicited. Smoking and use of anticoagulants including herbal remedies are particularly relevant.
- Examine the patient for skin excess and for musculo-aponeurotic laxity (diastasis of the recti), and also scars.

TYPICAL TECHNIQUE

In general, abdominoplasty aims to remove redundant skin apparent when the patient is flexed 45° at the hip and should **not involve excessive tension** except in the lateral areas (lateral-tension abdominoplasty).

- Antibiotics, DVT prophylaxis according to local protocols and urinary catheter.
- A folding table is needed. Ensure that the placement of the hips is correct.
- Subcutaneous infiltration of 'tumescent solution' (not to turgor) reduces blood loss.
- Use a lower incision within the pubic hairline 5–7 cm above the anterior vulval commissure and bevel the

Table 10.2 Matarasso classification of patients with reference to treatment of abdominal tissue excess. Liposuction is suitable for those with >3 cm fat on pinching and have good skin recoil and no rectus diastasis

Type	Features	Treatment
I	Excess fat only	Liposuction
II	Mild skin excess Infra-umbilical divarication	Mini abdominoplasty, infra-umbilical plication and liposuction
III	Moderate skin excess Divarication above and below	Mini abdominoplasty, plication above and below umbilicus + liposuction
IV	Severe skin excess Severe rectus divarication	Standard abdominoplasty + sheath plication + liposuction

upper skin flap edge. The incision lines and expected scar lines should be discussed with the patient; they can be tailored to their preferred types of underwear/swimwear to a certain extent.

- There is an **inherent length mismatch** in the upper and lower incisions. The classic '**Regnault open W**' aimed to counteract some of this and is still popular but still tends to produce dog ears. The upper flap can be 'ruched' to shorten it. More modern incisions include the U-M abdominoplasty (Ramirez) or W-M that aims to match incision lengths better. The trend is to modify the incision particularly laterally for cosmesis and to provide a degree of anterolateral thigh lift. Watch for the **lateral cutaneous nerve of the thigh** in the lateral part of the incision.
- Raise the abdominal flap as needed. Leaving the flimsy fascia overlying the rectus sheath (fascia of Gallaudet) may help reduce seroma; other strategies including **quilting sutures**.
  - Quilting sutures are independent of **progressive tension sutures** that are placed at 1–2 cm intervals between the underside of the flap and the abdominal muscle/fascia used to distribute tension away from the skin closure.
- **Plicate the rectus sheath** if there is any diastasis, with two continuous sutures (e.g. looped nylon) – one above and one below the umbilicus to avoid umbilical strangulation. Additional paramedian and transverse plication may be helpful in some patients. Plication seems to increase post-operative pain; some inject bupivacaine locally.
- Fold the table and excise the excess tissue. The elevated flap is split vertically and held with towel clips, whilst the lateral parts are adjusted. The skin is closed in layers but without excessive tension. The superficial fascial system (SFS) should be closed separately.
- The umbilicus is brought out through the flap (positioned at the level of the iliac crests), and the stalk is fixed to the fascia (to sink it) with a half-buried mattress (knot in umbilicus). Defat the flap in the midline below the umbilicus.
  - There are different types of incision to create the desired shape, e.g. reverse omega or 'smiley' with a superior flap (some suggest insetting the flap into an incision along the top of the umbilicus).

- The use of drains is common, though some have suggested that the use of quilting/'adhesion' sutures obviates this need (Arantes HL, *Aesth Plast Surg*, 2010), whilst others disagree (Ovens L, *Eur J Plast Surg*, 2009).
- Binders/compression garments are worn for support for at least 2 weeks. No heavy lifting is advised for 6 weeks.

VARIANTS

- **A mini-abdominoplasty** removes infraumbilical skin excess without the need to reposition the umbilicus. It is a less extensive procedure overall with a shorter scar but probably less effective too. Rectus plication with heavy non-absorbable sutures can be performed below and above the umbilicus (with endoscopic assistance).
- Somewhere in between, a **'limited' abdominoplasty** (Wilkinson TS, *Aesthet Plast Surg*, 1994) can be performed and the umbilicus is 'floated' by detaching at the fascia, moving downwards ~2 cm – this will be useful in patients with some upper abdominal laxity and a high umbilicus.
- **Belt lipectomy** is indicated for those with more extensive encircling bulk, e.g. after MWL, and provides an element of thigh/buttock lift. This necessitates several changes in operative positions including supine and lateral decubitus.
  - Use the **fleur-de-lis** technique for those with vertical skin excess; this is particularly suited to MWL patients (see below).
- **Reverse abdominoplasty** using a W-shaped inframammary incision (Baroudi R, *Plast Reconstr Surg*, 1979) has been suggested for central or upper abdominal laxity that is not adequately managed by a standard abdominoplasty.
  - It is often combined with an upper body lift and breast reshaping; de-epithelialised upper abdominal skin can be used for augmentation (~80–100 mL of tissue). 'Breast suspension test', where lifting up of the breasts results in a good/satisfactory abdominal shape, may identify suitable candidates.
    - There are several variants of this, e.g. **AMBRA** (augmentation mammoplasty by reverse abdominoplasty) – Zienowicz (2009) describes

the use of de-epithelialised tissue below the level of the IMF that is split like barrel staves and rolled under the breast tissue.

- It may be an option for those with cholecystectomy scars.

DOG EARS

According to some, dog ears arise due to the length mismatch between the upper and lower incisions; they can be reduced at the cost of a longer scar, whilst Momeni (*Ann Plast Surg*, 2008) uses fat excision in his 'rising sun' abdominoplasty to reduce dog ears by bevelling the resection to cut more fat than skin and subcutaneous fat trimming. The theory is that a dog ear is a convex contour deformity; emptying out the fat should flatten out the dog ear without the need to excise skin.

The skin is closed with a continuous subcutaneous suture causing **pleating** similar to a Lejour mammoplasty, resulting in a shorter scar (relies on skin contraction). The 'rising sun' aspect of this operation comes from taking bigger bites in the lower wound laterally to pull edges in laterally, and to reduce tension in the central portion, where bigger bites are taken from the upper wound.

COMPLICATIONS

- Early
  - Umbilical necrosis.
  - Flap necrosis (especially in smokers), wound dehiscence/infection (10%).
  - Haematoma, seroma (up to 24%). Pitanguy says that the keys to less seroma are avoiding desiccation, meticulous haemostasis and adequate drainage; the actual effects of this are unproven, though it seems to be good surgical practice.
  - Injury to lateral cutaneous nerve (10%).
  - TECs approximately 0.1%. Death, though rare, may result from PE.
- Late
  - Scarring and altered sensation; revisional surgery may be needed, e.g. for dog ears (up to a third).

The overall complication rate is ~30%, with 5% being major. Abdominoplasty patients are rather uncompromising, and there is significant post-operative dissatisfaction usually associated with dog ears, residual fullness and unnatural umbilicus appearance. Male abdominoplasty patients are more likely to be dissatisfied, which may be due in part to less realistic expectations, as well as due to their thicker, less elastic skin and having a larger amount of intra-abdominal fat.

Abdominoplasty: Risk factors, complication rates, and safety of combined procedures. (Winocour J, *Plast Reconstr Surg*, 2017)
This was a prospective study of 25,478 patients who were included in a national insurance database with abdominoplasty performed by board-certified plastic surgeons (2008–2013). Sixty-eight had combined procedures such as liposuction, breast surgery or body contouring. Complications included haematomas (31.5%), infections (27.2%) and suspected/confirmed TECs (20.2%).

The multivariate analysis found that having combined procedures, being male, being older than 55 years old and obesity were risk factors for complications (4% overall). The risk of complications for abdominoplasty alone was 3.1%, increasing to 10.4% in combination with liposuction and body contouring.

HIGH-LATERAL-TENSION ABDOMINOPLASTY

High-lateral-tension (HLT) abdominoplasty was described by Lockwood T in 1995. The technique is based on the belief that **epigastric skin excess is primarily horizontal, whilst infraumbilical skin excess is vertical.** The aim is to reduce central tension, which would tend to pull up the mons and over-flatten the centre, making it look odd. To this end, less skin is removed centrally and more removed laterally compared with a traditional abdominoplasty. This results in an **oblique lift vector** giving better waist definition and an element of lift to the anterior and lateral thigh (Figure 10.11).

- **Pattern** – lateral extent not so wide (i.e. shorter scar) and run up almost vertically to the superior excision.

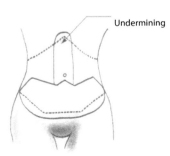
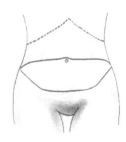

High-lateral-tension abdominoplasty

Traditional abdominoplasty

Figure 10.11 High-lateral-tension abdominoplasty – undermining is restricted to the paramedian area for muscle plication. High-lateral-tension and traditional. HLT abdominoplasty was derived from body lift techniques. Ted Lockwood (1945–2005).

Basically, flex patient, split flap in the centre and put in holding sutures at lateral ends and centre directly up and then trim, bevelling to allow excision of more deeper tissue. Lateral dog ear correction.

- **Subcostal undermining is minimised**. Dissection is limited to the central column ~7 cm wide over rectus to allow repair.
- **Closure in layers** – tension in SFS with interrupted non-absorbable, e.g. Ethibond, and then dermal layer and subcutaneous.
  - **SFS** (Lockwood TE, *Plast Reconstr Surg*, 1991) is the connective tissue network from the subdermis to the muscle fascia (i.e. a block of tissue, not a film/layer) that is formed of thin horizontal membranous sheets separated by fat but interconnected vertically (female) or obliquely (male).
- **Disadvantages** – more complex/takes longer, and more excision of skin laterally means that patients need to wait longer before they can stand upright. Scar is more irregular due to pleating; lateral ends are longer and higher a bit like a French cut.

FLEUR-DE-LIS ABDOMINOPLASTY

The fleur-de-lis (French for 'lily flower') abdominoplasty is an abdominoplasty with a component of vertical skin resection and is particularly used in MWL patients. The central resection pattern is akin to a long triangle that is narrowed inferiorly or like a truncated vertical ellipse.

Fleur-de-lis abdominoplasty: A safe alternative to traditional abdominoplasty for the massive-weight-loss patient. (Friedman T, *Plast Reconstr Surg*, 2010)
The rectus plication and resection of the transverse component is performed first, and then towel clips are used to judge the vertical tissue excess, which is then removed by excising to just below the xiphisternum. There should be **minimal undermining** to maximise the number of perforators to the skin flaps. The superficial fascial system is closed and the umbilicus set in the incision line without excising additional skin to reduce widening. The authors reported a minor complication rate of 26.3% and a major complication rate of 5.6%.

PREGNANCY

Abdominoplasty is generally not advisable when the patient plans to become pregnant in the near future. Apart from the effects on the aesthetics – re-expansion and further laxity – there is concern that the reduced abdominal wall compliance may pose risks to both the mother (fascial tears, organ compression) and the child (this has not been borne out).

Pregnancy after abdominoplasty. (Menz P, *Plast Reconstr Surg*, 1996)
Pregnancy after abdominoplasty is possible, but where midline rectus sheath plication has been performed, the pregnancy should be closely monitored, with delivery by an elective Caesarean section.

- Borman (*Plast Reconstr Surg*, 2002) also reported a successful pregnancy in a patient who became pregnant 2 months after surgery.
- Nahas (*Aesth Plast Surg*, 2002) reported on a patient who had an uneventful pregnancy 2.5 years after abdominoplasty with correction of rectus diastasis. A CT scan after the pregnancy demonstrated that the correction was intact.

BODY CONTOURING AFTER MASSIVE WEIGHT LOSS (MWL)

MWL has been variably defined as a weight loss of more than 100% above the patient's ideal weight or 100 pounds of weight loss. In general, contouring surgery should not be offered until 6 months to a year after the patient has achieved his or her ideal weight; partly this allows metabolic and hormonal homeostasis to be achieved – wound healing during the anabolic phase is compromised.

The patient should also be psychologically stable and willing to **trade skin excess for scars**, through multiple operations and the gamut of complications. The ideal candidate for body contouring is a patient who has attained a stable weight but has excessive skin laxity of the lower trunk and thighs. A body lift is usually defined as treating multiple areas in one operation, especially buttocks, medial thighs and flanks. Those who still have significant firm fat deposits are not good candidates for contouring surgery.

- Examine patients from behind, the sides and in front for contour and swelling. The diving position is a good way to see the abdominal excess.
- **Thickness of subcutaneous fat** – those with a thick subcutaneous fat layer are best pretreated with liposuction 3–6 months before excisions/lifts, or preferably, more weight loss.
- **Skin laxity** of thighs (gently push up) >8 cm laterally and >6 cm medially will be suitable for thigh lifts. Skin laxity of the abdomen; checking for hernia and diastasis.
- MWL patients have poor skin quality generally, and the fat has poor vascularity; wound healing problems are not uncommon.
  - Likely to have iron and vitamin B_{12} deficiency.
  - Four percent have low albumin.

THIGH LIFTS

Medial thigh lifts are generally less effective compared to lateral lifts – whilst a lateral thigh lift will improve the buttocks and most of the thigh, a medial lift will generally only lift the upper inner thigh (and may cause wide scars and vulvar distortion). An abdominoplasty will pull up on the anterior and medial thigh as a 'side effect'.

Fatty deposits in the lateral thigh and buttock area are best treated with liposuction unless there is a large excess of skin that should be excised. The medial thigh however does not respond well to liposuction (multiple fascial connections, less skin recoil) and lifts work better, though the patients need to be warned about the inferior displacement of pubic hair and scar.

Complications associated with thigh lifts include haematomas, infections and oedema (preserving more tissue over the femoral triangle may preserve more lymphatics) – patients should wear compression stockings.

CIRCUMFERENTIAL/BELT LIPECTOMY

MWL patients tend also to have excess tissue in the buttocks, lateral trunk and back rolls that are generally **not well managed by a standard abdominoplasty** alone (may actually make it worse). Lockwood combined the belt abdominoplasty with a medial thigh lift for a 'lower body lift', whilst others have described single-stage total body lifts, although the surgery takes 8–12 hours and (auto)-transfusions are usually necessary.

- Make the preoperative markings with the patient standing up and check by placing the patient in the operative position(s); they are only guides and can be changed intraoperatively. Some choose to prep the patient once from nipples to knees before induction of anaesthesia, whilst others choose to do it part by part. The sequence of the surgery varies according to individual surgeons, but it does impact on the amount of resection that is possible in each area as taking more from one part makes it more difficult for tissue to be resected from the others.
- Mark the midlines and the suprapubic crease above the pubic hairline (some use a wide-open W, with a central peak and the troughs dipping 2–3 cm below, which may provide an element of perineal lift) to join the ASIS laterally. This is taken around the back to meet above the natal cleft.
- The line of closure, which should be hidden by the patient's underwear/swimwear, is agreed after discussion with the patient. Generally, once you have **decided where you want the scar to lie**, then keeping a marking pen at the level of the scar, pull upwards (the patient or an assistant can help); the pen will now mark the lower limit of your excision. The superior resection line can be gauged by pinching the tissue excess to meet the lower line. It is important to have the patient **bend slightly away** to avoid over-resection. Over-resection of the back, say, may mean that the patient will be in difficulties with sitting, e.g. on the toilet.
- The posterior markings are made to meet in an arrowhead at the anterior axillary line, whilst the superior line meets the abdominoplasty markings. In general, the skin of the back and sides is **not elevated significantly**.
- Incisions should be **bevelled out to reduce the dead space**; some suggest leaving more deep fat posterior to the ASIS in particular. Tissue is closed in layers, including the SFS.

- When the patient is supine, the abdominoplasty is performed, often a fleur de lis.
- Some tools may help speed up closure, e.g. V-Loc barbed sutures, Insorb vicryl staples.

POST-OPERATIVE CARE

- Patients should not move until fully awake; early ambulation on the first or second post-operative day is then encouraged. The patient can slowly straighten after 1 week and return to normal activities after 4–6 weeks.
- Drains are usually kept in until 25–30 mL/day. However, even if there is still significant drainage at 2 weeks, the drains are usually removed, and compression/aspiration is used to manage any collections. There seems to be a higher risk of seromas with the posterior resections; quilting sutures may help.
- The use of compression garments/binders is not universal, but many use them for up to 6 weeks.

Complications include skin dehiscence (especially midline buttock and laterally), seroma and skin necrosis. The risk of complications increases in smokers and those who are overweight (BMI > 35) – in high-risk patients, it may be safer to stage surgery, performing abdominoplasty separately from a thigh/buttock lift.

BRACHIOPLASTY

The resection of the excess skin and fat that hangs from the arm is a common operation. A pinch test determines the amount to be removed, and the scar is placed inferiorly where it is usually well hidden. The resection should be judged intraoperatively – from the first anterior incision, the posterior flap is slowly elevated before committing to the second incision line; avoid undermining beyond the resection margins. Staging the procedure, temporarily closing the skin envelope, reduces swelling that may hinder closure.

The excision is often carried over onto the lateral chest wall; a Z-plasty placed in the axilla reduces the volume of the axilla and prevents webbing deformities. Large truncal rolls may need to be addressed with an upper body lift.

The most commonly injured structure is **the medial cutaneous nerve of the forearm** that runs close to the basilic vein and becomes superficial to the deep fascia proximal to the elbow as high as the mid-arm; the other superficial nerve is the inter-costobrachial. Wound dehiscence is not uncommon particularly after concomitant liposuction.

AFTER CARE

- Support garments. Seromas may be more common after using UAL.
- No lifting for 1–2 weeks (they are allowed to carry a kettle).
- No sports/exercise for 6 weeks.
- Bruising expected for several weeks; scar maturation takes 1–2 years.

11

General plastic

I. GENERAL COMPLICATIONS

ANAESTHETIC COMPLICATIONS

Major complications (approximately 1 in 1500):

- Airway – spasm, aspiration
- Circulation – excessive blood loss can cause hypovolaemia leading to arrhythmias, myocardial infarction and cerebrovascular accidents. DVT and PE can also occur.
- Common minor side effects include sore throat, nausea, vomiting and delayed recovery.

BLEEDING

Many reasonably well-conducted studies suggest that for **minor surgery**, continuing anticoagulant medication is safe and not associated with increased incidence of complications (Shalom A, *Ann Plast Surg*, 2003), although what actually constitutes 'minor' is rather arbitrary. In general, cutaneous procedures such as skin cancer excision are considered low risk and the potential for local control reduces concerns further.

- Studies often suffer from non-comparable patient populations as aspirin takers are often older and may have conditions that potentiate aspirin affects, e.g. liver disease.
- Oral anticoagulation is usually given for AF, prosthetic heart valves and previous thromboembolic disease. The risks of TECs (stroke and myocardial infarction) from stopping warfarin or aspirin are 1 in 6000 and 1 in 20,000, respectively, those with thromboembolic events including CVA/TIA in the previous 3 months are at highest risk.

- More time may be needed for intraoperative haemostasis, and pressure dressings may be a wise precaution. The role of vasoconstrictors is debatable, whilst the role of fibrin sealants is not established except, perhaps, for dental extractions.
- Those undergoing major surgery should take the last dose of warfarin on the evening of day 6, then LMWH is started on the morning of day 3 and continued until day 1, i.e. day before surgery.

  - For high risk of bleeding, the final LMWH dose should be a half dose. Those on unfractionated heparin instead should stop it 4–6 hours prior to surgery. INR should be checked on the day before surgery, vitamin K is given if INR >1.5.
  - The timing of heparin resumption depends on the type of surgery; maintenance dose warfarin can usually be resumed on the evening of the surgery or the next day.

HERBAL MEDICATION AND PLASTIC SURGERY

- **Ma-huang** (ephedra) is often in slimming preparations and is a sympathomimetic with positive inotropic and chronotropic effect. It can also interact with anaesthetic agents, causing severe hypotension. Stop 24 hours prior to surgery.
- **Glucosamine and chondroitin** are often taken together by sufferers of osteoarthritis and may also cause hypoglycaemia. They should be stopped 2 weeks before elective surgery.
- **Gingko biloba** has antiplatelet activity possibly through modulation of nitric oxide and anti-inflammatory pathways. It should not be combined with anticoagulants and should be stopped 36 hours before surgery.

- **Ginseng** (can also cause hypoglycaemia and hypertension) may have antiplatelet effects and should be stopped 1 week before surgery.
- **Garlic** is often taken to 'treat' atherosclerosis and hyperlipidaemia. The active ingredient is **allicin** that inhibits platelet aggregation; it should not be taken with anti-coagulants and should be stopped 1 week before surgery.
- **St John's wort** is said to be effective for depression and anxiety, which is possibly related to inhibition of monoamine oxidase. It may cause hypotension with GA and serotonergic syndrome, if taken with SSRIs. It should be stopped 1 week before surgery.
- **Ginger** may prolong bleeding by inhibiting thromboxane synthetase. Stopping 2 weeks before surgery is advised.
- **Vitamin E** affects platelets particularly in those who are already 'abnormal', e.g. diabetics. It may also delay wound healing. Stopping 2 weeks before surgery is recommended.
- **Fish oil** (eicosapentaenoic acid) should be stopped 3 weeks before surgery.

SUTURING

OPTIMISING RESULTS

- Minimise infection risk – asepsis, prophylactic antibiotics, if required; minimise preoperative stay; shave just before surgery, if required.
- Respect RSTLs – these tend to lie perpendicular to the direction of pull of the underlying muscles. On the face, they are sometimes called wrinkle lines (see below) and can be made more obvious by asking the patient to contract their muscles. When incision lines running parallel to RSTLs cannot be made, they should be curved/wavy or a series of Z-plasties.
- Everted edges will flatten gradually, whereas inverted edges tend to remain inverted and look unattractive. To promote skin eversion, simple interrupted stitches should be placed, so that the needle enters and exits the skin perpendicularly; occasional mattress sutures may help.

TYPES OF STITCHING

The numbering of sutures refers to their size; originally, there were sizes 0–3, but with advances in production, thinner sutures had to be denoted with an extra '0', e.g. 6/0, which is finer than 3/0.

- **Simple interrupted** stitches are simple and precise. Simple apposition of skin edges is sufficient; tension should be taken up by deeper layers.
- **Mattress sutures** (vertical or horizontal) are good for eversion, particularly where the skin is thin and unsupported. Horizontal mattress sutures are useful in the scalp with fewer problems with hairs getting into the wound, but can cause more ischaemia of the skin in between.

- **Subcuticular sutures** do not leave stitch marks, but it can be more difficult to be as precise as simple interrupted sutures. The half-buried mattress is useful, as it leaves a knot and suture tract only on one side of the wound, which can be useful in suturing around the NAC, e.g. suture marks will then only be left on the darker and uneven areolar side.
- **Alternatives to sutures:**
  - **Skin glue**. The first formulation was methyl-2-cyanoacrylate, but it turned out to be histotoxic and is no longer used, whilst some longer alkyl chain compounds were strongly pro-inflammatory. The wound is sealed (able to shower immediately and supposedly sealed off from bacteria from 72 hours); it cannot be combined with topical creams or ointments.
  - **Steristrips**. They offer less support than sutures and are less useful in uneven wounds, oozy wounds. Erythema (may be mistaken for 'allergy') or even blistering may occur, particularly in the elderly with overzealous closure.
  - **Staples**.

CLOSING DIFFICULT WOUNDS

Difficulty of closure is often an issue with flap donor sites. A number of suggestions have been described in the literature in order to avoid skin grafts, etc. Many of these techniques may create significant tension, causing pain and some necrosis. They are thus relatively contraindicated in those with peripheral vascular disease or in smokers.

- **Cross-suturing** has been described to reduce the size of donor defect after harvest of radial forearm flaps, which can then be covered with a smaller skin graft (Moazzam A, *Br J Plast Surg*, 2003); it creates dog ears that resolve.
- **Bootlace suturing** – the wound edges are undermined for 1–2 cm and a series of 1-0 nylon sutures on a large needles are passed across the wound taking 1–2 cm bites. These sutures cinched down to bring the wound edges together and tied together. The traction sutures are tightened further every couple of days.
  - **VADER** (vacuum-assisted dermal recruitment) combines bootlace like suturing with NPWT to reduce oedema and wound bacterial counts and facilitate movement of wound edges. The sutures are tightened when the NPWT dressing is changed.
- **Proxiderm™ device** – a plastic bridge with tissue hooks.
- **TopClosure®** – similar to plastic ties.

II. SKIN GRAFTS

Karl Thiersch (1822–1895) was the first to introduce a reliable method of harvesting thin skin (1886). Gibson was the first to describe second set rejection. See also 'Burns'.

CLASSIFICATION OF SKIN GRAFTS

Skin grafts can be classified in many ways, for example according to

- Thickness/composition – split thickness, full thickness, composite (more than one type of tissue)
- Origin – autograft, allograft, xenograft

THICKNESS OF GRAFTS

Skin grafts consist of epidermis and a variable amount of dermis. Depending on the amount of dermis taken, skin grafts can be classified as follows:

- **Partial thickness or split skin grafts (SSG, Thiersch graft)**. The graft can be taken by hand with a Watson skin graft knife or by a powered dermatome. The thickness of the graft can be assessed by its translucency and bleeding pattern from the donor – fine punctuate bleeding suggests a thin graft has been taken. The thicker the SSG is, the slower it will take, until it resembles an FTSG. The donor site will heal by virtue of the appendigeal structures in the dermis – the epidermis is reformed but the dermis remains thinned. Thus, whilst repeated harvest from the same donor site is possible, dermis is removed each time reducing healing potential.
  - Excess skin graft may be stored in a fridge at 4°C for up to 2 weeks (or kept in a specific medium for several weeks, or in liquid nitrogen for much longer, but these later options are generally impractical).
- **Full thickness skin grafts (FTSGs)**. The epidermal layer often sloughs off, if the graft is thick and the dermis remodels itself over 6 weeks or so. Quilting should be done carefully, as recipient site bleeding can be a disaster, particularly under a sheet graft.
  - **Wolfe graft (1975) – classically post-auricular.**
  - The amount of available FTSG is limited; graft take is less reliable.
  - The appearance and functional performance of the graft are better, whilst the donor can be closed to a linear scar. The graft is more durable and general skin functionality is more likely to be preserved:
    - SSGs are typically dry and may require emollients. FTSGs retain some sweat glands, and when reinnervated, their function approaches that of the recipient.
    - Sebaceous glands tend to retain characteristics of the donor; glandular function depends on glands in the graft itself being reinnervated by recipient site nerve endings.
    - Hair regrowth is possible to a certain extent, but follicles often extend into the subcutaneous fat layer, and thus will often be transected during harvest. Maintaining the follicles will require a graft thickness that will not 'take' reliably.
    - There is less overall contraction.

There are many different strategies for dressing the SSG donor site, and though the healing times may be similar, other factors such as patient comfort and fewer dressing changes may be significant factors.

- **Alginates** (with their supposed haemostatic function) will dry and peel off with healing; however, the dried block of material can be uncomfortable.
- **Film dressings such as Tegaderm** are more **comfortable**. However exudate may accumulate underneath and may need to be changed frequently in the first few days.
- **Hypafix** has been used as a retention dressing (for donor and graft sites), particularly in Australia. It is a one-way stretch, semiporous polyester material with polyacrylate adhesive; it can be sterilised either by gamma irradiation or autoclaving (dressings with water-based adhesives cannot). The areas can be gently washed and then patted/air-dried. It is removed by soaking with an oil-based liquid over approximately 1 hour, or just left to fall off as the skin re-epitheliases. Fewer dressing changes are needed, but there is no easy way to inspect the graft underneath.

SKIN GRAFT TAKE

The skin has been detached from its blood supply, which must be re-established before necrosis sets in. The take of skin grafts is traditionally described as consisting of four phases: adherence, plasmatic imbibition, revascularisation and remodelling.

- **Adherence** – fibrin bonds form between the graft and the recipient bed leading to adherence, but can be disrupted by shear forces, etc. (see below). By the end of the third day, there is ingrowth of collagen from these fibroblasts (and formation of vascular channels) that strengthens the attachment.
- **Plasmatic imbibition** – the breakdown of intracellular proteoglycans in graft cells leads to more osmotically active subunits, causing absorption of interstitial fluid by osmosis, and thus graft swelling and oedema.
- **Revascularisation** – the circulation to a skin graft is restored after 4–7 days with thicker grafts taking longer as might be expected. Two of the mechanisms put forward to explain the restoration of a blood supply include pre-existing blood vessels linking up with graft vessels (inosculation) or ingrowth/formation of new vessels (neovascularisation); they may co-exist. Lymphatic circulation is restored after approximately 1 week.
- **Remodelling/graft maturation**
  - **Appendages** – regeneration can occur especially of sweat glands and hair follicles. Hair is usually noticeable after 14 days in well-vascularised FTSGs; however, full thickness grafts tolerate ischaemia poorly and may lose appendages.

- **Re-innervation** – nerves enter existing neurilemmal sheaths (thus more in FTSG). Sensory re-innervation of SSGs occurs faster (from 3 to 4 weeks onwards) than FTSGs but will probably be less complete. Final sensation may approximate that of the adjacent skin, i.e. **recipient,** unless the bed is severely scarred. Another qualifier is the availability of end organs in the grafts, e.g. Meissner's corpuscles are only found in glabrous skin.
- **Sympathetic innervation** of sweat glands can be re-established and the resultant **sweating activity tends to parallel the recipient site** (e.g. emotion vs. temperature) rather than the donor site.
- **Pigmentation** – pigment changes in skin grafts are usually temporary, but good colour match can be achieved with carefully selected donor sites. The occurrence of hyperpigmentation can be reduced somewhat by avoiding ultraviolet stimulation of melanocytes. Hyperpigmented grafts may be treated by dermabrasion with superthin overgrafts.
  - Colour match for the pinker skin of the face is best achieved with skin from the head (and scalp), whilst the neck/supraclavicular area is still acceptable – skin from below the level of the clavicle should be avoided.
- **Contraction.** Although usually undesirable, e.g. ectropion from cheek SSGs, some contracture may be beneficial, e.g. on the fingertip, to draw sensate skin over the tip.
  - **Primary contraction** is the immediate contraction or recoil due to elastin fibres in the dermis and thus is greater in FTSG (~40% vs. ~10%).
  - **Secondary contraction** (from day 10 and continues for up to 6 months): the recipient bed, not the skin graft, is the site of contracture. Thicker grafts contract less as dermal elements are said to inhibit myofibroblast contraction. Other factors that decrease graft contracture include a rigid recipient site (e.g. periosteal bed leads to little contracture compared with mobile areas) and greater percentage graft take/less meshing (leaving fewer areas that need to heal by secondary intention).

SKIN GRAFT FAILURE TO TAKE

The recipient bed must be vascular enough to support the graft. Complete graft failure is usually due to placing the graft upside down (shiny side is the 'dermal' side).

- **Shear** – repeated movement between the graft and the recipient site. The use of tie-over dressings is common (and many different methods have been described); NPWT may be useful for fixation in more complex situations.

- **Haematoma/seroma** – the fluid raises the graft away from the vascular bed severely limiting the passive transfer of nutrients by increasing the diffusion barrier. Although the dermal component of the graft is haemostatic, it will not stop more profuse bleeding, and making fenestrations in the graft either by hand or by machine meshing allows drainage of potential collections, but will leave unattractive marks.
- **Infection** – e.g. bacterial collagenases. Streptococcal infection (classically group A β-haemolytic) is regarded as particularly deleterious to skin grafting.
- **Unsuitable bed** (avascular), e.g. **bare** bone, cartilage, tendon.

It is 'traditional' to inspect the graft on the fifth post-operative day, but inspecting earlier may allow collections or other minor problems to be detected and treated in good time – small collections may be carefully 'rolled out'. There is some evidence that overall survival is improved. With a cooperative patient, an **exposed graft** may be an option and the graft can be inspected continuously with collections rolled out as needed.

AFTERCARE

- Avoid UV exposure to reduce hyperpigmentation.
- Use emollients to moisturise grafts until sebaceous activity returns.
- Use pressure garments if hypertrophic scarring occurs.

COMPOSITE GRAFTS

A composite graft is a graft that contains a combination of tissues, such as skin, fat and sometimes cartilage. It is used when extra tissues/function such as support is needed, e.g. using auricular skin and cartilage to replace nasal defects.

Like simple (skin) grafts, they do not have their own blood supply and must be nourished by passive means. The central thickness and presence of a cartilage component for example, limits the effectiveness of passive transfer; consequently, composite grafts get a significant portion of their nourishment along the edge of the graft. The upper limit is usually regarded as 1–1.5 cm as then no tissue will be more than 5 mm from an edge (i.e. the nutrient supply). There is some evidence that **post-operative cooling** to reduce the temperature by 5–10°C for 3 days may actually enhance healing, contrary to the conventional practice of keeping them warm.

- Composite grafts are less successful in smokers, irradiated skin and diabetics. The data on hyperbaric oxygen (HBO) are inconclusive (and would be impractical to use routinely).
- They often go through a series of colour changes; the initially white graft acquires a pale pink tinge about 6 hours later; there is some congestion/cyanosis by the end of the first day that gradually pinks up over the next week.

- They are particularly useful in alar reconstructions. Native skin can be used as a turnover flap to increase vascular contact, although this means that defect will be larger than before.
- The survival of any cartilage component may be improved by adding a larger skin island, i.e. most of it is an FTSG. With a modified composite graft (Chandawarkar RY, *Br J Plast Surg*, 2003), part of the skin is de-epithelialised and inserted as a 'dermal pedicle' into a pocket adjacent to the defect.

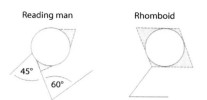

Figure 11.1 Reading man flap (a type of unequal Z-plasty) for closure of circular defects. It sacrifices less healthy tissue (ratio 1:2.5 approximately) than a rhomboid flap.

III. LOCAL FLAPS AND Z-PLASTY

TYPES OF LOCAL FLAP

Flaps should be raised to include at least full thickness skin to reduce secondary contraction, whilst taking care to avoid including too much bulk/fat that would impede flap movement; in practice, the flap includes the **subdermal plexus** along with a little subcutaneous fat.

FLAP MOVEMENT

Local flaps basically move via advancement, rotation or often a combination of the two.

- **Rotation flap** – a semicircular flap that rotates about a pivot point through an arc of rotation into an adjacent defect. The donor site either closes directly (buttock rotation flap) or with a skin graft (e.g. scalp rotation flap). Back cuts and lengthening the leading edge are often useful.
  - The defect is often converted into an isosceles triangle with its apex pointing towards the centre of the circle that the rotation flap is part of.
- **Advancement flap** – a flap that moves forwards without rotation or lateral movement, e.g. V–Y, Y–V flaps. Rectangular advancement flaps usually require excision of Burow's triangles.
  - Karl Burow was a nineteenth century German surgeon.
- **Transposition flap** – a flap that moves laterally about a pivot point into an adjacent defect, e.g. Limberg flap (1963), bilobed flap, reading man flap (Figure 11.1), Z-plasty (see below), larger flaps (Figure 11.2) such as posterior thigh flap for ischial sores. A hatchet flap is probably a combination of rotation and transposition; it can be likened to a rotation with a large back cut. The Dufourmentel flap (1962) is a bit more versatile than the Limberg; it can deal with rhomboids with a range of angles and is less likely to cause a dog ear.
  - **Interpolation** – a flap that moves laterally about a pivot point into a defect that is not immediately adjacent to it, e.g. nasolabial island flap to the nasal tip and a deltopectoral flap to the head and neck. Some describe this as an islanded flap.

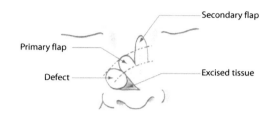

Figure 11.2 Bilobed flap for reconstruction of a nasal defect (Zitelli modification). The smaller angle between defect and adjacent flaps is about 45°, which reduces the size of the standing cone. Secondary flap is longer and thinner. It may cause alar rim retraction and should not be used if the rim is less than 10 mm away from the defect.

Z-PLASTY

This technique involves the transposition of two adjacent triangular flaps, and at the completion of the transposition, the 'Z' has rotated by 90°. All limbs of the 'Z' must be of equal length, though the angles (between 30° and 90°) do not have to be the same (this asymmetric variety is sometimes referred to as the skewed Z-plasty). Although it had been described before, the geometry was worked out by Limberg in 1929. Z-plasties are useful to

- **Transpose normal tissue** into a critical area, e.g. return a vermilion step into alignment.
- **Break up a linear scar** and **change the direction** of a scar.
- **Lengthen a scar**, e.g. burn scar contracture, lip lengthening with the Tennison cleft repair.
- **Treat a web.** Some authors emphasise that the problem is multiplanar.
  - 'Bridle scar' is a scar that bridges across a hollow, e.g. jaw to neck. It can be deep or shallow. The aim is to lengthen the scar to allow it to sit into the hollow, i.e. a fusiform excision with Z-plasties – single large Z-plasty if deep, multiple small Z-plasty if shallow.

Tip necrosis may occur particularly in previously burnt/scarred skin; using wide or rounded tips may help in addition to careful tissue handling, and avoid directly suturing the tip, using glue or steristrips instead.

The **actual length gain** (Table 11.1) is less than the theoretical length gain due to the viscoelastic properties of skin. In clinical practice, 60° permits a maximal length gain

Table 11.1 Effect of the angle of Z-plasty flaps and the theoretical length gains

Angle of flaps (°)	Theoretical gain in length (%)
30	25
45	50
60	75
90	100

whilst still allowing easy transposition of the two triangles. The tension required to close a 90°–90° Z-plasty is 10 times that required to close a 30°–30° Z-plasty, though to reduce this tension, the 90°–90° Z-plasty could be divided into four flaps, each with an angle of 45°.

Greater gain in length is achieved by one large Z-plasty than by multiple small Z-plasties whose total central limb length is equal. Although length gain is additive, the field of tension exerted by each Z-plasty affects the neighbouring flaps and thereby reduces the actual overall length gain. Furthermore, lateral skin availability may be limited, so a single large Z-plasty may not always be practical. In addition, in axillary surgery, the 'unwanted' transposition of hair-bearing skin is reduced with smaller multiple flaps.

Some thoughts on choosing the Z-plasty. (Hudson DA, *Plast Reconstr Surg*, 2000)

Multiple Z-plasties:

- **Z-plasties in series** – the central flaps tend to develop a square shape and do not interdigitate easily. This technique may be better applied to a long scar with less lateral tissue available (e.g. correcting volar skin shortage associated with Dupuytren's contracture).
  - **Double opposing Z-plasty** – a Z-plasty in reverse follows a Z-plasty; this produces triangular flaps that interdigitate easily.
- **Four-flap Z-plasty** – wide flaps of either 90° or 120° are bisected into two sets of flaps. This produces good length gain, equal to that of two individual 45° or 60° Z-plasties (100% and 150%), but the flaps are easier to transpose as triangles. There are two possible end results depending on which triangle moves the least. It represents **two Z-plasties in parallel** and is better applied to a short scar with a greater amount of lateral tissue available, e.g. deepening a **web space**. Adding another triangle of the outside of each side produces a six-flap Z-plasty (described by Mir L, *Plast Reconstr Surg*, 1973).
  - **Five-flap Z-plasty** – a double opposing Z-plasty that incorporates a V–Y advancement and is otherwise known as a **'jumping man flap'**. The length gain of 125% is better than a double opposing Z-plasty alone but has less lengthening than a four-flap Z-plasty for a given scar length.
- **'Single' limb Z-plasty** – used to introduce a triangular flap of skin into an area of skin shortage, it breaks up the contracted scar but does not offer the mechanical advantages of the Z-plasty.

The **W-plasty** involves excision of tissue and should not be used if there has been significant tissue loss already. It also lengthens the scar. The base of the last triangle at each end is at a right angle to the final scar. The segments are 5–7 mm and should be shorter at both ends to reduce dog ears.

IV. PEDICLED AND FREE FLAPS

BLOOD SUPPLY OF THE SKIN

Flaps can be harvested in part due to the rich vascularity of skin, which is **in excess of its nutritional needs** and is related to its other functions such as thermoregulation.

CUTANEOUS ARTERIES

The arterial supply of the skin comes from

- Direct branches of segmental arteries (concentration of direct cutaneous perforators near axial lines and intermuscular septae)
- Perforating branches from nutrient vessels supplying deep tissues especially muscle, i.e. indirect

Plexuses are formed at different levels:

- Subepidermal
- Dermal
- Subdermal
- Fascial
- Subfascial

There are anastomoses between neighbouring cutaneous arteries:

- **True anastomoses** do not have a change in calibre, e.g. labial arteries across midline, less common.
- **Choke vessels** have reduced calibre or are closed under normal circumstances, but dilate to restore blood flow to areas of flap ischaemia.

The vascular territories (angiosomes) of the body. (Taylor GI, *Br J Plast Surg*, 1987)
Three-dimensional blocks of tissue supplied by a single artery and its venae comitantes are called **angiosomes** and venosomes, respectively. Adjacent angiosomes are connected by true anastomoses (see above) or small calibre choke vessels; thus, flaps can be larger than one angiosome as choke vessels allow perfusion from adjacent angiosomes.

- If one source vessel is small, the adjacent source vessel is usually large – 'law of equilibrium', e.g. patterns of arteries supplying facial skin; when the facial artery is small, the transverse facial is larger. This compensation is less evident across the midline.
  - Chiu (*Rhinology*, 2009)

DELAY PHENOMENON

This term is used to describe the practice of elevating part of a flap (and thus dividing part of its vascular supply) for the purpose of expanding the territory prior to further elevation and definitive transfer. The mechanism underlying this is not fully understood.

- Conditions the flap to survive with reduced blood flow (metabolic adaptation to hypoxia)
- Partially sympathectomises the flap to facilitate opening of choke vessels and angiogenesis
- Choke vessel hypertrophy and hyperplasia, maximal at 48–72 hours
- Vascular reorientation along the longitudinal axis of the flap

Tissue expansion (TE) is considered a type of delay, whilst the delay phenomenon is also exploited in flap prefabrication.

- The optimal timing for a delay procedure remains controversial – from at least 2 weeks or just over 1 week, Atisha (*Ann Plast Surg*, 2009) reported an average of 38.92 days between delay surgery (ligation of inferior epigastric arteries) to pTRAM, the main indication being large tissue requirements.
- One method of assessing the effect on vascularity involves injecting 20 mL 5% fluorescein IV and then observing the pattern of yellow–green fluorescence under UV light (Wood's lamp) in a darkened room. ICG fluorescence offers a newer alternative.

SKIN FLAPS – MATHES AND NAHAI CLASSIFICATION

- **Direct cutaneous flaps:**
  - Axial cutaneous arteries, e.g. groin, scapular area.
  - The horizontal cutaneous vessels travel in loose connective tissue rather than on the deep fascia. There is usually soft tissue laxity.
- **Fasciocutaneous flaps:**
  - The horizontal cutaneous vessels lie on the deep fascia, which is not strictly essential to the flap vascularity. However, it is difficult to separate the vessels off the fascia so it is safest to include the fascial layer in the flap.
  - The skin is relatively immobile over deep fascia, e.g. limbs, scalp.
  - Cutaneous nerves often travel parallel to vessels; hence, many fasciocutaneous flaps are neurosensory.
- **Septocutaneous flaps** – the perforators come from the subfascial source vessel and course along intermuscular septae, e.g. lateral arm flap ('in-transit perforators').
- **Musculocutaneous flaps** – occasionally perforators arise as indirect branches from muscle branches off the source vessel (gluteal area).

CLASSIFICATION OF FASCIOCUTANEOUS FLAPS

MATHES AND NAHAI

- Type A – Direct cutaneous perforator

- Type B – Septocutaneous perforator
- Type C – Musculocutaneous perforator

CORMACK AND LAMBERTY

- Type A – Multiple perforators
- Type B – Solitary perforator
- Type C – Segmental perforator

Classification of flaps according to their blood supply:

- **Random pattern flap** relies for its vascularity upon the vessels of the dermal and subdermal plexuses of the skin.
- **Axial pattern flap** is vascularised by vessels running longitudinally within it:
  - Direct cutaneous artery
  - Fasciocutaneous artery
  - Septocutaneous artery
  - Muscle perforators

BLOOD SUPPLY OF MUSCLES

MATHES AND NAHAI CLASSIFICATION

A dominant pedicle is defined as a vessel that can perfuse the whole muscle. If there is only one dominant pedicle, then this is critical to muscle survival; where more than one vessel is dominant, these are called major vessels.

Non-dominant or minor pedicle vessels cannot support the whole muscle on their own; they may be variable in number. Thus, muscle flaps need to be raised on dominant pedicles; a portion of the muscle can be based on a minor pedicle, but the whole muscle will not survive.

- **Type I – one dominant pedicle**, e.g. TFL (there is an additional minor pedicle to the inferior aspect, making it a type II flap), gastrocnemius.
- **Type II – dominant pedicle(s) plus minor pedicle(s)**, e.g. gracilis, soleus. This is the commonest type of muscle flap.
  - Delaying a type II muscle flap by ligation of a non-dominant vessel may improve survival.
  - A portion of the muscle can be based on a minor pedicle.
- **Type III – two dominant pedicles**, e.g. pectoralis minor, RA, temporalis, gluteus maximus (GM). Type III muscles are suited to a split design, e.g. pectoralis minor for facial reanimation, with slips to orbit and angle of the mouth.
  - Some surgeons propose ligation of the inferior epigastric pedicle some 10 days before harvesting of a superiorly pTRAM flap.
- **Type IV – segmental supply**, e.g. sartorius. Muscle will not survive if too many segmental vessels are divided.
- **Type V – one dominant plus segmental vessels**, e.g. LD, PM. Such flaps will survive if the dominant vessel is ligated as long as all/most of the segmental vessels are preserved, e.g. PM turnover flap for sternal defects.

Some have investigated the effects of delaying the LD by ligating the segmental perforator vessels, e.g. prior to harvest for cardiomyoplasty.

FREE AND PEDICLED FLAPS AND THEIR APPLICATION

HISTORY

There are many figures associated with microsurgery, but the notable ones include the following:

- Alexis Carrel, who described the **triangulation technique** in 1902; he was inspired in part by observing his aunts' embroidery skills. He was awarded a Nobel Prize in 1912 but is also criticised for lending support to Nazi principles of euthanasia.
- Jacobson used modified jewellers tools and existing ENT microscopes (1960) and coined the phrase 'microvascular'.

MICROSURGERY

A free flap is a composite block of tissue that is moved from a donor site to a distant recipient site where its circulation is restored by microvascular anastomosis. A pedicled flap keeps its circulation intact during transfer, which is thus limited by the vascular axis. Age (independent of comorbidities) is not a contraindication; the most deleterious conditions are PVD and renal disease.

- Care needs to be taken in patients who are **smokers**. Nicotine adversely affects the microcirculation; it is a potent vasoconstrictor, is thrombogenic and interferes with wound healing; the rate of partial muscle necrosis is doubled and skin loss/infection (30%) is increased. Overall, smoker status does not seem to affect the rate of total flap loss, suggesting that the anastomosis itself is not threatened. Smokers should be advised not to smoke for at least 2 weeks before and after surgery.
- **Radiotherapy** causes subendothelial proliferation and sclerosis that are permanent and progressive; surgery on acutely irradiated tissues should be delayed by 1 week for every week of radiation given. Irradiation can safely begin 2 weeks after surgery but will alter the shape and consistency of flaps, which can be a major issue in breast reconstructions.
- Those with arterial disease, such as peripheral vascular disease, have a greater risk of flap failure and patient death. Caution is also required in patients with collagen vascular disease and Buerger's disease.
- **Diabetics** have less of a microvascular problem than previously thought, and thus impaired wound healing aside, microsurgery is not contraindicated.
- **Steroids or chemotherapy** does not affect microsurgery per se but will adversely affect healing; in the latter, it is better to postpone surgery until the white blood cell count has returned to normal (usually 3–4 weeks later) or start the treatment 2 weeks after flap surgery.

Cigarette smoking, plastic surgery and microsurgery. (Chang LD, *J Reconstr Microsurg*, 1996)
Smoking may compromise healing at the flap–recipient interface and at the donor site. Smokers are advised to stop smoking for at least 3 weeks pre- and post-operatively for the vascular effects; stopping smoking will also benefit general cardiorespiratory function, as well as reduce cancer risk.

There is a thrombogenic state due to effects of smoking on

- Dermal microvasculature.
- Blood constituents.
- Vasoconstrictive prostaglandins – nicotine leads to increased TXA2 and decreased PGI2.

Carbon monoxide causes formation of COHb, which exacerbates tissue hypoxia and increased platelet adhesiveness. Overall, there are several adverse effects on surgical procedures:

- Those that involve extensive undermining, e.g. facelift surgery, and thus rely upon subdermal and dermal plexuses.
- Where a block of tissue depends upon a single vascular pedicle for survival, e.g. breast reduction, pedicled TRAM flaps.

Smoking one cigarette reduces blood flow velocity to the hand by 42% for up to 1 hour; thus, digital replants are at particular risk in smokers.

A meta-analysis (Sorensen LT, *Ann Surg*, 2012) found that tobacco smoking attenuates both the inflammatory and proliferative phases of healing (decreasing collagen production), with the latter less likely to recover on giving up smoking. Complications are more frequent in smokers (Sorensen LT, *Arch Surg*, 2012) – 4 weeks was recommended to reduce the incidence of surgical site infections (other complications were not significantly affected).

RECIPIENT VESSELS

The recipient vessels should be out of zones of injury or irradiation. Some degree of vessel diameter mismatch is not unusual, and differences of up to 2:1 can be dealt with easily:

- **End-to-side anastomosis** is useful for dealing size discrepancy, and it is as effective as end-to-end anastomosis. They seem to be less prone to kinking or spasm, but leaks tend to continue to bleed more.
- **Differential suturing**, cutting obliquely/spatulating or dilating. Larger discrepancies have increased risks of turbulent flow and thrombosis, and thus should be sutured end to side; if and only if this is not possible, then there is the 'lifeboat' of closing down the larger vessel end.
  - Couplers can be useful for moderate-size discrepancy in veins.
- **Avoid using atherosclerotic vessels**, if possible. Using double needle sutures allows the needle to pass

through the vessel wall inside out on both vessels. This reduces trauma to plaques, which would tend to lift off when the needle passes from out to in.

Vein grafts may be needed when there is insuffcient vessel length. The length of the vein graft does not seem to affect patency per se, but increasing the length increases the risk of thrombosis and kinking.

- Upper limb veins are less prone to spasm due to having less muscle in their walls (compared to lower limb).
- Mark ends carefully and be particularly wary of twisting.
- Avoid branches or valves if possible as the vessels tend to be thinner here.

SUTURES

Interrupted non-absorbable sutures are most commonly used.
Performing the anastomosis requires meticulous technique, in particular, limiting unnecessary manipulation of the vessels. Reduce shaking by resting your hands on a platform rather than trying to hold them in mid-air. The adventitia is trimmed (circumcised), and the vessel ends sutured without excess tension (aim to just see the thread through the vessel wall) using 8-0 to 11-0 non-absorbable monofilament sutures. Take bites of the vessel that are twice the thickness of the wall, aiming to use the minimal number of sutures whilst avoiding significant bleeding from the anastomosis. A 'neat' anastomosis that avoids irregular/unequal/oblique placement of sutures is less likely to have flow problems.

- Animal studies have shown that vessels can still grow after interrupted non-absorbable sutures.
  - Absorbable sutures have been used without significant differences.
- Continuous sutures compare well to interrupted sutures and are faster – there is, however, a tendency to constrict anastomoses, particularly venous ones.
- Alternatives to sutures have been described:
  - Cuffs/coupler/staplers, e.g. 3M coupler often used for veins – does tend to shorten the vessel and is less able to cope with greater degrees of size discrepancy.
  - Adhesives, e.g. fibrinogen not as versatile, lasers largely experimental.
  - Sleeve technique; telescope technique has lower patency rates (Sully L, *Plast Reconstr Surg*, 1982; O'Brien BM, Plast Reconstr Surg, 1990).
  - Fishmouthing (Turan T, *Plast Reconstr Surg,* 2001).

LINING OF THE MICROANASTOMOSIS

- Days 1–3 platelets. Aggregate at anastomosis site due to exposure of subendothelial tissues (especially collagen) to blood. It will not progress to fibrin deposition and thrombosis if there is no further exposure of the media or injury to the lumen.

- Days 4–14 pseudointima.
- Day 14 intima. Muscle layers also regenerate but never to preinjury state.

FLAP SELECTION

- The aim is to replace like with like: the types and volume of tissue required are determined by the defect.
  - Sensate or insensate
- Donor site availability (which may be an issue in burn reconstruction).
  - Ease of harvesting, including changes of position
- Recipient vessels available and matching to the length of pedicle needed.
- Have a lifeboat.

Maximum warm ischaemia times (maximum cold ischaemia):

- Jejunum less than 2 hours
- Muscle less than 2 hours (8 hours)
- Bone flaps less than 3 hours (24 hours)
- Skin and fascia 4–6 hours (12 hours – reports of successful digital replants up to 42 hours after)

ANAESTHESIA

- Keep the patient **warm and well filled** whilst avoiding vasoconstrictors.
- Muscle relaxation.
- Monitor volume status with urine output and haematocrit (0.30–0.35).
- Prevention of pressure sores.

FLAP MONITORING

Post-operatively keep the patient **warm, wet** (intravenous fluid is titrated to achieve an hourly urine output of 0.5–1 mL/kg depending on cardiac status) and **well** (good pain control, preoperative oral gabapentin reduces post-operative analgesia requirements; Chiu TW, *Hong Kong Med J,* 2012). Clinical monitoring remains the most commonly used and the most practical.

- Colour.
- Refill.
- Temperature.
- Bleeding on pinprick.
- Muscle contraction in muscle flaps is **not** a good parameter.

About 80%–90% of thromboses develop in the first 48 hours; deciding when to stop monitoring does depend on the progress of the patient and the state of the flap, but 3–4 days is reasonable. Head and neck reconstructions may be more liable to have delayed problems (possibly due to neck movements or previous irradiation), and monitoring for 5 days may be prudent in such cases.

Other methods of flap monitoring include the following:

- **Doppler signal** – the presence of neighbouring vessels can give misleading false positives; arterial signal may persist even if the vein is occluded. Some use implantable Doppler probes, e.g. Swartz (*Plast Reconstr Surg*, 1994), that may overcome some of these problems.
- **Temperature** (δ-T, i.e. the difference between the flap temperature and the control site temperature); >1.8°C difference is predictive (Khouri RK, *Plast Reconstr Surg*, 1992). A replanted digit with an absolute temperature less than 30°C is likely to have a problem with occlusion. Implantable probes are less liable to be influenced by the environment.
- **Oxygen saturation/pulse oximetry** can be useful in replants (Jones NF, *Plast Reconstr Surg*, 1992) and toe transfers but less useful in free muscle flaps.
  - **Transcutaneous oxygen saturation** – relative changes are more useful than absolute values.
- **Laser Doppler** techniques measure blood flow but only penetrate 1.5 mm; near-infrared spectroscopy has better penetration of ~2 cm (Vioptix) and gives continuous monitoring. False positives are possible.
- **Indocyanine green** (ICG) is cleared quickly.
  - **IV fluorescein and a Woods lamp** – the fluorescein takes 12–18 hours to clear; thus, it is not suitable for continuous monitoring, though using minidoses may be better.
- **Thermography** – there are small thermal cameras that can be attached to smartphones that are cheap and easy to use, but it has not been validated.
- **Microdialysis** – insertion of small catheters into subcutaneous tissue to measure metabolites such as glucose and lactate/pyruvate at intervals, e.g. every 30 minutes for the first day, then every hour for the next day, etc. A low glucose and high lactate are warning signs. Very limited clinical usage (Jyranki J, *Ann Plast Surg*, 2006).
- **pH monitoring** – a pH below 7.3 or a difference of >0.35 compared to control suggests a problem; the greater the difference and the faster it develops, the more likely it is an arterial problem.

Monitoring of buried flaps, e.g. in pharyngeal reconstruction, offers another challenge, and methods that have been described include the following:

- Implantable Doppler probes popularised by Swartz.
  - Han (*Int J Surg*, 2016) found increased free flap salvage but there was also significant number of false positives. They concluded that more studies are required.
  - Poder (*Eur Ann Otorhi nolaryngol Head Neck Dis*, 2013) – 81% vs. 60% salvage rate, for an average cost of 312 Eur per use. They did not comment on their false-positive rate, but did explain that it was part of the learning curve. They suggest that it is cost effective for them, but obviously it is relative to a unit's performance. It would make more sense

for surgeons with a higher complication rate than one with 1%–2% failure rate.

- Surface Doppler probe (with or without markings on the skin surface) – may be prone to misinterpretation due to interference from other vessels.
- Exteriorised segment of flap, e.g. skin, muscle or mucosa (in jejunal flaps), that may be incorporated into the skin closure or divided secondarily (Chiu T, *Surg Pract*, 2009).
- Window technique (Bafitis H, *Plast Reconstr Surg*, 1989).
- Exteriorised vessel stumps (Yang JC, *Ann Plast Surg*, 2007).
- Endoscopy (but not contrast swallows) for pharyngeal reconstructions.

CAUSES OF FREE FLAP FAILURE

- **Mechanical** – problem with anastomosis or pedicle such as kinking, twisting, stretching or compression, e.g. by haematoma or by brachytherapy tubes.
- **Hydrostatic**.
  - Inadequate perfusion (hypovolaemia, spasm, hypothermia).
  - Inadequate drainage (inadequate vein size, dependency, shunting via superficial system).
- **Thrombosis** – Heparinised saline (100 U/mL) is commonly used for irrigation intra-operatively.
  - Traumatised vessels due to overhandling or using vessels in a zone of injury. Needles that are overly large or placed obliquely may tear the endothelium.
  - Hypercoagulable states.
  - Reperfusion injury (prolonged ischaemia time) – consider fasciotomy for limb replants.
  - Prolonged spasm (2 hours or more) or desiccation may cause endothelial sloughing. Antispasmodics include
    - **Papaverine** (30 mg/mL) – salt of opium alkaloid that causes smooth muscle relaxation through a mechanism that is not entirely clear but possibly involves inhibition of phosphodiesterase and blockade of calcium channels. It precipitates on contact with heparin that may cloud the operative field but seems to be harmless, and can be easily flushed away.
    - Lidocaine 2% (some dispute this and use 4% or more) – membrane stabilisation by sodium channel blockade, produces potent local vasodilatation.
    - Verapamil – calcium channel inhibitor.

Drug-induced vasodilation. (Gherardini G, *Microsurg*, 1998)

Using a rabbit carotid artery model, the effects of varying doses of lidocaine and papaverine were tested. They found that 2% lidocaine by itself had little effect; 20% lidocaine, papaverine (undiluted, 30 mg/mL) or in combination with 2% or 20% lidocaine significantly increased flow after microanastomosis.

FLOW PROBLEMS

Venous problems are more common; **check for compression** from suture lines, dressings or haematoma. Changes due to venous congestion may be quickly irreversible – erythrocyte extravasation, with disruption of the endothelium and deposition of perivascular fibrin, and leading to thrombosis and shunting.

- **Check for twisting** of the vessels or anastomosis.
  - Re-do the anastomosis if necessary.
- A thrombus will be temporary **if there is continuous flow**; transient platelet thrombus is completely formed by 5 minutes and starts to disintegrate at 10 minutes, completely gone in 1 hour. Small vessels are more likely to occlude simply due to their size.
- **Rather than irrigating to clear the thrombus, some argue that it is better to open up the microanastomosis and to squeeze the flap to evacuate the clot.** This avoids the tendency of irrigation to push the thrombus further along the vessel.
  - Consider fibrinolytics if a thrombus is found (see below) noting that heparin by itself cannot clear a blocked anastomosis, and fibrinolytics may dissolve a thrombus but will not prevent it from reforming.

PHARMACOLOGY

There is a wide range of practice, and there is a lack of strong evidence to support one drug/protocol over another.

- **Clear thrombus.**
  - **Fibrinolytics**, e.g. streptokinase, urokinase and tPA, are used sparingly. They generate plasmin, which splits fibrin; effects are temporary and the thrombus will **reaccumulate** after the treatment is stopped; so **antiplatelet or heparin therapy is needed subsequently** to prevent reaccumulation.
- **Post-operative prevention of thrombus**.
  - **Dextran 40** is a volume expander with beneficial effects on microcirculation – theories for this include the negative charge on platelets reducing adhesiveness and inactivation of vWF. There is a small risk of anaphylaxis/allergy, and test doses are recommended, though not often followed. It is commonly used as a 250 mL bolus, followed by an infusion of 20 mL/hour (500 mL/24 hours). Although there were some good animal studies, clinical evidence remains lacking, particularly of its usefulness in uncomplicated anastomosis.
  - **Heparin LMWH** (thrombolytic) has a half-life of 4 hours, which is twice that of 'normal' heparin, and is 90% bioavailable (compared to 10%). It potentiates antithrombin III and reduces platelet adhesion. Some propose a dose of heparin before clamp release and it is sometimes used in salvage, but there is little indication for its use in routine cases; the risk of bleeding (and thrombocytopenia) generally outweighs the potential benefits.
    - Thrombin that is in a clot is effectively hidden from circulating heparin, i.e. **heparin cannot clear a blocked anastomosis by itself**.
    - Some studies show that fibrin aggregation is more important than platelets to thrombosis suggesting that heparin would be more important than, say, **aspirin**, whilst yet others suggest that platelets may be more important in arterial thrombus and fibrin in venous, and that combining the two may be beneficial.
- **Aspirin** inhibits the cyclo-oxygenase enzyme by non-reversible acetylation and thus reduces platelet aggregation. It is not that useful in microsurgery, and there are risks of ulceration, bleeding and nephrotoxicity.

The short answer is that no single drug treatment can be recommended based on solid evidence: either they have not been shown to significantly affect the outcome or they have potentially serious side effects/complications. There may be a role for their use in re-exploration/salvage but will not be suffcient by themselves to ensure success. Overall, in microsurgery, surgical techniques particularly the pedicle choice and position are likely to be much more important, and in re-exploration, the speed of the response is key.

THE NO-REFLOW PHENOMENON

This is the failure of a flap to perfuse after anastomoses, which has been shown to be technically satisfactory, i.e. patent (Ames A, *Am J Pathol*, 1968).

- Anaerobic metabolites build up in **ischaemic** tissue, and on re-establishing blood flow, **oxygen free radicals** are generated causing calcium influx, generation of inflammatory mediators and cell damage, i.e. reperfusion injury.
- 'No reflow' has been attributed to platelet aggregation, endothelial injury and intravascular thrombosis, blocking off the microcirculation. Fluid shifts into tissues (from failing cellular pumps) with arteriovenous (AV) shunting.
- HBO has been shown to be useful for salvaging failing flaps in some animal studies, but there are little clinical data on its role. This requires access to an HBO facility and can be costly. Complications are rare, but it may cause seizures due to oxygen toxicity and barotrauma to the middle ear and pneumothorax.

Leeches

From *laece*, meaning physician in old English.

Leeches are annelid worms with 'V'-shaped mouth parts. Their three jaws, each with >100 teeth, form a 'Mercedes Benz symbol' shape. *Hirudo medicinalis* is one of more than 700 species of annelids.

- **Hirudin** is secreted in leech saliva. It is the most potent natural thrombin inhibitor; recombinant hirudin, lepirudin, is available.
  - Hirudin binds activated thrombin; prevents fibrinogen from being converted to fibrin; blocks activation of factors V, VIII, XI and vWF; and decreases activation of tPA, protein C and plasmin. Hirudin prolongs thrombin-dependent coagulation tests, but there is no direct effect on platelets or endothelial cells.
- A leech attaches by the sucker on the caudal end, before biting with its 'Mercedes Benz' jaws. The **smallest leech** is usually the hungriest. It will actively ingest blood (~5 mL), followed by a passive ooze of 50–100 mL over the next day. Blood loss is more rapid in the early phase – 90% in the first 6 hours or so. Excessive blood loss is unusual.
  - The main indication is venous congestion in flaps or replants, temporising the situation until neovascularisation, which takes over 4–5 days. They can be ordered as required.
- The leech harbours *Aeromonas hydrophila* (facultative Gram-negative rod) in its gut, and there is a 20% risk of transmission to the patient, which increases with any regurgitation of blood (e.g. traumatic removal including the use of salt water to detach it). Therefore, the use of prophylactic antibiotics (third-generation cephalosporins, quinolones, e.g. ciprofloxacin or trimethoprim-sulphamethoxazole [TMP-SMX]) is advisable. It is contraindicated in the immunosuppressed.
- Leeches are meant to be used once only (killed in alcohol), though some authors have described the use of saline to cause regurgitation and allow re-use in the same patient.
- **'Poor man's leech'** (Goedkoop AY, *Eur J Plast Surg*, 2000) – in the absence of a supply of medicinal leeches, a small area of flap skin can be de-epithelialised to promote bleeding; 400 IU/mL heparin-soaked gauzes are replaced every half hour to encourage continued bleeding. 'Chemical leech' described by Barnett (*Br J Plast Surg*, 1989) and Yokoyama (*Plast Reconstr Surg*, 2007) involved the use of subcutaneous injections of heparin (1000U in 0.1 mL saline).

Muscle Flaps

Muscle-only flaps can provide a large surface area and volume coverage, whilst the donor site can still be closed directly. The flap tissue is well vascularised – a quality that is often said to aid in combating infection/treating infected defects.

- Some muscle flaps may be split to allow further customisation.
- Some may retain motor function for reanimation/restoring motor function, i.e. functional free muscle

transfer (FFMT). Terzis (*Hand Surg*, 1978) found that maximum working capacity after transfer was one-fourth of the original.

- Muscles shrink when detached but generally can be easily stretched back out. However, late atrophy may lead to gaps, e.g. when used for scalp reconstruction thus some recommend a degree of overlap.

FASCIOCUTANEOUS FLAPS

These are often used in the extremities (Pontén B, *Br J Plast Surg*, 1981). Their advantages include providing a thin, pliable, potentially sensate flap with a useful length/breadth ratio (~3:1). There is relatively little donor morbidity, but the donor site may need skin grafting.

PERFORATOR FLAPS

Taylor and Palmer identified 374 perforators to the skin with diameters greater than 0.5 mm, each a potential 'perforator flap' (2003). The perceived advantages of perforator flaps are of less donor site morbidity (due to sparing of muscles), earlier patient recovery as well as more versatility in flap design.

Perforator flap terminology

Direct and indirect perforator flaps. (Hallock GG, *Plast Reconstr Surg*, 2003)

A perforator flap is a flap of skin/fat supplied by a perforating branch of the source vessel, passing through deep tissues and fascia to supply the flap. Some have coined the phrase **'perforasome'** to describe the block of tissue supplied by one perforator vessel.

- **Indirect perforators** – the perforating vessel passes through muscle and fascia before supplying the flap tissue.
  - Muscle/musculocutaneous perforator – perforating vessel passes through muscle before supplying the flap tissue, e.g. DIEP flap, S-GAP flap and most ALT flaps.
  - Septal/septocutaneous perforator – perforating vessel passes along a fascial septum before supplying the flap tissue, e.g. the minority of ALT flaps.
- **Direct perforators** – these are perforators that pass from the source vessel directly through fascia (but not septum) to supply the overlying tissue (most axial pattern fasciocutaneous flaps of the extremities).

Not everyone agrees with the consensus.

FLAPS BASED ON NERVES

More specifically, these are flaps based on the vascular axis of nerves.

- **Cephalic flap** – this is based on the axis of the lateral cutaneous nerve of the arm, and also includes the cephalic vein.
- **Sural neurocutaneous flap** is a reverse/distal flow lateral FC flap based on miniscule branches from the sural artery that nourish the sural nerve.
  - This may be used for heel defects especially in diabetics with neuropathy where medial plantar artery/instep flaps would be less suitable. This will result in a loss of sensation around the lateral foot; the sural nerve is taken with the flap, not for sensation but for the vascular plexus around it; thus, calling this a neurocutaneous flap is probably a misnomer. Alternative terms include distally based superficial sural artery flap and described as a skin island flap supplied by the vascular axis of the sural nerve.
  - The flap is raised with a maximum length halfway up the leg, aligned along the axis of the short saphenous vein, which is included. It is based on perforators above the lateral malleolus, and the pedicle, which is adipofascial in nature, can be narrowed down. It is not necessary to see the perforators during surgery; rather dissection stops 7 cm above the lateral malleolus.

OTHER FLAPS

- **Bone flaps** – bone is harvested with endosteal and periosteal circulations maintained, and the flap heals in a similar manner to simple fractures at the flap-recipient interfaces and at the wedge osteotomies used to conform the donor bone.
- **Toe and joint transfers** – replace composite functioning tissues, e.g. in thumb reconstruction. The transferred tissue has sensory potential; the donor defect can usually be closed primarily. Toe pulp may be transferred independently.
- **Gastrointestinal flaps**, e.g. jejunal. Due to the high metabolic rate of the tissue, it is important to keep ischaemic time to a minimum to avoid mucosal sloughing. Caution is required in patients with a history of previous abdominal surgery.
- **Other specialised tissues** – vascularised nerves and vascularised tendons.
- **Prelamination** – skin graft, cartilage or other materials inserted into a flap territory, with the aim of creating a composite flap that is transferred later, vs.
- **Prefabrication** – introduction of vascular pedicle (wrapped in Gore-Tex or silicone) into an area that is mobilised after ~8 weeks maturation, i.e. fabrication of axial flap. Viewed another way, it is a way to utilise donor tissue that has the required qualities but not the axial supply. It can be combined with TE. Venous congestion is not uncommon, and overall, it is not used that often due to the wide choice of donor sites, except to make use of specific areas of skin lacking axial

vasculature, e.g. using temporal vessels to prefabricate a flap out of the upper neck skin for head and neck defects.

V. INDIVIDUAL FLAPS

SARTORIUS

Type – (Mathes 1981) Type IV muscle flap

- Blood supply – 6–11 segmental arteries enter the muscle, mostly medially; proximal branches come from the lateral circumflex femoral artery (LCFA), middle branches from the superficial femoral artery and distal branches from the proximal genicular branches of the popliteal artery. Each branch seems to supply distinct and separate territories; thus, sufficient pedicles must be preserved to ensure viability, which restricts the mobility. Wu (2005) found a consistent superior pedicle 6.5 cm below ASIS, entering the deep surface from the medial aspect.
- Attachment – from ASIS to the medial tibial condyle.
- Actions – it is a flexor and external rotator of the hip.

HARVESTING

There are several described variations on the use of the sartorius muscle:

- **Simple mobilisation** without detaching origin. This has been called a 'myoplasty', but the use of this term is inconsistent.
- Detach origin and advancement of muscle – **'transposition'**.
- Detach origin and rotate muscle medially/internally. This **sartorius 'twist'** aims to leave the posterior medial vessels untouched and preserve the vascular supply as much as possible.

ADVANTAGES

Harvest is technically straightforward, and no significant permanent functional loss is associated with its harvest. It has a robust blood supply derived from multiple vessels. It can be used to cover the femoral vessels after a groin dissection.

DISADVANTAGES

- One of the most common complaints is its limited size and thus its inability to fill large dead spaces.
- The muscle has a small arc of rotation, when pedicled.

GRACILIS

It is a type II muscle flap; the muscle arises from the inferior pubic ramus to the medial side of the subcutaneous surface of the tibia, just below and behind the sartorius insertion. The local use of the gracilis was first popularised by Orticochea. The muscle is thin and strap-shaped (4–8 cm wide, widest superiorly), as long as the thigh (approximately 40 cm). It is often easier to delineate and mark with the patient standing. The major pedicle comes from the medial branch of the circumflex femoral artery, and one or two minor pedicles from branches of the superficial femoral artery. The motor nerve comes from the anterior branch of the obturator nerve (runs between adductor longus and brevis) that divides before entry into muscle on its medial side, just superior to the vessels. It can thus be split readily, making it a classical choice for facial reanimation.

The overlying skin is thin but has thicker fat compared to ALT. Early reports with the myocutaneous flap showed high rates of partial (skin) flap necrosis when used for vaginal reconstruction; however, improved dissection techniques that preserve peri-gracilis perforators have yielded more reliable results and it is a common backup option in breast reconstruction. Other tips for reliability include avoiding use of the distal third and taking a bigger skin paddle, which can be wider than the muscle.

HARVESTING

- With the leg abducted and flexed at knee (frog leg), the muscle can be palpated along a line from the pubic tubercle to the medial tibial condyle with the paddle posterior to this and the long saphenous vein (may seem quite posterior).
- Entrance of the pedicle 9–10 cm from the pubic tubercle on the deep surface of the muscle.
- Raise the posterior 'V' end first to ensure that the flap is centred on muscle and adjust as needed.

ADVANTAGES

- Dissection is usually straightforward, and the single pedicle allows easy rotation into the wound.
- No significant functional loss; in fact, the potential for functional transfer is the most useful characteristic, e.g. for face/lower lip. However, up to 2 years may be needed for maximal power to be achieved in the transplanted muscle.

DISADVANTAGES

- The muscle volume is limited.
- Distal skin paddles are less reliable.
- Only 6% report persistent weakness (Carr MM, *Microsurgery*, 1995). Hypaesthesia along distal thigh, possibly due to injury to the cutaneous branch of the obturator nerve, is a common complaint. Patients generally do not complain about functional problems but more about the long and painful scars; thus, some have suggested endoscopy-assisted harvest through a 6.5 cm incision.

RECTUS ABDOMINIS

COMMON USES

Defects requiring muscle (it is between gracilis and LD in size) – functional segments may be raised by preserving the intercostal nerves. This segmental pattern of nerve supply does limit its usefulness in functional muscle transfer, though small strips can be used for facial reanimation.

- Lower and upper limb defects as a muscle flap (myocutaneous flap is usually too bulky).
- Breast reconstruction (TRAM pedicled or free, DIEP). See 'Breast reconstruction'.
- Perineal/groin reconstruction (inferiorly pedicled).

Type: Type III (two dominant pedicles) muscle flap. The muscle is embryologically derived from segmental anterior mesodermal somites, thus explaining its segmental innervation T7–12. The muscle has distinctive tendinous intersections to which the anterior rectus sheath is firmly adherent; there is one intersection at the umbilicus, one at the xiphisternum and one in between (occasionally also below).

- Blood supply – larger pedicle (2–4 mm diameter) comes from the inferior epigastric artery; from the external iliac artery, it anastomoses with the superior epigastric (1–2 mm) via two or three vessels. There are small segmental branches entering the deep surface from the lower six intercostal arteries (travelling with the accompanying intercostal nerves).
  - The flap **can be delayed** by dividing one set of vessels.
  - The DIEA arises 1 cm above the inguinal ligament and enters the muscle on its deep lateral surface midway between the umbilicus and the pelvic crest (i.e. roughly at the level of the arcuate line).
  - There are an average of 5.4 (2–8) large perforators (>0.5 mm) per side, mostly within 4 cm of the umbilicus particularly lateral and inferior. It is important to note that smaller perforators may not actually reach the skin, but terminate at the level of the deep fat layer instead.
- Attachment – from the pubic crest/symphysis to the xiphoid and fifth to seventh costal cartilages. The pyramidalis muscle arises from the pubic crest and blends with its counterpart at the linea alba 4 cm above its origin.
- Action – it flexes the trunk (first 30–40°, lumbar and thoracic spine) and raises the intra-abdominal pressure.

HARVESTING

For a VRAM, an elliptical skin island 2 cm on either side of the rectus sheath can be harvested and closed; it is common to use a fascia sparing technique. The abdomen is closed in layers; some recommend the use of figure-of-eight sutures to repair the fascia, whilst others prefer mesh, in selected cases.

Robotic harvest of the muscle-only flap has been described (Ibrahim AE, *Semin Plast Surg*, 2014).

ADVANTAGES

- The flap is easily harvested and is reliable with a low failure rate.
- Although the muscle may be relatively thin, the overlying skin and fat can give it substantial bulk.

DISADVANTAGES

The significant donor site morbidity (herniation or bulging) and functional loss. See 'Breast reconstruction'.

- Obese patients may be unsuitable for a TRAM because of reduced reliability of the elongated para-umbilical perforators in supplying the skin.

TENSOR FASCIA LATA

Type – Type I muscle flap (one vascular pedicle, although smaller pedicles may supply the inferior portion, making it Type II in 20% cases)

- Blood supply – the ascending branch of LCFA enters the deep surface approximately 9 cm below ASIS after running in between RF and vastus lateralis (VL).
- Attachment – from the ASIS, the outer lip of the anterior iliac crest and fascia lata to the iliotibial tract (ITT).
- Action – it helps stabilise and steady the hip and knee joints by putting tension on the ITT. It also contributes to flexion at the hip, with abduction and medial rotation.

HARVESTING

The pedicled flap can be raised either as an MC or FC flap; the muscle can be dissected off the iliac crest to allow a greater arc of rotation. The axis of the flap lies along a line from the greater trochanter to the patella. The skin flap can be raised to within 8 cm of the knee joint (a longer flap requires delay as the distal part is essentially 'random' in nature).

- The 'TFL skin only' flap is the skin island based on the ascending branch of the LCFA, which runs transversely. The skin perforators are usually of a decent size and may travel through the muscle necessitating some intramuscular dissection. It is an option when the typical ALT perforators are too small for use.

ADVANTAGES

- The large skin paddle (up to 15 cm) is durable.
- The muscle is supposedly 'expendable', but there are reports of lateral knee destabilisation. The functional deficit may be reduced if the distal cut-end of fascia is sutured to the VL.

DISADVANTAGES

- Skin grafting of the donor is usually required if the defect is wider than 10 cm. When used as a transposition flap, there is often a big dog ear.

- The skin bridge between the donor and the defect often needs to be sacrificed.
- The deeper fascial layer of the flap may reduce proper adherence to the bed of the defect.

LATISSIMUS DORSI (SEE 'BREAST RECONSTRUCTION')

COMMON USES

- As an islanded pedicle flap, it may be used for chest wall, breast, shoulder, back and neck reconstruction. It can also provide a functional muscle flap for proximal upper limb reconstruction.
- As a free flap, it is often used for defects of the scalp and lower limb. A larger flap can be raised by also harvesting the SA ± rib.

Type – type V muscle flap.

- Blood supply – The dominant pedicle is the **TDA**, which is the continuation of the subscapular artery from the third part of the axillary artery – this passes through the **triangular space** (2 cm above the upper end of the posterior axillary crease, when viewed from the front: teres minor [some say subscapularis], teres major and long head of triceps) to gain the posterior axilla. The artery and (usually) single vein are ~2 mm in diameter.
  - The flap may still be harvested in some cases if the **TDA has been divided** previously; the vessels should be assumed to have been divided during an axillary dissection unless specifically mentioned.
- Attachments – The muscle arises from a broad origin stretching from the spinous processes from T7 downwards, and then across to the posterior superior iliac crest. It runs superomedially to converge upon the bicipital groove of the humerus; it forms the posterior axillary fold.
- Action – It is innervated by the thoracodorsal nerve (C6,7,8 – posterior cord of brachial plexus) and on contraction extends and adducts at the shoulder and also medial rotation of the humerus. The best way to test its function is to palpate the lower border during resisted adduction. There does not seem to be any difference in shoulder strength when one muscle has been harvested (Laitung, *Br J Plast Surg*, 1985).

SURFACE MARKINGS

- Skin defects of 8 × 15 cm can usually be closed primarily. Depending on the reconstructive requirements, the skin paddle can be placed anywhere over the muscle and up to 4 cm beyond, although it will become increasingly 'random'.
- Inferiorly the muscle thins out and becomes 'fascia-like' about 5 cm above the posterior iliac crest; this portion can be included, but the blood supply can be precarious and cannot reliably support the overlying skin. The upper lateral two-thirds has more perforators

from the muscle; medial and inferior skin paddles are supposedly less reliable.

- The operative markings are posterior axillary fold, angle of scapula, spinous processes from T6 to sacrum and posterior iliac crest. The true anterior border of the muscle **is 2–3 cm anterior to where you think you feel it** with the pinch/grasp test; a common mistake is to make the incision too posterior.

HARVEST

The patient is placed in a mid-lateral position with arm abducted to 90°. The borders of the skin paddle are incised, bevelling edges outwards; usually the upper border is developed first, then sweeping downwards to avoid inadvertent elevation of the SA, which is intimately associated with the deep surface of the muscle from its scapular attachment to the ninth rib.

- Identifying the vessels after delineating and retracting the anterior border is the key to the operation. Next, identify the SA and divide the pedicle to the lower half (upper half via lateral thoracic arteries). After the LD is separated from its distal attachments, it will shorten and widen but can be stretched out.
- The branch to the SA may be divided along with the circumflex scapular artery for greater pedicle length.
- Seroma is fairly common and some recommend quilting sutures to reduce its incidence.

OTHER POINTS

- **Reverse/turnover flaps** – the entire muscle can be raised based on the secondary lumbar perforators (ninth intercostal downwards), and transected distal to the thoracodorsal vessels. In selected cases, the thoracodorsal vessels can be preserved to allow supercharging.

RADIAL FOREARM FLAP

The radial forearm flap (RFF) is a fasciocutaneous flap (type C), typically used as a free flap but can be pedicled or distally based (best pivot point is about 2–3 cm proximal to the wrist) with reversed flow from the ulnar artery via the palmar arches. The ulnar artery is the main supply to the superficial palmar arch, which is the major supply to the digits.

- Theoretically, the entire forearm skin can be elevated on the radial artery, e.g. phalloplasty. A smaller flap is a common choice in oral cavity reconstruction. The RFF is the archetypal 'Chinese flap' and was brought to the United Kingdom by David Soutar in 1983.
  - The RFF can also be used as a flow-through flap due to its vascular anatomy.
  - A 10–12 cm segment of the lateral cortex of radius can be harvested (between pronator teres and brachioradialis insertions) if required. However, it is one of the worst choices for bone and is not suitable for osteointegration.

- The palmaris longus can be included, e.g. in lower lip reconstruction as a sling.
- The use of this flap is contraindicated where **Allen's test** indicates poor perfusion by the ulnar artery (7–12 seconds, 15% do not have complete palmar arches); some have suggested reconstruction of the artery with reversed cephalic or saphenous vein grafting. Note that the ulnar artery may be superficial in ~9% of patients and thus vulnerable during RFF harvesting.

SURFACE MARKINGS

The non-dominant forearm is usually preferred.

- Generally, the most distal parts of the forearm over the wrist crease are not harvested.
- The radial artery may be palpated at the wrist and traced proximally beneath the brachioradialis to the antecubital fossa (a Doppler probe may help). It is useful to mark out tributaries of the cephalic vein.
  - There are some concerns about possible relative arterial overload with the RFF; some suggest reducing this by using end-to-side anastomoses, bypass/flow through or an AV shunt.
  - Either the venae comitantes (VC, which can be small, ~1.3 mm) or the superficial veins (usually cephalic) can be used for microanastomosis. The cephalic vein often communicates with the VCs near the antecubital fossa, and this can drain the whole flap; some advise against anastomosing both venous systems, due to the possible risk of reduced flow leading to thrombosis, but this is not borne out in practice.

OPERATIVE TECHNIQUE

- The use of an arm tourniquet is common but not universal; some inflate without exsanguination to make the veins more pronounced whilst stopping arterial bleeding.
- Several methods have been described to raise the skin flap. Some points:
  - Preserve paratenon where possible particularly on FCR; exposed tendons should be covered with muscles if possible.
  - On the radial side of FCR, the dissection proceeds from superficial to the tendon to a deeper plane to **ensure fascial continuity** between vessels and skin paddle.
  - Care should be taken to avoid injury to the superficial branches of the radial nerve on the radial edge. If the flap is intended to be sensate, then either the medial or lateral cutaneous nerves of the forearm can be included.
- The **donor site is the main perceived disadvantage** with this flap; it can be poor in young or obese patients. It is usually closed with a skin graft (non-take is most

common over the FCR tendon), but many alternative techniques are described in the literature.

- Graft take can be improved using tie-over dressings, including NPWT.
- Bilobed flap based on the ulnar side (Hsieh CH, *Plast Reconstr Surg*, 2004) – pivot point 8 cm proximal to pisiform where a consistent perforator usually lies. First lobe perpendicular to the line from the pivot point to the furthest point of the defect; second lobe less than 90°, as long but narrower (one-half to two-thirds).

COMPLICATIONS

These are mostly related to the donor site, in particular grafting; SSG is more reliable than FTSG.

Other complications include the following:

- Tendon adhesion 19%−33%.
- Reduced wrist movement in up to 26%.
- Ischaemia, cold intolerance.
- Dysaesthesia from injury to sensory nerves 30%; patients should be counselled to **expect loss**.
- Fracture in up to 20% after bone removal with increased risk in postmenopausal women. The risk can be decreased by avoiding sawing the bone at right angles and prophylactic plating. The radius needs to be protected for 6 weeks.

SCAPULAR AND PARASCAPULAR FLAPS

The scapular flap is a (fascio)cutaneous flap based upon the horizontal or transverse branch of the **circumflex scapular artery** (CSA) from the subscapular artery (direct from the axillary artery in 3%), which emerges through the triangular space. The artery roughly divides the scapula into two halves; the average pedicle length is 4–6 cm with a 1.5–3 mm diameter artery with two large but thin-walled VCs. It can be traced back to the axilla to include the subscapular artery, if necessary, for extra length (up to 20 cm).

There may be effects on the shoulder function, but this can be improved by post-operative physiotherapy.

SURFACE MARKINGS

The maximum dimensions allowing primary closure are ~10 × 20 cm in the average-sized person. A bilateral scapular flap that crosses the midline can be harvested but requires two anastomoses and has been used for total face reconstruction (Angrigiani C, *Plast Reconstr Surg*, 1997).

The flap can be raised without fascia (suprafascial) or with bone from the scapula or in combination with other flaps on the **subscapular artery axis** such as LD or SA with or without rib for large composite defects.

- The free scapular flap was first described by Gilbert (*Plast Reconstr Surg*, 1982). It is a thin versatile flap with large quantities of good quality skin that is easy to raise; it is often used in limb resurfacing and facial reconstruction (poor colour texture match), but having to **reposition patients** adds to the operative time and is the main disadvantage.
  - Scapular (transverse) branch runs parallel to the spine of the scapula, but 2 cm below it; the skin flap can extend across the midline.
  - **Urbaniak rule of 2's** – medial end 2 cm from spinous processes, lateral 2 cm above the axilla at the position of the triangular space, superiorly 2 cm from the spine and inferiorly 2 cm above the angle. In practice, flaps well beyond these limits can be harvested with few functional problems.
  - Bony stock (14 cm × 3 cm) is inferior to the fibula (non-segmental supply), though it may permit osteointegration in males, but probably not females.
  - The best indication is for bone defect associated with a large soft tissue defect **with the bony requirements being secondary**.
- The **parascapular flap** can be harvested on the descending branch of the CSA that courses down the lateral border of the scapula.
- Pedicled scapular flaps are useful for axillary burn contractures; some describe a technique of passing the flap through the triangular space to extend the effective pedicle length.
  - **Bilobed parascapular/scapular flaps** with the common base centred over the triangular space. Vertical flap should be longer than horizontal secondary flap, which should be approximately half the width. The distal part of the vertical flap is usually closed directly.
  - The actual advantages of a bilobed flap over a single flap are unclear, but supposedly it offers more mobility in a larger flap (to cover axillary defects up to 10 cm wide) and allows mobilisation of more posterior areas, which are more likely to be unburnt. However, there is less mobility overall in burn tissue, and even if it looks only 'slightly' scarred, it may be under significant tension and the donor site defect significantly enlarges after flap harvest.

TECHNIQUE

- Mark scapula landmarks (if done preoperatively, the patient's position needs to be identical to the operative) position. Locate the **triangular space** above the posterior axillary fold; Doppler ultrasound can also be used.
- With the patient in the **prone or (mid-)lateral position,** elevation progresses in the bloodless plane superficial to the deep fascia of infraspinatus.
  - CSA is usually easily seen, but is vulnerable to damage, as it runs around the lateral edge of the scapula. The triangular space has fibrous fat that needs to be dissected gently. If necessary, the teres major can be released to improve exposure and then sutured to the teres minor. Muscle branches can be sacrificed.

- **To harvest bone** – lateral scapula from single CSA or lateral scapula with two branches – CSA and angular artery. Lateral scapula bone can be harvested up to 1.5 cm thick, 3–4 cm wide and 10–14 cm long, often with double pedicles.

DEEP CIRCUMFLEX ILIAC ARTERY (DCIA)

The DCIA flap was first described by Taylor (*Plast Reconstr Surg*, 1979). It is based over the iliac crest and may include some of this bone (up to 7 cm). The DCIA is a branch from the lateral aspect of the external iliac artery 2 cm above the inguinal ligament that then skirts the inner pelvic rim deep to the fascia overlying iliopsoas muscles.

COMMON USES

As an osseocutaneous flap, it is perhaps most suited to the reconstruction of curved bone (though step osteotomies can be used for straightening, the fibular is preferred for straight bone), e.g. using **the ipsilateral hip for hemimandible** and composite intra-oral defects; the bone can be orientated at right angles to the skin. The flap provides a large amount of bone that permits osteointegration. However, the skin flap is bulky and relatively immobile and is often thought to be unreliable, in up to 30% (Kimata Y, *Clin Plast Surg*, 2003).

Complications include donor pain and herniae, so the donor site has to be carefully closed. The scar is relatively inconspicuous.

SURFACE MARKINGS

The cutaneous paddle (up to 14 × 27 cm) is centred on the iliac crest with two-thirds of its area lying above the iliac crest. It can be extended medially to the femoral vessels and laterally 8–10 cm away from the ASIS.

The skin perforators emerge in a row just above the inner lip of the iliac crest, commencing near the ASIS and emerging at 2 cm intervals; the largest perforator is usually the terminal branch or close to it, and pierces the abdominal wall muscles 1–2 cm above the iliac crest and 6 cm behind the ASIS. The pedicle length is on average 5–8 cm with large vessels of diameters 1.5–4 mm; the VCs run lateral to the external iliac artery and then cross either in front of (50%) or behind the artery as they ascend medially to join the external iliac vein. There is an ascending muscular branch from the pedicle 1–2 cm medial to the ASIS, which does not contribute to the skin or bone of the flap.

TECHNIQUE

- Use a handheld Doppler to locate the perforators. Harvest with a sandbag under the hip.
- The medial upper part of the flap is usually raised first, along with a segment of the anterior abdominal wall muscles, whilst identifying and preserving the superficial circumflex iliac vessels. The DCIA is

followed laterally maintaining a cuff of iliacus between the vessels and the bone. The inferior border is then raised cutting through TFL and the gluteal muscles as an outer muscle cuff. Since the bone is supplied from its medial cortex, it can be split to harvest this cortex alone whilst preserving the outer cortex.

- The upper cut edge of the abdominal wall muscle is re-attached to the pelvic side wall using strong nylon sutures anchored through the bone.
  - Refinements – avoiding harvest of muscle (perforator flap) will reduce the donor site morbidity and the bone can be combined with the groin flap skin paddle as a chimeric flap with a thinner skin island than the classical DCIA.

FIBULA

This flap is supplied by the peroneal artery, which arises from the posterior tibial artery (PTA) 2.5 cm below its origin (the popliteal artery divides into anterior and posterior tibial arteries at the level of the popliteus muscle).

The **peroneal artery** is in the posterior compartment along with the PTA, running beneath the attachment of flexor hallucis longus (FHL) posteromedial to the fibula and gives off muscle branches to flexor digitorum longus (FDL) and tibialis posterior (TP); other muscle branches wind around the fibula to supply peroneus longus (PL) and brevis, and a **nutrient branch** is given off to the fibula itself at the junction of the upper and middle third but can be sacrificed. The peroneal artery terminates as the lateral calcaneal artery and a perforating branch, which penetrates the interosseous septum to reach the anterior compartment to the anterior tibial artery.

The skin paddle can be quite large, but direct closure is only possible with 6–8 cm. There are three to four septocutaneous perforators running in the intermuscular septum between the PL and the soleus around the **middle third** of the fibula. Sometimes the perforators arise from the muscular branches of the peroneal necessitating intermuscular dissection of the soleus. In up to 10%, the skin island over the fibula is supplied by a system of vessels separate from the peroneal artery and cannot be harvested together.

- Tan BK (Wong CH, *J Plast Reconstr Aesthet Surg*, 2009) described anomalous septocutaneous perforators to the skin paddle originating from the PTA. They remark that proximal perforators are less likely to arise from the peroneal artery.

COMMON USES

The fibula flap offers about 22–26 cm of the straight tubular bone; it is commonly used for **mandibular reconstruction** (sufficient to replace angle-to-angle defects) and segmental long bone defects, allowing weight bearing. Its use was first described by Taylor (*Plast Reconstr Surg*, 1975); it was first used for mandibular reconstruction by Hidalgo in 1989.

The rich periosteal supply allows the bone to be osteotomised to reconstruct angles and to be double-barrelled, keeping each segment at least 2–3 cm long.

- The fibula is too narrow to reproduce the full height of the mandible; it is usually placed inferiorly, which leads to a deficit at the top and a 'collapse' of the lip. The height can be increased by vertical distraction or by double barrelling. Shen (*J Plast Reconstr Aesthet Surg*, 2013) found that, on average, double barrelling could reconstruct an 8 cm gap.
  - Dental implants require 6–7 mm of healthy bone.

SURFACE MARKINGS

- Mark out the fibula head and lateral malleolus, and draw the line along the **posterior border** of the bone, which forms the axis of the skin paddle with most perforators at the junction of the upper and middle third.
- Mark a line 4–6 cm distal to the fibula head as the site of proximal osteotomy (distal to the common peroneal nerve; the nerve may be palpable as it travels forwards over the neck of the fibula to divide in the substance of the PL into branches – superficial to peroneal compartment and deep to anterior compartment). Maintain at least 5 cm proximal to the lateral malleolus to avoid disrupting the ankle joint. Ankle weakness may be due to excessive bony resection or detachment of muscles (FHL, FDL and TP).

Technique

Some suggest using the left leg as it is used less, e.g. in driving (Figure 11.3).

- The lateral approach is most common. The patient is placed in a supine position with the hip raised with pad under buttock and then flexed 120°. A thigh tourniquet (not universal) is inflated to 300 mmHg.

- The skin paddle is raised from anterior and then posterior borders, preserving the (posterior) intermuscular septum with the septocutaneous perforators, which are then traced to the posteromedial surface of the fibula.
- The peroneal muscles are retracted anteriorly, and dissected from the anterolateral surface of the fibula, leaving the periosteum and a thin muscle layer. Then the anterior septum of the lateral compartment, extensor hallucis longus and TP are transected in turn. The interosseous membrane is divided when it is reached.
- The distal osteotomy is performed and the peroneal vessels emerging from the lower border of the FHL are ligated. Early osteotomy facilitates the soft tissue dissection particularly freeing the anteriomedial surface. The proximal osteotomy will allow more room for further mobilisation. The pedicle vessels can be rather short – discarding some proximal bone (possibly sacrificing the nutrient branch) will 'lengthen' the pedicle.
  - The rare **peronea magna** or dominant peroneal artery with hypoplastic tibial vessels is something to be aware of but seems to be a very rare (<0.2%) phenomenon; elderly patients do seem to be more reliant upon the peroneal artery for supply to the foot.
  - Checking for palpable pedal pulses (dorsalis pedis and posterior tibial) seems to be an adequate preoperative screen in most; angiography may be indicated in selected patients, such as those with a history of trauma or with severe PVD.
- Wedge osteotomies can be performed whilst the flap is still attached by its pedicle; many prefer to do it on a side table. Nakayama (*Plast Reconstr Surg*, 2006) described out-fractures with opening osteotomies (and bone grafts) as an alternative to the conventional closing osteotomy after excision of a wedge.

It is important to realise that bony union in mandibular reconstruction does not take place at the speeds of, say, a fractured long bone. Union within 12 months is accepted as normal, whilst >12 months is delayed union. Good fixation is a slit between bone ends, whilst fair fixation is up to 3 mm gap (poor more than 3 mm). Osteointegration should be delayed for at least 6 months, usually for >1 year; its use after irradiation is relatively contraindicated (failure to integrate, failure to bear load), though some have suggested that HBO may help.

POST-OPERATIVE CARE

- Firm bandaging.
- Weight-bear with assistance after graft inspected (days 5–7); if skin grafts have not been used, then this can start after the second post-operative day.
- Partial weight-bearing for 3–4 weeks along with outpatient physiotherapy.

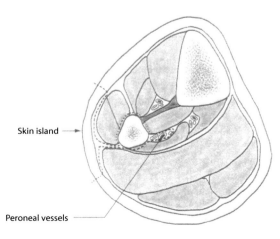

Skin island

Peroneal vessels

Figure 11.3 Cross section showing the tissues harvested during an osteocutaneous fibula flap. Skin island and peroneal vessels.

COMPLICATIONS

Patients generally do not have severe donor site morbidity, though some pain and discomfort are not uncommon and a grafted donor site can be rather unsightly; however, serious problems are generally uncommon.

- Ankle disruption and instability; seems to be a greater risk in children
- Peroneal nerve injury/infection, compartment syndrome
- Toe clawing

Quantitative assessments show that even patients without specific complaints may have measureable reduced hallux push-off force, an eversion torque deficit due to PL weakness that may potentially lead to progressive ankle instability and secondary ankle arthritis; mild medial ankle osteoarthritis was found in 70%, i.e. **most patients actually compensate well**. There have been attempts to reduce morbidity in children by replacing the segment with tricalcium phosphate, and although the bone regenerated radiologically, there were no detectable differences otherwise. Likewise, the effects of specific muscle strengthening programmes are unknown.

SERRATUS ANTERIOR

The serratus anterior (SA) muscle arises from the first to the eighth/ninth ribs; the upper half inserts into the deep aspect of the medial edge of the scapula, whilst the lower slips insert into the angle. When it contracts, it causes protrusion of the scapula and rotates the scapula upwards and outwards. It can be tested by pushing the outstretched hand against a wall – absence or denervation produces characteristic **winging**.

- The SA flap is a type III muscle flap – there are two dominant pedicles (the lateral thoracic artery to the upper part and the serratus branch of the TDA to the lower part). It can also be raised with some skin and rib.
- It is innervated by the **long thoracic nerve** (of Bell, C5, 6 and 7), which lies anterior to the artery but still **deep to the deep fascia**. The upper four muscle slips are innervated by C5, next two by C6 and the lowest two by C7 fibres – the lower half thus has an independent nerve and blood supply lending itself to easy splitting.

COMMON USES

The SA flap is most often used for coverage of defects of the head and neck and extremities. It may also be used as a functional flap for facial and hand reanimation.

TECHNIQUE

The incision parallels the eighth rib on the lateral chest side wall, curving superiorly to the axilla. Identify the anterior border of the LD and separate it from the posterior part of the SA under it; the anterior part is exposed by elevation of the overlying skin. Elevate the lower slips off their rib origins, tying off intercostal perforators unless the underlying bone is required.

The pedicle is traced superiorly; tying off the TDA (LD) and the CSA will provide a much longer pedicle (whole of the subscapular artery). The nerve is preserved if an innervated muscle is required – it is possible to separate out a discrete bunch of fascicles to the lower part of the muscle only.

LATERAL ARM FLAP

The lateral arm flap is a type C FC flap that is easy to make sensate. It is based upon the posterior radial collateral artery (PRCA) from the profunda brachii artery (it continues behind the lateral epicondyle to anastomose with the radial artery). The skin island is innervated by the lower lateral cutaneous nerve of the arm, a branch of the radial nerve that pierces the belly of triceps, whilst the upper cutaneous nerve of the arm is a terminal branch of the axillary nerve. There will be an area of numbness along the lateral forearm as a result of flap harvest. The pedicle has a diameter of 1–2 mm with a maximum length of 8 cm (requires some splitting of the lateral head of triceps).

COMMON USES

It provides a **thin flap** suited for soft tissue defects of the dorsal and volar surfaces of the hand. It is the classic choice for **covering tendons** due to deep fascial surface purportedly facilitating gliding.

Some variants have been described:

- **Extended lateral arm flap** – the flap can be extended distally beyond the classic boundaries. Dye and infusion studies have shown that the PRCA extends to 8 cm below, although others suggest that the PRCA itself does not extend beyond condyle – rather it anastomoses with an olecranon plexus, which supplies distal vessels that account for the bleeding that can be seen up to 12 cm beyond the elbow.
- **Distal lateral arm flap** – the flap is based on the lowest perforator found 4 cm above the epicondyle and can be innervated by including the PCNFA.
- **Lateral arm fascial free flap** – the fascia alone up to 12 × 9 cm can be transferred and is useful when a thin covering is required, e.g. ear reconstruction or for gliding around tendons.
- **It can also be raised with a piece of the humerus as an osseofasciocutaneous flap.**

OPERATIVE TECHNIQUE

The skin paddle lies on the **axis** of a line drawn between deltoid insertion and lateral epicondyle (LE), which also marks the position of the **lateral intermuscular septum** (anterior to the septum are biceps, brachialis, brachioradialis and ECRL, whilst posteriorly are lateral [above spiral groove] and medial [below groove] heads of triceps).

- A handheld Doppler probe can be used to determine the approximate position of the perforators before surgery; commonly, there are four significant perforators with the largest one approximately 10 cm proximal to the LE.
- A narrow sterile tourniquet can be used but is not necessary. The posterior incision is made first, and the flap is elevated forwards in the subfascial plane to the intermuscular septum, then it is dissected from the front. The **distal vessel is ligated** and the fascial septum progressively detached from the bone.
- The pedicle is followed proximally, a process that is made easier by incising the lateral head of triceps, taking care to preserve the radial nerve that lies between the brachialis and the brachioradialis, and the spiral groove.
- The radial nerve gives off the posterior cutaneous nerve of the arm, which runs through the flap; it innervates the skin on the back of the arm but must be taken in the lateral arm flap. Donor sites of up to 6 cm width will close directly.

GROIN FLAP

The groin flap is a cutaneous flap that can be used either free or pedicled. It is the archetypal axial pattern flap. The pedicle is the SCIA from the femoral artery at the medial border of the sartorius. The vessels have a narrow diameter, usually about 1 mm. There are paired VCs and often a direct cutaneous vein draining into the saphenous bulb.

COMMON USES

It is a versatile flap first described by McGregor (*Plast Reconstr Surg*, 1972) and can be used for a variety of defects such as the head and neck, chest and extremities. Flaps of up to 15 × 30 cm can be raised and closed directly leaving an inconspicuous linear donor site scar and is thus often described as being 'dispensable'. However, it can be quite bulky in obese patients. The main 'complaint' levelled at the flap is that the pedicle is small, short and inconsistent – **expect** anatomical variations.

TECHNIQUE

The long axis of the flap **parallels the inguinal ligament, running 2 cm below it**. The flap is raised from the lateral edge first (in the flank, the full thickness of fat need not be elevated but can be thinned to the dermis at this point) taking care to leave the lateral cutaneous nerve of the thigh. As the sartorius is reached, the fascia is included in the flap since this transmits a number of cutaneous perforators at this point. The superficial circumflex iliac vessels are on the underside of the flap and can be traced forwards. It can be useful to keep cutaneous veins as the primary or secondary system for outflow; preserve the inferior epigastric vein as it runs beneath the medial part of the flap since this has a sizeable tributary from the groin skin.

PECTORALIS MAJOR (PM)

This myocutaneous flap was first described by Ariyan (*Plast Reconstr Surg*, 1979) and was commonly used in head and neck reconstruction, though its use has declined after the introduction of free flaps.

- Blood supply – the muscle is supplied by the lateral thoracic arteries and the pectoral branch of the **thoraco-acromial trunk** (TAT, from the second part of the axillary artery) – the latter provides the flap pedicle that runs medially along a line drawn from the acromion to the xiphisternum after dropping down vertically to meet it.
  - The clavipectoral fascia transmits both the pectoral branch and the lateral pectoral nerve; it is 2–3 cm medial to the coracoid process. The pedicle bifurcates 2 cm from the origin into two branches: upper to clavicular head and lower to sternocostal head.
- Attachments – The muscle has sternocostal (upper six ribs) and clavicular heads, which combine to insert into the lateral lip of the bicipital groove of the humerus. The upper portion of the sternocostal is usually left intact.
- Action – The nerve supply comes from the medial and lateral pectoral nerves. The muscle forms the anterior border of the axilla and acts as a powerful adductor and medial rotator of the humerus.

TECHNIQUE

- The skin paddle is positioned medial to the nipple according to the reconstructive needs; in females, it is often better to position the paddle below the nipple. Making the island too medial may use skin that is more dependent on the IMA perforators; the TAT is actually orientated more towards the nipple.
- **A 'defensive' incision** is often used, even though the deltopectoral flap is a very uncommon option these days. Direct donor site closure is usually possible. The inferior portions of the flap are dissected first to define the lowest extent of the muscle to ensure that the skin island is located suitably. The dissection is continued to lift the muscle upwards when the pedicle is easily visualised.
- TAT perforator flaps have been described, e.g. hypopharyngeal reconstruction (Zhang YX, *Plast Reconstr Surg*, 2013).
- The Palmer and Bachelor modifications aimed to reduce the donor morbidity:
  - The upper portion of the sternocostal head is left intact.
  - The lateral pectoral nerve and as much as possible the medial nerve are left intact.

- The proximal portion of the pectoral branch before it enters the muscle is surrounded by loose areolar tissue and can be dissected off the muscle, and the islanded flap can be delivered through a 'buttonhole' in the muscle. This causes an increase in the pedicle length by about 4 cm (able to reach the oral cavity), a greater arc of rotation and less compromise of shoulder function.

ALTERNATIVES

- **Deltopectoral flap** (Bakamjian) is thin and pliable with a relatively straightforward harvest and is a useful salvage technique, but often needs grafting of the Donor. The multiple perforators restricts movement about the pedicle and the fact that it cannot be tunnelled leaves an unattractive dog ear. The standard DP flap can reach the ear and lower jaw.
- An **IMAP flap** that can be raised on any of the first four perforators (usually second) and provides enough tissue for the full height of neck and reaches the **angle of mandible**. Costal cartilages may be cut for more pedicle length. The random element beyond the deltopectoral groove can be included if it does not exceed 1:1 (or can be increased with delay, e.g. to reach jaw).
    - IMA runs 1–2 cm lateral to the sternal edge; the second perforator is usually the largest (about 0.8 mm with single dominant vessel 85%, whilst in females, the third and fourth IMAPs also fairly large). Perfusion tests have demonstrated that the IMA territory runs from the midline (very little flow occurs across to the other side) up to the anterior axillary fold, clavicle to xiphisternum.
- **Lateral thoracic artery flap** can be pedicled back just lateral to the TAT after cutting the pectoralis minor and the clavicular head of the PM and is said to reach the nasopharynx and zygoma.

SUPERIOR GLUTEAL ARTERY FLAP

This began as a type II muscle or myocutaneous flap.

- Blood supply – The GM muscle is supplied by both gluteal arteries. The **superior gluteal artery** (SGA) arises from the posterior branch of the internal iliac artery, whilst the inferior gluteal artery comes from the anterior branch.
- Attachment – The GM is a broad, flat sheet of muscle that lies most superficially in the buttock and crosses the gluteal fold at 45°, passing from the gluteal surface of the ilium, the lumbar fascia, the sacrum and the sacrotuberous ligament to the gluteal crest of the femur and the ITT.
- Action – Extends and externally rotates the femur, and acting through the fascia lata, it also supports the extended knee. The muscle is supplied by the inferior gluteal nerve only.

As the muscle itself offers little to the flap, it has largely evolved to a **perforator flap** with an inconspicuous donor site and no functional deficit:

- The pedicled S-GAP perforator flap is a good option for sacral pressure sores.
- The free S-GAP flap is recommended as a sensate flap for autologous breast reconstruction (Blondeel PN, *Br J Plast Surg*, 1999). However, the need to turn the patient during the operation is a disadvantage.

SURFACE MARKINGS

The SGA emerges from the pelvis through the greater sciatic foramen at a point between the upper third and lower two-thirds of a line connecting the posterior superior iliac spine (PSIS) and the greater trochanter. After it passes between the gluteus medius above and the piriformis below, it divides into deep and superficial branches. The flap may be drawn horizontally to conform to a bikini line.

TECHNIQUE

Incise around the skin flap margin down through the deep fascia. Dissect from the superior margin downwards over the upper GM to identify the SGA perforator(s), then split the muscle to see the pedicle emerging from between the gluteus medius and the piriformis. The inferior incision can then be completed.

TEMPOROPARIETAL FASCIAL FLAP

The temporoparietal fascia (TPF) is a large thin fascial sheet that covers the temporal, parietal and occipital areas of the scalp. It is an extension of the SMAS layer, passing from the face to the scalp, and continues above the temporal line as the galea aponeurosis, densely adherent to overlying skin/fat via connective tissue and separated by loose areolar tissue from the underlying pericranium. The temporalis muscle and temporalis fascia (deep temporal fascia) lie deep to the TPF inferior to the temporal line (Figure 11.4).

- The TPF flap can be used as a free or pedicled flap (the skin or underlying parietal cranial bone can be included). It is a very thin flap with cosmetic donor site unless there is male pattern baldness. It is often used in autologous ear reconstruction or upper limb reconstruction as it allows tendon gliding.
- It is supplied by large, anatomically consistent vessels with an artery of size of up to 2 mm (and vein >2 mm in diameter) from the superficial temporal artery, which can be palpated or identified by Doppler.
- The incision is made posterior to the pedicle at the level of the tragus; the pedicle is identified and traced superiorly. A skin paddle of up to 3 cm wide may be closed directly; transient alopecia has been observed.

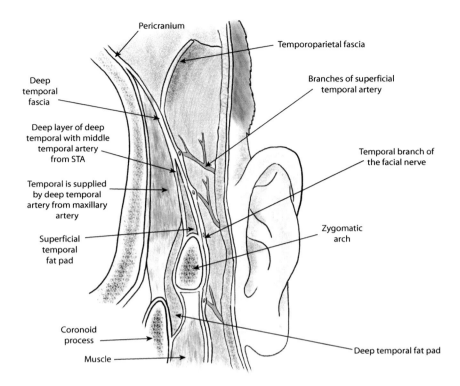

Figure 11.4 Cross section of the temporal region. The deep temporal fascia (sometimes called the temporal fascia proper) is split inferiorly into deep and superficial layers, encasing the superficial temporal fat pad. The TPF is continuous with the frontalis superiorly and the SMAS inferiorly. The temporal (frontal) branch of the facial nerve runs upwards over the zygomatic arch deep to/within this fascial layer.

Note that the temporal branch of the facial nerve passes from a point 0.5 cm below the tragus to 1.5 cm superior to the lateral brow.

- Just above the zygomatic arch, there are four fascial layers:
  - TPF.
  - Parotidotemporal fascia; covers the frontal branch.
  - Deep temporal fascia with deep and superficial components separated by a fat pad. Deep to this lies the temporalis muscle.

OMENTAL FLAP

This is a flap of the greater omentum (McLean DH, *Plast Reconstr Surg*, 1972), which is largely a mass of fat attached along the greater curvature of the stomach as far as the first part of the duodenum and loops down and backwards to attach to the transverse colon. It provides an extensive vascular film to restore moving tissue planes and supposedly delivers white cells making it useful in contaminated wounds. It has been used for certain purposes such as scalp reconstruction and filling in of contour deformities (Romberg's disease).

- The flap can be based on either of the **gastroepiploic arteries**, but usually the right-sided vessels (artery 2.8 mm, vein 3.2 mm are larger), providing a pedicle

roughly 3–4 cm in length; many side branches need ligating. The left pedicle involves more extensive dissection around the hilum of the spleen. Disadvantages are the need for laparotomy, and it is relatively contraindicated, if the patient has had previous surgery with adhesions. A (smaller) flap can be harvested endoscopically.

ANTEROLATERAL THIGH (ALT) FLAP

This is a fasciocutaneous flap based upon myocutaneous or septocutaneous perforators from the descending branch of the LCFA. It has become a workhorse flap in head and neck reconstruction in particular, including pharyngeal reconstruction as a tubed flap.

The flap provides a large skin paddle (which can be sensate) and can be used as a flow-through flap. When suitable perforator configuration/numbers permit, chimeric-type flaps with multiple skin islands or components, e.g. skin and muscle, can be harvested. The donor site morbidity is relatively minimal if direct closure is possible; compartment syndrome has been reported (Addison PD, *Ann Plast Surg*, 2008).

- Another concept is the **'mosaic flap'** (Koshima I, *Ann Plast Surg*, 1994) such as the anteromedial flap connected to the ALT at a muscle branch or the termination of the LCFA. This is particularly useful in re-do necks with a paucity of recipient vessels (Chiu T, *J Plast Reconstr Aesthet Surg*, 2013).

- The surface markings are fairly consistent; a line drawn from ASIS to the lateral border of the patella marks the lateral intermuscular septum between VL and rectus femoris, and most perforators are seen in the lateral inferior quadrant of a 3 cm circle centred on the midpoint of this line. The pedicle is at least 7–12 cm long with a 1.5–2.5 mm diameter artery.
- A more superiorly located flap based on the ascending/transverse branch of the LCFA is a 'lifeboat' if there are no 'typically' located perforators; otherwise, a medial thigh flap can often be raised.
- Pre-operative identification of the location of perforators is commonly performed with a hand held Doppler probe although some have documented experience with computed tomography angiography (CTA) or magnetic resonance angiography (MRA).
- The medial incision is made first down to the rectus femoris. Lateral subfascial dissection towards the intermuscular septum allows identification of the perforators, which are gradually traced back to the origin and may need significant intramuscular dissection (12% are septocutaneous according to Chen HC, *Clin Plast Surg*, 2003).

VI. TISSUE EXPANSION

TE aims to expand local skin allowing it to be used for reconstruction of nearby defects for the best match of colour, texture and hair-bearing quality (if needed) and is potentially sensate. The donor site can be closed directly under most circumstances.

HISTORY

- Neumann (*Plast Reconstr Surg*, 1957) expanded post-auricular skin for ear reconstruction with an air-filled subcutaneous implant.
- Radovan (1975) developed the silicone expander and used it to expand an arm flap to cover an adjacent defect (1976); it was later in breast reconstruction (Radovan C, *Plast Reconstr Surg*, 1982).
- At the same time, Austad (*Plast Reconstr Surg*, 1982) had done similar work in developing an implant independently. He demonstrated the histological changes accompanying TE in animals.

HISTOLOGICAL CHANGES

- **Epidermis thickens** due to cellular hyperplasia (the only layer/tissue that thickens), and there are increased mitoses in the basal layer. Rete ridges are less pronounced.
- Dermis thins despite increased dermal collagen that also realigns – fibrils straighten and become parallel.

- Rupture of elastin fibres.
- Appendages unaltered – thus hair density decreases and skin feels drier.
- Muscle thins – sarcomeres thin and become compacted. There are increased numbers of mitochondria.
- Adipose tissue atrophies with some permanent loss.
- Nerves – altered conductivity; decreased sensation in 50%. Expanded skin is often dry, pigmented with altered sensation.

A vascular capsule forms within a week; the increased vascularity (mostly at the junction of the capsule and normal tissue; Pasyk KA, *Clin Plast Surg*, 1987) makes tissue-expanded flaps more reliable and infections less 'critical' than with other foreign bodies. Lantieri LA (*Plast Reconstr Surg*, 1998) found an increased number of cells expressing VEGF. Two-thirds of the increase in tissue is due to visco-elastic deformation or 'creep'; one-third is true growth tissue that can be used for reconstruction.

Creep vs. stretch: A review of the viscoelastic properties of skin. (Wilhelmi BJ, *Ann Plast Surg*, 1998)
Skin is viscoelastic and responds to stretch in a characteristic manner.

- **Mechanical creep** is the elongation of skin under a constant load over time:
  - Collagen fibres stretch out and become parallel.
  - Elastin undergoes microfragmentation.
  - Water/interstitial fluid is displaced.
  - Some mechanical creep occurs during intra-operative TE and skin suturing under tension.
- **Biological creep** is the generation of **new tissue** secondary to a persistent chronic stretching force, i.e. the type of creep seen in pregnancy and conventional TE.
- **Stress–relaxation** describes the tendency for the resistance of the skin to a stretching force to decrease when held at a given tension over time, e.g. skin becomes tight when expanded, but by the next visit, it is no longer tight.

Molecular basis for tissue expansion: Clinical implications for the surgeon. (Takei T, *Plast Reconstr Surg*, 1998)
Mechanical strain was shown to induce transcription of cellular proto-oncogenes such as c-fos, c-myc and c-jun.

- **Up-regulation of growth factors** such as EGF, TGF-β and PDGF.
- **Deformational forces** acting on the cell membrane and disruption of integrins reduce cell–matrix adhesion.
- **Stretch-induced conformational changes of membrane proteins** cause opening of calcium channels leading to signal transduction and effects on the cytoskeleton (microfilament contraction) and

transduction pathways such as phospholipase C/protein kinase C.

- The actin cytoskeleton transmits mechanical forces intracellularly resulting in **mitosis** (growth and regeneration) via interaction with protein kinases, second messengers and nuclear proteins.

With TE, there is an increased rate of mitosis (up to 55% versus 5% in normal situation).

INDICATIONS

COMMON INDICATIONS FOR TE INCLUDE

- **Breast reconstruction** – expanders (usually placed subpectorally) can be used to expand the skin prior to replacement by a definitive implant. Alternatively, a permanent composite expander implant, e.g. Becker or McGhan, can be used to avoid additional surgery.
- **Scalp lesions**, e.g. alopecia. Expanders are placed in the subgaleal plane; initial expansion is typically difficult. It is common to base rotation or advancement flaps on named arteries such as temporal and occipital, taking care to orientate hair direction. It is possible to expand the remaining scalp to twice the size before thinning of hair is noticeable.
- Large cutaneous lesions such as **giant congenital melanocytic naevi** or **burn scars**.
- **Forehead expansion for nasal reconstruction** – critics suggest that this will lead to suboptimal results as the skin flap retracts.
- **Expanders** can be placed under planned skin flaps, e.g. groin or sometimes muscle flaps, e.g. PM or LD, to increase the amount of tissue that can be harvested, with added potential advantage of thinning out the muscle. FTSG donor sites can be expanded, either directly or by expanding the adjacent site, to facilitate closure of the donor site.
- **Prelaminated flaps**.

TECHNIQUE

The defect should be considered in terms of its shape and site, and the type of flap to be used. A significant disadvantage in the use of TE is the prolonged process needing two operations and multiple visits in between. Using multiple expanders could reduce the overall duration of expansion.

- **Position of incision**
  - Incision tangential to or just within lesion incision, which will be excised later. The incision is at the leading edge of the expansion zone.
  - **Remote** radial incisions (i.e. perpendicular to the direction of expansion) will tend to be under less tension with expansion and thus need less delay to allow for wound healing; however, using radial incisions usually means adding another scar.

Note that non-remote incisions will be in the expansion zone.
  - Commonly used to reduce complications in legs
- **Plane** – just above the muscle fascia, the subgaleal plane of the scalp and the subplatysmal plane of the neck. In the abdomen, the expander can be placed subcutaneously or between the obliques.
  - Make the largest pocket possible (>1 cm more than the expander base). A single large expander is preferable to several smaller expanders, but the space may not be available.
- **The port can be placed internally or externalised** (useful in children). A moderate amount of fluid (with or without methylene blue) is usually injected for an initial expansion that takes up the dead space. Expansion proper is commenced after 1–2 weeks and continues weekly (to the limits of patient pain tolerance and or blanching).

POTENTIAL DIFFICULTIES

- **Judging if the skin has been expanded adequately**. There are many different formulae that have been used to determine the amount of expanded skin, ranging from the simple, e.g. subtraction of the base size from the circumference of the expanded skin, to more complex mathematical formulae. For many practical reasons (leakage from port, stretchback, etc.), the actual tissue gained always seems to be less than predicted; thus, in practical applications, expanding just a bit more is always a safe practice.
  - **Leakage** from the injection dome or other parts may occur particularly if larger needles have been used. Some suggest using **Huber point needles** that are non-coring.
  - Rectangular expanders give the greatest amount of actual tissue gain vs. round expanders (40% vs. 25% of theoretical).
  - In practice, put in the largest expander that you can – the base should be two to three times that of the defect.
- **Using the expanded skin in the most efficient manner**. It can be difficult to convert a three-dimensional area of the expanded skin into a flap to cover what is usually a flat defect.
  - In most cases, simple rotation or advancement flaps are used.
  - **Unfolded box model** – It may be easier to visualise the expanded skin as five sides of a cube (minus the base) that can be split along its sides creating a flap as a chain of three 'squares' with the wings being positioned variably at these links. Theoretical concerns about the vascularity of distally based wings are not borne out in practice. The tissue can roughly be advanced by an amount twice the height of the expander.

- The capsule can be kept if there is sufficient tissue as it is extremely vascular; incision of the capsule (capsulotomy) adds a slight amount of mobility, whilst excision of the capsule (capsulectomy) increases the mobility further, also making it thinner and more compliant but risks compromising the vascularity.

COMPLICATIONS

TE does have a significant rate of complications:

- Extrusion and wound dehiscence
- Infection
- Rupture
- Migration – less with textured expanders

More difficulties may be encountered in

- Extremity expansion, especially lower limb; sural nerve neuropraxia
- Previously irradiated tissue
- Children, including the issue of port sites

Risk factors for complications for pediatric tissue expansion. (Friedman R, *Plast Reconstr Surg*, 1996)
The authors report on their experience with 180 expanders in children with an overall complication rate of 9%. Internal ports were associated with a higher complication rate (puncture). Overall, more complications were expected for burn scar surgery, soft tissue loss and age <7 years (perceived lack of cooperation).

Calvarial deformity and remodelling following prolonged scalp expansion in a child. (Calobrace MB, *Ann Plast Surg*, 1997)
The authors describe a 5 year old boy undergoing scalp expansion for burn scar alopecia over 15 months. A 3 cm deep depression had been created in the calvarium with bone lipping (deposition) at the margins, a deformity known as **saucerisation**. The changes were reversible and were fully remodelled by 6 months. Burn scar is unyielding and so may have transmitted more pressure to the calvarium in this instance.

TE IN THE LIMBS

Casanova (*Br J Plast Surg*, 2001) reviewed their use of 207 expanders in the lower limb. The complication rate was 15.5% (with expansion abandoned in 5%). Manders (*Plast Reconstr Surg*, 1988) reported a 50% infection rate. They suggested the following:

- Avoid bony areas, joints, scars or irradiated skin.
- Place expanders in a longitudinal direction above the muscle fascia; multiple expanders preferable.
- Use remote **radial incisions**, perpendicular to the long axis.

The high complication rates may be partly due to the vasculature in the leg, which is of the 'terminal' type with few axial vessels and a poorly formed subdermal plexus. Expansion below the knee is often a slower process and overall much less successful than in the thigh.

Vogelin (*Br J Plast Surg*, 1995) found high complication rates in situations such as PVD and infection, including osteomyelitis. They recommend that these problems should be treated with muscle flaps.

Tissue expansion at limb and non-limb sites. (Pandya AN, *Br J Plast Surg*, 2002)
In their practice, expanders are placed via short incisions, **radial to the direction of expansion**; intra-operative expansion is used to close the dead space. Adding methylene blue is useful to confirm correct needle placement in the port.

- Non-limb expansion mainly for breast reconstruction
- Limb expansion for post-traumatic scarring and other contour deformities

The commonest complications were infection and exposure of the expander. These were managed by hospitalisation, antibiotics and dressings until healed, and then further expansion was commenced if possible. Those unresponsive to conservative management had the expander removed after rapid expansion and the expanded tissue was used.

- Overall complication rate 27% in non-limb sites vs. 43% in limbs, especially lower.
- Despite the different complication rates, the authors report similar rates of **successful outcome** at limb and non-limb sites (83% and 86%, respectively).

The beginning of a new era in tissue expansion: Self-filling osmotic tissue expander. (Ronert MA, *Plast Reconstr Surg*, 2004)
These expanders are made from an osmotically active hydrogel and manufactured to 10% of its final volume. The expander gradually absorbs fluid to achieve a final size over 6–8 weeks, thus obviating the need for an inflation port, painful injections and regular clinic attendances for expansion.

- May be left in situ for up to 6 months before replacement
- Requires healthy skin/muscle coverage and thus unsuitable in previously irradiated areas

Osmotic expanders are not widely used but may be useful in paediatric patients particularly burns (Chummun S, *J Burn Care Res*, 2009) and clefts. Avoiding the need for regular injections is a major advantage, but many (Chummun S, *J Plast Reconstr Aesthet Surg*, 2010) suggest caution, given the high complication rate despite 'adequate precautions' and the **lack of control** over the expansion.

REFERENCES

Ablaza VJ. *Plast Reconstr Surg*. 1998;102:534.

Abubaker AO. *J Oral Maxillofac Surg*. 2001;59:1415.

Achar RA. *Acta Cir Bras*. 2014;29:125.

Achauer BM. *Lancet*. 1986;1:14.

Achauer BM. *Plast Reconstr Surg*. 1997;99:1301.

Achauer BM. *Plast Reconstr Surg*. 1999;103:11.

Adams WM. *Plast Reconstr Surg*. 1953;12:225.

Addison PD. *Ann Plast Surg*. 2008;60:635.

Agarwala SS. *J Clin Oncol*. 2004;22:2101.

Agrawal A. *Breast Cancer Res Treat*. 2007;103:1.

Ahn C. *Plast Reconstr Surg*. 1994;93:1481.

Akaishi S. *Ann Plast Surg*. 2008;60:445.

Al-Attar A. *Plast Reconstr Surg*. 2006;117:286.

Al-Ghazal SK. *Br J Plast Surg*. 1996;49:491.

Alconchel MD. *Br J Plast Surg*. 1996;49:242.

Alegre-Sanchez A. *Ped Dermatol*. 2017;34:619.

Allen EV. *Proc Staff Meet Mayo Clin*. 1940;15:184.

Allen RJ. *Ann Plast Surg*. 1994;32:32.

Allen RJ. *Plast Reconstr Surg*. 1995;95:1207.

Alnot JY. *Ann Chir Main*. 1985;4:11.

Alster TS. *Plast Reconstr Surg*. 1998;102:2190.

Alster TS. *Plast Reconstr Surg*. 1998;103:619.

Altintas MA. *Burns*. 2009;35:80.

Ambramson H. *J Pediatr Surg*. 2009;44:118.

Ames A. *Am J Pathol*. 1968;52:437.

Andel H. *Burns*. 2003;29:592.

Anderson ER. *Cochrane Database Syst Rev*. 2004; CD000163.

Anderson RL. *Arch Ophthalmol*. 1979;97:2192.

Anderson RR. *Science*. 1983;29:524.

Andraesen JO. *J Oral Maxillofac Surg*. 2006;64:1664.

Andrassy RJ. *Am J Surg*. 2002;184:484.

Angrigiani C. *Plast Reconstr Surg*. 1997;99:1566.

Arantes HL. *Aesth Plast Surg*. 2010;34:102.

Ardekani GS. *Plast Reconstr Surg*. 2009;123:112e.

Arden RL. *Arch Otolaryngo Head Neck Surg*. 1999;125:68.

Ardenghy M. *Ann Plast Surg*. 1996;37:211.

Ariyan S. *Plast Reconstr Surg*. 1979;63:78.

Ariyan S. *Plast Reconstr Surg*. 1983;72:468.

Ariyan S. *Plast Reconstr Surg*. 1995;96:1384.

Ariyan S. *Surg Oncol Clin N Am*. 1997;6:1.

Arnez ZM. *Clin Plast Surg*. 1991;19:449.

Arnez ZM. *Br J Plast Surg*. 1995;48:540.

Arnez ZM. *Br J Plast Surg*. 1999;10:82.

Arnez ZM. *Br J Plast Surg*. 2004;57:2.

Arnold PG. *Plast Reconstr Surg*. 1989;84:92.

Arons MS. *Br J Plast Surg*. 1998;51:570.

Arunachalam D. *Indian J Plast Surg*. 2011;17:184.

Asmussen S. *Burns*. 2013;39:429.

Atasoy E. *J Bone Joint Surg*. 1970;52:921.

Atisha D. *Ann Plast Surg*. 2009;63:222.

Atisha D. *Ann Plast Surg*. 2009;63:383.

Atkins JL. *Plast Reconstr Surg*. 2002;110:222.

Austad ED. *Plast Reconstr Surg*. 1982;70:704.

Austad ED. *Plast Reconstr Surg*. 2002;109:1724–1730.

Avni T. *Br Med J*. 2010;340:241.

Aydin F. *J Diabetes Res*. 2013;567834. https://doi.org /10.1155/2013/567834.

Aziz Z. *Cochrane Database Syst Rev*. 2015;9:CD002930.

Badger C. *Cochrane Database Syst Rev*. 2004;2:CD003140.

Badgwell B. *Ann Surg Oncol*. 2007;14:2867.

Bafaqeeh SA. *Br J Plast Surg*. 1998;51:508.

Bafitis H. *Plast Reconstr Surg*. 1989;83:896.

Bailey B. *Emerg Med J*. 2007;24:348.

Bajack AK. *Plast Reconstr Surg*. 2006;117:737.

Baker DC. *Aesthet Surg J*. 2001;21:14.

Balch CM. *Ann Surg Oncol*. 2000;7:87.

Balch CM. *Ann Surg Oncol*. 2001;8:101.

Balch CR. *Plast Reconstr Surg*. 1981;67:305.

Balch JM. *J Clin Oncol*. 2001;19:3635.

Balch JM. *J Clin Oncol*. 2009;27:6199.

Ballo MT. *Surg Clin North Am*. 2003;83:323.

BAPS/ BOA working party. *Br J Plast Surg*. 1997;50:570.

Baran R. *Brit J Dermatol*. 2007;157:149.

Bardach J. *Cleft Lip and Palate*. Polish Institute of Medical Publications. 1967.

Barkham MC. *J Plast Reconstr Aesthet Surg*. 2007;60:1269.

Barnett GR. *Br J Plast Surg*. 1989;42:556.

Baroudi R. *Plast Reconstr Surg*. 1979;2:368.

Barqouni L. *Cochrane Database Syst Rev*. 2014;6:CD008805.

Barret JP. *Burns*. 1999;25:509.

Bartels RJ. *Plast Reconstr Surg*. 1976;57:687.

Bartisich S. *Wounds*. 2012;24:51.

Bartlett SP. *Plast Reconstr Surg*. 1993;91:1208.

Baskett PJF. *Postgrad Med J*. 1972;48:138.

Bates SJ. *Plast Reconstr Surg*. 2009;124:128e.

Batta K. *Lancet*. 2002;9354:521.

Bauer SB. *Urol Clin N Am*. 1981;8:559.

Becker C. *Clin Plast Surg*. 2012;39:385.

Becker H. *Plast Reconstr Surg Global Open*. 2017;6:e1541.

Beer GM. *Br J Plast Surg*. 2004;57:12.

Benacquista T. *Plast Reconstr Surg*. 1996;98:834.

Bennett JE. *Plast Reconstr Surg*. 1957;20:261.

Bentolila V. *J Bone Joint Surg*. 1999;81:20.

Beriaghi S. *J Clin Ped Dentistry*. 2009;33:207.

Berkel H. *N Engl J Med*. 1992;326:1649.

Berman B. *J Am Acad Dermatol*. 2002;47:S209.

Bernstein EF. *Clin Dermatol*. 2006;24:43.

Bertelli G. *J Clin Oncol*. 1995;13:2851.

Berthe JV. *Plast Reconstr Surg*. 2003;111:2192.

Bhaskaranand K. *J Hand Surg Br*. 2002;27:229.

Bi Y. *Nat Med*. 2007;13:1219.

Biddulph SL. *Hand*. 1979;11:59.

Bigenwald RZ. *Cancer Epidemiol Biomarkers Prev*. 2008;17:706.

Biglioli F. *Plast Reconstr Surg.* 2012;129:852e.

Birdsell DC. *Plast Reconstr Surg.* 1993;92:795.

Bishop AT. *J Trauma.* 1986;26:201.

Bittar SM. *Plast Reconstr Surg.* 2012;129:1062.

Blanchard M. *J Plast Reconstr Aesth Surg.* 2012;65:1060.

Blomgren I. *Scand J Plast Reconstr Surg Hand Surg.* 1988;22:103.

Blondeel PN. *Br J Plast Surg.* 1999;52:104.

Blondeel PN. *Br J Plast Surg.* 1999;52:185.

Blondeel PN. *Br J Plast Surg.* 2003;56:266.

Blondeel PN. *Br J Plast Surg.* 2003;56:348.

Blondeel PN. *Clin Plastic Surg.* 2003;30:343.

Blundell JG. *J Bone J Surg.* 1964;46B:226.

Boccardo FM. *Lymphology.* 2009;42:1.

Bois E. *Int J Pediatr Otorhinolaryngol.* 2017;96:135.

Bonifazi E. *Ped Dermatol.* 2010;27:195.

Boorman JG. *Br J Plast Surg.* 1998;51:167.

Borisch N. *J Hand Surg Br.* 2003;28:450.

Borman H. *Plast Reconstr Surg.* 2002;109:396.

Bosch FX. *Int J Cancer.* 2005;114:779.

Bostwick J 3rd. *Clin Plast Surg.* 1979;61:27.

Bottomley A. *J Clin Oncol.* 2009;27:2916.

Bovill ES. *J Plast Reconstr Surg.* 2012;65:1390.

Boyd JB. *Plast Reconstr Surg.* 1995;95:1018.

Boyd JB. *Plast Reconstr Surg.* 2009;123:1641.

Bozikov K. *Ann Plast Surg.* 2009;63:138.

Bracka A. *Br J Urol.* 1995;76:31.

Bradley JP. *Plast Reconstr Surg.* 1999;103:351.

Bradley JP. *Plast Reconstr Surg.* 2006;118:1585.

Brain WR. *Lancet.* 1947;1:277.

Brauer JA. *Arch Dermatol.* 2012;148:820.

Braun M. *Can J Surg.* 1985;28:72.

Breidahl AF. *Br J Plast Surg.* 1996;49:46.

Breiting VB. *Plast Reconstr Surg.* 2004;114:217.

Breslow A. *Ann Surg.* 1970;172:902.

Breuninger H. *J Dermatol Surg Oncol.* 1991;17:574.

Brice G. *J Med Genet.* 2005;42:98.

British Association of Plastic, Reconstructive and Aesthetic Surgeons. *Standards for the management of open fractures of the lower limb.* 2009. Royal Society of Medicine Press.

Britto JA. *Br J Plast Surg.* 1998;51:343.

Broadland DG. *J Am Acad Dermatol.* 1992;27:241.

Brorson H. *Scand J Plast Reconstr Surg Hand Surg.* 1997;31:137.

Brouns F. *Eur J Surg Oncol.* 2003;29:440.

Broyles JM. *Plast Reconstr Surg.* 2012;129:874e.

Bryant H. *N Engl J Med.* 1995;332:1535.

Buckmiller LM. *Laryngoscope.* 2010;120:676.

Bull JP. *Ann Surg.* 1954;139:269.

Bulstrode NW. *Br J Plast Surg.* 2003;56:145.

Bulter T. *Eur J Clin Microbiol Infect Dis.* 2015;34:1271.

Burkhardt BR. *Plast Reconstr Surg.* 1995;96:1317–1325.

Burroughs JR. *Arch Facial Plast Surg.* 2006;8:36.

Burstein FD. *Ann Plast Surg.* 2000;44:188.

Byrd HS. *Plast Reconstr Surg.* 1989;76:159.

Byrd HS. *Plast Reconstr Surg.* 1996;97:928.

Byrd HS. *Plast Reconstr Surg.* 2000;106:1276.

Cacao FM. *Dermatol Surg.* 2009;35:629.

Calabrese L. *Acta Otorhinol Ital.* 2006;26:345.

Calder JS. *J Hand Surg Br.* 1998;23:147.

Calobrace MB. *Ann Plast Surg.* 1997;39:186.

Camilleri IG. *Br J Plast Surg.* 1998;51:181.

Campbell MJ. *Am J Surg.* 2010;199:636.

Campisi C. *World J Surg.* 2004;28:609.

Cannon CL. *Ann Plast Surg.* 2010;64:516.

Cantu G. *Oral Oncol.* 2006;42:619.

Caoutte-Laberge L. *Plast Reconstr Surg.* 2000;105:504.

Caprini JA. *Dis Mon.* 2005;51:70.

Cardenas-Camarena L. *Plast Reconstr Surg Glob Open.* 2017;5:e1539.

Carlson GW. *Plast Reconstr Surg.* 1996;97:460.

Carlson GW. *Ann Surg.* 1997;225:570.

Carr MM. *Microsurgery.* 1995;16:598.

Carta T. *Burns.* 2015;41:e11.

Casanova D. *Br J Plast Surg.* 2001;54:310.

Cascinelli N. *Lancet.* 1998;14:793.

Cascinelli N. *Sem Surg Oncol.* 1998;14:272.

Caterson SA. *J Reconstr Microsurg.* 2010;26:475.

Chakrabarti J. *Indian J Plast Surg.* 2009;42:36.

Chamorro M. *Br J Plast Surg.* 1993;46:426.

Champy M. *Zahn Mund Kieferheilkd Zentralbl.* 1975;63:339.

Chan YC. *J Am Acad Dermatol.* 2006;54:778.

Chana JS. *Br J Plast Surg.* 1997;50:456.

Chandawarkar RY. *Br J Plast Surg.* 2003;56:26.

Chang CS. *Plast Reconstr Surg.* 2014;134:511.

Chang JY. *Int J Radiat Oncol Bio Phys.* 2006;65:1087.

Chang LD. *J Reconstr Microsurg.* 1996;12:467.

Chang P. *J Burn Care Rehabil.* 1995;16:473.

Chang S. *Plast Reconstr Surg.* 2012;129:149.

Chao C. *Am J Surg.* 2002;184:520.

Chapman PB. *J Clin Oncol.* 1999;17:2745.

Chapman PB. *N Engl J Med.* 2011;364:2507.

Chaudhry AA, Baker KS, Gould ES, Gupta R. *Am J Roentgenol.* 2015;204:128.

Chen H. *Trauma.* 1997;43:486.

Chen HC. *Clin Plast Surg.* 2003;30:383.

Chen HC. *Burns.* 2009;35:857.

Cheng JC. *Clin Orthop Relat Res.* 1999;362:190.

Cheng MH. *Plast Reconstr Surg.* 2014;133:192e.

Chevray PM. *Plast Reconstr Surg.* 2004;114:1077.

Chin M. *Plast Reconstr Surg.* 1997;100:819.

Chin MS. *Plast Reconstr Surg Glob Open.* 2015;3:e591.

Chiu ES. *Plast Reconstr Surg.* 2003;112:628.

Chiu T. *World J Surg.* 2007;31:1941.

Chiu T. *Rhinology*. 2009;47:264.

Chiu T. *Surg Pract*. 2009;13:77.

Chiu T. *J Plast Reconstr Aesthet Surg*. 2013;66:1012.

Chiu TW. *Hong Kong Med J*. 2012;18:30.

Ch'ng S. *Hum Pathol*. 2008;39:344.

Choi JC. *Ophthal Plast Reconstr Surg*. 1997;13:259.

Chongchet V. *Br J Plast Surg*. 1963;16:268.

Choudhary S. *Plast Reconstr Surg*. 2003;111:576.

Chow SP. *J Hand Surg*. 1984;9:121.

Chummun S. *Br J Plast Surg*. 2001;54:476.

Chummun S. *Br J Plast Surg*. 2004;57:610.

Chummun S. *J Burn Care Res*. 2009;30:744.

Chummun S. *J Plast Reconstr Aesthet Surg*. 2010;63:2128.

Chung MH. *Ann Surg Oncol*. 2002;9:120.

Chung VQ. *Dermatol Surg*. 2006;32:193.

Chung YFA. *Brit J Surg*. 1999;86:661.

Cierny G. *Orthopedics*. 1984;7:1557.

Cioffi W. *J Trauma*. 1994;36:541.

Clark WH. *Cancer Res*. 1969;29:705.

Claro F Jr. *Br J Surg*. 2012;99:768.

Clary BM. *Ann Surg*. 2001;233:250.

Clay FS. *Am J Obstet Gynecol*. 2011;204:378.

Clough KB. *Ann Surg Oncol*. 2010;17:1375.

Coady MS. *Plast Reconstr Surg*. 1998;101:640.

Codner MA. *Plast Reconstr Surg*. 1995;96:1615.

Cody HS. *Ann Surg*. 1984;199:266.

Cohen MM Jr. *Am J Med Genet*. 1993;45:300.

Cohen MM Jr. *Sutural pathology*. In: Cohen MM Jr., MacLean RE, eds. *Craniosynostosis: Diagnosis, Evaluation, and Management*. New York: Oxford University Press; 2000b:95–99.

Cohen SR. *Plast Reconstr Surg*. 1991;87:1041.

Cohen T. *Am J Surg*. 2008;195:244.

Cohn BT. *Orthopedics*. 1986;9:124.

Cohn-Cedermark G. *Cancer*. 2000;89:1495.

Coleman DJ. *Br J Plast Surg*. 1991;44:444–448.

Coleman SR. *Plast Reconstr Surg*. 2007;119:775.

Collawn SS. *Plast Reconstr Surg*. 1998;102:509.

Collins J. *J Plast Reconstr Aesthet Surg*. 2012;65:864.

Collis N. *Br J Plast Surg*. 2005;58:286.

Colwell AS. *Plast Reconstr Surg*. 2004;113:1984.

Commons GW. *Aesthetic Plast Surg*. 2009;33:312.

Constantian MB. *Plast Reconstr Surg*. 1996;98:38.

Converse JM. *Proc R Soc Med*. 1942;53:811.

Converse JM. *Plast Reconstr Surg*. 1981;67:736.

Conway H. *Plast Reconstr Surg*. 1960;25:117.

Cook N. *Burns*. 1998;24:91.

Cordeiro P. *Head Neck*. 1994;16:112.

Cordeiro P. *Plast Reconstr Surg*. 1999;104:1314.

Cordeiro PG. *Plast Reconstr Surg*. 2002;110:1058.

Cordeiro PG. *Plast Reconstr Surg*. 2015;135:1509.

Cordova A. *J Plast Reconstr Aesthet Surg*. 2008;61:41.

Cosman B. *Plast Reconstr Surg*. 1961;27:225.

Cosman B. *Plast Reconstr Surg*. 1972;50:163.

Cosman B. *Clin Plast Surg*. 1978;5:389.

Cottle M. *Arch Otolaryngol*. 1960;72;11.

Cousley RR. *Br J Plast Surg*. 1997;50:536.

Crippa F. *J Nucl Med*. 2000;41:1491.

Cronin ED. *Plast Reconstr Surg*. 1988;81:783.

Cronin TD. *Am Surg*. 1951;17:419.

Crosby M. *Plast Reconstr Surg*. 2012;129:789e.

Cruz-Korchin N. *Plast Reconstr Surg*. 2003;112:1573.

Cucin RL. *CA Cancer J Clin*. 1981;31:281.

Culliford AT. *Ann Plast Surg*. 2007;59:18.

Cummings CW. *Ann Otol Rhinol Laryngol*. 1977;86:280.

Curreri PW. *J Trauma*. 1971;11:390.

Curtis RM. *J Bone Joint Surg Am*. 1973;55:733.

D'Andrea F. *Dermatol*. 200;204:60.

Damstra RJ. *Breast Cancer Res Treat*. 2009;113:199.

Dandurand M. *Eur J Dermatol*. 2010;16:394.

Dantzer E. *Br J Plastic Surg*. 2001;54:659.

Darzi MA. *Br J Plast Surg*. 1992;45:374.

Davis GM. *Plast Reconstr Surg*. 1995;96:1106.

Davis J. Reconstruction of the upper third of the ear with a chondrocutaneous composite flap based on the crus helix. In: Tanzer RC, Edgerton MT, eds. *Symposium on Reconstruction of the Auricle*. St. Louis: CV Mosby; 1974;24.

Day CL. *J Am Acad Dermatol*. 1993;28:281.

De Angelis B. *Int Wound J*. 2018 doi: 10.1111/iwj.12912.

De Benito J. *Aesth Plast Surg*. 2010;34:711.

De Boer M. *JAMA Oncol*. 2018;4:335.

De Bree R. *Head Neck*. 2007;29:773.

de Vooght A. *Plast Reconstr Surg*. 2003;112:1188.

de Vos RF. *JAMA*. 2010;303:144.

Deapen DM. *Plast Reconstr Surg*. 1992;89:660.

DeBaun MR. *Am J Hum Genet*. 2002;7:604.

DeCastro BJ. *J Urol*. 2008;179:1930.

DeFranzo AJ. *Plast Reconstr Surg*. 2001;108:1184.

Del Rosso JQ. *J Clin Aesthet Dermatol*. 2010;3:69.

Del Vecchio DA. *Plast Reconstr Surg*. 2012;130:1187.

Demling RH. *J Trauma*. 1980;20:242.

Demling RH. *J Burns Wounds*. 2005;4:e2.

Dean L. Allopurinol Therapy and HLA-B*58:01 Genotype. 2013 Mar 26 [Updated 2016 Mar 16]. In: Pratt V, McLeod H, Rubinstein W et al., editors. Medical Genetics Summaries [Internet]. Bethesda (MD): National Center for Biotechnology Information (US); 2012. Available from: https://www.ncbi.nlm.nih.gov/books/NBK127547/.

Denk MJ. *Cleft Palate Craniofacial J*. 1996;33:57.

Denkler K. *Plast Reconstr Surg*. 2001;108:114.

Desai MH. *Ann Surg*. 1990;211:753.

Desai MH. *J Burn Care Rehab*. 1991;12:540.

Devine JC. *Int J Oral Maxillofac Surg*. 2001;30:199.

Dewar DJ. *J Clin Oncol*. 2004;22:3345.

Dhepe NV. Scar reduction: principles and options. In: Lahiri K. (Ed). *Lasers in Dermatology*. New Dehli: Jaypee Brothers Medical Publishers Ltd; 2016.

Di Benedetto G. *Plast Reconstr Surg*. 1998;102:696.

Diao E. *J Hand Surg Am*. 1999;24:871.

Dierickx C. *Plast Reconstr Surg*. 1995;95:84.

Dinner M. *Ann Plast Surg*. 1983;11:362.

Disa JJ. *Plast Reconstr Surg*. 1998;101:979.

Donelan MB. *Plast Reconstr Surg*. 1995;95:1155.

Dorf DS. *Plast Reconstr Surg*. 1982;70:80.

Doting MH. *Eur J Surg Oncol*. 2002;28:673.

Doyle JR. Extensor tendons – acute injuries. In Green DP (Ed). *Operative Hand Surgery*, 3rd Edn. Churchill-Livingstone: New York, NY; 1993;2:1925.

Drosner M. *Med Laser Appl*. 2008;23:133.

Dublin BA. *Ann Plast Surg*. 1997;38:404–407.

Duckett JW. *Urol Clin N Am*. 1980;7:423.

Duckett JW. *Urol Clin N Am*. 1981;8:513.

Duffy SW. *J Med Screen*. 2010;17:25.

Duformentel C. *Ann Chir Plast*. 1965;10:227.

Dulguerov P. *Laryngoscope*. 1998;108:1692.

Dumville JC. *Cochrane Database Syst Rev*. 2013;CD010318.

Dunaway DJ. *Br J Plast Surg*. 1996;49:529.

Duymaz A. *Plast Reconstr Surg*. 2009;124:523.

Dziegielewski PT. *Oral Oncol*. 2010;46:612.

Earley MI. *Br J Plast Surg*. 1987;40:333.

Eastwood M. *Proc Inst Mech Eng H*. 1998;212:85.

Eaton RG. *J Bone Joint Surg*. 1973;55:1655.

Edsberg LE. *J Wound Ostomy Continence Nurs*. 2014;41:313.

Edwards-Jones V. *Burns*. 2003;29:15.

Egan CL et al. *J Am Acad Dermatol*. 1998;39:923.

Ehrlich HP. *Am J Pathol*. 1994;145:105.

Eilber FC. *Ann Surg*. 2003;237:218.

El Kollali R. *J Plast Reconstr Aesthet Surg*. 2009;62:1418.

Elder JS. *J Urol*. 1987;138:376.

Elliott LF. *Plast Reconstr Surg*. 1990;85:169.

Ellis E 3rd. *Oral Maxillofac Clin North Am*. 2009;21:163.

Emara TA. *Laryngoscope*. 2012;122:260.

Emmett AJJ. *Aust NZ J Surg*. 1981;51:576.

Erdmann D. *Br J Plast Surg*. 2002;55:675.

Erdmann MWH. *Br J Plast Surg*. 1997;50:421–427.

Erni D. *Br J Plast Surg*. 1999;52:167.

Esser JFS. *Dtsch Zschr Chir*. 1918;143:385.

Esser T. *Am J Obs Gynecol*. 2006;193:1743.

Evans DM. *Br J Plast Surg*. 1988;41:105.

Evans KC. *Int J Impot Res*. 2004;16:346.

Fabian TC. *Ann Surg*. 1994;219:643.

Faglia E. *Diabetes Care*. 1996;19;1338.

Failey CL. *Plast Reconstr Surg*. 2009;124:1304.

Fakhry C. *J Natl Cancer Inst*. 2008;100:261.

Falder S. *Br J Plast Surg*. 2003;56:571.

Fanning J. *Am J Obstet Gynecol*. 1999;180:24.

Farion KJ. *Cochrane Database Syst Rev*. 2002;CD003326.

Fattah A. *J Reconstr Aesthet Surg*. 2010;63:305–313.

Fazli M. *J Clin Microbiol*. 2009;47:4084.

Fearon JA. *Plast Reconstr Surg*. 1997;200:862.

Fehr B. *Dermatologica*. 1991;182:77.

Feldman KW. *Pediatrics*. 1983;71:145.

Fenig E. *Am J Clin Oncol*. 1999;22:184.

Fichtner J. *J Urol*. 1995;154:833.

Fichtner J. *J Urol*. 1995;172:1970.

Finley RK. *Surgery*. 1994;116:96.

Fiore M. *Ann Surg Oncol*. 2009;16:2587.

Fisher C. *Plast Reconstr Surg*. 2013;132:351.

Fisher DM. *Plast Reconstr Surg*. 2005;116:61.

Fitzgerald AM. *Br J Plast Surg*. 2000;53:690.

Fjortoft MI. *Neuroradiology*. 2007;49:515.

Flatt AE. Classification and incidence. In: Fatt AE, ed. *The Case of Congenital Hand Anomalies*. 2nd edn. St. Louis, Quality Medical Publishing Inc.; 1994;47.

Flatt AE. Cleft hand and central defects. In: *The Care of Congenital Hand Anomalies*. St. Louis: C. V. Mosby; 1977:265–285.

Flowers RS. *Aesth Plast Surg*. 1998;22:425.

Flugstad NA. *Aesthet Surg J*. 2016;36:550.

Fokin AA. *Chest Surg Clin N Am*. 2000;10:377.

Foroozan M. *Arch Dermatol*. 2012;148:1055.

Forslund O. *J Cutan Pathol*. 2003;30:423.

Foster RD. *Br J Plast Surg*. 1997;50:374–379.

Foucher G. *Plast Reconstr Surg*. 1979;63:344–349.

Foucher G. *J Hand Surg Am*. 1994;19:8.

Foustanos A. *Plast Reconstr Surg*. 2007;120:55.

Fraker DL. *Curr Treat Options Oncol*. 2004;5:173.

Francel TJ. *Plast Reconstr Surg*. 1992;89:478.

Friedman R. *Plast Reconstr Surg*. 1996;98:1242.

Friedman T. *Plast Reconstr Surg*. 2010;125:1525.

Fukano H. *Head Neck*. 1997;19:205.

Furlow LT. *Plast Reconstr Surg*. 1986;78:724.

Gabiani G. *Am J Pathol*. 1972;66:131.

Gabriel SE. *N Engl J Med*. 1994;330:1697.

Gaebler C. *J Trauma*. 1996;41:73.

Gandini S. *Int J Cancer*. 2008;122:155.

Garner WL. *J Burn Care Rehab*. 1993;14:458.

Gault DT. *Br J Plast Surg*. 1993;46:91.

Gear AJ. *J Oral Maxillofac Surg*. 2005;63:655.

Geissendorfer H. *Zentralbl Chir*. 1943;70:1107.

Gelberman RH. *J Bone Join Surg*. 1980;62:425.

Georgiannos SN. *Br J Plast Surg*. 2003;56:129.

Gerber B. *Ann Surg*. 2003;238:120.

Gerrand CH. *J Bone Joint Surg Br*. 2001;83:1149.

Gherardini G. *Microsurg*. 1998;18:90.

Gherardini G. *Plast Reconstr Surg*. 1998;102:473.

Giele H. *J Hand Surg Br*. 2002;27:157.

Gilbert A. *Plast Reconstr Surg*. 1982;69:601.

Gill PS. *Plast Reconstr Surg*. 2004;113:1153.

Gillies H. *J Roy Soc Med.* 1934;27:1382.

Gimbel MI. *Cancer Control.* 2008;15:225.

Gir P. *Plast Reconstr Surg.* 2012;130:249–258.

Godina M. *Plast Reconstr Surg.* 1986;78:285.

Godina M. *Plast Reconstr Surg.* 1991;78:28.

Goebel A. *Ann Intern Med.* 2010;152:152.

Goedkoop AY. *Eur J Plast Surg.* 2000;23:185.

Goes JCS. *Aesthet Surg J.* 2003;23:129.

Gold MH. *Am J Clin Dermatol.* 2003;4:467.

Goldstein EA. *J Speech Lang Hear Res.* 2007;50:335.

Gonzalez MH. *Plast Reconstr Surg.* 2002;109:592.

Gorgu M. *Eur J Plast Surg.* 2011;34:65.

Gosselin S. *Clin Toxicol* (Phila). 2016;54:899.

Graf R. *Aesth Plast Surg.* 2000;24:348.

Grant MP. *Clin Plast Surg.* 1997;24:539.

Grazer FM. *Plast Reconstr Surg.* 1977;59:513.

Green AC. *J Clin Oncol.* 2011;29:257.

Greuse M. *J Hand Surg Am.* 2001;26:589.

Griffiths RW. *Br J Plast Surg.* 1999;52:24.

Grobe A. *Int J Oral Maxillofac Surg.* 2011;40:685.

Grotting JC. *Ann Plast Surg.* 1991;27:351.

Grover R. *Burns.* 1996;22:627.

Grover R. *Br J Plast Surg.* 1998;51:51.

Grover R. *Br J Plast Surg.* 2001;54:481.

Grufferman S. *Cancer Causes Control.* 1993;4:217.

Gude W. *Curr Rev Musculoskelet Med.* 2008;1:205.

Gudi VS. *Br J Plastic Surg.* 2000;53:440.

Gudmundsson KG. *Scand J Prim Health Care.* 2001;19:186.

Gulec SA. *Nucl Med.* 2003;28:961.

Gulleth Y. *Plast Reconstr Surg.* 2010;126:1222.

Gunnarsson LG. *J Hand Surg.* 1997;22:34.

Gupta S. *Int J Dermatol.* 2001;40:349.

Gupta V. *Aesthet Surg J.* 2015;36:1.

Gustilo RB. *J Bone Joint Surg Am.* 1976;58:453.

Gustilo RB. *J Bone Joint Surg Am.* 1990;72:299.

Gutierrez JC. *Ann Surg.* 2007;245:952.

Gutowski KA. *Plast Reconstr Surg.* 2009;124:272.

Gylbert L. *Plast Reconstr Surg.* 1990;86:260.

Haddadin KJ. *Br J Plast Surg.* 2000;53:279.

Hakelius L. *Plast Reconstr Surg.* 1997;100:1566–1569.

Hall-Findlay E. *Plast Reconstr Surg.* 1999;104:748.

Hall-Findlay EJ. *Clin Plastic Surg.* 2002;29:379.

Haller JA Jr. *Ann Thorac Surg.* 1996;61:1618.

Hallock GG. *Plast Reconstr Surg.* 2003;111:855.

Hammond DC. *Plast Reconstr Surg.* 1999;103:890.

Hammond DC. *Plast Reconstr Surg.* 2012;129:1381.

Han HH. *Scientific World Journal.* 2014;482702.

Han S. *Plast Reconstr Surg.* 1999;104:389.

Han ZF. *Int J Surg.* 2016;32:109.

Handley JM. *J Am Acad Dermatol.* 2006;55:482.

Handoll HHG. *Cochrane Database Syst Rev.* 2004;3:CD004574.

Hansbrough JF. *Crit Care Med.* 1996;24:1366.

Har-Shai Y. *Plast Reconstr Surg.* 2003;111:1841.

Harlan JW. *Plast Reconstr Surg.* 2002;109:710. Change year

Harrah J. *Am J Surg.* 2000;180:55.

Harriger MD. *Transplantation.* 1995;15:702.

Harris I. *Injury.* 1993;24:565.

Hart DW. *Surgery.* 2001;130:396.

Hartrampf CR. *Plast Reconstr Surg.* 1982;69:216.

Hartrampf CR. *Plast Reconstr Surg.* 1985;76:563.

Hashim P. *Plast Reconstr Surg.* 2014;134:491.

Hatef DA. *Aesthet Surg J.* 2009;29:122.

Havenga K. *Eur J Surg Oncol.* 2003;29:662.

Hayes AJ. *Br J Surg.* 2004;91:673.

Hayes AJ. *Lancet Oncol.* 2016;17:184.

Haywood RM. *Br J Plast Surg.* 2003;56:689.

Hedelund L. *Lasers Med Sci.* 2010;25:749.

Heimbach D. *J Trauma Acute Care Trauma.* 1984;24:373.

Heinrichs HL. *Plast Reconstr Surg.* 1998;102:843.

Heliovaara A. *J Plast Surg Hand Surg.* 2017;51:52.

Hennekens CH. *JAMA.* 1996;275:616.

Henriksson TG. *Scand J Plast Reconstr Surg Hand Surg.* 2005;39:295.

Henry SL. *Plast Reconstr Surg.* 2008;122:1095.

Henry SL. *Plast Reconstr Surg.* 2010;125:210e.

Hensle TW. *J Urol.* 2002;168:1734.

Hernandez TL. *Obesity.* 2011;19:1388.

Herndon DN. *Ann Surg.* 1989;209:547.

Herndon DN, Tompkins RG. *Lancet.* 2004;363:1895.

Hester TR. *Plast Reconstr Surg.* 1982;69:226.

Hester TR. *Plast Reconstr Surg.* 1997;100:1291.

Hettiaratchy S. *Plast Reconstr Surg.* 2003;112:692.

Heywood AJ. *Br J Plast Surg.* 1991;44:183.

Hicks WL. *Head Neck.* 1997;19:400.

Hidalgo DA. *Plast Reconstr Surg.* 2005;115:1179.

Higgins TF. *Orthop Clin North Am.* 2010;41:233.

Higuera S. *J Plast Aesthet Surg.* 2009;62:1564.

Hildreth MA. *J Burn Care Rehabil.* 1990;11:405.

Hivelin M. *J Plast Reconstr Aesthet Surg.* 2012;65:1103.

Ho WS. *Dermatol Surg.* 2006;32:891.

Hodi FS. *N Engl J Med.* 2010;363:711.

Hodi FS. *J Clin Oncol.* 2013;31:3182.

Hodgson NC. *Am J Clin Oncol.* 2007;30:570.

Hoffman GL. *J Hand Eur Vol.* 2008;33:418.

Hogsberg T. *PLoS One.* 2011;6:e20492.

Holm A. *Acta Ortho Scand.* 1974;45:382.

Holm C. *Plast Reconstr Surg.* 2006;117:37.

Holstrom H. *Scand J Plast Reconstr Surg.* 1979;13:423.

Hong JP. *Plast Reconstr Surg.* 2004;113:1264.

Hong WK. *N Engl J Med.* 1990;323:795.

Honig JF. *Aesth Plast Surg.* 2009;33:302.

Howard BK. *Plast Reconstr Surg.* 1999;103:984.

Hsieh CH. *Plast Reconstr Surg.* 2004;113:1355.

Hsu TH. *J Cosmet Laser Ther.* 2017;19:275.

Hu Z. *Br J Surg.* 2017;104:836.

Huang AB. *J Comput Assist Tomogr*. 1998;22:437.
Huang C. *Wound Repair Regen*. 2014;22:462.
Huang JL. *Ann Plast Surg*. 1999;42:658.
Huang PP. *Ann Surg*. 1995;221:543.
Hudson DA. *Plast Reconstr Surg*. 1999;104:401.
Hudson DA. *Plast Reconstr Surg*. 2000;106:665.
Hueston JT. *Plast Reconstr Surg*. 1963;31:66.
Hueston JT. *Plast Reconstr Surg*. 1966;37:349.
Hughes KC. *Plast Reconstr Surg*. 1997;100:1146.
Hughes TM. *Br J Surg*. 2000;87:892.
Huikeshoven M. *N Engl J Med*. 2007;356:1235.
Hung TH. *Singapore Med J*. 2014;55:378.
Hunstad JP. *Ann Plast Surg*. 2011;67:423.
Hunt JA. *Plast Reconstr Surg*. 2003;112:606.
Hurteau JE. *Plast Reconstr Surg*. 1981;68:539.
Hurwitz DJ. *Plast Reconstr Surg*. 1981;68:521.
Hussain G. *Br J Plast Surg*. 2004;57:502.
Hussein R. *Ann R Coll Surg Engl*. 2005;87:171.
Hyakusoku H. *Plast Reconstr Surg*. 2009;123:360.
Hyldig N. *Brit J Surg*. 2016;103:477.
Hynes W. *Br J Plast Surg*. 1951;3:128.
Hyun SS. *Diabetes Metab Res Rev*. 2016;32:275.
Ibrahim AE. *Semin Plast Surg*. 2014;28:26.
Ibrahim I. *Ortop Traumatol Rehabil*. 2012;14:429.
Illouz GY. *Aesthet Plast Surg*. 2009;33:706.
Ingram JM. *Am J Obstet Gynecol*. 1981;140:867.
Inigo F. *Br J Plast Surg*. 1994;47:312.
Inigo F. *Br J Plast Surg*. 1996;49:452.
Iraniha S. *J Burn Care Rehab*. 2000;21:333.
Iseli TA. *Laryngoscope*. 2008;118:1781.
Iselin F. *J Hand Surg Am*. 1977;2:118.
Ishii H. *Plast Surg*. 2014;22:171.
Ishikawa S. *Ann Plast Surg*. 1988;20:485.
Iuchi M. *Burns*. 2009;35:288.
Jackson DMG. *Br J Surg*. 1953;40:588.
Jackson IT. *Ann Plast Surg*. 1983;11:533.
Jackson IT. *Clin Plast Surg*. 1985;12:711.
Jahss S. *J Bone Joint Surg*. 1938;20:178.
Jain A. *Laryngoscope*. 2015;125:1624.
Jakubietz MG. *Plast Reconstr Surg*. 2004;113:117e.
Jakubietz RG. *Microsurgery*. 2009;29:672.
James JIP. *Acta Ortho Scand*. 1962;32:407.
Janku F. *J Clin Oncol*. 2010;28:e15.
Jansen DA. *Plast Reconstr Surg*. 1998;101:361.
Jaqueti G. *Am J Dermatopathol*. 2000;22:108.
Jasim ZF. *J Am Acad Derm*. 2007;57:677.
Jelks GW. *Plast Reconstr Surg*. 1997;100:1262.
Jenkins SD. *Surgery*. 1983;94:392.
Jennings MB. *J Am Podiatr Med Assoc*. 2006;96:465.
Jeschke MG. *EBioMedicine*. 2015;2:1536.
Jewll M. *Plast Reconstr Surg*. 2011;127:253.
Jin Z. *J Androl*. 2011;32:491.
Johanssen K. *J Trauma*. 1990;30:568.

Jones BM. *Plast Reconstr Surg*. 2004;113:1242.
Jones NF. *Plast Reconstr Surg*. 1992;89:500.
Jorgensen B. *Int Wound J*. 2005;1:64.
Joss SK. *Am J Med Genet*. 2002;113:105.
Jull AB. *Cochrane Database Syst Rev*. 2012;CD005083.
    note spelling
Juma A. *Burns*. 1994;20:363.
Jyranki J. *Ann Plast Surg*. 2006;56:387.
Kaguraoka H. *J Thorac Cardiovasc Surg*. 1992;104:1483.
Kallen K. *Teratology*. 2002;66:185.
Kamer FM. *Laryngoscope*. 1984;94:391.
Kamolz LP. *Ann Burns Fire Disasters*. 2013;26:26.
Kandamany N. *Lasers Med Sci*. 2009;24:411.
Kang HC. *Radiat Oncol J*. 2014;32:156.
Kapetansky DI. *Plast Reconstr Surg*. 1971;47:321.
Kaplan EN. *Cleft Palate J*. 1975;12:356.
Kapp-Simon KA. *Cleft Palate Craniofac J*. 1998;35:197.
Karanas YL. *Plast Reconstr Surg*. 2003;111:1078.
Karsten A. *J Plast Surg Hand Surg*. 2017;51:58.
Katsaros J. *Br J Plast Surg*. 1985;38:220.
Kavanagh GM. *Br J Dermatol*. 2004;151:1093.
Kay AR. *Br J Plast Surg*. 1998;51:22.
Kay SP. *Br J Plast Surg*. 1998;51:43.
Kelahmetoglu O. *Plast Reconstr Surg*. 2015;136:440.
Keogh IJ. *Arch Otolaryngol Head Neck Surg*. 2007;133:997.
Kerrigan CL. *Plast Reconstr Surg*. 2013;132:1670.
Khan UD. *Aesth Plast Surg*. 2007;31:337.
Khayat D. *Cancer*. 2003;97:1941.
Khouri RK. *Plast Reconstr Surg*. 1992;89:495.
Khouri RK. *Plast Reconstr Surg*. 2012;129:1173.
Kim DY. *Ann Plast Surg*. 2003;51:636.
Kim DY. *Plast Reconstr Surg*. 2004;113:1668.
Kim IH. *Aesthet Surg J*. 2009;29:35.
Kim MR. *J Oral Maxillofac Surg*. 1992;50:1152.
Kim PJ. *Plast Reconstr Surg*. 2013;132:1569.
Kim PJ. *Plast Reconstr Surg*. 2015;136:657e.
Kim S. *Plast Reconstr Surg*. 2013;132:1580.
Kim YS. *J Plast Reconstr Aesthet Surg*. 2009;62:1347.
Kimata Y. *Clin Plast Surg*. 2003;30:433.
Kimball AB. *JEADV*. 2016;30:989.
Kimonis VE. *Am J Med Genet*. 1997;69:299.
Kind GM. *Clin Plast Surg*. Apr 2002;29:233.
King P. *Burns*. 2000;26:501.
Kinney BM. *Plast Reconstr Surg*. 1999;103:728.
Kinninmonth AW. *J Hand Surg Br*. 1986;11:261.
Kinsler VA. *Br J Dermatol*. 2009;160:143.
Kirschner RE. Speech outcome after cleft palte repair in
    patients with a chromosome 22q11 deletion. Presented
    at the *58th Annual Meeting of the American Cleft Palate-
    Craniofacial Association*, Minneapolis; 2001.
Kishi K. *Br J Dermatol*. 2009;161:345.
Kishi K. *Arch Facial Plast Surg*. 2012;14:116.
Kishore V. *Biomaterials*. 2012;33:2137.

Kjoller K. *Pediatrics*. 1998;102:1112.

Klein JA. *Dermatol Clin*. 1990;8:425.

Klein S. *N Engl J Med*. 2004;350:2549.

Knight SJ. *Developm Neuropsychol*. 2014;39:159.

Kohout MP. *Plast Reconstr Surg*. 1998;102:643.

Kohr D. *Pain*. 2009;143:246.

Kolde G. *Lancet*. 2003;9354:348.

Kolker AR. *Ann Plast Surg*. 2009;62:549.

Komanduri M. *J Hand Surg Am*. 1996;21:605.

Komorowska-Timek E. *Plast Reconstr Surg*. 2017;139:1e.

Kono T. *Br J Plast Surg*. 2001;54:640.

Kono T. *Ann Plast Surg*. 2005;54:487.

Koot VCM. *Br Med J*. 2003;326:527.

Koshima I. *Ann Plast Surg*. 1994;32:321.

Koshima I. *J Reconstr Microsurg*. 2003;19:209.

Koshima I. *Ann Plast Surg*. 2004;53:261.

Koshima I. *Plast Reconstr Surg*. 2006;118:1579.

Koulaxouzidis G. *J Plast Reconstr Aesthet Surg*. 2015;68:1262.

Kovalic JJ. *Int J Radiat Oncol Biol Phys*. 1989;17:77.

Kozin SH. *Plast Reconstr Surg*. 2015;136:241e.

Kraemer KH. *Arch Dermatol*. 1987;123:241.

Krag DN. *Surg Oncol*. 1993;2:335.

Kramer C. *Med Klin Intensivmed Notfmed*. 2016;111:708.

Kranke P. *Cochrane Database Syst Rev*. 2015;6:CD004123.

Kreis RW. *Burns*. 1993;19:142.

Kretschmer L. *Acta Oncol*. 2001;40:72.

Kretschmer L. *Melanoma Res*. 2002;12:499.

Kretschmer L. *Melanoma Res*. 2008;18:16.

Kriens OB. *Plast Reconstr Surg*. 1969;43:29.

Kroll SS. *Plast Reconstr Surg*. 1989;84:520.

Kroll SS. *Surg Gynecol Obstet*. 1991;172:17.

Kroll SS. *Br J Plast Surg*. 1998;51:503.

Kronowitz SJ. *Plast Reconstr Surg*. 2010;125:463.

Kua EH. *J Plast Reconstr Aesthet Surg*. 2011;64:e21.

Kumar P. *Br J Plast Surg*. 2002;55:616.

Kumar PA. *Br J Plast Surg*. 1995;48:83.

Kumar SP. *Indian J Palliat Care*. 2013;19:170.

Kuran I. *Plast Reconstr Surg*. 2000;105:574.

Kuriakose MA. *Curr Opin Otolaryngol Head Neck Surg*. 2009;17:100.

Kutler W. *J Am Med Assoc*. 1947;133:29.

Kwan P. *J Burn Care Res*. 2006;27:826.

Kwon DR. *Clin Rehab*. 2014;28:983.

Labbe D. *Plast Reconstr Surg*. 2000;105:1289.

Lai CS. *Ann Plast Surg*. 1989;22:495.

Lai CS. *Br J Plast Surg*. 1991;44:165.

Laitung JK. *Br J Plast Surg*. 1985;38:375.

Lalonde D. *J Hand Surg Am*. 2005;30:1061.

Lalonde D. *J Am Acad Orthop Surg*. 2013;21:443.

Lalonde DH. *Plast Reconstr Surg*. 2011;127:885.

Lam TK. *Melanoma Res*. 2009;19:94.

Lamberty BG. *Br J Plast Surg*. 1979;32:207.

Lane JE. *Pediatrics*. 2005;115:1312.

Langer I. *Ann Surg*. 2007;245:452.

Lantieri LA. *Plast Reconstr Surg*. 1998;101:392.

Lanz U. *J Hand Surg*. 1977;2:44.

Lassus C. *Plast Reconstr Surg*. 1996;97:373–380.

Lassus C. *Plast Reconstr Surg*. 2003;111:2200.

Laughlin RT. *J Orthop Trauma*. 1993;7:123.

Law NW. *Acta Chir Scand*. 1990;156:759.

Lawley LP. *J Eur Acad Dermatol Venereol*. 2010;27:320.

Lawrence WT. *Ann Plast Surg*. 1991;27:164.

Layland MK. *Laryngoscope*. 2005;115:629.

Lazar AJF. *Am J Path*. 2008;173:1518.

Lazzarini J. *Bone Joint Surg Am*. 2004;86:2305.

Leaute-Labreze C. *N Engl J Med*. 2008;358:2649.

Leckenby JI. *J Plast Reconstr Aesthet Surg*. 2012;68:603.

Lee AB. *Surgery*. 1976;80:433.

Lee DK. *J Foot Ankle Surg*. 2008;47:8.

Lee JT. *J Plast Reconstr Aesthet Surg*. 2007;60:1060.

Lee JY. *Am J Dermatopathol*. 2004;26:379.

Lee SJ. *J Cosmet Laser Ther*. 2013;15:255.

Lefaivre JF. *Plast Reconstr Surg*. 1997;99:629.

Leiter U. *Lancet Oncol*. 2016;17:757.

Lejour M. *Ann Chir Plast Esthet*. 1990;35:369.

Lejour M. *Plast Reconstr Surg*. 1994;94:100–114.

Lesseva MI. *Burns*. 1996;22:279.

Levin LA. *Ophthalmology*. 1999;106:1268.

Levine JJ. *JAMA*. 1994;271:240.

Lewis T. *J Athl Train*. 2014;49:422.

Li WL. *Tumor Biol*. 2014;35:7847.

Li YC. *Clin Exp Ophthalmol*. 2010;38:554.

Lille ST. *J Paediatr Surg*. 1996;31:1648.

Lim HY. *J Korean Assoc Oral Maxillofac Surg*. 2014;40:285.

Lin CH. *Plast Reconstr Surg*. 2009;123:1265.

Lin PY. *Microsurgery*. 2012;32:189.

Lin SJ. *Plast Reconstr Surg*. 2010;125:1146.

Lindner P. *Ann Surg Oncol*. 2002;9:127.

Lingam LK. *Br J Surg*. 1995;82:1343.

Lipworth L. *Ann Plast Surg*. 2007;59:119.

Lister G. *Emergency free flaps*. In Green DP (Ed.). *Operative Hand Surgery*, 2nd edn. Churchill Livingstone; 1988;1127.

Little JW. *Plast Reconstr Surg*. 1999;104:396.

Loch-Wilkinson A. *Plast Reconstr Surg*. 2017;140;645.

Lockwood TE. *Plast Reconstr Surg*. 1991;87:1009.

Lodi G. *Cochrane Database Syst Rev*. 2016; CD001829. update; Cochrane review (2016) found the vitamin A, beta carotene or bleomycin were not effective in preventing oral cancer in patients with leukoplakia.

Lohmander A. *J Plast Surg Hand Surg*. 2017;51:27.

Longaker MT. *Plast Reconstr Surg*. 1995;96:800.

Longhi P. *Onco Targets Ther*. 2008;1:1.

Lopez-Gutierrez JC. *Lymphat Res Biol*. 2012;10:164.

Lorenz HP. *Development*. 1992;114:253.

Losee J. *Plast Reconstr Surg.* 2000;106:1004.

Loth TS. *J Hand Surg Am.* 1986;11:388.

Luijendijk RW. *N Engl J Med.* 2000;343:392.

Lycka BAS. *Int J Dermatol.* 1989;28:531.

MacKinnon SE. *Plast Reconstr Surg.* 2000;107:1419.

Mackie RM. *Clin Exp Dermat.* 1991;16:151.

Madduri S. *J Control Release.* 2012;161:274.

Magnusson MB. *Eur J Vasc Endovasc Surg.* 2001;21:353.

Maguire S. *Burns.* 2008;34:1072.

Mahdavi-Mazdeh M. *Int J Organ Transplant Med.* 2013;4:72.

Mahmood U. *Arch Otolaryngol Head Neck Surg.* 2011;137:1025.

Malata CM. *Br J Plast Surg.* 1997;50:99.

Malata CM. *Br J Plast Surg.* 1997;50:600.

Malhotra AK. *Dermatology.* 2007;215:63.

Man LX. *Plast Reconstr Surg.* 2009;124:752.

Manders EK. *Plast Reconstr Surg.* 1988;81:208.

Mandrekas AD. *Plast Reconstr Surg.* 2003;112:1099–1108.

Manjulabai M. *Indian J Appl Res.* 2015;5:600.

Manske PR. *Plast Reconstr Surg.* 1993;91:196.

Manuskiatti W. *J Am Acad Dermatol.* 2010;63:274.

Marchac D. *Br J Plast Surg.* 1994;47:211.

Marchac D. *Plast Reconstr Surg.* 1995;95:802.

Margolis DJ. *Diabetes Care.* 2013;36:1961.

Marks R. *Lancet.* 1988;1:795.

Marrinam EM. *Cleft Palate Craniofac J.* 1998;35:95.

Marsden JR. *Br J Derm.* 2010;163:238.

Martin D. *Plast Reconstr Surg.* 1993;92:867.

Marvin R. *Am J Surg.* 2000;179:7.

Mathangi Ramakrishnan K. *Plast Reconstr Surg.* 1974;53:276.

Mathes SJ. *Clinical Atlas of Muscle and Musculocutaneous Flaps.* St. Louis: Mosby; 1979:91.

Mathieu D. *J Chir.* 1932;39:481.

Matsuo K. *Clin Plast Surg.* 1990;17:383.

Matthews MS. *Plast Reconstr Surg.* 1998;101:1.

Maubec E. *Melanoma Res.* 2007;17:147.

Mavili ME. *Plast Reconstr Surg.* 2000;106:393.

McCarthy JG. *Plast Reconstr Surg.* 1992;89:1.

McComb H. *Plast Reconstr Surg.* 1985;75:791.

McComb H. *Plast Reconstr Surg.* 1990;86:882.

McCord CD Jr. Lower lid blepharoplasty. In McCord CD Jr (ed). *Eyelid Surgery: Principles and Techniques.* Philadelphia: Lippincott-Raven; 1995;196.

McCulley SJ. *Br J Plast Surg.* 2005;58:889.

McGeorge DD. *Br J Plast Surg.* 1993;47:46.

McGregor AD. *Head Neck.* 1988;10:294.

McGregor IA. *Plast Reconstr Surg.* 1972;49:41.

Mcheik JN. *Plast Reconstr Surg Glob Open.* 2014;2:e218.

McInnes E. *Cochrane Database Syst Rev.* 2015;9:CD001735.

McKenna JK. *Dermatol Surg.* 2006;32:493.

McKenney MG. *Am J Surg.* 1996;171:275.

McKinney P. *Plast Recontr Surg.* 1996;98:795.

McKissock PK. *Plast Reconstr Surg.* 1972;49:245.

McLaughlin CR. *Br J Plast Surg.* 1954;7:274.

McLean DH. *Plast Reconstr Surg.* 1972;49:268.

McMasters KM. *J Clin Oncol.* 2001;19:2851.

McQueen MM. *J Bone Joint Surg Br.* 1996;78:99.

McQueen MM. *J Bone Joint Surg Br.* 2000;82:200.

Mehendale FV. *Cleft Palate Craniofacial J.* 2004;41:368.

Mehrara BJ. *Plast Reconstr Surg.* 1998;102:1805.

Meir DB. *J Urol.* 2004;171:2621.

Meier S. *Onkologie.* 2004;27:145.

Mellor RH. *Microcirculation.* 2010;17:281.

Mendelson B. *Aesthetic Plast Surg.* 2012;36:753.

Mennen U, Wise A. *J Hand Surg.* 1993;18B:416.

Menz P. *Plast Reconstr Surg.* 1996;98:377.

Messeguer F. *Actas Dermosifiliogr.* 2013;104:53.

Messina A. *Plast Reconstr Surg.* 1993;92:84.

Meyer M. *Br J Plast Surg.* 1991;44:291.

Micheals BM. *Plast Reconstr Surg.* 1997;99:437.

Michel JL. *Eur J Dermatol.* 2003;13:57.

Michelet FX. *J Oral Maxillofac Surg.* 1973:1:79

Mihara K. *Burns.* 2012;148:E1.

Miles BA. *J Oral Maxillofac Surg.* 2006;64:576.

Millard DR. *Plast Reconstr Surg.* 1960;25:595.

Millard DR. *Plast Reconstr Surg.* 1971;37:324.

Miller AP. *Plast Reconstr Surg.* 1995;95:77.

Miller AS. *Plast Reconstr Surg.* 1998;102:2299.

Millers JA. *Ann Thorac Surg.* 1984;38:227.

Milroy WF. *NY State J Med.* 1892;56:505.

Mir L. *Plast Reconstr Surg.* 1973;52:625.

Mitra A. *Plast Reconstr Surg.* 2004;113:206.

Mladick RA. *Plast Reconstr Surg.* 1971;48:219.

Moazzam A. *Br J Plast Surg.* 2003;56:695.

Modi S. *Indian J Med Microbiol.* 2014;32:137.

Moehrle M. *Dermatol Surg.* 2003;29:366.

Moffat CJ. *QJM.* 2004;97:431.

Moloney D. *Br J Plast Surg.* 1996;49:409.

Molsted K. *J Plast Surg Hand Surg.* 2017;51:64.

Momeni A. *Ann Plast Surg.* 2008;60:343.

Monafo WW. *J Trauma.* 1970;10:575.

Monteiro JA. *Eur J Int Med.* 1995;6:209.

Moon HK. *Plast Reconstr Surg.* 1998;82:815.

Moritz AR. *Am J Pathol.* 1947;23:695.

Morton DL. *Arch Surg.* 1992;127:392.

Morton DL. *Ann Surg.* 2003;238:538.

Morton DL. *Br J Dermatol.* 2004;151:308.

Morton DL. *N Engl J Med.* 2006;355:1307.

Morton DL. *N Engl J Med.* 2014;370:599.

Motamed S. *Br J Plast Surg.* 2003;56:829.

Motley R. *Br J Plast Surg.* 2003;56:85.

Moustoukas M. *Plast Reconstr Surg.* 2012;129:585e.

Movassaghi K. *Aesthet Surg J.* 2006;26:687.

Muir TM. *Clin Radiol.* 2010;65:198.

Mulhall JP. *J Urol.* 2006;175:2115.

Muneuchi G. *Ann Plast Surg.* 2005;54:604.

Munir A. *Ann Plast Surg.* 2006;57:374.

Muramatsu K. *Br J Plast Surg.* 2004;57:550.

Mureau MA. *J Urol.* 1996;155:703.

Murrell GAC. *J Hand Surg.* 1991;16:263.

Murthy J. *Indian J Plast Surg.* 2009;42:116.

Mustardé JC. *Plast Reconstr Surg.* 1967;39:382.

Mustoe T. *Aesthet Plast Surg.* 2008;32:82.

Mustoe TA. *Plast Reconstr Surg.* 2002;110:560.

Myckatyn TM. *Plast Reconstr Surg.* 2017;139:11.

Nahabedian MY. *Plast Reconstr Surg.* 2005;115:436.

Nahabedian MY. *Plast Reconstr Surg.* 2002;110:466.

Nahas FX. *Aesth Plast Surg.* 2002;26:284.

Nahhas AF. *J Clin Aesthet Dermatol.* 2017;10:37.

Nakajima T. *Br J Plast Surg.* 1996;49:178.

Nakayama B. *Plast Reconstr Surg.* 2006;117:1980.

Namiki T. *Case Rep Dermatol.* 2016;8:75.

Narahari R. *Cochrane Database Syst Rev.* 2008;1: CD006934.

Narayanan K. *Injury.* 1996;27:449.

Nasr A. *J Ped Surg.* 2010;45:880.

Nasser M. *Cochrance Database Syst Rev.* 2008;CD006703.

Nassif PF. *IX International Facial Nerve Symposium.* 2009, Rome, Italy.

Neovius EB. *Head Neck.* 1997;19:315.

Neri I. *Pediatr Dermatol.* 2017;35:11117.

Netscher DT. *Plast Reconstr Surg.* 2000;105:1628.

Neumann CG. *Plast Reconstr Surg.* 1957;19:124.

Neumuller J. *Clin Immunol Immunopathol.* 1994;71:142.

Ngan PG. *Ann Plast Surg.* 2009;63:135–137.

Ninkovic M. *Br J Plast Surg.* 1995;48:533–539.

Ninkovic M. *Plast Reconstr Surg.* 1998;101:971.

Norgaard M. *Urology.* 2009;74:583.

Nyren O. *Br Med J.* 1998;316:417.

Obagi ZE. *Dermatol Surg.* 1999;25:773.

Ogawa R. *Plast Reconstr Surg.* 2003;111:547.

Ogawa R. *Ann Plast Surg.* 2007;59:688.

Ogawa R. *Plast Reconstr Surg.* 2009;62:660.

Oh TS. *J Plast Reconstr Aesthet Surg.* 2013;66:243.

Ohshiro T. *Laser Ther.* 2016;25:99.

Oishi SN. *Plast Reconstr Surg.* 2002;109:1293.

Ongodia D. *J Maxillofac Oral Surg.* 2014;13:99.

Ono I. *Burns.* 1995;21:352.

Ono I. *Br J Plast Surg.* 1996;49:564.

Orlando R. *Br J Clin Pharmacol.* 2003;55:86.

Orr DJA. *Br J Plast Surg.* 1997;50:153.

Ortega VG. *J Craniofac Surg.* 2015;26:e507.

Orticochea M. *Plast Reconstr Surg.* 1968;41:323.

Osler T. *J Trauma.* 2010;68:690.

Ostad A. *Dermatol Surg.* 1996;22:921.

O'Brien BM. *Plast Reconstr Surg.* 1990;85:562.

O'Toole G. *Burns.* 1998;24:562.

Ovens L. *Eur J Plast Surg.* 2009;32:177.

Owsley JQ. *Plast Reconstr Surg.* 1996;98:1.

Ozmen S. *Aesth Plast Surg.* 2001;25:432.

Ozog DM. *Arch Dermatol.* 2011;147:1108.

Pabari A. *Tech Hand Surg.* 2011;15:75.

Pacifico MD. *J Plast Reconstr Aesthetic Surg.* 2007;60:455–464.

Padua L. *Clin Neurophysiol.* 2000;111:1203.

Paige KT. *Plast Reconstr Surg.* 1998;101:1819.

Pajkos A. *Plast Reconstr Surg.* 2003;111:1605.

Palao R. *Br J Plastic Surg.* 2003;56:252.

Pallua N. *Plast Reconstr Surg.* 2003;111:1860–1870.

Pallua N. *Plast Reconstr Surg.* 2005;115:1837.

Palmer KT. *Best Pract Res Clin Rheumatol.* 2011;25:15.

Palmieri B. *Breast Cancer Res Treat.* 2005;91:283.

Pan SC. *Burns Trauma.* 2013;1:27. Year

Panchapakesan V. *Aesth Plast Surg.* 2009;33:49–53.

Pandya AN. *Br J Plast Surg.* 2002;55:302.

Panje WR. *Otolaryngol Clin North Am.* 1982;15:169.

Pannucci CJ. *J Am Col Surg.* 2011;212:105.

Papazian MR. *J Oral Maxillofac Surg.* 1991;49:1059.

Pape SA. *Burns.* 2001;27:233.

Pappas DC. *Ear Nose Throat J.* 1998;77:914.

Paradisi A. *Cancer Treat Rev.* 2008;34:728.

Park C. *Plast Reconstr Surg.* 2018;3:713.

Parker TL. *J Am Acad Dermatol.* 1995;32:233.

Parkhouse N. *Br J Plast Surg.* 1985;38:306.

Parrett BM. *Burns.* 2010;36:443.

Pasyk KA. *Clin Plast Surg.* 1987;14:435.

Patel ND. *Am J Neuroradiol.* 2011;32:1703.

Patrizi A. *J Clin Pharmacol.* 2009;49:872.

Paulowski BR. *Head Neck.* 2004;26:625.

Peach AH. *Br J Plast Surg.* 1999;52:482.

Pederson WC. *Plast Reconstr Surg.* 2001;107:823.

Peeters R. *Burns.* 1988;14:239.

Pelissier P. *Plast Reconstr Surg.* 2003;111:2223.

Pellino G. *Int J Surg.* 2014;12:S64.

Penn J. *Plast Reconstr Surg.* 1955;16:76.

Perel P. *Cochrane Database Syst Rev.* 2013;2:CD000567.

Perkins DJ. *Br J Plast Surg.* 1995;48:546.

Perkins DJ. *Br J Plast Surg.* 1996;49:214.

Perko M. *J Maxillofac Surg.* 1979;7:76.

Petti S. *Oral Oncol.* 2009;45:340.

Perras C. *Aesthetic Plast Surg.* 1990;14:81.

Pierik FH. *Environ Health Perspect.* 2004;112:1570.

Pierrefeu-Lagrange AC. *Ann Chir Plast Esthet.* 2006;51:18.

Piggott TA. *Br J Plast Surg.* 1995;48:127.

Pitman GH. *Clin Plast Surg.* 1996;23:633.

Piza-Katzer H. *Br J Plast Surg.* 2003;56:365.

Platt AJ. *Burns.* 1998;24:754.

Poder TG. *Eur Ann Otorhinolaryngol Head Neck Dis.* 2013;130:79.

Pontén B. *Br J Plast Surg.* 1981;34:215.

Popov V. *Plast Reconstr Surg.* 2004;113:222.

Poswillo D. *Oral Surg Oral Med Oral Pathol.* 1973;35:302.

Potter LP. *J Dermatolog Treat.* 2007;18:46.

Prabhakar H. *Cochrane Database Syst Rev.* 2015;CD010645.

Pribaz J. *Plast Reconstr Surg.* 1992;90:421.

Pribaz JJ. *Plast Reconstr Surg.* 1997;99:1868.

Price G. *Eur J Plast Surg.* 2016;39:99.

Price HN. *Clin Dermatol.* 2010;28:293.

Pruzinsky T, Cash TF. Understanding body images. In Cash TF and Pruzinsky T (eds). *Body Image: A Handbook of Theory, Research, and Clinical Practice.* New York: Guilford Press; 2002;3–12.

Puckett CL. *Aesth Plast Surg.* 1990;14:15.

Qian JG. *J Plast Reconstr Aesthet Surg.* 2010;63:1003.

Quaba AA. *Br J Plast Surg.* 1990;43:24.

Quaba O. *Br J Plast Surg.* 2008;61:712.

Quinn JV. *Ann Emerg Med.* 1993;22:1130.

Quinn MJ. *J Hand Surg Am.* 1996;21:506.

Rabie A. *J Craniofac Surg.* 2011;22:1466.

Radovan C. *Plast Reconstr Surg.* 1982;69:195.

Raff T. *Burns.* 1997;23:313.

Raine C. *Br J Plast Surg.* 2003;56:637.

Ramakrishnan VV. *Ann Plast Surg.* 1997;39:241.

Ramasastry SS. *Plast Reconstr Surg.* 1991;87:1.

Ramirez O. *Plast Reconstr Surg.* 1995;96:323.

Ramirez OM. *Plast Reconstr Surg.* 1990;86:519.

Rapaport DP. *Plast Reconstr Surg.* 1995;96:1547.

Rautio J. *J Plast Surg Hand Surg.* 2017;51:14.

Rawlingson A. *Burns.* 2003;29:631.

Regnault P. *Plast Reconstr Surg.* 1980;65:840.

Reinisch JF. *Plast Reconstr Surg.* 2001;107:1570.

Reitsma JH. *Cleft Palate Craniofac J.* 2012;49:185.

Rheinwald JG. *Cell.* 1975;6:331.

Richards AM. *Burns.* 1997;23:64.

Rietjens M. *Breast.* 2007;16:387.

Riggotti G. *Plast Reconstr Surg.* 2007;119:1409.

Riker AI. *Expert Opin Bio Ther.* 2007;7:345.

Rinkel WD. *J Plast Reconstr Aesthet Surg.* 2012;66:151.

Rinker B. *Ann Plast Surg.* 2010;64:579.

Ritz M. *Aesth Plast Surg.* 2005;29:24.

Rizzo C. *Dermatol Surg.* 2009;35:1947.

Robbins TH. *Plast Reconstr Surg.* 1977;59:64.

Robert C. *N Engl J Med.* 2011;364:2517.

Roberts G. *J Trauma Acute Care Surg.* 2012;72:251.

Robertson AG. *Br J Plast Surg.* 1985;38:314.

Rockwell WB. *Plast Reconstr Surg.* 2000;106:1592.

Roderheaver GT. In Krasner D, Kane D (eds). *Chronic Wound Care: A Clinical Source Book for Healthcare Professionals,* 2nd Edn. 1997;97–108.

Rodrigues M. *Dermatol Surg.* 2015;41:1179.

Rogers GF. *J Plast Reconstr Aesthet Surg.* 2013;66:e90.

Rogers SN. *J Oral Maxillofac Surg.* 2003;61:174.

Rogers SN. *Head Neck.* 2004;26:54.

Rohrich RJ. *Plast Reconstr Surg.* 1995;95:580.

Rohrich RJ. *Plast Reconstr Surg.* 2000;105:202.

Rohrich RJ. *Plast Reconstr Surg.* 2003;111:909.

Rohrich RJ. *Plast Reconstr Surg.* 2003;112:259.

Rohrich RJ. *Plast Reconstr Surg.* 2006;118:1631.

Rohrich RJ. *Plast Reconstr Surg.* 2007;120:312.

Roldan JC. *Plast Reconstr Surg.* 2007;120:1231.

Ronert MA. *Plast Reconstr Surg.* 2004;114:1025.

Rose JK. *Burns.* 1997;23:S19.

Rosenberg L. *Burns.* 2004;30:843.

Rosental SR. *Burns.* 1959;8:215.

Ross GL. *Ann Surg Oncol.* 2004;11:690.

Ross JR. *Sports Health.* 2011;3:431.

Roth JH. *Can J Surg.* 1988;31:19.

Rousseau AF. *Clin Nutr.* 2013;32:497.

Rowe DE. *J Dermat Surg Oncol.* 1989;15:315.

Rowlatt U. *Virchows Archiv.* 1979;381:353.

Rubin A. *Plast Reconstr Surg.* 2002;109:1463.

Rubin JP. *Plast Reconstr Surg.* 1999;103:990–996.

Rubin JR. *Plast Reconstr Surg.* 2012;129:1029.

Rubin LR. *Plast Reconstr Surg.* 1986;77:41.

Rubin LR. *Plast Reconstr Surg.* 1974;53:384.

Ruhl CM. *Laryngoscope.* 1997;107:1316.

Ryan CB. *Semin Intervent Radiol.* 2014;31:167.

Saadi A. *J Cancer Therap.* 2013;4:1490.

Saar JD. *Plast Reconstr Surg.* 2000;106:125.

Safarinejad MR. *Int J Impot Res.* 2004;16:238.

Saffar P. *Ann Chir Main.* 1982;1:276.

Saffle J. *J Burn Care Res.* 2007;28:382.

Sakamoto N. *Ann Surg Oncol.* 2009;16:3406.

Sakellarides HT. *J Hand Surg.* 1996;21:63.

Saleh DB. *J Plast Reconstr Aesthet Surg.* 2014;67:1009.

Saleh M. *J Bone Joint Surg.* 1995;77:429.

Salgarello M. *Plast Reconstr Surg.* 2012;129:317.

Salvatori P. *Acta Otorhinilaryngol.* 2007;27:227.

Samartzis DD. *Spine.* 2006;31:E798.

Sammut D. *J Hand Surg Br.* 1999;24:64.

Sanchez-Guerrero J. *N Engl J Med.* 1995;332:1666.

Santanelli F. *Plast Reconstr Surg.* 2002;109:2314.

Santanelli di Pompeo F. *Plast Reconstr Surg.* 2014;134:871e.

Sarkar A. *Indian J Plast Surg.* 2014;47:381.

Sawada Y. *Burns.* 1997;23:55.

Saxton-Daniels S. *Arch Dermatol.* 2010;146:1044.

Schachter J. *N Engl J Med.* 2015;372:2521.

Schaverien MV. *J Plast Reconstr Aesthet Surg.* 2012;65:935.

Scheepers JH. *Br J Plast Surg.* 1992;45:529.

Scheflan M. *Plast Reconstr Surg.* 1981;68:533.

Scheflan M. *Ann Plast Surg.* 1983;10:24.

Schepull T et al. *Am J Sports Med.* 2011;39:38.

Schessel ES. *Br J Plast Surg.* 2001;54:439.

Schiavon M. *Plast Reconstr Surg.* 1995;96:1698.

Schlenz I. *Plast Reconstr Surg.* 2005;115:743.

Schmitt AR. *Mayo Clin Proc.* 2018;93:877.

Schneider WJ. *Br J Plast Surg.* 1977;30:277.

Schulman NG. *Plast Reconstr Surg.* 2004;114:44.

Schwacha MG. *Burns.* 2003;29:1.

Schwartz MS. *Mov Disord.* 1998;13:188.

Schweckendiek W. *Cleft Palate J.* 1978;15:268.

Schweitzer TP. *J Hand Surg Am.* 2004;29:407.

Sebastin SJ. *Plast Reconstr Surg.* 2011;128:723.

Segmuller G. *Handchirurgie.* 1976;8:75.

Seidenberg B. *Ann Surg.* 1959;149:162.

Seki T. *Int J Burn Trauma.* 2014;4:40.

Semb G. *Cleft Palate Craniofac J.* 1991;28:21.

Semple JL. *Plast Reconstr Surg.* 1998;102:528.

Senchenkov A. *J Surg Oncol.* 2007;95:229.

Senior M. *Plast Reconstr Surg.* 2000;106:224.

Serra MP. *Ann Plast Surg.* 2010;64:275.

Seyhan T. *Ann Plast Surg.* 2008;60:673.

Sgouros S. *J Craniofac Surg.* 1996;7:284.

Shah M. *J Cell Sci.* 1994;107:1137.

Shah JP. *Cancer.* 1990;66:109.

Shah S. *Head Neck.* 2001;23:954.

Shaked G. *Burns.* 2007;33:352.

Shalom A. *Ann Plast Surg.* 2003;50:296.

Shamberger RC. *J Pediatr Surg.* 1988;23:615.

Shamseddine AI. *Eur J Gynaecol Oncol.* 1998;19:479.

Sharif HS. *Am J Roentgenol.* 1990;154:989.

Sharma D. *J Gynecol Surg.* 2008;24:61.

Sharpe DT. *Br J Plast Surg.* 1981;34:97.

Shasha D. *Otolaryngol Clin North Am.* 1998;31:803.

Shaw WC. *J Oral Maxillofac Surg.* 2001;29:131.

Shenaq SM. *J Reconstr Microsurg.* 1989;5:63.

Sheridan R. *J Burn Care Rehab.* 1995;16:602.

Sheridan RL. *J Burn Care Res.* 2000;21:S234.

Shibata M. *J Bone Joint Surg.* 1998;80:1469.

Shons AR. *Plast Reconstr Surg.* 2002;109:383.

Shprintzen RJ. *Cleft Palate J.* 1978;15:56.

Shridarani SM. *Ann Plast Surg.* 2010;64:355.

Shum C. *J Bone Joint Surg.* 2002;84A:221.

Shumaker HB. *Arch Surg.* 1963;86:3847.

Shumaker PR. *J Trauma Acute Care Surg.* 2012;73:S116.

Shumrick KA. *Arch Otolarygngol Head Neck Surg.* 1992;118:373.

Shuster BA. *Plast Reconstr Surg.* 1995;96:1012.

Sigurdson L. *Plast Reconstr Surg.* 2007;119:481–486.

Silverstein MJ. *Arch Surg.* 1988;123:681.

Silverstein MJ. *Cancer.* 1990;66:97.

Simmons RM. *Ann Surg Oncol.* 2002;9:165.

Simmons RM. *Ann Plast Surg.* 2003;51:547.

Simon BE. *Plast Reconstr Surg.* 1973;51:48.

Simunovic F. *Plast Reconstr Aesthet.* 2012;66:187.

Singer A. *J Burn Care Rehab.* 2002;23:361.

Singh KP. *Burns.* 1998;24:733.

Skoog T. *Acta Chir Scand.* 1963;126:453.

Sladden MJ. *Cochrane Database Syst Rev.* 2009; CD004835.

Sladden MJ. *Med J Aust.* 2018;208;137.

Slade DE. *Br J Plast Surg.* 2003;56:451.

Slavin SA. *Plast Reconstr Surg.* 1998;102:49.

Sloan JP. *J Br Hand Surg.* 1987;12:123.

Smith DL. *West J Med.* 1986;144:478.

Snodgrass W. *J Urol.* 1994;151:464.

Snyderman RK. *Plast Reconstr Surg.* 1960;25:253.

Soejima O. *J Hand Surg Am.* 1995;20:801.

Soldin MG. *Br J Plast Surg.* 2000;53:434.

Soldin MG. *Br J Plast Surg.* 2004;57:143.

Sommerlad B. *Plast Reconstr Surg.* 2003;112:1542.

Sommerlad BC. *Plast Reconstr Surg.* 2003;112:331.

Sonmez A. *Plast Reconstr Surg.* 2003;111:2230.

Sood S. *J Laryngol Otol.* 2016;130:S142.

Sorensen LT. *Arch Surg.* 2012;147:373.

Sorensen LT. *Ann Surg.* 2012;255:106.

Soutar D. *Br J Plast Surg.* 1983;36:1.

Southern SJ. *Injury.* 1997;28:477.

Spahn DR. *Transfus Med Hemother.* 2015;42:110.

Spear SL. *Plast Reconstr Surg.* 2003;112:905.

Spear SL. *Plast Reconstr Surg.* 2006;118:136S.

Spinelli HM. *Atlas of Aesthetic Eyelid and Periocular Surgery.* New York: Elsevier Ch.; 2004;4:58–70.

Springer A. *Eur Urol.* 2011;60:1184.

Stark RB. *Plast Reconstr Surg.* 1962;29:229.

Stavrianos SD. *Br J Plast Surg.* 1998;51:584.

Stein J et al. *Hand Surg Am.* 1998;23:1043.

Steinmann G. *Br J Anaesth.* 2005;95:355.

Stevenson TR. *Plast Reconstr Surg.* 1987;79:761.

Stokes RB. *Plast Reconstr Surg.* 1998;102:761.

Stolz W. *Eur J Dermatol.* 1994;4:521.

Stoppa RE. *World J Surg.* 1989;13:545.

Storch CH. *Br J Dermatol.* 2010;163:269.

Storm-Versloot MN. *Cochrane Database Syst Rev.* 2010;3:CD006478.

Stranc MF, Robertson GA. *Ann Plast Surg.* 1979;2:468.

Streeter GL. *Contrib Embryol.* 1930;22:1.

Strombeck JO. *Br J Plast Surg.* 1960;13:79.

Stromberg J. *J Hand Surg.* 2016;41:873.

Su C. *Plast Reconstr Surg.* 1995;96:513.

Suarez C. *Head Neck.* 2007;30:242.

Subramanian S. *Bull World Health Organ.* 2009;87:200.

Sullivan SR. *Ann Plast Surg.* 2009;62:144.

Sully L. *Plast Reconstr Surg.* 1982;70:186.

Sutherland AB. *Burns.* 1976;2:238.

Swanson E. *Plast Reconstr Surg.* 2011;128:182e.

Swartz WM. *Plast Reconstr Surg.* 1994;93:152.

Sweeny L. *J Cutan Pathol.* 2012;39:603.

Sweetland S. *Brit Med J.* 2009;339:b4583.

Symmer W St C. *Br Med J.* 1968;3:19.

Taams KO. *J Hand Surg Br.* 1997;22:328.

Tajima S. *Plast Reconstr Surg.* 1977;60:256.

Takei T. *Plast Reconstr Surg.* 1998;102:247.

Takeishi M. *Plast Reconstr Surg.* 1997;99:713.

Tamboto H. *Plast Reconstr Surg.* 2010;126:835.

Tan BK. *J Plast Reconstr Aesthet Surg.* 2009;62:690.

Tan ST. *Br J Plast Surg.* 1994;47:575.

Tan ST. *Plast Reconstr Surg.* 1997;99:317.

Tang C. *Plast Reconstr Surg.* 1999;103:1682.

Tanner JC Jr. *Plast Reconstr Surg.* 1964;34:287.

Taras JS. *J Hand Surg Am.* 2001;26:1100.

Tarone RE. *Plast Reconstr Surg.* 2004;113:2104.

Tashkandi M. *Ann Plast Surg.* 2004;53:17.

Taylor GI. *Plast Reconstr Surg.* 1975;55:533.

Taylor GI. *Plast Reconstr Surg.* 1979;64:595.

Taylor GI. *Br J Plast Surg.* 1987;40:113.

Taylor S. *J Burn Care Res.* 2014;35:S235.

Tebbets JB. *Plast Reconstr Surg.* 2001;107:1255.

Tebbetts JB. *Clin Plast Surg.* 2001;28:501.

Telfer NR. *Br J Dermatol.* 1999;141:415.

Telfer NR. *Br J Dermatol.* 2008;159:35.

Teloken C. *J Urol.* 1999;162:2003.

Tennison CW. *Plast Reconstr Surg.* 1952;9:115.

Terrell JE. *Laryngoscope.* 2000;110:620.

Terzis J. *Hand Surg.* 1978;3:37.

Terzis JK. *Plast Reconstr Surg.* 2000;105:1932.

Terzis JK. *Plast Reconstr Surg.* 2000;106:1097.

Tessier P. *J Maxillofac Surg.* 1976;4:69.

Thaunat O. *Plast Reconstr Surg.* 2004;113:2235.

Thibaudeau S. *J Plast Reconstr Aesthet Surg.* 2010;63:1688.

Thien TB. *Cochrane Database Syst Rev.* 2004;18:CD003979.

Thoma A. *Plast Reconstr Surg.* 2004;114:1137.

Thomas JM. *N Engl J Med.* 2004;350:757.

Thomas WO. *Plast Reconstr Surg.* 1993;91:1080.

Thompson CF. *Eur Arch Otorhinolaryngol.* 2013;270:2115.

Thomson CJ. *Plast Reconstr Surg.* 2007;119:260.

Thorek M. *NY Med J Rec.* 1922;116:572.

Tiernan E. *Burns.* 1993;19:437.

Tierney EP. *J Drugs Dermatol.* 2009;8:723.

Titley OG. *Br J Plast Surg.* 1996;49:447.

Tomaino M. *J Hand Surg Br.* 1998;23:50.

Tomaino MM. *Am J Orthop.* 2001;30:380.

Tompkins RG. *Ann Surg.* 1986;204:272.

Tonnard P. *Plast Reconstr Surg.* 2002;109:2074.

Tonnard P. *Aesthet Surg J.* 2007;27:188.

Topping A. *Br J Plast Surg.* 2004;57:97.

Torrente-Castells E. *JADA.* 2008;139:1625.

Torresan RZ. *Ann Surg Oncol.* 2005;12:1037.

Toth B. *Plast Reconstr Surg.* 1991;87:1048.

Trelles MA. *Lasers Med Sci.* 2013;28:375.

Trelles MA. *Rev Col Bras Cir.* 2013;40:23.

Trott SA. *Plast Reconstr Surg.* 1998;102:2220.

Tsoutos D. *J Burn Care Res.* 2007;28:530.

Tulley P. *Br J Plast Surg.* 2000;53:378.

Tung TH. *Plast Reconstr Surg.* 2001;107:1830.

Tupper JW. *J Hand Surg.* 1989;14:371.

Turan T. *Plast Reconstr Surg.* 2001;107:463.

Turegun M. *Burns.* 1997;23:442.

Turner-Warwick R. *J Urol.* 1997;158:1160.

Turvey TA, Gudeman SK. Nonsyndromic craniosynostosis. In: Turvey TA, Vig KWL, Fonseca RJ, eds. *Facial Clefts and Craniosynostosis: Principles and Management.* Philadelphia: WB Saunders; 1996:596–629.

Tuzuner S. *J Pediatr Orthop.* 2004;24:629.

Uchiyama K. *Head Neck.* 2002;24:451.

Ueda K. *Ann Plast Surg.* 1994;32:166.

Uppal RS. *Plast Reconstr Surg.* 2001;108:1218.

Urban M. *J Hand Surg Br.* 1996;21:112.

Urbaniak JR. *J Hand Surg Am.* 1981;6:25.

Van Dam H. *Plast Reconstr Surg.* 2004;113:2224.

van der Velde M. *Ann Plast Surg.* 2005;55:660.

van Geertruyden J. *J Hand Surg Br.* 1996;21:257.

Van Geest AJ. *Phlebologie.* 2003;32:138.

Van Leeuwen MCE. *Plast Reconstr Surg Glob Open.* 2015;3:e437.

Van Noort DE. *Plast Reconstr Surg.* 1993;91:1308.

van Nunen SA. *Arthritis Rheum.* 1982;25:694.

Van Wilgen CP. *Head Neck.* 2004;26:839.

Varenna M. *Rheumatology.* 2013;52:534.

Varghese BT. *Br J Plast Surg.* 2001;54:499.

Venkataswami R. *Plast Reconstr Surg.* 1980;66:296.

Vento AR. *Cleft Palate Craniofac J.* 1991;28:68.

Venus B. *Crit Care Med.* 1981;9:519.

Verghese J. *Muscle Nerve.* 2000;23:1209.

Vermeulen H. *Cochrane Database Syst Rev.* 2007;1:CD005486.

Vilain R. *Plast Reconstr Surg.* 1977;52:374.

Vincent JL. *Crit Care Med.* 2004;32:2029.

Vogelin E. *Br J Plast Surg.* 1995;48:579.

Vogelin E. *Br J Plast Surg.* 1998;51:359.

von Heimburg D. *Br J Plast Surg.* 1996;49:339–345.

Vourc'h-Jourdain M. *J Am Acad Dermatol.* 2013;68:493.

Vrdoljak DV. *Tumori.* 2005;91:177.

Vuylsteke RJ. *J Clin Oncol.* 2003;21:1057.

Wada J. *Ann Thorac Surg.* 1970;10:526.

Wagner JD. *J Surg Oncol.* 2001;77:237.

Waizenegger M. *J Hand Surg Br.* 1994;19B:750.

Wall SA. *Br J Plast Surg.* 1994;47:180.

Wallace JG. *Br J Plast Surg.* 1979;32:15.

Walton RL. *Plast Reconstr Surg.* 1998;102:358.

Walton RL. *Plast Reconstr Surg.* 2002;110:234.

Wang HJ. *Plast Reconstr Surg.* 1996;98:524.

Wang XQ. *Ann Plast Surg.* 2009;63:688.

Warden GD. *World J Surg.* 1992;16:16.

Wardill WEM. *Br J Surg.* 1928;16:127.

Warner E. *JAMA.* 2004;292:1317.

Wasiak J. *Cochrane Database Syst Rev.* 2006;CD005489.

Wasiak J. *Cochrane Database Syst Rev.* 2013;3:CD002106.

Watanabe IC. *Medicine.* 2015;94:e934.

Watson HK. *J Hand Surg Br.* 1997;22:5.

Weber D. *J Pediatr Urol.* 2009;5:345.

Wechselberger G. *Plast Reconstr Surg.* 2004;114:69.

Weedon D. *ANZ J Surg.* 2010;80:129.

Weerda H. *Laryngol Rhinol Otol* (Stuttg). 1979;58:242.

Wei FC. *Plast Reconstr Surg.* 2003;112:37.

Weiner D. *Plast Reconstr Surg.* 1973;51:115.

Weinstein JM. *Arch Dermatol.* 2003;139:207.

Weiss I. *Laryngoscope.* 2011;121:1642.

Wening JV. *Br J Clin Pract.* 1990;44:311.

Wheatley K. *Cancer Treat Rev.* 2003;29:241.

White RR. *Ann Surg.* 2002;235:879.

Wilhelmi BJ. *Ann Plast Surg.* 1998;41:215.

Willadsen E. *J Plast Surg Hand Surg.* 2017;51:38.

Willard WC. *Surgery.* 1992;175:389.

Wilkinson TS. *Aesthet Plast Surg.* 1994;18:49.

Wilmink H. *Plast Reconstr Surg.* 1998;102:373.

Wilson AD. *Injury.* 2004;35:507.

Wilson GR. *Ann Roy Coll Surg Engl.* 1988;70:217.

Wilson GR. *Br J Plast Surg.* 1994;47:175.

Wilson YG. *J Hand Surg.* 1993;18:81.

Winocour J. *Plast Reconstr Surg.* 2017;136:597e.

Winter G. *Nature.* 1962;193:293.

Withey S. *Br J Plast Surg.* 2001;54:716.

Woerderman L. *Plast Reconstr Surg.* 2006;118:1288.

Wolf K. *Plast Reconstr Surg.* 1996;97:641.

Wolpert L. *J Theor Biol.* 1969;25:1.

Wong C. *Plast Reconstr Surg.* 2010;125:772.

Wong CH. *Plast Reconstr Surg.* 2006;118:1224–1236.

Wong CH. *Plast Reconstr Surg.* 2007;119:1259.

Wong GB. *Plast Reconstr Surg.* 2001;108:1316.

Wootton CI. *Br J Dermatol.* 2014;170:239.

Wrye SW. *Plast Reconstr Surg.* 2003;111:113.

Wung JT. *J Pediatr Surg.* 1995;30:406.

Wynn J. *Thorax Cardiovasc.* 1990;99:41.

Xu W. *J Invest Dermatol.* 2014;134:1044.

Xue FS. *Br J Anaesth.* 1998;80:447.

Yamada K. *J Eur Acad Dermatol Venereol.* 2010;27:319.

Yamagami T. *Neurosurg Rev.* 1984;7:165.

Yamamoto Y. *Plast Reconstr Surg.* 1997;100:1212.

Yang JC. *Ann Plast Surg.* 2007;59:378.

Yelamos O. *JAMA Dermatol.* 2017;153:689.

Yildirim S. *Plast Reconstr Surg.* 2006;117:2033.

Yim H. *Burns.* 2010;36:322.

Yim KK. *Plast Reconstr Surg.* 2004;114:107.

Yokoyama T. *Plast Reconstr Surg.* 2007;119:1284.

Yonehara Y. *Br J Plast Surg.* 1998;51:356.

Yoshida T. *Br J Plast Surg.* 1998;51:103.

Young D. *Br J Surg.* 1961;48:514.

Ysunza A. *Plast Reconstr Surg.* 2001;107:9.

Ysunza A. *Plast Reconstr Surg.* 2002;110:1401.

Yu P. *Plast Reconstr Surg.* 2002;109:610.

Yu SY. *Plast Reconstr Surg.* 2007;120:1240.

Yuen AP. *Head Neck.* 2009;31:765.

Yuryeva KS. *Biochem Moscow.* 2014;8:336.

Zagars GK. *Cancer.* 2003;97:2544.

Zallen RD. *J Oral Surg.* 1975;33:431.

Zancolli EA. *Surg Radiol Anat.* 1986;8:209.

Zancolli EA. *J Hand Surg.* 1988;13:130.

Zannis J. *Ann Plast Surg.* 2009;62:407.

Zenn MR. *Plast Reconstr Surg.* 2009;123:1648.

Zhang DZ. *PLoS One.* 2016;17:e0151627.

Zhang YX. *Plast Reconstr Surg.* 2013;131:759e.

Zhu ZX. *Burns.* 2003;29:65.

Ziade M. *J Plast Reconstr Surg.* 2013;66:209.

Zide MF. *J Oral Maxillofac Surg.* 1983;41:89.

Zide MF. *Clin Plast Surg.* 1989;16:69.

Zins JE. *Plast Reconstr Surg.* 1983;72:778.

Zitelli JA. *Arch Dermatol.* 1989;125:957.

Zocchi M. *Aesthet Plast Surg.* 1992;16:287.

Zufferey J. *Eur J Plast Surg.* 1988;11:109.

Index

Page numbers followed by f and t indicate figures and tables, respectively.